Pediatric clinical
gastroenterology

Pediatric clinical gastroenterology

ARNOLD SILVERMAN, M.A., M.D.

Director of Pediatrics, Denver General Hospital;
Professor of Pediatrics, University of Colorado
Health Science Center, Denver, Colorado

CLAUDE C. ROY, M.D., F.R.C.P.(C)

Director, Pediatric Research Center,
Hôpital Sainte-Justine, Montreal;
Professor of Pediatrics, University of Montreal,
Montreal, Quebec, Canada

Third edition

with **548** illustrations

The C. V. Mosby Company

ST. LOUIS • TORONTO • LONDON   1983

MOSBY

A TRADITION OF PUBLISHING EXCELLENCE

Editor: Karen Berger
Assistant editor: Theresa Van Schaik
Editing supervisor: Peggy Fagan
Manuscript editor: Carl Masthay
Book design: Kay M. Kramer
Production: Jeanne A. Gulledge

THIRD EDITION

The C.V. Mosby Company
11830 Westline Industrial Drive, St. Louis, Missouri 63141

Library of Congress Cataloging in Publication Data

Silverman, Arnold, 1933-
    Pediatric clinical gastroenterology.

    Rev. ed. of: Pediatric clinical gastro-
enterology / Claude C. Roy, Arnold Silverman,
Frank J. Cozzetto. 2nd ed. 1975.
    Includes index.
    1. Pediatric gastroenterology.   I. Roy,
Claude C., 1928-   . II. Roy, Claude C.,
1928-   .   Pediatric clinical gastroenterology.
III. Title.   [DNLM: 1. Gastrointestinal diseases—
In infancy and childhood.   WS 310 S587p]
RJ446.S47   1982   618.92′3   82-7949
ISBN 0-8016-4623-5   AACR2

C/CB/B   9   8   7   6   5   4   3   01/B/039

**To
Children**

Preface to third edition

Since publication of our second edition 8 years ago, we have witnessed a host of new developments in the field of pediatric gastroenterology. Important contributions have come from both pediatric gastroenterology and liver units from around the world. Most noticeable has been the continued thrust to define those aspects of gastroenterology unique to pediatrics while validating the data using age-related groups. As a result, the pediatric literature abounds with articles relating to gastrointestinal topics. This underscores the importance as well as the quality of the work, which is being recognized by editors of leading scientific journals. In addition, a number of new textbooks devoted entirely to specific subjects of pediatric gastroenterology have appeared in the last 5 years. Three excellent texts dealing exclusively with pediatric liver disease (Alagille, Mowat, and Chandra), one text on diseases of the small intestine in childhood (Walker-Smith), and two dealing with nutrition of infants and children (Suskind and Lebenthal) have been published. Of note is the publication of the first few issues of *Pediatric Gastroenterology and Nutrition,* which will have an impact on the specialty. In this third edition, we have attempted to blend this explosion of new knowledge into our 15 years of clinical experience in pediatric gastroenterology, necessitating complete revisions of many chapters and extensive changes in others. Especially notable are changes contained in those chapters dealing with immunology and the gut, diarrheal disorders, esophageal disorders, digestion and absorption of carbohydrates, fat and protein, inflammatory bowel diseases, liver disorders in children, management of portal hypertension, and nutritional care. Herein one will recognize alterations in our clinical approach, or new therapeutic challenges and prognostic considerations different from those previously considered. Throughout this third edition one will also find an abundance of new figures and tables, with updated and significantly expanded reference lists.

In the past 7 years we have also seen a variety of investigative modalities applied with greater confidence to the pediatric patient with gastrointestinal conditions. The important contribution of the newer fiberoptic instruments in the evaluation of gastrointestinal disorders of children is incorporated wherever applicable, as has the use of ultrasound, computerized tomography, and the new low-radiation isotopes employed in radionuclide scintigraphy.

Once again we have tried to maintain our previous commitment to present the subject of pediatric gastroenterology in a clinically oriented manner. It is our desire that the book continue to be practical and useful to all pediatric caregivers requiring additional information about gastrointestinal function in health and disease. However, we have also felt a growing responsibility to the expanding number of trainees entering into the field of pediatric gastroenterology, especially over the past 5 to 8 years. Therefore we considered it appropriate, even in a general text of this type, to enlarge sections dealing with pathophysiologic mechanisms, make mention of provocative but not necessarily proved theories, point out controversial areas of treatment, and include new, though rare, entities. It is our hope that these efforts will further stimulate our younger colleagues to critical thinking while suggesting areas needing additional research activity.

Needless to say, an undertaking of this magnitude requires the support and encouragement of many individuals to whom we owe a special debt of gratitude and thanks. We are particularly indebted to the administration at the Denver Department of Health and Hospitals, to Doctor Luc Chicoine, Director of the Department of Pediatrics at the University of Montreal, to the pediatric staff at Denver General Hospital, and to colleagues of the pediatric GI Unit at Hôpital Sainte-Justine, Doctors Claude Morin and Andrée Weber, for giving us the opportunity to undertake and complete this task. Warm thanks are also extended to our pediatric surgical colleagues J.R. Lilly, J.D. Burrington, Eli Wayne, Hervé Blanchard, and Arié Bensoussan; pediatric radiologists John Campbell, Carol Rumack, and Gilles Perreault; pathologists Blaise Favara, Donald Clark, and Pierre Brochu; medical photographers and illustrators George Silver, Nancy McPherson, Patricia Jones, Robert Leblanc, Denise Collins, Jacques Doyon, and

Richard Veillette. We would like to recognize especially the superb contributions of Andrea Bond, Guy Lepage, and Liette Chartrand and those of Jan Walters, Rita Hidalgo, and Danielle St-Cyr Huot, medical secretaries of extraordinary skill, perseverance, and patience.

Finally and most importantly, an expression of sincere gratitude, love, and reverence to our wives and children, who for the third time demonstrated patient understanding, support, and encouragement during this long rewriting period.

Arnold Silverman, M.D.
Claude C. Roy, M.D.

Preface to second edition

Rapid advances in pediatric gastroenterology since the publication of the first edition would have been sufficient reason for putting together this undertaking. We have also been prompted by the fact that with the increased recognition of gastroenterology as a pediatric subspecialty, there is an even more pressing responsibility for it to contribute to the practice of pediatrics. It is our desire for this second edition to demonstrate our strong feeling that pediatric gastroenterology should not isolate itself from general pediatrics, a process we see happening with increased concern between other pediatric subspecialties and the private office.

The present undertaking aims at bringing to family physicians and pediatricians recent concepts, information, and personal experience in a rapidly expanding field. The book has been extensively revised and expanded. It continues to reflect our own practice of gastroenterology. New entities, therapies, and procedures are described. Certain sections are now covered in much greater detail in order to correct deficiencies brought to light by kind reviewers, colleagues, and house staff. References have all been updated and augmented. A much greater emphasis has been placed on exploring pathogenic mechanisms. The many hours of discussion and the long road from drafts to manuscript have never been allowed to detract us from the original orientation of the book; practicality and immediate usefulness.

Special thanks and gratitude are presented to the following friends and colleagues: William Davis and John Campbell, radiologists at The Children's Hospital, Denver; Gilles Perreault and Jacques Boisvert, radiologists at Hôpital Sainte-Justine, Montreal; John Taubman, radiologist at Colorado General Hospital; Blaise Favara and Georges Berdnikoff, pathologists at The Children's Hospital, Denver, and Hôpital Sainte-Justine, respectively; Claude L. Morin and Reuben S. Dubois, our partners in gastroenterology; J.C. Ducharme, F. Guttman, S. Youssef, J.D. Burrington, and E. Wayne, pediatric surgeons; F. Desmarais-Lamothe, nutritionist at Hôpital Sainte-Justine; J. Doyon, M. Boisseau, D. Collins, J. Barbour, and G. Silver, medical photographers; M. Gagnon, H. Tapps, and N. McPherson, medical artists; Liette Chartrand, Guy Lepage, and Simone Roy; Phyllis Hamilton and Elaine Blain, medical secretaries "extraordinaires."

Finally, we feel greatly indebted to our wives for their supportive posture of patients and understanding during this long rewriting period.

Claude C. Roy
Arnold Silverman
Frank J. Cozzetto

Preface to first edition

By this undertaking, we hoped to fill a definite need, but even within a subspecialty area one quickly realizes how difficult it is to write a textbook without losing the original intent; that of practicality and immediate usefulness.

The physician who cares for children soon realizes that gastrointestinal complaints, with or without underlying disease, demand a sizable proportion of his time, either by telephone conversation or by direct patient contact; yet a textbook that deals entirely with this subject is not presently available. Besides its possible usefulness in office practice, such a text should also be helpful to hospital-based physicians, since as many as 10% of hospitalized pediatric patients have complaints of a gastrointestinal nature upon admission.

Hopefully, this book can bridge the gap between the general discussions of gastrointestinal problems in pediatric textbooks and the standard gastroenterology texts that, even if otherwise encyclopedic in scope, give but casual reference to the problems as they apply to the pediatric population.

Pediatric gastroenterology is coming of age as a subspecialty. Increased interest and momentum in the field are attested to by the recent publications of periodic bibliographic reviews of major pediatric gastroenterologic entities (Morin, C., and Davidson, M.: Gastroenterology **52:**565-586, 713-726, 1967; Silverberg, M., and Davidson, M.: Gastroenterology **58:**229-252, 1970). These reviews have not only provided a most useful tool for expanded reading in this field but have also alerted gastroenterologists to the spectrum of gastrointestinal problems encountered only in the pediatric age group.

In hope of reaching the physician involved in the care of children and of providing him with the most useful type of gastroenterologic information, we have stressed the methods of collecting and interpreting clinical data. The latter can then be used to suggest a group of possible causative or associated diseases to be supported or ruled out by appropriate laboratory tests, x-ray studies, and investigative procedures. Therapeutic strategy has been dictated by safety and practicality. As for prognosis, we have tried to cumulate and compound personal experience in various centers and available statistics.

Wherever appropriate we have included many observations and bedside tips gathered over the years by continued exposure to these particular conditions. Within this framework the book may properly serve as a useful guide for pediatricians, general practitioners, family practice physicians, and house staff.

Emphasis throughout is clinical, whether it be in discussion of common or uncommon entities. Some sections will seem surprisingly lengthy in view of the infrequent occurrence of the diseases discussed. Our intention was not to allocate space strictly on the basis of incidence and relative importance. Unknown pathogenesis, disagreements on clinical features, difficulties attached to the diagnostic approach, and nonspecific or erratic therapeutic effectiveness were, in our minds, sufficient excuses to justify a comprehensive and organizational approach to the specific topic or disease entity. Titles of chapters have been arbitrarily assigned in a problem-oriented way. This not only reflects our method of considering and classifying specific entities but better serves to attract attention to the more common problems. For some categories, the problem-oriented heading yields better to general diagnostic approach in the work-up of such patients than does an anatomic heading.

The book is organized into three major sections and can be used in several ways. The first section deals with symptoms and signs that have gastrointestinal significance. Here the reader is instructed in techniques of information gathering that permit rapid sorting of possible gastrointestinal diseases and conditions that properly belong to the pediatric age group. Awareness of a symptom, a physical sign, or an agglomeration of signs and symptoms should get the reader to the specific entity, provided he considers these clinical features as having gastrointestinal significance. Each entity is then discussed in the major section of the text. As suggested, emphasis is on the clinical approach to the problem, yet whenever basic concepts of biochemistry or physiology seem helpful in understanding the pathogenesis of the entity in question, they are incorporated into the discussion. Where treatment of a disease entity is discussed, specific details and options are included to permit the physician to give complete medical care to the patient. The third section of the book is devoted to a description and discussion of the procedures that have proved reliable and that we presently use. In addition, a description and interpretation of useful diagnostic laboratory tests are included. Last, a discussion of the nutritional care of the child, including specialized diets, is provided for completeness.

Commonly used drugs and dosages are included throughout. The references cited are primarily recent rather than "classic." In this regard, an effort has also been made to select those that should be easily available to most medical libraries.

Where roentgenologic diagnosis is referred to, it is intended only as a guide in the appropriate use of roentgenologic examinations. It cannot substitute for the services of a trained pediatric radiologist. Minor variations in techniques as well as subtleties of interpretation often are of enormous significance.

Similarly, the role of the pathologist in the proper handling and evaluation of histologic material is critical to gastroenterologic disorders. Much reliance is also placed upon the results and interpretation of laboratory investigations of these patients, and here the role of the clinical pathologist can assume major importance. One needs to encourage mutual friendship and enthusiasm among these specialty areas, particularly for problems related to the gastrointestinal system. This will result in the best diagnosis and treatment.

Special expressions of gratitude are extended to the following colleagues and friends who were so generous with their time and talent: Parker Allen and William Davis, radiologists at The Children's Hospital, Denver; Jacques Boisvert and Gilles Perreault from the X-ray Department at Hôpital Sainte-Justine; Blaise Favara and Ralph Franciosi, pathologists at The Children's Hospital, Denver; Ilona Kerner, pathologist at Hôpital Sainte-Justine; Reuben S. Dubois and Claude L. Morin, pediatric gastroenterologists; Janice Dodds, nutritionist, B.F. Stolinsky Laboratories, University of Colorado Medical Center; Nile Root, Jacques Doyon, André Brisset des Nos, and Michael Boisseau, medical photographers; Georgianna Starz, A. Baum, and Madeleine Gagnon, medical artists; Eliane Blain, Audrey County, Martha Hodgkinson, and Mary Richardson, secretaries and typists.

We feel indebted to the staff at The Children's Hospital, Denver, the Hôpital Sainte-Justine, and the University of Colorado Medical Center for having facilitated our efforts by carrying an extra work load and for sustaining our enthusiasm.

Arnold Silverman
Claude C. Roy
Frank J. Cozzetto

Contents

Part I

COMMON GASTROENTEROLOGIC SYMPTOMS AND SIGNS

1 Symptoms

History taking is an extraordinary investigative technique that constitutes the most important part of the clinical evaluation of patients with gastrointestinal complaints. Its value, however, depends not only on the sophistication and experience of the historian but also on the ability and willingness of the patient to describe subjective manifestations of bodily dysfunction. The necessity of interposing a third person between the clinician and the young patient can be a handicap. In fact, a mother will often underestimate or overestimate symptoms according to her own experiences with such complaints. These, in turn, may be subconsciously manipulated by the physician in an effort to make them seem more typical and thereby fit a preconceived diagnosis.

Much of the physician's history taking also occurs by telephone conversation in which interposed third-party evaluations of the symptomatic child can vary from complete accuracy to total unreliability. Not only are such conversations time-consuming, but too often they fail to completely alleviate the physician's or the parent's concern. The ineffective attempt at information gathering can be attributed to the physician's lack of skill or experience with this technique or simply to his being too busy to spend much time with seemingly minor complaints.

No doubt the effectiveness of history taking is related to one's interest in and knowledge of a given subject, whereas familiarity with the varied modes of presentation of a particular illness requires a personal discipline in, if not a fascination for, this aspect of medicine. Attentive eyes and ears can make every exposure to a patient become a learning experience, and with such experience comes the skill to effectively obtain needed information, rapidly yet accurately, even over the telephone. The systematic gathering of information can allow the physician to sort quickly through the diagnostic possibilities that are potentially responsible for a given complaint. The use of this valuable technique is demonstrated whenever possible in the following discussions of symptoms that have gastrointestinal significance.

In the office or in the hospital setting, where more time can be allotted to history taking, the story should be obtained perferably in the child's words, with the physician listening attentively. The conversation can be encouraged to follow productive lines concerning onset, course of the illness, rhythmicity of symptoms, and repercussions of the disease on the patient's physical and mental health.

The importance of a careful, painstaking interrogation of the patient or of his mother is further emphasized by the relative freedom from positive, observable physical signs in a number of pediatric patients with gastrointestinal manifestations. On the other hand, many children have subjective complaints caused by physiologic disturbances of the gastrointestinal tract that actually represent a secondary response to extraintestinal disease (referred pain).

The relationship of each symptom to the onset of the chief complaint or of the present illness should be established before a careful record is made of dietary, growth, and development history.

The systematic review of gastrointestinal symptoms will force a reappraisal and a more precise characterization of symptomatic sensations. It will also enable the clinician to decide whether the ambiguities noted during the recording of the history of the present illness relate to the underlying disease or to communication problems. When two clinicians obtain a different history from the same patient, it is often assumed that the patient is unreliable. In fact, the fault often lies with the examiners. This problem can be avoided if the same physician takes a second history and actually considers each contact with his patient as an opportunity to gather additional information.

FAILURE TO THRIVE

It is surprising how often the pediatrician rather than the parent will be the first to recognize that the infant or child is failing to thrive. Indeed, it is uncommon for the parent to present the child to the physician with the complaint that he is not gaining weight or growing properly. On the other hand, concern about poor appetite or the quality of diet is frequent. This phenomenon is further emphasized by a study at the University of Colorado Medical Center in Denver, caring primarily for indigent patients. Though evidence of failure to thrive was detected in 50% of all hospitalized pediatric patients less than 2 years of age, only 5% of these patients had failure to thrive as the primary admitting diagnosis. Similar figures have subsequently been reported from large pediatric centers located in Boston, Buffalo, and Pittsburgh.

Perhaps the most important reason that parents are unable to appreciate this condition is that failure to thrive evolves as a gradual deceleration from an established pattern rather than as a sudden event. Therefore the subtle slowing of rate of gain and growth (as opposed to absolute loss of weight or no growth) is not appreciated in the close day-to-day relationship between mother and child. Certainly, there are instances in which delay in diagnosis is the result of parental denial that anything is wrong with the child or simple acceptance that the child is small.

The routine use of growth charts for recording heights, weights, and head circumference permits the physician to quickly appreciate and confirm the impression that his patient is failing to thrive. By definition, the infant or child who shows a persistent deceleration from his established pattern or who falls consistently below the third percentile for height and weight is failing to thrive. Early recognition and prompt nutritional rehabilitation is critical, especially for the very young infant (less than 4 months) in whom pronounced protein-calorie malnutrition may result in irreversible damage to the central nervous system with resulting developmental and mental delays.

If failure to thrive is suspected by routine plotting of the measurements of weight, height, and head circumference, then additional manipulations of the data are suggested by Wilkins. That method involves first plotting the measurement of height, weight, and head circumference on standard growth charts. One then finds the age at which these values lie in the fiftieth percentile and transposes these fiftieth-percentile ages to a graph on which the abscissa is the chronologic age (months, years) and the ordinate is the developmental age (months, years). Deviations from normal (represented by a diagonal line) and from each of the plotted parameters become quickly apparent, and one of three basic patterns will be derived by application of this technique to the child who fails

to thrive. These observations can begin the sorting process for the physician in his efforts to establish a specific diagnosis.

Pattern I. Subnormal head circumference, weight and height proportionately reduced

This category includes a fairly large group of children who fail to thrive but are the easiest to recognize clinically (Fig. 1-1). These children are often described as the "funny-looking kids" (FLK), with microcephaly, developmental retardation, and seizures a frequent part of the complex. These children may have suffered from infections acquired in utero (such as rubella, cytomegalovirus, toxoplasmosis), whereas others suffer the severe impact of intrauterine growth retardation from a number of different causes. Perinatal insults resulting in birth asphyxia, severe prematurity, and hypoglycemia are contributory factors in others. Chromosomal anomalies (trisomy 13-15, 17-18, 21) are occasionally responsible but fortunately are uncommon. Despite nutritional intervention, infants who are small for gestational age in all parameters of growth are more than likely to remain small throughout childhood.

Pattern II. Normal or enlarged head circumference, weight only slightly reduced or at times proportionate to height

This category is primarily represented by children who have constitutional dwarfism, the so-called structural dystrophies, or an endocrinopathy (Fig. 1-2). Additional measurements of body proportions, such as span (fingertip to fingertip of outstretched arms) and ratio of upper segment to lower segment (top of pubic symphysis to heel), may be useful for better appreciation of the disproportions of skeleton often representative of this category.

Bone age examination by roentgenographic means usually involve the wrist or hemiskeleton depending on the patient's age. This study will not only evaluate skeletal maturity compared to the average but may also show evidence of metabolic defects. Comparison of the subject's chronologic age with respective height age (median age for patient's height) and skeletal maturation (bone age) permits sorting of this particular group of "failure-to-thrive" patients into three major subsets. The most common finding is that where bone age is nearly equal (or only slightly delayed) to the patient's height age, and it almost always suggests "constitutional" short stature, especially in

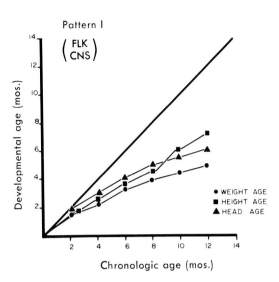

Fig. 1-1. Retardation of weight, height, and head circumference.

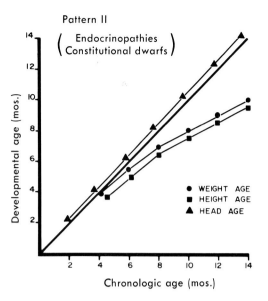

Fig. 1-2. Retardation of height greater than weight and normal head circumference.

an otherwise well infant or child. In such cases deceleration of growth rate, and occasionally of weight, becomes apparent between 8 to 15 months of age. Additional diagnostic considerations when bone age is equal to or slightly less than height age include chronic disease states, metabolic disturbances, and occasionally primary central nervous system disorders. When the subject's bone age is equal to his chronologic age, yet height age is retarded, such a child has a genotype for short stature (familial) and will in fact grow to be a small adult. In most cases, the final adult height in such individuals can be gleaned from application of mean parent height figures. Lastly, when bone age is significantly more delayed than the patient's height age, one must consider an underlying endocrine disorder, with hypothyroidism being the most common condition to explain these findings. Other possibilities include hypopituitarism, somatotropin or somatomedin deficiency, maternal deprivation syndrome (deprivation dwarfism), and in some cases severe malnutrition or chronic disease.

Pattern III. Normal head circumference, weight reduced out of proportion to height

The majority of patients failing to thrive will reflect pattern III, with malnutrition being the main underlying cause (Fig. 1-3). Malnutrition may result from (1) caloric intake inadequate for patients' needs, the most common problem; (2) ex-

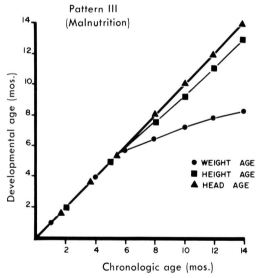

Fig. 1-3. Retardation of weight with near normal height and head growth.

cessive caloric losses from gastrointestinal disease; or (3) impaired peripheral utilization. Seldom will only a single cause for malnutrition be present, but rather a definite interplay among these three will be found. In addition, a group of external forces (environmental, social, cultural) are frequently woven into the reasons for failure to

Table 1-1. Etiologic factors leading to maternal deprivation (social, cultural, environmental, intrapsychic, and so on)

Infant of low birth weight	Mother of young age (less than
Child of unwanted sex	16 years)
Child born out of wedlock	Mother inadequately mothered
Marital discord	as a child
Unsupportive husband	Mother out of touch with reality
Too many children, especially	Psychoneurotic conflict
if under 2 years	Poor self-esteem
Inadequate income	Poor ability to relate to others
Alcoholic spouse	Limited ability to perceive
No husband	needs of others
Unwanted pregnancy	Limited capacity for concern
Appearance of child	Depression

thrive caused by malnutrition. For some time there was a controversy as to whether the psychosocial impact of *maternal deprivation* leads directly to malnutrition or whether caloric deprivation is the important denominator in the deprivation syndrome. Most workers presently agree that caloric deprivation is the single most important factor leading to malnutrition in this syndrome.

Since the majority of children with a diagnosis of failure to thrive suffer from malnutrition (pattern III), proper history taking and physical examination will be required for determination of the most likely cause for this problem. It is good practice to rely at times on a period of hospitalization for nutritional rehabilitation, limited laboratory tests, and simple observations of the child's feeding habits and of parent-child interaction before a specific diagnosis can be made.

Inadequate intake of calories

Because inadequate intake of calories is the most common specific problem, the physician should spend time in careful questioning of the parent about the particulars of the child's diet. Too often, the parent and even the physician are likely to consider the formula as the reason for the child's not doing well. The fact that an infant is failing to gain weight while receiving a standard formula that is quantitatively adequate should prompt the physician to do more than change the feedings. Healthy infants and children show a steady weight gain and growth, and alterations in this dynamic state should suggest to the physician who cares for children that something is abnormal with his patient and not with the formula.

As an office procedure, infants being breast fed may require weighing before and after nursing to convince the mother (and the physician) that the child is not receiving adequate volume and, therefore, calories. This may come as a great surprise to some mothers who will claim that their breasts are engorged and that the milk just seems to drip freely from the nipples. The story that these infants seem satisfied and need to be awakened for feedings is also obtained frequently. They seem to starve without complaint. Provided that the infant's oral (sucking) needs are fulfilled, it would appear that the body metabolism of these calorically deprived infants adjusts to the compromised caloric intake. A similar phenomenon has been documented in older children with marasmus. Observing the mother during nursing of the infant can provide valuable information to the physician regarding the mechanics of the feeding, sucking, and swallowing action of the infant as well as the mother-child relationship. It is not surprising to see a deceleration of weight gain in infants exclusively breast fed by 6 months of life.

If the infant is being *formula fed,* specific questions should be asked about *dilution.* How much formula is put in each bottle? How much is left after feeding, is discarded, is reused? How many bottles are taken day and night? These questions sometimes need to be asked before one can be certain of the quantity of formula consumed. Often a discrepancy will be found when the subject is approached from different aspects.

The type of feeding (breast or formula), amount of formula, dilution, and frequency offered are aspects of feeding practices that are subject to definite social, cultural, religious, and environmental influences. The recent popularity of dietary cults and use of strict vegetarian diets by both nursing and nonnursing mothers may compromise the infant's overall caloric intake and introduce specific vitamin-deficiency states.

Some mothers are unwilling to nurture their infants, whereas others are unable to do so because of underlying psychiatric disorders. Another group is simply unaware of what constitutes mothering. Evidence of maternal deprivation as a factor in malnutrition may be gained when one finds other physical signs of neglect or battering. Dirty skin with bruises, sores, severe diaper rash, and so forth should make the physician suspicious. Dirt under the nails of hands and toes is commonly found in neglected infants. The social history may quickly yield important information to explain the reasons for inadequate caloric intake. Sometimes there simply is not enough money in the house to buy adequate food supplies.

A list of etiologic risk factors in maternal deprivation syndromes appears in Table 1-1.

Other clues suggesting neglect and particularly sensory deprivation include developmental motor and language delays, apathy, and, in extreme cases, evidence of infantile autism.

The association of a malnutrition pattern of failure to thrive, with short stature, voracious appetite, abdominal distention, and delayed osseous maturation constitutes the entity of "deprivation dwarfism."

There are documented cases in which seemingly adequate amounts of qualitatively acceptable foods are offered, and yet caloric intake is inadequate. In this group are infants and children with neurologic and neuromuscular disorders affecting their ability to coordinate the acts of deglutition, sucking, and swallowing (such as familial dysautonomia, Werdnig-Hoffmann paralysis, Möbius syndrome, Krabbe's disease, and Tay-Sachs disease).

Intermittent periods of anorexia are very common in pediatric patients, but persistent apathy toward eating may be seen in children with acute and chronic infection, malignancy, collagen disease, genitourinary disease, central nervous system disease, and gastroenterologic conditions. Emotional problems may lead to anorexia. Some of these conditions give rise to anemia, which secondarily can affect caloric intake. Zinc deficiency may result in loss of taste discrimination and thereby perpetuate the anorexia. Easy tiring, fatigue, and anorexia may diminish caloric intake

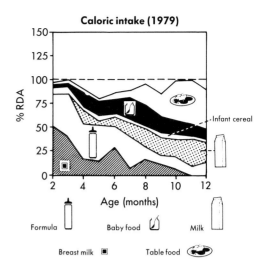

Fig. 1-4. Percentage of recommended daily allowance (RDA) from usual components of the infant's diet up to 12 months. (From Johnson, G.H., Purvis, G.A., and Wallace, R.D.: Nutrition Today **16:**4, 1981, with permission.)

in patients with cardiovascular disease, especially those with congenital cyanotic heart disease.

Iatrogenic causes of infantile malnutrition need also to be considered when therapeutic interventions involve prolonged use of "therapeutic fasting" for treatment of diarrhea states. Elimination diets employed in suspected cases of "food allergy" may also result in caloric insufficiency for the infant and young child. Fig. 1-4 shows the relative percentage of recommended daily allowance fulfilled by various foodstuffs in the infant's diet after the first year of life. It is important to note that milk represents 25% of the child's caloric intake at 1 year of age.

Excessive caloric losses

If it can be established that caloric intake is adequate, the physician should try to determine whether the calories being ingested are indeed available to the body for utilization or they are being lost for some reason after being ingested.

There are several ways in which ingested calories can be lost, the most obvious being the act of excessive *regurgitation* or *vomiting,* or both, rendering net caloric intake inadequate for growth. The conditions responsible for these symptoms are described in a subsequent section.

One must be sure to recognize in children *rumination,* a symptom stemming from an abnormal psychosocial interplay between mother and infant. This diagnosis may not become apparent until observations of the mother-child relationship can be made in a hospital setting and the infant can be closely observed after feedings for peculiar tongue movements characteristic of this condition. Caution needs to be exercised, however, that all organic possibilities have been eliminated when one makes the diagnosis of *rumination syndrome*. For example, this diagnosis may be incorrectly entertained in an infant with a brainstem glioma and more commonly in infants with gastroesophageal reflux associated with a sliding hiatal hernia.

Malabsorptive states, be they primary or secondary, need to be considered when intake seems adequate in a child who fails to thrive. Here faulty digestion or absorption or superimposed intestinal losses are at fault. More common entities such as cystic fibrosis, milk-protein intolerance, celiac disease, disaccharidase deficiency, immunologic deficiency states, parasitic infestation, hepatobiliary disease, inflammatory bowel disease, and congenital anatomic defect of the bowel (kinking, short-circuiting, and so forth) and chronic malnutrition itself need consideration. Most of these entities have in common the symptom of *diarrhea* and will receive attention under this heading elsewhere. Fortunately, many of these conditions are indicated by other important clues in the patient's history and obvious physical findings that can aid in early diagnosis.

Impaired or excessive utilization

Many diseases in children seem to affect the peripheral utilization of calories. Caloric utilization at a cellular level may be either inadequate (impaired) or excessive, depending on the underlying problem. Chronic infection, chronic renal disease, malignancy, cyanotic heart disease, anemia, and inborn errors of metabolism such as glycogen storage disease, galactosemia, fructose intolerance, and phenylketonuria may impair peripheral utilization of foodstuffs. Hyperthyroidism, diencephalic syndrome, and hyperkinesia affecting some children with cerebral dysfunction (minimal brain damage, athetoid cerebral palsy) may increase metabolic rates, and the children will fail to thrive even though they are ingesting a caloric intake that may in fact be more than adequate for their age and size. Additional clues to most organic causes just mentioned should be available from careful history taking and the physical examination.

Diagnostic approach

Despite a physician's comprehensive approach to information gathering from medical, social, and cultural spheres, the specific cause for failure to thrive may not be apparent. In this case, the response of the infant to a period of hospitalization, with a week's trial of simple nutritional rehabilitation, will often make possible a specific diagnosis. Caution should be used when one is ordering the diet for such a child. The malnourished child may have trouble tolerating formulas containing a high carbohydrate concentration, especially if the sugar is lactose. This may be overcome when certain special formulas (Pregestimil or Nutramigen) are used. It is also wise to employ a period of renutrition for the malnourished patient before entering into an extensive series of laboratory tests. Interpretation of data obtained from absorption studies in malnourished patients may be difficult. Compounding the caloric deprivation by enforcing long periods of fasting for certain tests of absorption may be detrimental to the patient. Careful bookkeeping of daily food intake and weights and close observation of feeding techniques are essential during the period of hospitalization. The patient's response to hospitalization may permit the physician to sort out major groups or causes.

If the intake has been *adequate* and the child *gains,* a faulty feeding technique or a disturbed infant-mother relationship should be suspected. In such cases a team approach is recommended and should involve support for both the mother and child. Not infrequently, the staff will include a hospital nutritionist, pediatric social worker, psychologist, and physical and recreational therapists to further complement the efforts of physician and nursing staff. Follow-up study often utilizes a home stimulation program. In difficult situations, placement in foster care is required.

If intake is *adequate* but *no weight gain* ensues when caloric intake is commensurate with the infant's ideal weight for present height, a loss of calories from vomiting, malabsorption, or an abnormal peripheral utilization should be strongly suspected. If the intake is *inadequate,* the individual entities previously discussed should be ruled out.

Many laboratory procedures can be eliminated

by proper interpretion of the infant's history and observation of the response to a period of nutritional rehabilitation. This has been repeatedly emphasized over the years. A recent study found only 18% of cases of failure to thrive to have an organic basis. Over 50% of cases responded simply when the infant was offered an adequate caloric intake. Selection of laboratory studies most appropriate for each of the patterns of failure to thrive that have been discussed are listed below.

Laboratory studies in failure to thrive

Routine in all cases
1. Complete blood count
2. Urine analysis and culture

Pattern I
1. Viral culture (CMV) of throat and urine
2. TORCH titers
3. VDRL
4. Serum pH, Mg^{++}, K^+, HCO_3^-, Cl^-, BUN, Ca^{++}, $PO_4^=$
5. Roentgenogram of skull and long bones; bone age
6. Urine amino and organic acids
7. Chromosome study if dysmorphic
8. CT scan of brain if central nervous system findings present in history or physical examination

Pattern II
1. Bone age (wrist or hemiskeleton) depending on age of patient
2. Roentgenograms of long-bone epiphyses
3. Thyroid studies
4. Growth hormone and somatomedin levels

Pattern III
1. History of inadequate intake
   a. Serum electrolytes, Ca^{++}, $PO_4^=$
   b. Arterial blood gas determination
   c. Liver function studies, serum protein electrophoresis
   d. Chest film, ECG
   e. Intravenous pyelogram
   f. Thyroid studies
   g. Serum zinc levels
   h. Urine organic acids
   i. Chromosome study if dysmorphic
   j. Brain CT scan
2. Excessive caloric losses by vomiting
   a. Serum electrolytes, pH, Ca^{++}
   b. BUN, creatinine
   c. Roentgenograms: esophagogram, upper gastrointestinal series, skull film
   d. Spinal fluid analyses
   e. Urine organic acids
   f. Blood ammonia
   g. Brain CT scan
3. Excessive caloric losses by diarrhea
   a. Sweat chloride determination
   b. 72-hour stool fat, D-xylose absorption test, breath H_2 test
   c. Stools for pH, blood, and presence of reducing substances
   d. Immunoglobulins
   e. Stool culture and examination for parasites, leukocytes
   f. Peroral small-bowel biopsy
   g. Upper gastrointestinal series, small-bowel follow-through
   h. Barium enema
   i. Thyroid studies
   j. Urine catecholamines, vanillylmandelic acid (VMA), serum vasoactive intestinal peptides (VIP), prostaglandins

It is obvious that the approach to the child who fails to thrive necessitates a comprehensive understanding of infant growth and development, infant nutrition, psychosocial interchange between mother and child, an awareness of external influences (racial, religious, cultural), and a long list of possible pathologic disorders that at times are responsible for this condition. A systematic approach utilizing simple techniques such as growth charts and observations in the hospital will place the physician very close to the specific cause in surprisingly short order. At times, specific laboratory tests will confirm the presence of a suspected underlying condition.

REFERENCES

Ashworth, A., Bell, R., James, W.P.T., and Waterlow, J.C.: Calorie requirements of children recovering from protein-calorie malnutrition, Lancet **2**:600-603, Sept. 14, 1968.

Fleisher, D.R.: Infant rumination syndrome, Am. J. Dis. Child. **133**:266-269, March 1979.

Hannaway, P.J.: Failure to thrive: a study of 100 infants and children, Clin. Pediatr. **9**:96-99, Feb. 1970.

Horner, J.M., Thorsson, A.V., and Hintz, R.L.: Growth deceleration patterns in children with constitutional short stature: an aid to diagnosis, Pediatrics **62**:529-534, 1978. Pediatr. **70**:317-324, March 1967.

Kerr, M.A.D., Bogues, J.L., and Kerr, D.S.: Psychosocial functioning of mothers of malnourished children, Pediatrics **62**:778-784, Nov. 1978.

Krieger, I.: Food restriction as a form of child abuse in ten cases of psychosocial deprivation dwarfism, Clin. Pediatr. **13**:127-133, Feb. 1974.

Krieger, I., and Whitten, C.F.: Energy metabolism in infants with growth failure due to maternal deprivation, undernutrition, or causes unknown. II. Relationship between nitrogen balance, weight gain, and postprandial excess heat production, J. Pediatr. **75**:374-379, Sept. 1969.

Sills, R.H.: Failure to thrive: the role of clinical and laboratory evaluation, Am. J. Dis. Child. **132**:967-969, Oct. 1978.

Silver, H.K., and Finkelstein, M.: Deprivation dwarfism, J. Pediatr. **70**:317-324, March 1967.

Wilkins, L.: The diagnosis and treatment of endocrine disorders in childhood and adolescence, ed. 3, Springfield, Ill., 1965, Charles C Thomas, Publisher, Chapter 9.

SPITTING, REGURGITATION, AND VOMITING

The physician who is involved in child care is unlikely to have a day in his practice in which some parent does not express worry about an infant's spitting, regurgitation, or vomiting.

The symptoms of spitting and regurgitation are nonspecific and therefore carry variable significance. Vomiting, however, has a different connotation and is potentially more worrisome to the physician.

Spitting, regurgitation, and particularly vomiting may be the earliest manifestation of a wide range of significant disease states and therefore the physician who approaches this constellation of symptoms solely by ordering rapid formula changes is foolishly ignoring the real problem. A certain sequence of questioning can rapidly provide the physician with information useful not only in helping him appreciate the significance of these symptoms but also at times in permitting him to establish the proper diagnosis.

The age and sex of the child should be immediately established. The physician should then carefully ascertain from proper questioning of the mother whether the child is spitting, regurgitating, or truly vomiting. In any case it is wise to inquire about the child's state of health. Has he been losing or gaining weight? Is there an underlying condition known to the parent which may predispose the child to these symptoms? Is there an intercurrent illness? What is the *nature of the vomitus?* Is it curdled milk or undigested or unaltered food? Is bile or blood present? How soon after a feeding does the vomiting or regurgitation occur? Does positioning make a difference? Information regarding the *diet* is often needed; in particular, one should inquire about the *quality, quantity, and frequency of feeding,* especially in the young child. It may be necessary to ask about the technique of feeding.

Last, but not least, inquiry into the psychosocial dynamics of the household should be made. Frequently, the physician will realize that the source of concern for the symptom in a well child is coming from other members of the household. The anxiety of the mother may be compounded by the presence of an immature husband or a nagging grandmother. In this environment, simple spitting in a colicky infant may progress to a severe case of maternal deprivation. It is not unlikely that rumination may spring from such a relationship.

Attention to the complaint, awareness of its possible significance, and reassurance when needed will usually suffice as treatment.

Spitting and regurgitation

In the absence of improper feeding techniques, simple spitting or regurgitation in a thriving infant is most often caused by *gastroesophageal reflux* (chalasia). The problem is self-limited and is seldom encountered after the child is walking. On the other hand, the infant who is spitting or regurgitating but appears to be ill or is not gaining well needs closer scrutiny, for significant pathologic states may be responsible for this condition. Failure to appreciate the potential medical significance of these associated findings may be disastrous. The possibility of sepsis, meningitis, chronic subdural hematoma, hydrocephalus, adrenal insufficiency, or pyelonephritis should be entertained and attended to promptly if these symptoms are evident in an acutely ill neonate or infant. A similar mode of presentation may occur early in the course of *pyloric stenosis* or in *peptic disease* of the infant or small child. Though vomiting rather than spitting is the more common complaint in these conditions, spitting and regurgitation may dominate the early clinical picture.

Spitting or regurgitation with *choking* may reflect structural or neuromuscular disorders of the esophagus. A host of inborn errors of metabolism (phenylketonuria, maple syrup urine disease, methylmalonic acidemia, urea cycle disorders) may also be responsible for these symptoms and require proper screening of blood and urine specimens for specific diagnosis. Other metabolic and endocrine disorders, such as galactosemia, diabetes insipidus, hypercalcemia, renal tubular acidosis, and lactic acidosis, may become evident in a similar manner. Rarely, a brainstem glioma may become manifest with bulbar signs of regurgitation, choking and aspiration.

Vomiting

Vomiting entails forceful ejection of stomach contents; it has greater potential significance than spitting and therefore should be properly differentiated from spitting at the time of history taking. Again, the physician must know quickly whether the small infant or child is well or unwell, gaining or losing weight, and so forth. Since vomiting may reflect the severe expression of any of the aforementioned possibilities, priority should be given again to those entities that are common and potentially life threatening. The infant who experiences recurrent vomiting and is not gaining or is unwell needs to be seen by the physician.

As an acute episode, vomiting may be the first and only manifestation of acute gastroenteritis. Parenteral infections, central nervous system disease (meningitis, subdural effusion, hydrocephalus), peptic disease, salt-losing adrenogenital syndrome, and inborn errors of metabolism may need to be ruled out, especially the latter group if associated with developmental delays or a seizure disorder.

Vomiting and feeding difficulties with inborn errors of metabolism*

Disorders of ammonia cycle metabolism
Phenylketonuria
Maple syrup urine disease
Hypervalinemia
Hyperlysinemia
Ketotic hyperglycinemia
Methylmalonic aciduria
Propionic acidemia
Butyric/hexanoic acidemia
Isovaleric acidemia
Lysosomal acid phosphatase deficiency
Wolman's disease
Fructose 1,6-diphosphatase deficiency
Fructose intolerance
Galactosemia
Glycogen-storage disease type I
Congenital diabetes

If the child is not acutely ill, poor feeding technique and psychosocial problems in the environment may be responsible. Projectile vomiting of nonbilious gastric contents in a first-born male will be easily recognized as the result of *hypertrophic pyloric stenosis,* especially if peristaltic waves are seen and a palpable mass is present. This same complex would also accompany an *antral* or *channel ulcer.* Vomiting and failure to thrive are exceptional as the severe expressions of chalasia and are more likely caused by a *hiatal hernia* or another esophageal disorder. *Milk protein allergy* and *lactose intolerance* may produce vomiting, and other manifestations of these conditions should be sought. Beware of the infant who vomits breast milk, for a pathologic cause is usually responsible for this symptom.

*Courtesy Serge Melançon, Hôpital Sainte-Justine, Montreal.

Finally, an infant with bilious vomiting should be considered as having *sepsis* or an *intestinal obstruction* until proved otherwise. Such a child will need immediate attention for prompt diagnosis and treatment. Frequently, roentgenographic support is needed for diagnosis. Simple scout films of the abdomen will demonstrate obstructions of the intestine. Contrast-medium studies of the esophagus, stomach, and intestine are needed to show partial obstructions and malfunctions. Scout-film evidence of low obstruction usually indicates need for a barium enema.

In the newborn, vomiting may indicate special types of obstruction, but the approach is the same—scout films to locate the probable general level and then contrast studies from above, if a high-level and from below, if a low-level obstruction is suspected. Added helpful findings may be noted, such as skeletal abnormalities associated with definite gastrointestinal lesions (duplications) or soft-tissue calcifications.

Although some 50% of infants have spitting, regurgitation, or vomiting as an isolated complaint, less than 5% have significant underlying disease. The majority simply reflect a combination of physiologic immaturity of the gastroesophageal junction, improper feeding techniques, or a disturbed relationship between the infant and his mother.

Vomiting in the older child is most often attributable to gastritis, gastroenteritis, hepatitis, or pneumonia, and is usually a self-limited problem. On rare occasions, it may herald the development of Reye's syndrome, be the dominating symptom of increased intracranial pressure (tumor), the superior mesenteric artery syndrome, or a symptom of Crohn's disease of the stomach or small bowel, or evolve into a syndrome called "cyclic or periodic vomiting." This latter condition is most often a psychophysiologic disorder rather than the forerunner of migraine disease, but organic disease needs to be ruled out. We have seen recently two children with cyclic vomiting caused by intermittent obstruction at the ureteropelvic junction, presumably the result of congenital stenosis.

DIARRHEA

The physician who cares for children is frequently called on to cope with the symptom of diarrhea, which in simplistic terms can be thought of as an increase in frequency of defecation or a change in character of the stool. The number of entities that may be responsible for this symptom is large, and therefore the physician must be able to quickly employ systematic information gathering to help determine the most likely cause. Depending on seasonal variations of illness, 10% to 50% of his calls may relate to this symptom. Therefore he must quickly size up the urgency of the situation and decide on a course of action.

Prompt inquiry as to the age of the child should be made, for the threat of rapid dehydration and acidosis from diarrhea of any cause is greater for the young infant. Therefore this complaint should not be taken lightly when it develops in the very young infant. In addition, the age of the child is important because a number of disease states that manifest themselves as diarrhea are unique to the small infant.

The physician should also establish whether the symptom of diarrhea represents a sudden change (acute) or whether it actually has been going on for some time (chronic). Rapid elimination of possible causes will be facilitated when one simply knows the child's age and whether the diarrhea is acute or chronic.

Acute diarrhea

A list of the more common causes of acute diarrhea in children is given in the following outline.

Causes of acute diarrhea in children

Previously well child
  Contaminated foodstuffs
  Constipation with encopresis
  Emotional stress (spastic colon)
  Parasites
  Poisons (Iron, arsenic, insecticides)
  Specific food intolerances
Sick child
  Enteral
    Antibiotics
    Appendicitis
    Bacterial and viral gastroenteritis
    Carbohydrate intolerance (acquired)
    Hirschsprung's disease
    Inflammatory bowel disease
    Milk protein allergy
    Necrotizing enterocolitis
    "Nonspecific" gastroenteritis
    Pseudomembranous enterocolitis—antibiotic-associated
  Parenteral
    Upper respiratory tract infection (otitis media)
    Urinary tract infection
    Adrenal insufficiency

General information

Is the child ill or not? Acute diarrhea commencing as part of an associated illness is an extremely common mode of presentation for viral or bacterial gastroenteritis and can simply be established if one inquires about fever, abdominal pain, and vomiting. Information about a similar illness in other family members is helpful. However, it is possible for acute infectious diarrhea to occur without other associated symptoms.

In the absence of symptoms suggestive of an acute illness (viral gastroenteritis) in either the patient or his immediate family, other possible causes of acute diarrhea should be considered in the differential diagnosis. For example, *foods recently introduced* into the diet may cause acute diarrhea, as may *contaminated foods,* which should be suspected if similar symptoms occur in the other members of the family.

A precise *description of the stools* can be helpful when one is considering acute diarrheal diseases. Clues to a specific diagnosis may come from information about the frequency and size of the stool, water content, presence or absence of blood or mucus, color (green, black, pale), or odor (foul, acid, rank). This information can tell the physician much about the severity of the illness and its possible cause.

The physician should also inquire about the likelihood that a *toxic substance* may have been ingested or inhaled. Heavy metals (arsenic, iron) and the phosphorylated hydrocarbons (Parathion, Malathion) are common household products that can produce acute diarrhea. Finally, the possibility of a *parasitic infection* (giardiasis, amebiasis) should be considered if the child resides in, or has recently visited, an area known to be endemic for these organisms.

Newborn period

As previously mentioned, the neonate with acute diarrhea will need rapid and accurate assessment of his condition. In years past a common and worrisome cause was pathogenic *Escherichia coli.* In the neonate, illness caused by this microorganism is characterized by passage of large, watery, explosive stools that seldom contain blood and often are greenish. The child may develop acidosis with severe dehydration within hours. Epidemics in nurseries for the newborn have been catastrophic. One should suspect this organism as causative in any neonate who develops diarrhea shortly after being discharged from a newborn nursery.

Less commonly, shigellas, salmonellas, and *Campylobacter* may be the organisms responsible for diarrhea during the newborn period. An abrupt onset of loose, watery stools containing flecks of blood is the typical mode of presentation for these pathogens in neonates.

A fulminating diarrhea that becomes bloody in a neonate should make the physician consider *necrotizing enterocolitis,* which can also be a complication of *Hirschsprung's disease.* This may be the likely diagnosis in the patient with Down's syndrome who suddenly develops diarrhea. Necrotizing enterocolitis without an underlying cause occurs in the premature infant more often than in a full-term child. *Klebsiella* organism is often found in stool and blood cultures.

On rare occasions, we have seen children with either *salt-losing adrenogenital syndrome* or *congenital adrenal hypoplasia* present with an acute fulminating diarrhea during the first month of life. Additional clues to this diagnosis may be found at physical examination (pigmentation and virilization). Adrenal insufficiency should also be suspected when the usual therapeutic measures fail to control the vomiting and diarrhea or when there are characteristic electrolyte abnormalities (low sodium and high potassium).

The awareness that in the neonate abdominal distention and watery diarrhea containing flecks of blood may be the first expression of *severe bovine milk protein hypersensitivity* should prompt the physician to order a formula change (Nutramigen, Pregestimil). Since a similar intolerance to soy protein is highly likely in infants sensitized to bovine milk protein, it is best to avoid any soy-based formula products, at least initially. A positive family history of bovine milk allergy may eliminate unnecessary investigations of the child and permit a rapid diagnosis and institution of proper therapy.

Congenital lactase deficiency or glucose-galactose malabsorption may appear early in life as watery, acid, explosive diarrhea without blood or other systemic signs. These rare possibilities should be given priority in a child developing severe diarrhea exclusively on a breast milk diet. Intermittent, colicky diarrhea that produces loose, greenish stools and occurs in a breast-fed infant may occasionally result from *maternal ingestion of iron* or iron-containing prenatal vitamins. Symptoms may promptly abate on the mother's discontinuance of use of the medication.

Infancy

After the neonatal period has passed, acute diarrhea is most likely produced by viruses or bacteria. *Viral gastroenteritis,* typically characterized by the development of vomiting, diarrhea, and crampy abdominal pain, is not difficult to diagnose in the older child and often can be controlled by diet and symptomatic therapy. Again, the diagnosis of viral gastroenteritis is facilitated by the presence of additional signs or symptoms that suggest a viral respiratory infection or by the presence of a similar illness in the family.

Bacterial enteritis, such as that caused by *Shigella,* in the small child often has an abrupt onset with high fever, chills, and explosive, watery stools containing flecks of blood and mucus. The child looks toxic and may even have a convulsion, causing one to mistakenly consider meningitis. Not infrequently, the diagnosis first becomes obvious during the spinal tap, when suddenly the patient will pass several explosive, watery stools. Dehydration and acidosis may ensure rapidly. *Salmonella* may cause an illness with a mode of onset similar to that of *Shigella;* however, the child generally appears less toxic though the stools have the same features as *Shigella* diarrhea. *Campylobacter*-caused diarrhea needs to be considered. Parasitic infections, especially those caused by *Giardia,* need consideration if the child spends much of his waking time in a day care center or other crowded environment.

School-age child

In the older child, acute diarrhea may herald an acute appendicitis, regional enteritis, or toxic megacolon of chronic ulcerative colitis. Any of these, and others, may mimic acute viral gastroenteritis.

Last but not least, an acute episode of diarrhea may usher in any one of a number of conditions discussed in the section concerning chronic diarrhea. Here a specific diagnosis may be delayed until the clinical syndrome becomes more apparent to the parents and the physician.

Chronic diarrhea

When the physician learns that the diarrhea has been of a chronic nature, a different priority of questions will be necessary to delineate or define which one of a large number of possible conditions is responsible for this symptom. Some are listed on the next page.

Causes of chronic diarrhea in children

Well child

  Carbohydrate intolerance in the older child (primary
    or postinfectious)
  Dietary indiscretions
  Irritable bowel syndrome
  Constipation with encopresis
  Parasites
  Polyposis

Sick child (not thriving)

  Abetalipoproteinemia
  Acrodermatitis enteropathica
  Blind or stagnant loop syndrome
  Carbohydrate intolerance in the young child (primary
    or postinfectious)
  Carcinoid
  Celiac disease
  Chronic pancreatitis
  Cystic fibrosis
  Enterokinase deficiency
  Exocrine pancreatic hypoplasia
  Familial chloride diarrhea
  Ganglioneuroma, ganglioneuroblastoma
  Hyperthyroidism
  Immune deficiencies
  Inflammatory bowel disease (ulcerative colitis, Crohn's
    disease)
  Intractable diarrhea of infancy
  Lymphangiectasis
  Maternal deprivation syndrome
  Milk protein intolerance
  Pancreatic tumors (non–beta cell types)
  Polyposis
  Protein-calorie malnutrition
  Short-bowel syndrome
  Upper small bowel contamination
  Whipple's disease

Diagnosis of these diseases is often dependent on acquisition of an accurate and comprehensive history since many patients with chronic diarrhea have few if any positive physical findings. However, there are times when the carefully performed physical examination will permit detection of those subtle findings that aid in establishing the specific cause of chronic diarrhea.

The *age of the child at which the symptoms began* is most informative. Next in importance is specific information about the well-being of the child: Has he been *gaining and growing,* or has he been *failing to thrive,* or, indeed, has he been *losing weight* during the course of the diarrhea?

Probably 95% of pediatric cases of chronic diarrhea can be attributed to fewer than half a dozen entities. The most common cause of continuous or intermittent diarrhea in a thriving patient be-

tween the ages of 6 months and 3 years is the *irritable bowel syndrome* (nonspecific diarrhea of infancy and childhood). It is not uncommon for this entity to start or be exacerbated by an intercurrent infection such as gastroenteritis. Stools are often passed during the earlier part of the day, after meals, and frequently after the ingestion of cold liquids. They are seldom passed during sleep. One should also consider an osmotic diarrhea from overfeeding as an explanation for diarrhea in a young infant who appears well nourished.

When diarrhea persists after a bout of acute gastroenteritis in an otherwise well child, one might suspect *acquired disaccharidase (lactase) deficiency* or *milk protein intolerance* as the cause.

In contrast to the just-mentioned entities that affect children who generally appear well, the onset of diarrhea that occurs before the age of 1 year and is associated with failure to thrive is likely to result from only a few but serious conditions. One may need additional history taking for making a specific diagnosis in this patient group.

Knowledge of the *sequence* of introduction of all food products into the diet of the infant and their temporal relationship to the diarrhea is essential. If the physician can establish that chronic diarrhea has occurred in an infant who receives only breast milk, the child may have *congenital lactase deficiency* or possibly *glucose-galactose malabsorption.* A similar diagnosis is tenable if the infant is taking lactose-containing formula as his entire diet. In contrast, the infant who has been receiving breast milk exclusively and then develops diarrhea after starting to receive solid foods (cereals and fruits) is not likely to have lactose intolerance but may have *sucrase-isomaltase deficiency.* However, if diarrhea commences when he begins eating applesauce but by history he has previously been tolerating table sugar on his cereal, he probably has an idiosyncrasy to applesauce rather than congenital sucrase deficiency. Specific questions as to the character of stools can be helpful. Stools of patients with disaccharidase deficiency states are usually loose, watery, and acid, and frequently they cause severe diaper rash.

Similarly, the child whose diarrhea began before the introduction of wheat-containing cereals (mixed or high-protein) to his diet is not likely to have celiac disease. Sometimes it is difficult to unravel the problem. For example, the infant with chronic diarrhea who improves when fed soybean protein formula is often considered an allergic child. In fact, he may have bovine milk protein allergy, lactase deficiency, or both, as his underlying problem, for these conditions will simultaneously be improved by this particular formula change. Soybean formulas (and others) not only eliminate dietary bovine proteins from the diet but also are lactose-free. Therefore it behooves the physician to become thoroughly acquainted with the contents of the proprietary formulas (Chapter 28), since random formula changes may not be helpful. Too often, they are made in an unscientific manner. It is extremely common to hear a mother list a long sequence of formula changes previously employed in an attempt to correct the diarrhea of her infant. These maneuvers often fail because therapy is oriented toward a change in the proprietary name of the formula rather than toward a qualitative composition change.

Caloric deprivation is inevitable with the use of dilute formulas or "clear liquids" and may usher in the syndrome of *intractable diarrhea of infancy,* which not infrequently requires sustained hospital confinement and prolonged use of total parenteral nutrition and generates monumental hospital charges.

The infant or child less than 1 year old with chronic diarrhea and failure to thrive should be suspected of having *cystic fibrosis.* Helpful clues sometimes present include a history of chronic cough (especially at night), a previous episode of pneumonia or rectal prolapse, and a family history of the disease. Stools of the patient with cystic fibrosis are characteristically large, foul, oily, foamy, and pale, reflecting the presence of significant steatorrhea.

A similar symptom complex (diarrhea, cough, and failure to thrive) is now recognized as the earliest expression of an *immune deficiency disease,* and specific laboratory tests will be needed for diagnosis. Another likely cause of diarrhea and failure to thrive of children less than 1 year old is *celiac disease.* Gluten enteropathy or celiac disease should be suspected when the physician can establish that the diarrhea and failure to thrive began *after* the introduction of wheat-containing foods. Again, the stools contain much fat and are described as large, pale, foamy, and greasy as well as extremely offensive. Celiac disease has many modes of presentation and expression, and diarrhea is only one of them. An awareness of physical features typical of celiac disease may aid in diagnosis.

In recent years, the *maternal deprivation syndrome* has been described as a cause of failure to thrive in the young child. It may mimic cystic fibrosis or celiac disease in that the appearance of the child and his stool characteristics may be identical to those typical of the other diseases. Where severe poverty exists, *protein-calorie malnutrition* can become evident through chronic diarrhea and failure to thrive.

In addition to the aforementioned entities, there still remain several conditions that can cause diarrhea and failure to thrive in the young child. These diagnoses are difficult to make because the patient's history is usually nonspecific and physical findings are few. These include *Giardia* infestation in endemic areas, ganglioneuroma, exocrine pancreatic insufficiency (noncystic fibrosis), and Whipple's disease. *Anatomic abnormalities* of the gastrointestinal tract, such as congenital short bowel, a blind or stagnant loop secondary to kinking of the the bowel, or malrotation, may be rare causes of chronic diarrhea and failure to thrive.

Other conditions causing similar symptoms in the young child can be identified or made evident by specific physical findings. The child will be recognized as having *acrodermatitis enteropathica* by the distributions of lesions around his mouth and anus. Likewise, the problem of chronic diarrhea in a child with *abetalipoproteinemia* (Bassen-Kornzweig syndrome) can be recognized, for physical findings of this syndrome include cataracts, ataxia, and mental retardation. *Intestinal lymphangiectasis* should be considered when a lymphedematous limb and pitting edema are noted in a child with chronic diarrhea.

The onset of chronic diarrhea in the school-age child should make the physician suspect a different group of diseases. Here, careful attention to presence or absence of associated symptoms and qualitative aspects of the stools will again help the physician to arrive at an early and correct diagnosis.

The *irritable bowel syndrome* is an uncommon cause of chronic diarrhea in a child older than 3 years, but the adult counterpart of spastic colon disease may also occur in the young school-age child. Fortunately this entity can be recognized on the basis of certain consistent features. First, the child is usually well. Second, functional diarrhea as seen in the irritable colon syndrome seldom awakens the child from a sound sleep, whereas inflammatory bowel disease often does. Finally, the stools may be loose, explosive at times, but they seldom contain blood.

One should also consider *constipation with en-*

copresis in a well child with chronic diarrhea, and the diagnosis is easily confirmed by rectal examination.

Lower abdominal pain relieved by defecation, intermittent fever, anorexia, weight loss, recurrent stomatitis, uveitis, growth failure, and arthralgias are consistent with *Crohn's disease.* The presence of these findings should be both inquired about and looked for when chronic diarrhea occurs in the child older than 5 years. In *ulcerative colitis,* the passage of loose stools with blood and mucus is typically accompanied by tenesmus and cramps; fever, weight loss, and anemia are commonly noted as associated features.

Chronic diarrhea may be an unusual but early complaint related to *hyperthyroidism.* Knowledge of associated symptoms may be obtained by history taking, and diagnosis can usually be made at physical examination. Late in the course of *chronic fibrosing pancreatitis,* chronic diarrhea may dominate the clinical picture. The onset of diarrhea with or without cramps in a teenager may be the first clue to *polyposis,* which requires prompt diagnosis. Intermittent or continuous abdominal pain associated with chronic diarrhea has been seen in rare cases of *Zollinger-Ellison syndrome, carcinoid,* or *intestinal lymphosarcoma.* It is extremely rare for gallbladder disease or chronic liver disease to produce chronic diarrhea without there being other associated findings. Roentgenographic examinations seldom are useful in diagnosis of acute diarrhea; even for chronic diarrhea, their diagnostic usefulness is much less than for gastrointestinal bleeding. However, diagnosis of colitis, localized enteritis, specific lesions such as fistulas, short-bowel syndrome, or intestinal lymphangiectasis can be made by proper roentgenographic examinations. Special tests, including the induction of dysfunction with the use of specific materials mixed with barium, as well as isotope excretion studies, have specific uses.

CONSTIPATION OR OBSTIPATION

A decrease in frequency of defecation, a change in the consistency of the stool, and painful defecation are common complaints. Although constipation occurs frequently during infancy and childhood, it seldom carries significant medical importance for the patient in this age group. The magnitude of this complaint is often determined by familial, cultural, and social factors that are likely responsible for the genesis and progression of this symptom.

In distinct contrast, constipation or obstipation during the newborn period is always significant until proved otherwise. Most nursery personnel are instructed to inform the responsible physician of any newborn infant who fails to pass meconium within the first 24 hours of life. This observation may be the first clue that intestinal obstruction exists. However, passage of meconium does not rule out high or low obstruction. Abdominal distention, bile-stained vomitus, and respiratory distress more commonly accompany the failure to pass meconium when lower bowel obstruction exists. The *meconium plug syndrome, Hirschsprung's disease, small left-colon syndrome, atresia, stenosis,* and *anorectal anomalies* are distinct possibilities. *Functional ileus of the newborn* may need to be considered in a smaller infant who experienced transient respiratory distress after delivery. These infants may not pass meconium during the first 24 hours and often regurgitate their early feedings. Preliminary roentgenograms of the abdomen usually show low obstruction, and barium enemas are safe and diagnostically helpful in most of the aforementioned conditions.

After the immediate newborn period has passed, constipation in the neonate may be dietary in origin. The most common specific cause is the early introduction of solid foods, particularly refined cereals (rice and oatmeal) and yellow vegetables (carrots, squash, sweet potatoes). Excessive intake of cow's milk or a change from breast feeding to formula feeding may result in passage of decreased numbers of firm, dry stools. The parent may relate that the infant is fussy, colicky, and gassy. Blood streaking may be noted on the outside of the formed stool.

The infrequent passage of bowel movements occurs in some breast-fed infants, presumably because of the lack of residue. An interval of 3 to 21 days has been observed in some cases in the absence of abdominal distention, or vomiting, and with minimal fussiness. The addition of bulk to the diet, such as cereal products or Metamucil, or offering a proprietary milk formula supplement usually cures the "constipation."

When the physician is first informed of the symptom of constipation, he should always try to establish whether this is an isolated problem in a well child or part of a larger symptom complex. Adherence to this rule will protect the physician against missing certain diagnoses. Although a change in stool pattern toward constipation occurs most often in the well child as a consequence of dietary manipulations, it may be the first symptom of serious metabolic or endocrine disorders to be appreciated by the mother. *Congenital hypothyroidism, diabetes insipidus, renal tubular acidosis,* and *hypercalcemia* are entities of which constipation may be the earliest symptom most concerning the parent. The physician should acquaint himself with other aspects of these entities so that proper questioning of the parent permits him to dismiss or consider these diagnoses as causes of constipation.

There are other reasons for which the physician should not dismiss this complaint lightly. Constipation in the young infant may be the first clue that future problems related to bowel function are likely. Even at this early age, physiologic factors that eventually are responsible for excessive dehydration of stool and the subsequent development of obstipation and fecal soiling are operative. Therefore infrequent evacuation of small, pelletlike stools during early life may *not* be normal but rather a consequence of a functional distal obstructive phenomenon.

To many physicians and parents, constipation means difficulty in passing stool, be it hard and formed or even soft. Not infrequently, the small infant may seem to have much difficulty in passage of such a soft, normal-sized stool. He is noted to struggle, squirm, and turn purple before passing his stool. Once the physician has obtained this information about the consistency and size of the stool, he is in a better position to explain these observations to the worried parent. Some infants seem to have a temporary imbalance or disorganization of autonomic input to the colon, rectum, and anal sphincter accounting for the apparent difficulty in passing even a soft stool. The condition is temporary and generally needs no treatment. Some authors have likened this problem to the spastic-colon syndrome of adults, in which increased resting tone in the spastic distal segment acts as a "cork in the rectum." Anticholinergic drugs and anal dilations have been used as modes of therapy, but watchful waiting and reassurance work as well. In fact, some people think that the infant is struggling to withhold stool because the act of defecation is uncoordinated and therefore painful. At best, this remains conjectural.

Besides inquiring about the well-being of the child, the associated symptoms, and the consistency of the stool, the physician may want to know about the relative size of the constipated stool. Passage of large-caliber stools is presumptive evidence that no distal anorectal anomaly exists, and for all practical purposes excludes entities such as Hirschsprung's disease, anal stenosis or stricture, or a perineal fistula associated with an anorectal anomaly. Later in childhood, when constipation becomes severe, the passage of stools capable of stopping the toilet plumbing promptly rules out congenital malformation of the large bowel as likely causes of this symptom.

Episodes of constipation may recur frequently during the first year of life. Most often, changes in environment, dietary factors, or an intercurrent illness may be responsible for temporary bowel dysfunction.

Anal fissures may lead to painful defecation and assume importance in the etiology of stool holding, even in the young child. Therefore, it is worthwhile to inquire about the presence of blood streaking on the outside of the stool. Anal fissures may often be seen simply when the buttocks and anal ring are spread; most commonly, they occur dorsally or ventrally. They may be found even though a history of blood streaking is not obtained from the parent. Local treatment and use of stool softeners usually alleviate the problem.

Habitual constipation may develop as a consequence of coercive efforts toward toilet training, when psychosocial factors interact and play a large contributory role. A family history of constipation may also be present. This condition may go on to become severe constipation with impaction. When a child is beyond the toilet-training age, the parent will infrequently find it necessary to pay attention to the frequency or consistency of the child's stool. Fecal soiling develops, and this complaint may be the first clue that the child has been severely constipated. Nocturia, through reduction of bladder capacity and relaxation of the internal urethral sphincter or recurrent urinary tract infections may be another consequence of constipation and may provide an important clue. The child suffering from *encopresis,* a fairly common pediatric condition, will need proper treatment and frequent revisits to prevent the emotional trauma that invariably accompanies this state.

Constipation is unlikely to be an isolated, single symptom of a metabolic or endocrine disorder or of another gastrointestinal disorder. Hypothyroidism, diabetes insipidus, intestinal pseudo-obstruction syndrome, colonic tumors, and even early inflammatory bowel disease and celiac disease may all initially produce a change in bowel habit but are easily recognized by other clinical features.

It is not uncommon for the school-age child to become constipated without experiencing associated symptoms. This usually develops when the urge to defecate comes at an inopportune time, such as during playtime or school hours; the child will choose to suppress the urge and make every effort to withhold defecation. Yet most of these children are never troubled by the consequences of this decision. In the older child, functional or habitual constipation is easily differentiated from aganglionosis by barium enema. As previously indicated, an evaluation of the urinary tract may be a valuable adjunct in the diagnostic work-up of patients with chronic constipation, since abnormalities of the lower urinary tract are frequently present.

FECAL SOILING (ENCOPRESIS)

Fecal soiling resulting from incontinence is a frequent complaint. Most often it develops in a previously well child who has been completely toilet trained. In others, effective toilet training has never been achieved, and they continue to soil.

The most common cause of this socially embarrassing situation is simply severe constipation, usually with impaction and painful defecation. Direct questioning of the parent concerning the child's bowel habits may give misleading information. Not only can parents misinterpret the child's daily visit to the bathroom as synonymous with "regularity," but they may in fact misinterpret fecal soiling as diarrhea. Since most of these children are beyond the toilet-training age, the parents seldom feel the need or have the desire to inspect the nature of the child's stool.

A delay in bringing this symptom to the attention of the physician is also common. At first, the child may attempt to conceal this problem by rinsing out his underwear, hiding it, or actually disposing of it. He may use the underwear of siblings if it is available. The parents may contribute to the delay by taking a punitive approach to the child in an attempt to deal with the symptom rather than the cause. At times, the cause is mistakenly assumed to arise from a recent psychologic conflict between child and parent, with fecal soiling the only effective weapon of the child.

The physician should not contribute to the delay once the complaint has been brought to his attention. Once informed of this symptom, he should promptly examine the child. As suggested, a delay has already occurred, and the psychoso-cial impact from parents and peers has already led to unfortunate consequences for the child.

Careful questioning of the child or parent will usually reveal information suggesting severe constipation as the underlying cause. Obstipation, painful defecation, fissures, occasional passage of a very large diameter stool, and urinary frequency are generally part of the symptom complex. Some degree of anorexia, abdominal pain, distention, and irritability may also be commented on by child or parent.

The presence of a sausage-shaped abdominal mass arising from the pelvis or over the course of the colon will be found on examination of the abdomen. Careful examination of the anus should include simple inspection of its location and contractile response to stimulation with a sharp object. The perianal skin is often irritated and inflamed. Digital examination will usually indicate normal sphincter tone, and shortly beyond the internal sphincter a large, firm fecal impaction will be found, confirming the diagnosis.

The institution of proper therapy for this condition will invariably render the young patient very grateful and appreciative.

At times, the problem of fecal incontinence will be deeply rooted in psychologic difficulties, and the patient will need both medical and psychiatric attention to attain continuous success.

When fecal continence has never been achieved, several other diagnostic possibilities exist. The presence of a neurologic disorder with or without constipation should be carefully considered. Chronic constipation with an impaction and encopresis is particularly frequent in association with a primary disorder of the central nervous system and mental retardation. Incomplete toilet training may be an early clue to a local *neurologic lesion* such as diastematomyelia, myelomeningocele, or tumor of the cauda equina. In addition, an anatomic or functional problem interfering with the mechanism of defecation may be at fault. Such an example may be seen in a patient with an anorectal anomaly in whom a perineal fistula may be mistaken for the normal anal opening. There are some children in whom failure to complete toilet training results from the presence of a rectal impaction, and confirmed soiling is involuntary. Fecal soiling on a voluntary basis in an otherwise physically normal child who has never been trained often reflects a severe psychologic disorder.

JAUNDICE

During the newborn period, when the development of jaundice is common, icterus is quickly recognized by personnel involved in newborn care. There are occasions subsequent to the newborn period when the physician caring for children will be presented with the complaint that the patient, or at least part of him, appears yellow. Many times, however, the jaundice develops in a slow and insidious fashion, thereby causing some delay in its recognition. It is not uncommon for a friend, a relative or even the physician to recognize it first and inform the patient that he appears jaundiced, whereas it is unusual to have the patient express this finding as an isolated event. Depending on the underlying cause of the jaundice. there will usually be other signs and symptoms evident to the physician that may help him establish a correct diagnosis.

In any and all circumstances, it is best to consider the appearance of jaundice as an abnormal event that demands explanation for its development, and specific treatment when indicated. Therefore, all patients with jaundice should be examined, and proper laboratory investigations should be made to aid in establishing a diagnosis.

The mechanisms responsible for the development of jaundice basically affect bilirubin (1) production, (2) hepatocyte uptake, (3) intrahepatocyte binding, (4) conjugation, (5) secretion, and (6) excretion. As is often the case, more than one mechanism can be involved or affected by the time the disease in question reaches full clinical expression. For example, simple bilirubin overload from hemolysis may cause hepatocellular injury or bile ductule injury, which then affects transport, secretion, or excretion. On the other hand, bilirubin excretion defects may result in impairment of uptake and transport of bilirubin. In addition, hepatocellular injury may shorten red cell survival, thereby adding to the overload and uptake difficulties.

Neonatal period

As with most other symptoms in children, it is generally easier to consider the neonatal period separately, since many diseases are unique to this particular age group. These are listed in Table 1-2. Several immediate and concerning possibilities should promptly come to mind once the physician has been informed that jaundice has developed in the newborn infant. First, is a *hemolytic condition* at fault and is there a possibility that kernicterus will develop as a consequence of the hyperbilirubinemia? Second, is *sepsis* possibly responsible for the jaundice? Third, is the jaundice an expression of an underlying *genetic, metabolic,* or *endocrine disorder* (such as galactosemia, fructose intolerance, tyrosinemia, hypothyroidism) for which early recognition and proper treatment will prevent irreparable damage?

Laboratory investigations begin the sorting process for possible causes, since the physical examination is seldom rewarding other than for jaundice, signs of anemia, and possibly hepatic and splenic enlargement. The major division of likely causes of jaundice is determined according to whether the hyperbilirubinemia is predominantly *unconjugated (indirect-reacting)* or is of the mixed or combined type. In the latter case, a variable but substantial part of the total bilirubin will be represented by the *conjugated (direct-reacting) fraction.*

Unconjugated hyperbilirubinemia

Information regarding the clinical condition of the jaundiced neonate should be sought immediately because a delay in the diagnosis of neonatal sepsis is often disastrous. In particular, unconjugated hyperbilirubinemia that develops in a newborn infant who is lethargic, feeds poorly, is vomiting, and has a high-pitched cry and a poor Moro reflex probably indicates sepsis. Blood, urine, throat, cerebrospinal fluid, umbilical cord, and stool cultures and studies should be done promptly, and antibiotics given at once. The mother's experience of prolonged ruptured membranes, long labor, and difficult delivery frequently correlates positively with neonatal sepsis. Neonatal meningitis and pyelonephritis should be considered and ruled out. It should be pointed out that severe neonatal infections may also produce a cholestatic picture (hepatocellular and canalicular), resulting in an elevated bilirubin of the mixed type, mimicking other entities that produce chronic obstructive jaundice.

Fortunately most cases of unconjugated hyperbilirubinemia in the neonate occur in a well infant and are caused by one of several mechanisms, including a maturation delay in hepatic glucuronyl transferase primarily responsible for the condition of *physiologic jaundice* of the newborn infant. Jaundice of this type appears during the second or third day of life and is generally mild and self-

Table 1-2. Some causes of jaundice of the neonate

Predominantly indirect reacting hyperbilirubinemia		Predominantly direct or mixed reacting hyperbilirubinemia	
Hemolytic	**Nonhemolytic**	**Intrahepatic**	**Extrahepatic**
Sepsis	Physiologic jaundice of	Sepsis	Biliary artresia
Isoimmunization	newborn	Pyelonephritis	Choledochus cyst
Hemoglobinopathies	Breast milk	Syphilis	Bile plug syndrome
Red blood cell	hyperbilirubinemia	Alpha-1-antitrypsin	Cholelithiasis
defects	Sulfonamide drugs,	Neonatal hepatitis	Perforation of bile ducts
	salicylates, novobiocin	Congenital fructose intoler-	
	Crigler-Najjar syndrome	ance	
	Gilbert's disease	Galactosemia	
	Large hematomas	Tyrosinemia	
	Gastrointestinal bleeding	Cystic fibrosis	
	Cretinism	Niemann-Pick disease	
	High small-bowel	Rotor syndrome	
	obstruction	Dubin-Johnson syndrome	
	Hypertrophic pyloric	Severe hemolytic disease	
	stenosis	("inspissated bile	
	Lucey-Driscoll syndrome	syndrome")	
		Paucity of the interlobular	
		bile ducts	
		Toxoplasmosis	
		Rubella	
		Histoplasmosis	
		Herpesvirus	
		Varicella	
		Enteroviruses	
		Drugs	
		Toxins	
		Byler's syndrome	
		Parenteral	
		hyperalimentation	
		Congestive heart failure	
		Hypoplastic left heart	
		syndrome	
		Postnecrotizing	
		enterocolitis,	
		gastroschisis, ruptured	
		omphalocele	
		Neonatal hypopituitarism	

limiting. However, the physician should be reluctant to make this diagnosis until he is certain that an isoimmunization caused by ABO, Rh, or other factors does not exist. The absence of anemia in the jaundiced newborn infant generally excludes other nonisoimmunizing hemolytic states such as congenital spherocytic hemolytic anemia, nonspherocytic hemolytic anemia, glucose-6-PD deficiency, and hereditary elliptocytosis as causes for the hyperbilirubinemia.

There still remain several conditions that can cause unconjugated hyperbilirubinemia in the well neonate. Since the discovery that a factor in mother's milk is capable of inhibiting glucuronyl transferase, *breast-milk hyperbilirubinemia* has been diagnosed with increasing frequency. The physician should specifically inquire whether *drug-induced* causes are possibly responsible for elevation of the indirect bilirubin fraction. Such drugs as vitamin K analogs, sulfonamides, salicylates, and novobiocin may lead to hyperbilirubinemia either by increasing hemolysis or by competing for albumin-binding sites. An easily recognized but seldom suspected condition capable of causing significant neonatal jaundice of this type is a large *enclosed hemorrhage* (cephalhematoma, retroperitoneal hemorrhage). In the neonate, other less common causes for predominance of unconjugated bilirubin include the familial entities of *Crigler-Najjar syndrome* and *Gilbert's disease*.

Crigler-Najjar syndrome is fortunately quite rare. If this syndrome is absent from the family history, the diagnosis of type I disease is seldom made before the development of neurologic defects and kernicterus. An early (during the first 24 hours) rapid increase of unconjugated bilirubin in the absence of hemolytic component should always make one suspicious of this possibility.

Prolonged elevation of the level of indirect bilirubin is frequently seen in *congenital cretinism*, though the diagnosis should be apparent from other clinical findings. The same would apply to the jaundice noted in patients with *pyloric stenosis* or *high small-bowel obstruction*, in which an elevated level of indirect bilirubin can be present in some 30% of cases.

Mixed or combined elevation of bilirubin ("obstructive" jaundice)

Under normal conditions, the clearance of bilirubin follows a series of sequential but independent physiologic processes of hepatic uptake, intrahepatocyte binding and transport, conjugation, canalicular secretion, and excretion of bilirubin. The sensitivity of this process is such that a disruption of one step is likely to affect adversely one or more of the other steps involved in bilirubin clearance, a situation that accompanies a number of pathologic states. Indeed, it is common to find an elevated level of both the direct- and the indirect-reacting fractions of serum bilirubin in disease states that affect this physiologic process.

During the neonatal period, the development of jaundice characterized by a mixed elevation of serum bilirubin occurs in a limited number of conditions falling under the broad heading of "cholestatic syndromes of the neonate" (Chapter 19). The most likely differential diagnosis will be between *extrahepatic biliary atresia* and *neonatal infectious* or *"idiopathic" hepatitis*. At times, severe hemolytic disease may rapidly promote a large bilirubin overload to the liver cells and excretory biliary system, which results in bile stasis and canalicular plugging. Therefore persistent hyper-

bilirubinemia of the mixed type may persist for as long as 4 to 12 weeks in severe cases of hemolytic disease, and this possibility should be ruled out by means of laboratory investigations including blood typing, Rh-factor determinations, and Coombs' test. Obstructive jaundice developing in the presence of hemolytic disease has been called the *inspissated bile syndrome*, but recent evidence suggests that some cases probably are caused by superimposed neonatal hepatitis. The associated physical findings of hepatosplenomegaly can be explained by extramedullary hematopoiesis or neonatal hepatitis. In the absence of hemolytic disease, a similar clinical picture may be secondary to a temporary impairment of biliary secretion, and this condition has many causes, collectively grouped under the heading *"intrahepatic cholestasis of the newborn."*

The major diagnostic dilemma to be considered in a neonate with persistent obstructive jaundice is whether the jaundice is caused by surgical or nonsurgical causes. Differentiation between these groups of diseases on clinical grounds or laboratory investigations or both remains extremely difficult and is discussed at length in Chapter 19.

Jaundice after the first month of life

It is not uncommon for the physician to first recognize the presence of jaundice at the 4- to 6-week examination of the infant. He should again inquire about the type of feeding, noting whether the stools are golden yellow to green in color and the urine clear, whether the infant is pale or anemic or both, whether there is a presence or absence of hepatosplenomegaly. This information should help differentiate possible causes of the hyperbilirubinemia. The most common cause at this age seems to be breast-milk hyperbilirubinemia. On the other hand, pale stools and dark urine are common to all forms of obstructive jaundice and therefore constitute helpful information, with biliary atresia and neonatal hepatitis being by far the most likely causes.

Jaundice after 6 months of age

After the first few months of life have elapsed, the most frequent cause of jaundice is *acute viral hepatitis*. The syndrome of anorexia, fever, vomiting, abdominal pain, darkening of the urine, and passage of clay-colored stools is familiar to most physicians as being compatible with type A viral hepatitis. Hepatitis from virus B produces a similar symptom complex and may be suspected in children born to carrier mothers or whose underlying condition increases their exposure to parenterally administered blood products (hemophilia, open-heart surgery, hemodialysis).

The teenager who becomes jaundiced should be questioned about the use of parenterally administered illicit drugs (heroin, Methedrine, "speed"). Male homosexuals are also at increased risk to develop hepatitis. They often know of friends who have recently been jaundiced and who could have been responsible for transmission of the disease.

A young female teenager who develops jaundice and has a history of intermittent arthritis, acne, perhaps amenorrhea, and fatigue may prove to have *chronic active hepatitis*. One should not limit this diagnosis to the adolescent age group, since this entity also occurs in young children. Acute, icteric hepatitis in any child should also make the physician consider a potentially treatable cause for this illness, such as *Wilson's disease* or, again, *galactosemia*. Presence of jaundice in a patient with exudative tonsillitis, adenopathy, or splenomegaly probably points to *infectious mononucleosis* as a cause for the jaundice.

Gallbladder disease (cholecystitis, cholelithiasis) can be the cause of jaundice in a pediatric patient. Many will have an underlying hemoglobinopathy (sickle-cell disease, thalassemia, spherocytic hemolytic anemia), but symptoms of colicky pain in the right upper quadrant, with or without fever, generally facilitate proper diagnosis. The triad of colicky abdominal pain, jaundice, and right upper quadrant mass, especially in a young girl, is compatible with a *choledochus cyst*.

Prolonged obstructive jaundice may result from other unusual anatomic aberrations of the biliary tree *(duplication cyst)*. Congenital narrowing or stricture of the common duct may slowly lead to the development of jaundice, pruritus, and pain in the right upper quadrant. Jaundice, pruritus, and xanthomas are frequently seen in the patient with *hypoplasia of the intrahepatic bile ducts*. This condition may be sporadic or familial, with neonatal hepatitis believed responsible for many former cases.

Rarely, tumors of the peritoneal cavity, biliary tree, or head of the pancreas may cause obstructive jaundice in children. *Intraduodenal leiomyomas* or *lymphosarcomas* that obstruct the ampulla

of Vater have been a cause of obstructive jaundice in some patients.

Intermittent, mild, unconjugated hyperbilirubinemia associated with nonspecific illness and abdominal pain will be recognized as *Gilbert's disease*. Mild, conjugated hyperbilirubinemia in a well patient may be caused by Dubin-Johnson or Rotor's syndrome. Confirmation of disease can be confirmed by family history, laboratory findings, and liver biopsy; the last is usually diagnostic. In rare cases, we have seen jaundice secondary to liver disease precede the bowel symptoms in *chronic ulcerative colitis. Drug-induced* and *toxic liver injuries* from a large variety of agents are possible causes of jaundice in children and will need consideration in the history taking.

HEMATEMESIS

Vomiting of blood is a frightening experience for both the child and his parent and will be brought to the physician's attention with great dispatch. Once again, the physician needs information that will permit him to correctly ascertain the urgency of the situation as well as the possible cause of the symptom. It is again apparent that the likelihood of a specific diagnosis for a given symptom is very age dependent within the pediatric population. This is well exemplified by the complaint of hematemesis, and common features of this symptom are outlined in Table 1-3.

Hematemesis noted shortly after birth (within the first 12 to 24 hours) may be the regurgitation of *material blood swallowed* during delivery. Since the quantity of blood may be sizable, prompt determination by means of the Apt-Downey test (Chapter 30) for the presence or absence of fetal hemoglobin in the vomitus is essential. Meanwhile, the physician should seek information that might suggest other likely causes for hematemesis in the newborn infant. Does the infant appear pale or ill? Was the labor difficult and prolonged? Were the maternal membranes ruptured for a long time? Is neonatal sepsis or meningitis a possibility? Has the baby been lethargic, irritable, or regurgitating? Is there fever or jaundice?

This line of questioning rapidly gives the physician a clue to possible source and perhaps cause of bleeding in the upper gastrointestinal tract. *Stress gastric ulcers* or a *hemorrhagic gastritis* may be a cause of hematemesis in the newborn infant and is most likely to occur in infants born after diffi-

Table 1-3. Causes of hematemesis in children

Entity	Age	Amount	Clinical features	Cause	Diagnostic means
Swallowed maternal blood	Newborn	Variable	Appears well	Delivery	Apt-Downey test
Stress ulcer	Newborn and older child	Large	Sick, pale appearance; shock	CNS disease, sepsis, difficult perinatal period	Upper GI series, nasogastric tube
Hemorrhagic gastritis	Newborn	Large	Sick, pale appearance; shock	CNS disease, sepsis, difficult perinatal period	Nasogastric tube, endoscopy
Hemorrhagic disease of the newborn	Newborn	Variable	Melena; skin or umbilical bleeding	Vitamin K deficiency, clotting disorders, liver disease	Coagulation studies
Gastric volvulus	Infancy	Small	Intermittent vomiting Abdominal pain	Congenital defect Eventration of diaphragm	Upper GI series
Peptic disease	Any age	Large	Appears well; vomiting, pain, anemia	Duodenal or antral ulcer	Upper GI series, endoscopy
Esophageal varices	Any age	Large	Well or ill appearance	Portal hypertension	Esophagography, esophagoscopy
Peptic esophagitis	Any age	Small	Vomiting, dysphagia, failure to thrive	Hiatal hernia, severe chalasia	Esophagography, esophagoscopy
Foreign body	Infant and older child	Small	Abdominal pain Dysphagia	Pin, coins, soda can pull-tab	Plain films of chest, abdomen Esophago-gastroscopy
Gastric outlet obstruction	Any age	Small	Vomiting, failure to thrive	Hypertrophic pyloric stenosis, antral ulcers, pyloric webs or diaphragm	Upper GI series
Erosive gastritis or esophagitis	Any age	Small	Vomiting, pain, dysphagia	Acids, alkalis, iron, aspirin	History of ingestion, endoscopy
Gastritis	Any age	Small	Protracted vomiting	Gastroenteritis	History, endoscopy
Mallory-Weiss	Preschool to adolescence	Moderate to large	Retching Vomiting	Increased intraluminal pressure	Esophagoscopy
Swallowed blood	Any age	Moderate to large	Nausea, nasal bleeding	Ear, nose, throat, or dental bleeding	History

cult labor or in those developing sepsis or neonatal meningitis.

Another likely cause of hematemesis is *hemorrhagic disease* of the newborn infant, and therefore the physician will need to pursue this possibility with additional questioning. Is there a generalized bleeding diathesis manifested in the infant? Does the child show petechiae or ecchymoses of the skin? Are there any signs of intracranial or pulmonary hemorrhage? Has blood been passed per rectum? Before delivery was the mother receiving medications such as aspirin, anticoagulants, or anticonvulsants? Was infant or mother given vitamin K? Is there a family history of bleeding disorders?

Other than for swallowed maternal blood as a cause of hematemesis, the physician should view with alarm this symptom in the neonate. Besides the above possibilities, virus-caused *neonatal hepatic necrosis* is often made evident by severe gastrointestinal bleeding, many times in the absence of significant icterus.

Results of the gastrointestinal series usually are normal in the newborn bleeder, and the tests are done mostly to rule out ulcer. Duplications and hiatal hernia are the most common lesions in the few patients in whom it is abnormal.

Beyond the newborn period and during the next year, hematemesis is most likely to occur from a limited number of diseases. The vomiting of a large amount of usually bright red blood most often is caused by a bleeding *duodenal* or *gastric ulcer*. History of frequent vomiting suggests peptic disease. A predisposing condition, such as a recent burn (Curling's ulcer), central nervous system injury, or an infection (Cushing's ulcer), makes peptic disease a likely explanation for bleeding. An unusual cause of large amounts of hematemesis in this age group may be a foreign body ulcerating the esophageal or gastric mucosa.

A large hematemesis may be caused by esophageal varices in this age group, and we have seen this complication in infants less than 1 year of age on several occasions. Therefore it is still worthwhile to inquire about conditions predisposing the patient to *portal hypertension* (intrahepatic or extrahepatic). A history suggestive of omphalitis, sepsis, diarrhea with shock, neonatal hepatitis, exchange transfusions, umbilical vein catheterization, and so on may antedate portal hypertension in such children.

More often the amount of blood noted in the vomitus is small (streaks, dropperful, spoonful) and is most likely to be described as dark brown or black (coffee-ground vomitus). This type of hematemesis rarely occurs spontaneously and is frequently related to an ongoing illness or predisposing abnormality.

Peptic esophagitis and *gastritis* are the most likely causes for this type of bleeding. *Sliding hiatal hernia,* severe *chalasia, hypertrophic pyloric stenosis, pyloric webs, diaphragms,* or *antral ulcer* leads to vomiting and reflux esophagitis. Proper roentgenographic studies are needed for precise

diagnosis. Routine roentgenograms of chest and abdomen may show foreign objects and occasionally demonstrate a hiatal hernia or a duplication. Portions of the skeleton included may give evidence of anemias, leukemia, or one of the metabolic diseases. Barium studies will diagnose with certainty any localized lesions and are highly accurate in the identification of most of the lesions just listed.

A patient suffering *protracted vomiting* during an acute viral illness may develop hematemesis of the coffee-ground type. Injudicious use of aspirin in the small child may result in erosive gastritis and bleeding. Ingestion of corrosive substances such as strong acids, alkalis, or iron may cause esophageal or gastric hemorrhage.

In the slightly older child (from 3 to 5 years) hematemesis of a large amount of bright red blood usually comes from *esophageal varices* and possibly from a *bleeding duodenal ulcer*. If the child has been asymptomatic, it is more likely that the blood is from varices than from ulcers. However, the physician might want to inquire about recent nosebleeds, tonsillectomy, adenoidectomy, or even dental work that might have caused unnoticed bleeding. A rare nasopharyngeal hemangioma may present with hematemesis.

The possibility that esophageal varices are the source of the bleeding may be enhanced by the answers to the questions alluded to earlier, which have bearing on causes for intrahepatic or extrahepatic portal hypertension. Since some forms of portal hypertension may be familial (congenital hepatic fibrosis, cystic fibrosis, Wilson's disease, alpha-1-antitrypin–deficiency cirrhosis, galactosemia, Rendu-Osler-Weber disease, porphyria), an inquiry into the family history is worthwhile.

Hematemesis may also arise from rare esophageal tumors (leiomyoma, hemangioma) or gastric tumor (leiomyoma, leiomyosarcoma, lymphoma, inflammatory polyps, or hamartomas). Again, the esophageal disorders discussed for the younger child may cause bleeding. An underlying predisposition to bleeding, such as hemophilia, leukemia, thrombocytopenia, or aplastic anemia, may manifest itself by hematemesis, but this is unusual. Small amounts of coffee-ground material in the vomitus are seen with viral gastritis or after aspirin ingestion.

In the older child, painless hematemesis of a large amount is also likely to stem from esophageal or gastric varices resulting from portal hypertension. Older children are usually symptomatic from peptic disease, and hematemesis, when it occurs in these patients, is usually the result of a bleeding ulcer.

Vomiting of blood remains a worrisome symptom regarding which the physician must be prepared to act promptly. The condition of the patient must be quickly assessed and the necessary preventive, supportive, and diagnostic measures (fiberoptic endoscopy) undertaken with minimal delay. Sudden onset of severe bleeding may be an indication for arteriography, which often pinpoints the bleeding site but must be done before barium from a gastrointestinal series obscures the areas. Adequate history taking greatly facilitates diagnosis and can alleviate some initial worry engendered by this symptom.

BLOOD IN THE STOOLS AND RECTAL BLEEDING

The passage of blood rectally is an alarming finding that will promptly be brought to the physician's attention in almost all cases. An exception might be the teenager who, after noticing the blood in stools, may be too frightened to divulge this occurrence to anyone. Selective questioning of the mother or child will quickly provide the necessary information to help the physician narrow down possible causes of rectal bleeding. This is necessary because the number of conditions associated with blood in the stools is impressive (Table 1-4).

The first question to be asked is the *age* of the patient; certain conditions associated with rectal bleeding are specific for certain age groups (newborn, infant, preschool child, and school-age child to teenager). Next in importance is some rough estimate of the *quantity of blood* seen: Are there streaks, drops, a teaspoonful, or a cupful of blood? The *condition of the patient* will provide information that aids in sorting out the various possibilities: Is the child sick? Are there associated symptoms such as abdominal pain, pallor, constipation, diarrhea, fever or vomiting? The *location of the blood in relation to the stool* also gives important information in aiding the attempt to localize the site of the origin of bleeding: Is it on the outside only, or is it mixed into stool? Knowing the *color of the blood* may be helpful, but caution is needed in interpreting this information: In particular, is it bright red, dark red, or tarry? Ask the parent or the child whether he is *sure it is blood,*

keeping in mind that the effects food coloring, beets, Kool-Aid, gelatin desserts, ampicillin, lincomycin, and other substances can simulate rectal bleeding.

Rushing the child to the hospital for roentgenographic examination of the colon in hope of quick diagnosis should not be a substitute for proper history taking or physical examination, since positive studies are not very frequent and the procedure may serve only to delay diagnosis. Scout films of the abdomen are helpful only if there is an associated obstructive lesion or perforation. However, intussusception cannot be ruled out by means of this method with any degree of certainty. As was noted previously, localized lesions causing bleeding in the upper gastrointestinal tract usually can be seen by contrast roentgenography. A few more are found at follow-through studies of the small bowel. Barium enema will demonstrate most local colon lesions causing rectal bleeding. Meckel's diverticulum is diagnosed by radioisotope scan or by exclusion of other causes more often than by direct demonstration of the diverticulum.

The occurrence of abdominal cramps accompanying bleeding, especially during the first 2 years of life, suggests *intussusception*. Barium enema is performed as an emergency procedure for diagnosis and results in hydrostatic reduction of the intussusception, with cure in about 80% of the patients.

Newborn infant

In the newborn infant, passage of blood in the stool has a limited number of causes, some of which are unique to this age group.

Maternal blood swallowed by the neonate during the course of labor and delivery is often passed in the first few days of life and may appear as bright red or dark red blood in the infant's stools. It can be easily be identified as of maternal origin by results of the Apt-Downey test of a sample of stool (Chapter 30).

Bright red or dark red blood mixed in and about the stools may be a manifestation of *hemorrhagic disease of the newborn*. This condition usually starts between the second and fifth days of life, when bleeding into many other parts of the body usually becomes apparent. Since hemorrhage in the newborn infant may be caused by a variety of conditions, a complete investigation of the clotting factors will be needed for specific treatment. Prolongation of the infant's prothrombin time be-

Table 1-4. Clinical clues to the causes of rectal bleeding

Entity	Age	Amount; appearance	Clinical features	Cause	Diagnostic means
Swallowed blood	Newborn	Variable; tarry to dark red	Appears well	Delivery	Apt-Downey test
Hemorrhagic disease of newborn	Newborn	Large; red to tarry	Hemorrhages elsewhere	Clotting disorders, vitamin K deficiency, others	Coagulation studies; prothrombin time and PTT, platelet count, others
Stress ulcer	Newborn to any age	Large; red to black	Shocklike, pale, sickly appearance	Difficult labor and delivery, CNS injury, sepsis	Nasogastric tube; upper gastrointestinal series normal or abnormal
Hemorrhagic gastritis	Newborn	Large; red to black	Shocklike, pale, sickly appearance	Stressful labor and delivery	Nasogastric tube; normal upper gastrointestinal series
Necrotizing enterocolitis	Newborn	Variable; red to currant jelly	Prematurity, diarrhea, sickly appearance	Hirschsprung's disease, prematurity, Shwartzman phenomenon	Palpation of abdomen, scout films of abdomen
Acute colitis	Any age	Variable; red	Sickly, toxic appearance, diarrhea, abdominal pain	Infection, allergy, isosensitization, chronic ulcerative colitis, chronic active hepatitis, ischemia	Proctoscopy, biopsy, barium enema
Infectious diarrhea	Any age	Small; red	Diarrhea, fever	Bacterial (*Salmonella, Shigella,* pathogenic *Escherichia coli), Campylobacter,* viral, or parasitic infection	Stool cultures
Milk-protein (bovine or soy) intolerance	Neonate and infant	Occult to small; red	Colic, diarrhea, vomiting, edema, rhinitis, asthma, atopic dermatitis	Cow's milk or soy protein intolerance	Dietary changes, administration of steroids
Midgut volvulus	Neonate	Variable; red to tarry	Shock, bile-stained vomitus, pain, obstruction	Malrotation with malfixation of mesentery	Upper gastrointestinal series, barium enema
Anal fissure	Infant	Small; red	Constipation, rectal pain	Constipation	Inspection of anus, anoscopy
Cryptitis, proctitis	Any age	Small; red	Colicky episodes, rectal pain, diarrhea	Gastroenteritis, ulcerative colitis, Crohn's disease, venereal disease	Stool culture, proctoscopy
Polyps	Any age	Small to moderate; red	Absence of pain; mucus, intermittent diarrhea	Idiopathic, genetic, or familial	Proctoscopy, barium enema, upper gastrointestinal series

Table 1-4. Clinical clues to the causes of rectal bleeding—cont'd

Entity	Age	Amount; appearance	Clinical features	Cause	Diagnostic means
Intussusception	Usually less than 2 years	Variable; red, currant jelly, tarry	Colicky pain, abdominal distention, vomiting, "knocked-out" look	Idiopathic; polyps, Meckel's diverticulum, lymphonodular hyperplasia, tumors	Barium enema
Intestinal parasites	Any age	Occult to small; red	Diarrhea, cramps, weight loss	Amebiasis, *Trichuris,* hookworms, others	Proctoscopy and biopsy; stool examination for eggs; barium enema
Meckel's diverticulum	Usually less than 2 years	Large; red to tarry	Usually absence of pain; pale, shocklike appearance; anemia	Congenital	Laparotomy, radioactive scan
Duplications	Usually less than 2 years	Variable to large; red to tarry	Mass, intestinal obstruction, rarely pain	Congenital	Upper gastrointestinal series, barium enema, radioactive scan, laparotomy
Nodular, lymphoid hyperplasia	Usually less than 2 years	Small; red	Appears well, postinfection diarrhea	Disrupted mucosa, idiopathic, immune deficiency states	Proctoscopy, biopsy, barium enema
Hemangiomas and telangiectasia	Any age	Occult to large	Absence of pain; mucocutaneous lesions; hemihypertrophy	Congenital	Physical examination, selective angiography, laparotomy
Peptic ulcer	Any age (most 5 to 15 years)	Occult to large; tarry	Epigastric pain	Idiopathic; CNS disease, steroids, burns, sepsis	Physical examination, upper gastrointestinal series, endoscopy
Henoch-Schönlein purpura	3 to 10 years	Small to large; red to tarry	Abdominal pain, vomiting, arthritis, purpura, hematuria	Idiopathic	Physical examination, upper gastrointestinal series, barium enema
Chronic ulcerative colitis	Any age (most 10 to 19 years)	Small to occult; red	Abdominal pain, tenesmus, diarrhea	Idiopathic	Proctoscopy, rectal biopsy, barium enema
Crohn's disease	Most 10 to 19 years	Occult to small, sometimes large; red	Abdominal pain, diarrhea, anorexia, weight loss	Idiopathic	Proctoscopy, upper gastrointestinal series, barium enema
Esophagitis	Any age	Occult to small	Dysphagia, vomiting, heartburn	Hiatal hernia, pyloric outlet obstruction	Esophagography, esophagoscopy, upper gastrointestinal series
Esophageal varices	Any age (most 3 to 5 years)	Large; tarry	Hematemesis, signs of portal hypertension	Cirrhosis or portal vein obstruction	Esophagography, esophagoscopy

Continued.

Table 1-4. Clinical clues to the causes of rectal bleeding—cont'd

Entity	Age	Amount; appearance	Clinical features	Cause	Diagnostic means
Hemorrhoids	Adolescent	Small; red	Pain on defecation	Constipation, perianal disease, portal hypertension, Crohn's disease	Anoscopy, digital examination
Foreign body	Toddler to school age	Variable; red	Rectal pain	Irritation effect of foreign body	Digital examination, proctoscopy, roentgenography
Hemolytic-uremic syndrome	Usually under 5 years	Small to large; red	Postdiarrhea, edema, hematuria	Postgastroenteritis effect (?), platelet thrombi (?)	Laboratory studies, barium enema, rectal biopsy
Antibiotic-associated colitis	Any age	Occult, small to moderate; red	Diarrhea, abdominal distention, cramps, recent use of antibiotic	Almost any antibiotic, especially ampicillin, cephalosporins in children	Stool culture Presence of *Clostridium difficile* toxin in stool

cause of vitamin K deficiency may at times be the problem. Aspirin, cephalothin (Keflin), phenobarbital, or phenytoin taken by the mother before delivery may predispose an infant to this condition or to thrombasthenia. Much less often is gastrointestinal bleeding the result of a specific disorder of the clotting mechanism. In addition, rectal bleeding may be seen in infants with *congenital thrombocytopenic purpura* from a variety of underlying causes.

The possibility of *stress gastric ulcers* or *hemorrhagic gastritis* should be considered when rectal bleeding is detected in a new-born infant whose mother experienced a difficult labor and delivery. We have also seen stress ulcers as a complication of sepsis and neonatal meningitis. Blood from the site may be quite large in quantity and may pass quickly through the gastrointestinal tract, thereby appearing bright or dark red in color rather than tarry. The infant may also suffer abdominal distention, suggesting perforation, in which case he may become pale and have a shocklike appearance.

Bloody stools discharged by the toxic newborn infant who is distended and vomiting or has diarrhea or suffers both should make the physician suspect *necrotizing enterocolitis* or *infectious diarrhea* (bacterial), and the specific causes should be quickly sought through proper culture tests and roentgenographic examination.

Acute ulcerative colitis and so-called *milk colitis*

have been reported to occur in the newborn infant, and frequent stools containing bright red blood may be the only manifestation. A positive family history is helpful. Again, prompt diagnosis may be lifesaving.

Infant (under 6 months)

The leading cause of rectal bleeding in infants past the newborn period and in children is *anal fissure*. Careful questioning of the mother will permit proper diagnosis of this frequent condition in almost all cases. The blood is always of small amount, is red in color, and most often appears as a strip on the outside of the stool in an otherwise well child. A drop or so of bright red blood may follow passage of the stool and may color the toilet water, diaper, or toilet tissue. A history of constipation is frequently obtained, and the passage of a large stool or hard stool causing some discomfort or frank pain is commonly associated with the presence of an anal fissure.

Cryptitis or *proctitis* may be cause for small amounts of bright red blood to be present both on and within the stool and should be considered especially if it occurs in conjunction with gastroenteritis.

Infectious diarrhea is another common cause of rectal bleeding, and the diagnosis should be apparent by the associated symptoms. The small amount of blood is mixed in with the stool. Shigellas, salmonellas, or *Campylobacter* are likely causes if the diarrhea is severe and watery and the child toxic. However, it is not uncommon for presumed virus-induced diarrhea to mimic these findings.

In the very young infant, bloody stools may be the first clue to severe *cow's milk protein intolerance*. The stools are loose and frequent and may be frankly bloody. Eczema, colicky pain, abdominal distention, and vomiting may be part of this symptom complex. That other members of the family suffer milk intolerance is helpful information and seems to carry greater significance if the maternal side of the family is affected.

Toddler to preschool child

After anal fissures, the next most frequent noninfectious cause of rectal bleeding in children of preschool age is *juvenile polyps*. A well child passing small amounts of bright red blood mixed with, as well as on the outside of, the stool is likely to have juvenile polyps. This diagnosis may be made by proctosigmoidoscopy or barium enema or both. Polyps associated with the *Peutz-Jeghers syndrome* can lead to occult blood loss. It should be suspected when the typical mucocutaneous pigmentation is noted during physical examination.

On the other hand, the passage of a large amount of bright to dark red blood by a well child suggests the presence of a *Meckel's diverticulum* until proved otherwise. This is an especially likely diagnosis if the child is less than 2 years of age and the blood loss was of sufficient magnitude to make him appear pale, if not frankly shocklike.

The passage of a dark red (currant jelly) stool or clots of blood by an infant or toddler experiencing intermittent crampy abdominal pain is most likely the result of *intussusception*. A barium enema should be done as quickly as possible after this diagnosis is suspected.

Bright red blood per rectum may occur in a child with *single* or *multiple hemangiomatoses* or from bowel *telangiectasia* associated with the Rendu-Osler-Weber, Klippel-Trenaunay, or Turner syndrome. The diagnosis of these conditions can often be made on the basis of other physical signs or their presence in the family history. Gastrointestinal bleeding from *duodenal ulcers* is an uncommon mode of presentation in this age group and, in our experience, remains a rare cause of this finding. Vomiting is much more common.

Duplications of the bowel containing heterotopic gastric mucosa may occur anywhere along the gastrointestinal tract and give rise to the painless passage of dark or red blood rectally. At times, duplication cysts may be felt by abdominal palpation, or they may be apparent as space-occupying lesions shown by roentgenograms of the abdomen.

Another cause of rectal bleeding to be considered in the young child experiencing crampy abdominal pain is *Henoch-Schönlein anaphylactoid purpura*. We have seen several instances in which the gastrointestinal component preceded the skin purpura or hematuria by as many as 7 to 10 days. An acute colitis-like picture may precede or complicate the *hemolytic-uremic syndrome*. Development of abdominal cramps, diarrhea, and abdominal distention and the finding of bright red blood in the stools of a child who is taking or has just completed a course of oral antibiotics may be attributable to *antibiotic-associated colitis*. This condition can develop after the use of most antibiotics, with ampicillin being the most frequently incriminated in the pediatric age group. Diagnosis can easily be made by proctoscopy, which permits direct viewing of the whitish to yellow plaque-like lesions scattered on normal or abnormal rectal mucosa. The stool will be positive for *Clostridium difficile* toxin.

School-age child

In children of school age, the sudden appearance of small or moderate amounts of bright red or dark red blood mixed into loose, frequent stools may result from *ulcerative colitis* or *Crohn's disease*. Systemic signs, arthritis, uveitis, and tenesmus may be present to support this diagnosis. Final confirmation will depend on proctosigmoidoscopy, biopsy, and specific radiography.

Parasitic infestations such as amebiasis may mimic the presentation of inflammatory bowel disease, and careful examination of both the stool and biopsy specimen will be needed for diagnosis.

The passage of dark blood or tarry stools most often indicates bleeding originating from the upper intestinal tract. The physician, however, should be aware that blind adherence to this rule may be dangerous. We have all seen large amounts of blood arising from the esophagus, stomach, and duodenum stimulate peristalsis and result in rapid transit of the blood. In these cases, the blood may appear unchanged in the stool. On the other hand, we have seen blood from the distal small bowel and the proximal large bowel appear quite tarry.

Melena in a young child is suggestive of an esophageal, gastric, or duodenal cause. If a history of vomiting, choking on solids, or dysphagia is present, *peptic esophagitis* resulting from *hiatal hernia* is a good possibility. The vomitus at times may contain flecks of blood.

A large tarry stool in a young child is likely to be the first clue that *portal hypertension* exists. If this occurs in association with hematemesis, the bleeding is certainly coming from the upper gastrointestinal tract. The history and physical examination may show evidence of chronic liver disease. Splenomegaly may be the only physical finding in an otherwise well child in whom *prehepatic portal hypertension* is the cause of the bleeding from esophageal varices. Careful questioning about the neonatal course (omphalitis, sepsis, umbilical vein catheterization) may yield vital information to support this diagnosis.

Again, tarry stools and anemia in the young infant who is vomiting may be caused by *peptic disease,* whereas in the older child the history of epigastric pain and tenderness makes the diagnosis a bit easier.

Rarely, a *foreign body* either swallowed by mouth or inserted into the rectum may be a cause of rectal bleeding. Tumor, leiomyoma, sarcoma, lymphoma, and adenocarcinoma are likewise rare causes of rectal bleeding in pediatric patients.

Melena in a teenager with some diarrhea may be caused by polyps found in conjunction with *familial polyposis* or *Gardner's syndrome.*

Fissures and *hemorrhoids* are unusual causes of rectal bleeding in the older child or teenager and may easily be found on direct inspection or anoscopy. Their occurence even in the absence of diarrhea should make the physician suspect Crohn's disease of the bowel. Portal hypertension from any cause will also need to be considered.

Finally, the physician must recall that in 25% of pediatric patients with rectal bleeding, no diagnosis will be forthcoming even after careful history taking, physical examination, laboratory and roentgenographic studies, and even laparotomy.

ABDOMINAL PAIN

Under the best of circumstances a precise diagnosis for the cause of abdominal pain may be difficult and elusive. Several important factors are responsible. Abdominal pain may be nonspecific, and, indeed, it may originate from a number of possible sites. The physician is thereby compelled to consider those *pain-sensitive structures,* be they

intra-abdominal or extra-abdominal, that may refer pain to the abdomen. Failure to appreciate the concept of referred pain is often responsible for missed diagnosis.

It would be nice if the characteristics of the pain were always useful information, but unfortunately individual reactions to the sensation of pain are quite variable and at times confuse or mislead the physician in his evaluation of this symptom. This difficulty is compounded for those who care for children by third-party involvement; the young infant or child who lacks adequate verbal expression is at the mercy of the parent for recognition and accurate evaluation of his distress.

Despite these handicaps, most physicians are able to successfully differentiate between pain that indicates surgical treatment and pain warranting medical treatment. This ability is often acquired through clinical experience. However, more effective and accurate methods may be afforded through the systematic gathering of specific information. Such an approach will allow the less experienced physician to sort through the possibilities and sift out the most likely abnormality provoking this symptom.

The specificity of certain conditions for both *age and sex* of the child is extremely useful information. The potential urgency of the complaint can often be assessed when one simply inquires whether the symptom is *new (acute)* or *recurrent (chronic).* The *medical history* is important, especially if there exists an underlying condition having the potential to produce abdominal pain, either acutely or chronically. The *time and mode of onset* of abdominal pain may provide helpful clues, as can the location, character, duration, and radiation of the pain.

Equally as important is information that helps establish whether the patient is *well or unwell:* Has the pain begun during an intercurrent illness? Is there fever, respiratory signs, vomiting, diarrhea, urinary symptoms, or other symptoms? Is the pain influenced by respiration, defecation, urination or vomiting? Is the pain related to any recent trauma? Has there been any previous abdominal surgery? Bolstered by this kind if information, the physician will be in a more favorable position from which he may arrive at an accurate diagnosis.

Neonate and infant

To most parents, an infant who cries is either hungry or in pain. If he fails to quiet down and be comforted after a feeding, it is commonly assumed that he has a "stomachache." Indeed, the small infant (2 to 8 weeks of age) who otherwise seems well but has spells of crying accompanied by flexing of the legs or a distended or taut abdomen is most likely experiencing *colic* as the cause of his "stomachache." The mother may say that the child is very gassy and seems temporarily improved after passing some flatus. The child usually has these symptoms during a particular segment of the day and generally can be comforted if held, rocked, or taken for a walk or ride. However, the mother should be instructed to look for other simple, but less common, explanations for the child's discomfort, such as an *incarcerated umbilical* or *inguinal hernia,* penetrating *open diaper pin, discolored scrotal sac* (torsion of a testicle), *occlusive hair* wrapped around a finger or toe, or signs of *anal fissures.* Transient abdominal discomfort in a previously well neonate may indeed be caused by a mild viral gastroenteritis. It is also reassuring to the physician to know that the infant is moving all limbs and that so-called *missed trauma* is probably not causing his discomfort. Colicky behavior that is more constant may be an early expression of milk-protein (bovine) intolerance or at other times may simply result from overfeeding.

Although many theories have been put forth to explain the causative mechanism for this common and distressful symptom, a temporary disorder of propulsive peristalsis (contraction-relaxation phenomenon) either in the small or large bowel is a most likely candidate. A temporary imbalance of autonomic input or an uncoordinated response of the infant's intestines could result in painful sensations from this vulnerable and frequently stressed structure.

The sudden onset of severe abdominal pain in the slightly older infant (typically from 6 to 24 months of age) may be the first symptom of an *intussusception.* This may occur in a previously well child, or it may occur during or after an intercurrent infection (diarrhea). The child may experience a relief between peristaltic waves typical of the episodic nature of the pain of intussusception. Pallor and vomiting are not frequently seen during the episodes of pain. Some children are lethargic after episodes of pain and have a "knocked-out" look.

One cannot justify waiting for abdominal distention, bile-stained vomitus, or a currant-jelly stool before acting. Once this diagnosis is entertained, a barium enema becomes a mandatory procedure.

Colicky crying and vomiting of bile-stained material should be regarded as signs of intestinal obstruction until proved otherwise. In a neonate between 1 and 3 days old, a midgut *volvulus* is very likely the cause, though *stenoses, duplications,* and *incarcerated hernias* are other possibilities. Occasionally an infant with prepyloric *channel or antral ulcers* may have abdominal pain and vomiting as his entire symptom complex. A few cases of *sigmoid volvulus* have also caused acute abdominal pain and may be misdiagnosed as "simple colic" until barium enema during a pain episode is obtained.

Preschool child

The physician should be concerned if a child between 2 and 5 years old has abdominal pain, and he should be very reluctant to accept a psychogenic origin for this complaint.

Once again, an acute onset of pain in association with other symptoms of gastroenteritis (fever, vomiting, diarrhea) is easily diagnosed and is self-limited. However, the physician should seek additional information before accepting this explanation. Most important is to determine (1) where the pain is located, (2) how long it has been in that location, and (3) whether it is intermittent or constant. Most parents are concerned that the child has *acute appendicitis,* the hallmark of which remains persistent localized pain and tenderness in the right lower quadrant. Anorexia, fever, and vomiting are helpful clues at times in making this diagnosis, but the physician cannot always rely on their presence.

The sudden onset of abdominal pain and vomiting may again be suggestive of gastroenteritis, but not infrequently they will be the initial complaints of a child suffering *pneumonia.*

It is worthwhile to recall that the farther away the abdominal pain is from the umbilicus, the greater the chances are that an organic intra-abdomonial condition is the difficulty. Epigastric and upper quadrant pain can be caused by peptic disease or liver or gallbladder disease but most often will be caused by *hydronephrosis* or *pyelonephritis.* Therefore questions about frequency of urination, dysuria, hematuria, and enuresis are important, as is examination of the freshly voided urine. Vague, periumbilical pain may be the only manifestation of genitourinary disease. This mode of presentation is more frequent in girls than in boys simply because the incidence of genitourinary disease is greater in girls than in boys.

Unusual causes of abdominal pain in the preschool child can be *inflammatory bowel* disease, *choledochal cysts, cholelithiasis, hepatic tumors,* acute or chronic *pancreatitis,* recurrent *intussusception, intermittent volvulus,* or inflammatory complications of a *Meckel's diverticulum. Diabetes* and *rheumatic fever* can give rise to severe, recurrent abdominal pain, especially early in the course of illness.

Child 6 to 18 years of age

In the school-age or teen-age patient, the diagnosis of an acute abdominal condition requiring immediate operation is made easier for the physician. The history is more reliable and the symptom complex conforms more to the classic description of the acute abdomen for a patient at these ages than for a younger child. The cooperation of the patient during the physical examination is obviously very helpful. Again, most patients suffering abdominal pain do not require surgery. The pain is vaguely periumbilical, generally crampy, and intermittent and is relieved by treatment of the symptoms. The concern for appendicitis and for other causes of an acute condition affecting the abdomen should remain great, and inquiry as to location and persistence of the pain should be made. *Mittelschmerz* in the teen-age girl should be considered in the differential diagnosis and can be recognized by the temporal relation of pain to the menstrual cycle. Pelvic inflammatory disease stands high on the list of priorities.

Chronic recurrent abdominal pain occurs in some 10% of school-age children, and the pain in fewer than one in 10 of these children has a definite organic cause. Such entities as peptic disease and inflammatory bowel disease are less frequent than genitourinary disease as possible causes of the abdominal pain. Rarely gastric or small-bowel polyps are responsible for episodes of recurrent intussusception as a manifestation of Peutz-Jeghers syndrome. Usually this complaint occurs in an otherwise well child and has psychosocial significance. The physician is cautioned against complacency when he hears that a child is having recurrent abdominal pain, since that child may later manifest an organic disease that requires immediate diagnosis and treatment. The physician should always consider each episode as a separate entity, especially if the pattern of the attack is different.

Since roentgenographic examinations are frequently relied on to aid in the specific diagnosis of abdominal pain, some additional comments pertaining to these procedures are necessary. As noted in the preceding discussion, the implications of abdominal pain differ according to age group, acuteness of onset, severity, and accompanying symptoms. The need for and the value of roentgenographic examination vary accordingly. For example, scout-film examination of older children with acute renal colic is frequently accurate in detecting opaque stones, and intravenous urography is yet more accurate in detecting ureteral obstruction.

The sudden onset of cramps during the first 2 years very often signifies intussusception and requires a barium enema for confirmation. However, for repeated or chronic abdominal pain, especially after the first few years of age, gastrointestinal roentgenography is seldom helpful in diagnosis. Statistically, it is better to examine the urinary tract first. In the gastrointestinal tract, once the possibility of ulcer is excluded, the attention is focused on the terminal ileum, since Crohn's disease is one of the most common causes of chronic pain that can be diagnosed by roentgenographic examination.

When pain is the only symptom, plain films are seldom of value except to show obvious lesions such as opaque calculi and appendicoliths and associated findings such as localized ileus or perforation.

ABDOMINAL ENLARGEMENT

It is as common for the examining physician to first notice that a child's abdomen is distended or enlarged as it is for the parents to bring it to the physician's attention. The former is more likely to be the case if the enlargement has been painless, slow, and insidious rather than acute and rapid in its onset. The more common causes are presented in the outline below.

Causes of abdominal distention in children
Intestinal causes
Obstruction, partial or complete
   Incarcerated hernia
   Malrotation with volvulus
   Intussusception
   Hirschsprung's disease
   Stenosis and atresia
   Duplication
   Appendiceal abscess
   Tumor
   Bezoar

    Sigmoid volvulus
    Imperforate anus
    Tracheoesophageal fistula
  Intestinal pseudo-obstruction syndrome
  Malabsorption syndromes
  Chronic constipation, fecal impaction
  Aerophagy
Extra-intestinal causes—structural abnormalities
  Wilms' tumor
  Neuroblastoma
  Liver tumor
  Storage disease (hepatosplenomegaly)
  Hydronephrosis
  Pancreatic cyst
  Skeletal muscle defect
  Peritoneum (mesenteric cyst)
  Gallbladder disease (choledochus cyst, hydrops)
  Urinary bladder disease (retention)
  Hydrometrocolpos (imperforate hymen)
  Ovarian cyst or tumor
Ascites
  Portal hypertension
    Extrahepatic disease (portal vein occlusion)
    Cirrhosis
    Hepatic vein occlusion (Budd-Chiari syndrome)
  Thrombosis of inferior vena cava
  Pancreatitis
  Acute peritonitis
  Acute glomerulonephritis
  Chronic renal disease
  Protein-losing enteropathies
  Constrictive pericarditis
  Cardiac failure
  Nutritional protein deficiency
  Intraperitoneal tumor
  Chylous ascites, lymphatic obstruction

The physician should recall that for most children, from birth to preschool age, it is normal to have a somewhat prominent abdomen, an appearance that relates to the typical but normal lordotic posture. Indeed, a scaphoid abdomen in the newborn infant is worrisome because *diaphragmatic hernia* or *esophageal atresia* may exist. After the age of 5 years, it is rare for the contour of the abdomen to extend above an imaginary line drawn from the xiphoid process to the symphysis pubis when the child is supine. However, the physician should always insist on seeing the child when the possibility of abdominal enlargement exists.

A major consideration is whether the abdominal enlargement is associated with signs of *intestinal obstruction*. Thus inquiry has to be made as to the presence or absence of pain, vomiting (especially bile-stained), and the recent passage of stool.

Specific causes of intestinal obstruction are somewhat age-dependent. *Incarcerated inguinal hernia, malrotation with volvulus, intussusception,* and *Hirschsprung's disease* are more common causes in the infant less than 2 years of age, whereas *incarcerated hernia* and *appendiceal abscess* are the most common causes after 2 years of age.

The most frequent causes of abdominal enlargement in the patient who has no signs of intestinal obstruction but has subjective and objective evidence of malabsorption are *cystic fibrosis* and *celiac disease.*

When no preexisting disease is known, careful history taking and physical examination are needed. Often, more specific questioning will be needed after the patient has been examined. Solid masses responsible for abdominal enlargement are often caused by *hydronephrosis, hepatomegaly,* or *splenomegaly.*

An abdominal mass in a young infant is secondary to *hydronephrosis, neuroblastoma,* or *Wilms' tumor,* in that order of frequency. *Polycystic kidney disease* may also produce abdominal enlargement and be confused with hepatosplenomegaly on physical examination.

Storage diseases, hematologic conditions, liver disease with portal hypertension, and *portal hypertension* without liver disease are frequent causes of hepatosplenomegaly. *Hepatomas, hamartomas* and *cysts of the liver* may initially enlarge the abdomen.

Other abnormal intra-abdominal structures that give rise to this condition may be fluid-filled *duplications* of the bowel, *mesenteric cysts, hydrometrocolpos, ovarian cysts,* or even a *distended bladder.* These last three conditions can be strongly suspected in a patient with a distended abdomen when a mass rising up from the pelvis can be palpated.

At times, the abdominal enlargement results from fluid accumulation that may be hepatic, pancreatic, urinary tract, lymphatic, or mesenteric in origin. Ascites with hepatosplenomegaly may be of sudden onset and may reflect *hepatic vein occlusion (Budd-Chiari syndrome).* Nonchylous abdominal fluid accumulating in a patient having neither liver nor pancreatic disease is most often caused by hypoalbuminemia. Periorbital or pretibial edema is usually present when abdominal distention from ascites is secondary to hypoproteinemia. In the absence of proteinuria, or *protein malnutrition,* a gastrointestinal or cardiac cause should be sought. Because digestive (pancreatic), absorptive (celiac), or increased (exudative enteropathy) losses may be involved, a history of other symptoms of cystic fibrosis or celiac disease should be sought in these patients.

If chylous fluid is found when paracentesis is performed, *intestinal lymphangiectasis* is the most likely possibility. Lymphedema of a limb noted in association with abdominal enlargement may permit one to determine the abnormality before paracentesis or intestinal biopsy is performed. Cardiac failure with or without constrictive pericarditis may also result in ascites.

Finally, abdominal enlargement may be caused solely by air-filled loops of bowel, in which case the abdomen is tympanitic and has no palpable mass and no demonstrable fluid wave. *Aerophagy, constipation,* and *fecal impactions* are common causes. *Tracheoesophageal fistula* of the H type may first be suspected if a distended abdomen is associated with air-filled loops.

Sometimes no pathogenic cause will be found. Poor posture, weak abdominal muscles, or a large diastasis recti will prolong this childish abdominal profile. However, the physician is cautioned against making these diagnoses solely by telephone conversation with the mother.

Roentgenographic examination of the patient with abdominal enlargement is often necessary, and plain films of the abdomen (supine, erect, and decubitus) usually provide the key to diagnosis. If the gut is distended, the pattern can be identified as nonobstructive (ileus of extraintestinal cause) or as mechanical obstruction, with the approximate level demonstrated. If the gut is not distended, one may see free fluid or one or more localized masses. The nature of the mass is delineated by its effect on normal structures. Usually contrast-medium studies, starting with intravenous urography (and sometimes arteriography) followed by barium studies of the gastrointestinal tract, will localize the mass well enough to permit identifying its origin and often provide exact diagnosis. Free fluid usually is readily apparent on the original scout films, particularly if special positioning is used. Radioisotope imaging and ultrasound are useful adjuncts when the patient with abdominal enlargement is studied.

DYSPHAGIA

In the broadest sense, we prefer to include any disability of sucking and swallowing in the defi-

nition of dysphagia. Difficulty in swallowing is truly an alarming symptom whether beginning during the newborn period or during later life. Prompt attention to this complaint should be given so that a specific diagnosis can be made and proper treatment started when indicated.

Deglutition involves the careful neuromuscular integration of the acts of sucking, swallowing, and breathing; dysphagia may arise from impairment of any one of these functions.

There are two broad categories into which this symptom may be divided, regardless of the age at which it becomes manifest: (1) structural abnormalities of the oropharynx, esophagus, or thorax, which are usually congenital but may be acquired, and (2) neurologic or neuromuscular disorders, which are congenital, developmental, or acquired.

Sometimes specific entities may fit either of these two categories. A partial list of causes of dysphagia appears in the outline below. Some are discussed in detail in other sections dealing with specific esophageal disorders (Chapter 6).

Causes of dysphagia in children*

Malformations
  Congenital anatomic defects
    Choanal atresia
    Cleft lip and palate
    Submucous cleft
    Macroglossia, cysts, lymphangioma
    Micrognathia, Pierre Robin syndrome
    Temporomandibular joint ankylosis
    Pharyngeal cyst or tumor
    Laryngeal cyst, epiglottic cyst or tumor
    Esophageal atresia, stenosis, web, diverticulum, duplication
    Tracheoesophageal fistula
    Hiatal hernia
    Paraesophageal hernia
    Abnormalities of great vessels, aberrant right subclavian artery, vascular rings, double arch, and others
  Acquired anatomic lesions
    Infectious: stomatitis, esophagitis (herpesvirus, candidiasis)
    Allergic: stomatitis, esophagitis (Stevens-Johnson syndrome)
    Corrosive: stomatitis, esophagitis (lye, iron, bleaches), Crohn's disease of esophagus
Neuromuscular and neurologic disorders
  Delayed maturation, prematurity, mental deficiency, normal variation
  Cerebral palsy

*Modified from Illingsworth, R.S.: Arch. Dis. Child. **44:**655, 1969.

Bulbar and suprabulbar palsy

Werdnig-Hoffmann disease

Dysautonomia (Riley-Day syndrome)

Prader-Willi syndrome, or hypogonadism, hypomentia, hypomentia, hypotonia, obesity (HHHO)

Cornelia de Lange syndrome

Chalasia or achalasia

Cricopharyngeal incoordination

Chronic idiopathic intestinal pseudo-obstruction syndrome (CIIPS)

Collagen disease (dermatomyositis, scleroderma)

Demyelinating disease

Lipidoses

Tetanus

Guillain-Barré syndrome (acute infectious polyneuritis)

Myasthenia gravis

Muscular dystrophy

Möbius syndrome

The physician may be able to anticipate disorders of deglutition in the newborn by simple history taking. Polyhydramnios in the mother may suggest esophageal atresia, as well as other *high small-bowel anomalies* in the infant. *Maternal myasthenia gravis* may lead to temporary dysphagia in the newborn. *Premature* infants may have temporary neuromuscular disorders of deglutition. Difficulties in feeding are complicated by respiratory distress or simple fatigue in the small infant. That an *analgesic* was given to the mother just before delivery should alert the physician to possible difficulties with early feeding of the neonate.

Most anatomic variants of the oropharynx are obvious during physical examination at the time of birth, as are some neuromuscular disorders. Before the infant is fed, the examining physician may recognize some degree of *respiratory distress* as the earliest sign of an abnormality related to sucking and swallowing. Life-threatening breathing difficulties beset infants with Pierre Robin syndrome, choanal atresia, laryngeal or pharyngeal tumors, macroglosia, and esophageal atresia. Accumulated oral mucus cannot be easily disposed of by the neonate, and choking, respiratory distress, and aspiration may ensue.

The initial feeding of the infant may produce the first clue to an underlying problem when poor or feeble sucking efforts are noted. Also, incoordination of sucking and swallowing, with choking and respiratory distress, may occur. Feeding difficulties reported by nursery personnel may give early evidence of delayed maturation or underlying neuromuscular impairment. The so-called sleepy infant who refuses to suck or fails to suck energetically fits this category; he can take only a few sucks without resting to seemingly catch his breath. Nasal regurgitation without associated vomiting is likewise abnormal.

After the neonatal period has passed, neuromuscular causes of dysphagia are generally more apparent because other signs of the primary disorder can usually be found. Delayed development, failure to thrive, microcephaly, severe hypotonia or spasticity, seizures, typical facies, and other disorders are found in varying degrees and are easily recognized.

Some anatomic lesions do not become symptomatic until after the neonatal period. Difficulty with swallowing and choking on solid foods, episodes of pneumonia, and rattling or wheezing respiration may go on for several months before their cause is recognized as *vascular compression of the esophagus, esophageal duplication,* or *cricopharyngeal incoordination.* Brainstem tumor must also be considered when these symptoms are present.

Progressive dysphagia occurring in a child who fails to thrive and has a history of persistent regurgitation and vomiting should make one suspect *esophageal stenosis.* Usually a sliding *hiatal hernia* will lead to peptic esophagitis and an acquired stenosis. Congenital esophageal stenosis is rarely seen.

Dysphagia after the *ingestion* of corrosive alkali (Drano), bleaches, or iron preparations usually implies progressive esophageal stenosis. Herpesvirus or *Candida* infection should be considered when dysphagia develops in an immunecompromised host.

In the older child, dysphagia may result from *achalasia;* it may be an early clue to a systemic *collagen disease* (dermatomyositis, scleroderma); or it may be a rare consequence of *inflammatory bowel disease* (Crohn's disease). Difficulty with swallowing may on occasion be an early symptom of *chronic idiopathic intestinal pseudo-obstruction syndrome* (CIIPS). Thyroiditis, mediastinal masses, foreign bodies, esophageal progression of lesions in Stevens-Johnson syndrome, epidermolysis bullosa, brain tumors, and demyelinating diseases may produce dysphagia.

The etiologic diagnosis for dysphagia should not be delayed. Malformations of the mouth and pharynx are usually detected at birth during routine examination of these structures. One can establish patency of the oronasal pharynx by passing a catheter through each naris into the stomach. Choanal atresia, obstructing pharyngeal masses, and esophageal atresia are thus quickly ruled out. Observation of the infant during feeding gives invaluable information regarding the vigor of the suck and coordination of sucking, swallowing, and breathing. It is said that the infant who can tolerate either breast or bottle feeding in the lateral recumbent position has normal oral and pharyngeal function.

Most lesions arising from malformations can be demonstrated radiographically. Lateral views of the neck use the contrast of air passages to show some lesions, whereas others require opaque contrast media. Cineradiography of the infant swallowing a contrast medium from a feeding bottle demonstrates functional defects, often quite accurately. Pharyngolaryngoscopy and esophagoscopy may be needed, as well as esophageal motility and manometric studies in selected cases.

PRURITUS

In the absence of an allergic predisposition, pruritus is a very unusual presenting symptom in children. However, this symptom does, at times, have gastrointestinal significance for the child, as it does for the adult.

Pruritus associated with liver disease, no longer believed to be exclusively related to elevated levels of circulating bile acids, occurs early in the course of obstructive disease of the hepatobiliary tract. Fortunately, a proper diagnosis is easily made in most cases, since jaundice is an accompanying feature of pruritus. Children with chronic cholestasis from any cause are likely to have bothersome pruritus. In the first few months of life it is most commonly seen in children with *idiopathic neonatal hepatitis, paucity of the interlobular bile ducts,* and *extrahepatic biliary atresia.* They are irritable and restless, and excoriated skin is frequently noted on physical examination. Itching may be so distressing that the child's pinching of and digging into the skin may lead to noticeable bruising. The diagnosis of extrahepatic biliary atresia is usually made before the child is 3 months old. Paucity of the interlobular bile ducts may not always be so apparent because signs can be mild or absent during the first year. Only when severe pruritus or xanthoma, or both, develop does the physician suspect the correct diagnosis.

Episodes of itching in children may accompany other infrequent entities capable of completely or partially obstructing bile excretion, such as *cho-ledochus cyst, cholelithiasis, ascending cholangitis, drug-induced cholestatic hepatitis, pericholangiolitic hepatitis, parasitic infestation, obstructing lesion of the ampulla of Vater* (lymphoma, leiomyoma), *stricture of the common bile duct,* and *hematobilia.* Any of these entities may then lead to a regurgitation of biliary excretory products into the circulation, causing symptomatic pruritus. Again, jaundice is usually noted, making diagnosis easier, and a palpable mass should be sought in the right upper quadrant, especially if the child is female. An underlying hemolytic condition may be known; this raises the possibility of obstructing gallstones as cause for the symptom. The patient's recent travel to areas of the country or world endemic for certain parasites (*Ascaris,* liver flukes, and others) may be useful information.

Anemia, weight loss, anorexia, and abdominal pain may arise from tumors in the region of the ampulla of Vater. We have seen two children with pruritus and minimal abnormalities of liver function tests who proved to have *sarcoma botryoides* of the common duct. Severe itching may be a symptom of *carcinoid syndrome* or *mastocytosis,* both of which are extremely rare in children. Chronic renal disease and uremia may be made evident by anicteric pruritus, and careful attention to the genitourinary system is needed. Occult lymphomas (Hodgkin's disease, lymphosarcoma) may also have generalized pruritus as an initial symptom.

RECURRENT FEVERS OF UNKNOWN CAUSE

Recurrent fevers may originate from pathologic states of the gastrointestinal tract, and specific diagnosis may be elusive and difficult. Though admittedly uncommon in children, certain gastrointestinal problems may masquerade as fever of undetermined origin (FUO) for some time before other symptoms become manifest.

Recurrent bouts of fevers associated with cough, bronchitis, or bronchopneumonia may actually have their origin in the upper intestinal tract. Incoordination of sucking and swallowing may lead to aspiration pneumonia, as may *tracheoesophageal fistula without atresia.* Less noticeable episodes of aspiration may occur in children with *thoracic vascular abnormalities* that partly obstruct the esophagus. Regurgitation and vomiting from *hiatal hernia* may occur in a subtle manner and also result in aspiration pneumonia. The malformations just mentioned are not difficult to recognize in that the associated symptoms, physical findings, and chest roentgenogram should give evidence of abnormality of the oropharyngeoesophageal pathway. Proper roentgenologic studies with contrast material should facilitate making any one of these diagnoses.

Episodes of recurrent and low-grade fevers may be the only symptom of a *hepatic pyogenic* or *amebic abscess,* or secondarily infected *hepatic cyst.* Hepatic abscesses have several sources, but some 50% are idiopathic. The major clinical symptom is fever, which may be abrupt, high (from 100° to 105° F.), continuous, intermittent, or remittent. Chills may or may not be present. After an unpredictable period of time (from 10 days to 3 weeks), additional clues may become manifest, the most important being pain over the area of the liver, which make diagnosis less difficult. Anorexia, malaise, and others occur but are not specific enough to be helpful. Hepatic cysts (congenital or acquired) are usually sterile, but at times they are capable of eroding into the biliary system and become contaminated. Amebic abscesses caused by *Entamoeba histolytica* are being reported with greater frequency and may also initially produce low-grade fevers. Symptoms of liver involvement may begin months or years after the episode of intestinal amebiasis, and therefore it is most uncommon for these patients to have experienced recent diarrhea. Again, pain in the right upper quadrant eventually occurs, making diagnosis a bit easier.

The younger child with *chronic active hepatitis* may have a prolonged febrile course with minimal physical signs of hepatic dysfunction. *Hepatic cirrhosis* and *"granulomatous hepatitis* of unknown origin" may produce a prolonged febrile illness.

What needs to be emphasized concerning this group of entities is that the physician should consider the liver as a source of infection causing fevers of unknown origin. Proper roentgenograms and specialized techniques such as liver scans and arteriography are very helpful. Results of liver-function tests may vary from entirely normal to modestly abnormal.

Continuous, remittent, or intermittent fevers may accompany other nonspecific symptoms of *Crohn's disease* such as anorexia, malaise, and fatigue. Abdominal pain with or without diarrhea may not be part of the original complaints. Careful questioning about the frequency and consistency of the stools may yield important information. What is considered an abnormal stool pattern by the physician may have been considered normal by the patient. In the investigation of fevers of unknown cause, studies of the upper gastrointestinal tract and the small bowel are essential. Since the colon may also be involved or may, in fact, be the only area of involvement, a barium enema is indicated in all cases in which Crohn's disease is believed to be causative.

Occasionally *Salmonella infections* will be the cause of persistent fevers, and diarrhea will not necessarily ensue. Stool culture test and studies of febrile agglutinins should obviously be part of the investigation. This organism and others may secondarily infect an unsuspected tumor, and the resulting fever then leads to diagnosis of the tumor.

Sometimes, persistent temperature elevation follows a transient episode and nonlocalizing abdominal pain. A variable period of time may pass before adequate localization of the underlying process permits diagnosis on physical examination. An *intra-abdominal abscess,* most often from an undiagnosed ruptured appendix, may at times become evident in this manner. Pain in the right lower quadrant or pelvis may be noted on abdominal and rectal examination. A barium enema or intravenous pyelograms may show disturbances of these structures.

Lymphoma of the gastrointestinal tract, a rare disorder, may become evident through fever of unknown origin. This mode of presentation is said to occur in less than 5% of such cases. *Brucellosis* or *familial Mediterranean fever* with polyserositis may also become apparent in this manner.

The gastrointestinal tract may be the source of undiagnosed fevers and should always be considered a possible source as long as the diagnosis remains in doubt.

Although from 5% to 8% of patients will escape specific diagnosis for their recurrent episodes of fever, the physician should also consider *factitious fever* as a possible cause before stopping his pursuit of a diagnosis.

2 *Physical signs*

It may seem embarrassing, belittling, or trite to continually emphasize to physicians the value of a carefully performed, complete physical examination, but the need continues. The development of a personal discipline in the art of physical examination that allows students of medicine to see what they are looking at, to feel what they are touching, and to hear what they are listening to can be made much easier if they can learn first by observing the "masters" and then by repeatedly practicing these techniques zealously.

There are times when an incomplete examination of the patient results in missed physical signs and consequently a missed diagnosis. At other times, a physical sign is recognized, but its significance is not appreciated. For the purposes of our discussion, we will assume that a careful examination of the patient has been done, and what follows in this chapter is, then, an outline of physical findings that have gastrointestinal significance. These features can be found during the examination of the pediatric patient, be he ill or well.

That a large number of physical signs indeed have potential gastrointestinal importance again reinforces the need for careful examination of the patient. Sometimes, these signs are in accord with a diagnosis already made on the basis of the patient's symptoms and history, whereas at other times, physical findings themselves will make a diagnosis possible or will at least narrow down the number of possibilities to be considered when the diagnosis is not apparent by the history alone.

MEASUREMENTS AND VITAL SIGNS

Measurements and graphic representation of height, weight, head circumference, temperature, pulse, and blood pressure are invaluable in pediatrics and should be recorded for every patient who visits the physician's office. Occasionally, for example, even the rare neuroblastoma is capable of causing chronic diarrhea and may first be suspected when an elevated blood pressure is documented. Differentiating the well child from the sick one, or the acutely ill from the chronically ill, or

recognizing that a child is failing to thrive is achievable if the physician uses methodical (graphic), repeated evaluation of growth and nutrition.

TOTAL PATIENT OBSERVATION: "LOOK, DON'T TOUCH"

The examination of the patient should always start with a period of observation—simply watching the child and paying attention particularly to his *general appearance*. An immediate assessment of the child's state of health can often be made at a single glance. Is he fat, skinny, tall, short, clean, dirty? Does his face look normal in view of his inheritance and age? What position does he assume? Is he quiet or active? Are his speech, affect, and neuromotor development normal for his age?

The *facies* should be noted, for a diagnosis can be made by recognition of a characteristic facial appearance. The *proportions* of the patient, particularly the head, trunk, and limbs, may give early clues to failure to thrive, malabsorption states, endocrine problems, and others. The state of *nutrition* should be noted and an attempt made to differentiate acute malnutrition from chronic malnutrition. Differentiating normal nutrition from overnutrition may also be important at times.

These preexamination observations may also reveal important information about *mentality, speech* and *motor development,* and the *mother-child relationship.*

SKIN

No other system of the body contains more potential clues for specific gastrointestinal diagnoses than does the skin. On the other hand, some findings in the skin are specific for diseases that have as part of their total expression gastrointestinal symptoms. Recognition of such findings can then permit the proper diagnosis, which, in turn, accounts for the symptom in question. Careful, thorough, methodical observation and examination of the entire body should be standard procedure in any complete physical examination. The infant or child should be *completely undressed,* though gowns may be used as indicated for temporary cover.

The *hair* and the *nails* should be included in the examination of the skin.

Skin

Color (pigmentation)—adrenogenital syndrome, Addison's disease, neurofibromatosis, Wilson's disease, Hartnup's disease

Pallor—gastrointestinal bleeding from esophagus to anus, gastrointestinal allergy

Jaundice—hepatobiliary diseases, pancreatic diseases, tumors; genetic, metabolic, and endocrine entities

Carotenemia—anorexia nervosa, hypervitaminosis A, hypothyroidism, diabetes mellitus, nephrosis

Periorbital edema—Wilson-Lahey syndrome, protein-losing enteropathies

Perioral rash—acrodermatitis enteropathica, malabsorption states, syphilis

Perioral freckling—Peutz-Jeghers syndrome

Rose spots—typhoid fever

Diaper dermatitis—deprivation syndrome, dysgammaglobulinemia, disaccharidase deficiencies

Spider angioma—cirrhosis

Petechiae—portal hypertension, Henoch-Schönlein purpura, hemolytic-uremic syndrome

Ecchymosis—portal hypertension, Henoch-Schönlein purpura, malabsorption syndromes

Café-au-lait pigmentation—neurofibromatosis

Urticaria—lymphomas, mastocytosis

Erythema nodosum—chronic ulcerative colitis, Crohn's disease

Telangiectasia—Rendu-Osler-Weber disease, ataxia-telangiectasia

Hemangiomas—Rendu-Osler-Weber disease, hemangioendothelioma of liver

Lipomas—Gardner's syndrome

Dilated veins—constrictive pericarditis, hormone-secreting ganglioneuromas

Varicella lesions—Reye's syndrome

Bullae—dermatitis herpetiformis, epidermolysis bullosa

Tanning of the dorsum of hands—Hartnup's disease

Tanning of the anterior tibial skin—Wilson's disease

Scratch marks—hepatobiliary disease (intrahepatic or extrahepatic)

Xanthoma—biliary obstruction (intrahepatic or extrahepatic)

Webbing of neck—Turner's syndrome

Nails

Clubbing (with or without cyanosis)—Crohn's disease, liver disease, celiac disease, cystic fibrosis

Pitting, spooning—anemia

Hair

Color change—protein calorie malnutrition, marasmus, protein-losing enteropathies

Abnormal texture—hypothyroidism, malabsorption states, protein-losing enteropathies, Menkes' "kinky-hair" syndrome

Sparseness—protein calorie malnutrition, trichotillomania, acrodermatitis enteropathica

NODES

Lymph nodes in children should be sought by gentle palpation in the following areas: postauricular, suboccipital, submandibular, anterior and posterior cervical, axillary, epitrochlear, and inguinal.

Adenopathy—infectious mononucleosis, typhoid fever, histiocytosis X

Lymphoid hypoplasia—dysgammaglobulinemia, intestinal lymphangiectasia

HEAD

Careful recording of head growth is mandatory in the young infant. Sequential measurements of head circumference often provide valuable diagnostic information, especially when they are compared with the patient's height and weight curves.

Microcephaly—failure to thrive, congenital rubella, toxoplasmosis, cytomegalic inclusion disease (neonatal hepatitis), inborn errors of metabolism, birth hypoxia or asphyxia

Hydrocephalus—failure to thrive, diencephalic syndrome, syphilis, postmeningitis, encephalitis

Craniotabes—malabsorption syndromes, hypervitaminosis A

Bruits—Rendu-Osler-Weber disease, chronic liver disease

Bulging fontanel (pseudotumor cerebri)—hypervitaminosis A, rapid protein renutrition

EYES

A difficult but important part of the physical examination is a satisfactory appraisal of a child's eyes. Inspection of the conjunctiva, sclerae, and iris and evaluation of pupil response can be facilitated by use of distraction techniques. Vision may be tested in young infants when their awareness of the environment and pupillary response to light are noted. The importance of careful inspection of the iris, lens, and fundus is obvious. At times, sedation and eye medication to dilate the pupils may be needed to permit better viewing of the fundi. *Fields of vision* may be grossly evaluated by confrontation techniques.

Corneal ulcer—familial dysautonomia (Riley-Day syndrome)

Telangiectasia—ataxia-telangiectasia

Iritis—Crohn's disease, chronic ulcerative colitis

Uveitis—Crohn's disease, chronic ulcerative colitis

Xerophthalmia—malabsorption syndromes

Kayser-Fleischer rings—Wilson's disease, chronic cholestasis

Cataracts—Basscn-Kornzwcig syndrome, Wilson's disease, galactosemia

Papilledema—hypervitaminosis A, cystic fibrosis

Defects in field of vision—diencephalic tumors

Posterior embryotoxon—arteriohepatic dysplasia (Alagille's syndrome)

NOSE AND SINUSES

One should observe whether the patient can take air through the nasal passages without difficulty. With one naris occluded and the mouth closed, the patient is instructed to breathe. The opposite naris is then occluded, and the procedure is repeated. Use of the nasal speculum will generally permit detection of the cause of most obstructions.

Polyps—cystic fibrosis

Palpation of the maxillary sinuses by finger tapping may permit detection of underlying inflammation. Pinching or squeezing the bridge of the nose may help indicate presence of ethmoidal infection.

Sinusitis—hypogammaglobulinemia

MOUTH

A careful look at the perioral area, buccal and alveolar mucosa, teeth, tongue, tonsils, palate, and posterior pharynx takes little time and may be diagnostically helpful. An illuminated tongue blade holder is invaluable for this part of the examination.

Pigmentation of the lips—Peutz-Jeghers syndrome

Pigmentation of the gums—adrenogenital syndrome, plumbism, adrenal insufficiency

Cheilosis—malabsorption syndrome

Rhagades—syphilis

Candidiasis (thrush)—immunity defects

Hemangioma—Rendu-Osler-Weber disease

Aphthous stomatitis—Crohn's disease

Gingival inflammation—Wilson's disease, Crohn's disease

Absence of taste buds—dysautonomia

Fetor—hepatic coma

Glossitis—vitamin B_{12} deficiency, Crohn's disease, celiac disease

CHEST

The format of inspection, palpation, percussion, and auscultation may not be easy to follow when the chest of a child is being examined. If the child is quiet, the examiner should attempt to auscultate the chest first and then go on to the other maneuvers if crying ensues. A number of gastrointestinal diagnoses may be suspected by examination of this region of the body.

Increased anteroposterior diameter—cystic fibrosis, immunity defects

Increased respiratory rate—ascites, tracheoesophageal fistula, anemia, chronic liver disease

Gynecomastia—cirrhosis, hepatoma

Costal rosary—malabsorption syndromes, deprivation syndromes

Asymmetrical expansion—diaphragmatic hernia, cystic fibrosis, pleural fluid, neuroblastoma, duplication cyst

Abnormal breath sounds (rales, rhonchi, wheezes, with or without diminished transmission of sound)—cystic fibrosis, pancreatitis with pleural effusion, chylothorax, protein-losing enteropathy, immunity defects

Bowel sounds—diaphragmatic hernia, eventration

Bruits—Rendu-Osler-Weber disease, cirrhosis

Murmurs—liver disease, anemia

Kussmaul's respiration—Reye's syndrome, diabetic ketoacidosis, hepatic failure

HEART

The same sequence of inspection, palpation, percussion, and auscultation is required to detect abnormalities, but only a few gastrointestinal diseases will affect the heart.

Shift of mediastinum—diaphragmatic hernia

Signs of pericardial effusion—lymphangiectasia, protein-losing enteropathy, amebiasis

High output murmurs—cirrhosis, anemia

Cardiomegaly—protein-losing enteropathy, anemia

Levocardia—polysplenia syndrome

ABDOMEN

With young children, the abdomen can be best evaluated if it is the first area examined, since it requires no instruments that may frighten them. A thorough examination cannot be done if the child is tense or crying, and therefore mother's lap is invariably more reassuring to the child than is the examining table with its noisy paper cover. Despite all precautions and mollifying attempts, it is often necessary to reexamine the abdomen repeatedly during periods of relative calm. Distracting tactics (using a toy or a bottle to suck on) can be helpful. The infant's hands can be occupied with tongue blades or a small tape measure.

Simple inspection

Simple inspection of the child's abdomen is often instructive. One should observe the shape or contour of his abdomen, for his abdominal musculature is thinner than the adult's. Until the age of about 11 to 13 years, the child has a lordotic stance that gives him a potbellied appearance when he is standing. However, when the child is supine, the abdomen should not appear convex after 5 or 6 years of age. A scaphoid abdomen in the newborn infant is suggestive of an underlying abnormality such as a diaphragmatic hernia or an esophageal atresia without a fistula or with a proximal fistula.

Distention of the abdomen is usually caused by air, fluid, or a mass, but it may also be secondary to an atonic abdominal musculature. *Transillumination* can help in differentiating cystic from solid masses. *Respiration* is abdominal in the pediatric patient; therefore, if the abdominal wall fails to move during respiration, an acute condition of the abdomen requiring surgery is likely to be at hand, though a large amount of air or ascitic fluid can also limit abdominal excursions. The umbilical area is observed for the presence of a small hernia so common in young children. The hernia can be particularly large in association with chronically distended abdomens. Granulomas, a polypoid mass, or a discharge should be looked for in the umbilical region. The examiner should look for *distended veins* and ascertain the direction of blood flow within them. Blood flow in the veins is cephalad in patients suffering portal hypertension. A number of prominent collateral veins radiating from the umbilicus (caput medusae) can be seen when cirrhosis is present. Peristalsis is easily seen if the examiner's eye is at the level of the abdomen. Peristalsis may be seen normally in thin, malnourished infants, but it is otherwise considered indicative of an obstruction lesion.

Auscultation

Since palpation may alter peristaltic sounds and render sound appraisal impossible, auscultation should be done first. *Peristaltic sounds* have a metallic, short tinkling quality and are heard every 10 to 30 seconds. Since they may be of low intensity, one must listen carefully. The absence of peristaltic sounds is significant and is good evidence for an ileus. Interpretation of peristaltic sounds that are increased in intensity or frequency is fraught with difficulty.

Percussion

A *tympanitic sound* in a distended abdomen signifies that gas is present; it is common with aerophagy, obstruction, or ileus. A distended abdomen with little tympany is suggestive of presence of fluid or solid masses. A *fluid wave* is difficult to elicit, whereas a *shifting dullness* is comparatively easy. An area of dullness is delineated with the patient in one position and is found again after his position has changed. Percussion assessment of liver size is particularly valuable when liver size is in doubt after palpation alone. Recent information suggests that the percussible upper border in the midclavicular line is between the fourth and sixth intercostal spaces, the majority being in the fifth space.

Palpation

Satisfactory palpation requires both the skill of the examiner and the cooperation of a relaxed patient. There are many ways of distracting the pediatric patient in order to get relaxation of the anterior abdominal muscles. In the young infant, flexion of the legs on the abdomen is helpful. Flexion of the knees likewise gives the desired result in older children. Quiet conversation with the patient distracts him and may also work nicely. Asking the child to "suck in his tummy" to make his abdomen "skinny" is much more effective than requesting deep breaths when palpating the liver, spleen, or other intra-abdominal structures. In a crying child, one can distinguish between a soft and a hard abdomen by feeling immediately on inspiration. However, when a thorough examination is necessary and is rendered impossible through voluntary tensing of the abdominal musculature, intramuscular meperidine hydrochloride sedation (Demerol) 1 mg/kg is recommended.

One should always inquire as to the presence of pain and its location before proceeding. Palpation should always start in an area that is removed from the zone of maximum subjective pain and proceed from the groin upward. First, one palpates gently and superficially with a balottement effort of the fingers. This will minimize discomfort and permit the detection of enlarged solid organs such as the liver and spleen or of masses close to the surface. The first question the examiner must ask himself is whether the *abdomen is soft or hard*. The abdomen that remains tense during both respiratory phases is pathologic. The young child often employs breath holding as a means of guarding his abdomen. A feeling of noticeable rigidity or resistance to pressure is indicative of an acute condition of the abdomen. *Tenderness* is noted, and the point of maximal tenderness is determined when the patient's face is watched in response to the examination of specific areas. Asking the child to point out with one finger the area of tenderness is helpful. Also of great help is a one-finger palpation of each quadrant. Tenderness can be further localized when pain on rebound is noted. The examiner places one hand deep in the abdomen away from the suspected area of tenderness and quickly removes his hand; the child then points to the area originally under suspicion. Intra-abdominal tenderness can be distinguished from muscle tenderness when the child is asked to raise his head and then is palpated. This maneuver increases superficial muscle tenderness.

Poorly localized areas of abdominal tenderness are commonly caused by a number of medical conditions, which have been enumerated in the section on abdominal pain in Chapter 1.

During the first 6 months of life, the palpable edge of the liver extends from 1 to 3 cm below the right costal margin in the midclavicular line. It seldom exceeds 2 cm in the child from 6 months to 4 years of age. Older children should not have a liver edge palpable for more than 1 to 2 cm below the thoracic cage unless the upper edge is percussible below the sixth intercostal space. One can be certain of enlargement of the liver only when it is striking; subtleties of hepatomegaly are more difficult to discern.

The spleen can be palpated from 1 to 2 cm below the left costal margin during the first few weeks of life. A spleen tip is not considered an abnormal finding in otherwise well infants and young children. Palpation of solid masses often requires palpation deeper than for either the liver or the spleen. The spleen border is best palpated using gentle ballottement. Masses such as the tumor of pyloric stenosis or the sausage-shaped mass of intussusception can be particularly difficult to detect. Examination of the abdomen should include maneuvers to palpate the kidneys.

Scaphoid abdomen (newborn)—diaphragmatic hernia, eventration of diaphragm

Distention (after 5 years of age)—malabsorption syndromes, masses, aerophagy, constipation

Visible peristalsis—pyloric stenosis, antral ulcers, Hirschsprung's disease, partial obstructions

Venous pattern—portal hypertension

Differential percussion note—celiac disease, cystic fibrosis

Bruits (Cruveilhier-Baumgarten murmur)—portal hypertension

Cullen's sign, Turner's sign—pancreatitis

Hepatomegaly—hepatic tumors, hepatobiliary disease, tumors, cysts, storage disease, abscesses

Splenomegaly—portal hypertension, infectious mononucleosis, cysts, hepatitis, storage diseases

Mass—duplications, liver abscess, cysts

Ascites—cirrhosis, lymphangiectasia, protein-losing enteropathy, pancreatitis

Peritoneal signs—peritonitis, polyserositis, pneumonia

Abnormal bowel sounds—peritonitis, obstruction, gastroenteritis

Hernia

INGUINAL REGIONS AND GENITALIA

Aware of Osler's classic saying, "the abdomen extends from the neck to the knees," the physician should pay particular attention to the inguinal and femoral regions for the presence of a gonad or a hernia that may give rise to symptoms of an acute condition of the abdomen.

Clitoral enlargement—adrenogenital syndrome

Scrotal edema—chylous ascites, protein-losing enteropathy

Testicular mass—cystic fibrosis, histiocytosis X

Hernia

Rectovaginal fistula—imperforate anus

ANUS AND RECTUM

Simple inspection of the perianal area should be part of any examination. Attention should be paid not only to the position of the anus but also the perianal skin. Gently spreading the buttocks will show anal abnormalities.

Digital rectal examination should be made, with attention to sphincter tone and presence and consistency of the stool and any other masses. This procedure is best done with the child supine and his legs flexed. In small infants the fifth finger will usually be accepted without difficulty, and in older children (more than 6 months) the index finger may be used. The fecal material on the finger cot should be promptly checked for presence of blood.

LIMBS AND JOINTS

A surprising number of physical findings having gastrointestinal significance may be found by careful examination of limbs and joints.

Asymmetry—lymphangiectasia

Lymphedema—lymphangiectasia

Pitting edema—protein-losing enteropathy

Thrombophlebitis—chronic ulcerative colitis

Arthritis—Crohn's disease, chronic ulcerative colitis, chronic active hepatitis, hepatitis virus B disease

Widened epiphyses—malabsorption syndromes

Pigmentation (hands, anterior tibial skin)—Hartnup's disease, Wilson's disease

Clubbing of nails—Crohn's disease, celiac disease, cirrhosis, cystic fibrosis

NEUROLOGIC EXAMINATION

Probably the most difficult and at times the most neglected part of the examination is a careful neurologic investigation, which can yield clues to a number of gastrointestinal diagnoses.

Sucking and swallowing disorders—brainstem tumors

Ataxia—malabsorption syndromes, Hartnup's disease, abetalipoproteinemia (Bassen-Kornzweig syndrome), chronic vitamin E deficiency

Tremors—Wilson's disease

Dystonia—Wilson's disease

Dysarthria—Wilson's disease, ataxia-telangiectasia

Confusion—Reye's syndrome, hepatic coma

Posturing (decerebrate, decorticate)—Reye's syndrome

Papilledema—cystic fibrosis, anemia, hypervitaminosis A

Areflexia—vitamin E deficiency

Hyperreflexia—hepatic coma, Reye's syndrome

Babinski's reflex—Reye's syndrome, hepatic coma

Asterixis—hepatic coma

Ophthalmoplegia—vitamin E deficiency

Part II

DISEASE ENTITIES

3 *Gastrointestinal emergencies of the neonate*

NEONATAL INTESTINAL OBSTRUCTION

Intestinal obstruction is the most frequent gastrointestinal emergency that requires surgery during the neonatal period. Early recognition is essential since (1) significant increase in mortality is noted when surgery is delayed in conditions associated with a mechanical obstruction, (2) when unnecessary operation is performed, or (3) when proper medical management is not given to those neonates who present with a functional type of intestinal obstruction. The differential diagnosis of neonatal intestinal obstruction is extensive (see list below). However, a careful maternal and perinatal history in conjunction with close attention to the presence and the severity of a few major intestinal and extraintestinal signs and symptoms will usually lead to the diagnosis, which then requires to be validated by appropriate roentgenograms.

Familial and perinatal history

The clinical assessment of the neonate with intestinal obstruction would be incomplete without a good genetic history. Information should be obtained concerning consanguinity and the outcome of previous pregnancies with regard to birth weight, inborn errors, and gross anatomical defects. A maternal history of diabetes, a systemic infection, or an intrauterine infection during pregnancy may orient toward a functional type of obstruction associated with the small left colon syndrome or sepsis. An account of events that may have complicated labor and delivery, and of drugs administered, may also help the clinician in placing his patient in the large category of neonates, particularly those of low birth weight, who have no anatomical defect but who have a paralytic type of ileus. On the other hand, a family history of cystic fibrosis, Hirschsprung's disease or of multiple system anomalies in siblings or close relatives suggests a mechanical type of obstruction.

Causes of neonatal intestinal obstruction

Mechanical
Atresias, stenosis, webs, and diaphragms
Malrotation with or without volvulus
Abnormal intraluminal contents
Meconium ileus and meconium plug syndrome
Lactobezoars with enteral feeding of 24 kcal/30 ml of formula for infants of low birth weight
Hirschsprung's disease: classical and segmental
Congenital abdominal wall defects: gastroschisis and omphalocele
Anorectal anomalies
Duplications
Perforation of the gastrointestinal tract secondary to an obstructive or inflammatory process
Incarcerated hernia: diaphragmatic, inguinal, internal
Segmental dilatation of the small bowel or of the colon
Megacystis-microcolon-hypoperistalsis syndrome
Neonatal primary chronic adynamic bowel
Functional
Necrotizing enterocolitis (initial stage)
Immaturity of neural plexus in infants of low birth weight
Pseudo-Hirschsprung's disease
Respiratory distress syndrome
Small left colon syndrome
Infections
   extra-abdominal: sepsis, meningitis, pneumonia
   intra-abdominal: primary peritonitis, appendicitis, cholecystitis
Toxemia of pregnancy
Maternal drugs (opiates, ganglion-blocking agents, magnesium sulfate)
Central nervous system damage or depression
Hypothyroidism

Polyhydramnios

Amniotic fluid is continuously swallowed by the fetus and is absorbed through the gastrointestinal tract. The presence of more than 2000 ml of amniotic fluid may denote inability of the fetus to swallow (anencephaly) or else the presence of an intestinal obstruction high in the gastrointestinal tract (esophagus, pylorus, duodenum, proximal jejunum). The overall incidence of polyhydramnios is said to be close to 50% in cases of high intestinal obstruction. Its prevalence and degree tends to be lower in lesions affecting the jejunum and is not usually present in lesions affecting the ileum, colon, and rectum.
Antenatal detection of life-threatening fetal dis-

orders by amniocentesis has proved increasingly important and effective not only for the termination of pregnancy in selected cases but also for ensuring that the high-risk mother is given appropriate obstetric and neonatal care. The analysis of amniotic fluid in experimentally produced intestinal atresias has not revealed significant alterations of composition; however, in humans with duodenal and ileal atresias a thirtyfold increase in bile acid concentration has been reported. A decrease in amniotic fluid disaccharidase activity may also prove to be a useful approach.

In the latter part of pregnancy, the presence or suspicion of polyhydramnios is an indication for ultrasonography. It will show an echofree sonolucent area and can demonstrate the presence of fetal intestinal obstruction such as duodenal atresia, malrotation with jejunal atresia, gastroschisis and Hirschsprung's disease.

Abdominal distention

The presence of a scaphoid abdomen is usually picked up early in the nursery and is diagnostic of a diaphragmatic hernia or an esophageal atresia without a fistula or with a proximal tracheoesophageal fistula. Abdominal enlargement is usually noted within the first 12 to 48 hours in babies with an intestinal obstruction, but it tends to be mild at birth, unless there is a ruptured viscus or an extraintestinal mass (hepatosplenomegaly, mesenteric cyst, renal tumor, or hydronephrosis). A functional type of obstruction usually becomes manifest after the first 48 hours of life and tends to be milder.

The higher the obstructive lesion in the gastrointestinal tract, the more rapid is the development of abdominal distention. However, it tends to be less severe in proximal than in distal mechanical obstructions. Protuberance of the epigastrium is suggestive of duodenal obstruction.

Intermittent distention favors a partial obstruction but may also be compatible with hypoperistalsis or with the various causes of paralytic ileus noted in the previous list. Vomiting or the presence of a nasogastric tube will decrease abdominal distention and may detract from a diagnosis of obstruction. Since abdominal distention usually gives rise to difficult breathing and to respiratory distress when it is severe, the clinician may focus his attention away from an intra-abdominal problem.

Bilious vomiting

Although excessive mucus noted at birth suggests a tracheoesophageal fistula, an intestinal obstruction should be suspected in the delivery room if a nasogastric tube brings back more than 25 ml or if gastric contents are bile tinged. Vomiting is a symptom common to all patients suffering obstruction. If it occurs at or soon after delivery, one should consider a high complete occlusion. A delayed onset favors a distal obstruction. Since obstruction proximal to the ampulla of Vater is relatively rare once esophageal atresia has been ruled out, bilious vomiting even in the presence of a normal-appearing abdomen is indicative of a mechanical intestinal obstruction until proved otherwise.

Failure to pass meconium or obstipation

Close to 95% of neonates evacuate meconium within the first 24 hours of life. The failure to pass meconium is often the first sign of intestinal obstruction. However, newborns with atresia normally evacuate meconium, especially if the obstruction is situated high in the gastrointestinal tract. Figures of 30% and 20% have been cited for those with duodenal atresia and jejunoileal atresia, respectively.

The clinician should pay close attention to the description of the evacuations. If, after 36 hours, only white mucoid material or small discrete amounts of meconium have been passed, the diagnosis of obstruction should be entertained. Obstipation occurring after normal evacuation of meconium and within a few days after initiation of oral feedings in a sick premature infant whose abdomen is distended can occur during the initial stage of necrotizing enterocolitis because of paralytic ileus. The importance of obstipation as a clinical sign in sorting out neonates with obstruction takes on added significance when poor feeding, vomiting, and abdominal distention are also present.

Other clues

Identification of associated anomalies constitutes a useful diagnostic tool and should also be used in the design of the strategies of intervention. The high incidence of trisomy 21 (30%), prematurity (25% to 50%), and major congenital anomalies (30%) is particularly striking in duodenal atresias. Prematurity is also frequent in jejunoileal atresia, but severe malformations (heart, kidney, skeleton, central nervous system) are less common except in babies with multiple small-bowel atresias. The VACTERL (formerly Vater) syndrome, an aggregation of anomalies including vertebral defects, anal defects, tracheoesophageal atresia with esophageal atresia, radial dysplasia, and renal defects, poses a particularly challenging problem and alerts one to the need for a thorough clinical assessment of the neonate with intestinal obstruction. The presence of an omphalocele or a gastroschisis calls for immediate surgery; however, the common association of severe extraintestinal anomalies with the former and jejunoileal and colon atresias in the latter should be kept in mind. All neonates with ileal atresias, antenatal volvulus, microcolon, or the meconium plug syndrome should be checked for cystic fibrosis. Hirschsprung's disease should be ruled out in babies with trisomy 21 who are obstipated.

Physical findings

Close inspection of the distended abdomen may reveal a purplish discoloration of the abdomen in cases of perforation with peritonitis or necrotizing enterocolitis with peritonitis. Active peristalsis of distended loops is likely to be seen and heard in mechanical obstructions. A silent abdomen for a period of 5 minutes is a good sign of peritonitis or a paralytic ileus. If crying invariably accompanies light palpation, an "acute abdomen" is likely; however, the absence of abdominal rigidity does not rule out peritonitis. A mass in the abdomen orients toward meconium ileus or a volvulus and is a red flag for an immediate work-up. Copious amounts of meconium found on rectal examination argue against a complete obstruction, whereas explosive passage of gas and stools suggests Hirschsprung's disease. The passage after a rectal examination or a contrast enema of sticky plugs of mucus and meconium followed by flatus and fluid meconium is diagnostic of either the meconium plug or the small left colon syndrome.

Close monitoring of the baby suspected of intestinal obstructionn is critical. The neonate who "does not look well" requires special attention. Lethargy, fluctuation of body temperature, regurgitation and vomiting, grunting respirations, unexplained acidosis, and evidence of vasomotor collapse are indicative of complications of mechanical intestinal obstruction but are also associated with some entities responsible for paralytic ileus. However, it is worth noting that a large number of neonates with a functional type of obstruction have few symptoms other than abdominal distention, failure to pass more than small amounts of meconium, and some vomiting.

X-ray findings

As soon as intestinal obstruction is suspected, roentgenograms of the chest and abdomen are in order. Supine, upright, and lateral views are obtained. Swallowed air will normally reach the rectum within 6 hours. However, in small prematures or in neonates with central nervous system depression or damage, progression may be slower. A gasless abdomen may be seen in severely dehydrated infants or in neonates receiving high concentrations of oxygen because it is absorbed and washes out nitrogen. The presence of a nasogastric tube may also decrease the usefulness of the air pattern as a diagnostic tool. In such cases, gastric contents should be removed and replaced with 10 to 20 ml of air.

Two air-filled cavities with fluid levels, the "double-bubble" sign, is diagnostic of duodenal obstruction but not necessarily of atresia. This should be followed by the administration of a small amount of barium by tube to establish the diagnosis of malrotation with bands, annular pancreas, or volvulus. Two or three dilated loops beyond the jejunum indicate a jejunal obstruction. In cases where only partial obstruction is present, introduction of air may improve the diagnostic value of the films. An abdomen containing many loops of dilated bowel indicates ileal atresia or meconium ileus. Because it is difficult to distinguish gas-filled colon from gas-filled small bowel, a barium enema is essential for identification of colonic atresia. It will also establish the presence of a microcolon diagnostic of a lower small-bowel obstruction. The colon may have a normal caliber in total aganglionosis and may not show the narrowed segment of Hirschsprung's disease. Scout films taken daily and showing failure of evacuation of barium in a full-term newborn is of great value. The meconium plug syndrome is recognized by a normal-sized colon and is frequently (25%) the initial manifestation of Hirschsprung's disease and less often cystic fibrosis.

The presence of bubbly granular density suggests meconium ileus. Dilated loops and pneumatosis (bubbles or layers of gas in the wall of the bowel) are diagnostic of necrotizing enterocolitis. Frcc air will indicatc a pcrforation that occurred postnatally, whereas soft-tissue masses or calcifications with or without free fluid are associated with prenatal perforation and meconium peritonitis. Scout films may also identify lactobezoars reported in the stomach and small bowel of prematures fed LBW casein formulas at 24 kcal/30 ml on a continuous basis.

Management

As soon as the diagnosis of obstruction is suspected, a nasogastric tube is inserted to provide appropriate drainage of air and secretions. Special emphasis is placed on thermoregulation during transport and during blood and roentgenographic studies. Proper oxygenation and prompt correction of fluid losses, electrolyte imbalances, and acid-base disturbances are essential. Hypoproteinemia is commonly seen in low birth weight infants with intestinal obstruction because of losses through the obstructed bowel. Salt-poor human albumin constitutes a good substitute for plasma and is of great value in the preoperative phase. Peripheral parenteral nutrition is recommended for a few days in babies who are severely malnourished and whose underlying surgical condition does not require immediate operation. Antibiotics are not routinely recommended unless sepsis or peritonitis is present.

REFERENCES

Bell, R.S., Graham, C.B., and Stevenson, J.K.: Roentgenologic and clinical manifestations of neonatal necrotizing enterocolitis, Am. J. Roentgenol. Radium Thermal Nucl. Med. **112**:123-134, 1971.

Bell, M.J., Ternberg, J.L., Feigin, R.D., and others: Neonatal necrotizing enterocolitis, therapeutic decisions based upon clinical staging, Ann. Surg. **187**:1, 1978.

Benirschke, K.: Neonatal enterocolitis, Am. J. Dis. Child. **126**:15, 1973.

Davis W.S., and Allen, R.P.: Conditioning value of plain film examination in diagnosis of neonatal Hirschsprung's disease, Radiology **93**:129-133, 1969.

Delèze, G., Sideropoulos, D., and Paumgartner, G.: Determination of bile acid concentration in human amniotic fluid for prenatal diagnosis of intestinal obstruction, Pediatrics **59**:647-650, 1977.

Dudgeon, D.L., Coran, A.G., Lauppe, F.A., and others: Surgical management of acute necrotizing enterocolitis in infancy, J. Pediatr. Surg. **8**:607-614, 1973.

Erenberg, A., Shaw, R.D., and Yousefzadeh, D.: Lactobezoar in the low birth weight infant, Pediatrics **63**:642-646, 1979.

Frantz, I.D., L'Heureux, P.L., Engel, R.R., and Hunt, C.E.: Necrotizing enterocolitis, J. Pediatr. **86**:259-263, 1975.

Guttman, F.M., Garance, P.H., Blanchard, H., and others: Multiple atresias and a new syndrome of hereditary multiple atresias involving the gastrointestinal tract from stomach to rectum, J. Pediatr. Surg. **8**:633-640, 1973.

Heyman, M.B., Berquist, W.E., Fonkalsrud, E.W., and others: Esophageal muscular ring and the VACTERL association: a case report, Pediatrics **67**:683-686, 1981.

Hopkins, G.B., Gould, V.E., Stevenson, J.K., and Oliver, T.K.: Necrotizing enterocolitis in premature infants, Am. J. Dis. Child. **120**:299-332, 1970.

Horvat, J.M., and Wilkinson, A.W.: Functional intestinal obstruction in the neonate, Arch. Dis. Child. **45**:800-804, 1970.

Joshi, V.V., Draper, D.A., and Bates, R.D.: Neonatal necrotizing enterocolitis: occurrence secondary to thrombosis of abdominal aorta following umbilical arterial catheterization, Arch. Pathol. **99**:540-543, 1975.

Kosloske, A.M.: Necrotizing enterocolitis in the neonate, Surg. Gynecol. Obstet. **148**:259-269, 1979.

Lee, T.G., and Warren, B.H.: Antenatal ultrasonic demonstration of fetal bowel, Radiology **124**:471-474, 1977.

Lloyd, J.R., and Clatworthy, H.W. Jr.: Hydramnios as an aid to the early diagnosis of congenital obstruction of the alimentary tract: a study of the maternal and fetal factors, Pediatrics **21**:903-909, 1958.

Mizrahi, A., Barlow, O., Berdon, W., and others: Necrotizing enterocolitis in premature infants, J. Pediatr. **66**:697-705, 1965.

Moore, T.C.: Gastroschisis and omphalocele: clinical difference, Surgery **82**:561-568, 1977.

Morin, P.R., Potier, M., Dallaire, L., and others: Prenatal detection of intestinal obstruction: deficient amniotic fluid disaccharidases in affected fetuses, Clin. Genet. **18**(3):217, 1980.

Polin, R.A., Pollack, P.F., Barlow, B., and others: Necrotizing enterocolitis in term infants, J. Pediatr. **89**:460-462, 1976.

Rodin, A.E., Nichols, M.M., and Hsu, F.L.: Necrotizing enterocolitis occurring in full term infants at birth, Arch. Pathol. **96**:335-338, 1973.

Roy, C.C., Morin, C.L., and Weber, A.M.: Gastrointestinal emergency problems in paediatric practice, Clin. Gastroenterol. **10**:225-230, 1981.

Santulli, T.V., Schullinger, J.N., Heird, W.C., and others: Acute necrotizing enterocolitis in infancy, Pediatrics **55**:376-387, 1975.

Stewart, D.R., Nixon, G.V., Johnson, D.G., and Condon, V.R.: Neonatal small left colon syndrome, Ann. Surg. **186**:741-745, 1977.

Talbert, J.L., Felman, A.H., DeBusk, F.L.: Gastrointestinal surgical emergencies in the newborn infant, J. Pediatr. **76**:783-797, 1970.

Temtamy, S.A., and Miller, J.D.: Extending the scope of the VATER association: defunction of the VATER syndrome, J. Pediatr. **85**:345-349, 1974.

Touloukian, R.J.: Neonatal necrotizing enterocolitis, Surg. Clin. North Am. **56**:281-298, 1976.

Touloukian, R.J.: Intestinal atresia, Clin. Perinatol. **5**:3-18, 1978.

Touloukian, R.J., and Hobbins, J.C.: Maternal ultrasonography in the antenatal diagnosis of surgically correctable fetal abnormalities, J. Pediatr. Surg. **15**:373-377, 1980.

Wrobleski, D., and Wesselhoeft, C.: Ultrasonic diagnosis of prenatal intestinal obstruction, J. Pediatr. Surg. **14:**598-600, 1977.

Zachary, R.B.: Intestinal obstructions, Prog. Pediatr. Surg. **2:**57-72, 1971.

Esophageal atresia and tracheoesophageal fistula

The lung bud is a median ventral outgrowth of the foregut. With the lengthening of the distal portion of the pharynx, the lung bud is carried caudally. The lumen of the single tube thus produced has the shape of a narrow, laterally compressed slit. The division is accomplished by the folding in of the lateral walls of the single tube until they meet and fuse, thus turning the slitlike cavity into two tubes, the esophagus dorsally and the trachea ventrally. An arrest or an alteration of the division process readily leads to anomalies. Tracheoesophageal fistula may occur at any level below the larynx, but the most common site is at or just above the tracheal bifurcation. More commonly, the esophagus is closed just above the fistula.

Incidence

There are striking variations in the incidence reported, but, in general, it stands between 1 in 3000 and 1 in 4500 newborn infants. Familial cases are exceptional. Furthermore, since both concordance and discordance for the entity has been seen in monozygotic twins, it is unlikely that genetic factors are important.

Types of anomaly

More than 85% of the congenital anomalies of the esophagus are characterized by a blind pouch of the upper esophagus, with a lower segment in communication with the trachea near its bifurcation. Two forms of esophageal atresia lead to the absence of air throughout the gastrointestinal tract. In these cases, both ends of the esophagus end blindly, or, more rarely, only the upper segment communicates with the trachea. A double tracheoesophageal fistula may take off from two blind esophageal pouches. A fistula may occur without atresia, in which case the fistula is usually higher than that seen when there is atresia.

Because much confusion has arisen from the many classifications, an anatomic description has been proposed (Fig. 3-1).

Associated malformations

More than 40% of the patients have associated anomalies. By far the most frequent malformations are cardiovascular. Coarctation of the aorta, vascular ring, and patent ductus arteriosus are common and are more likely in premature infants than in full-term infants. Attention has been drawn to the association of vertebral defects, anal atresia, tracheoesophageal fistula with esophageal atresia, renal defects, and radial limb dysplasia (the VACTERL association). In all cases of imperforate anus, esophageal atresia should be ruled out because it remains the most commonly (10%) associated digestive anomaly. In cases of esopha-

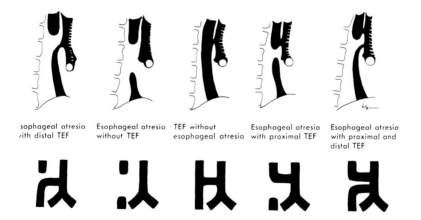

sophageal atresia / with distal TEF

Esophageal atresia without TEF

TEF without esophageal atresia

Esophageal atresia with proximal TEF

Esophageal atresia with proximal and distal TEF

Fig. 3-1. Tracheoesophageal anomalies. A schematic outline and description of the relationship between the trachea, esophagus, and fistula are much more helpful than the classifications formerly advocated. (Modified from Holder, T.M., and Ashcraft, K.W.: Ann. Thorac. Surg. **9:**445-467, 1970.)

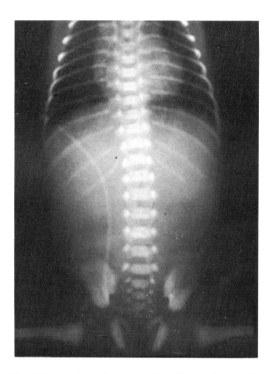

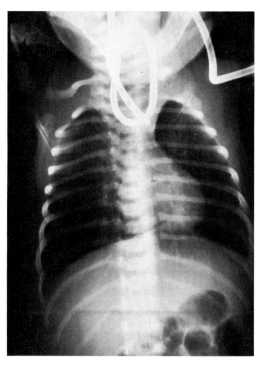

Fig. 3-2. Esophageal atresia without a tracheoesophageal fistula. The abdomen is gasless.

Fig. 3-3. Esophageal atresia with a distal tracheoesophageal fistula. Curling of the catheter may lead the physician away from a diagnosis of esophageal atresia unless an roentgenogram is taken or the pH of the contents of the upper esophageal pouch is measured.

geal atresia the incidence of imperforate anus is estimated at 7% to 10%. One report shows a high incidence of malrotation (8%) and of duodenal anomalies (6%). It strongly advocates initial abdominal roentgenograms to rule out duodenal obstruction. Urologic and neurologic anomalies are described less frequently. Prematurity, which is present in 30% of cases, and associated malformations particularly affect the ultimate prognosis. These should be carefully looked for in every patient.

Clinical findings

Polyhydramnios is frequently noted during the third trimester of pregnancy and at delivery. The first clue to diagnosis is excessive mucus around the neonate's mouth; saliva collects in the pouch of the atretic esophagus and froths around the mouth and nose. With the first feeding, the triad of choking, coughing, and cyanosis becomes apparent. Respiratory distress supervenes as a consequence of pneumonia and atelectasis.

Esophageal atresia without a tracheoesophageal fistula (Fig. 3-2) or with a proximal fistula is suggested by inability to swallow, a scaphoid abdomen, and radiographic evidence that the gastrointestinal tract is devoid of air. Aspiration of saliva or food will lead to pneumonia. In esophageal atresia with a distal tracheoesophageal fistula or with a double one, excessive oral mucus and prompt regurgitation of food through the nose and mouth are rapidly followed by severe respiratory difficulties characterized by coughing, aspiration, and the development of chemical pneumonitis and atelectasis. In the case of a single fistulous tract without atresia, there are few swallowing difficulties, but repeated bouts of coughing and aspiration are the main problem. It is important to remember that, although in all other types of fistula the signs occur shortly after birth, a tracheoesophageal fistula without esophageal atresia may not produce symptoms until the infant is several months old, or even later. We have been impressed with the intermittency and the range of symptoms in

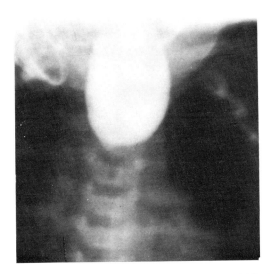

Fig. 3-4. Esophageal atresia. The medium-filled blind upper esophageal pouch usually reaches the level of the third thoracic vertebra.

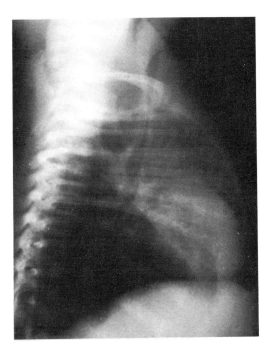

Fig. 3-5. Esophageal atresia. This newborn presented with excessive salivation, regurgitation of clear fluids, and a scaphoid abdomen. A lateral view shows the upper blind esophageal pouch filled with air.

the same patient from time to time. Nursery personnel may report that the baby cannot suck properly, swallows wrong, coughs after feedings, or becomes breathless after taking a few ounces.

Diagnosis

Since there is a significant prognostic advantage in making a diagnosis before respiratory complications occur, it has been suggested that every newborn be screened at birth by having a tube passed into the stomach. It is mandatory that all newborn infants with excessive mucus have a semirigid rubber catheter (8 F) passed through the length of their esophagus. Because the catheter may become curled (Fig. 3-3), it is well to aspirate some of the fluid and verify its pH. The obstruction usually lies within 10 cm of the nares (Fig.3-4). Because pneumonia is three times as likely to develop when a radiopaque material is introduced into the upper esophageal pouch, routine use of this material has fallen into disrepute. Small amounts (0.5 to 1 ml) of a dilute barium mixture may be used in the event that a lateral view fails to show the blind esophageal pouch. It can also be useful in the rare case (1% or 2%) of esophageal atresia with proximal tracheoesophageal fis-

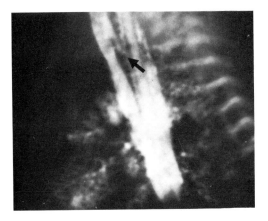

Fig. 3-6. Tracheoesophageal fistula without esophageal atresia. Reverse filling of the esophagus demonstrates a fistulous tract that runs obliquely cephalad from the esophagus to the trachea, *arrow*. The medium has filled the trachea and runs out into the lungs. The anatomic configuration of this H type of tracheoesophageal fistula illustrates why it is often so difficult to demonstrate a fistula.

tula. Since perforation of the pharynx in the new-born may clinically mimic esophageal atresia (Fig. 6-4), careful interpretation of roentgenograms taken with radiopaque material can protect these neonates from an unnecessary surgical procedure. At times, the diagnosis first becomes apparent when a roentgenogram of the chest taken for respiratory distress reveals dilatation of the esophagus with air and secretions on the lateral film (Fig. 3-5). When esophageal atresia has been demonstrated, air in the stomach is pathognomonic of a fistulous tract with the lower esophageal segment (the most common type). A tracheoesophageal fistula without atresia may be more difficult to demonstrate because of intermittent patency related to its size and obliqueness. However, rapid instillation of watery opaque medium through a catheter placed just below the middle of the esophagus will usually result in enough reversed filling to show the fistula (Fig. 3-6). Occasionally, lateral chest roentgenograms taken while the infant is crying can show air distention of the esophagus. When symptoms compatible with the diagnosis are present, at least three negative esophagograms, performed in the manner described above, should be done before the diagnosis is ruled out.

Management

Preoperative measures. Once the diagnosis is made, a 12 F Replogle catheter is placed in the proximal esophageal pouch under gentle suction. The head and thorax are elevated at 20 degrees with the baby in an Isolette with oxygen. Hydration should be maintained parenterally, and antibiotics should be prescribed. Performing a gastrostomy, with the patient receiving local anesthesia within a few hours of diagnosis, will prevent further reflux of gastric juice and more extensive lung damage. A Pezzer catheter is used to facilitate gastric drainage through the gastrostomy. Air should be used to irrigate the gastrostomy tube. The use of hyperalimentation can permit the surgeon to temporarily defer repair until the severe pulmonary complications or other surgically correctable anomalies have been attended to.

A primary repair is preferred in all infants with adequate esophageal segments regardless of associated anomalies or low birth weight. However the repair is not performed until the infant's condition is stable and respiratory complications have been corrected. Any life-threatening anomaly that is

Table 3-1. Colonic prostheses in 17 patients at Hôpital Sainte-Justine, Montreal*

Features of procedure	Number of patients
Indications	
Intractable esophageal strictures from caustic burns	5
Esophageal atresia	
Without fistula	7
With fistula	
Where anastomosis could not be done	3
Where anastomosis was done	2
Types of replacement	
Right colon	5
Transverse colon	4
Jejunum	3
Ileocolic	3
Gastric tube	2
Functional esophageal results	
Excellent	5
Dysphagia	
For meat only	4
For all solids	4
Gastrointestinal and growth complications	
Diarrhea	6
Deceleration of growth curve in post-operative follow-up (mean, 5 years) of 8 patients	4

*From Blanchard, H., Roy, C.C., Collin, P.P., and others: Can. J. Surg. **15:**137-145, 1972.

amenable to surgical correction or palliation is treated. Procedures designed at staging the repair result in complications as many as or more than those occurring after a primary repair.

Indications for "staging" the surgical correction are now restricted to the group of patients in whom the proximal and distal pouches are widely separated. They are closely monitored and kept on sump suction and gastrostomy decompression. Nutritional needs are met by peripheral or central parenteral nutrition. In our hands attempts at elongation by daily bougienage are not very satisfactory. After making sure that there is a distal esophageal pouch, one should attempt an approximation of the two pouches at 5 to 6 weeks of age.

Primary repair is particularly difficult in esophageal atresia without fistula, or with a proximal fistula, because of the long distance between the esophageal segments. However, there are reports of successful anastomosis after progressive elongation of the upper pouch and also of the distal pouch, but this approach has been largely unsuccessful in our hands. Despite notable advances in surgical techniques for primary repair, some patients still require reconstructive procedures. Colonic interposition has given satisfactory results but is not without complications (Table 3-1).

An alternative method to esophageal substitution is the gastric tube. In contrast to colonic interposition, it can be used in the presence of colonic or anal anomalies. There are none of the ischemic problems associated with the colon, and the gastric tube can be fashioned to the length necessary. Like the colon, the gastric tube has no intrinsic peristalsis and will not empty in a horizontal position. Propping of infants is necessary after meals. Leaks or strictures, or both, at the cervical anastomosis can be expected in more than 50%, but they are easily treated.

Postoperative measures. The gastrostomy should be kept draining to a bedside bottle for the first 24 hours, but no suctioning should be done and no irrigation or feedings given initially. Later, if the baby's condition permits, gastric feedings should be started. The tube can be kept open with periodic instillation of 2 to 4 cc of air. Upper pouch suctioning can be done effectively through a nasal catheter marked at the time of surgery so that the tip of the catheter does not lie against the anastomotic site. When definitive surgery has been done, feedings through the gastrostomy should not be started until residual gastric contents are minimal and one is certain that there is no other site of obstruction distally. Initial feedings should be small and should consist of 5% glucose, after which a dilute milk formula may be given through a vented drip bulb. Oral feedings are best put off until the tenth day after operation.

Complications

An anastomotic leak is frequent, occurring in 5% to 10% of cases, even under the best of circumstances. It is a consequence of undue tension, ischemia, or local infection. The associated mortality was around 50% when the transpleural approach was used. It is almost nil with the extrapleural technique. All oral feedings are to be withheld, gastric suction through a gastrostomy is carried out, and feedings can be safely administered through a small inlying duodenal tube with a continuous infusion pump.

Roentgenograms of the esophagus taken within the first weeks of a primary repair usually show a narrowing at the anastomotic site. If stenosis is associated with dysphagia, bougienage of the anastomotic site is done. Stridor may result from tracheal compression secondary to distention of the proximal esophagus with air and secretions. Protracted bougienage then becomes necessary.

All patients with atresia of the esophagus have a derangement of the normal motility, especially in the distal half of the esophagus. Peristalsis may be reversed or disorganized. Varying degrees of dysphagia are present as a result of this abnormal motility, which is usually well tolerated by the patient. Distal esophageal incompetence is present in most patients and may result in reflux esophagitis, recurrent stricture, nocturnal regurgitation, and aspiration pneumonia. Bethanechol therapy has been used successfully in a few cases, but an antireflux procedure (Nissen's fundoplication) may be necessary.

Prognosis

Management of esophageal atresia remains a monumental challenge to even the most experienced surgical, medical, and nursing personnel. Survival is related to birth weight, associated congenital malformations, and delay in making the diagnosis. The survival rate of patients who are receiving the best of care and who are without severe associated respiratory problems or congenital malformations is close to 100% in full-term infants.

In babies whose birth weight is below 2000 gm and in whom there are severe pulmonary problems or congenital anomaly, the mortality may be up to 40%.

REFERENCES

Abrahamson, J., and Shandling, B.: Esophageal atresia in the underweight baby: a challenge, J. Pediatr. Surg. **7:**608-613, 1972.

Anderson, K.D., and Randolph, J.G.: Gastric tube interposition: a satisfactory alternative to the colon for esophageal replacement in children, Ann. Thorac. Surg. **25:**521-525, 1978.

Andrassy, R.J., and Mahour, H.: Gastrointestinal anomalies associated with esophageal atresia or tracheoesophageal fistula, Arch. Surg. **114:**1125-1128, 1979.

Cozzi, F., and Wilkinson, A.W.: Low birth weight babies with esophageal atresia or tracheo-oesophageal fistula, Arch. Dis. Child. **50:**791-795, 1975.

Ducharme, J.C., Bertrand, R., and Debie, J.: Perforation of the pharynx in the newborn, a condition mimicking esophageal atresia, Can. Med. Assoc. J. **104:**785-787, 1971.

German, J.C., Mahour, G.H., and Woolley, M.M.: The twin with esophageal atresia, J. Pediatr. Surg. **14:**432-435, 1979.

Holder, T.M., Cloud, D.T., Lewis, J.E., and Pilling, G.P.: Esophageal atresia and tracheoesophageal fistula: a survey of its members by the Surgical Section of the American Academy of Pediatrics, Pediatrics **34:**542-549, 1964.

Howard, R., and Myers, N.A.: Esophageal atresia: a technique for elongating the upper pouch, Surgery **58:**725-727, 1965.

Koop, C.E., Schnaufer, L., and Broennle, F.M.: Esophageal atresia and tracheoesophageal fistula: supportive measures that affect survival, Pediatrics **54:**558-564, 1974.

Parker, A.F., Christie, D.L., and Cahill, J.L.: Incidence and significance of gastroesophageal reflux following repair of esophageal atresia and tracheoesophageal fistula and the need for anti-reflux procedures, J. Pediatr. Surg. **14:**5-10, 1979.

Quan, L., and Smith, D.W.: The Vater association, J. Pediatr. **82:**104-107, 1973.

Shermeta, D.W., Whitington, P.F., Seto, D.S., and Haller, J.A.: Lower esophageal sphincter dysfunction in esophageal atresia: nocturnal regurgitation and aspiration pneumonia, J. Pediatr. Surg. **12:**871-876, 1977.

Strodel, W.E., Coran, A.G., Kirsh, M.M., and others: Esophageal atresia, Arch. Surg. **114:**523-527, 1979.

Pyloric atresia

Pyloric atresia represents about 1% of all intestinal atresias. Close to two thirds of cases consist of an internal web or diaphragm, which may give rise to a complete or partial gastric outlet obstruction. Other types consist of an atretic segment bridging two blind ends or of a complete segmental defect. The patient presents in the first few days with nonbilious vomiting. A single gastric bubble (Fig. 3-7) is seen on roentgenographic examination when the obstruction is complete. Perforation of the stomach and pneumonia from aspiration have been reported. Treatment is surgical. There are reports of four patients with pyloric atresia and epidermolysis bullosa.

REFERENCES

Bell, M.J., Ternberg, J.L., Keating, J.P., and others: Prepyloric gastric antral web: a puzzling epidemic, J. Pediatr. Surg. **13:**307-313, 1978.

Shafie, M.E., Stidham, G.L., Klippel, C.H., and others: Pyloric atresia and epidermolysis bullosa: a lethal combination in two premature newborn siblings, J. Pediatr. Surg. **14:**446-449, 1979.

Tunnell, W.P., and Smith, E.I.: Antral web in infancy, J. Pediatr. Surg. **15:**152-155, 1980.

Congenital duodenal obstruction: intrinsic

Intrinsic duodenal obstruction is usually caused by atresia in which the lumen is obliterated. At times, a complete gap between the two bowel ends may be found. Stenosis and the presence of a diaphragm restricting the duodenal lumen constitute

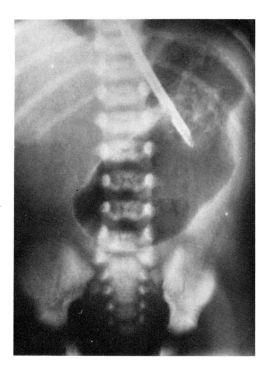

Fig. 3-7. Pyloric atresia with the typical air-distended stomach and the absence of gas elsewhere in the gastrointestinal tract.

other causes of intrinsic obstruction. (Fig. 3-8). Both atresias and stenoses may affect the duodenum proximal to (20%) or distal from (80%) the ampulla of Vater. The incidence in Australia has been estimated to be 1 per 4100 live births.

Clinical findings

Complete obstruction (atresia). Vomiting begins within a few hours after birth or after the first feedings. Since most atresias involve the postampullary duodenum, the vomitus is usually bilious. Distention is limited to the epigastrium. Meconium may be normally passed. Jaundice occurs in more than one third of cases and a history of polyhydramnios in 50%. Fig. 3-9 shows an example of the frequent association between duodenal atresia and severe congenital anomalies (30%). The high incidence of prematurity (25% to 50%) and trisomy 21 (20% to 30%) is particularly striking.

Partial obstruction (stenosis or diaphragm). When duodenal obstruction is partial, the symptoms of obstruction are intermittent and may fail to appear for weeks, months, or years. Even though a postampullary location of the stenotic area is usual, the vomitus does not always contain bile.

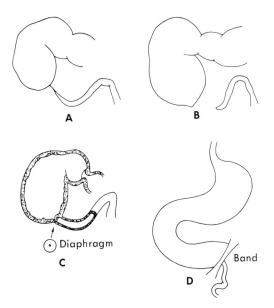

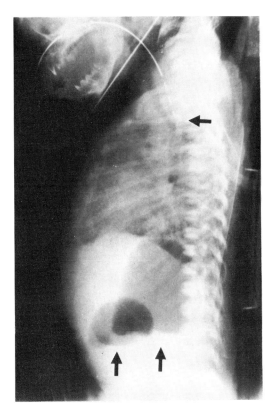

Fig. 3-8. Congenital duodenal obstruction. **A,** Duodenal atresia with obliteration of the lumen. **B,** Duodenal atresia with a complete gap between the two bowel ends. **C,** An imperforate web or diaphragm may mimic duodenal atresia. There are signs of partial obstruction when the diaphragm has a small central opening. **D,** When rotation stops and the cecum lies anterior to the superior mesenteric artery, peritoneal bands extend from the cecum and right colon to the right upper quadrant of the abdomen. These bands form dense adhesions binding the colon and duodenum together. They are particularly dense over the duodenum, and extrinsic obstruction is often produced.

Fig. 3-9. Duodenal atresia. This premature infant was admitted for imperforate anus and excessive salivation. The lateral film shows a blind proximal esophageal pouch diagnostic of esophageal atresia, *arrow*. In addition, this patient had a duodenal atresia, illustrated by the "double bubble" sign, *lower arrows*.

Diagnosis

Clinical and roentgenographic findings cannot do more than indicate either partial or complete duodenal obstruction. Roentgenograms of the abdomen usually show gastric and duodenal gaseous distention proximal to the atretic site (Fig. 3-10). Air may also be seen in the portal vein or in the biliary tract. When protracted vomiting and dehydration occur, there may be little air in the stomach; it is then advisable to instill 10 cc of air in the stomach to elicit the typical roentgenographic pattern. Total absence of gas from the intestinal tract distal to the obstruction is suggestive of atresia or an extrinsic obstruction severe enough to completely occlude the lumen. On the other hand, air scattered in the lower part of the bowel may indicate a partial duodenal obstruction of either intrinsic or extrinsic variety. A contrast study is indicated only in these other cases. Once the

study has been completed, the contrast material should be removed through a nasogastric tube.

Treatment

In all duodenal obstructions, intermittent suction should be carried out and the infant kept in an Isolette. Fluid, protein, and electrolyte replacement should precede surgery, which can usually be performed within a few hours after the diagnosis is established. At operation, a thorough exploration is necessary, not only to find the cause of the obstruction, but also to make sure that no additional abnormality is present lower in the gastrointestinal tract.

Prognosis

Mortality (35% to 40%) is significantly increased by prematurity, trisomy 21, and associated congenital anomalies.

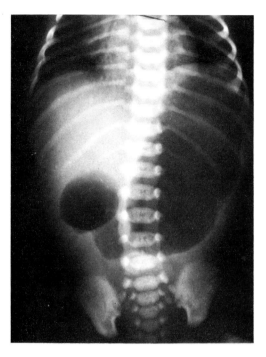

Fig. 3-10. Duodenal atresia with the characteristic gastric and duodenal gaseous distention proximal to the atretic site, the "double bubble" sign.

Congenital duodenal obstruction: extrinsic

The extrinsic variety of duodenal obstruction occurs more commonly in males. It is usually secondary to congenital peritoneal bands (Fig. 3-7, *D*) with or without associated malrotation. It may also occur with an annular pancreas or with a duplication of the duodenum. More rarely, an incomplete rotation of the duodenojejunal loop can result in redundancy and kinking of the duodenum or jejunum (Fig. 3-11) with partial upper intestinal obstruction noted in the presence of normal rotation of the colon. A preduodenal portal vein is no longer believed to be obstructive. An associated anomaly such as malrotation, atresia, or congenital diaphragm is responsible for the duodenal obstruction.

When the obstruction is complete, the symptoms and signs occur early and the clinical findings are those described for the intrinsic duodenal anomalies. The diagnosis is more difficult to make when there is only partial obstruction, since persistent regurgitation may be the only sign, though vomiting of bilious material is usually present. The gastrointestinal series demonstrates the site, severity, and probable cause of most partial obstructions of the duodenum. As a rule, such obstructions are considered significant only if there is enlargement proximal to the obstruction and delay in emptying of the medium.

REFERENCES

Braun, P., Collin, P.P., and Ducharme, P.C.: Preduodenal vein. A significant entity? Can. J. Surg. **17:**316-322, 1974.

Chamberlain, J.W.: Partial intestinal obstruction in the newborn due to kinking of the proximal small bowel, N. Engl. J. Med. **275:**1241-1242, 1966.

Esscher, T.: Preduodenal portal vein: a cause of intestinal obstruction, J. Pediatr. Surg. **15:**609-612, 1980.

Fonkalsrud, E.W., DeLorimier, A.A., and Hays, D.M.: Congenital atresia and stenosis of duodenum: a review compiled from the members of the Surgical Section of the American Academy of Pediatrics, Pediatrics **43:**79-83, 1969.

Girvan, D.P., and Stephens, C.A.: Congenital duodenal obstruction: a 20-year review of its surgical management and consequences, J. Pediatr. Surg. **9:**833-839, 1974.

Kraeger, R.R., Gromoljez, P., and Lewis, J.E.: Congenital duodenal atresia, Am. J. Surg. **126:**762-764, 1973.

Wayne, E.R., and Burrington, J.D.: Extrinsic duodenal obstruction in children, Surg. Gynecol. Obstet. **136:**87-91, 1973.

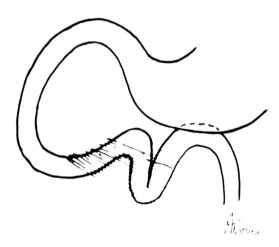

Fig. 3-11. Kinking of the duodenum. Partial obstruction may be secondary to kinking of the duodenum. The exact pathogenesis of this entity is unknown, but it is believed to be a developmental defect. (Modified from Chamberlain, J.W.: N. Engl. J. Med. **275:**1241-1242, 1966.)

Congenital duodenal web or diaphragm

Intrinsic duodenal obstruction may be secondary to a web or diaphragm (Fig. 3-8, *C*). Since the web or diaphragm may assume a preampullary

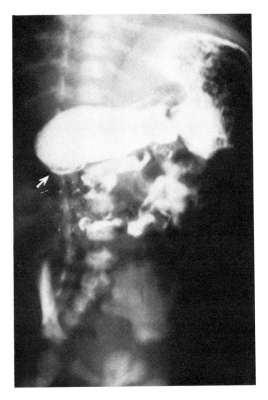

Fig. 3-12. Windsock deformity of the duodenum in an infant with vomiting and failure to thrive. Note the thin stream of barium taking off from the greatly distended first part of the duodenum, *arrow.*

or postampullary position, the vomitus may or may not contain bile.

The onset of symptoms may be delayed, sometimes for years, since the web may be perforate and permit passage of the upper duodenal contents. When there is an aperture in the web, the classic double bubble of dilated stomach and duodenum may be absent. The associated dilatation of the duodenum is not a manifestation of the true level of obstruction, since the thin duodenal web can be easily ballooned and pushed distally (Fig. 3-12). Attention has been drawn to the danger of constructing a duodenojejunostomy downstream from a duodenal diaphragm.

As in other entities responsible for intrinsic and extrinsic congenital duodenal obstruction, associated malformations are common. The diagnosis of a duodenal web or diaphragm may be missed because of the severity of other gastrointestinal anomalies such as malrotation, anorectal malformations, and Hirschsprung's disease.

REFERENCES

Lynn, H.B.: Duodenal obstruction: atresia, stenosis and annular pancreas. In Ravitch, M.M., Welch, K.J., Benson, C.D., Aberdeen, E., and Randolph, J.G., editors: Pediatric surgery, ed. 3, Chicago, 1979, Year Book Medical Publishers.

Richardson, W.R., and Martin, L.W.: Pitfalls in the surgical management of the incomplete duodenal diaphragm, J. Pediatr. Surg. **4:**303-312, 1969.

Rowe, M.I., Buckner, D., and Clatworthy, H.W.: Windsock web of the duodenum, Am. J. Surg. **116:**444-449, 1968.

Swartz, R.M., Hunter, M.T., and Hartz, C.R.: Reoperation for congenital duodenal diaphragm, Ann. Surg. **177:**441-447, 1973.

Annular pancreas

The pancreas develops from two entirely distinct entodermal outgrowths, known as the dorsal and the ventral pancreas, which fuse to make a single organ. The ventral pancreatic bud is bilobate. The left bud normally degenerates; if it persists and develops into its own pancreatic lobe, it grows around the left side of the duodenum to join the other two parts of the pancreas in the dorsal mesentery (Fig. 3-13). The presence of an annular pancreas may be regarded, in a significant number of cases, as a sign of failure of segmental duodenal development. Coexistent duodenal atresia, malrotation with bands, and duodenal diaphragm are described frequently. Histologically, there may be penetration of the duodenal wall by pancreatic tissue, leading to the intermingling of pancreatic tissue with the muscular coat of the duodenum.

Clinical findings

The annular pancreas may not constrict the duodenum at all or may be associated with partial or complete duodenal obstruction. Trisomy 21 and severe congenital anomalies of the gastrointestinal tract occur frequently in association with an annular pancreas. As with other obstructive lesions affecting the neonate, polyhydramnios often develops during the pregnancy. The roentgenographic pattern is that of a partial or complete duodenal obstruction. Supine, upright, and lateral films show an obstruction in the second portion of the duodenum. If air does not outline the stomach, it may be instilled by use of a nasogastric tube (Fig. 3-14).

Attention needs to be drawn to the occasional late onset of symptoms associated with this anomaly. A recent review of 15 cases from the Mayo Clinic reveals that 6 were neonates and 9 were

Fig. 3-13. Annular pancreas. There is complete obstruction in the second portion of the duodenum; pancreatic tissue has grown around the duodenum. It must be pointed out that, in most cases, an annular pancreas is a sign of an intrinsic duodenal anomaly rather than the cause of a duodenal obstruction. (Modified from Snyder, W.H., and Chaffin, L.: Malrotation of the intestine. In Mustard, W.T., and others, editors: Pediatric surgery, ed. 2, Chicago, 1969, Year Book Medical Publishers, Inc.)

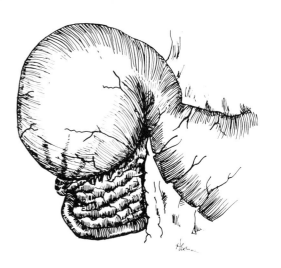

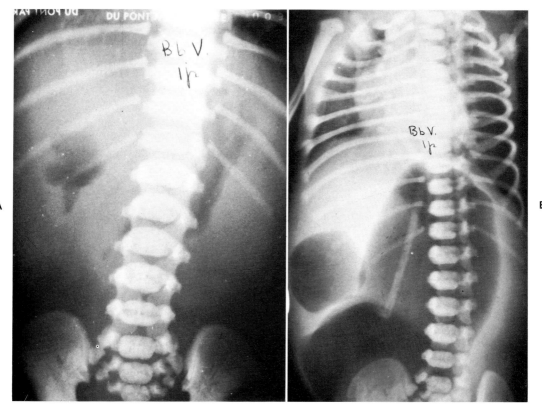

Fig. 3-14. Annular pancreas. "Double bubble" is secondary to an annular pancreas. The obstruction was relieved by a laterolateral duodenojejunostomy. **A,** Note how the typical x-ray pattern of a duodenal obstruction disappears with nasogastric suction. **B,** Protracted vomiting may decrease gastric and duodenal air to such an extent that the classic "double-bubble" pattern may not be evident unless air is injected.

adults. Complaints in the latter were intermittent epigastric discomfort, which usually was relieved by vomiting. Upper gastrointestinal roentgenograms showed narrowing of the second portion of the duodenum in seven of eight patients. One patient had a duodenal ulcer. In adults, the incidence of major anomalies associated with annular pancreas stands at around 10%.

Treatment

Because of the high incidence of associated duodenal anomalies, the patient with signs of upper bowel obstruction and an annular pancreas is likely to have an intrinsic anomaly of his duodenum or perhaps an associated malrotation with volulus. The operation of choice is either a duodenostomy or a duodenojejunostomy. No attempt should be made at operative dissection or division of the pancreatic annulus.

REFERENCES

Elliott, G.B., Kliman, M.R., and Elliott, K.A.: Pancreatic annulus: a sign or a cause of duodenal obstruction, Can. J. Surg. **11**:357-364, 1968.

Feuchtwanger, M.M., and Weiss, Y.: Side to side duodenoduodenostomy for obstructing annular pancreas in the newborn, J. Pediatr. Surg. **3**:398-401, 1968.

Kiernan, P.D., ReMine, S.G., Kiernan, P.C., and Remine, W.H.: Annular pancreas, Arch. Surg. **115**:46-50, 1980.

Longo, M.F., and Lynn, H.B.: Congenital duodenal obstruction: review of 30 cases encountered in a 30-year period, Mayo Clin. Proc. **42**:423-430, 1967.

Wayne, E.R., and Burrington, J.D.: Extrinsic duodenal obstruction in children, Surg. Gynecol. Obstet. **136**:87-91, 1973.

Malrotation with or without volvulus of the midgut

Anomalies of intestinal rotation and fixation occur in somewhat less than 1 per 6000 live births. They represent the fourth commonest major gastrointestinal malformation after tracheoesophageal anomalies, imperforate anus, and intrinsic duodenal obstruction. Malrotation of the intestine is related to the abnormal movement of the intestine around the superior mesenteric artery during embryologic development. It can be best understood if one follows the rotation of the two ends of the intestinal tract, that is, the proximal duodenojejunal loop and the distal cecocolic loop, around the superior mesenteric artery (Fig. 3-15).

Normally, the midgut extends from the duodenojejunal junction to the middle of the transverse colon and is supplied by the superior mesenteric

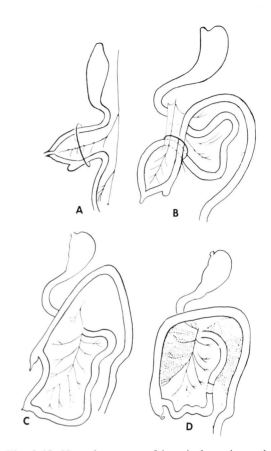

Fig. 3-15. Normal progress of intestinal rotation and fixation. **A,** The midgut is developing in its extracoelomic position. It is supplied by the superior mesenteric artery and divided into an upper limb (duodenojejunal loop) and a lower limb (cecocolic loop). **B,** Around the tenth week of embryonic life, a 270-degree counterclockwise rotation takes place around the superior mesenteric artery as the midgut gradually returns to the coelomic cavity. The duodenojejunal loop lies posterior to the cecocolic loop and under the superior mesenteric artery (SMA). The duodenum is pushed to the left of the SMA as the small intestine is withdrawn first. **C,** The cecum and right colon return to the left side of the abdominal cavity and pass anterior and above the SMA. **D,** This is the stage of descent of the cecum into the right lower quadrant and the stage of fixation and fusion of the mesentery from the ligament of Treitz and downward to the right lower quadrant. (Modified from Gross, R.E.: The surgery of infancy and childhood, Philadelphia, 1953, W.B. Saunders Co.)

artery. It returns to an intra-abdominal position during the tenth week of embryonic life while the root of the mesentery rotates 270 degrees in a counterclockwise direction. This causes the colon to cross ventrally; the cecum moves from left to right and descends in the right lower quadrant, where it is fixed posteriorly. The duodenum crosses dorsally to become partly retroperitoneal.

Pathologic anatomy

Rotation of the duodenojejunal segment and of the cecocolic segment is sequential. Arrest of rotation at various times may affect either or both of these segments. In the latter case, the nonrotation often leads to volvulus of the midgut (duodenum to midtransverse colon), since it hangs on a single pedicle consisting of the duodenum, the midtransverse colon, and the superior mesenteric vessels, which may twist and lead not only to complete duodenal obstruction but also to infarction of the entire midgut.

A second clinical aspect of nonrotation or incomplete rotation is that it leads to partial or complete duodenal obstruction by peritoneal bands. The most commonly reported ones result from abnormal fixation of the duodenum associated with malrotation of the colon and the presence of the cecum in the upper quadrant of the abdomen to the left of the duodenum. The bands extend from the cecum across the descending part of the duodenum to the right paravertebral gutter. In the second variety, the colon has rotated normally but the hepatic flexure of the colon is higher than normal and lies medial to the duodenum, which is compressed by bands originating from the hepatic flexure. In cases where the duodenojejunal loop has failed to complete its rotation while the cecocolic loop assumes its normal position and fixation, the duodenum and ligament of Treitz remain to the right of the midline. Bands usually obstruct the distal portion of the third part of the duodenum. This anomaly of rotation may also lead to kinking of the duodenum. A final variety of bands occurs in the absence of any error of rotation of either the duodenum or colon. It is considered to represent hypertrophy of the hepatoduodenal ligament, which obstructs the duodenum at the junction of its first and second portions.

Clinical findings

Of symptomatic cases, 80% have evidence of high intestinal obstruction within the first 3 weeks of life. Characteristically these newborn infants will retain food for the first 24 to 48 hours, and then vomiting will occur and become bilious. Abdominal distention localized to the upper abdomen is a frequent finding, and visible peristaltic waves can occur. In addition to intestinal obstruction, volvulus will lead to signs of vascular obstruction of the midgut manifested by melena, currant-jelly stools, and, eventually, sepsis, perforation, and peritonitis.

The association of malrotation with annular pancreas, congenital atresia, or stenosis of the duodenum is seen in 25% of cases. Nonrotation is also associated with midgut volvulus found in patients with omphaloceles, with gastroschisis, with hernias through the foramen of Bochdalek, and occasionally with jaundice when the common bile duct is twisted. Extraintestinal malformations are rather frequent, with congenital heart disease being the most common.

One fifth of cases will develop symptoms after the first month of life or during childhood or even adulthood. Chronic intermittent crampy abdomi-

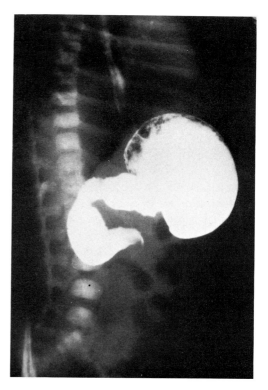

Fig. 3-16. Volvulus of the midgut. Opaque medium was used to demonstrate the stomach, duodenum, and twisted site of obstruction at the ligament of Treitz.

nal pain may be the presenting symptom along with bouts of vomiting and chronic constipation. In one series, it accounted for 10% of all infants and children treated for malrotation. Less frequently, the clinical picture is that of abdominal distention involving particularly the upper abdomen and a "celiac-like" syndrome secondary to chronic lymphovenous obstruction. Alternating bouts of diarrhea and evidence of malabsorption and malnutrition dominate the clinical picture, and there is a history of feeding problems during the first few months of life.

Anomalies of intestinal rotation are commonly found at autopsy, but most patients remain asymptomatic throughout their lifetime. Therefore the mere presence of these lesions is not an indication for surgery.

Diagnosis

The clinical history and physical findings are extremely important if an early diagnosis is going to be made. One must look assiduously for any signs of intestinal obstruction appearing during the newborn period.

In volvulus of the midgut, the plain films may be normal. In some, the obstruction near the ligament of Treitz is sufficiently severe to produce some gaseous distention of the stomach and duodenal loop, usually with some gas scattered lower in the abdomen. In contrast, patients with atresia of the duodenum show much more enlargement of the first part of the duodenum and no gas at all in the bowel distal from it. The upper gastrointestinal series in midgut volvulus shows obstruction, often with a twisted contour in a narrow area near the duodenojejunal juncture, with little or no medium passing beyond (Fig. 3-16). When this is found, the diagnosis must be volvulus of the midgut, and operation is urgent. Congenital bands and malrotation without volvulus rarely produce the same picture and can be differentiated only surgically. Since the mortality from volvulus of the midgut is still about 35%, it is imperative that patients who suddenly begin vomiting bile be examined radiographically as an emergency procedure. Emergency surgery should be done when the examination indicates that volvulus is the problem. A barium enema may show malrotation of

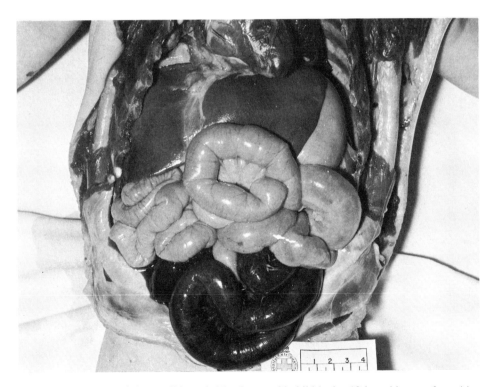

Fig. 3-17. Volvulus of the small bowel. The 2-year-old child had a 12-hour history of vomiting and abdominal pain and distention; he was dead on arrival. Postmortem examination failed to find an anatomic explanation for the extensive area of small bowel twisted around its mesentery.

the colon, but it is of confirmatory value only and does not substitute for the upper series.

Bands may produce transverse indentations on the duodenum without causing obstruction. In rare cases, they may lead to kinking of the proximal small bowel and partial intestinal obstruction. Some are associated with malrotation. Few ever produce significant obstructions. Barium enema demonstration of failure of complete descent of the cecum is of no significance at any age, since it is highly unlikely to become symptomatic. Some degree of malrotation is common in the newborn infant, gradually becoming anatomically more normal within a few weeks.

Small intestinal volvulus may occur in the absence of malrotation. In a few cases, there is no apparent cause (Fig. 3-17). In most, however, twisting or knotting of the bowel can be traced to congenital defects (Meckel's diverticulum with persistence of omphalomesenteric remnants, mesenteric cyst, and duplication of the small bowel) to acquired conditions (adhesions) as in Fig. 3-18, or to factors that may increase intestinal mobility and ease of rotation (long mesentery).

Midgut volvulus is one of the most catastrophic diseases of the newborn period. The ischemia caused by the volvulus often involves the entire segment of the intestine in the territory of the superior mesenteric artery (from the ligament of Treitz to the midtransverse colon). In such circumstances, one first reduces the volvulus by turning the entire small bowel in a counterclockwise direction until the transverse colon and cecum are anterior to the pedicle of the midgut. Ladd's bands are then divided. The next step is to assess the viability of the intestine and abide by the principle that unless there is a perforation, apparently compromised intestine should not be resected. A "second-look" operation is recommended 36 to 48 hours after the initial procedure. During this interval, parenteral antibiotics, oxygen, and blood are administered. Low molecular weight dextran (dextran 40), 10 ml/kg every 6 hours, has been advocated. It is said to improve the microcirculation and prevent extension of venous thromboses. It has been the experience of all groups that this second-look policy saves bowel that would have previously been resected.

Ladd's procedure, which consists in dividing adhesions and bands after derotation of the bowel, is a standard procedure. There have been heated discussions whether intestinal fixation should be carried out in the hope of decreasing the chances

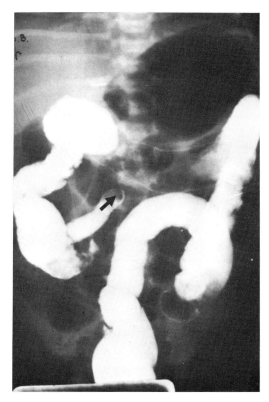

Fig. 3-18. Volvulus without malrotation. The barium column has outlined a normally placed colon and has undergone reflux in the terminal ileum. The area of obstruction is tapered and has a twisted appearance, *arrow*. This 1-day-old infant had abdominal distention and respiratory distress. Meconium was passed. There were numerous adhesions in the peritoneal cavity. A 25 cm segment of necrotic small bowel had to be resected.

(10%) of recurrence of intestinal obstruction. A long-term study has shown that this is of no benefit and is therefore unnecessary.

Prognosis

The prognosis during the newborn period is guarded. The incidence of associated severe congenital anomalies is frequent. Intestinal necrosis, gangrene, and perforation with generalized peritonitis is a rather frequent complication when volvulus is present. The mortality is about 15%.

Unfortunately, malrotation with volvulus leads commonly to resections of the absorptive apparatus that are so extensive as to compromise for long periods and sometimes permanently any possibility of sustaining nutrition and growth by the oral route. It is the entity most commonly responsible for the short-bowel syndrome (see Chapter 10).

REFERENCES

Berdon, W.E., Baker, D.H., Bull, S., and Santulli, T.V.: Midgut malrotation and volvulus, Radiology **96:**375-384, 1970.

Chamberlain, J.W.: Partial intestinal obstruction in the newborn due to kinking of the proximal small bowel, N. Engl. J. Med. **275:**1241-1242, 1966.

Firor, H.V., and Harris, V.J.: Rotational abnormalities of the gut, Am. J. Roentgenol. Radium Ther. Nucl. Med. **120:**315-321, 1974.

Janik, J.S., and Ein, S.H.: Normal intestinal rotation with nonfixation: a cause of chronic abdominal pain, J. Pediatr. Surg. **14:**670-674, 1979.

Krasna, I.H., Becker, J.M., Schwartz, D., and Schneider, K.: Low molecular weight dextran and reexploration in the management of ischemic midgut-volvulus, J. Pediatr. Surg. **13:**480-483, 1978.

Pochaczevsky, R., Ratner, H., Leonidas, J.C., and others: Unusual forms of volvulus after the neonatal period, Am. J. Roentgenol. Radium Ther. Nucl. Med. **114:**390-393, 1972.

Stauffer, U.G., and Hermann, P.: Comparison of late results in patients with corrected intestinal malrotation with and without fixation of the mesentery, J. Pediatr. Surg. **15:**9-12, 1980.

Steiner, G.M.: The misplaced caecum and the root of the mesentery, Br. J. Radiol. **51:**406-413, 1978.

Stewart, D.R., Colodny, A.L., and Daggett, W.C.: Malrotation of the bowel in infants and children: a 15 year review, Surgery **79:**716-720, 1976.

Verma, T.R., and Bankole, M.A.: Lymphovenous obstruction in anomalous midgut rotation, Arch. Dis. Child. **48:**154-157, 1973.

Congenital jejunal and ileal obstruction

Jejunoileal atresias occur more frequently (2:1) than duodenal atresias, but they may occur together. Their incidence varies from 1 in 400 to 1 in 1500 live births. Complete occlusion of the lumen is much more common than stenoses are; the latter account for only 5% of cases. The incidence of multiple atresias varies from 6% to 20% according to authors. Atresia of the proximal jejunum and of the distal ileum account for more than two thirds of cases.

Arrest in growth at the solid stage may result in atresia of the duodenum, but there is considerable evidence that this is not the cause of atresia in the jejunum and ileum. Operating room findings suggest vascular insufficiency, and the malformation has been reproduced in unborn animals by ligation of superior mesenteric vessels so that vascular insufficiency is maintained in utero. Observations are that the bowel distal to the site of atresia frequently contains bile. The latter is not secreted until the end of the first trimester, an indication suggesting that jejunoileal atresia may occur relatively late in the course of fetal development. The description of jejunal atresia in twin premature infants with evidence of congenital rubella introduces another dimension to the pathogenesis—virus-induced vascular lesions.

In at least three reports of cases of multiple atresias, vascular lesions were absent whereas inflammatory lesions were prominent. In some cases the inflammatory process was both acute and chronic. The chronic pathologic lesions led to the formation of pseudopolyps, septal, corklike atresias, a sieve-like appearance, and intraluminal and intramural calcifications. This evidence suggests that, although jejunoileal atresias are the likely result of vascular insufficiency, certain forms could be the consequence of an intrauterine inflammatory process of unknown origin.

About 5% to 9% of children with jejunoileal atresia have cystic fibrosis, and close to 15% have an associated intestinal malrotation. Trisomy 21 occurs in less than 1% of cases. A number of other anomalies have been described. As in duodenal atresia, low birth weight newborns are particularly susceptible to small-bowel atresia.

Clinical findings

Hydramnios can be documented in perhaps one fourth of the cases. Amniotic fluid is reported as "meconium stained" and likely results from vomiting in utero. Vomiting of bile-stained material usually starts within the first 24 hours of life. In protracted cases the vomitus may become fecal and lead to aspiration pneumonia. Abdominal distention is more frequently present than that with duodenal obstruction. Perforation may occur. The passage of small amounts of green-colored meconium does not rule out intestinal atresia. However, in most cases only a modest amount of green mucoid material is evacuated, especially if the lower part of the ileum is involved. Jaundice characterized by an elevation of indirect-reacting bilirubin is reported in a third of cases of jejunal atresia and in 20% of those with ileal involvement. Symptoms tend to develop earlier in patients with an upper type of atresia than in those with a lower one.

Atresia, stenosis, and diaphragms in multiple sites are well known, and the intestine may take on the appearance of a string of sausages. The incidence of multiple sites of involvement in jejunoileal atresia ranges from 6% to 29% in reported series. An autosomal recessive mode of inheritance has been suggested in a few families. Our experience with 10 cases suggests that extensive segments of duodenum, jejunum, and ileum may be involved and that in certain cases the colon may also be affected.

Multiple small-bowel atresias*
(Number of patients: 10)

Birth weight: 6 under 2500 gm
Perinatal history:
  Hydramnios (3)
  Green amniotic fluid (2)
  Jaundice (4)
Onset of symptoms: 3 to 78 hours
Area involved:
  Jejunum and ileum (3)
  Duodenum, jejunum, and ileum (2)
  Stomach to rectum (5)
Length of involvement: 15 cm to total small bowel
  in addition to duodenum or colon, or both
Associated major anomalies: 4 cases

Another unusual group of patients are those with "apple-peel" atresia or "Christmas-tree" deformity. They present with jejunal atresia near the ligament of Treitz, a shortened bowel, the absence of a mesentery, and the helical coiling of hypoplastic loops distal to the atresia. These loops are precariously supplied in a retrograde fashion by anastomotic arcades from the ileocolic, right colic, or inferior mesenteric artery. Low birth weight, an increased number of associated anomalies, and a familial pattern are recognized in the 45 cases reported so far. Less than 50% survive the immediate postoperative period.

Patients with jejunal or ileal stenosis may develop symptoms of partial intestinal obstruction at birth, within the first few weeks of life, or much later. The stenotic area may be limited to a diaphragm or a narrow band or may extend over a long segment. Intermittent bouts of abdominal pain, vomiting and distention are suggestive, particularly when associated with failure to thrive. Jejunoileal stenoses may be the result of necrotizing enterocolitis rather than that of an intrauterine vascular accident or inflammatory process.

X-ray findings

Scout films of the abdomen of patients with atresia will show dilated loops of small bowel and the absence of colonic gas (Fig. 3-19). Intraluminal calcifications may indicate that an antenatal volvulus has taken place or that multiple atresias are

*Courtesy F.M. Guttman and others, Hôpital Sainte-Justine, Montreal.

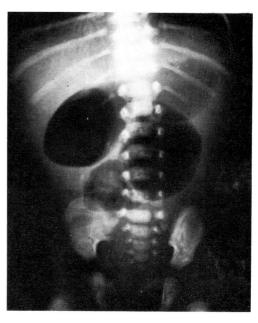

Fig. 3-19. Atresia of the jejunum. In addition to the gas-filled stomach, there are two grossly distended bowel loops, and then no gas is visible in the rest of the abdomen. This is pathognomonic of a high atresia of the jejunum, since there is too great a length of gas-distended bowel for the atresia to be in the duodenum.

present. Peritoneal calcifications (more than 10%) signifies that there is meconium peritonitis, the result of intrauterine bowel perforation. Depending on the level of atresia, the barium enema may show a restricted caliber of the colon, which is appropriately called a disuse microcolon. Relating the level of intestinal obstruction to the caliber of the colon at birth has been most helpful in giving diagnostic signficance to the finding of a microcolon. In esophageal and duodenal obstruction, the colon caliber is always normal. Since the production of succus entericus and meconium by the small bowel is believed to influence the caliber of the colon, the length of small bowel distal from the obstruction can be ascertained preoperatively by the findings at barium enema. A number of cases of jejunal and ileal atresias have been associated with a normal colon, though in low ileal obstructions (meconium ileus or atresia) a microcolon is invariably found (Fig. 3-20).

There is usually no indication to perform upper gastrointestinal contract studies in instances of complete obstruction. In cases of stenoses suggested by a partial obstruction, barium meal with small bowel follow-through is indicated.

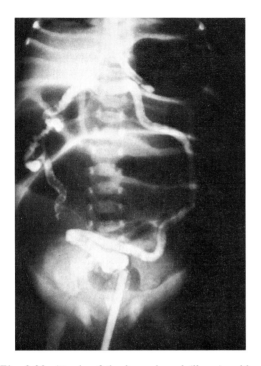

Fig. 3-20. Atresia of the lower bowel (ileum), with a barium enema showing a microcolon of disuse. The large number of bowel loops indicates a low obstruction. The small-diameter colon proves that the obstruction is antenatal and must be either an atresia or meconium ileus.

Differential diagnosis

The differential diagnosis of stenoses should include Hirschsprung's disease; paralytic ileus secondary to sepsis, gastroenteritis, or pneumonia; midgut volvulus; duplications, and meconium ileus. In the last condition, the initial manifestation of cystic fibrosis can be found in association with intestinal atresia. Every patient with an ileal atresia should later be tested for cystic fibrosis. The meconium obtained at surgery should be examined for the presence of excessive amounts of albumin and for proteolytic enzymes.

Jejunoileal atresia may coexist with malrotation as well as with meconium ileus secondary to cystic fibrosis. The incidence probably stands at 10% for the coexistence of jejunoileal atresia with malrotation or with meconium ileus.

Treatment

Surgical intervention is mandatory. Immediate decompression of the gastrointestinal tract should be done and intravenous fluids given. An end-to-end small-bowel anastomosis is the accepted tech-

nique. Careful attention should be paid to the possibility of stenotic segments or mucosal diaphragms. Saline solution should be injected to rule them out. In cases of multiple atresias involving a modest segment, it is preferable to sacrifice some length of bowel and have a single anastomosis. When multiple atresias involve a large proportion of the small bowel, multiple limited resections become necessary.

Prognosis

The prognosis is adversely affected by delay in diagnosis, prematurity, or the presence of an associated major congenital malformation.

The chances of survival are about 65% to 75% in cases of a single atresia. It is poorer when multiple atresias are present, since the length of uninvolved small bowel ma► be incompatible with survival.

REFERENCES

Abrams, J.S.: Experimental intestinal atresia, Surgery **64:**185-191, 1968.

Berdon, W.E., Baker, D.H., Santulli, T.V., and others: Microcolon in newborn infants with intestinal obstruction, Radiology **90:**878-885, 1970.

Clerc, G., Mathieu, P., Bientz, J., and others: Le syndrome "apple peel small bowel" ou syndrome du grêle en colimaçon, Chir. Pédiatr. **20:**191-195, 1979.

DeLorimier, A.A., Fonkalsrud, E.W., and Hays, D.M.: Congenital atresia and stenosis of the jejunum and ileum, Surgery **65:**819-827, 1969.

Esterly, J.R., and Talbert, J.L.: Jejunal atresia in twins with presumed congenital rubella, Lancet **1:**1028-1029, 1969.

Guttman, F.M., Garance, P.H., Blanchard, H., and others: Multiple atresias and a new syndrome of hereditary multiple atresias involving the gastrointestinal tract from stomach to rectum, J. Pediatr. Surg. **8:**633-640, 1973.

Martin, C.E., Leonidas, J.C., and Amoury, R.A.: Multiple gastrointestinal atresias with intraluminal calcifications and cystic dilatation of bile ducts: a newly recognized entity resembling "a string of pearls," Pediatrics **57:**268-271, 1976.

Rittenhouse, E.A., Beckwith, J.B., Chappell, J.S., and others: Multiple septa of the small bowel: description of an unusual case with review of the literature and consideration of etiology, Surgery **71:**371-379, 1972.

Santulli, T.V., Chen, C.C., and Schullinger, J.N.: Management of congenital atresia of the intestine, Am. J. Surg. **119:**542-547, 1970.

Shafie, M.E., and Rickham, P.P.: Multiple intestinal atresia, J. Pediatr. Surg. **5:**655-659, 1970.

Teja, K., Schnatterly, P., and Shaw, A.: Multiple intestinal atresias: pathology and pathogenesis, J. Pediatr. Surg. **16:**194-199, 1981.

Zerella, J.T., and Martin, L.W.: Jejunal atresia with absent mesentery and a helical ileum, Surgery **80:**550-553, 1976.

Congenital colonic atresia or stenosis

Less than 10% of intestinal atresias or stenoses are in the colon. Colonic atresia may be associated with a similar defect in the small bowel. Of reported colon atresias, 10% to 20% coexist with other gastrointestinal anomalies. Major abdominal wall defects and malformation of the genitourinary system are also described as associated congenital anomalies. Cases of colonic stenosis are equally divided between those affecting the colon proximal to and distal from the splenic flexure. For some authors, rectal atresia, traditionally described as a form of congenital anorectal anomaly, belongs to colonic atresia and stenosis, since it is not believed to be of embryologic origin.

As in other forms of atresia and stenosis of the intestine, colonic involvement is believed to represent the result of vascular injury or accident to the fetal intestine rather than an embryonic malformation. Interference with the mesenteric blood supply or thromboembolic episodes are postulated causes. These mechanisms may be at play either prenatally or early in the neonatal period. Gross and microscopic findings from relatively short or long colonic segments are those of inflammatory, necrotic, and fibrotic changes. They are the result of necrotizing enterocolitis (Fig. 3-21).

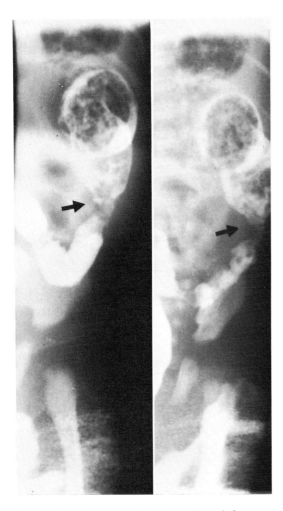

Fig. 3-21. Colonic stenosis. The newborn infant was admitted with abdominal distention, obstipation, and vomiting. Barium enema was compatible with Hirschsprung's disease. However, ganglion cells were present on a rectal suction biopsy. At operation, there was a 2 cm long segment of stenotic distal colon, *arrow*. Histologic examination of the resected segment showed extensive inflammatory changes compatible with the cicatricial stage of a vascular or infectious insult.

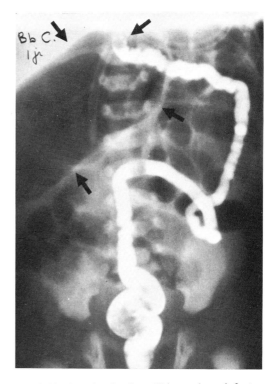

Fig. 3-22. Atresia of colon. This newborn infant was admitted with signs of intestinal obstruction. Enema shows an abrupt arrest of the barium column in a microcolon. Surgical findings were those of an atretic 2 cm segment of midtransverse colon. Arrows outline dilated proximal colon.

Clinical findings

Failure to pass meconium, obstipation, abdominal distention, and vomiting are signs of atresia during the neonatal period. In cases of colonic stenosis, failure to thrive and diarrhea may predominate. Abdominal radiographs will show absence of air in the affected part of the colon; however, a barium enema is necessary because air-filled small bowel and colonic loops are indistinguishable (Fig. 3-22).

Treatment

A colostomy should be done, and eventually the affected segment of colon must be resected.

REFERENCES

Boles, E.T., Vassy, L.E., and Ralston, M.: Atresia of the colon, J. Pediatr. Surg. **11**:69-74, 1976.

Erskine, J.M.: Colonic stenosis in the newborn: the possible thromboembolic etiology of intestinal stenosis and atresia, J. Pediatr. Surg. **5**:321-333, 1970.

Heydenjek, J.J., and Van Der Riet, R.G.S.: Atresia of the colon: a review of the literature with a report of two cases, S. Afr. Med. J. **47**:1965-1966, 1973.

Hirschsprung's disease

A more complete description of Hirschsprung's disease appears in Chapter 14. Aganglionic megacolon accounts for 20% to 25% of cases of neonatal intestinal obstruction. It occurs in 1 in 5000 live births. This section is limited to the discussion of the findings (Table 3-2) that may help the physician make the diagnosis in the newborn, keeping in mind that Hirschsprung's disease is uncommon (less than 3%) in low birth weight newborns and that it is frequently (up to 25%) associated with trisomy 21. Features of trisomy 21 should be looked for.

Table 3-2. Clinical findings in the neonate with Hirschsprung's disease

Delay in the passage of meconium	95%
Evidence of a lower intestinal obstruction, complete or partial (abdominal distention, bilious vomiting, respiratory distress)	50%
Obstipation with abdominal distention; failure to thrive, followed by vomiting or diarrhea, or both	25%
Intestinal perforation (appendiceal and cecal) with peritonitis	4%

Based on data from Swenson, O., Sherman, J.O., and Fisher, J.H.: J. Pediatr. Surg. **8**:587-594, 1973.

Mode of presentation

Most cases of Hirschsprung's disease have symptoms within the first week of life, but they are not always recognized. Only 5% of neonates with the disease are known to pass meconium within the first 24 hours. Abdominal distention, respiratory distress, and bilious vomiting are regular features in most cases. Severe intractable diarrhea with toxemia, dehydration, and shock is also likely to occur as a dreaded complication of this disease (enterocolitis).

Less often, at birth or within a few days, there are signs of complete intestinal obstruction with absent bowel sounds and peritonitis. Three-way abdominal roentgenograms show the presence of free air, and surgical exploration permits identification of a cecal, appendiceal, or colonic perforation. The clinical picture is therefore that of a distal obstruction that may mimic perfectly ileal atresia. More commonly, though, the symptoms are not as pronounced as they are in this latter entity.

In other cases, the disease may present as a meconium plug syndrome. Symptoms disappear after the passage of flatus and meconium, often brought about by an enema, a rectal thermometer, or an examining finger. Invariably, however, and in contrast to uncomplicated meconium plug syndrome, the symptoms recur within a few days. The physician contacted over the phone regarding the infant's obstipation may be tempted to change the formula or prescribe stool softeners or enemas. Meanwhile, abdominal distention may set in, followed by vomiting or Hirschsprung's enterocolitis.

Diagnostic approach

All full-term infants who fail to pass meconium spontaneously or pass it sparingly should be watched closely. Hirschsprung's disease should be ruled out in all cases of low intestinal obstruction, in all cases of meconium plug syndrome not followed by the regular daily passage of stools, and in all cases of unexplained cecal, appendiceal, or colonic perforation.

The x-ray diagnosis rests on the demonstration of a persistent, irregularly margined, narrow segment starting just above the rectal ampulla (which may be of normal diameter). It may extend only a few centimeters, or it may run the length of the entire colon and part of the small bowel. Above the narrowed segment, the colon is dilated to varying degrees and may fill the entire abdomen. Usually, microscopic examination indicates that the zone of aganglionosis extends several centimeters up into the dilated portion. During the first few days of the infant's life, it is often difficult to demonstrate the narrow spastic segment. Failure of satisfactory evacuation of the barium should lead the physican to take simple abdominal roentgenograms on subsequent days. Aganglionosis of the entire colon may result in a slightly reduced diameter and frequently in a shortened total length producing the so-called question-mark deformity. The appearance of ''jejunalization'' of the colon may be suggestive of total aganglionsis. A significant number of newborn infants with the meconium plug syndrome later show a classic aganglionic megacolon, and, with this fact in mind, it is good practice to do a recheck barium enema on all such patients with bowel difficulties.

The pathologic proof of the diagnosis of Hirschsprung's disease can be obtained with a rectal biopsy. If the clinical picture is suggestive, suction mucosal biopsies should be obtained. The presence of ganglion cells and the absence of increased nerve fibers documented by acetylcholinesterase staining in specimens taken 2.5 to 3 cm proximal to the anal margin for all practical purposes excludes the diagnosis. We have totally dispensed from doing full-thickness rectal biopsies. Rectal manometry may show the characteristic failure of relaxation of the internal sphincter but should not be substituted for the histologic diagnosis because the test is unreliable during the first few days after birth.

Anorectal anomalies
Embryology

Anorectal anomalies probably occur once in every 3000 to 5000 live births and are somewhat more common in males. The embryologic events that lead to the development of the lower rectum, urogenital tract, and anus take place between the fourth embryonic week and the sixth month. The urorectal septum divides the cloaca into a ventral part, or the urogenital sinus (bladder and urethra), and a dorsal portion, or the hindgut (rectum). However, this septum divides the cloaca only as far down as the pubococcygeal line. Before completion of the separation of the gut from the urinary tract through lateral ingrowths of mesoderm, the hindgut, destined to become the upper part of the anal canal, moves caudally and posteriorly. It will eventually join the lower part of the anal canal.

The cloacal membrane disappears as the urorectal septum progresses downward, a development that both the urogenital sinus and the hindgut to open separately. The anal membrane, which is the posterior part of the cloacal membrane, disappears a short time after the anterior part of the cloacal membrane (the urogenital membrane). Anal tubercles converge and encircle the termination of the hindgut. The central depression thus created is called the ''proctodeum'' and forms the lower portion of the anal canal. The anal opening is thus dependent on the anal tubercles rather than on the anal membrane, which has already disappeared by that time. Although rudimentary or functionally absent in many cases, the external sphincter develops in its normal position independently, even in cases of extensive anomalies of the anal tubercles.

X-ray findings

A lateral view taken with the infant held in upside-down position for 3 to 5 minutes, his legs at right angles to the trunk and a radiopaque marker fixed to the usual location of the anus, will demonstrate the position of the end of the bowel (Fig. 3-23). It may also show air in the bladder fistulas and the presence of sacral or lower vertebral anomalies. The interpretation of the roentgenogram should take into account the fact that sometimes 24 hours must elapse before air progresses to the most distal part of the bowel. Air may be significantly decreased if a fistula is present. Finally, a distal accumulation of meconium may prevent a true outline of the distal intestinal pouch. The roentgenogram of the distal end of the bowel may be outlined either by the nasogastric instillation of 15 ml of diatrizoate methylglucamine (Gastrografin) or by the direct injection of contrast medium into the blind pouch. The addition of an organic dye such as indigo carmine may give visual evidence of an otherwise unsuspected rectourinary fistula.

Air seen below an imaginary line traced between the lower part of the pubic bone and the inferior margin of the lower sacral segment (pubococcygeal line) suggests a low-positional anomaly (anal agenesis) that can be surgically approached through the perineum. However, high lesions can also exist with gas shadows distal to the line. Air above the pubococcygeal line signals a high-positional anomaly (rectal agenesis). Since a large percentage of the high anomalies are associated with genitourinary fistulas connected to

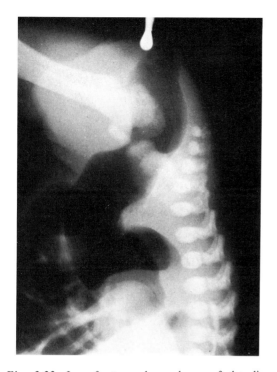

Fig. 3-23. Imperforate anal membrane of the diaphragm type demonstrated with the patient in an upside-down position. Air has reached the skin. When air does not reach the skin, the film taken with the patient in this position should be interpreted with caution, since the atresia may be as high as the film would suggest or it may be much lower, with impacted meconium filling the gap.

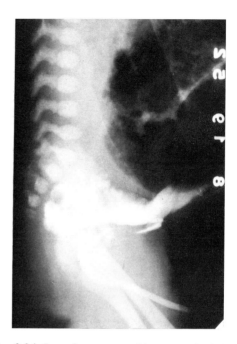

Fig. 3-24. Imperforate anus with rectourethral fistula. The anterior tract of medium is the urethra leading to the bladder. The posterior one is the fistula through which most of the medium has gone to fill the blind rectal pouch and mix with the stool.

the rectal segment, a retrograde urethrogram in the male and a urethrogram and vaginogram in the female are required to demonstrate the fistula (Fig. 3-24). These studies can also establish the level of the blind pouch. Calcium visible on the scout films in the rectal area is a strong indication that a rectourethral fistula is present, since meconium appears to calcify more readily when it is in contact with urine. Intravenous pyelography should always be carried out in children with anorectal anomalies.

Clinical findings

Inspection of the perianal area at the time of birth is essential. Fig. 3-25 illustrates the various types of anorectal anomalies and Fig. 3-26 the fistulas associated with them.

Anal stenosis. Anal stenosis is manifested by a very small anal aperture filled with a dot of meconium. Defecation is difficult, and there may be ribbonlike stools. The abdomen can be distended; fecal impaction and secondary megacolon may supervene. Onset of symptoms varies with the severity of the stenosis. The diagnosis cannot be made on the basis of a history of straining at defecation. It has to be objectively documented by the presence of a tight and small anal aperture. This malformation accounts for perhaps 10% of cases of anorectal anomalies. It can be treated with digital dilatations, which may need to be continued for a few months. If the anorectal stenosis is extensive, it may be necessary to excise the fibrous tissue and mobilize the rectum so that it can be brought down and sutured to the lower part of the anal canal or the perineal skin. The good prognosis is related to the fact that the rest of the anorectal region is normal.

Imperforate anal membrane. Imperforate anal membrane, or covered anus, becomes evident during the neonatal period when the infant fails to pass meconium. A greenish, bulging membrane is seen. Through this membrane there may be a small fistulous tract running forward to the midline of the scrotum, and this should be looked for. Exci-

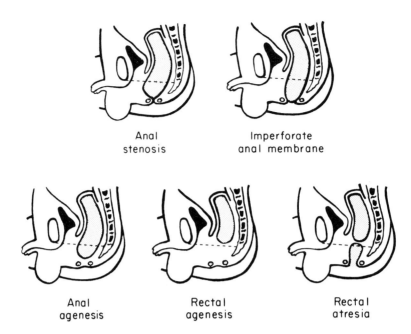

Anal   Imperforate
stenosis   anal membrane

Anal   Rectal   Rectal
agenesis   agenesis   atresia

Fig. 3-25. Types of anorectal anomalies. The fistulas have not been drawn in. *Stippled line,* Projection of the puborectalis sling. This imaginary line on a roentgenogram, joining the lower part of the pubic bone and the sacrococcygeal junction, is usually a valuable method of dividing anorectal anomalies into "low" and "high" anomalies. *Anal stenosis* is difficult to diagnose since the only finding is a tight anal canal. *Imperforate anal membrane* is reportedly a rare anomaly easily diagnosed and treated. *Anal agenesis* is by far the most common anomaly. Note that the rectum ends blindly below the pubococcygeal line. The location of associated fistulas, when present, helps to establish the diagnosis of this "low" anomaly. *Rectal agenesis* is a "high" anomaly that is most commonly associated with a fistula in both males and females. *Rectal atresia,* a rare anomaly, is difficult to diagnose because of the normal-appearing anus. There are no associated fistulas.

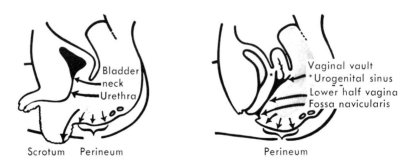

Bladder
neck
Urethra

Vaginal vault
Urogenital sinus
Lower half vagina
Fossa navicularis

Scrotum   Perineum   Perineum

Fig. 3-26. Fistulas associated with anorectal anomalies. In the male, the anoperineal fistulas may be located anywhere on the perineum anterior to the anal dimple. Anobulbar and anourethral fistulas are rare and, when present, are seen in " low" anomalies. The frequently encountered rectourethral fistula and the rare rectovesical one are seen in "high" anomalies. In the female, anoperineal fistulas may open up in the perineum or in the fourchette. Rectovestibular fistulas can be associated with either a "high" or a "low" anomaly. Rectovaginal or rectocloacal fistulas are always associated with "high" anomalies. (Modified from Bill, A.H.: The colon and rectum. In Cooke, R.E., editor: The biologic basis of pediatric practice, New York, 1968, McGraw-Hill Book Co.)

sion of this thin skin lid usually leads to normal bowel and sphincter function. Occasionally, the anus may remain patulous and leak small amounts of mucus. Differentiation of this entity from cases of anal agenesis with an anal cutaneous fistula or without a fistula must be made.

Anal agenesis. Anal agenesis results from the defective development of the anus. Consequently, the bowel extends below the pubococcygeal line. The anal dimple is always present. When the baby strains, the area bulges forward. Puckering can be seen when the external sphincter contracts in response to stimulation of the area. Intestinal obstruction may be the mode of presentation if there is no associated fistula. The fistulas, when present, may be perineal or vulvar in the female and perineal or urethral in the male. A cutaneous collection of meconium in thickened perineal skin is an important physical finding.

Rectal agenesis. Rectal agenesis and anal agenesis together account for more than 75% of anorectal anomalies. Rectal agenesis is the more difficult to treat because fistulas are usually present. Since the rectal pouch lies at or above the pubococcygeal line, rectal agenesis is an anomaly situated high in contrast to anal agenesis, an anomaly situated low. The anal dimple, which is evident in anal agenesis cannot be identified in the high anomalies, and the fistulas are never visible on inspection of the perineum.

Fistulas in the female may be vestibular, high or low in the vagina, or cloacal. In this last variety, the fistula enters a urogenital sinus (Fig. 3-26), which is a common passageway for the urethra and vagina. In the male, fistulas are rectourethral or rectovesical. All patients with high anomalies should be treated with a colostomy during the neonatal period. An abdominoperineal procedure should be carried out when the infant weighs between 20 and 25 pounds.

Rectal atresia. Rectal atresia is still classified as a high anorectal anomaly without fistula. There are indications that at least the incomplete type does not have an embryonic origin but may be secondary to enterocolitis or a vascular insult. In the complete type, intestinal obstruction is present in a newborn infant with a normal anus. The blind low segment or severe stricture lies just above the level of the levator ani muscle.

Family history and associated anomalies

Although anorectal anomalies are among the more common congenital defects, a familial incidence is rarely mentioned. There are fewer than 20 families with two or more members affected. A mother-daughter and father-son occurrence has been reported. A new autosomal dominant syndrome consisting of imperforate anus, triphalangeal thumbs, other bony anomalies of the hands and feet, and sensory nerve deafness has been recognized in a few families.

At least 50% of the patients have concomitant congenital malformations (Table 3-3). They tend to be more frequent in cases where the rectal pouch lies above the puborectalis sling and adversely affect the prognosis (Table 3-4). Only a small percentage of the mortality can be ascribed to the imperforate anus itself and its local complications. The most common associated congenital malformations involve the genitourinary tract, the skeletal, central nervous, and cardiovascular systems, and the gastrointestinal tract. Esophageal atresia is certainly the most frequent associated anomaly involving the gastrointestinal tract; other anomalies include small and large bowel atresias, annular pancreas, malrotation, and duplication. Of significance in terms of risk and ultimate prognosis is the fact that 25% of cases are found in low birth weight infants.

Management

On being confronted with a newborn who has no obvious anal opening, one needs to pass a

Table 3-3. Congenital malformations in 230 cases of imperforate anus at Hôpital Sainte-Justine, 1957 to 1975

Vertebral malformations	177
Genito-urinary malformations	33
Esophageal atresia	22
Extremities	11
Myelomeningocele	9
Congenital heart disease	8
Trisomy 21	7
Cloacal exstrophy	6
Intestinal malrotation	5
Omphalocele	4
Bronchial cyst	2
Duodenal atresia	2
Meckel's diverticulum	2
Pulmonary agenesis	1
Cleft palate	1

Courtesy B. Dandurand, J. Boisvert, and P.P. Collin, Montreal.

Table 3-4. Congenital malformations and
mortality in 230 cases of imperforate anus at
Hôpital Sainte-Justine, 1957 to 1975

	Number	Congenital malformations (%)	Mortality (%)
Low anomalies (translevator)	162	48	16
High anomalies (supralevator)	68	86	41

Courtesy B. Dandurand, J. Boisvert, and P.P. Collin, Montreal.

catheter in the stomach to rule out an associated
esophageal atresia with or without a fistula because this associated anomaly is present in 5% of
cases. A flat film of the abdomen will eliminate
duodenal atresia. A urinalysis should be performed, and the sediment examined for the presence of meconium cells, which would point to a
rectourinary fistula.

Close inspection of the perineum may give clues
as to the level of the anomaly. A dimpled area
indicates a low-lying rectal pouch. The dimple
usually lies anterior to the normal position of the
anus; it is present in 50% of cases and usually is
associated with a tiny opening, which on probing
may yield some meconium. This opening may
sometimes be found along the raphe of the scrotum or in the vulva.

If no orifice is visible, roentgenologic studies
should be done to help determine the level of the
rectal pouch. When roentgenograms reveal a low
pouch, a primary anoplasty is attempted. Should
no bowel be evident, a colostomy is carried out.
In cases where the films suggest a pouch lying
more than 2 cm from the skin, a colostomy is
done and subsequently an investigation is carried
out to rule out a fistula. An intravenous pyelogram, a voiding cystourethrogram, and opacification of the colon distal to the colostomy are indicated.

Definitive surgical procedures are carried out
between 6 to 10 months of age. In boys with low-
lying anomalies in whom the level of air is within
1.5 cm of the anal dimple and without evidence
of a rectobulbar fistula, a perineal anoproctoplasty
is carried out. Male infants with a pouch lying
above the puborectalis sling undergo abdominoperineal repair and closure of the associated rectourethral or rectovesical fistula (Fig. 3-26). In fe-

male infants, fistulas are almost invariably present
in both low- and high-lying anomalies; therefore
vaginoscopy, cystoscopy, intravenous pyelogram,
voiding cystourethrogram, and contrast study of
the colon distal to the colostomy should be carried
out. However an anoplasty can correct the low-
lying fistulas. A pull-through procedure is required for the high-lying anomalies with their associated rectovaginal and rectocloacal fistulas (Fig.
3-26).

Prognosis

Birth weight and associated anomalies are more
important factors influencing prognosis than are
the type of anorectal anomaly and the presence or
absence of a fistula–though the overall mortality
may be around 20%, it can be as high as 55% in
the small premature infants and in newborn infants with associated anomalies. On the other hand,
it is as low as 4% in infants weighing more than
4 pounds and having few or no associated congenital defects.

The functional results in terms of control of
feces, flatus, and urine are far better in the low-
lying anomalies than in those in which the distal
end of the bowel stays above the pubococcygeal
line, since these latter anomalies frequently have
associated fistulas and sacral and nerve deficits and
require complex surgical procedures.

Fecal incontinence

It is essential to tell parents that toilet training
is likely to be delayed. Urinary control will approximate the normal timing unless a neurogenic
bladder is present. However bowel control is a
problem. Table 3-5 shows that good results (occasional soiling) were obtained in roughly 90% of
children with low anomalies and in only a little
more than 50% of those with high anomalies (rectal agenesis and rectal atresia).

Most patients have a decreased awareness of
rectal fullness and have a very short warning period. This sensory defect tends to improve with
age, and most children will show a gradual improvement with the development of continence.
Those without appreciation of sensation to impending defecation usually have significant defects in the puborectalis sling of the levator ani
muscle. On the other hand, good continence is
possible in children who have grossly defective
internal and external sphincters, but with a functioning puborectalis sling. Studies show that in
the high-lying anomalies (rectal agenesis) both

Table 3-5. Continence achieved by 191 patients

	Good	Fair	Poor
Anal stenosis	14	1	0
Imperforate anal membrane	17	0	0
Anal agenesis	68	5	4
Rectal agenesis	40	20	18
Rectal atresia	2	1	1

From Kieswetter, W.B.: In Ravitch, M.M., and others: Pediatric surgery, ed. 3, Chicago, 1979, Year Book Medical Publishers.

sphincters are rudimentary and therefore functionally absent; furthermore, the levator ani musculature is abnormal. In the low-lying anomalies (anal agenesis and imperforate anal membrane), the internal sphincter is absent and the external sphincter is rudimentary. The levator ani, however, is normal in most of these cases.

The approach to the child who is incontinent after treatment for a high-lying anomaly is centered around making sure that there is a functional puborectalis sling and that the rectum has been brought down through it. A rectal examination and a manometric study should be done. Reoperation may be necessary after this assessment. In cases where the puborectalis sling is not functional, bilateral gracilis transplants can be carried out at around 6 years of age. The decision to do a permanent colostomy should not be made until after puberty. Motivation to achieve continence increases with age, and biofeedback training may be a very useful adjunct (see Chapter 14).

REFERENCES

Kieswetter, W.B., Bill, A.H., Nixon, H.H., and Santulli, T.V.: Imperforate anus, Arch. Surg. **111:**518-525, 1976.

Kiesewetter, W.B., and Chang, J.H.T.: Imperforate anus: a 5 to 30 year follow-up perspective, Prog. Pediatr. Surg. **10:**81-88, 1977.

Manny, J., Schiller, M., Horner, R., and others: Congenital familial anorectal anomaly, Am. J. Surg. **125:**639-640, 1973.

McGill, C.W., Polk, H.C., and Canty, T.G.: The clinical basis for a simplified classification of anorectal agenesis, Surg. Gynecol. Obstet. **146:**177-181, 1978.

Santulli, T.V., Kiesewetter, W.B., and Bill, A.H., Jr.: Anorectal anomalies: a suggested international classification, J. Pediatr. Surg. **5:**281-287, 1970.

Taylor, I., Duthie, H.L., and Zachary, R.B.: Anal continence following surgery for imperforate anus, J. Pediatr. Surg. **8:**497-503, 1973.

Townes, P.L., and Brocks, E.R.: Hereditary syndrome of imperforate anus with hand, foot and ear anomalies, J. Pediatr. **81:**321-326, 1972.

Wilkinson, A.W.: Congenital anomalies of the anus and rectum, Arch. Dis. Child. **47:**960-969, 1972.

Table 3-6. Pathologic features of 39 duplications in 37 children at The Children's Hospital, Denver

Abnormality	Number
Mucosal pattern	
Gastric mucosa (with peptic ulceration in 8/12)	12
Intestinal mucosa	10
Cuboid or columnar epithelium	13
Unidentified	4
Neurenteric cysts	2
Communication with adjacent gastrointestinal structure	
Single lumen with biliary tree	1
Single lumen with small bowel	2
Double-barrel lumen	1

Based on data from Favara, B.E., Franciosi, R.A., and Akers, D.R.: Am. J. Dis. Child. **122:**501-506, 1971.

Duplications of gastrointestinal tract

Duplications of the gastrointestinal tract are congenital malformations most often discovered during infancy. They may occur anywhere along the tract as spherical or tubular structures of various sizes and shapes. Duplications are found in direct contact with the tract and lined by an intestinal epithelium supported by smooth muscle. They are invariably on the mesenteric side of the gut, commonly share a muscular coat and mesenteric blood supply, and communicate with the adjacent gastrointestinal structure (Table 3-6). The intestinal epithelium is either of the same type as that seen in the area of the gastrointestinal tract from which it originates, or else it is gastric mycosa, which may cause peptic ulceration, bleeding and perforation. Some duplications are attached to the spinal cord and are associated with the presence of hemivertebrae (Fig. 3-27, *A*). The embryologic implications of these neurenteric cysts remain

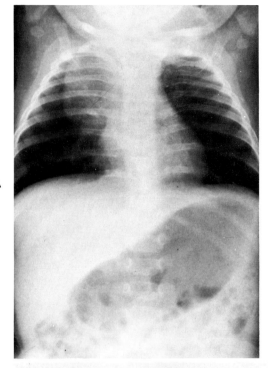

A

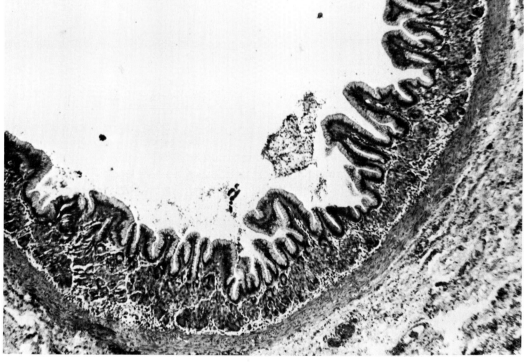

B

Fig. 3-27. Thoracic neurenteric cyst. **A,** Tomogram showing a right superior mediastinal mass associated with extensive broadening of the spinal canal and vertebral anomalies extending from C7 to T4. This 4-month-old infant, after a traumatic skull fracture, developed respiratory distress, which led to the identification of the mediastinal mass and of the vertebral anomalies. **B,** The large spherical structure in **A** was distended with opalescent fluid, and it was attached to both the esophagus and the spinal cord. The cross section showed a normal gastric mucosa, muscularis mucosae, submucosa, and muscular layers.

Table 3-7. Distribution of and malformations associated with 37 cases of duplications at The Children's Hospital, Denver, 1942 to 1970

Feature	Number
Topographic distribution	
Tongue	1
Esophagus	6
Stomach	3
Duodenum	4
Jejunum	6
Ileum	14
Cecum	2
Ascending colon	1
Rectosigmoid	1
Biliary tree	1
Associated malformations (14 of 37 cases)	
Cardiovascular	4
Tracheoesophageal fistula	2
Vertebral anomalies	4
Omphalocele	1
Malrotation	1
Short small bowel	2
Small-bowel atresia or stenosis	6
Imperforate anus	1

Courtesy B.E. Favara, R.A. Franciosi, and D.R. Akers.

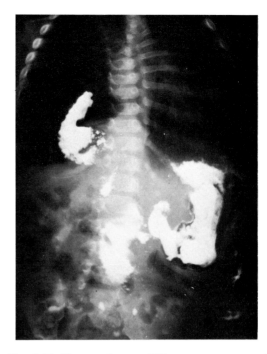

Fig. 3-28. Neurenteric cyst. This cyst was connected with the duodenum through the diaphragm and is shown filled with medium. Note the vertebral body malformations, which are associated with neurenteric cysts but not with other types of duplications.

controversial. The notochord arises from the ectoderm and grows into the entodermal layer. The notochordal plate is eventually extruded from the entoderm into the mesoderm. If, during the process of extrusion of the notochordal plate, there is incomplete separation from the entoderm, the primitive gut may be drawn up into a diverticulum. Since vertebral development is dependent on the notochord, an abnormal attachment of the notochord to the gut will interfere with the growth of vertebrae.

A number of pathogenic schemes have been described to explain duplications of the gastrointestinal tract. Aberrant recanalization of the gut, persistence of fetal enteric diverticula, notochordal maldevelopment, and, more recently, a vascular occlusive event have all had proponents. According to the vascular theory, intrauterine ischemic infarction occurs and may lead to intestinal atresia, stenosis, or short bowel. It may also give rise to an enteric duplication in the event that a fragment of intestine is spared necrosis, is nourished by adjacent vasculature, and develops on its own. The fact that duplications are occasionally associated with atresia, stenosis, and short bowel (Table 3-7) would seem to support this explanation.

Spherical duplications are much more common than the tubular ones. Most duplications are noncommunicating, but when there is a lumen between the adjacent bowel and the duplication, enteric contents are present. Duplications usually contain fluid and sometimes blood if necrosis has taken place or if heterotopic gastric mucosa is identified (Fig. 3-27, *B*).

Abdominal duplications are much more frequent than the thoracic ones, which are usually attached to the esophagus. Some thoracic duplications may originate from an abdominal structure such as the stomach, duodenum, or small bowel, and they are known as thoracoabdominal duplications (Fig. 3-28). Most abdominal duplications are attached to the ileum. Gastric, pyloric, duodenal, jejunal, gallbladder, and biliary tract duplications are much less common (Fig. 3-29). Duplications of the colon and rectum account for close to 10% of the total. In rare cases, the tubular or cystic type is seen in the ascending or transverse colon. The commonest type involves the rectum

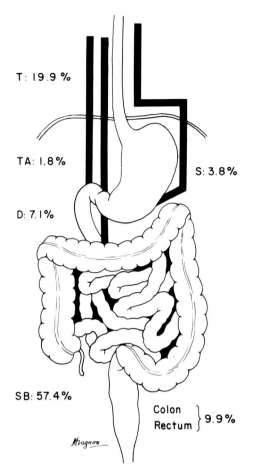

Fig. 3-29. Topographic distribution of duplications based on a composite analysis of 800 reported cases. *T,* Thoracic; *TA,* thoracoabdominal (black lines running through diaphragm); *S,* stomach; *D,* duodenum; *SB,* small bowel. (Modified from Daudet, M., Chappuis, J.-P., and Daudet, N.: Ann. Chir. Infant. *8:*5-17, 1967.)

Table 3-8. Symptomatology of 37 cases of duplication at The Children's Hospital, Denver

Symptom	Number of patients
Intestinal obstruction	10
Abdominal pain	8
Abdominal mass	7
Gastrointestinal bleeding	5
Intussusception	3
Respiratory distress	3
Incidental finding at laparotomy	1

Courtesy B.E. Favara, R.A. Franciosi, and D.R. Akers.

In typical cases, the physical examination indicates a rounded, smooth, freely movable mass. Roentgenograms of the abdomen may demonstrate a noncalcified mass displacing the intestine or compressing the stomach. With involvement of the end of the small bowel, a duplication can trigger an intussusception. Those lesions that are long, tubular duplications of the bowel, especially colonic lesions, often become infected and dilated. They may then obstruct the adjoining colon. When a connection exists, it is usually through a small proximal communication. Duplication cysts of the esophagus or thoracoabdominal duplications, which can become evident within the first few days of life, produce respiratory distress as a result of tracheal and pulmonary compression.

Diagnosis

The preoperative diagnosis can be difficult. Duplication is a likely diagnosis in a newborn infant who has signs of intestinal obstruction and an abdominal mass. However, in most cases it is not that simple, since hemorrhage, peritonitis, intussusception, partial intestinal obstruction, or a malabsorption syndrome (Fig. 3-31) may be the mode of presentation.

The roentgenographic findings seldom help the physician to make the diagnosis except in the rare cases in which opacification of the duplication is possible. Usually the roentgenographic evidence is presumptive; there are signs of obstruction or extrinsic compression (Fig. 3-32).

Treatment

Surgery is usually performed for partial intestinal obstruction, an abdominal mass, peritonitis through a perforation, intussusception, volvulus, or a severe intestinal hemorrhage. When there is

and causes constipation and sometimes obstruction. Because of its location behind the rectum, it may be confused with a presacral teratoma. There are a number of reports of complete duplication of the colon, anus, bladder, urethra, and external genitalia.

Clinical findings

Symptoms usually start in early infancy, though they may not develop for months or years, or the patient may even remain asymptomatic throughout life (Table 3-8). Distention, colicky pain, rectal bleeding, partial or total intestinal obstruction, or an abdominal mass may be the initial complaints (Fig. 3-30). Rare cases of pyloric duplications may mimic hypertrophic pyloric stenosis.

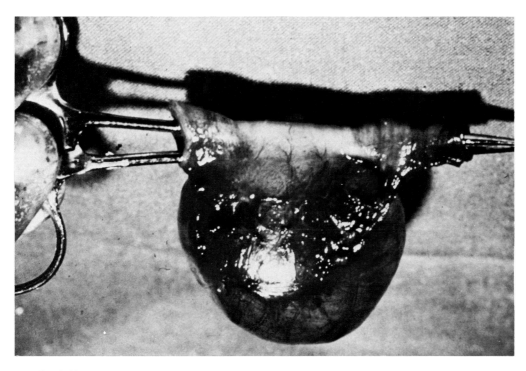

Fig. 3-30. Ileal duplication of noncommunicating type, removed from a 6-month-old infant who suddenly suffered abdominal distention, bilious vomiting, and a mass in the right lower quadrant.

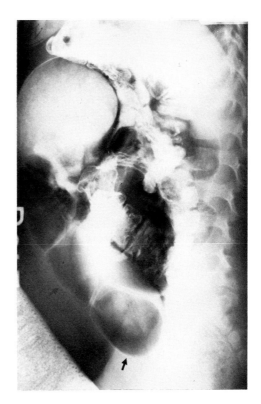

Fig. 3-31. Lateral view of a large communicating small bowel duplication, *arrow*, in a 2-year-old child who presented a clinical picture suggestive of celiac disease.

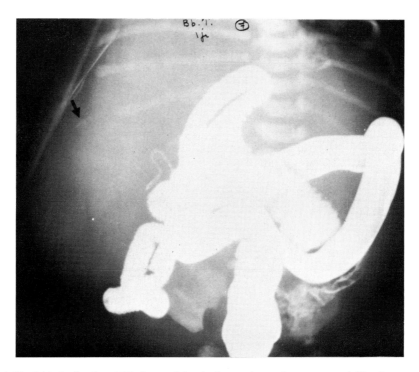

Fig. 3-32. Ileal duplication. This large abdominal mass has a few sparse calcifications, *arrow.*
The barium enema shows a well-opacified appendix high in the right flank and close to the
midline. Cyanosis and abdominal distention were noted at birth; these were rapidly followed by
bilious vomiting. At operation, a sausage-shaped duplication was found on the distal part of the
ileum, and there was partial malrotation.

complete duplication of the colon, resection of the
second colon is usually not possible and only the
second rectum is removed to relieve the obstruction. The associated genitourinary anomalies are
treated only if necessary.

REFERENCES

Beardmore, H.E., and Wigglesworth, F.W.: Vertebral anom-
    alies in alimentary duplications, Pediatr. Clin. North Am.
    2:457-474, 1958.
Daudet, M., Chappuis, J.-P., and Daudet, N.: Symposium sur
    les duplications intestinales, Ann. Chir. Infant. **8:**5-80, 1967.
Favara, B.E., Franciosi, R.A., and Akers, D.R.: Enteric du-
    plications: 37 cases, a vascular theory of pathogenesis, Am.
    J. Dis. Child. **122:**501-506, 1971.
Grosfeld, J.L., O'Neill, J.A., and Clatworthy, H.W.: Enteric
    duplications in infancy and childhood, Ann. Surg. **172:**83-
    90, 1970.
Kottra, J.J., and Dodds, W.J.: Duplication of the large bowel,
    Am. J. Roentgenol. Radium Ther. Nucl. Med. **113:**310-
    315, 1971.
Pruksapong, C., Donovan, R.J., Pinit, D., and Heldrich, F.J.:
    Gastric duplication, J. Pediatr. Surg. **14:**83-85, 1979.
Ravitch, M.M.: Duplications of the alimentary canal. In Rav-
    itch, M.M., Welch, K.J., Benson, C.D., Aberdeen, E., and
    Randolph, J.G., editors: Pediatric surgery, ed. 3, Chicago,
    1979, Year Book Medical Publishers.

Meconium ileus
General comments

Meconium ileus most frequently occurs as a
complication of cystic fibrosis. It may also occur
in patients without cystic fibrosis (10%). The inspissation of meconium associated with cystic fibrosis starts before birth, with several factors
probably contributing to this event. Abnormality
in viscosity of meconium has been reported. It may
result from several factors that can alter the physicochemical properties of the meconium, such as
macromolecules, which are derived primarily from
swallowed amniotic fluid and which escape digestion in the face of pancreatic achylia. Meconium
from most patients is typified by decreased to absent trypsin and chymotrypsin activity; it readily
precipitates with trichloroacetic acid because of its
high albumin content. In addition, the hyposecretion of water, electrolytes, and resulting thick mucus (Fig. 3-33) in patients with cystic fibrosis
probably contributes to the inspissation of meconium. This reduced fluid contribution from pancreas, biliary system, and intestine into the lumen

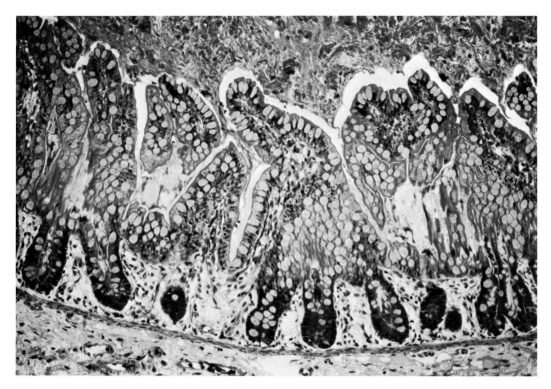

Fig. 3-33. Meconium ileus associated with cystic fibrosis. Microscopically, glands in the resected segment of ileum share some of the features characteristic of other exocrine glands. There are an abnormal number of goblet cells and a significant dilatation of the glands, with inspissation of secretions.

of the gut may be a simple yet important explanation for the physical properties of the meconium. The frequent roentgenographic findings (50%) of distention without air-fluid levels may also be explained by this hyposecretion theory. Further desiccation of the meconium probably occurs from intestinal reabsorption, since the mucus in these patients is hyperpermeable to water, and explains the pelletlike meconium plugs found in the distal ileum. More tenacious, puttylike meconium is found in the dilated proximal segment; it is sometimes mixed with air, which accounts for its bubbly roentgenographic appearance.

Evidence for antenatal intestinal obstruction is supported by the findings of hypertrophy of the muscular layers of the bowel, a high incidence (33%) of associated intra-abdominal complications, and a microcolon of disuse. The associated findings of volvulus, atresia, gangrene, meconium peritonitis, pseudocysts, and others are the result of a local ischemic phenomenon or twisting of the meconium-filled bowel loops occurring at various times during gestation. However, roughly two

thirds of cases are uncomplicated. The obstruction is maximal in the middle and distal parts of the ileum. The bowel wall is hypertrophied, dilated, congested, and packed with sticky meconium. Distal to the obstruction the ileum is smaller in caliber and pale and contains pellets of gray mucus as does the small unused microcolon.

Clinical features

The newborn infant with meconium ileus becomes symptomatic within the first 24 to 48 hours of life. Signs of intestinal obstruction develop with abdominal distention, poor eating, and bile-stained vomitus. Rectal passage of meconium is scant or absent. Besides distention, the flanks may be full, and peristalsis can be seen on the abdomen. A palpable mass of dilated, meconium-filled bowel loops or a pseudocyst may be felt. A history of hydramnios is not common (10%).

The symptom complex is likely to evolve before the first 24 hours of life have elapsed if an associated intra-abdominal complication exists, such as atresia, volvulus, or perforation. Abdominal

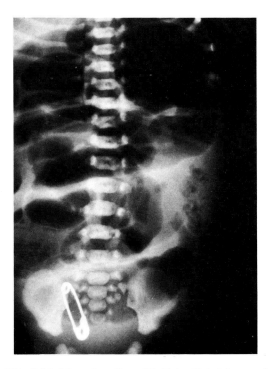

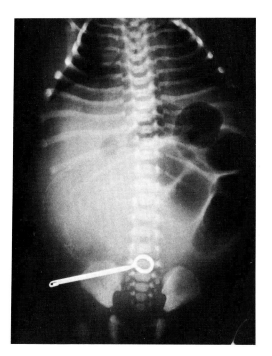

Fig. 3-34. Meconium ileus. Multiple dilated loops of small bowel and several areas of tiny air bubble formation point to a low mechanical intestinal obstruction, associated with meconium ileus. The small bubbles are seen only occasionally in atresia without meconium ileus.

Fig. 3-35. Atresia of the jejunum with intestinal perforation. The several dilated loops on the left side are diagnostic of a complete bowel obstruction somewhere in the middle portion of the small bowel. The opacity occupying the right abdomen is partly calcified and is diagnostic of a meconium peritonitis secondary to a perforation. The absence of free air is an indication that the perforation occurred before birth and that the inflammatory reaction sealed the communication between the intestinal tract and the peritoneal cavity.

distention with prominent venous circulation increases rapidly and causes respiratory difficulties. Vomiting is impressive. An antenatal perforation may be suspected if the abdomen is tympanitic or if ascites is present. Sudden deterioration, distention, and tympany are suggestive of postnatal perforation.

Diagnosis

Radiographic examination. Newborn infants with bile-stained vomitus need emergency radiographic examinations. The typical roentgenographic findings from three-way studies of the abdomen in patients with uncomplicated meconium ileus include uneven distention of bowel loops, paucity of air-fluid levels, and a bubbly granular density somewhere in the lower abdomen (Fig. 3-34). The finding of a microcolon of disuse on barium enema rules out volvulus resulting from malrotation and also the meconium plug syndrome. These roentgenographic findings, in conjunction with a family history of cystic fibrosis, give very strong evidence of meconium ileus. Remember,

however, that ileal atresia without cystic fibrosis may give rise to similar findings (Fig. 3-35). If a family history cannot be obtained, reliance solely on these findings for the diagnosis of uncomplicated meconium ileus is unwise.

Meconium ileus with complications may not always be indicated roentgenographically. Volvulus may be present and yet give a roentgenographic picture of uncomplicated meconium ileus. However, air-fluid levels are frequently seen if atresia coexists, whereas free peritoneal air is present in recent perforation. Calcifications (10% to 25%) may be luminal or extraluminal and always signify prenatal meconium peritonitis. A recent paper suggests that calcifications are more likely to occur in cases where the meconium ileus is not associated with cystic fibrosis. Firm testicular masses containing calcific densities evident on the roentgenogram are the result of prenatal meconium peritonitis and may occur with or without meconium ileus.

Sweat test. Since neonates produce little or no sweat, the test is unreliable during the first weeks of life. Three tests yielding chloride concentrations above 60 mEq/L performed at 4 to 6 weeks of age are diagnostic. All cases of meconium plug syndrome, volvulus, meconium peritonitis, and ileal atresia should be tested to rule out cystic fibrosis.

BM (Boehringer-Mannheim) test. This paper strip test has been extensively used for the screening of cystic fibrosis. It is positive when albumin is present at a concentration exceeding 20 mg/gm of meconium, which normally contains less than 3 mg/gm. However false-positive and false-negative results have been reported. It should not be relied on to establish the diagnosis of cystic fibrosis.

Treatment

Surgical intervention is mandatory in all complicated cases of meconium ileus as well as in those where calcifications are present. Resection of nonviable segments and a Roux-en-Y anastomosis with a distal ileostomy is the treatment of choice. It permits extraperitoneal closure of the ileostomy after a week of irrigations initiated during the surgical procedure. Irrigating solutions that have been shown to be effective and well tolerated are Tween 80 (1% in Tyrode's solution) or Mucomyst (acetylcysteine) at a concentration of 4%. The latter is also given by mouth postoperatively at a dose of 5 ml every 6 hours. It is recommended to administer a meglumine diatrizoate (methylglucamine diatrizoate, Gastrografin) enema on the third or fourth postoperative day to remove any remaining meconium and make sure that the distal part of the ileum is patent.

In cases of uncomplicated meconium ileus, conservative management can be attempted and is expected to be successful in 60% of cases. Diagnostic criteria of uncomplicated meconium ileus are hard to define in certain cases. So, in doubtful cases, surgery should be performed. Cases of uncomplicated meconium ileus are milder: the infant may pass some meconium before suffering distention; there is no evidence of volvulus, atresia, or peritonitis; and the baby does not look very ill. Successful medical management of such patients has followed the rectal administration of Gastrografin enemas, which are effective in causing the osmotic dislodgment of the meconium plugs.

Preparation of the patient before an enema is administered is extremely important to prevent untoward consequences. Meglumine diatrizoate (Gastrografin) has an osmolality of 1900 mOsm/L and can rapidly decrease the plasma volume and increase hematocrit and the osmolality of the serum. An osmotic diuresis may further deplete the plasma volume. Therefore, before use of this technique, preexisting dehydration must be treated and an increased intravenous fluid rate continued during and after the enema. Close monitoring of fluid balance (hematocrit, serum electrolytes and osmolality, intake and output, and so on) will prevent any deleterious effects of this procedure.

The following technique is used: full-strength Gastrografin is slowly allowed to flow retrograde under fluoroscopic control through a Foley catheter. The solution is allowed to run slowly into the distal ileum. A second enema is given 24 and 48 hours later, but this is rarely necessary. Oral feedings are offered within 48 hours if signs of obstruction have disappeared. *N*-Acetylcysteine (4%), 5 ml, is given every 6 hours by gastric tube for the first 5 days. Pancreatic extracts are added to the feedings.

Prognosis

Nonoperative management is associated with few or no deaths when cases are well screened before medical treatment is initiated and when they are monitored closely. In cases of simple meconium ileus, which is treated surgically, the mortality is low (less than 20%), but it goes up to 40% in babies with complicated meconium ileus. Since most cases of meconium ileus are caused by cystic fibrosis, the long-term prognosis will depend more on the severity of the pulmonary disease than on anything else. In the absence of cystic fibrosis, patients with meconium ileus have a good survival rate.

REFERENCES

Bowring, A.C., Jones, R.F.C., and Kern, I.B.: The use of solvents in the intestinal manifestations of mucoviscidosis, J. Pediatr. Surg. **5**:338-343, 1970.

Dolan, T.F., and Touloukian, R.J.: Familial meconium ileus not associated with cystic fibrosis, J. Pediatr. Surg. **9**:821-825, 1974.

Donnison, A.B., Shwachman, H., and Gross, R.E.: Review of 164 children with meconium ileus seen at Children's Hospital Medical Center, Boston, Pediatrics **37**:833-850, 1966.

Leonidas, J.C., Berdon, W.E., Baker, D.H., and Santulli, T.V.: Meconium ileus and its complications: a reappraisal of plain film roentgen diagnostic criteria, Am. J. Roentgenol. Radium Ther. Nucl. Med. **108**:598-609, 1970.

Noble, H.H.: Meconium ileus. In Ravitch, M.M., Welch, K.J., Benson, C.D., Aberdeen, E., and Randolph, J.G., editors: Pediatric surgery, ed. 3, Chicago, 1979, Year Book Medical Publishers.

Noblett, H.R.: Treatment of uncomplicated meconium ileus by Gastrografin enema: a preliminary report, J. Pediatr. Surg. **4:**190-197, 1969.

Poole, C.A., and Rowe, M.I.: Distal neonatal intestinal obstruction: the choice of contrast material, J. Pediatr. Surg. **11:**1011-1015, 1976.

Prosser, R., Owen, H., Bull, F., and others: Screening for cystic fibrosis by examination of meconium, Arch. Dis. Child. **49:**597-601, 1974.

Rowe, M.I., Furst, A.J., Altman, D.H., and Poole, C.A.: The neonatal response to Gastrografin enema, Pediatrics **48:**29-35, 1971.

Stephan, U., Busch, E.W., Kollberg, H., and Hellsing, K.: Cystic fibrosis detection by means of a test-strip. Pediatrics **55:**35-38, 1975.

PERFORATIONS OF THE GASTROINTESTINAL TRACT

Close to 60% of neonatal spontaneous gastrointestinal perforations involve the stomach or the duodenum (Table 3-9). Intestinal perforation has the same clinical mode of presentation whether the stomach, duodenum, jejunum, ileum, or colon is involved. Recent evidence convincingly indicates that the underlying lesions and etiologic factors are identical no matter where the perforation occurs.

Pathogenesis

At this time, the theory of gastric congenital muscular defects as cause appears largely dispelled in favor of ischemic necrosis, which, in turn, leads to acute gastric or intestinal ulcerations and perforations in the newborn infant. In a series of 126 patients with neonatal perforations of the gastrointestinal tract, 81% had suffered a definite asphyxial insult prenatally, at birth, or in the early postnatal period. In 67.2% of cases, maternal complications were noted. There was unequivocal evidence of asphyxia in the 61 of 68 infants who did not survive. Lesions were identified not only in the gastrointestinal tract beyond the punched-out areas of ulceration but also in the brain, adrenals, heart, kidney, and liver. The current hypothesis is that, in response to asphyxia, there is a selective circulatory ischemia in the gastrointestinal tract to protect the infant's brain and heart. The persistent intramural spasm of arterioles in the mesenteric circulation leads to acute ulcerations, bleeding, and perforations.

Ischemic necrosis may also explain the so-called stress ulcers, and it is known to be an important triggering factor in necrotizing enterocolitis of the newborn. Sepsis is a likely consequence of a generalized peritonitis complicating a perforation.

Clinical findings

In utero intestinal perforations are frequently associated with perinatal complications such as abruptio placentae.

A number of gastrointestinal anomalies and disease conditions are responsible for an intrauterine perforation and will give rise to meconium peritonitis.

Perforation of appendix
Intestinal atresia or stenosis
Malrotation with volvulus
Perforation of Meckel's diverticulum
Meconium ileus
Internal hernia
Idiopathic perforation of stomach and duodenum
Thrombosis of intestinal vascular supply
Intestinal duplication
Intussusception
Hirschsprung's disease

Table 3-9. Gastrointestinal perforations in the newborn from a survey of world literature up to 1969 and figures of The Children's Hospital of Michigan up to 1967

	Patients		Survivors	
	Number	**(% of total)**	**Number**	**(%)**
Gastric	251	(48.7)	62	(24.7)
Duodenal	50	(9.7)	19	(38)
Small intestine	59	(11.5)	18	(30.5)
Colon	125	(24.3)	29	(23.2)
Undetermined	30	(5.8)	19	(63.3)
Total	515*		147	(28.5)

*Exclusive of perforations occurring in the course of necrotizing enterocolitis. From Lloyd, J.R.: In Ravitch, M.M., and others: Pediatric surgery, ed. 3, Chicago, 1979, Year Book Medical Publishers.

Most of these conditions will require an operation after birth but in situations where the perforation has occurred more than a few days before delivery, sealing of the tear (Fig. 3-35) and sometimes short circuiting of the obstruction have occurred. Calcifications are said to indicate that the perforation antedates delivery by at least 10 days.

Most perforations occurring postnatally in the absence of a specific obstructive lesion are the result of the ischemic bowel syndrome discussed above. Lloyd reports that the average age of his 126 patients was 3.7 days (range 12 hours to 18 days). All neonates asphyxic at birth had evidence of perforation by the fifth day. Sick newborn infants and prematurely born infants are more prone to develop intestinal perforation. Usually, affected newborn infants appear normal at birth. Refusal of feeding is followed by vomiting that may contain blood. The abdomen becomes rapidly distended; dyspnea and cyanosis frequently ensue and are followed by a state of shock. A routine three-way roentgenogram of the abdomen will show free air under the diaphragm (Fig. 3-36).

The gastric air bubble is absent when the perforation is large, especially if it is gastroduodenal. Calcifications indicate that perforation occurred prenatally. A high incidence of colonic perforation has been reported in newborn infants who have had exchange transfusions. Rectosigmoid perforation is also known to occur after the injudicious use of thermometers, rectal tubes, or enemas, and in one series accounted for 13% of neonatal intestinal perforations.

Treatment

Fluid and electrolyte imbalance should be corrected while the abdomen is decompressed by nasogastric suction. Volume-replacement antibiotic therapy and prevention of hypothermia and of anoxia are essential measures. The perforation is repaired surgically only after critically ill infants have shown significant improvement.

Prognosis

The prognosis is usually very poor (Table 3-9). The interval between the onset of symptoms and

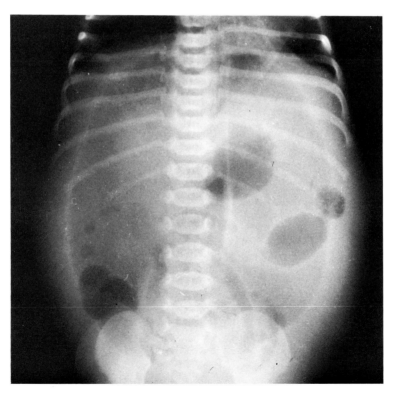

Fig. 3-36. Neonatal peritonitis. This film of a supine newborn infant suffering respiratory distress from abdominal distention shows air in the peritoneal cavity, giving rise to the classic football sign. The falciform ligament is outlined.

definitive treatment, the duration of hypoxia, and the degree of prematurity influence the outcome.

REFERENCES

Barlow, B., and Santulli, T.V.: Importance of multiple episodes of hypoxia or cold stress on the development of enterocolitis in an animal model, Surgery **77:**687-691, 1975.

Emmanuel, B., Zlotnik, P., and Raffensperger, J.G.: Perforation of the gastrointestinal tract in infancy and childhood, Surg. Gynecol. Obstet. **146:**926-928, 1978.

Fonkalsrud, E.W., and Clatworthy, H.W.: Accidental perforation of the colon and rectum in newborn infants, N. Engl. J. Med. **272:**1097-1100, 1965.

Hardy, J.D., Savage, T.R., Shirodaria, C., and others: Intestinal perforation following exchange transfusion, Am. J. Dis. Child. **124:**136-141, 1972.

Harrison, M.W., Connell, R.S., Campbell, J.R., and Webb, M.C.: Microcirculatory changes in the gastrointestinal tract of the hypoxic puppy: an electron microscope study, J. Pediatr. Surg. **10:**599-604, 1975.

Lloyd, J.R.: The etiology of G.I. perforation in the newborn, J. Pediatr. Surg. **4:**77-84, 1969.

Lloyd, J.R.: Gastrointestinal perforations of the newborn. In Ravitch, M.M., Welch, K.J., Benson, C.D., Aberdeen, E., and Randolph, J.G., editors: Pediatric surgery, ed. 3, Chicago, 1979, Year Book Medical Publishers.

Touloukian, R.J.: Gastric ischemia: the primary factor in neonatal perforation, Clin. Pediatr. **12:**219-223, 1973.

PERITONITIS

Perforation of the gastrointestinal tract leads to peritonitis. If the perforation has occurred before birth, the abnormal communication between the lumen of the bowel and the peritoneal cavity may already have closed, thus leading to a chemical peritonitis. Meconium peritonitis associated with prenatal intestinal perforation may present as meconium ascites. In these cases the abdomen is distended with meconium-stained ascitic fluid, as pseudocyst formation, or as areas of abdominal calcification between matted loops of distended bowel (Fig. 3-35). It usually leads to intestinal

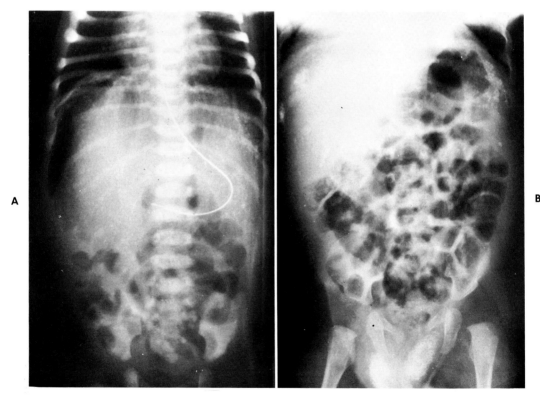

Fig. 3-37. Neonatal peritonitis secondary to necrotizing enterocolitis with colonic perforation. This 3-day-old infant suddenly developed abdominal distention and bilious vomiting. **A,** Film of the abdomen shows free air in the subphrenic space. In addition, there are numerous disseminated small foci of calcification. **B,** Two months later, note the striking scrotal calcifications. The meconium peritonitis was secondary to a perforation of the transverse colon.

obstruction. The list of conditions associated with meconium peritonitis appears on p. 84. When the prenatal gastrointestinal perforation does not seal itself, a secondary bacterial peritonitis will result. Most cases of postnatal peritonitis are bacterial.

Clinical findings

Failure to pass meconium, obstipation, abdominal distention, and vomiting are the common initial symptoms. A history of polyhydramnios is obtained in cases of high intestinal obstruction. Shock, cyanosis, dyspnea, and grunting respirations inevitably follow. Newborn infants with peritonitis rarely are hyperthermic. In many critically ill infants sclerema neonatorum is present.

Diagnosis

Roentgenograms may show a pneumoperitoneum, which can give rise to the so-called football sign (Fig. 3-36). Abdominal or scrotal calcifications (Fig. 3-37) without free air are diagnostic of a sealed-off meconium peritonitis.

Most cases of bacterial peritonitis are the result of a postnatal perforation secondary to an obstructive anomaly, to an ischemic lesion, or to necrotizing enterocolitis (Fig. 3-37). Less commonly it is the result of either meconium peritonitis, traumatic perforation of the rectum, or sepsis.

Management and prognosis

Neonatal peritonitis is the most lethal complication of congenital intestinal obstruction. Delay in diagnosis and prematurity are associated with a 90% mortality. Systemic antibiotics, nasogastric suction, adequate oxygenation, and the correction of shock, hypothermia, and electrolyte and acid-base disturbances are essential to the successful treatment of the underlying condition, which is generally surgical.

Rarely, neonatal peritonitis is not associated with an intestinal perforation and is primary. Umbilical sepsis is a common predisposing cause. Within the first 2 weeks of life, a periumbilical inflammation or a purulent discharge is noted. Abdominal distention, vomiting, and distended abdominal veins are followed by ileus. Abdominal roentgenograms show air fluid levels, and peritoneal aspiration helps establish the diagnosis. Nonoperative management is advocated if perforation can be confidently excluded.

REFERENCES

Duggan, M.B., and Khwaja, M.S.: Neonatal primary peritonitis in Nigeria, Arch. Dis. Child. **50:**130-132, 1975.

Fonkalsrud, E.W., Ellis, D.G., and Clatworthy, H.W.: Neonatal peritonitis, J. Pediatr. Surg. **1:**227-239, 1966.

Germain, M., Jezequel, C., and Contel, Y.: Les péritonites néonatales; á propos de 15 observations, Ann. Pediatr. (Paris) **15:**725-738, 1968.

Martin, L.: Meconium peritonitis. In Ravitch, M.M., Welch, K.J., Benson, C.D., Aberdeen, E., and Randolph, J.G., editors: Pediatric surgery, ed. 3, Chicago, 1979, Year Book Medical Publishers.

NECROTIZING ENTEROCOLITIS

Necrotizing enterocolitis (NEC) in the newborn infant is an acute fulminating disease associated with focal or diffuse ulceration and necrosis of the

Table 3-10. Surveys on the incidence of necrotizing enterocolitis

Intensive care units	Year	Number of cases per 1000 admissions	Number of cases per 1000 live births
USA and Canada (No 31)*	1975-1977	24	1.2‖
McMaster University† (University Hospital)	1973-1975	33	—
University of Alberta‡	1975-1977	19	2.0
(Royal Alexandra Hospital)	1978	—	3.6
University of Montreal§	1974-1977	10	—
(Ste-Justine)	1978	20	—

*Sweet, A.Y.: In Brown, E.G., and Sweet, A.Y., editors: Neonatal necrotizing enterocolitis, New York, 1980, Grune & Stratton, p. 11.
†Yu, V.Y.H., and Tudehope, D.I.: Med. J. Aust. **1:**688, 1977.
‡Moriartey, R.R., and others: J. Pediatr. **94:**295, 1979; Finer, N.N., and Moriarty, R.R.: J. Pediatr. **86:**170, 1980.
§Teasdale, F., and others, Can. Med. Assoc. J. **123:**387, 1980.
‖Figure based on an estimate that 5% of live births are admitted to intensive care units.

lower small bowel and of the colon. The ileum is the most common site of the disease. In close to three fourths of cases there are lesions in the colon, with the following distribution in decreasing order of frequency: ascending colon, cecum, transverse colon, and rectosigmoid. The stomach and upper small bowel are rarely affected.

Necrotizing enterocolitis is an epidemiologic enigma in that it only became a major clinical problem in the mid-1960s. In the past decade it has become a notorious major illness. Table 3-10 reports data on the current incidence in North America. The disease seems less frequent in Scandinavia and Holland where the lowest infant mortalities are recorded. There is no seasonal pattern and both sexes are equally affected. Isolated gastric, appendiceal, and colonic perforations could share the same pathogenesis, which is discussed on p. 84. Necrotizing enterocolitis complicating a lower bowel obstruction, such as Hirschsprung's

disease or meconium ileus, is described with these entities. There are now reports of necrotizing enterocolitis occurring after major surgery, as after open-heart surgery, correction of gastroschis, and imperforate anus. The interval between the operation and the diagnosis varied from 3 days to 4 months.

Pathogenesis

There is no single etiologic factor. It is probably multifactorial, but the cascade-like sequence of events that produces the disease is still hypothetical (Fig. 3-38).

Known and hypothetic pathogenic factors
(Fig. 3-38)

Risk factors. NEC is primarily seen in low birth weight newborns. On review of seven recently reported series accounting for more than 350 cases, it is apparent that more than 50% of cases occur

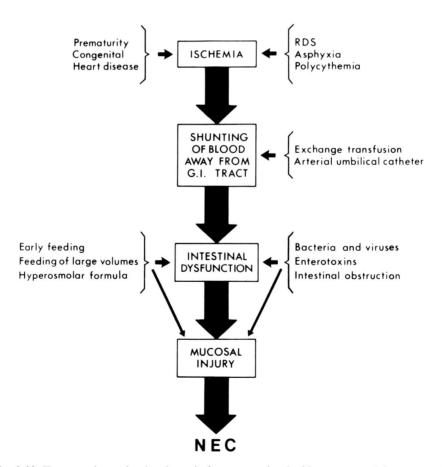

Fig. 3-38. Known and postulated pathogenic factors associated with acute necrotizing enterocolitis, *NEC.*

in babies weighing less than 1500 gm, 30% in those with a birth weight between 1500 and 2500 gm, and 20% in neonates weighing more than 2500 gm. Neonates whose weight is appropriate for gestational age are more vulnerable. Between 15% and 20% of cases are seen in babies who are small for gestational age.

Exchange transfusions, umbilical arterial catheters, perinatal asphyxia, respiratory distress syndrome, polycythemia, and congenital heart disease are well-known risk factors. However, a few studies have shown that birth weight, gestational age, Apgar scores, respiratory distress syndrome, and other perinatal risk factors do not differ from those of control groups.

Ischemia. The decrease in mesenteric flow as a concomitant of asphyxia in animals and the histologic findings of ulceration and necrosis (Fig. 3-39) have given strong support to a selective circulatory ischemia of the gut wall as an essential component of the disease. The decrease in perfusion observed with asphyxia is attributable to actual physiologic shunting of blood away from the gastrointestinal tract and toward more vital areas. This phenomenon is similar to the "diving reflex" seen in aquatic mammals. It could account not only for the postnatal development of acute NEC but also for congenital segmental stenoses and atresias of the gastrointestinal tract, the likely result of intrauterine asphyxia.

The role of both arterial and venous umbilical catheters in disruption of the hemodynamics of the splanchnic circulation is difficult to assess. The relationship of NEC with umbilical vein catheterization and exchange transfusion is irrefutable. The catheter residing in the portal vein increases portal vein pressure. The role of arterial catheters is less certain. It is nevertheless recommended to position them in the aorta, with the tip lying at a level below the origin of the renal arteries.

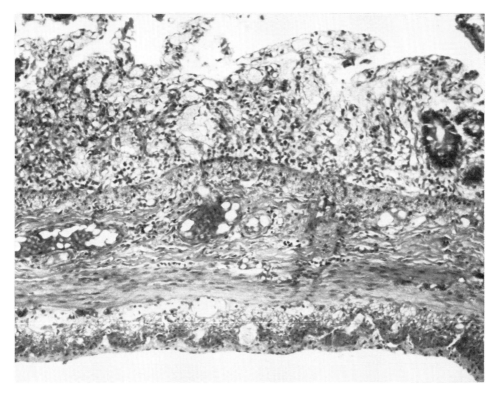

Fig. 3-39. Ileal segment removed from a neonate with necrotizing enterocolitis. Note the totally necrotic mucosa. The epithelium and the villi have been sloughed off. The lamina propria is infiltrated by inflammatory cells and collections of bacteria. Note on the right a relatively intact crypt.

Infection. There is abundant evidence that altered intestinal function and an injured mucosa through ischemia could not by themselves lead to NEC, and intestinal bacteria play an important role. A recent report from the Middle East attracts attention to NEC occurring in older children (45 days to 2 years) as a sequel to gastroenteritis. There is experimental evidence in rats that colonization of the ischemic bowel is essential. Clinical studies have long documented outbreaks of NEC. In some epidemics no microorganisms have been found, whereas in others, they have been associated with coxsackievirus B$_2$, *Klebsiella, Salmonella,* pathogenic *Escherichia coli,* and *Clostridium.* When clostridia are found, the disease tends to be more severe and even fulminant. Because of the frequency of *Clostridium difficile* in the feces of neonates, two studies of 42 patients with NEC involved a specific search for *Clostridium difficile,* and none were found. On the other hand, the toxin was found in 5 of 20 cases from one nursery. Other endotoxins may also be involved and could well explain the frequent occurrence of shock and of liver dysfunction.

The normal gramnegative flora of the bottle-fed neonate *(E. coli)* may play a secondary role by invading the gut wall, producing an infection that in turn leads to the typical accumulation of gas, which dissects the bowel wall (pneumatosis) and mesentery and may invade the portal vein. A sizable proportion (30%) of intramural gas is hydrogen (H$_2$), the product of bacterial metabolism. Decreased mucosal resistance through lack of mucosal immunity may be a compounding factor accounting for systemic invasion of the sick infant by his own normal flora. Nevertheless, close attention to hand-washing technique before one handles neonates at risk and isolation of cases of NEC are believed to be wise precautions until more is known of the relationship between infection and NEC.

Nutrition. Most babies developing NEC have been fed either clear fluids or formula before developing symptoms. A survey of close to 300 cases reveals that feeding had been started before the onset of the disease in 97%. In 80% of neonates the initial symptons of NEC occur within the first 3 days of initiation of oral feedings; in a series of 80 cases, more than a third were symptomatic within 24 hours. Infants who develop the disease within the first week have generally been fed earlier. Feeding a premature infant within the first 48 hours after birth seems to be an important risk factor.

The volume and the type of feeding have also been the subject of some scrutiny. One group found that those premature infants on daily formula increments of 20 to 50 ml/kg more at risk than those on the 10 ml/kg schedule. This needs further examination.

Because of the experimental study in rats showing the protective effect of mother's milk, the presumption has been that breast milk decreases the risk of NEC. The immune properties (humoral antibodies and cellular components) of human milk and its low pH protect against proliferation of gramnegative pathogens and invasion are well known. However, at least three studies have failed to show a demonstrable protective effect. One group explained the negative results by suggesting that a decline in cellular components is associated with refrigeration of human milk and that isolation of the infant from his mother prevents milk antibodies from being specifically directed against the intestinal flora normally shared by the mother and her infant.

Additional studies are necessary in this important area as the relationship between feeding and NEC has not been confirmed by some groups. Nevertheless it seems prudent to retard enteral feeding, to give small amounts, and, if possible, to offer human milk to babies at risk.

Table 3-11. Clinical course of necrotizing enterocolitis

	Perinatal period	Latent period	Acute illness	Late symptoms
Premature infant	Respiratory distress Apnea Asphyxia Exchange transfusion	24 hours to 3 weeks	Abdominal distention Vomiting Rectal bleeding Perforation Peritonitis Sepsis, shock	Strictures in ileum or colon

Modified from Touloukian, J., Posch, J.N., and Spencer, R.: J. Pediatr. Surg. **7:**194-209, 1972.

Clinical course and findings

Classically, symptoms are noted within the first 5 days of life, though they may occur as early as the first day and as late as the fourth week after birth (Table 3-11). An early onset of disease tends to be more severe and more acute. The infant is usually premature and the product of an abnormal gestation or of a complicated delivery. Resuscitation measures were probably necessary at birth, or the infant develops respiratory distress syndrome. Over the next few days feedings are poorly tolerated. Regurgitation and vomiting are followed by abdominal distention and hematochezia. Diarrheal stools are not frequent (25%) during the initial stage of the disease, since obstructive phenomena predominate. Within a few hours, there is evidence of perforation and peritonitis. Lethargy, severe acidosis, sepsis, disseminated intravascular coagulation, and shock rapidly supervene. In other cases, the course is not so fulminating, the baby is lethargic and feeds poorly, mild upper abdominal distention is noted, and bloody diarrhea is usually seen, followed by ileus. A few days later, intestinal perforation and peritonitis are detected, or else there is gradual clearing of symptoms.

Initially physical findings are most often dominated by the overall picture of a sick-looking baby with a moderately distended but soft abdomen. Fullness may be palpated in one area of the abdomen, and it may be tender. A purplish discoloration in one area of the abdomen, usually around the umbilicus, is indicative of an intraperitoneal hemorrhage. In certain cases, the abdominal wall may become ecchymotic and necrotic. This is an indication of an underlying perforation with peritonitis.

In certain cases, it is likely that the disease has run its course before birth. Perforation is then diagnosed within a few hours after birth. In others, the first symptoms are those of a partial obstruction in the distal small bowel or colon and may occur later in the neonatal period or after a few months. At surgery, a localized segment of bowel is stenotic and its mucosa is ulcerated (Fig. 3-21).

X-ray diagnosis

Roentgenographic findings must be interpreted in the light of clinical findings. When the clinical picture is typical, the purpose of the roentgenographic examination is to determine the presence and extent of complications. The classic findings in advanced cases include the presence of the bubbly or of the linear type of pneumatosis intestinalis (Fig. 3-40), the demonstration of gas in the portal system, and free air in the peritoneal cavity. A significant number of cases will be missed if the presence of intramural air is judged essential to make the diagnosis. On the other hand, overdiagnosis is likely in centers where nonspecific roentgenographic signs are accepted. A recent paper emphasizes the interobserver variability in the roentgenographic diagnosis of babies with clinical evidence of NEC.

An early roentgenographic diagnosis that could confirm a clinical picture compatible with incipient or mild NEC would be of great help. Progress has been made in that direction. In one series, 87% presented with early roentgen features before definitive diagnosis. These features include ileus with moderate distention, irregular and scattered bowel loops, loss of bowel-wall definition through edema, and finally the presence of fluid-filled loops and peritoneal fluid.

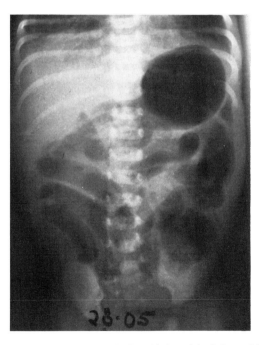

Fig. 3-40. This 5-day-old low birth weight infant with respiratory distress presented with abdominal distention, vomiting, and ileus. The pattern is abnormal. There is both dilatation and edema of the bowel loops. Note the bubbly appearance, particularly in the left lower quadrant, and a widespread linear type of pneumatosis.

Pathology findings

The particular vulnerability of the distal small intestine and colon to NEC is believed to be caused by the anatomic dissimilarity in the bowel supply. There is a single arcade of vessels in the upper jejunum, and it progresses to four levels of arcades in the terminal ileum. The low flow state in the gastrointestinal tract may be associated with vasospasm and thromboembolic phenomena. This leads to a type of mucosal necrosis that simulates autolysis in postmortem examinations. Hemorrhage, thrombosed veins, and infarction of the full mucosal width may progress to involve the entire bowel wall. Pneumatosis intestinalis is seen. It is characterized by gas cysts in the submucosa and subserosa, as well as in the mesentery (Figs. 3-41 and 3-42).

When there are late manifestations of the disease, we have been impressed with the fact that there seems to be ongoing chronic inflammatory changes along with extensive fibrosis of the submucosal and muscular layers, which accounts for the lesions of stenosis or atresia.

Treatment

As soon as the diagnosis of NEC is entertained, oral feedings should be withheld, and nasogastric suction and intravenous fluids should be started before a roentgenogram is taken. Parenteral antibiotics are indicated. Since the intestinal flora is clinically and experimentally an important pathogenic factor, oral antibiotics have been used in addition to the systemic antibiotics, but they have generally not been shown to be useful. Flat films of the abdomen are recommended every 8 to 12 hours for the first few days to detect early perforation and to follow the roentgenologic course of the disease. Nasogastric suction is stopped when roentgenograms no longer demonstrate pneumatosis and when the gastric return is small and clear-colored. Feedings are resumed gradually after a period of about 10 days of medical therapy.

Any evidence of rapid clinical deterioration (acidosis and thrombocytopenia), intestinal perforation (free air), or peritonitis (tenderness, rigidity, edema, and discoloration of the abdominal wall) constitutes an indication for immediate operation. The operative procedure may be a resection with primary anastomosis in the rare cases when the lesion or lesions are localized. When the process is extensive, the guiding principle is to resect only unquestionably necrotic or perforated

bowel. When there is doubt about the viability, a second-look operation should be planned. In desperately ill neonates with perforations, peritoneal drainage under local anesthesia appears to be warranted as a temporizing procedure. Subsequent surgery is reported to be necessary in two thirds of cases. The overall mortality of 46% in 15 cases treated with this regimen is comparable to that (45%) in 33 cases who underwent a laparotomy. Primary anastomosis is advisable if a perforation is high in the gastrointestinal tract. In other cases a simple resection with a temporary ileostomy or colostomy is advisable and should be left in place for at least 2 months. The stoma should not be closed until a barium enema rules out a stricture. However, not all strictures warrant surgery; it should be reserved for those who are symptomatic and show evidence of intestinal obstruction (Fig. 3-43).

Total parenteral nutrition is not infrequently needed for the small infant who requires an ileostomy. After discharge, neonates with NEC must be followed closely for signs of perforation or partial obstruction. These complications can occur as late as 3 to 5 months after an acute bout of NEC (Fig. 3-43).

In terms of prevention, the following recommendations are made:

1. Delay oral feedings for 5 to 7 days in low birth weight newborns with a history of perinatal asphyxia.
2. Hypertonic (hypercaloric) formulas are not recommended in sick newborns.
3. In the presence of significant polycythemia (hematocrit over 75%), consider a small phlebotomy and exchange transfusion with plasma by way of a peripheral vein.
4. Encourage mothers of low birth weight newborns to provide fresh breast milk.
5. Arterial umbilical catheters should lie in the aorta below the takeoff point of the renal arteries.
6. Venous umbilical catheters should not be positioned in the portal vein for an exchange transfusion.

Complications

Acute. Sepsis is said to be present in 60% of cases. Peritonitis is an acute complication that occurs in the 20% to 30% who develop an intestinal perforation. Abscesses, meningitis, and disseminated intravascular coagulation (DIC) are other complications related to infections. Bleeding is a usual gastrointestinal manifestation, but unfortunately it may also occur elsewhere (central ner-

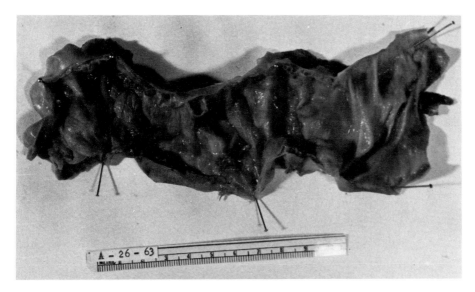

Fig. 3-41. Most common cause of pneumatosis is necrotizing enterocolitis. This segment of small bowel shows a number of air pockets dissecting its wall. In this case gas extended well into the mesentery and omentum.

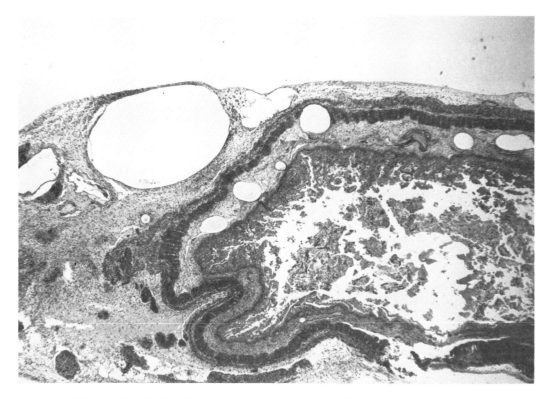

Fig. 3-42. All the classical features of necrotizing enterocolitis are seen in this specimen of a resected segment of descending colon. There is extensive necrosis of the mucosa and submucosa with involvement of the muscular layers in some areas. Gas cysts are noted in the submucosa as well as in the serosa and mesentery. A few thrombosed veins are identified.

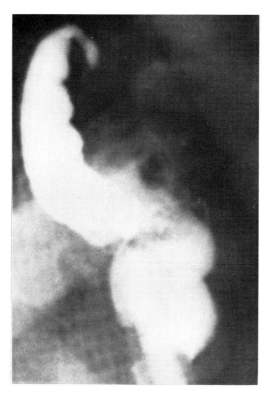

Fig. 3-43. Barium enema in a 5-month-old boy who had necrotizing enterocolitis during the first week of life. Four months after recovery from the acute phase of the disease, the mother noted progressive constipation, abdominal distention, and failure to thrive. The roentgenographic findings are those of a tight area of stenosis at the junction between the sigmoid and the descending colon.

vous system, kidney, and so on) and is indicative of disseminated intravascular coagulation or thrombocytopenia (less than 50,000). The overall incidence of these two problems may be as high as 60%. Fresh frozen plasma (10 ml/kg), platelet concentrate, or an exchange transfusion are in order if the above measures are not effective. Shock with metabolic complications such as hypoglycemia and acidosis is usual in the severe forms of the disease. The frequency of perforations is variable.

Chronic. The incidence of strictures or atresias after acute NEC is said to be between 18% and 25%. The time interval is variable; in most cases, the condition becomes detectable within 60 days. We have seen an interval as long as 1 year between the initial insult and the onset of obstipation and partial colonic obstruction. The majority (60%) occur in the left colon, especially at the

splenic flexure, but the distal ileum and other segments of colon may also be involved. All patients treated for NEC should have a barium enema 3 weeks after reinstitution of feedings.

Prognosis

In a large survey of 31 intensive care units in the USA and Canada the overall death rate in 798 cases seen between 1975 and 1977 was 29.3%. Sweet pointed out that 1 in 100 to 1 in 200 deaths probably result from NEC annually in the USA.

The prognosis is adversely affected by the degree of prematurity and ongoing problems with ventilation. Neonatologists at Hôpital Sainte-Justine have attracted attention to the fact that early-onset NEC is associated with a much poorer prognosis than the late-onset (more than 7 days) form of the disease. The mortality was 32% in the former group versus 12% in the latter. The rate of survival is much better in full-term infants and in those whose disease has been triggered by an exchange transfusion.

REFERENCES

Amoury, R.A., Goodwin, C.D., McGill, C.W., and others: Necrotizing enterocolitis following operation in the neonatal period, J. Pediatr. Surg. **15**:1-8, 1980.

Barlow, B., Santulli, T.V., Heird, W.C., and others: An experimental study of acute neonatal enterocolitis: the importance of breast milk, J. Pediatr. Surg. **9**:587-597, 1974.

Bell, M.J., Feigin, R.D., and Ternberg, J.L.: Changes in the incidence of necrotizing enterocolitis associated with variation of the gastrointestinal flora in neonates, Am. J. Surg. **138**:629-631, 1979.

Brown, E.G., and Sweet, A.Y., editors: Neonatal necrotizing enterocolitis, New York, 1980, Grune & Stratton.

Cashore, W.J., Peter, G., Lauermann, M., and others: Clostridia colonization and clostridial toxin in neonatal necrotizing enterocolitis, J. Pediatr. **98**:308-311, 1981.

Frantz, I.D., L'Heureux, P., Engel, R.R., and others: Necrotizing enterocolitis, J. Pediatr. **86**:259-263, 1975.

Hutter, J.J., Jr., Hathaway, W.E., and Wayne, E.R.: Hematologic abnormalities in severe neonatal necrotizing enterocolitis, J. Pediatr. **88**:1026-1031, 1976.

Janik, J.S., and Ein, S.H.: Peritoneal drainage under local anesthesia for necrotizing enterocolitis perforation: a second look, J. Pediatr. Surg. **15**:565-568, 1980.

Kliegman, R.M., Pittard, W.B., and Fanaroff, A.A.: Necrotizing enterocolitis in neonates fed human milk, J. Pediatr. **95**:450-453, 1979.

Kogutt, M.S.: Necrotizing enterocolitis of infancy: early roentgen patterns as a guide to prompt diagnosis, Radiology **130**:367-370, 1979.

Mata, A.G., and Rosengart, R.M.: Interobserver variability in the radiographic diagnosis of necrotizing enterocolitis, Pediatrics **66**:68-71, 1980.

Moriartey, R.R., Finer, N.N., Cox, S.F., and others: Necrotizing enterocolitis and human milk, J. Pediatr. **94**:295-296, 1979.

Rodin, A.E., Nichols, M.M., and Hsu, F.L.: Necrotizing enterocolitis occurring in full-term neonates at birth, Arch. Pathol. **96**:335-338, 1973.

Schwartz, M.Z., Richardson, C.J., Hayden, C.K., and others: Intestinal stenosis following successful medical management of necrotizing enterocolitis, J. Pediatr. Surg. **15**:890-899, 1980.

Stein, H., Beck, J., Solomon, A., and others: Gastroenteritis with necrotizing enterocolitis in premature babies, Br. Med. J. **2**:616-619, 1972.

Stevenson, J.K., Oliver, T.K., Graham, B., and others: Aggressive treatment of neonatal necrotizing enterocolitis: 38 patients with 25 survivors, J. Pediatr. Surg. **6**:28-35, 1971.

Stone, H.H., Webb, H.W., and Kovalchik, M.T.: Pneumatosis intestinalis of infancy, Surg. Gynecol. Obstet. **130**:806-812, 1970.

Takayanagi, K., and Kapila, L.: Necrotizing enterocolitis in older infants Arch. Dis. Child. **56**:468-471, 1981.

Teasdale, F., Le Guennec, J.-C., Bard, H., and others: Neonatal necrotizing enterocolitis: the relation of age at the time of onset to prognosis, Can. Med. Assoc. J. **123**:387-390, 1980.

Tonkin, I.L., Bjelland, J.C., Hunter, T.B., and others: Spontaneous resolution of colonic strictures caused by necrotizing enterocolitis: therapeutic implications, Am. J. Roentgenol. **130**:1077-1081, 1978.

Touloukian, R.J., Posch, J.N., and Spencer, R.: The pathogenesis of ischemic gastroenterocolitis of the neonate: selective gut mucosal ischemia in asphyxiated neonatal piglets, J. Pediatr. Surg. **7**:194-205, 1972.

Virnig, N.L., and Reynolds, J.W.: Epidemiological aspects of neonatal necrotizing enterocolitis, Am. J. Dis. Child. **128**:186-190, 1974.

FUNCTIONAL INTESTINAL OBSTRUCTION IN THE NEONATE

Close to 95% of normal neonates evacuate meconium within the first 24 hours of life, and the failure to pass meconium is often the first sign of intestinal obstruction. However, the passage of meconium may occur in neonatal intestinal obstruction; this is usually seen when the level of obstruction is situated high in the intestinal tract. The two other classic signs of lower obstruction are abdominal distention and bile-stained vomitus. This triad of symptoms may be seen in the absence of organic lesions in 20% of neonates.

The pathogenic mechanisms leading to functional intestinal obstruction can be grouped under two main headings: disturbance of intestinal peristalsis and abnormal meconium. Although meconium ileus associated with cystic fibrosis and Hirschsprung's disease would theoretically fall under these two headings, they are excluded from the present discussion. Following is a list of complications of pregnancy and delivery as well as factors that have been associated with the development of the syndrome.

Pathogenesis and factors associated with functional intestinal obstruction

"Abnormal" meconium
    Meconium plug syndrome
    Non–cystic fibrosis meconium ileus
Disturbance of peristalsis
    Immaturity of neural plexus in the small premature infant
    Small left colon syndrome (often in infants of diabetic mothers)
    Sepsis
    Respiratory distress syndrome
    Maternal drugs (opiates, ganglionic blocking agents, $MgSO_4$)
    Hypothyroidism

Although there has been increased recognition of this entity during the past years, there remain a significant number of neonates in whom the pathogenesis of functional obstruction is hypothetical and multiple factors may be involved.

Clinical findings

The symptoms and signs associated with meconium ileus are discussed on p. 80. Neonates with non–cystic fibrosis meconium ileus have typical signs of lower small-bowel obstruction and cannot be distinguished clinically from those in whom the ileus is the initial manifestation of cystic fibrosis. It is estimated that perhaps 10% of cases of meconium ileus occur in the absence of mucoviscidosis. Small premature infants are particularly vulnerable, but we have seen the syndrome in full-term infants.

Patients with functional intestinal obstruction usually present with failure to pass meconium (small amounts of mucus may be passed), abdominal distention, and bile-stained vomitus. Some have few symptoms, and their clinical course tends to be less severe than in patients with organic intestinal obstruction. The onset is usually within the first 3 days of life, and half are premature infants. A history of toxemia of pregnancy, maternal drugs, sepsis, maternal diabetes, and respiratory distress syndrome is common. Hypothyroidism is also reported.

X-ray findings

There is usually uniform gaseous distention of the whole intestine, except in neonates with non—

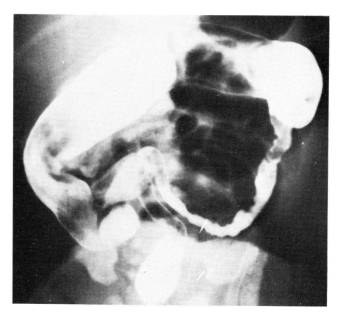

Fig. 3-44. Small left colon syndrome, shown in barium enema roentgenogram carried out in a low birth weight newborn who failed to pass meconium. He was born after 38 weeks of gestation from a diabetic mother. The meconium in the rectal ampulla was whitish and "sticky." Rectal suction biopsies showed normal ganglion cells.

cystic fibrosis meconium ileus. Upright films in the supine and erect positions are useful diagnostic aids. There is usually a lack of fluid levels in the distended loops of bowel, in contrast to what is generally seen when obstruction is secondary to an organic cause (except cystic fibrosis meconium ileus). When a lower colonic obstruction is present, as in the meconium plug syndrome, which is discussed below, mottled densities (meconium) may be seen in the rectosigmoid.

Small left colon syndrome

At times, the barium enema radiograph may show a greatly diminished caliber of the colon from anus to splenic flexure, with a sharp zone of transition at that level. The colon proximal to the splenic flexure is always dilated and distended with meconium that is easily evacuated and does not seem abnormally viscid. Fluid levels may occasionally be seen. These roentgenographic features (Fig. 3-44) have been identified as the small left colon syndrome.

An unusually high percentage of these patients are infants of diabetic mothers. There is also a high frequency of prematurity, twinning, and delivery by cesarean section. Nonoperative treatment is indicated for the small left colon syn-

drome because normal bowel action is usually established within a few days. Close surveillance of these patients is in order because perforation of the cecum and of the colon have been reported.

Conservative management requires a barium enema that is usually curative. Saline enemas and eventually Gastrografin enema can be administered. If the latter is unsuccessful and if persistent cecal distention is seen, a colostomy is in order. Hirschsprung's disease should be ruled out in all cases with persistence of symptoms after the diagnostic barium enema. The left colon is not expected to regain its normal caliber until a few weeks or months.

Paralytic ileus versus immaturity of neural plexus

A certain percentage of neonates with functional intestinal obstruction have been shown to have an increased proportion of small immature ganglion cells in their intermyenteric plexus, which could account for the functional difficulties. Because the process of maturation of ganglion cells progresses in a cephalocaudad direction, the ratio of mature (large multipolar cells) to immature cells is always greater proximally than distally during fetal development. These considerations suggest that the aganglionosis-like syndrome, the small left colon syndrome, and the meconium plug syndrome have the same underlying pathogenesis—immaturity of the neural plexus.

In other cases, particularly in neonates with infection, respiratory distress, and asphyxia, there is no evidence for delayed maturation of the neurologic apparatus of the large bowel. Paralytic ileus is probably secondary to a number of humoral and metabolic factors. Hypermagnesemia has been described as a cause of functional obstruction in neonates from toxemic mothers given magnesium sulfate.

Differential diagnosis and management

One must always maintain a high degree of suspicion and be aware of nonsurgical conditions that can present with intestinal obstruction. Necrotizing enterocolitis must stand high on the list of differential diagnoses because the perinatal factors involved are very similar.

Feedings can be continued, but careful observation is essential in the neonate who fails to pass meconium and who shows moderate abdominal distention, if distention becomes severe or if vomiting occurs, feedings should be stopped and neogastric suction started. All newborns who fail to pass meconium within the first 24 hours should have films of the abdomen, a careful rectal examination, and a small saline enema.

If normal flow of meconium does not follow or fails to relieve symptoms, a barium enema should be done.

In cases of functional intestinal obstruction, particularly those involving small premature infants (less than 1500 gm) and neonates with sepsis or with respiratory distress, the colon is easily filled with barium, but evacuation is delayed for as long as 3 to 5 days. Further testing to rule out Hirschsprung's disease is indicated and includes histochemistry (acetylcholinesterase) on mucosa obtained by a rectal suction biopsy and a manometric study. Normal relaxation of the internal sphincter rules out aganglionosis. However the absence of relaxation has little significance because there is a high incidence of false-negative results during the first week of life especially in low birth weight infants.

Prognosis

Death may occur from aspiration into the respiratory tract or from unnecessary surgery in a sick premature infant. In general, the prognosis is excellent with supportive nutritional care, since features of obstruction resolve spontaneously within a few days.

REFERENCES

Bughaighis, A.G., and Emery, J.L.: Functional obstruction of the intestine due to neurological immaturity, Progr. Pediatr. Surg. **3**:37-52, 1971.

Cain, A.R.R., Deall, A.M., and Noble, T.C.: Screening for cystic fibrosis by testing meconium for albumin, Arch. Dis. Child. **47**:131-132, 1972.

Davis, W.S., and Campbell, J.B.: Neonatal small left colon syndrome, Am. J. Dis. Child. **129**:1024-1027, 1975.

Dolan, T.F., and Touloukian, R.J.: Familial meconium ileus not associated with cystic fibrosis, J. Pediatr. Surg. **9**:821-831, 1974.

Howat, J.M., and Wilkinson, A.W.: Functional intestinal obstruction in the neonate, Arch. Dis. Child. **45**:800-804, 1970.

Le Quesne, G.W., and Reilly, B.J.: Neonatal radiology: functional immaturity of the large bowel in the newborn infant, Radiol. Clin. North Am. **13**:331-342, 1975.

Nixon, G.W., Condon, V.R., and Stewart, D.R.: Intestinal perforation as a complication of the neonatal small left colon syndrome, Am. J. Roentgenol. **125**:75-80, 1975.

Philippart, A.I., Reed, J.O., and Georgeson, K.E.: Neonatal small left colon syndrome: intramural not intraluminal obstruction, J. Pediatr. Surg. **10**:733-738, 1975.

Rickham, P.P.: Intraluminal intestinal obstruction, Progr. Pediatr. Surg. **2**:73-82, 1971.

Shigemoto, H., Seisaburo, E., Isomoto, T., and others: Neonatal meconium obstruction in the ileum without mucoviscidosis, J. Pediatr. Surg. **13**:475-479, 1978.

Sokal, M.M., Koenigsberger, M.R., Rose, J.S., and others: Neonatal hypermagnesemia and meconium plug syndrome, N. Engl. J. Med. **286**:823-825, 1972.

Vanhoutte, J.J., and Katzman, D.: Roentgenographic manifestations of immaturity of the intestinal neural plexus in premature infants, Radiology **106**:363-367, 1973.

MECONIUM PLUG SYNDROME

The meconium plug syndrome is an uncommon and relatively benign form of functional intestinal obstruction in the newborn infant. It is discussed separately because it can also be the mode of presentation of Hirschsprung's disease. Close to 50% of patients with the meconium plug syndrome have subsequently been shown to have Hirschsprung's disease. The association between the meconium plug syndrome and cystic fibrosis is also well recognized.

The inspissated meconium mass has a rubbery consistency and therefore lacks the flow characteristics of normal meconium. It is not clear whether this represents a primary abnormality of the meconium itself, a decrease in intestinal mucolytic enzymes, or reduced distal colonic motil-

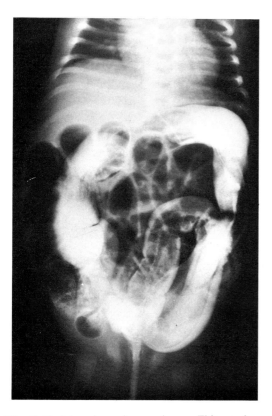

Fig. 3-45. Meconium plug syndrome. This newborn infant failed to pass meconium and developed abdominal distention and vomiting. The barium enema shows a colon of normal caliber. The radiopaque medium has infiltrated between the colonic wall and the meconium mass. The infant was subsequently proved to have Hirschsprung's disease.

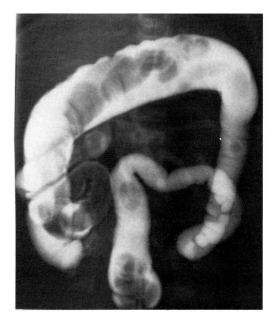

Fig. 3-46. Extensive distribution of large meconium plugs throughout an otherwise normal colon. Formation of these plugs is the likely result of deficient peristalsis. Once formed, they may very well be responsible for the obstructive phenomenon in a colon endowed with mature neural plexuses. In this case the barium enema was curative.

ity that permits excessive desiccation of the plug. Recent reports favor an unrecognized immaturity of the intramural ganglion cells as a likely cause of this condition in cases unassociated with aganglionosis. Once formed, they may obstruct an otherwise normal colon capable of propulsive peristalsis.

Clinical features

Both the full-term newborn and the premature infant can be affected. Evidence of low intestinal obstruction usually becomes apparent by the second day of life. Little or no meconium is passed during this time. Abdominal distention is usually followed by bile-stained vomitus, and dehydration may ensue. Inspection of the abdomen may reveal dilated loops, and peristaltic waves may be seen. Rectal examination is important in that the anal canal may seem small and empty of meconium.

In other cases, within the first 5 cm beyond the mucocutaneous junction, the finger may feel a hard mass impacted in the rectum. Digital stimulation may result in the sudden passage of a meconium cast along with much gas. Small plugs may continue to be passed for another 24 hours. If clinical signs of obstruction are present, roentgenographic studies should be made promptly, regardless of whether meconium has been passed spontaneously or after digital examination.

Diagnosis

Routine three-way abdominal films will show signs of low colonic obstruction. Airfluid levels may be present, a presacral intraluminal mass is outlined by gas anteriorly, and its presence is confirmed by a lateral film. A barium enema performed slowly and under low pressure reveals a normal-sized colon, with the barium surrounding and outlining the meconium mass (Fig. 3-45). Most often the plug is found on the left side of the colon, though at times it may extend to the cecum (Fig. 3-46). The enema can dislodge the plug, and meconium is passed during evacuation of the medium. The roentgenographic appearance of a normal colon at this time does not rule out Hirschsprung's disease.

Treatment

In mild cases, digital rectal examination is therapeutic. The barium enema will dislodge the meconium plug in all but a rare case. Occasionally, it may be necessary to administer a Gastrografin enema to promote complete passage of the plug.

Prognosis

For most of these patients, normal bowel function begins after passage of the plug, and stools are then passed without difficulty. However, the physician should consider that coexistent aganglionosis may exist (Fig. 3-45) and should keep in touch with parents of these babies regarding bowel function. The development of constipation or diarrhea in the subsequent few weeks is a definite indication for a repeat barium enema, a rectal suction biopsy, and a manometric study to rule out Hirschsprung's disease. A sweat test is also in order.

REFERENCES

Ellis, D.G., and Clatworthy, H.W.: The meconium plug syndrome revisited, J. Pediatr. Surg. **1**:54-61, 1966.

Leeuwen, G. van, Riley, W.C., Glenn, L., and Woodruff, C.: Meconium plug syndrome with aganglionosis, Pediatrics **40**:665-666, 1967.

Le Quesne, G.W., and Reilly, B.J.: Neonatal radiology: functional immaturity of the large bowel in the newborn, Radiol. Clin. North Am. **13**:331-338, 1975.

Pochaczevsky, R., and Leonidas, J.C.: The meconium plug syndrome: roentgen evaluation and differentiation from Hirschsprung's disease and other pathologic states, Radiology **120**:342-352, 1974.

Swischuk, L.E.: Meconium plug syndrome: a cause of neonatal intestinal obstruction, Am. J. Roentgenol. Radium Ther. Nucl. Med. **103**:339-346, 1968.

Taybi, H., and Patterson, J.: Plain film diagnosis of meconium plug syndrome: presacral mass, Radiology **104**:113-114, 1972.

NEONATAL PRIMARY CHRONIC ADYNAMIC BOWEL

Hirschsprung's disease is the most common form of chronic functional intestinal obstruction in the neonate. Well-defined clinical entities representative of temporary large-bowel dysfunction include the small left colon syndrome and the meconium plug syndrome. Rare cases with either small immature ganglion cells, or increased or decreased ganglion cells, have been labeled "pseudo-Hirschsprung's disease." The observations that are the subject of this section are concerned with functional obstruction involving the small bowel or the large bowel, or both.

In seven infants, an autosomal recessive mode of inheritance was found. Associated anomalies include short small bowel, malrotation, and pyloric hypertrophy. Other reports describe infants without associated gastrointestinal anomalies but with severe genitourinary manifestations, the megacystis-microcolon-hypoperistalsis syndrome. These male neonates have severe abdominal distention and bilious vomiting. There is a small-bowel ileus and a small microcolon of disuse. The genitourinary anomalies become clinically manifest by a large central mass (flaccid bladder) and bilateral flank masses (hydronephrotic kidneys).

In another category are neonates in whom the sole manifestation is the failure of peristalsis in both the small and large bowel. These unfortunate babies become symptomatic shortly after birth. Small amounts of meconium may be passed. The abdomen is strikingly distended, and bilious vomiting precludes oral feedings. Ganglion cells are present and manometric studies reveal normal relaxation of the internal sphincter. In those cases in whom silver staining of the biopsy specimen or of autopsy material has been carried out, a striking reduction or else total absence of argyrophil neurons have been noted in the myenteric plexus. Argyrophil cells comprise 5% to 20% of the total number of neurons; the processes of these cells run in the plexus along with extrinsic sympathetic and parasympathetic fibers. This network is believed to be responsible for the control of peristalsis by modulating the secretion of neurotransmitters originating from the argyrophobe cells.

There is no satisfactory treatment for this disorder. Although segmental resections, jejunostomies, and continuous enteral alimentation have led to long-term survival in one patient, the prognosis is very poor unless a life-long commitment to parenteral nutrition can be made.

REFERENCES

Byrne, W.J., Cipel, L., Euler, A.R., and others: Chronic idiopathic intestinal pseudo-obstruction syndrome in children: clinical characteristics and prognosis, J. Pediatr. **90**:585-589, 1977.

Duhamel, J.F., Ricour, C., Dupont, C., and others: L'adynamie intestinale chronique primitive à révélation néonatale, Arch. Franc. Pédiatr. **37**:293-297, 1980.

Ehrenpreis, T.H.: Pseudo-Hirschsprung's disease, Arch. Dis. Child. **40:**177-179, 1965.

Puri, P., Lake, B.D., and Nixon, H.H.: Adynamic bowel syndrome: report of a case with disturbance of the cholinergic innervation, Gut **18:**754-759, 1977.

Tanner, M.S., Smith, B., and Lloyd, J.K.: Functional intestinal obstruction due to deficiency of argyrophil neurones in the myenteric plexus, Arch. Dis. Child. **51:**837-841, 1976.

Wiswell, T.E., Rawling, J.S., Wilson, J.L., and Pettett, G.: Megacystis-microcolon-intestinal hypoperistalsis syndrome, Pediatrics **63:**805-808, 1979.

CONGENITAL DIAPHRAGMATIC HERNIA

Between the eighth and tenth weeks of fetal life, the diaphragm is formed and the coelomic cavity is divided into its abdominal and thoracic components. During this same stage of morphogenesis, the gastrointestinal tract undergoes its major development, elongating into the umbilical pouch and rotating on its return to the abdominal cavity. An alteration in these two closely interrelated processes leads to a diaphragmatic hernia, which can be secondary either to a posterolateral defect in the diaphragm (foramen of Bochdalek) or, more rarely, to a retrosternal defect (foramen of Morgagni). Less than 2% of cases are secondary to a retrosternal defect. In the posterolateral variety, about 85% to 90% involve the left leaf of the diaphragm. The incidence of diaphragmatic hernia is 1 in 4000 live births. Eventration of the diaphragm is not strictly speaking, a hernia but is considered here because the clinical picture may be quite similar. A leaf of the diaphragm is ballooned out through a diminution of muscular elements (Fig. 3-47). Agenesis of the left hemidiaphragm is a rare congenital anomaly associated with the same clinical picture as the one associated with a Bochdalek hernia. Hiatal hernia is discussed in Chapter 6.

Clinical features

Signs and symptoms vary with the size and location of the hernial defect. Hernias through the foramen of Bochdalek are large and therefore cause early and severe symptoms. In 90% of cases the small bowel is involved; in 50% the liver is also included. At birth, the infant may appear normal, but as gas fills the herniated bowel, dyspnea and cyanosis develop. The abdomen is scaphoid (Fig. 3-48), and a rocking type of respiration is noted. There is dullness to percussion, and breath sounds are absent on the affected side. The point of maximal cardiac impulse is displaced, and circulatory disturbances can accompany the mediastinal shift. Although signs of respiratory distress predominate there may also be evidence of intestinal obstruction.

Generally speaking, the symptoms associated with a right posterolateral defect are less severe. The reason is that in such cases a portion of the liver is also herniated and prevents, to some extent, bowel from occupying the right side of the chest (Fig. 3-49).

Although most hernias through the foramen of Bochdalek have no sac, the much rarer retrosternal diaphragmatic defect through the foramen of Morgagni usually has a true membranous sac. The latter somehow limits the amount of herniated bowel, and therefore few cardiorespiratory symptoms or none are seen. Symptoms of partial large bowel obstruction have been described (Fig. 3-50).

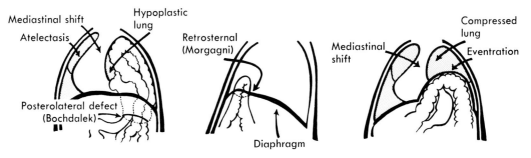

Fig. 3-47. Congenital diaphragmatic hernias. Most diaphragmatic hernias are secondary to posterolateral defects (Bochdalek), and 80% involve the left leaf of the diaphragm. Eventration is not a true hernia, since there is no actual hernial orifice, but the resulting elevation of the diaphragmatic leaf may lead to symptoms similar to those encountered in true hernias. (Modified from Bill, A.H., Jr., and Laroye, G.J.: Northwest Med. **65:**555-560, 1966.)

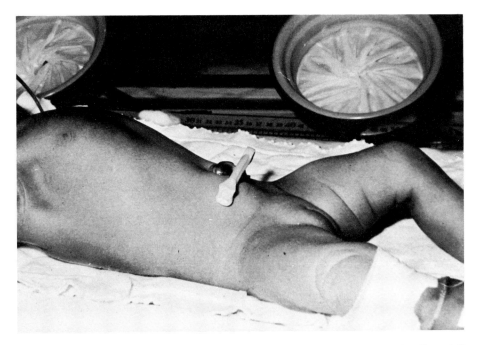

Fig. 3-48. Diaphragmatic hernia. Within a few minutes after birth, swallowed air fills and distends the gastrointestinal tract. A scaphoid abdomen indicates either a high obstructive lesion (esophageal atresia without a fistula or with a proximal fistula) or a large diaphragmatic hernia, with which a significant proportion of the abdominal structures are in the chest.

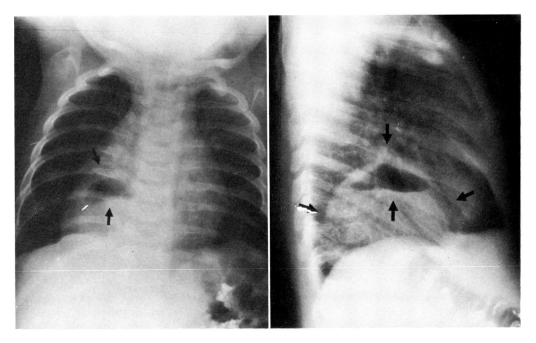

Fig. 3-49. Diaphragmatic hernia through a right posterolateral defect. Hernias through the foramen of Bochdalek on the right are uncommon and are generally less extensive; the liver can prevent the hernia from being as extensive as in the left-sided defect. Arrows point to an intrathoracic structure containing air.

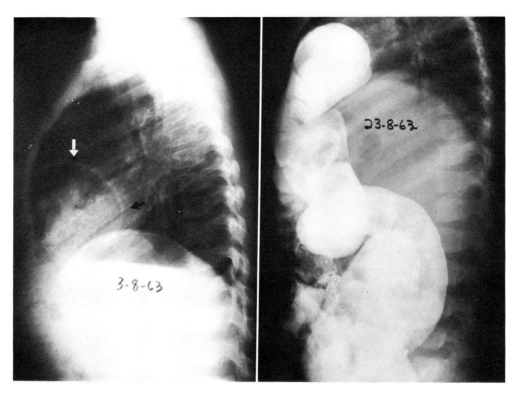

Fig. 3-50. Hernia through the foramen of Morgagni. A well-defined globular mass containing air and liquid or solid material is present in the retrosternal area, *arrows*. The barium enema shows a loop of colon herniating through the hiatus of Morgagni. This 3½-year-old child had recurrent episodes of abdominal pain associated with obstipation and vomiting.

Associated anomalies

The significance of diaphragmatic hernia in terms of survival is related to the secondary effects on respiratory function. The presence of a space-occupying lesion in the chest results in mediastinal shift and bilateral pulmonary compression. More importantly, however, the herniated abdominal contents prevent differentiation of the lung buds, and pulmonary hypoplasia results. A true maturational arrest in lung development has been demonstrated. Several studies have shown a decrease in lung weight and in pulmonary vessels, which show thickening of their muscle coat. In physiological terms, these defects are associated with pulmonary hypertension leading to shunting through the ductus arteriosus, reduction in biventricular emptying, and cardiac enlargement. In addition there is evidence of abnormal pulmonary vascular reactivity, which contributes significantly to ventilatory failure. Pulmonary hypoplasia is more severe in left posterolateral defects because the her-

niated mass is larger. Pulmonary hypoplasia is not a feature of hernias through the foramen of Morgagni or of eventration.

The presence of midgut in the chest entails the absence of normal mesenteric fixation and the diagnosis of malrotation. Intestinal obstruction may therefore be secondary to a volvulus or to peritoneal bands.

Diagnosis

The newborn who has bouts of cyanosis, dyspnea, feeding difficulties, and dextrocardia has diaphragmatic hernia until proved otherwise. Roentgenograms permit confirmation of the diagnosis. Gas-filled bowel and often stomach are seen in the thorax, with collapse of the lung and displacement of the mediastinum. There is a clear continuation of gas shadows between abdomen and chest. Blood gases (arterial) show acidosis, a low Po_2 and a high Pco_2.

Eventration of the diaphragm should be differentiated from paralysis of the diaphragm secondary to phrenic nerve involvement. Under fluoroscopy, patients with eventration do not have the typical paradoxical movement of the paralyzed diaphragmatic leaf.

Management

As soon as the diagnosis is made, attention should be drawn to the relief of respiratory distress through the administration of oxygen and the decompression of the stomach, with a nasogastric tube providing constant suction. Positive-pressure breathing may be required. It should not be given by face mask for fear of further compressing the lung by increasing the air content of the herniated portion of the gastrointestinal tract. Endotracheal intubation is essential, and great care should be exercised in positive-pressure ventilation because of the risk of pneumothorax in the contralateral lung.

Operation should be performed as soon as possible. In hernias through the foramen of Bochdalek, the abdominal approach will permit exploration for the presence of a volvulus or of peritoneal bands. In addition, because the abdominal cavity is of restricted capacity, stretching of abdominal musculature may be carried out. When the abdominal cavity is too small to accommodate the herniated contents, the skin alone may be closed initially.

Although some hernias of the foramen of Morgagni may give rise to few symptoms, it is recommended that they all be treated surgically. As for eventration of the diaphragm, surgical treatment is recommended only if symptoms are severe. A transthoracic approach is used for the imbrication of the eventrated leaf of the diaphragm.

The hypoplastic lung should not be expanded beyond its capacity. Continuous suctioning of the pleural space through an endothoracic intercostal catheter connected to a low-level water seal usually leads, within days or weeks, to the complete filling of the pleural space by the fully expanded lung. Emphysema is common for the first few days postoperatively. Incomplete aeration of a lobe may persist for as long as a year. Blood gas studies should be frequently monitored for assessment of pulmonary function.

Pulmonary hypertension often leads to shunting through the ductus arteriosus, which fails to close, or through the foramen ovale. Pharmacologic efforts have been recently utilized to decrease pulmonary hypertension.

There are a few reports showing that tolazoline is an effective pulmonary vasodilator in patients with congenital diaphragmatic hernia. However others report a variable response and disquieting side effects (gastrointestinal bleeding, hypotension, thrombocytopenia).

Despite improvement in anesthetic, respiratory, and surgical management, the mortality has not improved in the past two decades and is still very high (30% to 60%). The "hidden" mortality has decreased because fewer infants die before being treated. Diagnosis is made earlier, and transport and resuscitation of these critically ill neonates are also contributory. However, this has not changed the overall mortality because more victims of this severe anomaly die of ventilatory failure. Successful management depends as much on the postoperative management as on the surgical procedure. A transient period of satisfactory respiratory exchanges often takes place postoperatively, but unfortunately it is commonly followed by intense pulmonary vasospasm, a right-to-left shunt, progressive deterioration, and death.

A pharmacologic approach to the treatment of pulmonary hypertension offers the best hope of improving the prognosis. Tolazoline and other alpha-blockers, prostaglandins, and hydralazine in combination with diazoxide are some of the drugs being investigated.

Studies carried out 6 to 12 years after hernia repair have shown, despite normal roentgenographic appearance, residual defects in ventilatory function.

REFERENCES

Baran, E.M., Houston, H.E., Lynn, H.B., and O'Connell, E.J.: Foramen of Morgagni hernias in children, Surgery **62:**1076-1081, 1967.

Bloss, R.S., Aranda, J.V., and Beardmore, H.E.: Congenital diaphragmatic hernia: pathophysiology and pharmacologic support, Surgery **89:**518-524, 1981.

Chatrath, R.R., Shafie, M.E., and Jones, R.S.: Fate of hypoplastic lungs after repair of congenital diaphragmatic hernia, Arch. Dis. Child. **46:**633-635, 1971.

Dibbins, A.W., and Wiener, E.S.: Mortality from neonatal diaphragmatic hernia, J. Pediatr. Surg. **9:**653-662, 1974.

Eichelberger, M.R., Kettrick, R.G., Hoelzer, D.J., and others: Agenesis of the left diaphragm: surgical repair and physiologic consequences, J. Pediatr. Surg. **15:**395-397, 1980.

Harrison, M.R., Bjordal, R.I., Langmark, F., and Knutrud, O.: Congenital diaphragmatic hernia: the hidden mortality, J. Pediatr. Surg. **13:**227-230, 1978.

Kerr, A.A.: Lung function in children after repair of congenital diaphragmatic hernia, Arch. Dis. Child. **52:**902-906, 1977.

Lister, J.: Recent advances in the surgery of the diaphragm in the newborn, Progr. Pediatr. Surg. **2:**29-39, 1971.

Moodie, D.S., Telander, R.L., Kleinberg, F., and Feldt, R.H.: Use of tolazoline in newborn infants with diaphragmatic hernia and severe cardiopulmonary disease, J. Thorac. Cardiovasc. Surg. **75:**725-730, 1978.

Pearl, W.: Gastrointestinal complications of tolazoline therapy [letter], J. Pediatr. **91**(6):1025-1026, 1977.

Raphaely, R.C., and Downes, J.J.: Congenital diaphragmatic hernia: prediction of survival, J. Pediatr. Surg. **8:**815-823, 1973.

Reale, F.R., and Esterly, J.R.: Pulmonary hypoplasia: a morphometric study of the lungs of infants with diaphragmatic hernia, anencephaly, and renal malformations, Pediatrics **51:**91-96, 1973.

Wayne, E.R., Campbell, J.B., and Burrington, J.D.: Eventration of the diaphragm, J. Pediatr. Surg. **9:**643-651, 1974.

4 *Intestinal obstruction of infancy and childhood*

Failure of progression of intestinal contents may result from a mechanical obstruction or inadequate activity of intestinal muscles. There are many mechanical causes of intestinal obstruction (Table 4-1). They can be broken down in terms of (1) intraluminal obstruction by foreign bodies, bezoars, fecaliths, and others, and (2) encroachment of the lumen by extrinsic compression or disease of the bowel wall.

Nonmechanical obstruction is referred to as ileus. The likely cause of ileus is an increased sympathetic discharge with hyperpolarization of smooth muscle cells. It is not known whether this is mediated through extrinsic nerves or whether local reflexes could cause inhibition of the normal tonic and phasic activity that regulate bowel motility. Humoral factors could also be implicated in certain instances of paralytic ileus. A wide variety of clinical conditions give rise to adynamic ileus in infants and children (Table 4-1).

Ileus may follow trauma to the abdomen, and it is always present after surgical manipulations requiring the opening of the peritoneal cavity. A peritoneal insult by hydrochloric acid, blood, pancreatic enzymes, or microorganisms, as occurs in solid or hollow viscus rupture, perforation, or infection, leads to adynamic ileus. Severe electrolyte disturbances, particularly those associated with severe potassium depletion, decrease intestinal motility and cause intestinal ileus. Any disorder that compromises the arterial blood supply or interferes with venous blood return may give rise to intestinal ileus. Sepsis, pneumonia, pyelonephritis, primary peritonitis, and pelvic inflammatory disease are some of the infections often responsible for ileus. Renal or gallbladder stones and diabetic acidosis are rarer etiologic conditions.

Clinical findings

Classically, acute mechanical intestinal obstruction becomes manifest by the onset of colicky abdominal pain, nausea and vomiting, abdominal distention, and constipation.

In cases of ileus, pain is not an outstanding feature. When present, it is duller and more diffuse. Discomfort usually results from the abdominal distention, and there is obstipation. Vomiting is often the first sign of a high obstruction; it occurs later in lower obstructions. Obstipation and constipation become obvious late in upper bowel obstructions. In fact, a child with a high obstruction can pass stools for a day or two. Furthermore, it is not exceptional to see a young infant with peritonitis have diarrheal stools.

Physical findings vary with the age of the child and the nature and duration of the underlying disease. Tachycardia, fever, and dehydration favor an acute mechanical obstruction secondary to an inflammatory process or complicated by necrosis or peritonitis, or both. Abdominal distention is minimal or absent if the obstruction is high in the small bowel. Peristaltic waves characteristic of small bowel obstruction may be seen through a thin abdominal wall. An abdominal mass should be carefully sought. The abdomen of the child may be difficult to examine because of pain, rebound tenderness, and guarding, which indicate peritoneal irritation or involvement. Bowel sounds may be absent in long-standing obstruction with peritonitis. Early on, they may be high pitched and tinkling. In cases of ileus, there is mild or severe abdominal tenderness but no rigidity or involuntary guarding. Bowel sounds are absent. Gaseous distention develops and leads to the sequestration of extracellular fluid and protein in the adynamic intestine. Dehydration and shock may supervene.

X-ray diagnosis

Mechanical intestinal obstruction leads to dilatation of the segments above the occlusion and accumulation of gas and fluid. Airfluid levels are best demonstrated with the patient in decubitus and erect positions with anterior and lateral projections. The stepladder distribution of distended small bowel loops is a classic pattern for small bowel obstruction. The colon is usually devoid of gas after complete obstruction of the small intestine. In cases of colonic obstruction, there is distention of the large bowel proximal to the level of the obstruction and of the small bowel as well. Although the widely spaced haustral markings in the

Table 4-1. Intestinal obstruction of infancy (beyond the neonatal period) and childhood

Mechanical obstruction		Paralytic ileus
Intraluminal	**Extraluminal (bowel-wall disease or extrinsic compression)**	**Paralytic ileus**
Foreign body	Hernia	Trauma, surgery
Bezoar	Intussusception	Perforation of a hollow viscus
Fecalith	Volvulus	Rupture of a solid viscus
Gallstone	Duplication	Hypokalemia
Parasite	Stenosis	Shock, intravascular coagulation, mesen-
Meconium ileus equivalent	Adhesions	teric arterial or venous thrombosis
Tumor	Granulomatous process	Renal or gallbladder stones
	Infection and abscess formation	Diabetic acidosis
	Tumor	Sepsis, pneumonia
	Mesenteric cyst	Severe gastroenteritis in the young infant
	Superior mesenteric artery syn-	Pyelonephritis
	drome	Pelvic inflammatory disease
		Primary peritonitis

dilated, gas-filled colon should help differentiate it from the pattern of closely spaced small bowel loops, this differentiation is often impossible to make, particularly in young infants. Adynamic ileus usually gives rise to dilated air-filled loops or to air-fluid accumulation in both large and small bowel.

In cases where abdominal scout films fail to distinguish colonic from small intestinal obstruction, a carefully performed barium enema will establish the diagnosis. A barium meal can help distinguish mechanical obstruction from paralytic ileus, but it is contraindicated until colonic obstruction can be ruled out.

Treatment

Therapy consists in correcting fluid and electrolyte imbalance, with constant anticipation of current losses, which can be extraordinarily large. Protein depletion can rapidly lead to shock. Young infants should always receive plasma or salt-poor albumin when mechanical intestinal obstruction is present.

Alleviating vomiting and attending electrolyte losses are essential and can be achieved by gastric or small bowel decompression. A soft 10 F rubber catheter is used for intermittent suction, preventing swallowed air from gaining access to the small and the large bowels. If distention is already quite advanced, respiratory distress and shock can occur. In such cases, duodenal or small bowel de-

compression is sometimes necessary and can be done with the introduction of a small Cantor tube (12 F). A rectal tube may be very helpful, particularly in cases of adynamic ileus.

The specific surgical and nonsurgical therapeutic measures appropriate to the various conditions leading to intestinal obstruction during infancy and childhood are dealt with further in this chapter and elsewhere in the book.

INTUSSUSCEPTION

With incarcerated inguinal hernia, intussusception is the most frequent cause of intestinal obstruction during infancy. Half of the cases occur in the first year of life and the majority of the others in the second year; rare cases have been reported in the first week of life. The condition is three times more common in males. In most instances, the intussusception starts at a point immediately proximal to the ileocecal valve. Thus, at the onset, the invagination is ileocecal: tension on the mesentery is readily established. Invagination further into the colon is known as ileocolic and is by far the most frequent. Other forms include ileoileal and colocolic. The apex of the intussusception is usually found at the level of the hepatic or splenic flexure, or in the midtransverse colon. More rarely it progresses down the descending colon or even protrudes through the anus. As a result of the invagination and impairment of venous return, swelling begins promptly and is

Table 4-2. Age of patients with intussusception and relationship to associated intestinal lesions

Age	Number	Incidence of observed lesions
1-12 months	198 (52.4%)	Meckel's diverticulum: 21 cases
		Ileal polyp: 1 case
1- 2 years	96 (25.4%)	Ileal granuloma: 1 case
2- 3 years	36 (9.5%)	None
3- 6 years	36 (9.5%)	None
> 6 years	12 (3.2%)	Lymphosarcoma: 6 cases
	378	

From the data of Wayne, E.R., Campbell, J.B., Kosloske, A.M., and Burrington, J.D.: J. Pediatr. Surg. **11:**789, 1976.

rapidly followed by hemorrhage, incarceration with necrosis, eventual perforation, and peritonitis.

Etiology

There is considerable current interest in the etiology of intussusception. Overall statistics indicate a specific lesion or disease triggering the intussusception in only 5% or 6% of cases. Table 4-2 attracts attention to the relative importance of specific intestinal lesions in different age groups. Lymphosarcoma in the Denver series is the most frequent (50%) anatomic lesion causing intussusception in children over 6 years of age. Other described lead points besides Meckel's diverticulum, lymphosarcoma, polyps, and lymphoid hyperplasia, include appendiceal stumps, heterotopic pancreatic nodules or gastric mucosa, hemangiomas, parasites, and foreign bodies.

The occurrence of intussusception in patients with cystic fibrosis is relatively common and usually is related to inspissated fecal material in the terminal ileum, appendix, and colon. Henoch-Schönlein purpura with intestinal involvement is a well-known disease associated with intussusception. The relationship of intussusception with hyperplastic Peyer's patches secondary to viral infections has been confirmed. The John Hopkins group reports that 21% of their patients had either otitis media or an upper respiratory infection. Grossly enlarged mesenteric lymph nodes are said to be present in more than a third of the cases without an associated intestinal lesion. The role of adenoviruses in the pathogenesis is further supported by the description of identical twins who presented with intussusception within 24 hours and who had adenoviruses in their appendix and lymph nodes. A study from Japan has convincingly implicated the human rotavirus as an etiologic agent

in a number of cases. Confirmation of this finding is awaited.

Interestingly, some patients suffer small bowel intussusception immediately after an abdominal procedure has been performed. The cause is not clear but is probably related to disturbances in intestinal motility.

Clinical features (Figs. 4-1 and 4-2)

Classically, intussusception occurs in thriving previously healthy infants. However, in one series, 7% of patients had had a attack 10 days to 6 months previously. The affected infant, usually between 3 and 12 months of age, suddenly develops abdominal pain, screams, and draws up his knees. Vomiting occurs soon afterward. He may pass a single normal stool, evacuating the colon distal to the apex of the intussusception. Bouts of colicky pain occur at more or less regular intervals. Vomiting continues. Initially quite normal between episodes of pain, the infant gradually becomes apathetic. A striking degree of lethargy and irritability associated with vomiting may suggest encephalitis as alterations of consciousness ("knocked-out look") may overshadow to a considerable extent the classic intestinal manifestations. Currant jelly bowel movements are noted, especially when diagnosis has been delayed. Severe prostration and fever supervene. The abdomen is tender and becomes distended; on palpation, a sausage-shaped tumor may be found in the upper abdomen (50%), and the right lower quadrant feels strangely empty. With perforation, the pain rapidly decreases in intensity, and signs of peritonitis are noted.

Although the triad of colicky abdominal pain, vomiting, and bloody stools is typical, it is rarely present early (10% in a recent series). All too often the diagnosis of intussusception is not enter-

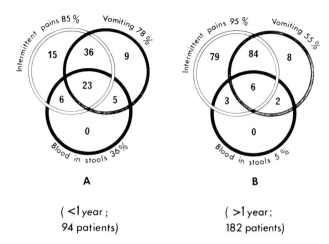

Fig. 4-1. Cardinal symptoms associated with intussusception. The symptoms are grouped according to the age of the patients. (From Gierup, J., Jorulf, H., and Livaditis, A.: Pediatrics **50:**535-546, 1972.)

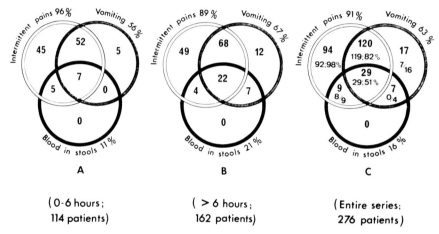

Fig. 4-2. Cardinal symptoms associated with intussusception. The symptoms are grouped according to the time interval between onset of symptoms and the initial consultation. (From Gierup, J., Jorulf, H., and Livaditis, A.: Pediatrics **50:**535-546, 1972.)

tained until bloody stools appear. Abdominal pain may be absent in 13% to 18% cases. Diarrhea may be present and be nonspecific enough to suggest gastroenteritis. Similarly, the constipation noted in 20% of cases may lead the physician astray. The intussusception may persist for several days without creating the picture of complete intestinal obstruction. In these chronic cases, the symptoms may be recurrent attacks of colicky abdominal pain with occasional vomiting. Bouts of chronic constipation or of diarrhea may also occur. Such a clinical picture usually indicates chronic recurrent intussusception with spontaneous reduction (Fig. 4-3).

Diagnosis and treatment

Serious consequences attend the failure to promptly make a diagnosis. It is therefore essential that one closely watch a patient whose aggregation of symptoms does not fit the classic picture. Colicky abdominal pain associated with vomiting constitutes sufficient subjective evidence to warrant close observation and investigation.

As soon as the diagnosis of intussusception is suspected, the child is taken to the x-ray department and, at the same time, is scheduled in the operating room.

Although approximately one third of the patients with intussusception show the intussuscep-

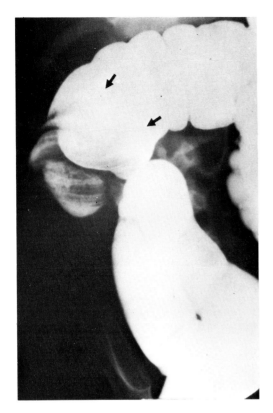

Fig. 4-3. Recurrent bouts of intussusception. A 2-year-old child had a history of six individual bouts of abdominal pain, blood-tinged diarrhea, vomiting, and a 10-pound weight loss during a period of 4 months. A sausage-shaped mass was palpable in the epigastric region. The barium enema shows absence of filling of the ascending colon at the hepatic flexure and the typical "coiled-spring" appearance with a good outline of the intussusception head.

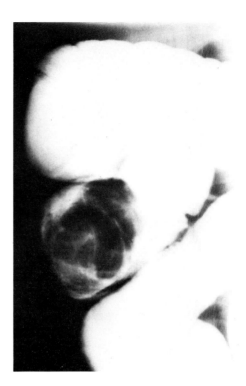

Fig. 4-4. Intussusception. The barium surrounds the intussuscepted mass and demonstrates the classic "coiled-spring" appearance.

tion outlined by colon gas or show evidence of intestinal obstruction in the scout film, the diagnosis must be confirmed by barium enema (Fig. 4-4). No special technique or apparatus is used. The intussusception may be found anywhere from the anus back to the low ileum, but most of them are seen in the transverse colon.

Hydrostatic reduction. Nasogastric suction and intravenous administration of blood or albumin are started. Although some centers advocate sedation or even general anesthesia, we use neither in preparation for hydrostatic reduction, which over the past decade has been the treatment of choice. Most centers report a success rate of at least 75%. The diagnostic enema is merely continued, and the intussusception is observed intermittently with the fluoroscope until the mass completely disappears in the ileum and a long segment (at least

several loops) of ileum becomes filled with barium. Frequently this is accomplished in a few minutes, but occasionally it takes as long as half an hour.

It is our practice to attempt hydrostatic reduction in almost every patient except in those with evidence of peritonitis. Primary operation is also advised when plain abdominal roentgenograms show evidence of intestinal obstruction. According to the Cincinnati group, this may be an indication that the involved bowel may be incarcerated and gangrenous. The age of the patient and the duration of symptoms were not predictive of a complicated intussusception in that series. Significant amounts of bleeding, evidence of intestinal obstruction, or any deterioration of the patient's clinical condition warns us to make the attempt brief and to send the patient quickly to surgery if success is not obtained within a few minutes. The risk of missing a lead point by barium reduction is insignificant, since those cases usually are irreducible.

The success rate in achieving satisfactory hydrostatic reduction is related in part to the experience of the radiologist. The duration of symptoms decreases the chances of successful reduction (more than 48 hours).

1. No attempt should be made at hydrostatic reduction if there are clinical signs of perforation or shock.
2. The barium solution should be allowed to drip by gravity through a Foley bag catheter inserted into the rectum from a height not exceeding 3½ feet above the fluroscopic table.
3. There should be no manipulations of the abdomen during the hydrostatic reduction under fluoroscopic examination for fear of further increasing intraluminal pressure and increasing the risk of perforation.
4. If at any point during the reduction attempt absolutely no progress is made for several minutes, the attempt should be abandoned. The barium is siphoned out by lowering of the barium reservoir to the floor, which allows the infant to evacuate, and two more attempts at reduction can be made. Progress, even if slow, is an indication to continue; on the other hand, arrest of the barium column for 10 minutes is an indication to terminate the attempt.
5. On reduction, there should be free reflux of barium into the ileum to rule out the possibility of a persistent ileoileal intussusception. Because of the amount of barium present, small bowel opacification is often better documented in a film taken after evacuation and should be repeated 24 hours later. Since recurrences are more likely to occur within 36 hours after reduction, we keep the patients in the hospital for 2 or 3 days. It has been recommended that an upper gastrointestinal series be performed after the barium is evacuated in older children (more than 6 years of age), even if the intussusception has been completely reduced.

Surgical treatment. For patients with intussusception for whom hydrostatic reduction is not suitable or for those in whom it is unsuccessful (25%), surgery is performed as soon as an adequate preparation of the patient has been carried out.

Surgery is indicated when, despite apparent complete reduction, the patient's clinical improvement is in doubt. Surgery should also be done when intussusception recurs after barium enema reduction, especially in older children in whom the incidence of a pathologic lesion acting as a lead point is higher. At Hôpital Sainte-Justine in Montreal, lead points were found in 11 out of a recent series of 12 patients suffering intussusception after the age of 4 years. When no specific cause is found to explain the recurrence, the subsequent recurrence rate after surgery is not any different from that reported after barium enema reduction alone (4% to 10%).

Prognosis

Intussusception is uniformly fatal if reduction is not accomplished. Overall mortality stands at around 1% or 2%.

REFERENCES

Bergdahl, S., Hugosson, C., Lauren, T., and Söderlund, S.: Atypical intussusception, J. Pediatr. Surg. **7:**700-705, 1972.

Bjarnason, G., and Pettersson, G.: The treatment of intussusception: thirty years' experience at Gothenburg's Children's Hospital, J. Pediatr. Surg. **3:**19-23, 1968.

Ein, S.H., and Stephens, C.A.: Intussusception: 354 cases in 10 years, J. Pediatr. Surg. **6:**16-27, 1971.

Gierup, J., Jorulf, H., and Livaditis, A.: Management of intussusception in infants and children: a survey based on 288 consecutive cases, Pediatrics **50:**535-546, 1972.

Hutchison, I.F., Olayiwola, B., and Young, D.G.: Intussusception in infancy and childhood, Br. J. Surg. **67:**209-212, 1980.

Konno, T., Suzuki, H., Kutsuzawa, T., and others: Human rotavirus and intussusception [Letter to the editor], N. Engl. J. Med. **297:**945, 1977.

McGovern, J.B., and Gross, R.E.: Intussusception as postoperative complication, Surgery **63:**507-513, 1968.

Ravitch, M.M.: Intussusception. In Ravitch, M.M., Welch, K.J., Benson, C.D., Aberdeen, E., and Randolph, J.G., editors: Pediatric surgery, ed. 3, Chicago, 1979, Year Book Medical Publishers, Inc.

Rosenkrantz, J.G., Cox, J.A., Silverman, F.N., and Martin, L.W.: Intussception in the 1970's: indications for operation, J. Pediatr. Surg. **12:**367-373, 1977.

Singer, J.: Altered consciousness as an early manifestation of intussusception, Pediatrics **64:**93-95, 1979.

Thomas, G.G., and Zachary, R.B.: Intussusception in twins, Pediatrics **58**(5):754-756, 1976.

Wayne, E.R., Campbell, J.B., Burrington, J.D., and Davis, W.S.: Management of 344 children with intussusception, Radiology **107:**597-601, 1973.

Wayne, E.R., Campbell, J.B., Kosloske, A.M., and Burrington, J.D.: Intussusception in the older child: suspect lymphosarcoma, J. Pediatr. Surg. **11:**789-794, 1976.

Yoo, R.P., and Touloukian, R.J.: Intussusception in the newborn: a unique clinical entity, J. Pediatr. Surg. **9:**495-498, 1974.

INGUINAL HERNIA

A peritoneal sac precedes the testicle as it descends from the genital ridge to the scrotum. The lower portion of this sack (processus vaginalis) envelops the testis to form the tunica vaginalis, and the remainder normally atrophies.

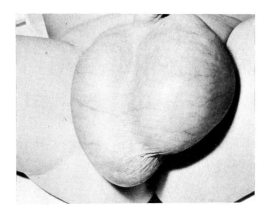

Fig. 4-5. Inguinal hernia. Both large bilateral hydroceles appeared gradually in a young infant during a period of a few weeks. They were not tender nor reducible and did transmit light. The mother reported that the "testes were larger" when the child cried. Since the history was that of a communicating hydrocele, surgery was recommended.

The processus vaginalis is said to be patent in 57% of 1-year-old children examined after death; it provides, therefore, the congenital defect leading to the indirect type of inguinal hernia seen in children. A hernia does not exist, however, unless some parts of the abdominal contents are pushed into the open sac.

Persistence of the processus vaginalis becomes manifest as a mass in the inguinal region when an abdominal structure or peritoneal fluid is forced into the scrotum (Fig. 4-5). In some cases, peritoneal fluid may become trapped in the tunica vaginalis of the testis (noncommunicating hydrocele). If the processus vaginalis remains open, peritoneal fluid (hydrocele of the spermatic cord, or the canal of Nuck in the female), or an abdominal structure may be forced into it (indirect inguinal hernia). The content of the hernia sac is usually the small intestine. The appendix and Meckel's diverticulum are occasionally found. Of note is the observation that, of 94 cases of acute appendicitis occurring in the first 30 days of life, 27 were found in a hernial sac and 18 of these were incarcerated. They all occurred in boys. In girls, it is common to find a fallopian tube and ovary. It is important to note that about 2% of phenotypic females with an inguinal hernia have a feminizing testis. The gonad can be palpated in the labium.

Most inguinal hernias are of the indirect type. Direct inguinal hernias are rarely seen in children. They are usually large and have been described in association with exstrophy of the bladder and in infants after repair of an indirect inguinal hernia.

Indirect inguinal hernias occur much more frequently in boys than in girls (8:1), but this ratio decreases to 4:1 in infants. Hernias may be present at birth; close to 40% become apparent before the age of 6 months. The frequency of hernias is increased in prematures (5%). The incidence is reportedly very high (30%) in infants of very low birth weight weighing less than 1000 gm. Increased intra-abdominal pressure (ascites) is also a very strong predisposing factor. Inguinal hernia is important because it is the most common cause of intestinal obstruction in infants from the end of the first week of life to the age of 4 months, after which age it is second only to intussusception.

Clinical features

There are no symptoms associated with an empty hernial sac. In most cases, the hernia is manifested as a painless inguinal swelling that is classically absent when the child is sleeping and increases in size when he strains and coughs. Careful inspection of both sides of the groin will indicate a small lump beneath a thick layer of adipose tissue. Mild external pressure is sufficient to bring about reentry of the herniated bowel into the abdominal cavity. Physical findings are quite often nonexistent, and one is forced to rely on parental observation of the hernia.

When the contents of a hernial sac cannot be reduced, the hernia is said to be incarcerated. In children, changes in the blood supply and partial or complete intestinal obstruction almost invariably follow incarceration. The clinical features in such cases (25%) are more striking. There is a sudden appearance of a mass in the groin or scrotum. Tenderness and pain in that area lead to intermittent or continuous crying. Nausea, vomiting, and abdominal distention are commonly present.

Hernia is much less frequent in girls. However, in those who do suffer hernia, incarceration is much more frequent than in boys.

Differential diagnosis

An inguinal mass may represent lymph nodes. A hydrocele of the cord is not tender, is not reducible, does transmit light, and is oblong in shape. An undescended testis may be moved along the canal into the upper part of the scrotum. Torsion of the cord or of the appendix testis is more frequent in the undescended testis and may be difficult to differentiate clinically from an incarcerated

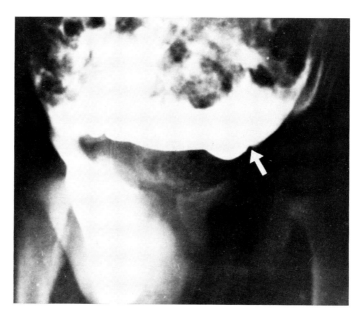

Fig. 4-6. Herniography demonstrating a right inguinoscrotal hernia-hydrocele. There is no hernia on the left. *Arrow,* Notch formed by the impression of the recurrent epigastric vessels marking the medial border of the hernial sac. (Courtesy F.M. Guttman, J.C. Ducharme, and R. Bertrand, Hôpital Sainte-Justine, Montreal.)

hernia. A hydrocele around the testis is most commonly of the communicating type and is almost always associated with a hernia.

Treatment

Repair of a hernia should be carried out as soon as possible, unless prematurity or other conditions preclude surgery. There is still some controversy as to the advisability of exploration of the opposite side. Because the processus vaginalis is patent in the contralateral side in close to 80% during the first 3 months and in more than 50% up to the age of 16, many centers explore the asymptomatic side. However a contralateral hernia occurs over the next few months or years in only 18% to 20% of cases. Consequently the justification for bilateral repair is still contested. A recent long-term study of 160 infants with an inguinal hernia has revealed that 29% developed a hernia on the opposite side during a mean follow-up period of 20 years. Age at the time of the initial repair had no influence, but the patient's chance of requiring contralateral repair went up to 41% if the first operation was for a left-sided hernia and came down to 14% in the case of an initial right-sided hernia.

Inguinal herniography can be used to detect the children with a unilateral inguinal hernia who have a contralateral patent processus vaginalis. The experience at Hôpital Sainte-Justine in Montreal, with more than 1000 cases, is that this technique accurately and safely identifies children who have a hernia by history alone and those who are potential candidates for bilateral repair. Essentially, the technique delineates radiographically the patent processus vaginalis after the injection of contrast material into the peritoneal cavity (Fig. 4-6). Girls with inguinal hernias should have a biopsy of the gonad in the hernial sac and also buccal smears to rule out a feminizing testis.

Incarcerated inguinal hernias occur most often during the first 6 months of life. Manipulative reduction with gentle digital pressure can be attempted after sedation of the child with intramuscular administration of 1 mg/kg of meperidine and placing him in a Trendelenburg position with an ice bag on the affected side. Herniotomy should then be carried out after 48 hours. This conservative treatment is contraindicated if the incarcerated hernia has led to continuous crying, vomiting, distention, and local redness and edema or if bloody stools are noted. In such a situation, surgery should be carried out on an emergency basis.

REFERENCES

Bar-Maor, J.A., and Zeltzer, M.: Acute appendicitis located in a scrotal hernia of a premature infant, J. Pediatr. Surg. **13:**181-182, 1978.

Guttman, F.M., Bertrand, R., and Ducharme, J.C.: Herniography and the pediatric contralateral hernia, Surg. Gynecol. Obstet. **135:**531-555, 1972.

Harper, R.G., Garcia, A., and Sia, C.: Inguinal hernia: a common problem of premature infants weighing 1000 grams or less at birth, Pediatrics **56:**112-115, 1975.

James, P.M.: The problem of hernia in infants and children, Surg. Clin. North Am. **51:**1361-1370, 1971.

Kuhn, J.P.: Herniography in perspective, Am. J. Dis. Child. **131:**1206-1208, 1977.

McGregor, D.B., Halverson, K., and McVay, C.B.: The unilateral pediatric inguinal hernia: should the contralateral side be explored, J. Pediatr. Surg. **15:**313-317, 1980.

Rowe, M.I., and Clatworthy, H.W.: The other side of the pediatric inguinal hernia, Surg. Clin. North Am. **51:**1371-1376, 1971.

Srouji, M.N., and Buck, B.E.: Neonatal appendicitis: ischemic infarction in incarcerated inguinal hernia, J. Pediatr. Surg. **13:**177-179, 1978.

Viidik, T., and Marshall, D.G.: Direct inguinal hernias in infancy and early childhood, J. Pediatr. Surg. **15:**646-647, 1980.

INTERNAL HERNIA

Internal hernias are much rarer in the pediatric age group than in adults. They usually become evident as intestinal obstructions or as peritonitis in the first few months of life. In older infants and in children, the symptoms may mimic recurrent bouts of intussusception or recurrent abdominal pain.

Whereas most adult internal hernias are paraduodenal, the common ones in children are retrocecal or transmesenteric. The former is brought about by the herniation of small bowel loops behind the cecum through a breach in the posterior attachment of the ascending colon. The roentgenogram may show small bowel lying to the right of the ascending colon and pushing it medially. In the transmesenteric variety, the small bowel herniates through a breach in the mesentery. There is usually abdominal distention localized in the upper half of the abdomen. A flat film may show bunched upper small bowel loops distended by air and fluid in the upper abdomen and no air present in the rest of the small bowel and colon.

The association of internal hernias with cystic fibrosis and ileal atresia has been reported.

REFERENCES

Deffrenne, P.: Les hernies internes du nouveau-né et du nourrisson, Ann. Chir. Infantile **11:**319-328, 1970.

Moore, T.C.: Internal hernia with high jejunal obstruction in infancy due to adhesions from antenatal meconium peritonitis, J. Pediatr. Surg. **8:**971-972, 1973.

Murphy, D. A.: Internal hernias in infancy and childhood, Surgery **55:**311-316, 1964.

Touloukian, R.: Miscellaneous causes of small bowel obstruction. In Ravitch, M.M., Welch, K.J., Benson, C.D., Aberdeen, E., and Randolph, J.G., editors: Pediatric surgery, ed. 3, Chicago, 1979, Year Book Medical Publishers, Inc.

Zer, M., and Dintsman, M.: Incarcerated "foramen of Winslow" hernia in a newborn, J. Pediatr. Surg. **8:**325, 1973.

PERITONITIS
Primary peritonitis

Primary peritonitis is an acute inflammatory process of the peritoneal cavity for which local spread from inflammation or perforation of an intra-abdominal viscus cannot be demonstrated.

Incidence and pathogenesis

The incidence of primary peritonitis has decreased with the advent of antibiotics. It currently accounts for fewer than 1% of "acute abdomens" in pediatric hospitals. A 10-year survey of 26 cases in Cleveland reports 6 cases in the first 2 months of life. The average age of the 20 others was 8.5 years. There were two times more girls than boys in the former group, whereas in the latter the ratio was 1.2 to 1 in favor of girls. Gram-negative bacteria accounted for 70% of the infecting organisms. The most commonly cultured organism from the ascitic fluid was *Escherichia coli.* Streptococci and pneumococci were grown from only five and four cases, respectively. This is in contrast with earlier reports showing that the predominant organisms were either pneumococci or streptococci.

Half of the infants had extensive pneumonias. Associated diseases and infections in the other group included urinary tract infection in 10 cases, nephrotic syndrome in four, postnecrotic cirrhosis in three, hydronephrosis, cystic fibrosis, and adrenogenital syndrome in one patient each. Other series have underscored the particular risk for primary pneumococcal peritonitis in nephrotics and infants and children after a splenectomy. The incidence of primary peritonitis in adult cirrhotics with ascites reaches 10%; it is certainly much lower in children, but we have seen cases in biliary cirrhosis as well as in post necrotic cirrhosis. The diagnosis should also be entertained in patients with decreased immunologic competence, inborn or acquired, and in those with a focus for bacteremia such as a central catheter. There is still some controversy concerning the pathogenesis of primary peritonitis though hematogenous spread is probably involved in most cases.

Clinical findings

No matter what the underlying illness or state of health, the onset is usually rapid, with severe abdominal pain, vomiting, and prostration. The child is toxic. The temperature is septic in type and may be as high as 104° or 105° F. The pulse rate is rapid and the respirations shallow.

There is usually abdominal distention, diffuse tenderness, and rigidity or a doughy resistance similar to the peritoneal signs associated with pancreatitis. Free fluid may be elicited from the patient with nephrosis or cirrhosis. Rectal examination indicates tenderness. Diarrhea sometimes occurs, particularly in the young patient. In contrast to the ileus associated with a perforated appendix, bowel sounds may still be audible in these patients.

Diagnosis

A history of nephrosis, splenectomy, or chronic liver disease should alert the clinician to the possibility of primary peritonitis. A significant degree of proteinuria may help in the identification of the rare cases of nephrosis presenting initially with primary peritonitis.

The physical signs can be very similar to those associated with appendicitis or pelvic inflammatory disease. However, the white blood cell count is much more elevated (from 20,000 to 50,000). One should entertain the diagnosis in the child with peritoneal signs developing in less than 24 hours who is suspected of a urinary tract infection. A gram stain and culture of the urine should be done immediately.

The differential diagnosis includes familial Mediterranean fever and idiopathic panniculitis because peritonitis is the most common initial manifestation of these entities. A few milliliters of cloudy peritoneal fluid may be obtained from a patient with these diseases, but the Gram stain and the culture are negative for organisms.

Treatment

A diagnostic paracentesis can be safely made in all patients in whom primary peritonitis is suspected. It should be the procedure leading to the diagnosis. Normally ascitic fluid contains less than 300 leukocytes and 75 polymorphonuclear cells per cubic millimeter. The presence of red blood cells is indicative of a bloody tap and invalidates these normal values.

In the absence of specific clinical and radiological signs (free air, calcifications, localized air-fluid levels) indicative of peritoneal sepsis, conservative management is in order. A rational choice of the appropriate antibiotic or antibiotics to be administered intravenously is made on the basis of the Gram stain and of cultures. The Gram stain is helpful in 50% of cases, and cultures of the organism can be expected to grow in 90% of cases. If the gram stain is unrewarding, the combination of ampicillin, clindamycin, and gentamicin is advocated before the results of peritoneal, urine, and blood cultures are available.

Prognosis

Before the antibiotic era, 50% to 100% of such patients died. The prognosis at the present time is good except in the primary peritonitis associated with postnecrotic cirrhosis, in which the pneumococcal infection is likely to be associated with the end stage of liver disease.

REFERENCES

Conn, H.O.: Spontaneous bacterial peritonitis: multiple revisitations [editorial], Gastroenterology **70**:455-457, 1976.

Epstein, M., Calia, F.M., and Gabrizda, G.J.: Pneumococcal peritonitis in patients with postnecrotic cirrhosis, N. Engl. J. Med. **278**:69-73, 1968.

Fowler, R. Jr.: Primary peritonitis: changing aspects 1956-1970, Aust. Pediatr. J. **7**:73-83, 1971.

Golden, G.T., and Shaw, A.: Primary peritonitis, Surg. Gynecol. Obstet. **135**:513-516, 1972.

Harken, A.H., and Shochat, S.J.: Gram-positive peritonitis in children, Am. J. Surg. **125**:769-772, 1973.

McDougal, W.S., Izant, R.J., and Zollinger, R.M.: Primary peritonitis in infancy and childhood, Ann. Surg. **181**:310-313, 1975.

Sohar, E., Gafni, J., Pras, M., and Heller, H.: Familial Mediterranean fever, Am. J. Med. **43**:227-253, 1967.

Tal, Y., Berger, A., Abrahamson, J., and others: Intestinal obstruction caused by primary adhesions due to familial Mediterranean fever, J. Pediatr. Surg. **15**:186-187, 1980.

Secondary peritonitis

An inflammatory response to bacteria, bile, or pancreatic enzymes is set up in the peritoneal cavity as a consequence of an abscessed or ruptured intra-abdominal viscus.

Pathophysiology

If the inflammatory process is not promptly localized, the entire peritoneal surface becomes involved. Since this surface can approximate one half the body's surface, it provides a large exudative area that may rapidly lead to the sequestration of a significant amount of extracellular fluid in the peritoneal cavity. A further cause of reduction of circulatory volume and shock is the increased loss of body fluids in the distended lumen of the adynamic bowel. The patient looks ill and rapidly becomes toxic.

Peritonitis produces pain. There are signs of generalized or localized tenderness. The abdominal wall protects against any movement of the inflamed visceral and parietal peritoneal surfaces by "muscular guarding," and the child assumes a "position of comfort" that will reduce to a minimum intra-abdominal pressure changes. Vomiting will precede stool changes. Small, loose stools may initially be passed but will be followed by signs of paralytic ileus, abdominal distention, and complete cessation of evacuation of stools and of expulsion of gas.

Etiology

In general, peritonitis secondary to perforations of enteric organs are attributable to congenital or acquired mechanical obstructions in infants, whereas infections or an inflammatory process are etiologic in children. Most cases of secondary peritonitis occur during the first months of life. A rough compilation of recent series reveal that 60% are caused by necrotizing enterocolitis and 20% to a spontaneous perforation of the stomach. In childhood, there is a much higher incidence of perforation of the appendix and secondary peritonitis in boys. Peritonitis may also be secondary to trauma or foreign-body rupture of a hollow viscus. More rarely, peptic ulcer, cholecystitis, pancreatitis, volvulus, intussusception, strangulated hernia, Meckel's diverticulum, mesenteric cyst, duplications of the gastrointestinal tract, trauma, regional enteritis, or chronic ulcerative colitis will lead to peritonitis.

The invading bacteria are usually enteric organisms; the ability of the host to localize the infection is dependent to some extent on the number of organisms spilled into the peritoneal cavity, but perhaps more importantly on the age of the patient. That localization is less likely to take place in infants and young children than in older people has been attributed to the former's relatively shorter omentum. If localization occurs, it is likely to be appendiceal, pelvic, subhepatic, or subphrenic.

The microbiology of intra-abdominal sepsis depends on the nature of the microflora of the perforated organ. In contrast to that of patients with primary peritonitis, multiple aerobic and anaerobic organisms are grown from most (65% to 75%) cases. The most frequently identified aerobes include *Escherichia coli, Klebsiella, Proteus,* and *Enterobacter. Bacteroides fragilis* is the major representative of the anaerobic flora. The same types of bacteria are isolated from abcesses in different intra-abdominal locations.

Clinical findings

The signs are those of a ruptured viscus and of an underlying obstructive or inflammatory process complicated by a severe degree of toxemia. The patient suffers restlessness, irritability, chills, and a high fever. Abdominal pain is diffuse; however, in the child with appendicitis or an obstructive intestinal lesion, such as volvulus or intussusception, perforation may bring about a relative and short-lived diminution of the severity of abdominal pain.

The child looks anxious, the pulse is rapid, and respiration may be quite superficial from splinting of the diaphragm. There is abdominal rigidity and rectal tenderness. At times, containment of the peritoneal suppuration may limit the tenderness to one particular area and permit palpation of an abdominal or rectal mass. When an abscess is formed, adjacent loops of bowel cover the area, limiting the extension of the infection. In older children, the omentum covers the abscess.

Clinical features of special intra-abdominal abscesses

In general, localized infections of the peritoneal cavity are indistinguishable from retroperitoneal abscesses. Intestinal obstruction is not necessarily complete, and abdominal findings in the absence of a mass are not always easily characterized. The evolution may be a course of several days or weeks, with periods of remission interspersed with exacerbations. Most commonly, there is a history of a recent abdominal operation or of abdominal symptoms treated with antibiotics.

Pelvic abscess. An appendiceal infection may give rise to a pelvic abscess with tenesmus, urinary frequency, constipation, or diarrhea.

Appendiceal abscess. The perforated appendix gives rise to a fever higher than that seen with acute appendicitis. Either generalized or localized peritonitis may develop. If localized, the para-appendiceal abscess may lessen in severity after a few days of antibiotic treatment and produce only mild pain. Symptoms may be related to the urinary tract. On physical examination, the right lower quadrant is tender, and a mass is palpated.

Subdiaphragmatic (subphrenic) abscess. A ruptured intra-abdominal viscus may lead to the formation of a subdiaphragmatic abscess. Respiratory signs predominate. There is splinting of the diaphragm, with reduced respiratory excursions, shoulder or back pain, and elevation of the diaphragm. There may be pleural fluid. A pocket of air can sometimes be seen below the diaphragm.

Diagnosis

Distinguishing between primary and secondary peritonitis is largely based on the patient's history. In the absence of a background suggestive of primary or secondary peritonitis, the differential diagnosis can often be impossible to make. Plain abdominal roentgenograms may help to localize the site of an intra-abdominal abscess, but ultrasonography and radioactive scanning greatly facilitate the diagnosis. Specimens of peritoneal fluid should be collected and transferred under appropriate conditions for aerobic and anaerobic culture. Blood cultures are important because they can be expected to be positive in a significant number of cases, particularly in infants where the incidence is about 30%.

Acute pelvic inflammatory disease is very difficult to differentiate from appendiceal infections. The patient may admit clandestine sexual experience only very reluctantly. It is helpful to remember that menstrual problems and the onset of symptoms during or right after a menstrual period are frequently documented in pelvic inflammatory disease.

When confronted with an "acute abdomen," it is essential that the clinician keep in mind the number of medical diseases in childhood that have components of abdominal pain severe enough to mimic peritonitis.

Mumps, diabetic ketoacidosis, acute rheumatic fever, Henoch-Schönlein purpura, sickle-cell anemia, hemophilia with retroperitoneal or intraperitoneal bleeding, pancreatitis, right lower-lobe pneumonia, herpes zoster, and lead poisoning are well-known causes of the "acute medical abdomen" giving rise to severe generalized abdominal pain. Special attention should be paid to acute pyelonephritis and the early stage of acute gastroenteritis (shigellosis and salmonellosis particu-

larly). Refer to the section on the "acute abdomen" at the end of this chapter for a more complete discussion.

Treatment

Adequate preoperative preparation is essential and is oriented toward rehydration, correction of blood volume, and gastric suction. Pain should be relieved with meperidine. As soon as the diagnosis is made, the combination ampicillin, clindamycin, and gentamicin should be started. When peritoneal and blood culture results become available, appropriate changes should be made if the data so indicate.

The operative management consists in removal or repair of the responsible abscessed or perforated viscus, drainage of the localized abscess, or, in the case of a generalized peritonitis, lavage with saline solution and antimicrobial agents. In certain circumstances, the nonsurgical management of gastrointestinal perforations is recommended. This approach consists in dependent peritoneal drainage carried out under local anesthesia and is reserved for those patients who are considered poor operative risks. This is particularly advocated in small very sick premature infants with perforation secondary to necrotizing enterocolitis.

The prevention of postoperative intra-abdominal sepsis depends primarily on good surgical technique but also on the nature of the underlying disease and its duration, as well as on the defense mechanisms of the host (nutritional and immune status). Antibiotic prophylaxis has a place in the prevention and should be given preoperatively and during the operation. They will provide adequate antibiotic tissue levels in infants and children suspected or identified as having an enteric perforation to prevent intraperitoneal spread, distant dissemination, and wound infections.

Prognosis

The mortality is probably less than 10%.

REFERENCES

Bell, M.J., Ternberg, J.L., and Bower, R.J.: The microbial flora and antimicrobial therapy of neonatal peritonitis, J. Pediatr. Surg. **15:**569-573, 1980.

Emanuel, B., Zlotnik, P., and Raffensperger, J.G.: Perforation of the gastrointestinal tract in infancy and childhood, Surg. Gynecol. Obstet. **146:**926-928, 1978.

Fock, G., Gästrin, U., and Josephson, S.: Appendiceal peritonitis in children, Acta Chir. Scand. **135:**534-538, 1969.

Holgersen, L.A., and Stanley-Brown, E.G.: Acute appendicitis with perforation, Am. J. Dis. Child. **122:**288-293, 1971.

Janik, J.S., and Ein, S.H.: Peritoneal drainage under local anesthesia for necrotizing enterocolitis perforation: a second look, J. Pediatr. Surg. **15**:565-568, 1980.

Leonidas, J.C., Krasna, I.H., Fox, H.A., and Broder, M.S.: Peritoneal fluid in necrotizing enterocolitis; a radiologic sign of clinical deterioration, J. Pediatr. **82**:672-675, 1973.

Makker, S.P., Tucker, A.S., Izant, R.L., and Heyman, W.: Nonobstructive hydronephrosis and hydroureter associated with peritonitis, N. Engl. J. Med. **287**:535-537, 1971.

McDougal, W.S., Izant, R.I., and Zollinger, R.M.: Primary peritonitis in infancy and childhood, Ann. Surg. **181**:310-313, 1975.

Nichols, R.L.: Infections following gastrointestinal surgery: intra-abdominal abscess, Surg. Clin. North Am. **60**:197-212, 1980.

Sells, C.J., and Loeser, J.D.: Peritonitis following perforation of the bowel: a rare complication of a ventriculoperitoneal shunt, J. Pediatr, **83**:823-824, 1973.

Shandling, B., Ein, S.H., Simpson, J.S., and others: Perforating appendicitis and antibiotics, J. Pediatr. Surg. **9**:79-83, 1974.

GASTRIC AND SIGMOID VOLVULUS

Volvulus of the small bowel occurring after the neonatal period in patients with anomalies of rotation (malrotation long mesentery), congenital defects (Meckel's diverticulum, persistent omphalomesenteric band, mesenteric cyst), or acquired conditions (adhesions), or, in rare cases, without apparent cause is discussed under the description of each entity.

Gastric volvulus

Acute gastric volvulus is one of the least common causes of alimentary tract obstruction in infants and children (51 cases up to 1981). The stomach rotates on itself about an axis joining the lesser and greater curvatures, with the pylorus going from right to left anteriorly and superiorly. Plain films showing a double fluid level or a medial "beak" of narrowing superiorly may suggest the diagnosis, which one can confirm by showing an "upside down" stomach with an obstructed distal segment (Fig. 4-7). Immediate surgery is indicated. At operation, mesenteroaxial volvulus is found and reduced. There are rarer instances of organoaxial volvulus where the stomach rotates around its long axis usually from left to right anteriorly. A third of cases occur in the absence of associated anomalies. The cause of this anomaly is unclear; it has been linked to prematurity and chronic respiratory problems in the face of large volumes of feedings. A recent series of 12 infants suggests that conservative management (orthostatic positioning and thickened feedings) may result in prompt disappearance of the symptoms. Absence or abnormal laxity of the gastrocolic and

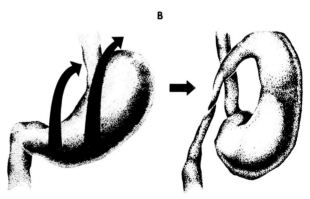

Fig. 4-7. Mesenteroaxial volvulus of the stomach. **A,** Upright anteroposterior roentgenogram of the abdomen showing a large air-fluid level, *clear arrows.* A beaklike projection of air is noted medially, *arrow.* The left hemidiaphragm is elevated. **B,** In mesenteroaxial volvulus, the stomach rotates anteriorly about the axis perpendicular to the long axis of the stomach. In other cases (not shown here) the stomach rotates about its long axis (organoaxial volvulus). (Courtesy J.B. Campbell, The Children's Hospital, Denver.)

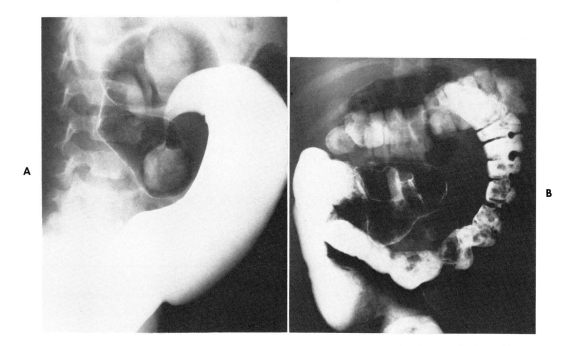

Fig. 4-8. Volvulus of the sigmoid in a 5-year-old boy with chronic constipation who had a sudden onset of colicky abdominal pain and nausea. The barium enema shows an incomplete obstruction of the sigmoid colon, which ends in a beaklike fashion, **A.** The postreduction film demonstrates a sigmoid colon lying in the right side of the abdomen and vulnerable to volvulus because of its increased length, **B.**

gastrosplenic ligaments has been noted. A further predisposing factor is eventration of the diaphragm or a previously repaired hernia of the left hemidiaphragm.

Although malrotation has been suggested as an etiologic factor, there is only a single report of this association. It concerns a 2-year-old child who suddenly developed abdominal pain and vomiting. At operation he had gastric volvulus, midgut volvulus, and pancreatitis.

Acute gastric volvulus will give rise to severe pain, upper abdominal distention, and retching. Vomiting may be scant or totally absent in cases where the volvulus is complete since there is occlusion of both the pylorus and cardia. Needle decompression may be necessary because a nasogastric tube cannot be passed. A challenging form of the disease is the chronic intermittent type of gastric volvulus. Intermittent upper abdominal pain with vomiting are the presenting symptoms. Gastropexy is curative.

Sigmoid volvulus

Although rare in children, sigmoid volvulus is a frequent cause of large bowel obstruction in adults. The sigmoid undergoes a counterclockwise rotation on itself, leading to obstruction of strangulation of the loop. Congestion and edema rapidly ensue and lead to gangrene if detorsion of the volvulus does not occur. It is much more frequent (6 to 1) in boys than in girls.

Clinical findings

The clinical picture is dominated by the occurrence of severe abdominal pain. That a child of school age has previously experienced a similar attack is not unusual. Chronic constipation is believed to be a predisposing factor (Fig. 4-8). It has been described in those with encopresis and with Hirschsprung's disease. We have also seen a few cases in whom a long redundant sigmoid colon was attributable to the consumption of a high-residue vegetarian diet. The sudden onset of cramping pain particularly in the lower abdomen of a child who is older than usual for intussusception suggests volvulus of the sigmoid. The abdominal pain starts abruptly, is usually colicky, and tends to increase as the sigmoid distends with air and fluid. Vomiting is commonly reported. On physical examination, the abdomen is distended and tender, and a mass may be palpable. The rectum is usually empty, and bleeding is uncommon. Signs of peritonitis may supervene after a few hours, but fortunately this complication is rare.

Plain films of the abdomen may show a dilated gas-filled loop of bowel and the absence of gas in the rectum. Use of a barium enema is usually necessary for diagnosis of this entity. Barium enema shows the sigmoid colon to have a more circular pattern than usual. At the junction of the sigmoid and the left colon, the column of barium stops as it tapers to a twisted point similar to the snakehead configuration seen in adults.

Treatment and prognosis

In children, the condition tends to develop rapidly, with a progressive or intermittent course. The physician's alertness to this condition is necessary for an early diagnosis.

Most of the cases of sigmoid volvulus can be reduced within a few minutes by the hydrostatic pressure of a barium enema. Sigmoidoscopy is commonly used in adults and successfully reduces the volvulus in two thirds of cases. Although the rate of recurrence is very high in adults, this does not seem to be the case in children. Elective sigmoid resection advocated for adults has no place for pediatric patients. Surgery should be reserved for patients in whom hydrostatic reduction is impossible and for those who have signs of peritonitis or perforation.

REFERENCES

Arnold, G.J., and Nance, F.C.: Volvulus of the sigmoid colon, Ann. Surg. **177:**527-537, 1973.
Asch, M.J., and Sherman, N.J.: Gastric volvulus in children: report of two cases, J. Pediatr. Surg. **12:**1059-1062, 1977.
Buts, J.P., Claus, D., Beguin, J.C., and Otte, J.B.: Acute and chronic sigmoid volvulus in childhood: report of three cases, Z. Kinderchir. Grenzgeb. **29:**29-33, 1980.
Campbell, J.B., Rappaport, L.N., and Sherker, L.B.: Acute mesentero-axial volvulus of the stomach, Radiology **103:**153-156, 1972.
Cole, B.C., and Dickinson, S.J.: Acute volvulus of the stomach in infants and children, Surgery **70:**707-717, 1971.
Dine, M.S., and Martin, L.W.: Malrotation with gastric volvulus, midgut volvulus and pancreatitis, Am. J. Dis. Child. **131:**1345-1346, 1977.
Eggermont, E., Devlieger, H., Marchal, G., and others: Chronic organo-axial twisting of the stomach in infants born prematurely and affected by chronic respiratory disease, Acta Paediatr. Belg. **33:**233-242, 1980.
Hunter, J.G., and Keats, T.E.: Sigmoid volvulus in children, Am. J. Roentgenol. Radium Ther. Nucl. Med. **108:**621-623, 1970.
Keramidas, D.C., Skondras, C., Anagnostou, D., and Voy-atzis, N.: Volvulus of the sigmoid colon, J. Pediatr. Surg. **14:**479-480, 1979.
Shepherd, J.J.: Treatment of volvulus of sigmoid colon: a review of 425 cases, Br. Med. J. **1:**280-283, 1968.
Wilk, P.J., Ross, M., and Leonidas, J.: Sigmoid volvulus in an 11-year-old girl, Am. J. Dis. Child. **127:**400-402, 1974.

ACUTE ABDOMINAL INJURIES

Trauma is the leading cause of death and disability in children. Accidents account for 40% of the annual deaths of children and adolescents in the United States. In addition to the 13,000 children killed annually, an estimated 100,000 are permanently disabled. Motor vehicles account for 40% of the fatalities.

Since accidental injuries and willful physical abuse by adults constitute an increasing problem in the pediatric population, the incidence of traumatic injury of the gastrointestinal tract is also climbing. In fact, abdominal trauma is documented in most children brought to the hospital after serious injury. Blunt abdominal trauma is the most common form of abdominal trauma and occurs in close to 5% of all childhood accidents.

Young children are especially susceptible to the effects of trauma. Intra-abdominal solid organs are proportionately of larger size and poorly protected by a flexible lower rib cage, a small pelvis, a thin abdominal wall, and relatively little perineal, omental, and mesenteric fat.

Neonatal period

Severe intra-abdominal injuries occurring during the newborn period are relatively rare. Postmortem studies in newborn infants show that a little more than 1% of neonatal deaths are attributable to the laceration of an intra-abdominal organ and hemorrhage. Listlessness, rapid respirations in conjunction with fullness of the abdomen, an abdominal mass, and a rapidly developing anemia are characteristic signs. The incidence of trauma increases in proportion to the size of the infant and would perhaps be more frequent in breech deliveries. A ruptured spleen usually gives immediate signs, though delayed rupture has been reported. Subcapsular hematomas of the liver secondary to a laceration of the liver are quite common, especially if there have been manual attempts at resuscitation. Kidney injuries give rise to retroperitoneal hematomas. Peritoneal taps are helpful in making a diagnosis, and emergency surgery is indicated. Iatrogenic injuries account for a small percentage of intra-abdominal injuries in this age group. Assisted ventilation may lead to gastric distention and rupture. Insertion of a thermometer or of a monitoring probe into the relatively short retroperitoneal canal carries a risk for perforation of the rectum.

Childhood

The peak age during which a child sustains abdominal trauma is between 6 and 8 years. In 65% of cases, the child is struck by a vehicle. Blunt abdominal trauma is, by far, the most common form of abdominal injury. Penetrating wounds are seen in less than 10% of cases. When trauma is isolated to the abdomen, it is the result of a fall in 80% of cases. In cases where multiple injuries are present, traffic accidents are the usual (60%) cause.

Adolescence

In the teen years, the peak incidence is between 15 and 18 years of age. Penetrating injuries (stab and gunshot wounds) outnumber blunt trauma. Close to 50% of cases are attributable to automobile accidents, with the adolescent being an occupant. Sports account for only a fifth of all injuries in this age group.

Clinical findings

Careful history taking is important when one is documenting the type of injury and its extent and severity, especially since, in most instances, there is little external evidence of internal injury.

An exact description of the accident will provide important clues. Falls against objects such as the handlebar of a bicycle or the edge of a table, a direct blow to the abdomen (head, foot, or fist) or visible extra-abdominal injuries all carry a risk for serious intra-abdominal injuries. In the case of the child who has been struck by an automobile, the speed of the vehicle and the site of the initial impact in relationship with the place where the body was found need to be documented.

The physical examination provides key information. It is on this basis that the decision for or against operative intervention is made. Overall inspection and assessment of the patient's condition are the most important initial steps. Vital signs, the level of consciousness, the type of breathing, evidence of splinting of the abdominal musculature, and the presence of abdominal distention or of a superficial injury to the abdomen should be monitored. The rib cage should be carefully examined, and bowel sounds will also provide an important clue. Palpation of the abdomen may be difficult and fail to yield information. A rectal examination will rule out intraluminal bleeding and a pelvic mass. Repeated examinations at close intervals by a skilled observer are the best available tool for proper diagnosis and treatment. It is more the regression or progression of signs from hour to hour than a certain constellation of physical signs that will establish the nature of the internal injury and the need for exploration.

A penetrating wound of the abdomen is an indication for a surgical intervention. A painful abdomen with localized or generalized guarding and vomiting usually indicates perforation of a hollow organ. In cases where there are signs of hemorrhagic shock, rupture of a solid viscus is likely.

Abdominal contusions. In a series of 418 cases of trauma from the Boston City Hospital, more than 40% of patients suffered abdominal contusions. The clinical findings can mimic a hollow-viscus rupture. Abdominal pain can be severe; there is vomiting, generalized tenderness, and sometimes rigidity, and bowel sounds are absent. The leukocyte count is usually high. The hematocrit reading is usually stable. What differentiates this entity from a major visceral injury is the fact that within a few hours there is pronounced improvement. The symptoms are presumably brought about by retroperitoneal bleeding or contusion to the abdominal wall musculature. Retroperitoneal hematoma is a frequent complication of severe abdominal trauma. It is usually associated with an injury to a retroperitoneal organ.

Spleen, liver, kidney, and pancreas injury. In all published series, injuries to solid organs outnumber by a wide margin those to hollow organs. Cumulative figures for two recently published large series show that, as a result of blunt trauma to the abdomen of 229 children and adolescents, the spleen was injured in 31%, the kidney in 29%, the liver in 25%, and the pancreas in somewhat less than 5% of cases. In penetrating trauma, injuries to the liver outnumber those to all other solid organs combined, by a ratio of 3 to 1.

Splenic rupture is the most frequent solid organ injury after blunt trauma. A blow over the left upper quandrant or the lower chest leads rapidly to an acute condition of the abdomen. Pain may radiate to the shoulder and neck. All the signs of an abdominal contusion are present. In addition, there is pronounced pallor and the rapid onset of circulatory collapse. In perhaps 15% of cases, the rupture is delayed. It is important to keep in mind the possibility of a ruptured spleen even though a few hours or days intervene between the trauma and the onset of symptoms. Pediatricians always express much anxiety about the dangers of traumatic splenic rupture in patients with splenomegaly. Recent information suggests that the added risk is small or nonexistent except in cases of an acute disease such as infectious mononucleosis.

Once the diagnosis of splenic rupture has been confirmed, there is no need to perform surgery unless hemorrhage is brisk and life-threatening. There are now several reports of nonsurgical management of ruptured spleens. If a laparotomy is done and limited splenic injuries are noted, partial splenectomy and suture of limited capsular tears are indicated. When removal of an injured spleen is necessary, patients should be counseled and given prophylaxis in view of the 1% to 2% incidence of overwhelming sepsis, which carries a mortality of more than 50%.

Kidney injuries give rise to pain and tenderness in the lumbar region. Hematuria is usually present. In a third of the cases, there is a rupture of the involved kidney. Rapid exploration is rarely necessary and over 75% of renal injuries will not require surgery.

The incidence of liver injury is high, and in all series they are associated with a high mortality (40%). Rupture of the liver constitutes an extreme emergency with a poor outlook in cases where the damage is extensive. Because of massive hemorrhage, over 30% of children die before reaching an emergency room. The right lobe is much more vulnerable than the left and accounts for 80% of cases. Pain may be accentuated with respiration and referred to the shoulder as the result of diaphragmatic irritation. Rebound tenderness and shock are usually present. A fluid wave may be elicited. The diagnosis may be extremely difficult in the absence of definite signs of hemorrhage or peritonitis. A peritoneal tap and lavage will confirm the diagnosis; large amounts of blood (more than 100,000 red blood cells per cubic milliliter) is an indication for an emergency laparotomy. It is only in highly selected cases that hepatic artery ligation or a lobectomy is indicated. Most hepatic injuries can be repaired with mattress sutures after ligation of bleeding vessels and débridement. In the stable patient, nonoperative management is in order because one report has shown that more than

50% of patients who were explored for liver injuries did not require surgical intervention.

The pancreas is deeply situated in the abdomen and, though relatively well protected, may be injured by a closed abdominal injury or as a consequence of a penetrating wound. In our experience, the most common cause of pancreatic injury is the result of trauma in the epigastrium by the handlebar of a bicycle. Closed wounds of the abdomen damage the pancreas by compressing it against the prominence of the vertebral column. As a result of damage, blood and pancreatic enzymes escape and pancreatitis develops. The resultant symptoms are persistent severe abdominal pain, bilious vomiting, and fever. The serum amylase level is high. Injury to the pancreas may not be suspected after a relatively mild trauma until, a few weeks later, symptoms of pseudocyst become apparent (p. 853).

Gastrointestinal tract. Solid organs such as the spleen, kidney, and liver are more commonly and more seriously injured than are the hollow organs. However, a penetrating injury or a trivial blow can lead to a rupture or a hematoma of a hollow viscus. Avulsion of the mesentery can also occur.

In order of frequency, the jejunum, ileum, and duodenum can be perforated. The signs are those of an acute abdomen. The duodenum in its fixed retroperitoneal portion is particularly vulnerable to

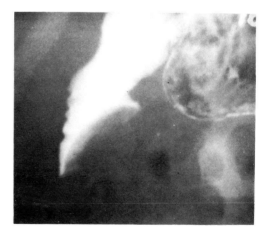

Fig. 4-9. Hematoma of the duodenum producing complete obstruction of the second portion of the duodenum by a smooth-margin, convex mass representing the localized intramural hematoma. Although a duplication cyst might produce a similar picture, the appearance is practically pathognomonic of posttraumatic hematoma of the duodenum.

the development of an obstructing intramural hematoma (Fig. 4-9), which may also occur in the ileum and the colon. Intramural hematomas in the duodenum or at the duodenojejunal junction are frequently seen in the battered child and in handlebar accidents. Although the classic story of sudden onset of vomiting after blunt trauma to the abdomen is highly suggestive of hematoma of the duodenum, a gastrointestinal series is needed to confirm the diagnosis. Also, that trauma has been sustained is frequently elicited only after the lesion has been demonstrated. The films show a rounded mass projecting from the wall of the descending portion of the duodenum, usually completely occluding the lumen. Patients with this condition should be treated conservatively for a week to 10 days. Later films usually show the gradual regression of the mass with reestablishment of luminal patency. A delay in the onset of symptoms of partial intestinal obstruction has been reported as a consequence of sealed localized perforations after seat-belt injuries.

Management

All children suffering abdominal trauma or serious injuries that may have resulted in the injury of abdominal structures should be admitted to an intensive care unit. The team responsible for the patient should be experienced in the management of such problems. An airway is provided when necessary; vital signs are recorded on a close time schedule. A large-caliber intravenous catheter should be promptly inserted for the rapid perfusion of fluids. A central venous pressure line should be introduced if hypovolemic shock is present or likely to occur and will be essential in the assessment of volume replacement. A nasogastric tube is used for continuous suction. If the patient is unconscious, a Foley catheter will facilitate making the hourly record of urine volume and the diagnosis of renal injuries.

Roentgenograms of the chest and abdomen should be made, enabling easy detection of diaphragmatic injury, intestinal obstruction, or pneumoperitoneum. The instillation of a few ounces of a dilute barium solution may prove the diagnosis of an intramural hematoma or of an abnormal C loop secondary to pancreatic injury. It is suggested that an intravenous pyelogram be done in all patients with hematuria.

Abdominal arteriography is a valuable tool. However, it has been largely replaced by abdominal scanning with ultrasound. An irregular contour or an echogenic mass surrounding and displacing the kidney, spleen, and liver suggests rupture and a hematoma. Radionuclide imaging has proved to be a valuable diagnostic tool for splenic hepatic and renal injuries.

Determination of the hematocrit value is one of the most important laboratory tests available, and the values should be determined serially. A falling hematocrit suggests active or recent blood loss; a rising reading after trauma may be a clue to the intraluminal or intraperitoneal sequestration of extracellular fluid or plasma in response to obstruction or peritonitis. The serum amylase level should be determined in all patients. High base-line values may be seen even though there is no pancreatic injury of consequence; however, serially recorded increasing values are indicative of serious pancreatic trauma. Abdominal taps should be done in all four quadrants if hemorrhage is suspected.

The decision to operate should be based on deteriorating clinical signs or a falling hematocrit reading or both. A rising amylase level is not sufficient indication for operation if the patient's condition is stable.

REFERENCES

Braun, P., and Dion, Y.: Intestinal stenosis following seat belt injury, J. Pediatr. Surg. **8:**549-550, 1973.

Dickerman, J.D.: Splenectomy and sepsis: a warning, Pediatrics **63:**938-941, 1979.

Dickerman, R.M., and Dunn, E.L.: Splenic, pancreatic and hepatic injuries, Surg. Clin. North Am. **61:**3-14, 1981.

Erkalis, A.J.: Abdominal injury related to the trauma of birth, Pediatrics **39:**421-424, 1967.

Feins, N.R.: Multiple trauma, Pediatr. Clin. North Am. **26:** 759-771, 1979.

Gornall, P., Ahmed, S., Jolleys, A., and Cohen, S.J.: Intraabdominal injuries in battered baby syndrome, Arch. Dis. Child. **47:**211-214, 1972.

Hood, J.M., and Smyth, B.T.: Nonpenetrating intra-abdominal injuries in children, J. Pediatr. Surg. **9:**69-77, 1974.

Mahow, G.H., Woolley, M.M., Gans, S.L., and others: Duodenal hematoma in infancy and childhood, J. Pediatr. Surg. **6:**153-160, 1971.

Sinclair, M.C., and Moore, T.C.: Major surgery for abnormal and thoracic trauma in childhood and adolescence, J. Pediatr. Surg. **9:**155-162, 1974.

Sinclair, M.C., Moore, T.C., Arch, M.J., and others: Injury to hollow abdominal viscera from blunt trauma in children and adolescents, Am. J. Surg. **128:**693-698, 1974.

Stewart, D.R., Byrd, C.L., and Schuster, S.R.: Intramural hematomas of the alimentary tract in children, Surgery **68:**550-557, 1970.

Talbert, J.L., and Rodgers, B.M.: Acute abdominal injuries in children, Pediatr. Ann. **5:**36-67, 1976.

SUPERIOR MESENTERIC ARTERY SYNDROME

The superior mesenteric artery may cause digestive symptoms in children of any age by compressing the third portion of the duodenum. In its final course to the ligament of Treitz, the duodenum passes upward from right to left across the aorta at the level of the second lumbar vertebra. It then runs behind and below the superior mesenteric artery. If the duodenum crosses higher than usual, if the artery originates from the aorta at a lower level than normal, or if its angle formed with the aorta becomes more acute, duodenal obstruction may occur.

Clinical findings

The syndrome occurs more frequently in teen-aged girls. It is characterized by postprandial epigastric discomfort and pain, distention, and bilious vomiting. The symptoms are relieved to a certain extent when the patient lies on the left side but more characteristically by the knee-chest position. Predisposing factors include prolonged supine rest, a body cast, traction for a spinal injury, or the postoperative phase of surgery for scoliosis.

Diagnosis

The clinical findings vary in their severity and may be atypical. An upright film of the abdomen may show a dilated stomach and duodenum with an abrupt cutoff or reduction of caliber just to the right of the third lumbar vertebra (Fig. 4-10). Under fluoroscopy, reverse peristalsis may be seen. The duodenal holdup of the opaque material may disappear when the patient is moved on his left side or face down. Angiography with lateral views will show a narrowed superior mesenteric artery to aortic angle.

Treatment

Once the disorder is recognized, and depending on the clinical condition of the patient, the initial treatment can be conservative in both the acute and the chronic forms. Nasogastric suction is followed a few days later by small, frequent, low-residue, soft feedings. The left lateral, prone, or knee-chest position is helpful at mealtime. Patients who do not respond to conservative measures require surgical treatment. More recently, duodenal and jejunal mobilization that removes the duodenum from its position beneath the superior

mesenteric artery has proved to be a very successful operative approach.

REFERENCES

Akin, J.T., Gray, S.W., and Skandalakis, J.E.: Vascular compression of the duodenum: presentation of ten cases and review of the literature, Surgery **79:**515-522, 1976.

Altman, D.H., and Puranik, S.R.: Superior mesenteric artery syndrome in children, Radiology **118:**104-108, 1973.

Appel, M.F., Bentlif, P.S., and Dickson, J.H.: Arterio-mesenteric duodenal compression syndrome: comparison of methods of treatment, South. Med. J. **69:**340-342, 1976.

Burrington, J.D., and Wayne, E.R.: Obstruction of the duodenum by the superior mesenteric artery—does it exist in children?, J. Pediatr. Surg. **9:**733-741, 1974.

Puranik, S.R., Keiser, R.P., and Gilbert, M.G.: Arteriomesenteric duodenal compression in children, Am. J. Surg. **124:**334-339, 1972.

RECURRENT OR CHRONIC INTESTINAL PSEUDO-OBSTRUCTION

Secondary intestinal pseudo-obstruction

This recurrent or chronic syndrome is characterized by a clinical picture of intestinal obstruction without evidence of an intraluminal or extraluminal cause of a lesion obstructing the bowel. It stimulates paralytic ileus, which is an acute form of intestinal pseudo-obstruction (see chart). Recurrent or chronic intestinal pseudo-obstruction may be primary or seconday. The following material lists disease conditions that can be associated with the secondary type of chronic intestinal pseudo-obstruction in the pediatric age group.

Idiopathic intestinal pseudo-obstruction

Patients with the primary type of chronic intestinal pseudo-obstruction have no underlying disease to explain their motility problem. The disease can either be familial or sporadic. Certain features such as a younger age at onset, gastric atony, and a more generalized type of dilatation, as well as a worse prognosis, have been reported to be more frequent in sporadic cases, but this has not been our experience.

Causes of secondary chronic intestinal pseudo-obstruction in infants and children

Collagen diseases
    Scleroderma, dermatomyositis, systemic lupus erythematosus
Myopathies
    Myotonic dystrophy
    Muscular dystrophy, Duchenne type
Disorders of intrinsic innervation of bowel
    Hirschsprung's disease

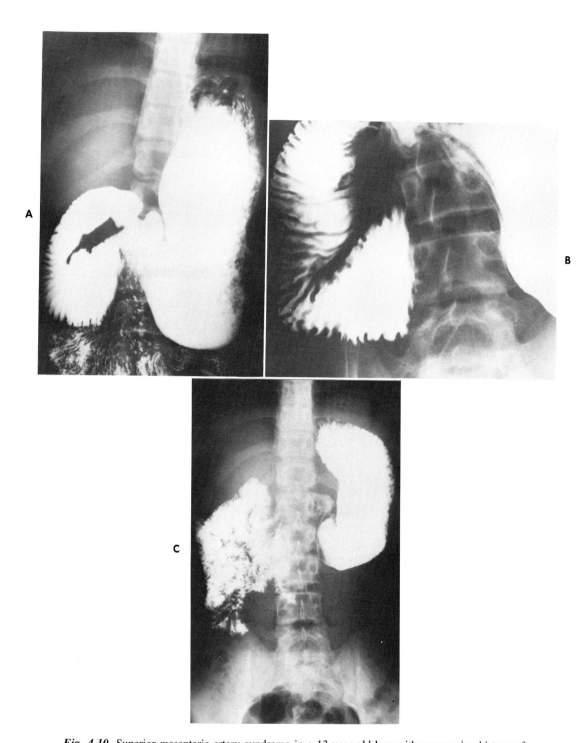

Fig. 4-10. Superior mesenteric artery syndrome in a 13-year-old boy with progressive history of abdominal pain, postprandial vomiting, and significant weight loss (15 pounds). Upper gastrointestinal roentgenogram shows, **A,** large fluid-filled stomach and dilated proximal duodenum with, **B,** obstruction to the right of the midline at the level of the third lumbar vertebra. To-and-fro churning of the contrast medium was noted in the proximal duodenum. **C,** Postoperative appearance of small bowel in which the duodenum has been mobilized and brought down from under the superior mesenteric artery.

Deficiency of argyrophil neurons in the myenteric
  plexus
Delayed maturation of myenteric ganglia
Ganglioneuromatosis in MEN (multiple endocrine
  neoplasia) type 2b
Chagas' disease
Neurofibromatosis
Endocrine and metabolic disorders
  Hypothyroidism
  Hypoparathyroidism
  Pheochromocytoma
  Hypercalcemia
  Diabetic visceroneuropathy
Miscellaneous
  Celiac disease
  Nontropical sprue
  Cathartic colon

The disease is not rare because close to 100 cases have been described, but it is not at all certain that it forms a single entity. There is much variation in the age of presentation, the severity of symptoms, the clinical course, and the areas of the gastrointestinal tract that are adynamic. On the other hand, the symptoms and the roentgenographic and manometric findings are quite similar. Pathologic studies have not been helpful in singling out a common cause. Both smooth muscle cells and neural plexuses are generally normal, but a deficiency of argyrophil neurons has been noted in neonates presenting as a typical Hirschsprung's disease or as a motility disorder involving the entire gastrointestinal tract. In other cases there is atrophy and degeneration of smooth muscle; it can involve both layers or only the internal one (Fig. 4-11). In yet another category, degenerative changes are described in the ganglion cells.

Clinical findings

The affected neonates present with abdominal distention, bilious vomiting, and obstipation. Small diarrheal stools usually supervene, but there is persistence of signs of intestinal obstruction and also an absence of bowel sounds. Rectal manometry will reveal a normal relaxation of the internal sphincter, and a biopsy will rule out the diagnosis of Hirschsprung's disease. Some cases are limited to the colon, whereas others involve both the small and the large bowel.

Most cases of idiopathic intestinal pseudo-obstruction become symptomatic during the first decade (Table 4-3). Abdominal distention and a flattening of the growth curve are the first signs. Attacks of abdominal pain associated with bilious

vomiting and chronic constipation then follow. The course is chronic and relentless though we have seen spontaneous remissions in two cases. As recurrent attacks of pseudo-obstruction become more frequent and last longer, malnutrition and starvation occur. Some patients have symptoms of urinary retention with enlarged bladders and vesicoureteral reflux.

We have been impressed by cardiovascular manifestations, which have not been noted in other reports, except for the one by Maldonado. Bradycardia, first-degree heart block, and even complete heart attack, necessitating a pacemaker, have been noted in a few patients (Table 4-3).

X-ray and motility studies

The stomach is generally spared, and the colon is much less commonly affected than the small bowel. The distal two thirds of the esophagus shows reduced to absent peristalsis with incomplete relaxation of the lower esophageal sphincter, indistinguishable from that seen in achalasia. Gastric motility and emptying are normal. The duodenum is strikingly dilated, and the folds appear prominent (Fig. 4-12). The rest of the small bowel is modestly dilated and usually is of normal caliber in its distal portion. Transit through the small bowel may require 3 or 4 days and lead to impaction. Motility studies of the proximal small bowel are abnormal. In cases with colonic involvement, the large bowel is dilated and redundant.

Laboratory findings

There is anemia, hypoalbuminemia, and steatorrhea. The contaminated small bowel syndrome is a constant finding. It can be proved by a positive breath test and the presence of up to 50% of free bile acids in the duodenal juice, which is grossly contaminated with the aerobic and anaerobic microflora of the lower intestinal tract.

Differential diagnosis

Scleroderma causes alimentary tract disturbances symptomatically and roentgenologically similar to idiopathic intestinal pseudo-obstruction. however, in the latter, the onset is much earlier, Raynaud's phenomenon is absent, and lesions are limited to the gastrointestinal tract.

Treatment

Most patients have had at least one surgical procedure for a bout of intestinal obstruction. Surgery has no place in the treatment of this disorder

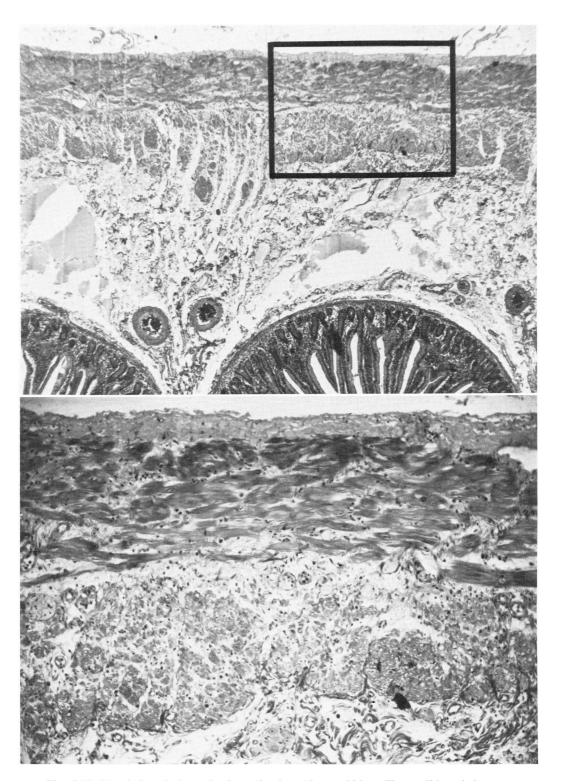

Fig. 4-11. Chronic intestinal pseudo-obstruction in a 15-year-old boy. The small bowel shows a relatively normal external muscle layer. However, the internal layer presents severe degenerative changes. There is extensive vacuolation and dropping out of muscle cells. Even in areas where muscle cells appear less severely affected, there are vacuoles, degenerated muscle cells, and some degree of lacy fibrosis.

Table 4-3. Idiopathic chronic intestinal pseudo-obstruction: experience with 7 patients at Hôpital Sainte-Justine

Mean age at onset	9 years (5½ to 16)
Family history	Three in one sibship
Gastrointestinal symptoms	Abdominal distention, constipation, diarrhea, vomiting, failure to thrive (6/7)
	Dysphagia (2/7)
Areas involved (roentgenograms and motility)	Esophagus and small bowel (7/7)
Malabsorption syndrome	Steatorrhea (6/7)
	Increased loss of bile acids (4/6)
	Contaminated small bowel (5/5)
	Abnormal Schilling test (2/6)
	Hypoalbuminemia (3/7)
Cardiac manifestations	Bradycardia (4/7)
	Complete heart block (2/7)
	Myocardial, sinoauricular node and coronary artery fibrosis at postmortem exam in 2
Evolution	Death after a mean survival of 8 years in 5
	Dysphagia in 1
	Remission in 1

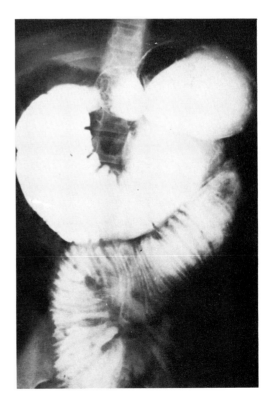

Fig. 4-12. Chronic idiopathic intestinal pseudo-obstruction in a 9-year-old girl with a 3-year history of abdominal pain, repeated attacks of intestinal obstruction, and severe malabsorption and malnutrition. The barium meal shows a striking degree of dilatation of the duodenum and jejunum. In this girl, the ileum was only minimally involved, and the colon was intact.

except in rare neonatal cases limited to the colon or in those where colonic involvement is severe.

Medical management is currently unsatisfactory because it is solely directed toward the relief of symptoms and the correction of malnutrition. The treatment of the contaminated small bowel syndrome with antibiotics is disappointing. Efforts to stimulate peristalsis with carbachol, betanechol, neostigmine, metoclopramide, cerulein, and cholecystokinin have all failed miserably.

The management of a bout of intestinal obstruction includes nasogastric suction, restriction of oral intake, and parenteral nutrition. When symptoms become chronic and unremitting, total parenteral nutrition through a central catheter becomes necessary. A home program using total parenteral nutrition then becomes the only solution for this otherwise fatal illness.

REFERENCES

Anuras, S., and Christensen, J.: Recurrent or chronic intestinal pseudo-obstruction, Clin. Gastroenterol. **10:**177-190, 1981.

Bouglé, D., Roy, C., Combes, J., and others: Bradycardia, complete heart block and arterial lesions in chronic idiopathic intestinal pseudo-obstruction (IIPO), Pediatr. Res. **15:**526, 1981 [abstract].

Byrne, W.J., Cibel. L., Euler, A.R., and others: Chronic idiopathic intestinal pseudo-obstruction syndrome in children: clinical characteristics and prognosis, Pediatrics **90:**585-589, 1977.

Carney, J.A., Go, V.L.W., Sizemore, G.W., and Hayles, A.B.: Alimentary tract ganglioneuromatosis: a major component of multiple endocrine neoplasia type 2B, N. Engl. J. Med. **295:**1287-1291, 1976.

Duhamel, J.F., Ricour, C., Dupont, C., and others: L'adynamie intestinale chronique primitive à révélation néonatale, Arch. Fr. Pediatr. **37:**293-297, 1980.

Hanks, J.B., Meyers, W.C., Andersen, D.K., and others: Chronic primary intestinal pseudo-obstruction, Surgery **89:**175-182, 1981.

Lewis, T.D., Daniel, E.E., Sarna, S.K., and others: Idiopathic intestinal pseudo-obstruction: report of a case with intraluminal studies of mechanical and electrical activity and response to drugs, Gastroenterology **74:**107-111, 1978.

Maldonado, J.E., Gregg, J.A., and Green, P.A.: Chronic idiopathic intestinal pseudo-obstruction, Am. J. Med. **49:**203-212, 1970.

Navarro, J., Boccon-Gibod, L., Sonsino, L., and others: Démembrement du cadre "pseudo-Hirschsprung," Arch. Fr. Pediatr. **37:**437-444, 1980.

Shaw, A., Shaffer, H., Teja, K., and others: A perspective for pediatric surgeons: chronic idiopathic intestinal pseudo-obstruction, J. Pediatr. Surg. **14:**719-727, 1979.

Schuffler, M.D., Lowe, M.C., and Bill, A.H.: Studies of idiopathic intestinal pseudo-obstruction. I. Hereditary hollow visceral myopathy: clinical and pathological studies, Gastroenterology **73:**327-338, 1977.

Schuffler, M.D., and Pope, C.E.: Studies of idiopathic intestinal pseudo-obstruction: family studies, Gastroenterology **73:**339-344, 1977.

Tanner, M.S., Smith, B., and Lloyd, J.K.: Functional intestinal obstruction due to deficiency of argyrophil neurones in the myenteric plexus, Arch. Dis. Child. **51:**837-841, 1976.

5

Abdominal wall developmental defects and omphalomesenteric remnants

GASTROSCHISIS

Before 1963, most physicians believed that gastroschisis simply represented an intrauterine rupture of an omphalocele. Since then clinical findings and embryologic studies have shown that gastroschisis and omphalocele are separate and distinct entities. However, there is still considerable controversy concerning the pathogenesis of these two major abdominal-wall developmental defects.

Gastroschisis is the herniation, without a covering sac, of variable lengths of the small intestine and, rarely of portions of the liver, through an abdominal wall defect. The defect is to the right of the umbilical cord, which has a normal insertion. One hypothesis is that the herniation into the amniotic cavity is secondary to a congenital abdominal wall defect. It occurs before the programmed herniation of the bowel normally occurs and is attributed to failure of formation of one of the lateral plates of the somatopleure. More recently, it has been suggested that gastroschisis is the result of an antenatal or perinatal tear or rupture through the membrane of a hernia of the umbilical cord with evisceration through the less well-supported and more vulnerable side of the umbilical hernia sac.

Clinical features

Most defects are on the right of the umbilical cord and vary from 2 to 15 cm in size.

The eviscerated mass of small bowel loops is adherent, edematous, and of a dark color. It is encased by a thick, gelatinous matrix with greenish fibrinous material. Peristalsis is absent. The mesentery is thick and edematous. The peritoneal cavity is relatively small. In such cases, the evisceration has presumably occurred early in pregnancy. In contrast to this antenatal type, the perinatal variety shows only a mild to moderate intestinal and mesenteric reaction, in which case the peritoneal cavity may be normal in size.

The incidence of prematurity is close to 60%, but that of associated malformations is relatively low (Table 5-1). There is little evidence that genetic factors play a role in the origin of gastroschisis. The risk of congenital abnormalities in future pregnancies appear to be very small. Most jejunoileal malformations are atresias or stenoses that may have been acquired as a result of ischemia and autoamputation in association with small strangulating defects or by intrauterine volvulus of eviscerated intestines. All patients have intestinal malrotation and some degree of shortening of the small bowel because of its prolonged contact with amniotic fluid. Experimentally, amniotic fluid has been shown to cause damage to myenteric ganglion cells and decrease acetylesterase and acetylcholinesterase activity. This may account for the disordered peristalsis.

Management

The newborn infant with gastroschisis should be operated on as soon as possible to prevent or minimize gross bacterial contamination. A one-stage intervention is possible only in the patients (10%) who have a normal-appearing herniated mass and in whom the peritoneal cavity can receive, without undue pressure, the extra-abdominal mass.

The majority of patients require staged procedures. The exposed viscera are supported and covered with sterile dressings, and a nasogastric tube is inserted. Antibiotics and intravenous fluids are given before surgery. The use of skin flaps are associated with a lower incidence of infection than that of prosthetic material such as Silon sheets for the creation of a pouch. However, tight closure and abdominal crowding should be avoided at all costs. A gastrostomy is also carried out during the initial surgical procedure. Subsequent operations aimed at gradual reductions of the pouch lead to a progressive enlargement of the abdominal cavity, permitting complete repair of the defect usually within 2 weeks.

A small number of patients with perinatal evisceration who can undergo primary repair can be fed early. A large number undergo staged procedures: they all require parenteral nutrition until the defect is finally closed. Because intestinal malfunction persists for long periods after gastros-

129

Table 5-1. Gastroschisis and omphaloceles: clinical differences

	Gastroschisis (%)	Omphalocele (%)
Prematurity	59	10
Associated malformations		
Gastrointestinal tract		
Jejunoileal	14	1
Nonjejunoileal	4	36
Cardiac	2	20
Others	11	34
Associated syndromes		
Lower midline syndrome	—	24
Upper midline syndrome	—	25
Beckwith-Weidemann	—	10

Data compiled by Moore, T.C.: Surgery **82**:561, 1977.

chisis repair, two thirds of cases of primary repair and 80% of the others are expected to require parenteral nutrition postoperatively for varying periods of time. Motility problems and poor absorption in the remaining bowel are indications for prolonged parenteral nutrition. Paralytic ileus may persist for weeks and sometimes for 3 to 4 months, but a real mechanical obstruction may occur and require reoperation. Wound infection, volvulus, bowel necrosis, constricting bands, and intestinal fistulas are some complications to be anticipated in cases treated with a Silon pouch.

Prognosis

Prematurity, infection, gangrenous small bowel requiring resection, paralytic ileus, and the short bowel associated with the defect are major problems that account for a mortality of 30%.

The low mortality of 6.2% has been recently reported in a series of 32 infants. These impressive results were achieved with the use of prosthetic material reserved to the rare cases where a primary skin flap closure could not be done. Secondary ventral hernia repair was done between 6 to 12 months of age.

Total parenteral alimentation is largely responsible for recent improvement of the prognosis by preventing the malnutrition secondary to severe intestinal malfunction associated with bowel changes. The intestinal dysfunction is characterized by poor peristalsis and diminished carbohydrate and fat absorption, as well as by some degree of protein-losing enteropathy. Normal intestinal function may not return before 6 months of age.

OMPHALOCELE

During the embryologic process of lengthening of the midgut, a ventrally directed loop, connected with the yolk sac by the short yolk stalk, is formed and extends into the umbilical coelom. Further longitudinal growth of the small bowel takes place in that herniated loop. Eventually, tightly coiled loops of small intestine fill most of the available space. At 10 weeks, with reduced growth of the liver and coincident expansion of the body walls, the coiled intestines are normally returned to the abdominal cavity. Anomalies (omphalocele and umbilical hernia) related to this extra-abdominal position of the intestines are the result of delayed migration of the coils of bowel from the umbilical coelom through failure of the normal morphogenesis of the folds comprising the ventral wall and failure of closure of the umbilical ring, respectively.

Clinical findings

An omphalocele may be evident as a slight enlargement of the base of the umbilical cord or as a convex disc of amniotic membrane above the abdominal wall. In such cases, the unwary obstetrician may clamp and divide both an isolated loop of bowel and the cord.

However, most patients with this condition have a much larger defect that is easily diagnosed. It may contain liver, spleen, and a large portion of the gastrointestinal tract (Fig. 5-1).

The umbilical cord usually is inserted into the sac and the umbilical vessels run radially within its wall. There is no deficiency of the abdominal wall other than that of the skin over the herniation

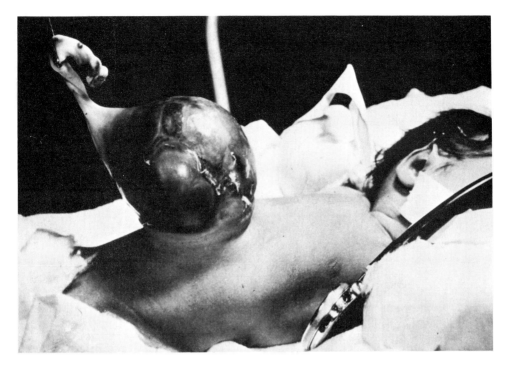

Fig. 5-1. This large omphalocele contained loops of small bowel, the spleen, and part of the liver. The transparent amniotic membrane leading to the cord permits the easy identification of its solid organ content. A staged repair was carried out.

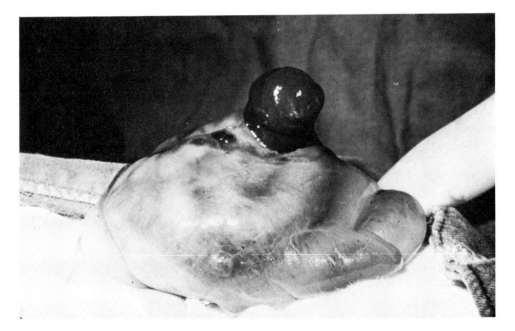

Fig. 5-2. Ruptured omphalocele. In this instance, the diagnosis of a ruptured omphalocele is easily made because the sac is clearly visible. The bowel loops protruding from the sac can be edematous and matted together and can mimic gastroschisis. However, ruptured omphaloceles always have a sac, whereas the rarer cases of gastroschisis do not. Furthermore, in gastroschisis, there is a normal cord insertion.

itself. The abdominal muscles are intact even when the sac is gigantic. Most have no fixation of their midgut and incomplete rotation, both of which expose them to volvulus. The intact omphalocele sac may rupture partially or completely either in utero, during labor, or after birth. The sac is thin and made up of a membrane composed of amnion externally and parietal peritoneum internally. In patients with a postnatally ruptured sac, the appearance of the intestine is essentially normal, whereas in those in whom the sac ruptured earlier, the eviscerated mass of the intestine is thickened, edematous, and matted together by a fibrinous material. Little peristalsis is seen, and the appearance of the eviscerated mass is the same as in a case of gastroschisis (Fig. 5-2).

The incidence of other gastrointestinal tract anomalies is high (Table 5-1). Omphaloceles are frequently seen in association with the lower midline syndrome (vesicointestinal fissure, imperforate anus, agenesis of the colon, and so on), the upper midline syndrome (sternal, diaphragmatic, pericardial, and cardiac defects), and the Beckwith-Weidemann syndrome (exomphalos-macroglossia-gigantism-hypoglycemia). Although no familial tendency has been confirmed, congenital anomalies have been reported in 40% of cases in first-degree relatives.

Treatment

When an infant with an omphalocele is first seen, the sac should be covered with moist gauze sponges and the abdomen wrapped without any pressure being applied on the herniated mass. Gastric suction is instituted to prevent an increase in the size of the omphalocele subsequent to accumulation of air in the bowel. At operation, the surgeon should carefully inspect the bowel to rule out bands, volvulus, and failure of rotation.

The one-stage repair can usually be accomplished when the defect at the base of the cord does not exceed 5 cm in diameter. In the ones exceeding this dimension, the abdominal cavity is too small to receive the eviscerated abdominal contents. Attempts at primary repair may lead to respiratory failure and compression of the inferior vena cava in the patient. Staged repair involves initially covering the sac with prosthetic material such as Silon, Dacron, Silastic, and siliconized Teflon. A recent paper suggests the use of Opsite, a polymer membrane believed to have an advantage over Silon in terms of infection.

Nonoperative management consisting of repeated painting of the sac with benzalkonium chloride (Zephiran Cl) or dilute alcohol may create a tough dry eschar, which will promote skin growth over the sac. This may be used in massive omphaloceles. Skin closure over the omphalocele is a good approach in certain cases. The ventral hernia can be repaired when the abdominal cavity has grown sufficiently to accommodate the viscera without creating too much intra-abdominal pressure.

Postoperative care greatly influences the prognosis. Because of the inevitable compression of herniated bowels returned to a small abdominal cavity, prolonged ileus is common. Oral alimentation is often precluded for prolonged periods of time. Parenteral alimentation is necessary in patients treated with the staged procedure by use of prosthetic material because no feeding is done until the sheeting is removed (2 to 3 weeks). In patients with ruptured omphaloceles that occurred prenatally, motility problems will preclude oral feedings and require prolonged parenteral nutrition.

Respiratory distress, infections, intestinal obstruction, gastroesophageal reflux, and inguinal hernia are some of the other postoperative problems, but most of the mortality (30%) is attibutable to associated malformations.

REFERENCES

De Vries, P.A.: The pathogenesis of gastroschisis and omphalocele, J. Pediatr. Surg. **15**:245-251, 1980.

Ein, S.H., and Shandling, B.: A new nonoperative treatment of large omphaloceles with a polymer membrane. J. Pediatr. Surg. **13**:255-257, 1978.

Fonkalsrud, E.W.: Selective repair of neonatal gastroschisis based on degree of visceroabdominal disproportion, Ann. Surg. **191**:139-144, 1980.

Girvan, D.P., Webster, D.M., and Shandling, B.: The treatment of omphalocele and gastroschisis, Surg. Gynecol. Obstet. **139**:222-224, 1974.

Mahour, G.H.: Omphalocele, Surg. Gynecol. Obstet. **143**:821-828, 1976.

Mahour, G.H., Weitzman, J.J., and Rosenkranz, J.G.: Omphalocele and gastroschisis, Ann. Surg. **177**:478-482, 1973.

Moore, T.C.: Gastroschisis and omphalocele: clinical differences, Surgery **82**:561-568, 1977.

Noordijk, J.A., and Bloemsma-Jonkman, F.: Gastroschisis: no myth, J. Pediatr. Surg. **13**:47-49, 1978.

Oh, K.S., Dorst, J.P., Dominguez, R., and Girdany, B.R.: Abnormal intestinal motility in gastroschisis, Radiology **127**:457-460, 1978.

O'Neill, J.A., and Grosfeld, J.L.: Intestinal malfunction after antenatal exposure of viscera, Am. J. Surg. **127**:129-132, 1974.

Schuster, S.R.: Omphalocele, hernia of the umbilical cord and gastroschisis, In Ravitch, M.M., Welch, K.J., Benson, C.D., Aberdeen, E., and Randolph, J.G., editors: Pediatric surgery, ed. 3, Chicago, 1979, Year Book Medical Publishers, Inc.

Shaw, A.: The myth of gastroschisis, J. Pediatr. Surg. 10:235-244, 1975.

Stringel, G., and Filer, R.M.: Prognostic factors in omphalocele and gastroschisis, J. Pediatr. Surg. **14:**515-519, 1979.

Towne, B.H., Peters, G., and Chang, J.H.T.: The problems of "giant" omphalocele, J. Pediatr. Surg. **15:**543-547, 1980.

UMBILICAL HERNIA

An umbilical hernia results from the incomplete closure of the fascia of the umbilical ring. It is much commoner in premature than in full-term infants. As many as 40% of black children under 1 year of age have detectable umbilical hernias.

Whereas major defects of the abdominal wall such as gastroschisis and omphalocele are developmental in origin, the etiology of umbilical hernia is much less clear. There is no doubt that increased intra-abdominal pressure from enlargement of an organ, a space-occupying lesion, gas, ascites, coughing, crying, or vomiting influences the closure and weakens the umbilical ring. Diseases such as cretinism, trisomy 18, and trisomy 13, along with Beckwith's syndrome and Hurler's syndrome, are often associated with umbilical hernia.

Clinical features

The size of the umbilical protrusion is variable. The underlying fascial defect varies from 0.5 to 4 cm. Herniated small bowel is usually easily reducible (Fig. 5-3).

Excessive thinning of the skin distended by the hernia and progressive enlargement of the fascial defects are reported very rarely unless there is increased intra-abdominal pressure from enlargement of an organ or from ascites. Incarceration is very rare (1 in 1500) in infants and children, and it tends to occur in smaller hernias.

Most umbilical hernias in children resolve by spontaneous and progressive closure of the ring. Fascial defects with diameter less than 0.5 cm almost always heal spontaneously before the patient is 2 years of age. With a ring between 0.5 and 1.5 cm in diameter, healing is usually complete by the age of 4 years. Those greater than 2 cm can still disappear without treatment but seldom before the child reaches school age.

Treatment

Surgery is advisable if the fascial defect still exceeds 1.5 cm at 2 years of age. A small hernia that has led to incarceration or to symptoms such as abdominal pain should be repaired. Similarly, it is suggested that even small hernias persisting until the child reaches school age are better treated surgically in view of the significant complication of incarceration in adults.

It has been suggested that adult and childhood hernias may be separate entities on the basis of anatomic differences and of a large preponderance in women. Furthermore, a recent study in black children suggest that half the hernias present at 4 to 5 years of age close spontaneously by 11 years of age. On the basis of this information on the natural history of the defect after entrance in school, the suggestion has been made that a hernia does not require surgery before puberty unless it is a cause of psychologic disturbance.

Reducing the hernia and then strapping the skin

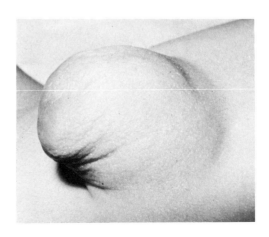

Fig. 5-3. Umbilical hernia. Large hernia in an infant without any associated malformations. The large underlying fascial defect (2 cm) is likely to close spontaneously. However, the natural history of the condition predicts that if the defect still exceeds 1.5 cm at 2 years, it is likely to be present by the time the child goes to school. Surgery is, therefore, advocated in such situations.

drawn together into a longitudinal fold over the umbilical ring does not accelerate the healing process; it only serves to keep the parents from looking at the protrusion.

REFERENCES

Angel-Lord, G.: Infantile umbilical hernia: to strap or not to strap, Med. J. Aust. **1:**83-85, 1971.

Hall, D.E., Roberts, K.B., and Charney, E.: Umbilical hernia: what happens after age 5 years, J. Pediatr. **98:**415-417, 1981.

James, P.M.: The problems of hernia in infants and adolescents, Surg. Clin. North Am. **51:**1361-1370, 1971.

Lassaletta, L., Fonkalsrud, E., Tovar, J.A., and others: The management of umbilical hernias in infancy and childhood, J. Pediatr. Surg. **10:**405-409, 1975.

Morgan, W.W., White, J.J., Stumbaugh, S., and Haller, J.A.: Prophylactic umbilical hernia repair in childhood to prevent adult incarceration, Surg. Clin. North Am. **50:**839-845, 1970.

Need, A.G.: Obstructed umbilical hernia in children: two case reports, Aust. Paediatr. J. **8:**152-154, 1972.

Walker, S.H.: The natural history of umbilical hernia, Clin. Pediatr. **6:**29-32, 1967.

MECKEL'S DIVERTICULUM

The vestigial remnant of the omphalomesenteric duct known as Meckel's diverticulum is the most frequent malformation of the gastrointestinal tract and is present in 1.5% of the population. Familial cases have been reported. The majority remain asymptomatic, and they are found twice as frequently in men as in women. Complications related to Meckel's diverticulum occur three to five times more frequently in males than in females. Heterotopic tissue, present in 50% of cases, is 10 times as likely to be found in symptomatic cases, most of which are seen in the first 2 years of life. Although the heterotopic mucosa is more likely to be gastric (80%), pancreatic tissue and jejunal and colonic mucosa can also be found in the diverticulum.

Meckel's diverticulum is located at the distal ileum, usually within 100 cm of the ileocecal valve. It always runs antimesenterically and has its own blood supply. Duplications and mesenteric cysts are located on the mesenteric side of the bowel. A few cases of large diverticula measuring up to 3.5 cm in diameter and 9 cm in length have been reported in newborns presenting with a palpable mass and intestinal obstruction. Although it has a wide base of 1 to 10 cm, the lumen of the diverticulum is usually narrower than that of the ileum (Fig. 5-4). Not infrequently its apex is connected to the umbilicus by a fibrous band or cord.

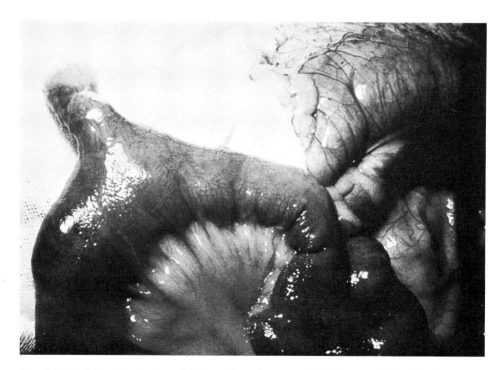

Fig. 5-4. Meckel's diverticulum. A history of previous rectal bleeding was elicited in this 2-year-old admitted for painless rectal bleeding and anemia.

Clinical features

Hemorrhage. Painless rectal bleeding is the chief complaint of symptomatic cases below 2 years of age. In certain instances the patient has experienced bleeding previously. Tarry stools are rare as the only evidence of bleeding, for in most cases, bright red blood or maroon stools are noted (Table 5-2).

Severe anemia or shock affects most of these children. Children who have previously experienced bleeding are likely to have bled within a year and in rather small amounts. Gastric mucosa with peptic ulceration is found in the Meckel's diverticulum of most cases presenting with hemorrhage.

Intestinal obstruction. It is the mode of presentation in 25% to 40% of cases and is attributable to intussusception, volvulus, torsion, or herniation of a loop (Table 5-3).

Intussusception. The diverticulum acts as the lead point. The early signs are those of ileocolic intussusception (Fig. 5-5), but the course is fulminant with severe early vomiting and rapid intestinal infarction. A mass is present on examination, and reduction of the intussusception by a barium enema is unsuccessful. More than half the cases occur in infancy.

Volvulus. Twisting of the bowel around a fibrous cordlike remnant of the omphalomesenteric duct extending from the tip of the diverticulum to the abdominal wall is common.

Other causes of obstruction. A loop of bowel may be caught across an obliterated omphalomesenteric (or vitelline) duct and become compressed. In other instances, herniation of a segment of bowel through a patent omphalomesenteric duct or through a hiatus created by a meso-diverticular band coursing from the base of the mesentery to the tip of the diverticulum is the cause of obstruction.

Diverticulitis. Diverticulitis is clinically indistinguishable from acute appendicitis. The pain is periumbilical early in the disease but may be to the right of the midline. Acute suppuration may lead to perforation and generalized perforation in the young infant. The presence of gastric ectopic mucosa probably makes a diverticulum more susceptible to infection because peptic ulcerations favor bacterial invasion, which is followed by necrosis and perforation in 25% to 50% of cases.

Diagnosis

The infant or young child who has a massive, painless bout of bright red or dark red rectal bleeding most likely has Meckel's diverticulum. A rectosigmoidoscopy should be done, as well as screening tests for bleeding disorders. A nasogas-

Table 5-2. Type of rectal bleeding observed in 43 cases of Meckel's diverticulum

Type of bleeding	Percent
Bright red	35
Bright red or dark red	12
Dark red	40
Dark red or tarry	6
Tarry	7

From Rutherford, R.B., and Akers D.R.: Surgery **59:**618-626, 1966.

Table 5-3. Complications in 311 cases of symptomatic Meckel's diverticulum

	Denver* (80)	Detroit† (115)	Paris‡ (116)	Percentage of total
Hemorrhage	43	47	35	40
Intestinal obstruction				
Intussusception	7	23	29	19
Torsion or vulvulus herniation	13	14	19§	15
Diverticulitis	4	24	13	13
Umbilical discharge	—	7	20	21

*Rutherford, R.B., and Akers, D.R.: Surgery **59:**618, 1966.
†Benson, C.D.: In Ravitch, M.M., and others: Pediatric surgery, ed. 3, Chicago, 1979, Year Book Medical Publishers, Inc.
‡Pellerin, D., Harouchi, A., and Delmas, P.: Ann. Chir. Infantile **17:**157, 1976.
§Five of these patients had umbilical discharge.

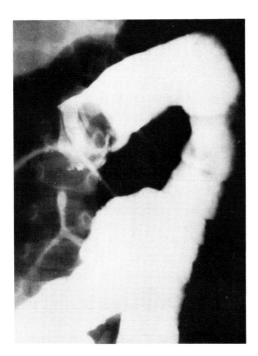

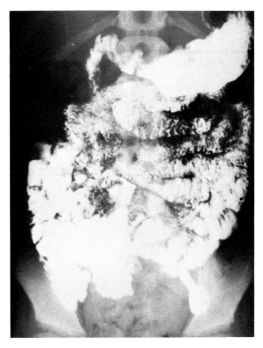

Fig. 5-5. Ileocolic intussusception in a 5-year-old with Meckel's diverticulum. The barium column is arrested at the midtransverse colon. Barium enema reduction was unsuccessful.

Fig. 5-6. Meckel's diverticulum. The clublike collection of barium in the left lower quadrant would be an unusual configuration for normal intestine and does represent a barium-filled Meckel's diverticulum. Small-bowel barium examination rarely demonstrates a Meckel's diverticulum.

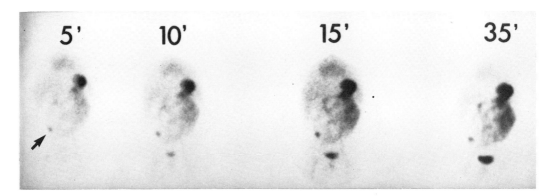

Fig. 5-7. Meckel's diverticulum. Within 5 minutes, the pertechnetate scan becomes positive, *arrow,* in the right lower quadrant of a 2-year-old child who had chronic rectal bleeding for a period of 3 months.

tric tube should be passed to rule out an upper gastrointestinal hemorrhage proximal to the ligament of Treitz.

An x-ray diagnosis can seldom be made (Fig. 5-6). Radionuclide imaging with ^{99m}Tc-pertechnetate scan is of value in delineating Meckel's diverticula with heterotopic gastric mucosa (Fig. 5-7). Cimetidine (1200 mg/1.73 m^2) given during the 24 hours before the examination increases the yield of positive scans. Since barium absorbs pertechnetate, barium contrast studies done previously may give rise to false-negative results. Other causes of a false-negative scan include concomitant inflammation with destruction of the heterotopic gastric mucosa. False-positive results are reported with hemangiomas, abdominal aneurysm, hydronephrosis, lymphoma, peptic ulcerations of the small intestine, Peutz-Jeghers syndrome, and small bowel intussusception or obstruction and may lead to unnecessary surgery. In our hands the pertechnetate scan has not proved to be a consistently reliable diagnostic tool. The decision to operate is largely based on the clinical features, and a positive scan provides supplementary evidence. A lateral scan should always be done to ensure that the focus of radioactivity is not in the bladder, ureters, or kidney.

Treatment

Preoperatively, attention should be directed to correction of the hypovolemic shock with blood and to the control of infection when an obstructive complication or inflammation is present. Cimetidine has been used successfully to stop the bleeding before the diverticulectomy is performed.

At operation, a close inspection of the ileum proximal to and distal from the diverticulum should be carried out, since heterotopic mucosa and ulcerations may be adjacent to the mouth of the diverticulum.

REFERENCES

Benson, C.D.: Surgical complications of Meckel's diverticulum. In Ravitt, M.M., Welch, K.J., Benson, C.D., Aberdeen, E., Randolph, J.G., editors: Pediatric surgery, ed. 3, Chicago, 1979, Year Book Medical Publishers, Inc.

Berquist, T.H., Nolan, N.G., Stephens, D.H., and others: Specificity of ^{99m}Tc-petechnetate in scintigraphic diagnosis of Meckel's diverticulum: review of 100 cases, J. Nucl. Med. **17:**465-469, 1976.

Collins, J.C.: Hemorrhage from a Meckel's diverticulum: one case with heterotopic gastric mucosa treated with cimetidine, Arch. Surg. **115:**83-84, 1980.

Graft, A.W., Watson, A.J., and Scott, J.E.S.: Giant Meckel's diverticulum causing intestinal obstruction in the newborn, J. Pediatr. Surg. **11:**1037-1038, 1976.

Martin, G.I., Kutner, F.R., and Moser, L.: Diagnosis of Meckel's diverticulum by radioisotope scanning, Pediatrics **57:**11-12, 1976.

Pellerin, D., Harouchi, A., and Delmas, P.: Le diverticule de Meckel: revue de 250 cas chez l'enfant, Ann. Chir. Infantile **17:**157-171, 1976.

Rutherford, R.B., and Akers, D.R.: Meckel's diverticulum, Surgery **59:**618-629, 1966.

Seagram, C.G.F., Louch, R.E., Stephens, C.A.: and Wentworth, P.: Meckel's diverticulum: a ten-year review of 218 cases, Can. J. Surg. **11:**369-373, 1968.

Tauscher, J.W., Bryant, D.R., and Gruenther, R.C.: False positive scan for Meckel's diverticulum, J. Pediatr. **92:**1022-1023, 1978.

OMPHALOMESENTERIC DUCT REMNANTS

At birth, the umbilical vessels and the urachus involute to become ligamentous remnants, whereas

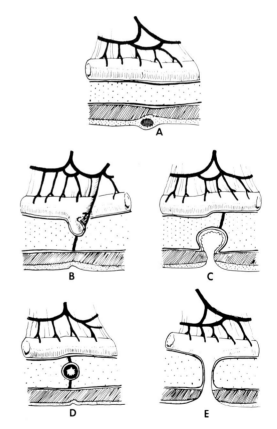

Fig. 5-8. Omphalomesenteric duct remnants. **A,** Umbilical granuloma. **B,** Meckel's diverticulum with a persistent omphalomesenteric band. **C,** Omphalomesenteric duct sinus and fistula. **D,** Cystic dilatation. **E,** Patent omphalomesenteric duct.

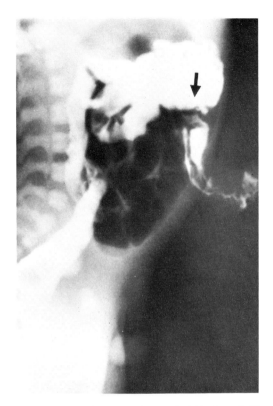

Fig. 5-9. Omphalomesenteric canal. This lateral film shows the persistence of the omphalomesenteric canal draining barium from the distal ileum, *arrow,* abnormally located high in the right upper quadrant. This patient had drainage of fecal material from his umbilicus but had no symptoms from the associated intestinal malrotation.

the omphalomesenteric duct normally leaves no evidence that it ever existed.

The *umbilical granuloma* (Fig. 5-8, *A*) is well known to the pediatrician and is represented by a small red mass of granulation tissue that, if left untreated, may become the seat of a low-grade infection. Applications of silver nitrate lead to complete healing. If, on the other hand, the lesion fails to respond and secrete mucus, an *umbilical polyp* is the likely diagnosis. It is made up of intestinal mucosa and is amenable to surgery.

Obliteration of the omphalomesenteric duct is completed within the first 8 weeks of gestation. Anomalous involution of this structure may give rise to *Meckel's diverticulum* or to Meckel's diverticulum *with a persistent omphalomesenteric band* (Fig. 5-8, *B*) attached to the anterior abdominal wall. In other cases, the band is attached to the anterior abdominal wall through an *omphalomesenteric duct sinus and fistula* (Fig. 5-8, *C*).

There is usually discharge of mucinous material from a structure that resembles a polyp or a granuloma. The sinus tract can usually be probed and opacified. A persistent omphalomesenteric band may, within its course to the abdominal wall, give rise to a *cystic dilatation* (Fig. 5-8, *D*) that may become quite large and give rise to lower intestinal obstruction between the third and fifth day of life. Bilious vomiting, abdominal distention, a palpable mass, roentgenographic evidence of a cystic formation with an air-fluid level, and a soap-bubble appearance are the important symptoms and signs. A persistent omphalomesenteric band is always a potential hazard, since the looping of bowel around this band can lead to a mechanical type of intestinal obstruction.

A *patent omphalomesenteric duct* (Fig. 5-8, *E*) allows communication between the umbilicus and the small intestine. There is a fecal discharge from the umbilicus. The duct can be opacified with contrast material through a small polyethylene catheter (Fig. 5-9).

REFERENCES

Benson, C.D.: Surgical complications of Meckel's diverticulum. In Ravitch, M.M., Welch, K.J., Benson, C.D., Aberdeen, E., and Randolph, J.G., editors: Pediatric surgery, ed. 3, Chicago, 1979, Year Book Medical Publishers, Inc.

Cross, V.F., Wendth, A.J., Phelan, J.H., and others: Giant Meckel's diverticulum in a premature infant, Am. J. Roentgenol. Radium Ther. Nucl. Med. **108:**591-597, 1970.

Grosfeld, J.L., and Franken, E.A.: Intestinal obstruction in the neonate due to vitelline duct cysts, Surg. Gynecol. Obstet. **138:**527-532, 1974.

PRUNE-BELLY SYNDROME

"Prune belly" is a descriptive term for a syndrome consisting of congenital hypoplasia of the striated muscles of the anterior abdominal wall along with patchy deficiency of smooth muscle in the pelvis, ureter, and bladder. It may also affect the developing renal parenchyma. Less than 5% of cases are found in girls who do not have the full-blown syndrome in that the defect is limited to the abdominal musculature. There is no known mendelian basis for transmission of the syndrome.

At birth the abdomen is shapeless, the skin hangs in wrinkled folds, and the flanks usually bulge. Severe phimosis preventing urination is seen in close to 50% of cases. A urachus may be present. The large kidneys, dilated tortuous ureters, and megacystis can be palpated and are diagnostic of obstructive uropathy, which affects 90% of cases. Associated malformations are invariably found and are most commonly musculoskeletal, gastrointestinal, and cardiac. There is usually malrotation, and it may lead to volvulus or obstruction by bands or atresia. Imperforate anus is also reported. In a recently published series of 45 cases the prognosis is that 20% of patients will die before the age of 1 year, 10% will survive to age 5, and 70% will reach adulthood.

REFERENCES

Harley, L.M., Chen, Y., and Rattner, W.H.: Prune-belly syndrome, J. Urol. **108:**174-176, 1972.

Welch, K.J.: Abdominal musculature deficiency syndrome (prune belly). In Ravitch, M.M., Welch, K.J., Benson, C.D., Aberdeen, E., and Randolph, J.G., editors: Pediatric surgery, ed. 3, Chicago, 1979, Year Book Publishers, Inc.

6 *Sucking and swallowing disorders*

At birth, all mammals are developmentally ready for feeding. The sucking reflex is a familiar index of neurologic maturity and integrity. Swallowing movements are present even in small premature infants. Sucking and swallowing difficulties may be secondary to malformations involving the palate, pharynx, tongue, or esophagus. They may result from primary muscle disorders in the oropharyngeal and esophageal areas. Finally, they may be related to primary disease of the central nervous system affecting the medulla and midbrain. A list of conditions leading to sucking and swallowing difficulties appears in Chapter 1.

INTEGRATION OF SUCKING, SWALLOWING, AND BREATHING

Sucking, swallowing, and breathing occur in a patterned sequence that is under medullary control. Sucking movements in a newborn infant are followed by swallows that inhibit respiration. With initiation of swallowing, respiration or expiration. There is an upward movement of the laryngeal-pharyngeal column, and the laryngeal lumen is closed as the epiglottis folds over its entrance. The final phase of swallowing involves relaxation of the cricopharyngeal muscle, which guards the upper end of the esophagus. The upper esophageal sphincter promptly recovers its normal tone, and the body of the esophagus undergoes peristaltic contraction, giving rise to a contractile wave moving toward the stomach. Shortly before the peristaltic contraction reaches the lower esophageal sphincter (LES), the cardia, which is normally closed, relaxes. Opening of the lower esophageal sphincter, which is contracted at rest, is closely coordinated with other events of the swallowing process. Relaxation of the lower esophageal sphincter represents transient inhibition of the constant discharge of its motor nerves by vagal stimulation induced by swallowing. There is reason to believe that relaxation could also be brought about by pressure-sensitive reflexes under the dependence of the intramural plexuses of the esophagus.

Because most of the esophagus is located in the thorax, where the pressure is lower than that in the pharynx and stomach, the esophagus is a low-pressure tube that must withstand entry of air from the pharynx and of gastric contents from the stomach by competent sphincters. During the first 6 months of life, a considerable amount of air fills the retrophyarnx during sucking and filling of the oral cavity and is propelled into the esophagus and stomach with each swallow. This explains why "burping" is necessary. The lower esophageal spincter is also somewhat handicapped. It maintains a poor tone in the face of a gradual increase of gastric-to-esophageal pressure gradient, which accounts for the regurgitations of the first 6 months.

Clinical findings

Because of the several conditions in which deglutition disorders can occur, careful history taking and physical examination are more important than the functional exploration of the swallowing mechanisms. Polyhydramnios is usually noted in esophageal atresia. Maternal myasthenia gravis may lead to temporary dysphagia in the newborn infant. Life-threatening breathing difficulties are seen in infants with Pierre Robin syndrome (glossoptosis, cleft palate, micrognathia), with choanal atresia, and with either layngeal, or pharyngeal tumors. Dysphagia in the neonate is commonly accompanied by respiratory distress. There is usually abundant mucus, since secretions cannot be swallowed and are often aspirated. More dramatic is the infant who chokes with his first feeding. It is helpful to have the mother relate how her infant feeds in comparison with her other children. Questioning related to feeding technique used and unusual sucking and swallowing patterns is mandatory.

Evidence of neurologic impairment is helpful when one is anticipating sucking and swallowing problems. The nursing personnel will be alerted by the "sleepy" newborn who refuses to suck, fails to suck energetically, or cannot make more than a few suckles before stopping to catch his breath. Nasal regurgitation associated with vomiting can be seen in normal infants, but it should alert the physician to esophageal disorder; in the absence of vomiting, nasal regurgitation is always abnormal. In cleft palate, the defect is obvious; however, when no anatomic defect is found, nasal regurgitation points to abnormal palatal and pharyngeal function. Past the neonatal period, developmental and neurologic abnormalities aid in making the diagnosis. In children with primary or acquired disease of the central nervous system, failure to thrive, recurrent pneumonia, and convulsions are often concomitants.

Diagnosis

Malformations of the mouth and pharynx are usually detected at birth. As a routine in the nursery, a catheter should be passed the length of each nasal passage. The anatomy of the floor of the mouth, tongue, mandible, palate, and hyoid bone should be carefully examined. The physician can evaluate the tone of lip closure and the negative pressure exerted on his finger while the neonate is sucking. The exploring finger will also permit assessment of the tonus of the soft palate.

At the first indication of dysphagia, the physician should bottle-feed the infant. This simple measure will give invaluable information concerning the quality of oral reflexes and the coordination of sucking, swallowing, and breathing. That the infant can breathe while sucking exonerates nasal passages and indicates that he can control the flow of the feeding with his tongue and soft palate. It is said that the infant who can drink and tolerate either breast or bottle feeding in the lateral recumbent position has normal oral and pharyngeal functions.

The extent of the exploration of the oropharyngeal and esophageal function should be dictated by the severity of the dysphagia or of the breathing difficulties. A lateral roentgenogram of the neck will yield a significant amount of information concerning anatomic structures. Use of the chest roentgenogram should be routine because of the ubiquitous aspiration pneumonias. The instillation of a thin solution of barium in the nasopharynx may yield precious information not obtainable otherwise. A cineradiographic study done with the infant in the supine position and swallowing a thin solution of flavored barium is the most important study. When the infant experiences breathing difficulties such as stridor, choking spells, and repeated pneumonias, hospitalization is mandatory. Pharyngolaryngoscopy, endoscopy of the esophagus, and esophageal motility and manometric studies should be carried out.

Treatment

In mild cases, instruction concerning feeding technique and reassurance will usually be sufficient. Infants' poor nipple prehension is a common complaint of the young, inexperienced mothers with engorged breasts. In bottle-fed infants, the use of soft nipples with adequate holes and of bottles in which air entry is adequate and the gentle rhythmic elevation of the baby's mandible are measures that will frequently be helpful to the small, weak neonate.

Whenever there is a discrete motor disability or an anatomic defect such as cleft palate, the feeding technique can safely introduce measures such as the Breck feeder or the compressible bottle, which will deliver formula to the mouth and pharynx. However, if there is a palatal paralysis or a posterior cleft, a palatal prosthesis should be used. It is worthwhile noting that in cases of Pierre Robin syndrome, feeding the infant in the prone position is beneficial. Infants with cleft palates, though, should be fed upright.

Whenever there is choking on feeding or evidence or history of aspiration or of inadequate pharyngeal emptying, as indicated by nasal regurgitation without vomiting, the oropharyngeal route should be bypassed by means of tube feeding or a gastrostomy.

Prognosis

Little can be done for the neonate with a primary disorder of the central nervous system who has sucking and swallowing difficulties. Surgical reconstructions are likely to lead to excellent results in cases in which congenital malformations are responsible for the problem.

REFERENCES

Christensen, J.: The controls of esophageal movement, Clin. Gastroenterol. **5**:15-27, 1976.

Cohen, S.: Medical progress: motor disorders of the esophagus, N. Engl. J. Med. **301**:184-192, 1979.

Ferguson, C.F.: Esophageal dysfunction and other swallowing difficulties in early life, Ann. Otol. Rhinol. Laryngol. **80**:1-8, 1971.

Grand, R.J., Watkins, J.B., and Torti, F.M.: Development of the human gastrointestinal tract, Gastroenterology **70**:790-810, 1976.

Reichert, T.J., Bluestone, C.D., Stool, S.E., Sieber, W.K., and Sieber, A.M.: Congenital cricopharyngeal achalasia, Ann. Otol. Rhinol. Laryngol. **56**:603-610, 1977.

Swischuk, L.E., Smith, P.C., and Fagan, C.J.: Abnormalities of the pharynx and larynx in childhood, Semin. Roentgenol. **9**:283-300, 1974.

ESOPHAGEAL DISORDERS

Esophageal disease in children presents certain problems of diagnosis because of the difficulty in obtaining a description of the pattern and sequence of symptoms, which could be more informative than the clues provided by roentgenology. A further problem has to do with the frequently associated respiratory symptoms that may attract one's attention to the larynx and trachea rather than to the esophagus. Esophageal atresia and tracheoesophageal fistula have already been discussed in the section dealing with gastrointestinal emergencies of the newborn infant.

Congenital esophageal stenosis and webs

The observation that strictures and stenosis of the esophagus occur early in the course of hiatal hernia has led to the idea that congenital esophageal stenosis is rare. Usually, the infant has no dysphagia until he reaches a few weeks or a few months of age. The gradual onset of dysphagia, vomiting, and repeated aspiration occurs as a result of inflammation and edema secondary to retention of ingested feedings proximal to the obstruction. In the majority of cases, the obstruction occurs between the middle and the lower third of the esophagus. Roentgenograms may show variable degrees of obstruction of the contrast material (Fig. 6-1). Treatment may necessitate a gastrostomy if bougienage proves impossible from above. There are reports of other forms of congenital esophageal stenosis. In these cases the resected strictures have been shown to contain ciliated pulmonary epithelium and tracheobronchial remnants.

Esophageal webs are rare and may be found when solid foods are first introduced (Fig. 6-2) or later. An esophageal muscular ring has been described in a 2 year old with some of the malformations described in the VACTERL syndrome (ventricular septal defect, anal atresia, tracheoesophageal fistula, radial anomalies).

Esophageal duplication

Duplication cysts of the esophagus and bronchial cysts produce symptoms related to the esophagus, but more strikingly to the airway (p. 78). Tachypnea and cyanosis are often present from birth. Patients may present with congenital laryngeal stridor. Swallowing difficulty, vomiting, and aspiration pneumonitis are less frequent. Esophageal duplications are cystic structures filled with

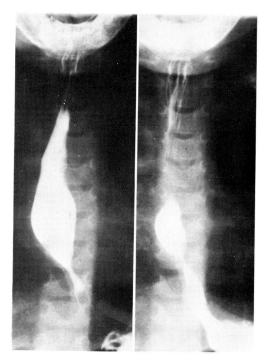

Fig. 6-1. Congenital stenosis of the esophagus. A 2-year-old child with a history of vomiting starting after the introduction of solid foods at the age of 6 months. Symptoms were intermittent initially. Six months before his admission, dysphagia was noted even with pureed foods. He had no anemia, no hematemesis, and no history of recurrent respiratory infections. A 1 cm long stenotic segment is present at the junction of the middle and distal thirds with proximal dilatation and stasis of food. There is no hernia or evidence of esophagitis. Endoscopic examination confirmed the x-ray findings and showed that the stenotic segment was easily distensible. A satisfactory result was obtained with bougienage.

fluid and localized in the posterior mediastinum (Fig. 6-3). The neurenteric type is always associated with vertebral body malformations. The histologic condition is that of a duplication of some portion of the gastrointestinal tract more frequently gastrogenic and enterogenic than esophageal.

Pseudoesophageal atresia

There are a number of cases of esophageal stenosis secondary to a traumatic injury of the hypopharyngeal mucous membranes and to the subsequent formation of a submucosal abscess extending in the proximal esophagus. We have had experience with 4 such cases. The condition may be easily mistaken for esophageal atresia. Shortly

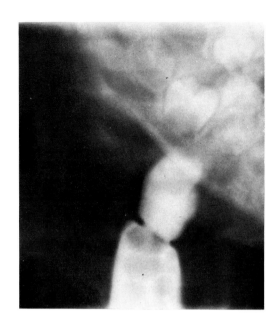

Fig. 6-2. Esophageal web or diaphragm. Obstruction may occur at a number of levels. The web or partial diaphragm may remain asymptomatic until a foreign body or food is trapped in it, producing a complete obstruction.

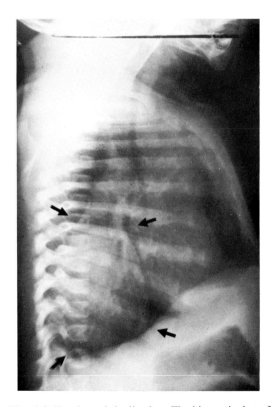

Fig. 6-3. Esophageal duplication. The history is that of a newborn with cyanosis at birth and respiratory distress. The lateral view shows a large mediastinal mass that, at surgery, proved to be an esophageal duplication, *arrows*. There was absence of vertebral lesions and no connection between the duplication and the spinal cord. Note the posterior displacement of the esophagus.

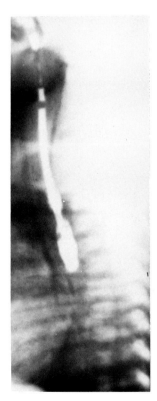

Fig. 6-4. Pseudoesophageal atresia. This roentgenogram shows a long, narrow column of barium behind the esophagus. It ends blindly at the level of the sixth and seventh thoracic vertebrae and is a submucosal canal that originates in the hypopharynx. The blind pouch of esophageal atresia usually ends at the level of the third thoracic vertebra, and its caliber is much larger. In this case, there was obstruction in the proximal third of the esophagus.

after birth or at least within the first 12 hours, there is hypersalivation and inability to swallow, and frothy and bloody secretions may be seen. The stenosis can be at the pharyngoesophageal junction or in the proximal third of the esophagus (Fig. 6-4). The injury is produced during the routine suctioning of secretions at birth and subsequent infection. Antibiotics and parenteral feeding is the treatment of choice. To prevent this condition, suctioning of the pharynx, esophagus, and stomach in neonates should be done with utmost care. The sterile catheter should be soft and rounded at the edges.

Diverticula of esophagus

Congenital diverticula with complete muscular walls localized above the cricopharyngeal fibers are rare and present in the neonatal period with the clinical picture of atresia of the esophagus. Diverticula can be associated with a tracheoesophageal fistula but are not likely to occur above an area of stenosis. A few cases of true diverticula without an underlying tracheoesophageal anomaly are described. Stridor, progressive dysphagia, and recurrent respiratory infections are the usual clinical manifestations.

Intramural diverticulosis is a rare condition characterized by the presence of numerous small flask-shaped diverticula distributed in the upper esophagus. Dysphagia is a presenting complaint. Areas of stenosis, chronic inflammatory changes, abnormal motor activity, and hiatal hernia are occasionally described. Only 3 cases of this condition of unknown cause are described.

Vascular compression of the esophagus

A duplicated aortic arch or a subclavian artery passing to the left of the aorta and behind the esophagus may also compress the esophagus. Dysphagia may not become evident for many years. Repeated bouts of aspiration pneumonia may be the initial complaint. The diagnosis is made by the demonstration of an indentation on the column of barium high in the thorax.

Acquired esophageal strictures

A restricted esophageal lumen may be secondary to peptic esophagitis, which is dealt with in detail on p. 153. In debilitated patients or in those on long-term antibiotic therapy or with immune deficiency states, candidal esophagitis may lead to symptomatic stricture formation (Fig. 6-5). It is

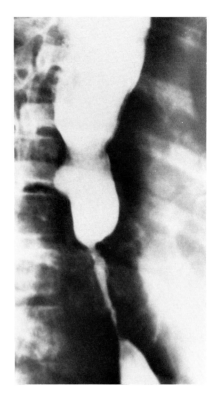

Fig. 6-5. Acquired esophageal stricture in an 8-year-old girl with severe juvenile diabetes and recent weight loss. Esophagoscopy revealed severe inflammation. *Candida albicans* was found in the biopsy material taken from this lesion.

also a common occurrence after anastomosis of esophageal stumps in patients with esophageal atresia. Most commonly, however, acquired esophageal stricture is secondary to chemical burns.

Because the epithelium of the esophagus is squamous, it may be seriously injured in patients suffering from epidermolysis bullosa. Of the six forms of the disease, the autosomal recessive variety most extensively involves the esophagus. The involvement may be noted at any age, but it usually occurs between 3 and 14 years of age. Bullae and inflammation are usually (50%) noted in the upper third of the esophagus. The resulting strictures can be weblike or be as long as 4.5 cm. Complete destruction of the esophagus requiring colonic interposition may be the result. Esophageal perforation may occur after attempts at dilatation of the strictures.

Perforations of esophagus

There are about 50 reports of spontaneous rupture of the esophagus in the neonatal period. In contrast to pseudoesophageal atresia, there is no history of vigorous suctioning and trauma to the hypopharnyx, cyanosis, and dyspnea. A right pleural effusion and a pneumothorax are noted within the first few hours after birth. The perforation is usually found on the right side of the distal esophagus close to the diaphragm, except when it is associated with the rarely reported esophageal ischemic lesions of necrotizing enterocolitis. The pathogenesis of this disorder is obscure though it has been reported in one case of cricopharyngeal incoordination and in association with a mucosal web, as well as in a case of duodenal atresia. In infants and children most perforations are the result of accidental trauma, extensive corrosive burns, foreign bodies, endoscopic procedures, or instrumental dilatations on a diseased esophagus.

REFERENCES

Atkins, J.P.: Some aspects of benign esophageal disease in children, Ann. Otol. Rhinol. Laryngol. **77:**883-891, 1968.

Beardmore, H.E., and Wiglesworth, F.W.: Vertebral anomalies and alimentary duplications; clinical and embryological aspects, Pediatr. Clin. North Am., pp. 457-474, 1958.

Braun P., Nussle D., Roy C.C., and Cuendet A.: Intramural diverticulosis of the esophagus in an eight-year-old baby, Pediatr. Radiol. **6:**235-237, 1978.

Ducharme, J.C., Bertrand, R., and Debie, J.: Perforation of the pharynx in the newborn: a condition mimicking esophageal atresia, Can. Med. Assoc. J. **104:**785-787, 1971.

Fonkalsrud, E.W.: Esophageal stenosis due to tracheobronchial remnants, Am. J. Surg. **124:**101-103, 1972.

Fritz-Mikulska, V.: Stenosis of the esophagus secondary to hypopharyngeal abcess in the newborn, Progr. Pediatr. Surg. **7:**1-25, 1974.

Girdany, B.R., Sieber, W.K., and Osman, M.Z.: Traumatic pseudodiverticulum of the pharynx in newborn infants, N. Engl. J. Med. **280:**237-240, 1969.

Heyman, M.B., Berquist, W.E., Fonkalsrud, E.W., and others: Esophageal muscular ring and the VACTERL association: a case report, Pediatrics **67:**683-686, 1981.

Hillemeier, C., Touloukian, R., McCallum, R., and Gryboski, J.: Esophageal web: a previously unrecognized complication of epidermolysis bullosa, Pediatrics **67:**678-682, 1981.

Langston, H.T., Tuttle, W.M., and Patton, T.B.: Esophageal duplications, Arch. Surg. **61:**949-956, 1950.

Lee, S.B., and Ruhn, J.P.: Esophageal perforation in the neonate: a review of the literature, Am. J. Dis. Child. **130:**325-329, 1976.

Lequien, P., Wurtz, A., Daltroff, G., and others: Perforation spontanée de l'oesophage chez le nouveau-né, Nouv. Presse Méd. **8:**687-689, 1979.

Lincoln, J.C., Deverall, P.B., Stark, J., and others: Vascular anomalies compressing the esophagus and trachea, Thorax **24:**295-306, 1969.

Ravitch, M.M.: Diverticulum of the esophagus. In Ravitch, M.M., Welch, K.J., Benson, C.D., Aberdeen, E., and Randolph, J.G., editors: Pediatric surgery, ed. 3, Chicago, 1979, Year Book Medical Publishers, Inc.

Chemical burns of the esophagus

The commonest cause of esophageal stricture in children is the accidental ingestion of strong corrosive agents. Over the past 6 years (1975 to 1980) the Poison Control Center at Hôpital Sainte-Justine examined 4985 children after the ingestion of drugs and household products. Corrosives were implicated in 831 cases. Eighty percent were below 3 years of age, and close to two thirds of the children were boys.

The short- and long-term morbidity and mortality associated with caustic burns are significant. Commonest of the chemicals ingested accidentally and resulting in burns of the mouth and esophagus are the alkali caustics such as sodium hydroxide or potassium hydroxide. These drain cleaners come in granular, paste or liquid form. The last, even if taken in very small amounts, cause the most extensive and the most severe injury. They are colorless and odorless and contain between 25% and 36.5% sodium hydroxide or potassium hydroxide. Weaker alkaline cleaning solutions commonly contain ammonia, which leads to lesser damage. Household bleaches made up of sodium hypochlorite are much less dangerous and account for two thirds of accidental ingestions of alkali at Hôpital Sainte-Justine. In a recent study from Pittsburgh of 200 cases of ingestion of liquid bleach, only one patient who drank 1 quart of liquid bleach suffered esophageal irritation.

A third group of cleaning products that deserve attention are the nonphosphate and the electric-dishwasher detergents, which can lead to corrosive gastritis and esophagitis. Acids are more likely to cause damage to the stomach and duodenum. Clinitest tablets and silver nitrate have recently become notorious offenders.

Contact of the caustic agent with the esophageal mucosa results in an intense inflammatory reaction, necrosis, and thrombosis of the vessels. Acids do not adhere very much to the esophageal mucosa and produce a coagulation necrosis with an overlying eschar, which gives some protection against a deeper injury.

Caustic burns may involve the mucosa alone, or they may be transmucosal or transmural, involving the periesophageal tissues and structures

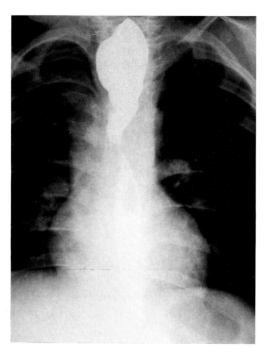

Fig. 6-6. Chemical burn of the esophagus. There is irregular constriction of the esophagus starting in the upper third. The corrosive esophagitis was transmural and involved the mediastinum. Note widening of the mediastinum resulting from mediastinitis.

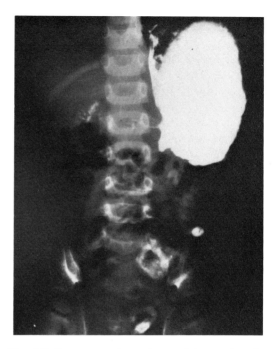

Fig. 6-7. Severe corrosive stricture of the antral region after the ingestion of a commercial drain cleaner containing 10 N HCl.

such as the mediastinum. In severe cases the burn may lead to perforation of the pleural (Fig. 6-6) or the peritoneal cavity, or both. This acute phase subsides within days, after which the child may become asymptomatic until at least the third or fourth week, when cicatrization takes place, leading to strictures.

Clinical findings

The history of ingestion and a brief examination of the mouth often make the diagnosis self-evident. However, in a significant number of cases, the mother can only surmise that the child has swallowed a chemical because of the presence of an overturned bottle or container near the child. The absence of oral lesions does not rule out the diagnosis of a chemical burn of the esophagus. In a recent series of children with esophageal lesions, 25% had no oropharyngeal burns. In a significant number of cases, particularly with acids, the mouth and esophagus may be spared. Location of the gastric injury is related to the position of the patient, the nature and form of the corrosive, and whether it was taken in the fasting or

fed state. Generally, corrosive gastritis is more noticeable in the antrum and in the greater curvature (Fig. 6-7).

Examination of the oral cavity usually reveals circumoral and glossal edema, erythema, ulcerations, and bleeding. Severe pain, refusal of fluids, and burns on the clothing, face, and hands are usually seen. At times, there may be shock; substernal or abdominal pain is indicative of mediastinal or peritoneal extension. Stridor or dyspnea is suggestive of aspiration of the chemical during swallowing.

Symptoms resulting from developing esophageal strictures can occur within 3 or 4 weeks of the accident but are, at times, so slowly progressive that stricture formation does not become symptomatic for many months or even years. Gradual dysphagia usually first appears for meat before becoming evident for all solids and eventually for liquids.

Roentgenograms usually show more severe strictures in the areas of anatomic narrowing, as in the cervical region, at the point at which the left bronchus crosses the esophagus (Fig. 6-8), and

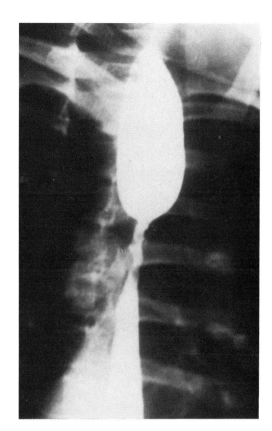

Fig. 6-8. Chemical burn and stricture formation caused by Clinitest tablet ingestion in a 2-year-old child.

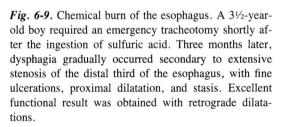

Fig. 6-9. Chemical burn of the esophagus. A 3½-year-old boy required an emergency tracheotomy shortly after the ingestion of sulfuric acid. Three months later, dysphagia gradually occurred secondary to extensive stenosis of the distal third of the esophagus, with fine ulcerations, proximal dilatation, and stasis. Excellent functional result was obtained with retrograde dilatations.

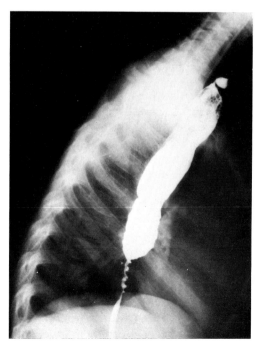

at the level of the cardia (Fig. 6-9). Strictures may extend throughout the esophagus or selectively affect any portion of the esophagus. Esophagoscopic findings are those of localized eschars. Later, the affected portion of the esophagus becomes shortened and narrowed. Severe shortening of the esophagus may lead to the development of hiatal hernia (Fig. 6-10).

Concomitant gastric involvement has been noted in 20% of patients with esophageal burns from lye. In case of acid ingestion, the esophagus is commonly spared and gastric burns may be seen. The corrosive gastritis may result in a perforation or, in less severe cases, widespread superficial lesions and eventually antral stenosis and pyloric obstruction.

Management

It is important to remember that burns of the mouth do not provide evidence that there is an esophageal burn; on the other hand, the absence of burns of the oral mucosa does not preclude esophageal involvement. For these reasons, it is mandatory to evaluate the extent and degree of the burns. Failure to recognize the seriousness of the accident and to provide adequate therapy may cause the patient problems of lifelong duration.

The immediate home care given for ingestion of lye should be familiar to all parents. Vomiting should not be induced either mechanically or pharmacologically. Water or milk can be used to dilute the corrosive. Milk of magnesia and antacids may neutralize a strong acid. Hospitalization is recommended even if there is only a reasonable doubt that an alkali (other than a liquid chlorine bleach) or a strong acid (oxalic, nitric, sulfuric, or hydrochloric) has been ingested. Intravenous fluids are started and hydrocortisone 10 mg/kg/day is administered. Close monitoring for laryngitis, mediastinitis, and peritonitis is essential. From 24 to 48 hours after admission, an esophagoscopy is performed under general anesthesia. In the absence of any visible lesions, the treatment is discontinued and the child is discharged. The instrument is never advanced beyond the first point of esophageal mucosal injury. If, on admission, roentgenograms show evidence of erosion into the mediastinum or peritoneum, antibiotics become mandatory.

Although it is true that a first-degree burn never results in strictures, the endoscopist can never decide on the depth on an esophageal burn. Therefore, whenever there is evidence of a lesion in the esophagus, treatment with corticosteroids (prednisone 1 mg/kg/day) is continued for 3 weeks before an esophagogram is taken. The decision to start dilatations is then made, and steroids are discontinued.

When there is severe involvement of the esophagus, management may also include a tracheostomy because of laryngeal edema. A gastrostomy may be required for feeding. Use of steroids is definitely contraindicated if roentgenograms show erosion into the mediastinum or peritoneum. As soon as he can tolerate liquids, the patient is made to swallow a No. 4 surgical thread, which is allowed to advance through the gastrointestinal tract and is used as a guide to bougies. If a gastrostomy is done for feeding purposes, it may be used as a means for retrograde, string-guided esophageal dilatations. In patients with esophageal lye strictures that are extensive or impenetrable or that require continuous dilation, colonic reconstruction of the esophagus is justified.

Prognosis

Experience shows that the long-term prognosis is significantly influenced by early treatment to prevent strictures and by frequent and aggressive follow-up evaluation of the need for esophageal dilatations. If liquid lye has been ingested, the lesions are extensive, severe, and difficult to dilate. The prognosis for bleach burns is substantially better than for those after lye ingestion. All children who have ingested bleach probably do not need to be put through the cortisone, antibiotics, and early dilatation routine. However, if there is extensive mucosal injury, the treatment advocated for lye should be given.

REFERENCES

Bernirschke K.: Time bomb of lye ingestion? Am. J. Dis. Child. **135:**17-18, 1981.

Butler, C., Madden, J.W., David, W.M., and Peacock, E.E.: Morphologic aspects of experimental esophageal lye strictures. II. Effect of steroid hormones, bougienage, and induced lathyrism on acute lye burns, Surgery **81:**431-435, 1977.

Chong, G.C., Beahrs, O.H., and Payne, W.S.: Management of corrosive gastritis due to ingested acid, Mayo Clin. Proc. **49:**861-865, 1974.

Haller, J.A., Andrews, H.G., White, J.J., and others: Pathophysiology and management of acute corrosive burns of the esophagus: results of treatment in 285 children, J. Pediatr. Surg. **6:**578-583, 1971.

Leape, L.L., Ashcraft, K.W., Scarpelli, D.G., and others: Hazard to health: liquid lye, N. Engl. J. Med. **284:**578-581, 1971.

Lowe, J.E., Graham, D.Y., Boisaubin, E.V., and Lanza, F.L.: Corrosive injury of the stomach: the natural history and role of fiberoptic endoscopy, Am. J. Surg. **137:**803-806, 1979.

Moriarty, R.W.: Corrosive chemicals: acids and alkalis, Drug Therapy (Hosp.), pp. 89-99, March 1969.

Stannard, M.W.: Corrosive esophagitis in children: assessment by the esophagram, Am. J. Dis. Child. **132:**596-599, 1978.

Esophageal dysfunction in collagen disease

The gastrointestinal tract is involved in 50% to 80% of patients with scleroderma. The corresponding figures in those with dermatomyositis is 60% and systemic lupus erythematosus 10% to 25%. There is absence of peristalsis in the distal two thirds of the esophagus, and the lower esophageal sphincter is patulous, leading to reflux esophagitis, candidiasis, and occasionally strictures. In dermatomyositis and systemic lupus erythematosus the motility disorder also affects the striated muscle portion of the esophagus. Symptoms include retrosternal burning pain and dysphagia for solid foods, but they are not invariably present. In a series of 12 children with scleroderma, only 4 had any symptoms referable to the esophagus.

REFERENCES

Clinical Conference, S.Cohen, moderator: The gastrointestinal manifestations of scleroderma: pathogenesis and management, Gastroenterology **79:**155-166, 1980.

Dabich, L., Sullivan, D.B., and Cassidy, J.T.: Scleroderma in the child, J. Pediatr. **85:**770-775, 1974.

Gastroesophageal reflux (GER)

The reflux of small amounts of gastric contents into the lower esophagus is very frequent. It occurs in all age groups and in most there are no associated symptoms. Reflux becomes symptomatic with increased frequency and duration of each reflux, with the type of material in reflux, and with a decrease in the intrinsic capacity of the esophagus to withstand attack by pepsin, hydrochloric acid, and bile acids. Heartburn with and without regurgitation is the hallmark of reflux. When lower esophageal sphincter incompetence is severe and permits free reflux or when there is an associated dysfunction of the upper esophageal function, regurgitation is also present.

Anatomic sphincter

The lower esophageal sphincter (LES) is distinguishable from the body of the esophagus in that its lumen is closed at rest and opens upon swallowing. Although a well-localized sphincteric

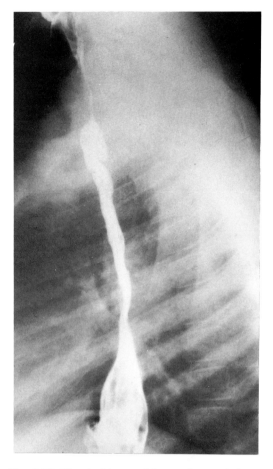

Fig. 6-10. Chemical burns of the esophagus. A 5-year-old boy suffered extensive lye burns of the esophagus. Gradual fibrosis has led to shortening of the esophagus and hiatus hernia. Colonic interposition had to be carried out eventually.

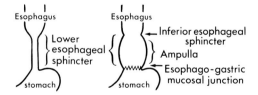

Fig. 6-11. The anatomy of the lower esophageal sphincter. It is closed at rest, *left.* When barium is given, the ampulla is dilated, *right.* Endoscopically the squamocolumnar junction (Z line) is easily identified, but it does not always correspond to the constriction noted at the diaphragmatic hiatus.

mechanism can be documented manometrically as a zone of high resting pressure, it has never been anatomically (Fig. 6-11) shown to correspond to a specific muscle sphincter. It is a "brilliant feat of engineering," since it forms a barrier preventing reflux from the supra-atmospheric pressure in the stomach to the subatmospheric pressure within the thoracic esophagus and yet permits evacuation of air and of gastric contents when this becomes necessary.

Developmental aspects of functional sphincter

The pressure zone detected with an assembly of pressure-sensing catheters inserted into the stomach and then gradually withdrawn averages 1 cm (0.75 to 2 cm) in children less than 3 months of age, 1.6 cm (0.75 to 3 cm) in those older than 1 year, and 3 to 4 cm in adults. The length of the high-pressure zone does not correlate well with sphincter competence, but there is a tendency for a shorter high-pressure zone in children with reflux.

Because 40% of newborns and infants regurgitate, there has been a long-standing interest in esophageal function in this age group. Prematures and newborns show poorly coordinated responses to swallowing with rapid biphasic and often non-peristaltic repetitive waves (tertiary waves). Although initial studies reported low LES pressures during the first few weeks of life, recent data with constantly perfused catheters show values of 46.3 ± 7.7 mm Hg. In 46 children younger than 1 year, a mean pressure of 43.4 ± 2.4 mm Hg was recorded; the corresponding value in 16 over 1 year of age was 30.6 ± 2.3 mm Hg.

Recent work in infants and children with gastroesophageal reflux shows that there are factors other than resting pressures that determine the competence of the LES. The mean LES pressures in infants and children with gastroesophageal reflux are lower than control values, but there is a lot of overlap. The majority have values within the range of pressures for their age group, but they tend to increase with age as the condition improves.

Physiological and pharmacological control of LES competence

An age-dependent rise in resting LES pressure was found in opossums and interpreted as the result of a reduced functional LES muscle mass and of a diminished responsiveness to neurohormonal stimulation. In adults with gastroesophageal reflux and low LES pressure the rise in pressure after the administration of gastrin, bethanechol, and metoclopramide is less than in controls. In contrast, the only study in children with gastroesophageal reflux shows a very good response of the

---

Table 6-1. Factors that alter basal LES pressure

	Increase	Decrease
Diet	Proteins	Fat
	Coffee	Chocolate
		Alcohol
Hormones	Gastrin	Glucagon
	Motilin	Secretin
		Cholecystokinin
		Progesterone
		Estrogens
Neural	Bethanechol	Nicotine (smoking)
transmitters,	Norepinephrine	Epinephrine
drugs, and	Phenylephrine	Isoproterenol
various agents	Acetylcholine	Salbutamol
	Serotonin	Dopamine
	Prostaglandin $F_{2\alpha}$	Prostaglandins E_1 and E_2
	Histamine	
	Cimetidine	
	Metoclopramide	
Operations	Fundoplication	Vagotomy

LES to bethanechol. This suggests that neurohormonal factors responsible for LES competence may be abnormal or late to mature. A list of dietary components, neural transmitters, hormones, and pharmacological agents known to affect basal sphincter pressure appears in Table 6-1.

Hiatus hernia and competence of lower esophageal sphincter

Although a significant number of infants and children with gastroesophageal reflux have a hiatus hernia, several experimental and clinical observations indicate that it does not cause gastroesophageal reflux. In a recent study, 41 of 52 children with gastroesophageal reflux were shown to have normal LES pressures for their age. Competence of the LES depends on its functional integrity rather than on its location. The so-called diaphragmatic pinchcock, the acute esophagogastric angle formed by the rosette of mucosa at the entrance of the esophagus into the stomach, and the phrenoesophageal membrane seem to play a minor role if any, as shown in animal models.

Sliding hiatus hernia (Fig. 6-12)

As implied in the previous section, the last several years have witnessed a destruction of the myth that hiatus hernia is a synonym for reflux. Although it is true that a significant percentage of infants and children with gastroesophageal reflux have a hernia (15% to 75%), a large number with a hernia are asymptomatic. Severe reflux symptoms occur in the absence of a detectable hernia. However, in a large (1000) adult series, patients with a hernia were 10 times more likely to have free reflux than those without a roentgenoologically demonstrable hernia. Among patients with gastroesophageal reflux, esophagitis correlates with

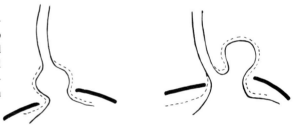

Fig. 6-12. Hiatus hernia. *Left,* Prolapse of both the abdominal esophagus and a portion of the stomach into the thoracic cavity. This is a sliding type of hernia, and it is by far the most common. *Right,* Paraesophageal hernia. The lower esophagus remains in its normal position, and a portion of the cardiac end of the stomach herniates through the hiatus alongside the esophagus.

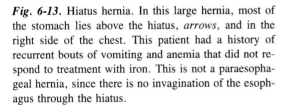

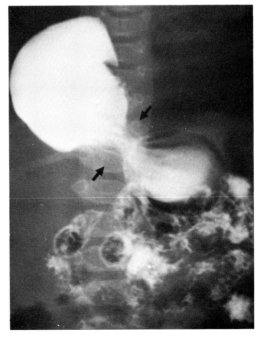

Fig. 6-13. Hiatus hernia. In this large hernia, most of the stomach lies above the hiatus, *arrows,* and in the right side of the chest. This patient had a history of recurrent bouts of vomiting and anemia that did not respond to treatment with iron. This is not a paraesophageal hernia, since there is no invagination of the esophagus through the hiatus.

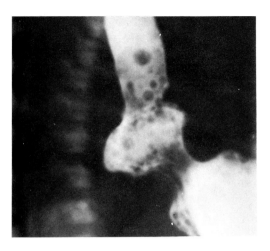

Fig. 6-14. Hiatus hernia. This small hernia showing little evidence of peptic esophagitis was not associated with any signs of gastrointestinal bleeding, failure to thrive, or aspiration pneumonitis. It was successfully treated medically. A hernia of this relatively small size often requires cinefluoroscopy because it may only be intermittently demonstrable.

spincter competence and not with the existence of a hernia.

X-ray diagnosis. The higher incidence of hiatus hernia in European centers was attributed to the fact that the radiologists were better at diagnosing them. American radiologists also started finding many hernias in hospitals where pediatricians held tightly to the belief that hernia was a synonym for reflux and kept returning infants to the radiologist with the note that three negative examinations were necessary to rule out a hernia. Certainly, when a large portion of the stomach is displaced into the chest (Fig. 6-13), the x-ray diagnosis is easy. The recognition of a small hernia is a problem. The presence of gastric folds, a mucosal notch, and a supradiaphragmatic nonperistaltic pouch are the usual criteria, but their interpretation is difficult (Fig. 6-14).

Endoscopy and manometry. Manometry can identify the exact location of the diaphragmatic opening because there is a change from positive

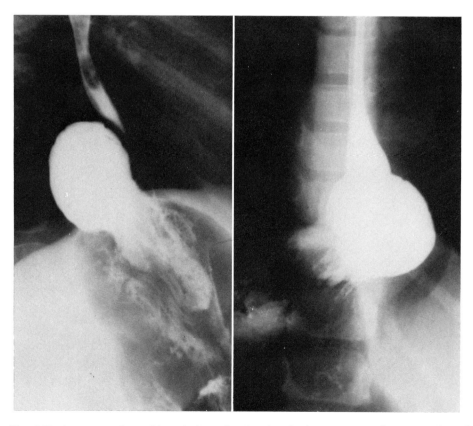

Fig. 6-15. Anteroposterior and lateral views showing the classic appearance of a paraesophageal hernia in a 5-year-old child with symptoms of abdominal pain and intermittent vomiting.

to negative deflection on inspiration when the pressure-sensitive catheters move up through the diaphragmatic hiatus. A second advantage over the x-ray examination is that the LES pressure zone can be located and is generally increased in length when a hernia is present. The endoscopist will note a segment of gastric mucosa distal from the Z line and proximal to the indentation caused by the diaphragmatic hiatus. A view from the cardia using a J-maneuver will show the widened opening of the diaphragm, and on inspiration gastric folds are noted to be sliding upward.

Pathogenesis and associated conditions. Sliding hernias can be detected within the first few weeks of life, and they are believed to be congenital. The theory of the so-called congenitally short esophagus as the cause of gastric herniation is no longer tenable. A certain number of sliding hernias can be acquired as a consequence of shortening of the esophagus, itself the result of esophagitis, stricture, and eventual cicatricial traction on the upper region of the stomach (Fig. 6-10). A higher incidence of hiatus hernia and gastroesophageal reflux is reported in cerebral palsy. Contortions of the head and neck and a torticollis-like head posturing in association with a hiatus hernia is known as Sandifer's syndrome. Correction of the hernia and of the associated reflux leads to clearing of the symptoms. The rumination syndrome characterized by the projection of gastric contents into the mouth and by regurgitation and rechewing followed by swallowing has also been reported as an important manifestation of hiatus hernia.

Clinical findings and treatment. The symptoms and signs of gastroesophageal reflux in infants and children with a hiatus hernia are identical to those in patients without an associated hernia. Management does not differ either. A discussion of clinical findings and treatment is found under chalasia. Surgical repair is reserved for the few patients who do not respond to medical management. Its purpose is not to "wrench a wandering pouch of stomach back down where it belongs" but to prevent reflux by a procedure that will increase the pressure at the esophagogastric juntion.

Paraesophageal hernia (Fig. 6-12)

This is a rare condition. The esophagus extends normally to the hiatus, but part of the stomach herniates alongside the esophagus (Fig. 6-15).

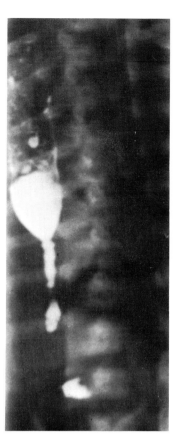

Fig. 6-16. Peptic esophagitis showing a narrow lower third of the esophagus with proximal dilatation. Note the ulcer crater at the junction of the dilated and constricted segments.

Paraesophageal hernias give rise to abdominal pain with distention and vomiting. The risk of strangulation and infarction is high. Surgery is advocated in all cases.

Chalasia

The term "chalasia," coined by Neuhauser and Berenberg in the early 1950s, applies to infants and children with clinically manifest gastroesophageal reflux but who do not have an associated hiatus hernia. It is a primary disorder of LES competence, but a recent paper suggests that infants with severe gastroesophageal reflux have a significantly delayed gastric emptying. This may contribute to their failure to thrive and pulmonary problems. Low pressures have also been found in the upper esophageal sphincter, but this has not been confirmed in infants and children.

Clinical findings. The symptoms attending the efflux of gastric contents from the stomach to the esophagus is impossible to document in infants but will give rise to chest pain and heartburn in older children. Regurgitation is the usual manifestation of gastroesophageal reflux, and it is effortless. In contrast, vomiting is caused by a problem below the diaphragm or by a central stimulation of the vomiting center. It is associated with contraction of abdominal muscles and leads to a powered projection of the gastrointestinal contents. Close questioning will often reveal that the feeding wells out initially and then the emesis becomes forceful. The regurgitated material nauseates the infant as it passes through the mouth and induces vomiting, which may even contain some bile.

In a small number of patients the amounts regurgitated are sufficiently large to impair weight gain and lead to failure to thrive. A significant degree of esophagitis may occur. This can bring about occult blood loss, iron-deficiency anemia, hematemesis, and esophageal strictures (Fig. 6-16). Inflammatory esophagogastric polyps constitute a rare complication of hiatal hernias with esophagitis. There have been 15 cases reported in adults as of 1979 and only two in the pediatric age group. We have personally seen three (Fig. 6-17). Attention is drawn to the relationship between gastroesophageal reflux and respiratory disease. Recurrent aspiration pneumonia, chronic cough, wheezing, and asthma-like attacks are reported. Respiratory complications are more likely to occur before 1 year of age. Apneic spells in the newborn and the sudden infant death syndrome (SIDS) have been ascribed to gastroesophageal reflux.

Unusual presentations include the rumination syndrome and Sandifer's syndrome (see hiatus hernia). Finger clubbing and a protein-losing enteropathy are reported with these two syndromes and regress after surgical correction of the reflux. Also, the incidence of symptomatic reflux is increased in conditions associated with central nervous system disease and mental retardation.

Diagnosis. The clinician confronted daily with babies who spit up must make a triage of those requiring investigation. Infants who are growing well and seem to suffer no ill effects from regurgitation should be left alone. A less-than-satisfactory weight curve, occult blood in the stools or vomitus, iron-deficiency anemia, repeated lower respiratory infections, a chronic cough, or wheezing in the infant with regurgitations should be investigated. Children with neurologic problems and normal children who are chronically symptomatic beyond the age of 2 years are at high risk for complications and deserve testing of their swallowing mechanism, esophageal peristalsis, and behavior of their gastroesophageal function. Although the presence of significant reflux in children attending our chest clinic has been disappointingly small, we are aware of reports showing the coexistence of pulmonary roentgenographic abnormalities in 76% of children with major reflux. The techniques used currently to evaluate LES competence include roentgenography, endoscopy, manometry, acid reflux test, extended pH monitoring of the distal esophagus, and gastroesophageal scintigraphy. They permit confirmation of the clinical evidence of reflux.

The *barium swallow* accurately identifies only 50% to 75% of symptomatic patients. Five grades of reflux are recognized:

Grade 1: reflux into the distal esophagus
Grade 2: reflux above the carina
Grade 3: reflux into the cervical esophagus
Grade 4: free reflux with a widely patent lower esophageal sphincter
Grade 5: reflux with aspiration

Endoscopy sometimes permits a diagnosis of esophagitis. Biopsies must provide histologic evidence. Since 20% to 25% of control subjects show epithelial alterations, the diagnosis of esophagitis should only be made when there are well-defined inflammatory changes.

Manometry remains a specialized technique, and its ability to identify children with major reflux on the basis of LES resting pressures has not been good. As stated previously, the overlap between refluxers with or without hernia and controls is considerable. A survey of the recent literature suggests that in children without gastroesophageal reflux the LES pressure should be above 15 mm Hg. A sleeve-sensor device allows continuous recording of LES pressure without the artifact introduced by axial sphincter movement. A recent study shows that one of the likely explanations for the poor correlation between gastroesophageal reflux and LES pressure is that inappropriate (unrelated to swallowing) relaxation of the sphincter may occur.

The *acid reflux test* (Tuttle's test) consists in instilling a calculated volume (300 ml/1.73 m^2) of 0.1N HCl through a nasogastric tube, which is

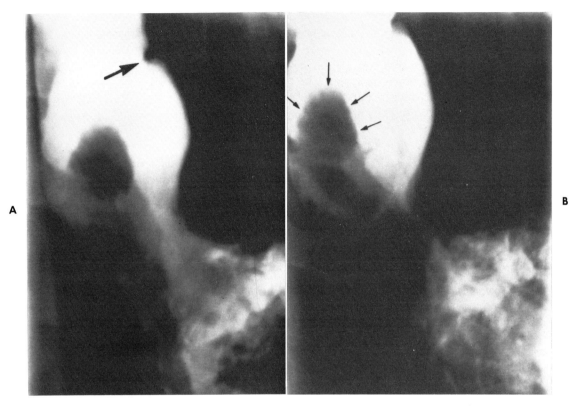

Fig. 6-17. Inflammatory esophagogastric polyp in a 14-year-old boy with steroid-dependent asthma associated with mild symptoms of gastroesophageal reflux. **A,** Roentgenogram shows reflux, a hiatal hernia, a Shatzki ring *(arrow),* and a large polyp. **B,** Film demonstrates more clearly the large polypoid mass, *arrows,* attached to a large gastric fold tapering into the stomach. This is a rare complication of a hiatal hernia. it was first reported in children by Jones, T.B., et al. (A.J.R. **133:**314-316, 1979), and we have seen three such cases in the past few years.

then removed before positioning of a pH probe with its tip at a level 87% of the distance from the nares to the LES. Monitoring of the pH is carried out with the patient in various positions with and without abdominal compression. Reflux is defined as a drop of intraesophageal pH to less than 4. Tuttle's test has been very accurate in its ability to confirm clincal reflux. Its main advantage is that in one study it has been predictive of the need for surgical correction. Tuttle tests were negative in those who responded to medical therapy.

Twenty-four-hour pH monitoring of the distal esophagus has proved both sensitive and specific in the detection of reflux. A flexible glass-tipped pH electrode 1.2 mm in diameter is passed through the nares and positioned at a level 87% of the distance from the nares to the LES. Records from patients kept supine at a 30 degree angle differ significantly from controls in the percentage of monitored time with pH below 4, the number of reflux episodes, and the duration of the longest episode of reflux. Recent information suggests that the difference in esophageal pH records between patients and controls is maximal during the first 2 hours after a low pH fluid such as apple juice is fed twice at a 4-hour interval. It quantitates the severity of reflux and may be used to assess the response to medical management. Overnight probing is particularly useful in patients with apneic spells or recurrent pulmonary infections.

Scintigraphic scanning represents a significant advance in that it is a noninvasive technique involving little radiation. It is more sensitive than roentgenography in the detection of severe reflux and reflux complicated by esophagitis and aspiration. One hundred microcuries of technetium (^{99m}Tc) sulfur colloid is instilled into the stomach followed by saline solution or 5% glucose (300 ml/1.73 m^2) through a nasogastric tube, which is then removed. The radioactivity is monitored over the esophagus and stomach with the patient in the upright and supine positions for 30 minutes each. Delayed images are obtained 4 and 24 hours later in an attempt to detect aspiration. One calculates the gastroesophageal reflux index by counting for each 30-second period the esophageal radioactivity and expressing it as a percentage of gastric radioactivity.

Management. The aim of the treatment is to protect the esophagus and eventually the lungs from contact with gastric contents and bile acids that undergo reflux from the duodenum while ensuring normal growth. One can accomplish this by strengthening the LES, neutralizing gastric acid, and decreasing gastric emptying time.

Diet. In infants, thickening the formula and decreasing the total amount offered at each sitting is usually helpful. A decrease in the fat content of the diet and avoidance of chocolate are advocated in children.

Orthostatic posturing. This traditional treatment has come under attack. Posturing the infant for a few hours after feedings or maintaining him at a 60 degree angle around the clock have been a mainstay of management for decades. The prone position at a 30 degree angle may be more favorable in terms of reflux episodes and acid clearance. In addition, the prone position facilitates gastric emptying. In older children, the head of the bed should be elevated by 20 to 30 cm.

Drug therapy. Bethanechol (8.7 mg/m^2/day), given every 8 hours in infants and 45 minutes before each meal in children, has been shown to be effective. It confirms an earlier manometric study documenting an increase in LES pressure in infants with gastroesophageal reflux given bethanechol (0.1 mg/kg) subcutaneously. It has also been shown to be effective in patients with LES incompetence after repair of esophageal atresia. Theoretically, metoclopramide should have the added advantage of not stimulating acid secretion, but the results with this drug in infants and children have been disappointing. Antacids (30 ml/1.73 m$_2$) and cimetidine (1200 mg/1.73 m$_2$/day) neutralize gastric acid and decrease hydrochloric acid secretion, respectively. This will not only protect the esophagus but may also lead to an increase in sphincter pressure through an increase in gastrin. We believe that cimetidine should only be used in situations where antacids prove ineffective.

Surgery. Fundoplication is a very effective procedure. Displacement below the diaphragm of a segment of distal esophagus and the wrapping of this segment with a cuff of stomach greatly improves the resting LES pressure as well as its responsiveness to drugs and hormones. Furthermore, the LES has been shown to relax on swallowing.

Indications for surgery include the following:
1. Persistent vomiting with failure to thrive after 2 to 3 months of intensive conservative management
2. Esophagitis refractory to medical treatment and the presence of strictures
3. History of a "near miss," apneic spells, and chronic recurrent pulmonary problems that are absolute surgical indications
4. Children with underlying central nervous system problems for whom medical management is likely to fail

Prognosis. The natural history of chalasia starting within the first few weeks is very favorable. Most (95%) get better without treatment and are asymptomatic by 6 to 9 months of age. When reflux is severe, the prognosis is good if proper management is instituted early. Eighty-five percent of infants begun on medical therapy before 3 months of age can be expected to be free of symptoms by 1 year of age, and 95% by the age of 2. The responsibility of the clinician is to identify early the infants at high risk for complications that can be life threatening or that can be associated with a significant morbidity. The success rate of medical management drops to 75% if treatment is initiated between 3 and 24 months and only 50% between 2 and 12 years of age.

REFERENCES

Arasu, T.S., Wyllie, R., Fitzgerald, J.F., and others: Gastroesophageal reflux in infants and children: comparative accuracy of diagnostic methods, J. Pediatr. **96:**798-803, 1980.

Boix-Ochoa, J., and Canals, J.: Maturation of the lower esophagus, J. Pediatr. Surg. **11:**749-756, 1977.

Bray, P.F., Herbst, J.J., Johnson, D.G., and others: Childhood gastroesophageal reflux: neurologic and psychiatric syndromes mimicked, J.A.M.A. **237:**1342-1345, 1977.

Casasa, J.M., Boix-Ochoa, J.: Surgical or conservative treatment in hiatal hernias in children: a new decisive parameter, Surgery **82:**573-575, 1977.

Carcassone, M., Bensoussan, A., and Aubert, J.: The management of gastroesophageal reflux in infants, J. Pediatr. Surg. **8:**575-586, 1973.

Cohen, S.: Developmental characteristics of lower esophageal sphincter function: a possible mechanism for infantile chalasia, Gastroenterology **67:**252-258, 1974.

Cohen, S.: Medical progress: motor disorders of the esophagus, N. Engl. J. Med. **301:**184-192, 1979.

Darling, D.B., McGauley, R.G.K., Leonidas, J.C., and Schwartz, A.M.: Gastroesophageal reflux in infants and children: correlation of radiological severity and pulmonary pathology, Radiology **127:**735-740, 1978.

Euler, A.R., Fonkalsrud, E.W., and Ament, M.E.: Effect of Nissen fundoplication on the lower esophageal sphincter pressure of children with gastroesophageal reflux, Gastroenterology **72:**260-262, 1977.

Euler, A.R., and Byrne, W.J.: Twenty-four hour esophageal intraluminal pH probe testing: a comparative analysis, Gastroenterology **80:**957-961, 1981.

Euler, A.R.: Use of bethanechol for the treatment of gastroesophageal reflux, J. Pediatr. **96:**321-324, 1980.

Forget, P.P., and Meradji, M.: Contribution of fiberoptic endoscopy to diagnosis and management of children with gastro-esophageal reflux, Arch. Dis. Child. **51:**60-66, 1976.

Forget, P., Devos, P., De Roo, M., and Eggermont, E.: Dynamic gastroesophageal scintigraphy in the investigation of GE reflux in children. (Submitted for publication.)

Friedland, G.W., Sunshine, P., and Zboralske, F.F.: Hiatal hernia in infants and young children: a 2 to 3-year follow-up study, J. Pediatr. **87:**71-74, 1975.

Herbst, J.J., Book, L.S., and Bray, P.F.: Gastroesophageal reflux in the "near miss" sudden infant death syndrome, J. Pediatr. **92:**73-75, 1978.

Hillemeir, A.C., Lange, R., McCallum, R., and others: Delayed gastric emptying in infants with gastroesophageal reflux, J. Pediatr. **98:**190-193, 1981.

Jones, T.B., Heller, R.M., Kirchner, S.G., and Greene, H.L.: Inflammatory esophagogastric polyp in children, A.J.R. **133:**314-316, 1979.

Kaye, M.D., and Showalter, J.P.: Pyloric incompetence in patients with symptomatic gastroesophageal reflux, J. Lab. Clin. Med. **83:**198-206, 1977.

Moroz, S.P., Espinoza, J., Cumming, W.A., and Diamant, N.E.: Lower esophageal sphincter function in children with and without gastroesophageal reflux, Gastroenterology **71:**236-241, 1976.

Murphy, W.J., and Gellis, S.S.: Torticollis with hiatal hernia in infancy: Sandifer's syndrome, Am. J. Dis. Child. **131:**564-565, 1977.

Nebel, O.T. and Castell D.O.: Inhibition of the lower esophageal sphincter by fat as a mechanism for fatty food intolerance, Gut. **14:**270-274, 1973.

Randolph, J.G., Lilly, J.R., and Anderson, K.R.: Surgical treatment of gastroesophageal reflux in infants, Ann. Surg. **180:**479-485, 1977.

Sondheimer, J.M.: Continuous monitoring of distal esophageal pH: a diagnostic test for gastroesophageal reflux in infants, J. Pediatr. **96:**804-807, 1980.

Werlin, S.L., Dodds, W.J., Hogan, W.J., and Arndorfer, R.C.: Mechanisms of gastroesophageal reflux in children, J. Pediatr. **97:**244-249, 1980.

NEUROMUSCULAR DISORDERS
Cricopharyngeal dysfunction

The upper esophageal sphincter is largely made up of the cricopharyngeal muscle and of circular upper esophageal muscle fibers. At rest, it remains closed and effectively separates the esophagus from the pharynx, thereby preventing eddying of air with inspiration. The upper esophageal sphincter not only prevents esophageal distention during respiration but also esophagopharyngeal reflux and eventual tracheobronchial aspiration. A recent study has shown that patients with heartburn and regurgitation differ from those without regurgitation in that they have hypotension in their upper esophageal sphincter. This has not yet been studied in infants and children. Relaxation of this sphincter normally occurs as a bolus reaches the posterior pharyngeal wall and precedes pharyngeal contractions above it. Functional obstruction at the level of the cricopharyngeal muscle leads to severe swallowing difficulties, pharyngeal dilatation, vomiting, nasal regurgitation, and aspiration pneumonia.

In the largest series reported to date in newborns, the symptoms started shortly after birth. Only four of the 15 infants did not have associated abnormalities, which were myelomingocele, microcephaly, arthrogryposis, and cerebral palsy with seizures. They improved with conservative management (gavage and posturing). In their hands, cricopharyngeal myotomy in two cases with central nervous disease led to very little improvement. Dilatations are not generally helpful. Other reports suggest that a cricopharyngeal myotomy should be performed in babies who have no underlying problem that could be responsible for the cricopharyngeal dysfunction.

Cineradiography, used as the infant drinks from a bottle of a barium mixture, demonstrates a persistent dorsal indentation at the level of the cricopharyngeal muscle (Fig. 6-18). Although transitory indentations are present in normal infants, persistence of the pattern in the presence of swallowing difficulties is significant. Aganglionosis of the wall of the upper third of the esophagus has been found in one such patient.

Oropharyngeal dysphagia does not necessarily imply cricopharyngeal dysfunction or incoordination. In familial dysautonomia the swallowing reflex is abnormal, but the cricopharyngeus muscle is normal. Impaired cricopharyngeal activity is re-

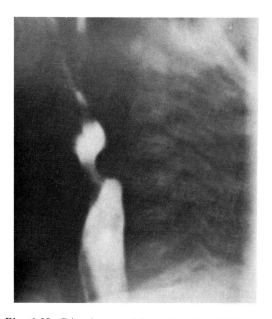

Fig. 6-18. Cricopharyngeal incoordination. Failure of relaxation of the cricopharyngeal muscle is demonstrated by a persistent posterior indentation usually at the level of the third to fourth cervical vertebrae. Lesser degrees of similar indentation, particularly those that are transitory, are seen frequently in normal children and cause no trouble.

ported in amyotrophic lateral sclerosis, thyrotoxic myopathy, myasthenia gravis, and muscular dystrophies, as well as in dermatomyositis and rarely in systemic lupus erythematosus. Patients with cricopharyngeus muscle disease will often say that food catches in their throat and that goes around and around without going down. In contrast to disorders of the lower esophageal sphincter, swallowing of solids is often easier than that of liquids in disorders of the upper esophageal sphincter.

REFERENCES

Bishop, H.C.: Cricopharyngeal achalasia in childhood, J. Pediatr. Surg. **9:**775-778, 1974.

Blank, R.H., and Silbiger, M.: Cricopharyngeal achalasia as a cause of respiratory distress in infancy, J. Pediatr. **81:**95-98, 1972.

Bluestone, C.D., Stool, S.E., Sieber, W.K., and Sieber, A.M.: Congenital cricopharyngeal achalasia, Ann. Otol. Rhinol. Laryngol. **56:**603-610, 1977.

Bondonny, J.M., Hehunstre, J.P., Diard, F., and Bechraoui, T.: L'achalasie du cricopharyngien: cause exceptionnelle de dysphagie du nouveau-né, Chir. Pédiatr. **20:**60-73, 1979.

Palmer, E.D.: Disorders of the cricopharyngeus muscle: a review, Gastroenterology **71:**510-519, 1976.

Achalasia

Esophageal achalasia is a disease of unknown cause characterized by the absence of peristalsis in the body of the esophagus and by failure of the lower esophageal sphincter to relax in a normal way in response to swallowing. For a long time lesions of Auerbach's plexus have been believed to be responsible for the motility disorder. Intramural nerve fibers are also involved. There is a deficiency of argyrophil ganglion cells which are believed to be essential for the coordination of peristalsis and for the stimulation of argyrophobe cells to release acetylcholine. Muscular changes are more discrete and are compatible with denervation atrophy. The significance of degeneration and disappearance of vagal nerve cells and fibers as well as of lesions in the dorsal vagal nucleus in the brainstem is a matter for speculation. As these changes are variable, the site of the primary lesion in achalasia remains controversial.

Dysphagia is the clinical manifestation of a range of primary functional esophageal motility disorders under which one also finds diffuse esophageal spasm, the esophageal involvement of idiopathic chronic intestinal pseudo-obstruction, and familial dysautonomia.

Clinical features

Achalasia of the esophagus is occasionally seen in children, but it is uncommon in children younger than 5 years of age. However, in two recent series totaling 37 cases, close to 25% of patients were younger than 5 years and four were below 2 years of age. Table 6-2 summarizes the clinical findings in the patients reported from the Children's Hospital Medical Center in Boston. Reports of familial cases have been infrequent. The rare gene appears to be transmitted in an autosomal recessive fashion. The history of difficulty in swallowing solid food is intermittent at first and often goes back for many years. These children are described as slow eaters consuming large amounts of fluid while eating. The symptoms are slowly progressive, and failure to thrive can be associated in long-standing cases. Typically, the dysphagia is manifested by retrosternal pain and frequent episodes in which food sticks in the throat or upper chest. The dysphagia is relieved by repeated swallowing movements or by regurgitation. Besides dysphagia and regurgitation, bouts of coughing and wheezing are reported, along with recurrent pneumonia, anemia, and weight loss.

Table 6-2. Clinical findings in 20 cases
of achalasia

Mean age: 9.5 years (1 to 15 years)
Interval between onset and diagnosis: 21 months
Regurgitation of undigested foods: 100%
Dysphagia: 80%
Substernal pain: 50%
Respiratory symptoms: 25%
Impairment of growth: 70%

From Azizkhan, R.G., and others: J. Pediatr. Surg. **15:**452,
1980.

Dysphagia is an occasional complaint postoperatively in children with esophageal atresia even if there is no stenosis at the anastomotic site. Esophageal motility studies show the typical pattern of achalasia. It is now apparent that these motility disturbances are uniformly present in all cases of esophageal atresia, though only a small percentage of them are symptomatic.

Diagnosis

The barium swallow shows a grossly dilated esophagus except for a narrowing at its distal end. The length of the narrowed segment is usually very short (Fig. 6-19). A cinefluoroscopic examination may show absence of normal peristalsis and failure of relaxation of the gastroesophageal sphincter.

The esophageal motility pattern confirms the abnormal peristalsis and malfunctioning of the lower esophageal sphincter. LES pressure at rest is twice that recorded in normals, and it does not relax to the level of gastric pressure during swallowing (Fig. 6-20). There are no true peristaltic contractions in the body of the esophagus, and the cardia is hypersensitive to gastrin. Injection of a small dose (2.5 mg) of methacholine (Mecholyl) subcutaneously, which does not influence the peristaltic activity of the normal esophagus, further disorganizes the altered motility pattern and is almost pathognomonic.

Differential diagnosis

Organic stricture of the lower end of the esophagus may cause diagnostic difficulties. Peptic esophagitis secondary to hiatal hernia is the most common cause of organic esophageal strictures during childhood and can be ruled out by esophagoscopy, roentgenograms, and manometric studies. Diffuse esophageal spasm characterized by

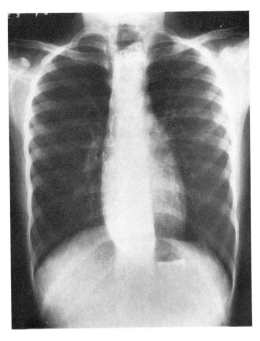

Fig. 6-19. Achalasia. Barium roentgenogram of the esophagus shows a narrowed distal esophagus with proximal esophagomegaly. This 8-year-old child was admitted with a 3-month history of dysphagia for solids, vomiting, and weight loss. At first, the symptoms were intermittent, and food sticking retrosternally was relieved by his drinking fluids after he swallowed each bolus of solid food. Later on, dysphagia became more severe, and at admission, even intake of milk led to vomiting. Fluoroscopy demonstrated noticeable delay in esophageal emptying. Manometric studies showed absence of peristalsis in the body of the esophagus; at the cardia, there was a zone of greatly increased pressure, which did not decrease with deglutition. The patient became asymptomatic after Heller's operation.

dysphagia and chest pain is said to occur in all age groups but is as yet unreported in children. It is believed to represent an incomplete form of achalasia, since the esophagus has some remaining normal motor function. Temporary achalasia of the newborn infant is radiograhically indistinguishable from the more permanent achalasia of the older child, but it is transitory and disappears spontaneously after a few weeks (Fig. 6-21).

After truncal vagotomy for peptic disease, a transitory type of achalasia is common. A megaesophagus with a smooth distal narrowing is seen in children with familial dysautonomia (Riley-Day syndrome), but esophageal peristalsis is preserved. In cases of idiopathic chronic intestinal

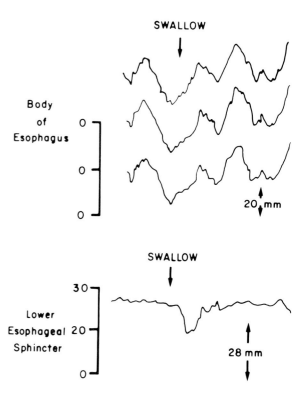

Fig. 6-20. Esophageal motility and manometry in achalasia. In this tracing, the tips of three catheters are located 5 cm apart in the body of the esophagus. There is a high resting pressure of 20 mm Hg. There are no true peristaltic waves in response to a swallow. Note the broad, low-amplitude simultaneous pressure waves. The lower esophageal sphincter shows a pressure of 28 mm Hg (N 6-8 mm) and only a small pressure fall in response to deglutition. This study was obtained in an 11-year-old boy with a 1-year history of progressive dysphagia. (Tracing courtesy André Archambault, gastroenterologist, Hôpital Maisonneuve, and consultant, Hôpital Sainte-Justine, Montreal.)

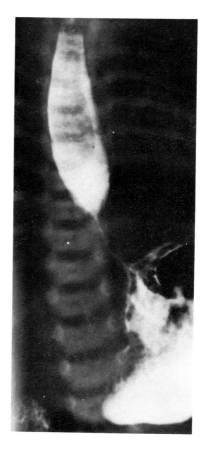

Fig. 6-21. Achalasia of the newborn infant. This transitory condition is of unknown origin and of little consequence. The only manometric study of esophageal motility in neonates has shown incoordination of the esophageal motor response to deglutition.

pseudo-obstruction, the smooth muscle portion (lower two thirds) of the esophagus shows no contractions with swallowing and there may be no relaxation of the LES. These same changes may be seen in scleroderma. Dysphagia is also a frequent complaint in dermatomyositis; it is much rarer in systemic lupus erythematosus.

Treatment

Partial destruction of the gastroesophageal sphincter achieved either by surgical myotomy or by instrumental stretching of the sphincter muscle reduces esophageal stasis and its clinical consequences but does not restore the disordered motility. In adults, a carefully performed forceful dilatation is advocated as the primary treatment in view of the low risk and the satisfactory long-term results after one or several dilatations. Although older children can be successfully dilated, only 25% can be expected to achieve relief of their symptoms and there is an ever-present risk of esophageal perforation.

The cumulative results of esophagomyotomy suggests that an excellent result can be expected in 85% of cases. The operation is safe and postoperative reflux esophagitis is rarely a problem. An antireflux procedure is therefore not necessary.

Prognosis

Because of the shorter duration of the illness in pediatric patients and because the proximal motility is less disturbed than in adults, the prognosis for return of the esophagus to normal caliber after surgery is very good.

Poorer results can be expected after forceful dilatation and surgery in long-standing cases with a decompensated and tortuous megaesophagus.

REFERENCES

Asch, M.J., Liebman, W., and Lachman, R.S.: Esophageal achalasia: diagnosis and cardiomyotomy in a newborn infant, J. Pediatr. Surg. **9:**911, 1974.

Azizkhan, R.G., Tapper, D., and Eraklis, A.: Achalasia in childhood: a 20-year experience, J. Pediatr. Surg. **15:**452-456, 1980.

Cohen, S., and Lipshutz, W.: Lower esophageal sphincter dysfunction in achalasia, Gastroenterology **61:**814-820, 1971.

Csendes, A., Valasco, N., Bragheto, I., and Henriguez, A.: A prospective randomized study comparing forceful dilatation and esophago-myotomy in patients with achalasia of the esophagus, Gastroenterology **80:**789-795, 1981.

Dayalan, N., Chettun, L., and Ramakrishnan, M.: Achalasia of the cardia in sibs, Arch. Dis. Child. **47:**115-118, 1972.

Elder, J.B.: Achalasia of the cardia in childhood, Digestion **3:**90-96, 1970.

London, F.A., Raab, D.E., Fuller, J., and Olsen, A.M.: Achalasia in three siblings, Mayo Clin. Proc. **52:**97-100, 1977.

Menzies-Gow, N., Gummer, J.W.P., and Edwards, A.M.: Results of Heller's operation for achalasia of the cardia, Br. J. Surg. **65:**483-485, 1978.

Soulier, Y., Lefort, C., Borde, J., and Valayer, J.: Le mégaœsophage idiopathique de l'enfant, Chir. Pédiatr. **20:**311-316, 1979.

Vantrappen, G., Janssens, J., Hellemans, J., and others: Achalasia, diffuse oesophageal spasm and related motility disorders, Gastroenterology **76:**450-457, 1979.

Vantrappen, G., and Hellemans, J.: Treatment of achalasia and related motor disorders, Gastroenterology **79:**144-154, 1980.

Vaughan, W.H., and Williams, J.L.: Familial achalasia with pulmonary complications in children, Radiology **107:**407-409, 1973.

Westley, C.R., Herbst, J.J., Goldman, S., and Wiser, W.C.: Infantile achalasia inherited as an autosomal recessive disorder, J. Pediatr. **87:**243-246, 1975.

7 *Disorders of stomach and duodenum*

HYPERTROPHIC PYLORIC STENOSIS

After inguinal hernia, congenital hypertrophic pyloric stenosis is the most common condition requiring surgery during the first few months of life. The cause of the increase in the size of the circular muscle of the pylorus is unknown. In certain studies of patients with pyloric stenosis, pyloric ganglion cells have been shown to be smaller and lacking in normal mitochondrial acitivty. Immaturity of the myenteric plexus perhaps accounts for a congenital inability of the pylorus to open, leading to the development of work-hypertrophied musculature. Hypergastrinemia has been reported but could not be confirmed by others. The likelihood that gastrin plays a role in the pathogenesis of the affection is remote because patients with Zollinger-Ellison syndrome have very high levels of gastrin and do not have hypertrophic pyloric musculature. Furthermore, the possibility that high gastrin concentrations in cord serum could be implicated has been dismissed.

The disease occurs in one of every 500 births. Males are affected four to five times more often than females. It is congenital in nature, often occurring in members of the same family or in family cluster. Twin studies have shown higher rate of concordance in both monozygotic and dizygotic twins. In close to 5% of cases, there is a positive family history of the disease in the father or in siblings. The risk to sons and daughters of affected mothers is 1:6 and 1:10, respectively. The reported increased incidence of the disease in firstborns and during the spring and fall months does not appear to be a generally accepted observation.

Clinical findings

The disease is more likely to affect a full-term infant than a premature infant (3%). The age of onset and the pattern of vomiting are more variable than is generally described. In the typical case, nonbilious vomiting begins between the second and fourth weeks of life and henceforth increases in frequency, becomes projectile, and may lead to complete obstruction by 4 to 6 weeks. There are a number of babies (10% to 20%) whose symptoms start at birth. Changes of formula have very little effect. Frequency of vomiting, which gradually becomes projectile, may be lessened temporarily by glucose-water feedings, but loss of weight becomes apparent as obstruction of the gastric outlet becomes more complete. There is yet a third category of patients who do well for the first few weeks of life but suddenly develop projectile vomiting leading to dehydration within a few days.

Diagnosis

The diagnosis can be made with a high degree of accuracy for the patient who has a history of progressive, nonbilious vomiting that becomes projectile and may be blood tinged. Constipation rapidly supervenes, leading occasionally to obstipation. Failure to gain weight is then followed by mild or pronounced weight loss. The infant is ravenously hungry and nurses avidly. The upper abdomen is distended, and gastric peristaltic waves are seen in practically all cases. An olive-sized tumor, which may be felt to the right of the umbilicus in most of the patients, is usually more readily palpable immediately after the infant has vomited. Dehydration, loss of skin turgor, fretfulness, and apathy may be present.

The vomiting leads to a metabolic alkalosis usually accompanied by severe potassium depletion. All patients should have electrolyte studies no matter how good the clinical picture is. Protracted periods of neonatal indirect-reacting hyperbilirubinemia described with pyloric stenosis remain unexplained. Electron microscopy of liver biopsy specimens has shown, in a small number of patients, dilatation of the endoplasmic reticulum. Hemoconcentration may be reflected by elevated hemoglobin and hematocrit values; serum chloride is low, and the pH of the blood is elevated. Urine is concentrated and alkaline, but it may be acid if potassium deficiency is severe.

X-ray and echographic diagnosis

Upper gastrointestinal series properly performed are very helpful. The examination should include a study of the esophagus so that a stricture, a hernia, and a significant degree of chalasia can be ruled out.

The diagnosis rests entirely on demonstration of an unchanging elongation and narrowing of the antrum and pylorus, the so-called string sign. The degree of narrowing depends on the severity of constriction of the lumen produced by the muscle hypertrophy. Hypertrophied muscle may indent the stomach and the base of the bulb (Fig. 7-1). Delayed emptying is an unreliable sign because it may be absent in less severe cases of true hypertrophic pyloric stenosis and may be present in normal patients as well as those with other diseases. Rapid emptying of the stomach does not exclude pyloric stenosis. Furthermore, if the antrum gradually tapers into the pyloric canal, pyloric stenosis may be missed. Attention has been recently drawn to atypical antropyloric deformities seen in cases of hypertrophic pyloric stenosis but easily mistaken for pylorospasm or a channel ulcer.

A recent report advocates a double-contrast study with manual compression to increase the accuracy of the examination. The stomach is aspirated through a nasogastric tube before introduction of a small amount of creamy barium. The patient is turned on his right side to coat the antrum and prepyloric region, and then a few milliliters of air are added until the antrum is adequately overdistended. Gentle epigastric pressure is then applied with a gloved hand. According to these authors pylorospasm and antral spasm can give rise to all the classic signs of the disorder. This technique is said to eliminate the false-positive and false-negative signs associated with the conventional barium study. It may more consistently demonstrate the ''figure-3'' sign produced by invagination of the pyloric mass into the antrum (Fig. 7-2).

Ultrasound demonstration of a thick hypoechoic ring in the region of the pylorus anterior to the right kidney and just medial to the gallbladder appears promising. In a series of 100 patients suspected of hypertrophic pyloric stenosis, 54 of 58 were confirmed at surgery, and there were only 4 (7%) false negatives and no false positives.

Differential diagnosis

The differential diagnosis should not be a problem. The absence of increased intracranial pres-

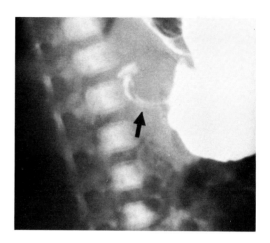

Fig. 7-1. Pyloric stenosis. This full-term firstborn infant suffered postprandial projectile vomiting starting at 6 weeks of age. Loss of weight, constipation, and dehydration subsequently became manifest. The barium meal shows an elongated and curved pyloric canal with the often described railroad sign, *arrow*. The duodenal bulb is normally shaped but poorly filled. Note indentation of the barium-filled antrum by the hypertrophied pyloric muscle.

sure and of virilization with hyperkalemia rule out intracranial lesions and congenital adrenal hyperplasia with adrenal insufficiency. In achalasia, the food is undigested; in annular pancreas, the vomitus almost always contains bile. Sepsis and infections of the urinary tract can easily be ruled out. In simple cases of pylorospasm there may be a delay in gastric emptying, but the elongated, narrow pyloric canal is not seen.

Other causes of obstruction of the gastric outlet include rare cases of complicated antral and channel ulcers and of congenital pyloric or prepyloric diaphragm and atresia. Benign tumors such as leiomyomas and ectopic rest tumors also may lead to symptoms remindful of pyloric stenosis. In these conditions, the age at onset and the x-ray findings are different. The prepyloric membrane, for instance, has a small opening so that the medium goes through and forms a small separate chamber just proximal to the pylorus.

Treatment

Surgical management. Pyloromyotomy is the treatment of choice but is not an emergency procedure and should be carried out when the dehydration and electrolyte abnormalities are corrected. Before surgery, a gastric tube should be

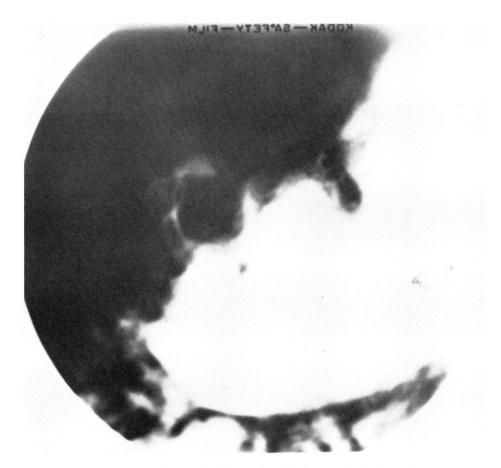

Fig. 7-2. Hypertrophic pyloric stenosis. Conventional barium study showing elongation of the pyloric canal, the double track, and the figure-of-3 sign.

passed into the stomach so that the gastric contents can be aspirated.

Because of the danger of entering the duodenal mucosa or of incompletely dividing the muscle fibers, it is important that the serosal incision be started on the proximal gastric side and extended toward the duodenum but not beyond the tumor mass. The division should be deepest on the antral aspect of the pylorus and shallower distally.

Glucose and saline feedings can usually be started 4 hours after surgery. Within 1 or 2 days, most infants can be fed milk every 4 hours.

Medical management. Medical management of hypertrophic pyloric stenosis has not gained much favor in North America. A few reports suggest that milder cases can be appropriately treated medically. Parenteral fluids are given if necessary, and gastric lavage with normal saline solution is carried out three times a day for 24 to 48

hours. Methscopolamine nitrate is administered intramuscularly at a dose of 0.12 to 0.15 mg every 4 to 6 hours until peristaltic waves and gagging subside. After 2 days, small amounts of 5% glucose are given orally every 4 hours, and methscopolamine nitrate is given by mouth 20 to 30 minutes before feedings.

In our experience, surgery is indicated in the majority of cases; medical management is probably useful in those milder cases in which the onset of symptoms or the recognition of the disease has been delayed beyond the age of 2 months.

Complications

Postoperative vomiting is rather common. Actually, many infants for whom operation has been successful exhibit some vomiting for the first 24 to 48 hours. During the first hours after operation, the physician should watch for signs of peritonitis associated with a perforated duodenum.

The persistence of severe vomiting beyond 5 days may indicate an inadequate division of the hypertrophied pylorus or adhesions around a so-called duodenal niche. In these cases, reoperation may be necessary.

There is no explanation for the continued vomiting of many infants surgically relieved of hypertrophic pyloric stenosis.

A recent study of 627 cases has shown that 13% had an associated gastroesophageal reflux. This may account for the fact that 1 in 4 had blood-tinged vomitus preoperatively as well as a high incidence of postoperative vomiting. Altered peristaltic activity has been demonstrated in the early postoperative period both roentgenographically and manometrically. However, the gastric motility pattern returns to normal within 5 days. It is important to keep in mind that roentgenographic studies performed after either surgical or medical therapy of hypertrophic pyloric stenosis reveal pretreatment findings with some persistence of the elongated canal.

REFERENCES

Bell, M.J.: Infantile pyloric stenosis: experience with 305 cases at Louisville Children's Hospital, Surgery **64:**983-989, 1968.

Benson, C.D.: Infantile hypertrophic pyloric stenosis. In Ravitch, M.M., Welch, K.J., Benson, C.D., Aberdeen, E., and Randolph, J.G., editors: Pediatric surgery, ed. 3, Chicago, 1979, Year Book Medical Publishers, Inc.

Boggs, T.R., Jr., and Bishop, H.: Neonatal hyperbilirubinemia associated with high obstruction of the small bowel, J. Pediatr. **66:**349-356, 1965.

Friesen, S.R., and Pearse, A.G.E.: Pathogenesis of congenital pyloric stenosis: histochemical analysis of pyloric ganglion cells, Surgery **53:**604-608, 1963.

Grochowski, J., Szafran, H., Sztefko, K., and others: Blood serum immunoreactive gastrin levels in infants with hypertrophic pyloric stenosis, J. Pediatr. Surg. **15:**279-282, 1980.

Huguenard, J.R., and Sharples, G.E.: Incidence of congenital pyloric stenosis within sibships, J. Pediatr. **81:**45-49, 1972.

Levine, G., Favara, B.E., Mierau, G., and others: Jaundice, liver ultrastructure, and congenital pyloric stenosis, Arch. Pathol. **95:**267-270, 1973.

Mellin, G.W.: Santulli, T.V., and Altman, H.S.: Congenital pyloric stenosis: a controlled evaluation of medical treatment using methylscopolamine-nitrate, J. Pediatr. **66:**649-657, 1965.

Pellerin, D., Bertin, P., and Tovar, J.A.: Reflux gastroœsophagien et sténose hypertrophique du pylore, Ann. Chir. Infant. **155:**7-14, 1974.

Schärli, A., Sieber, W.K., and Kiesewetter, W.B.: Hypertrophic pyloric stenosis at the Children's Hospital of Pittsburgh from 1912 to 1967: a critical review of current problems and complications, J. Pediatr. Surg. **4:**108-114, 1969.

Strobel, C.T., Smith, L.E., Fonkalsrud, E.W., and Isenberg, J.N.: Ectopic pancreatic tissue in the gastric antrum, J. Pediatr. **92:**586-588, 1978.

Swischuk, L.E., Hayden, C.K., and Tyson, K.R.: Atypical muscle hypertrophy in pyloric stenosis, Am. J. Radiol. **134:**481-484, 1980.

Werlin, S.L., Grand, R.J., and Drum, D.E.: Congenital hypertrophic stenosis: the role of gastrin reevaluated, Pediatrics **61:**883-885, 1977.

Yousefzadeh, D.K., Soper, R.T., and Jackson, J.H.: Diagnostic advantages of manual compression fluoroscopy in the radiologic work-up of vomiting neonates, J. Pediatr. Surg. **15:**270-278, 1980.

PEPTIC DISEASE

Childhood peptic ulcer is no longer considered a rare disease. The importance of peptic ulceration in infants, children, and adolescents is becoming more evident with increased awareness of peptic disease in this age group and a parallel improvement in diagnostic techniques. In particular, realization that the pattern of epigastric distress typical of adult peptic disease is not necessarily present in children has led to performance of proper diagnostic procedures. An increasing number of children with vague abdominal pain or gastrointestinal bleeding or both are now being diagnosed as having peptic disease.

The overall incidence of peptic disease in the pediatric age group is unknown. Of inpatient populations, it is estimated at 3.4 per 10,000 admissions. Peptic ulcers may occur at any age, but they are most frequent between the ages 12 and 18 years. Boys are affected twice as often as are girls, and the preponderance of boys over girls is greater in children older than 12 years. Up to the age of 6 years, the majority of ulcers are found in children in whom an underlying disease, a drug, or a toxic substance is known to be causally related. In the older age group, there are four primary ulcers for each secondary ulcer. In patients up to 6 years of age gastric ulcers are as common as duodenal ulcers, if not more so. In the 6- to 18-year-old group, duodenal ulcers outnumber gastric ulcers by 5 to 1.

There is a strong familial tendency in duodenal ulcer. About 50% of monozygous twins have shown concordance for duodenal ulcer, whereas only 14% of dizygous twins were concordant. A family history can usually be found in 25% to 50% of cases of duodenal ulcers. Patients are more often of HLA-B$_5$ type than expected. Duodenal ulcer and particularly their complications are notably common in people of blood group O. High levels of pepsinogen I tend to segregate as an autosomal dominant. Undoubtedly genetic factors play

Table 7-1. Gastric cells and their secretory products

	Cell type	Product
Oxyntic glands (corpus and fundus	Surface mucous cells	Mucus
	Mucous cells	Mucus and pepsinogens I
	Neck cells	None known
	Parietal cells	HCl and Intrinsic factor
	Chief cells	Papsinogens I
	Argentaffin cells	Serotonin, histamine
Antral glands	Surface mucous cells	Mucus
	Undifferentiated neck cells	None recognized
	G cells	Gastrin
	D cells	Somatostatin
	Pyloric glands	Mucus and pepsinogens I & II

Modified from Isenberg, J.I.: The parietal cell, Viewpoints on Digestive Diseases, vol. 7, no. 2, March 1978.

Table 7-2. Gastric acid secretion in infants and children after betazole stimulation

Mean age	Volume (ml/hr)	Mean titratable acid (mEq/hr)	Mean acid output (mEq/hr/kg)
1 day	3.3	8.1	0.01
4 weeks	3.1	26.4	0.02
12 weeks	13.4	34.8	0.10
16 weeks	44.0	41.6	0.08
24 weeks	64.0	49.2	0.17
> 4-9 years	42.5	114.2	0.24
>11 years and adults	143.2	91.2	0.19

Compiled by Grand, R.J., Watkins, J.B., and Torti, F.M.: Gastroenterology **70**:790, 1976, from studies carried out by Deren, Agunod, Rodbro, and others; see reference section.

an important part, but there are also strong environmental influences such as climatic conditions, dietary habits, and emotional strain.

Secretory mechanisms of stomach

The study of gastric function has been a topic of interest for the past century. Better understanding of gastric secretory mechanisms has led to improved strategies of intervention for peptic disease thanks to greater insight into the role of the autonomic nervous system, hormonal mechanisms, the number and functional capacity of oxyntic glands, and gastric circulation.

Ontogenesis. G cells, chief cells and parietal cells responsible for the secretion of gastrin, pepsinogen, and hydrochloric acid appear in the oxyntic glands during the early part of the second trimester (Table 7-1). At birth, the secretory activity is low despite hypergastrinemia. Within 48

hours there is a progressive increase in acid output. The close relationship present between parietal cell mass, acid output, and body weight is noted by the age of about 3 months (Table 7-2).

Pepsin and hydrochloric acid. Pepsinogen in the presence of acid (pH < 5.0) is converted to pepsin, which hydrolyzes proteins and polypeptides. Its main stimuli are food, cholinergic stimulation (hypoglycemia, gastric distention), histamine, and gastrin. Of interest in the pathogenesis of secondary ulcers is the observation that back-diffusion of hydrogen ions, the result of a disruption of the gastric mucosal barrier by agents such as aspirin, bile salts, and alcohol, stimulates pepsin secretion. Pepsinogen and pepsin form two main groups of proteins that can be measured in the serum. Pepsinogen I is secreted only by the cells in the oxyntic glands of the stomach, whereas pepsinogen II is also produced in the pylorus and

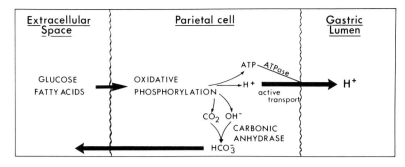

Fig. 7-3. The biochemical sequence of H^+-ion production by parietal cells.

in the duodenum. Specific radioimmunoassay values of pepsinogen I correlate well with gastric secretory capacity and vagal integrity. It is presently the best indirect test of gastric acid secretion.

Hydrochloric acid is secreted into the gastric lumen by parietal cells. Oxidative phosphorylation yields hydrogen ions, which are then transported out of the cell against an extraordinarily large concentration gradient (1 million to 1) by a special carrier system. For each hydrogen ion secreted, a molecule of carbon dioxide is converted to bicarbonate by the enzyme carbonic anhydrase and enters venous blood leaving the stomach (Fig. 7-3). This gives rise to the transient postprandial metabolic alkalosis known as the "alkaline tide." Gastric juice potassium (8 to 20 mEq/L) and chloride (170 mEq/L) concentrations are higher than in plasma and tend to parallel hydrogen-ion secretion.

Parietal cell mass and gastric circulation. There is a good correlation between the number of parietal cells and acid output. A higher parietal cell density per unit area is reported in newborns, but there is no information in infants or in children. It is estimated that the 1 billion acid-secreting cells occupy 35% of the oxyntic mucosa as opposed to 25% for the pepsinogen-secreting cells (chief cells). After vagotomy or antrectomy, the parietal call mass decreases, but also what is left has a decreased response to secretory stimulants. Patients with duodenal ulcers have twice the normal number of parietal cells, and they are abnormally sensitive to stimuli. There is evidence that chronic distention of the stomach may bring about an increase in the parietal cell mass. An adequate blood flow is essential for parietal cell response to food, gastrin, histamine, and vagal stimulation. Of interest is the information that inhibitors of gastric secretion such as secretin, glucagon, prostaglan-

dins, and cimetidine decrease gastric mucosal blood flow. Ischemia will invariably decrease acid output but will also render the mucosa more permeable to hydrogen in backdiffusion. Therefore a broken mucosal barrier is associated with many known causes of secondary or "stress" ulcers occurring in "low-flow" states.

Regulation of gastric secretion. A number of chemical messengers are closely interrelated and provide an integrated system closely regulating gastric secretion.

The *parasympathetic nervous system (vagus)* is a direct stimulant of the parietal cell mass through the release of acetylcholine and gastrin from G cells in the antrum. Antrectomy and anticholinergic drugs both decrease the vagal response stimulation.

Histamine is present in large quantities in oxyntic mucosa. It is produced by APUD cells (see Chapter 18) and its role has grown in importance with the discovery that histamine H_2 antagonists inhibit acid secretion stimulated not only by histamine but also by gastrin, insulin, coffee, and so on. The chemical and physiological mechanisms for the synthesis and release of histamine in the gastric mucosa are unknown. One explanation is that histamine is not released by other stimulants but sensitizes parietal cells to other stimuli. This "permissive" hypothesis explains the fact that cimetidine blocks acid secretion produced in response to many stimuli.

Gastrin is the peptide hormone most clearly identified as an important stimulant of gastric acid secretion. Little gastrin (G-17) is six to eight times more potent than big gastrin (G-34) and is the most abundant form found in the antrum. However the serum immunoassay identifies more G-34 because of its slower catabolic rate. Gastrin is released by alkalinity of the antrum and by its direct contact with amino acids and peptides given orally. If given intravenously, amino acids increase acid output but there is no concomitant elevation of gastrin. The most effective blood-borne stimulant is calcium. Sham feeding, gastric distention, and insulin hypoglycemia are stimuli that suggest that there is a vagal cholinergic mechanism for the release of gastrin. The only known physiological inhibitor of gastrin release is acification of gastric contents below 3. Hormonal inhibitors include somatostatin and vasoactive intestinal polypeptide (VIP), but their role in normal physiology is obscure.

Variable degrees of escape from the negative-feedback inhibition of gastrin secretion by gastric acid is seen in several conditions. In the Zollinger-Ellison syndrome associated with gastrinomas, there is severe hypergastrinemia despite massive acid secretion. A lesser degree of escape occurs in antral G-cell hyperplasia, in duodenal ulcers with a large parietal cell mass, in long-standing pyloric obstruction, in patients with renal failure and during the first few months after a massive resection of the small intestine. Hypergastrinemia is reported in patients with endocrinopathies such as hyperparathyroidism and multiple endocrine neoplasia type I, as well as in rare cases of type II, pheochromocytoma and neurofibromatosis. Because of lack of parietal cell mass capable of secreting hydrochloric acid, hypergastrinemia is regularly seen in achlorhydric subjects who have primary pernicious anemia or atrophic gastritis with a spared antrum.

Hypergastrinemia is present in cord blood and is of fetal origin because gastrin concentrations are higher than those in the mother's blood. Continuous basal acid secretory studies have demonstrated hyposecretion of gastric acid for the first 5 hours of life despite hypergastrinemia. This is presumably attributable to the absence of gastrin receptors on parietal cells. Fasting gastrin concentrations are higher during the first 3 years of life than later (Table 7-3).

The prolonged postprandial increase of serum gastrin seen in adults also occurs in children. Gastrin concentrations are normal in children with primary gastric ulcers or in those with secondary ulcers associated with sepsis, trauma, and shock. Occasionally, the deeply penetrating ulcers seen after neurosurgical procedures or intracranial trauma may be accompanied by hypergastrinemia. Studies in children with duodenal ulcers show higher gastric acid secretion in response to Histalog but

Table 7-3. Fasting gastrin concentrations

Age (years)	Fasting gastrin values (pg/ml)
0-3	32.7 ± 22.3
3-6	20.9 ± 28.8
6-9	14.8 ± 14.3
9-12	20.5 ± 22.0
12-15	17.8 ± 22.3

From Janik, J.S., Akbar, A.M., Burrington, J.D., and Burke, G.: Pediatrics **60**:60, © 1977, American Academy of Pediatrics.

gastrin concentrations are normal or only moderately elevated (100 to 120 pg/ml). The main indication for the measurement of gastrin in children with peptic disease is suspicion of a Zollinger-Ellison syndrome, and in all instances where hypercalcemia is present.

Pathogenesis of peptic disease

Although gastric and duodenal ulcers are clinically indistinguishable, they are regarded as different. It has been suggested that they are different manifestations of the same disease as gastric and duodenal ulcers coexist more often than would be expected on statistical grounds. In addition, they both share symptoms identical to that of nonulcer peptic disease. The latter may well represent the initial and the healing phases of peptic ulcer disease; however, in certain instances, gastroduodenitis coexists with peptic ulcer disease.

Mucus and the gastric mucosal barrier. The dictum "no acid—no ulcer" still holds. Acid pepsin is essential for both ulcer and nonulcer peptic disease. A further unifying aspect of their pathophysiology is that of a decreased mucosal resistance to acid and pepsin. Mucus is a first line of defense, but a change in mucus is observed only in patients with a very high acid output (Zollinger-Ellison syndrome). In contrast to studies with aspirin, corticosteroids do not reduce the rate of secretion and viscosity of gastric mucus. The critical defense against autodigestion is maintenance of the normal gastric mucosal barrier. Disruption of the mucosal barrier allows greatly increased backdiffusion of hydrogen ions from the lumen into the mucosal cells, which are damaged in the process. This brings about a release of histamine, which in turn leads to vasodilatation and stimulates parietal cells to produce more acid and more pepsin (Fig. 7-4).

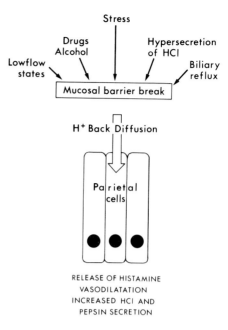

Fig. 7-4. Causes and effects of H$^+$-ion backdiffusion.

Factors leading to a breakdown of the mucosal barrier. When intraluminal concentrations of acid are increased to about twice the concentration (0.15 N HCl) that the secreting stomach can generate, the barrier may be broken. However, even low concentrations of hydrochloric acid will break the gastric barrier when a number of substances such as bile, bile salts, lysolecithin, alcohol, salicylate, or urea are placed in the stomach. A number of studies have shown that both gastric and duodenal ulcers are associated with an abnormal degree of duodenogastric reflux, which allows hydrolyzed lecithin (lysolecithin) and bile salts to disrupt the gastric mucosal barrier. The role of salicylates has been well studied. In contrast to studies in animals, both aspirin given parenterally and enteric-coated preparations are less frequently associated with chronic blood loss, acute erosive gastritis, and chronic gastric ulcer. Acetaminophen has minimal effects, whereas nonsteroid anti-inflammatory agents such as phenylbutazone, indomethacin, naproxen, and ibuprofen cause gastric damage. The changes associated with ibuprofen are milder and tend to occur with a higher dosage. Nonsteroid anti-inflammatory drugs inhibit prostaglandin (PG) synthesis. Prostaglandin inhibits gastric secretion and protects the mucosa against injury. The precise mechanism of cytoprotection is unknown, but "tightening" of the gastric mucosal barrier has been demonstrated.

Corticosteroids and stress ulcers. Although it is known from a number of reports that adrenocorticosteroid therapy is frequently complicated by the appearance or reactivation of peptic ulcers, the association is a weak one if one excludes patients who have a previous history of peptic ulcer disease or those who have had a kidney transplant. Although duration of corticosteroid therapy and daily dosage are not associated with a higher incidence of peptic ulcers, there is a close association between total dose of steroid administered and peptic ulcer in those patients who have been given more than 1000 mg. Of interest is the observation that large doses of steroids decrease the tissue levels of prostaglandins. Steroids inhibit phospholipase A responsible for the release of arachidonic acid (substrate for prostaglandin synthesis) from phospholipids. A number of disease conditions have been associated with peptic disease. Patients with cirrhosis, the nephrotic syndrome, or Crohn's disease are commonly hypoalbuminemic. In such circumstances a larger percentage of administered corticosteroids are unbound. It has been postulated that unbound corticosteroids could be more injurious to the gastric and duodenal mucosa. The incidence of peptic disease also appears to be increased in extrahepatic portal hypertension. Our clinical experience with three cases adds weight to experimental data showing that venous congestion alters the mucosal defenses against autodigestion.

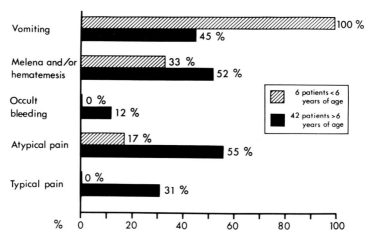

Fig. 7-5. Symptoms associated with primary ulcers in 48 children. (From Deckelbaum, R.J., Roy, C.C., Lussier-Lazaroff, J., and Morin, C.L.: Can. Med. Assoc. J. **111:**225-228, 1974.)

Stress ulcers usually appear in the corpus of the stomach and spare the antrum. They are less frequent in the duodenum. The lesions are generally erosions rather than frank ulcers. They are multiple and superficial and appear within hours of a serious insult. Conditions most frequently associated include extensive burns, brain injury, sepsis, severe respiratory insufficiency, and hypotension. Available information does not suggest that erosive gastritis is caused by a disruption of the gastric mucosal barrier, and there is no evidence that increased gastric acid secretion is implicated at least in the initial phase. The most attractive explanation is that focal mucosal necrosis results from an energy deficit, the result of a "low-flow" state.

Pathogenesis of duodenal ulcer

In contrast to gastric ulcer disease where there is low acid secretion and normal gastric emptying, duodenal ulcer disease is associated with the following abnomalities of gastric function:

1. Increased capacity to secrete acid and pepsin. The parietal mass and maximal acid secretion are usually twice normal.
2. Increased responsiveness to gastrin and pentagastrin.
3. Defective inhibition of gastrin release by secreted hydrochloric acid.
4. Abnormally rapid emptying of the stomach and therefore the loss of the buffering capacity of meals.

The influence of psychologic factors on the genesis of duodenal ulcers has been a topic of intense debate for the past 50 years and remains an open question. Certain personality characteristics are said to be more prevalent in patients with duodenal ulcer, and stress could contribute to the genesis and exacerbations of the disease. Two studies carried out many years ago in children with duodenal ulcers describe them as being commonly of high intelligence with a strong tendency to overachieve. They are said to internalize their aggressive feelings and are described as submissive. They were believed to handle feelings of anxiety and frustration with difficulty. A recent study has not found an obvious relationship between life-stress events and chronic gastric ulcer. However, there was no evaluation of personality, or coping style, or cognitive appraisal of the situation. We certainly have been impressed with identifiable events responsible for exacerbations of duodenal ulcer disease and its complications, but we are less certain about their role in the genesis of the first bout.

Clinical findings of peptic ulcer disease

Because symptoms and signs, as well as location and type, vary, it is best to group the clinical findings according to patient age. The relative frequency of symptoms associated with primary and secondary ulcers in the younger (1 month to 6 years) and older (6 to 18 years) age groups is shown in Figs. 7-5 and 7-6.

Neonatal period. In the neonate, duodenal ulcers are seen, but a gastric location is more common. Perforation is usually the first manifestation,

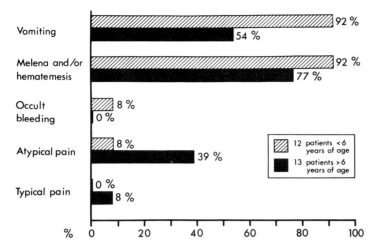

Fig. 7-6. Symptoms associated with secondary ulcers in 25 children. (From Deckelbaum, R.J., Roy, C.C., Lussier-Lazaroff, J., and Morin, C.L.: Can. Med. Assoc. J. **111**:225-228, 1974.)

though bleeding also occurs (Fig. 7-7). The gastric perforation usually takes place at or near the greater curvature. Necrotic changes can often be seen not only around the edges of the perforation, but also elsewhere in the stomach and gastrointestinal tract. The newborn with gastric perforation is commonly a premature infant who has a history of hypoxia. He may also have sepsis, hypoglycemia, respiratory distress syndrome, or a disorder of the central nervous system. Feeding tubes have also been implicated, as well as hypertrophic pyloric stenosis.

Age 1 month to 3 years. In infants past the neonatal period and up to the age of 3 years, symptoms of primary peptic disease include poor eating, vomiting, crying spells late after meals, abdominal distention or bleeding characterized by tarry stools, or hematemesis. However, ulcers in this age group are usually associated with an underlying illness such as encephalitis, meningitis, brain tumor, head injury, sepsis, and burns. It still remains to be determined whether the increased incidence of secondary ulcers associated with corticosteroid therapy can be accounted for by the effect of corticosteroids themselves or by the underlying illness for which they were given (Fig. 7-8). Secondary ulcers in this age group are as likely to be located in the duodenum as in the stomach. Primary ulcers, on the other hand, tend to be more frequent in the stomach. Generally speaking, secondary ulcers are very acute in their mode of presentation; rectal bleeding, hematemesis, or perforation may be the first symptoms.

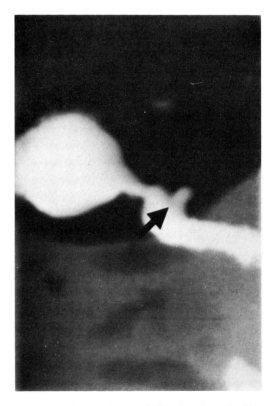

Fig. 7-7. Perforated duodenal ulcer in a 3-week-old infant, who presented with a 2-week history of postprandial vomiting and 2 days of abdominal distention, diarrhea, and lethargy. On admission, profuse hematemesis occurred, and hepatomegaly and ascites were noted. A perforated ulcer is identified on the anterosuperior aspect of the bulb, *arrow*. A diagnosis of galactosemia was made in this patient, who subsequently developed normally.

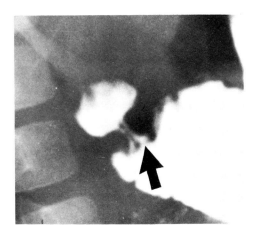

Fig. 7-8. Gastric ulcer. Upper gastrointestinal series in a young child with severe asthma who required daily corticosteroid therapy. He developed abdominal pain, hematemesis, and melena. The roentgenogram shows an antral ulcer, *arrow,* that persisted throughout the examination.

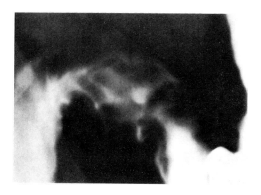

Fig. 7-9. Ulcer of the duodenum. The ulcer is demonstrated in the middle of the duodenal bulb as a white deposit of barium. This patient shows little bulb deformity.

Age 3 to 6 years. In children between 3 and 6 years of age, vomiting related to eating is always present. Periumbilical or generalized abdominal pain is common. The typical "ulcer pain" is related to meals. It is relieved by food and wakes the patient at night or in the early morning hours. Melena, hematemesis, and perforation are always present in secondary ulcers but are also part of the clinical picture in primary ulcers, though less commonly than in patients 1 month to 3 years of age. The stomach is as frequently involved as the duodenum, and the preponderance of males is evident when primary ulcers are considered. Overall, the incidence of ulcers in patients 3 to 6 years of age is lower than in the younger and older groups.

Age 6 to 18 years. School-age children and teenagers have clinical findings that are more typical of the syndrome described in adults. Despite the more typical symptoms, the interval between onset of symptoms and the establishment of a diagnosis is in excess of 10 months. Secondary ulcers are outnumbered by primary ulcers in a ratio of 1:6. As in the other age groups, secondary ulcers are found as frequently in the stomach as in the duodenum. In addition to the acute underlying illnesses responsible for secondary ulcers, certain chronic diseases are frequently found in children with peptic disease, namely chronic obstructive lung disease (though ulcers are rare in cystic fibrosis), rheumatoid arthritis, nephrotic syndrome,

extrahepatic portal hypertension, cirrhosis of the liver, and Crohn's disease of the upper small bowel. The association between peptic disease and a gastrin-secreting tumor is discussed in the section on the Zollinger-Ellison syndrome.

The male/female ratio tends to increase with age; the overall figure in the group is 3½:1. Chronic peptic duodenal ulcers (Fig. 7-9) in a school-age children are far more frequent than gastric ulcers (7:1). The most common symptom is pain. Typically, it is a burning or gnawing sensation in the epigastrium, which tends to occur in the fasting state or at night and which is relieved by milk or food. If there is penetration of the viscus, radiation to the back or to either the left or right upper quadrants may be important. In other cases, it is a vague upper abdominal discomfort with little of the pain-food-relief characteristic sequence. In our experience, the majority of children fall in this last category, with only a third having the typical pain leading to an early diagnosis. Melena or hematemesis, or both, are noted in more than 50%, and occult bleeding and anemia without other identifiable symptoms occur in a surprising number. Vomiting is present in less than half the school-age children with peptic disease.

Diagnosis

The diagnosis of acute secondary ulcers (stress ulcers) should be suspected in any child with a severe underlying disease who suddenly presents with hematemesis, melena, or abdominal distention. Neonates and infants appear to be particularly vulnerable. Central nervous system disorders were documented in 10 of 26 cases in our recent series. The combination of corticosteroids and aspirin or the presence of leukemia or of a severe burn is also a good setup for an acute stress ulcer. Clinical recognition is difficult in the absence of a complication because of the common absence of pain.

Because of the large spectrum of symptoms associated with primary ulcers, the diagnosis depends primarily on the awareness of the physician. The differential diagnosis includes chronic idiopathic recurrent abdominal pain, irritable colon syndrome, esophagitis associated with hiatal hernia or free gastroesophageal reflux, chronic pancreatitis, cholelithiasis, and Crohn's disease of the upper small bowel. Peptic ulcer disease should be considered not only when there is an aggregation of suggestive symptoms but also in the following circumstances:

1. Chronic abdominal pain if it is present at night or in the early morning hours
2. Recurrent vomiting if related to eating
3. Anemia if occult blood is present in the stools
4. Vague gastrointestinal complaints in a patient with a positive family history for duodenal ulcer.

Nonulcer peptic disease

The relationship between gastroduodenal mucosal inflammation and peptic ulcer is unclear. We certainly frequently note gastroduodenitis in association with and in the proximity of gastroduodenal ulcers. In a recent adult series of 100 cases with symptoms of dyspepsia, more than 60% had classic manifestations of peptic disease. Symptoms were atypical in close to 40% and characterized by poorly localized nonperiodic pain, diffuse tenderness, nausea, sometimes vomiting, belching, bloating, excessive flatus, and loss of appetite. Twenty-five percent had peptic ulcer disease, 86% to 90% of whom had associated gastroduodenitis. In 59% no ulcers were seen and endoscopic findings revealed either acute (39%) or chronic (20%) gastroduodenitis. Of interest was the observation that it was clinically impossible to distinguish those with a crater from those with acute gastroduodenitis and that 81% of those with classic symptoms of peptic disease had an ulcer or acute inflammation, or both.

Thus it would appear that gastroduodenitis may be a component of the peptic ulcer spectrum. Gastroduodenal abnormalities may persist or become exacerbated as gastroduodenitis with or without an ulcer crater. Although few prospective studies are available, it would seem that more than 30% of patients with symptomatic duodenitis will develop a duodenal ulcer within 3½ years. Furthermore, a previous ulcer history can be elicited in a significant proportion of patients with gastroduodenitis. More work is needed in this area, but at the moment it would seem that nonulcer peptic disease represents the initial and healing phases of peptic ulcerations. In others, it constitutes an entity that, on clinical and probably pathogenetic grounds, is indistinguishable from peptic ulcer disease. Consequently, it warrants the same treatment.

Gastrin assays and gastric analysis. A fasting and a 60-minute postprandial gastrin level should be obtained in patients with peptic disease. In patients with duodenal ulcers the fasting levels are usually normal but the postprandial rise is generally greater than normal. Values in children with gastric ulcer or with gastritis and a healthy antrum may show high fasting values; this is a reflection of low rates of acid secretion. The main indication for obtaining gastrin determinations is to rule out the presence of a gastrinoma (see the Zollinger-Ellison syndrome section). It is well known that gastrin values are high in patients on cimetidine, and they tend to remain abnormal for as long as 2 weeks after the medication is stopped.

There are few indications for the execution of gastric acid secretion studies. They still have a place in recurrent peptic disease, in atrophic gastritis with or without pernicious anemia, and in the rare cases of hypersecretory syndromes.

After an 8-hour fast and discontinuation of antisecretory drugs for at least 48 hours, a size 10 to 12 Salem double-lumen tube is placed in the dependent part of the stomach. Continuous suction is applied while the patient lies on his left side. After removal of the residual gastric juice two or preferably four times, 15-minute collections are made. Pentagastrin given subcutaneously (6 µg/kg) is a safer stimulant than betazole (Histalog) (1 mg/kg). With the latter, an ampule of epinephrine 1:1000 should be kept at hand. Four 15-minute samples are again collected in ice-filled containers. Each sample is measured for volume, pH, and titratable acidity. The sum of the four

Table 7-4. Gastric acid studies in children with duodenal ulcer (DU)

Children	Acid output (mEq/kg/hr)			Authors
	BAO	MAO	PAO	
Controls	0.035	0.248	0.332	Christie and Ament (1976)
DU	0.064	0.486	0.507	
Controls	0.032	0.202	—	Ghai et al. (1965)
DU	0.043	0.300	—	
DU	—	0.330		Habbick et al. (1968)

basal samples corresponds to the basal acid output (BOA) in milliequivalents per hour (mEq/hr). The maximal acid output (MAO) corresponds to the sum of the four samples obtained after pentagastrin or betazole (Histalog). One calculates the peak acid output (PAO) by pooling the results of the two highest poststimulation samples and multiplying by 2. Until a few years ago, gastric acid output was believed to be helpful in establishing the long-term prognosis for duodenal ulcer.

Recent studies have failed to find a correlation between BAO and PAO with the incidence of complications (bleeding, perforation, stenosis) and with the need for surgical interventions. However, both BAO, MAO, and PAO acid values are higher in children with duodenal ulcers than in controls though there is some overlap.

X-ray studies

Roentgenographic signs of ulceration or of a deformity of the duodenal bulb may be present. Duodenal irritability is a frequent roentgenographic observation in asymptomatic children. In patients with severe degrees of duodenal irritability, an ulcer niche may not be demonstrated because barium is moved out of the bulb too rapidly or because a blood clot or fibrin may cover the ulcer. Nevertheless, the diagnosis of duodenal ulcer should not be made unless a persistent crater is demonstrated (Fig. 7-10). Deformity of the duodenal bulb without a crater is an indication of a previous ulcer and scar formation and does not necessarily indicate that an active ulcer is present. Coarsened mucosal folds in the duodenum are believed by some to represent so-called ulcer equiv-

alents, which should be treated as ulcer disease. Although this is probably true in some patients, a coarsened mucosal pattern may be seen in totally asymptomatic children and can therefore be considered only a variation of the normal under those circumstances.

In infants, ulcers are occasionally found in the pyloric region. The roentgenographic findings resemble those of pyloric stenosis. The muscular indentation in the barium-filled antrum of pyloric stenosis is absent, and usually a crater is visible as a persistent "spot" of barium.

In rare cases of hypertrophic pyloric muscles, the space left between muscle fibers disposed as an inverted V may be filled with contrast material and a niche that can easily be mistaken for a channel ulcer is created.

Primary gastric ulcers in children are located on the lesser curvature of the stomach. The crater is sharply delimited, and folds radiate to its edge (Fig. 7-11). A considerable degree of edema and inflammation is often present and leads to a partial or total outlet obstruction. Since peptic ulcer disease is accompanied by a significant degree of functional disorder, evidence of fasting hypersecretion and delayed emptying may not necessarily indicate structural changes in the pyloric or prepyloric area.

Stress ulcers are found as commonly in the stomach as in the duodenum. They are frequently multiple and may be present in both the stomach and the duodenum. The crater is usually shallow without underlying induration and hence is difficult to recognize roentgenologically. Double-contrast barium examinations have significant advan-

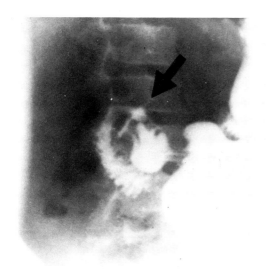

Fig. 7-10. Duodenal ulcer. A 70 mm spot film taken during a barium meal demonstrates a midbulbar niche measuring 4 mm, *arrow*. Note some edema of the folds converging toward the ulcer. The patient, a 10-year-old boy, had experienced crampy epigastric pain associated with anorexia and a 9-pound weight loss over a 3-week period. This was the fourth such episode in 3 years, two of them associated with significant bleeding necessitating transfusions. The prognosis in this patient is for continuing disease and for progressive resistance to medical management.

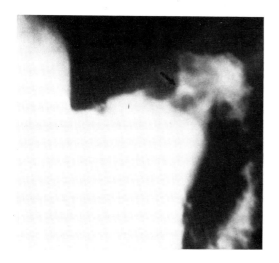

Fig. 7-11. Primary antral ulcer. *Arrow*, Crater with radiating gastric mucosal folds and surrounded by a thickened rim of edematous tissue. Vomiting was a prominent feature in this case.

tages for the demonstration of shallow ulcers and erosions. The technique permits imaging of the mucosa. It has been most helpful and can be carried out at the same time as the single-contrast examination. Air-contrast upper gastrointestinal roentgenograms are necessary for the diagnosis of bleeding acute gastrointestinal lesions, though the diagnostic accuracy is still far short of that obtained by endoscopy.

Panendoscopy

The barium roentgenographic examination remains the single most widely useful diagnostic tool. The advent of fiberoptic instruments adapted to pediatric needs make a significant contribution to the detection of peptic disease.

Studies correlating roentgenologic and endoscopic findings reveal that x rays can pick up two thirds of duodenal ulcers and more than half of gastric ulcers. In pediatric series close to half of gastric and duodenal ulcers may be missed by x rays. Furthermore, there is the occasional patient in whom a false-positive diagnosis of peptic ulcer disease is made when endoscopy is not available to confirm doubtful findings. Double-contrast barium studies are said to pick up close to 70% of patients with nonulcer peptic disease localized to the duodenum but only somewhat less than 40% of those with gastric lesions. The advantages of panendoscopy over roentgenographic studies are even more striking in cases of acute erosions associated with acute gastritis and stress ulcers. Endoscopy should always be complemented by biopsy specimens to confirm the endoscopic changes. Otherwise, a number of false-positive diagnoses will be made.

Although it is true that in the absence of endoscopic evidence, the presence of symptoms cannot be assumed to indicate the presence of peptic disease, we tend to be conservative. Endoscopy is indicated when roentgenographic findings are doubtful or absent in symptomatic patients. If after adequate treatment there is persistence of symptoms and yet there is roentgenographic evidence of healing, or else absence of symptoms and persistence of a crater, endoscopy should be carried out. Prompt and accurate identification of a bleeding site is an absolute indication for endoscopy (see section on upper gastrointestinal bleeding). The instrumentation and technique of esophagogastroduodenoscopy are described in Chapter 32.

Treatment

Chronic ulcer. Peptic ulcers in children have a strong natural tendency not only to heal spontaneously but also to recur. Although rest in a hospital bed is the only significant treatment shown to improve the rate of ulcer healing in adults, this kind of restriction is usually unnecessary for the child unless he has signs of gastric or duodenal obstruction, active bleeding, or perforation.

If there are signs of outlet obstruction, gastric suction should be carried out for a few days. Thereafter, hourly feedings are necessary initially and should be continued until pain has disappeared. Foods that cause the child to have pain should be avoided. In addition, beef broth, tea, coffee, spices, and carbonated beverages should be restricted because they enhance gastric secretion.

Diet. There is no evidence that hourly feedings of milk and cream as well as of a bland diet reduce gastric acidity or affect the rate of ulcer healing. In fact, it has been shown to stimulate acid secretion because of its calcium and protein content. Bedtime snacks stimulate the delivery of acid over the first part of the night and should be avoided. For the same reasons it is best to avoid between-meal snacking. Children adapt well to this dietary advice. Alcoholic beverages, aspirin, and other drugs that may damage the gastric mucosal barrier are contraindicated. As cigarette smoking is known to increase the incidence of duodenal ulcers and also decrease their healing rate, adolescents should be advised to stop smoking.

Antacids. Antacids are the preferred medication for the initial management of peptic disease. Although they are not much more effective than a placebo for the relief of symptoms, they promote the healing of duodenal ulcers. Liquids neutralize substantially more acid than tablets do. Aluminum hydroxide and magnesium hydroxide mixtures are best. Should constipation or diarrhea occur, the proportion of aluminum and magnesium can be changed to ameliorate tolerance. The recommended dosage is 30 ml/1.73 m^2 at 1 hour and 3 hours after each meal and at bedtime. We have been using Maalox II and Mylanta II; they both have a very high in vitro capacity to neutralize acid. The medication is continued for a period of 6 weeks and then gradually tapered. Within a week patients are generally symptom-free and healing is complete in 80% of cases within 6 to 8 weeks. To this regimen we sometimes add propantheline bromide (Pro-Banthine 0.25 mg/kg) at bedtime for children with duodenal ulcer. Anticholinergics decrease nocturnal acid secretion, but the dosage has to be adjusted so that the patient experiences tolerable side effects, otherwise it is ineffective. However the place of anticholinergic agents is controversial, except in cases with Zollinger-Ellison syndrome.

Cimetidine. H_2-receptor antagonists are potent inhibitors of acid secretion. They reduce basal acid secretion by 80% and can keep the stomach free of acid overnight. They will also suppress food-stimulated acid secretion by 70% to 80% for a 3-hour period. Cimetidine is absorbed rapidly and has a prolonged action when taken with a meal. If given to patients with chronic renal failure, the dosage of 300 mg/1.73 m^2 with meals and at bedtime should be reduced to the morning and evening dose. Its main side effects are gynecomastia (less than 5%), a rare occurrence of rashes, mental confusion that has been reported in elderly patients, and also a report of a decrease in the sperm count. The possibility that it could promote an increase in the parietal mass is the main drawback to its utilization. Rebound hypersecretion of hydrochloric acid is described as occurring after discontinuation of the drug. A new H_2-receptor blocker, ranitidine, appears to be more potent and longer acting than cimetidine. A healing rate of 92% has been obtained with a dosage of 100 mg twice a day with this inhibitor of acid secretion.

Cimetidine 300 mg just before retiring may be added to an antacid regimen if night pain occurs. Other indications in peptic disease are for those cases who fail to respond clinically, roentgenologically, and endoscopically to the more conservative but equally expensive antacids. Noncompliance to antacids has been a problem with children and adolescents. Cimetidine is a better choice in such circumstances. There is a small percentage of children who either remain symptomatic despite roentgenographic and endoscopic evidence of healing, or who are totally asymptomatic but in whom the ulcer is still visible. In such circumstances, we advocate a 6-week trial of cimetidine.

Cimetidine heals most duodenal ulcers, but a certain number relapse rapidly. By 6 months 70% to 80% have recurred. Maintenance therapy (400 mg twice a day) for a year does not totally protect; 10% to 25% have been reported to relapse. It is suggested that treatment forever (and ever and ever) beyond a year is unjustified for the time being, except in patients with gastrinomas. However, in selected adolescents with chronic duodenal ulcers and disabling pain, cimetidine may be a good alternative if surgery is refused or contraindicated because of an associated condition.

Surgical management of peptic ulcers is reserved for patients with complications of intractable pain, perforation, hemorrhage, and obstruction. Vagotomy with pyloroplasty has been shown to be a safe and consistently successful procedure in patients with duodenal ulcers unresponsive to medical management.

Series of pediatric patients recorded before the advent of cimetidine show that 25% to 40% required surgery because of complications or disabling pain. It is expected that this percentage range has now decreased significantly. A highly selective vagotomy and pyloroplasty is now advocated. The rate of relapse (6.6%) is no different from that after truncal vagotomy, and side effects such as diarrhea are much lower.

Acute ulcer. Any child with a major gastrointestinal hemorrhage should have a large-bore nasogastric tube inserted. If the bleeding is from the intestine, gastric drainage will be free from blood. On the other hand, if blood is present, the cause of bleeding should be identified by roentgenograms, panendoscopy, and, in certain instances, angiography. (See section on gastrointestinal bleeding, p. 181.) Repeated gastric irrigations with ice-cold water have a therapeutic effect. Maintenance of gastric suction is important until there is no further evidence of bleeding. It prevents gastric distention, which undoubtedly favors blood loss from an ulcer, and it permits a dynamic assessment of the blood loss.

The patient with a bleeding ulcer should be kept under close supervision. Vital signs, central venous pressure measurements, and hematocrit values should be the parameters determining the volume of blood to be transfused and indicating the necessity of emergency surgery in cases in which closure of the perforation or suture of the bleeding point may be lifesaving.

About 15% of children with primary peptic disease are admitted with a severe gastrointestinal hemorrhage as compared to 50% of those with secondary ulcers. Most stop bleeding on iced-fluid gastric lavage. Cimetidine (intravenously 300 mg/ 1.73 m^2) every 4 hours has been a precious adjunct in bleeding primary and secondary ulcers. However, its effectiveness has been reported to be much greater in gastric than in duodenal ulcers. A double-blind clinical trial has shown that cimetidine is effective in the prophylaxis of gastrointestinal bleeding after brain injury or surgery. Acute hemorrhagic gastritis and acute bleeding peptic disease can also be adequately controlled by an antacid drip (60 to 80 ml/1.73 m^2/hr) adjusted to keep the pH around 7.

Prognosis

The prognosis for the neonate with acute gastric perforation is poor and reflects the severity of the underlying disease bringing about the ulceration. In infants and children who develop an acute ulcer with initial symptoms of bleeding or perforation rather than typical ulcer pain, healing is the rule, though emergency surgery is at times necessary when perforation has occurred. Since stress ulcers are secondary, the prognosis is evidently affected by the precipitating disease.

The rate of complications (bleeding, perforation, obstruction) is said to be higher than in adults. Fifty percent of children and adolescents with peptic disease have a recurrence within a year and 70% have repeated relapses over the years.

In our study of children below the age of 6 years with primary ulcers (gastric and duodenal) with a mean follow-up study at 3.8 years, only 1 in 4 had a relapse. Much less encouraging were the results in the older age group (6 to 18 years), since two thirds had recurrences, with 12 of 19 requiring surgery. Fortunately, surgical results have been excellent in terms of symptoms and growth. The availability of potent and safe H_2-receptor antagonists have considerably decreased the indications for surgery. However, the benefits of a safe and effective surgical intervention in the young certainly outweigh the long-term inconveniences, cost, and disability associated with chronic relapsing peptic disease.

REFERENCES

Agunod, M., Yamaguchi, N., Lopez, R., and others: Correlative study of hydrochloric acid, pepsin, and intrinsic factor secretion in newborns and infants, Am. J. Dig. Dis. **14:**400-414, 1969.

Berstad, A., Kett, K., Aadland, E., and others: Treatment of duodenal ulcer with ranitidine, a new histamin H_2-receptor antagonist, Scand. J. Gastroenterol. **15:**637-639, 1980.

Chapman, M.L.: Peptic ulcer: a medical perspective, Med. Clin. North Am. **62:**39-51, 1978.

Christie, D.L., and Ament, M.E.: Gastric acid hypersecretion in children with duodenal ulcer, Gastroenterology **71:**242-244, 1976.

Curci, M.R., Little, K., Sieber, W.B., and Kiesewetter, W.B.: Peptic ulcer disease in children reexamined, J. Pediatr. Surg. **11:**329-335, 1976.

Deckelbaum, R.J., Roy, C.C., Lussier-Lazaroff, J., and Morin, C.L.: Peptic ulcer disease: a clinical study in 73 children, Can. Med. Assoc. J. **111:**225-228, 1974.

Deren, J.J.: Development of structure and function in the fetal and newborn stomach, Am. J. Clin. Nutr. **24:**144-159, 1971.

Donaldson, R.M.: Breakdown of barriers in gastric ulcer, N. Engl. J. Med. **288:**316-317, 1973.

Duane, W.C., and Wiegand, D.M.: Mechanism by which bile salt disrupts the gastric mucosal barrier in the dog, J. Clin. Invest. **66:**1044-1049, 1980.

Editorial: Duodenal-ulcer inheritance, Lancet **1:**650-651, 1979.

Editorial: Cimetidine for ever (and ever and ever), Br. Med. J. **1:**1425, 1978.

Euler, A.R., Byrne, W.J., Cousins, L.M., and others: Increased serum gastrin concentrations and gastric hyposecretion in the immediate newborn period, Gastroenterology **72:**1271-1273, 1977.

Feldman, E.J., and Sabovich, K.A.: Stress and peptic ulcer disease, Gastroenterology **78:**1087-1089, 1980.

Fisher, R.S., and Cohen, S.: Pyloric-sphincter dysfunction in patients with gastric ulcer, N. Engl. J. Med. **288:**273-276, 1974.

Garcia, J.C., Carney, J.A., Stickler, G.B., and others: Zollinger-Ellison syndrome and neurofibromatosis in a 13 year old boy, J. Pediatr. **93:**982-984, 1978.

Ghai, O.P., Singh, M., Walia, B.N.S., and Gadekar, N.G.: An assessment of gastric secretory response with "maximal" augmented histamine stimulation in children with peptic ulcer, Arch. Dis. Child. **40:**77-79, 1965.

Grand, R.J., Watkins, J.B., and Torti, F.M.: Development of the human gastrointestinal tract: a review, Gastroenterology **70:**790-810, 1976.

Greenlaw, R., Sheahan, D.G., DeLuca, V., and others: Gastroduodenitis: a broader concept of peptic ulcer ddisease, Dig. Dis. Sci. **25:**660-672, 1980.

Grosfeld, J.L., Shipley, F., Fitzgerald, J.F., and Ballantine, T.V.N.: Acute peptic ulcer in infancy and childhood, Am. Surg. **44:**13-19, 1978.

Habbick, B.F., Melrose, A.C., and Grant, J.C.: Duodenal ulcer in childhood, Arch. Dis. Child. **43:**23-27, 1968.

Halloran, L.G., Zfass, A.M., Gayle, W.E., and others: Prevention of acute gastrointestinal complications after severe head injury: a controlled trial of cimetidine prophylaxis, Am. J. Surg. **139:**44-48, 1980.

Johnson, P.W., and Snyder, W.H.: Vagotomy and pyloroplasty in infancy and childhood, J. Pediatr. Surg. **3:**238-245, 1968.

Karlstrom, F.: Peptic ulcer in children in Sweden during the years 1953-1962, Ann. Paediatr. **202:**218-232, 1964.

Konturek, S.J.: Secretory mechanisms of acid and pepsin. In Sircus, W., and Smith, A.N., editors: Foundations of gastroenterology, Philadelphia, 1980, W.B. Saunders Co.

Krasna, I.H., Schneider, K.M., and Becker, J.M.: Surgical management of stress ulcerations in childhood, J. Pediatr. Surg. **6:**301-306, 1971.

McGuigan, J.E., and Trudeau, W.L.: Differences in rates of gastrin release in normal persons and patients with duodenal-ulcer disease, N. Engl. J. Med. **288:**64-66, 1973.

McLeod, R.S., and Cohen, Z.: Highly selective vagotomy and truncal vagotomy and pyloroplasty for duodenal ulcer: a clinical review, Can. J. Surg. **22:**113-120, 1979.

Menguy, R.: The prophylaxis of stress ulceration, N. Engl. J. Med. **302:**461-462, 1980.

Moorthy, A.V., and Chesney, R.W.: Peptic ulcer in uremic children, J. Pediatr. **92:**420-421, 1978.

Nord, K.S., and Lebenthal, E.: Peptic ulcer in children, Am. J. Gastrol. **73:**75-80, 1980.

Peterson, W.L., Sturdevant, R.A.L., Frankl, H.D., and others: Healing of duodenal ulcer with an antacid regimen, N. Engl. J. Med. **297:**341-345, 1977.

Piper, D.W., McIntosh, J.H., Ariotti, D.E., and others: Analgesic ingestion and chronic peptic ulcer, Gastroenterology **80:**427-432, 1981.

Puri, P., and Boy, E.: Children with duodenal ulcers and their families, Arch. Dis. Child. **50:**485-486, 1975.

Raffensperger, J.G., Condon, J.B., and Greengard, J.: Complications of gastric and duodenal ulcers in infancy and childhood, Surg. Gynecol. Obstet. **123:**1269-1274, 1966.

Ravitch, M.M., and Duremdes, G.D.: Operative treatment of chronic duodenal ulcer in childhood, Ann. Surg. **171:**641-646, 1970.

Robb, J.D.A., Thomas, P.S., Orszulok, J., and Odling-Smee, G.W.: Duodenal ulcer in children, Arch. Dis. Child. **47:**688-696, 1972.

Robert, A.: Cytoprotection by prostaglandins, Gastroenterology **77:**761-767, 1979.

Rodbro, P., Krasilnikoff, P.A., and Christiansen, P.M.: Parietal cell secretory function in early childhood, Scand. J. Gastroent. **2:**209-213, 1967.

Royston, C.M.S., Polak, J., Bloom, S.R., and others: G cell population of the gastric antrum, plasma gastrin and gastric acid secretion in patients with and without duodenal ulcer, Gut **19:**689-698, 1978.

Tedesco, F.J., Goldstein, P.D., Gleason, W.A., and Keating, J.P.: Upper gastrointestinal endoscopy in the pediatric patient, Gastroenterology **70:**492-494, 1976.

Thomas, W.E.G.: Duodeno-gastric reflux: a common factor in pathogenesis of gastric and duodenal ulcer, Lancet **2:**1166-1167, 1980.

Thompson, W.O., Joffe, S.N., Robertson, A.G., and others: Gastroduodenitis: a broader concept of peptic ulcer disease, Dig. Dis. Sci. **25:**660-672, 1980.

Tudor, R.B.: Gastric and duodenal ulcers in children, Gastroenterology **62:**823, 1972.

ZOLLINGER-ELLISON SYNDROME

Zollinger-Ellison syndrome was first described as a triad consisting of a non–beta islet cell tumor of the pancreas, gastric hypersecretion, and severe atypical or intractable peptic ulcers. It is now known that all patients with this syndrome have high levels of circulating gastrin originating from a gastrinoma that is usually in the pancreas but, on occasion, can be found in the wall of the duodenum or of the stomach. As a result, the parietal cell mass is greatly expanded. The hypersecretion of gastric acid leads not only to peptic ulcer disease but also to functional and morphologic abnormalities of the small intestine. There is commonly evidence of duodenitis, and these lesions extend in the jejunum with mucosal erosions, stunting of villi, and acute inflammatory changes.

Gastrin not only has an effect on gastric acid secretion but also plays a major role in gastrointestinal functions. It stimulates gastric motility, pancreatic secretion of water and bicarbonate, pancreatic enzyme output, and biliary flow. It brings about a contraction of the cardia and a relaxation of the ileocecal valve.

The syndrome is rare in the pediatric population. Fewer than 25 cases have been described in children, with the youngest patient being a 5-year-old girl. The disease occurs more frequently in boys than in girls (4:1). Islet cell tumors of the endocrine organs, thyroid, adrenal, pituitary, and especially the parathyroid, have been associated with Zollinger-Ellison syndrome. So far, multiple adenomatosis has not been reported in children with Zollinger-Ellison syndrome. It has been observed in one child with the Marden-Walker syndrome. Half the islet cell tumors reported in the pediatric age group are malignant.

Clinical findings

The outstanding symptom of the Zollinger-Ellison syndrome, abdominal pain, is commonly accompanied by vomiting, passage of tarry stools, and occasional diarrhea and steatorrhea. The pain-food-relief pattern is usual. The symptoms either fail to respond or exacerbate despite medical treatment. Massive hematemesis, severe anemia, and perforations can occur.

In all pediatric cases described, the ulcers are either gastric, duodenal, or jejunal. Multiple ulcers are common. The stomach shows pronounced hypertrophy of the gastric rugae, and the duodenum is dilated and may be grossly deformed by cicatricial deformities. The presence of multiple atypically located ulcers or of giant ulcers is highly suggestive.

In the past few years it has become apparent that the textbook description of the Zollinger-Ellison syndrome is present in only 50% of adult cases. Clinical, roentgenographic and endoscopic findings are often those of ordinary peptic ulcer disease or of gastroduodenitis. This is the apparent result of the routine measurement of gastrin in patients with peptic disease. Although the immunoassay of gastrin is also widely used in the pediatric population, the Zollinger-Ellison syndrome remains a very rare entity, and it has features that are readily distinguishable from those of idiopathic peptic disease.

Gastrinemia and gastric acid studies

In the past decade the gastrin radioimmunoassay has made possible an earlier and more secure diagnosis of the disease than gastric acid studies could. Mean values in our laboratory are 35 pg/ml with a range 5 to 170 pg/ml. Hypergastrinemia can be divided into the following two groups:

Hypergastrinemia with normal or low gastric acid secretion
Atrophic gastritis with preserved antrum
Pernicious anemia
Pheochromocytoma
Hypergastrinemia with gastric acid hypersecretion
Zollinger-Ellison syndrome
Antral G-cell hyperplasia (never reported in children)
Protracted pyloric obstruction
Chronic renal failure
Short bowel syndrome (controversial in children)
Duodenal ulcer

Although fasting hypergastrinemia is reportedly unusual in patients with duodenal ulcers, we have seen a sizable proportion of children and adolescents with duodenal ulcers with gastrin levels between 150 and 250 pg/ml. Such values overlap with those of a small number of gastrinoma patients though the majority have a fasting gastrinemia of over 1000 pg/ml. The calcium infusion test is particularly useful when the diagnosis is in doubt. Calcium is administered at a dosage of 15 mg/kg over a 3-hour period. A two- to threefold increase of gastrin over basal values or over 500 pg/ml during the third hour is diagnostic because there is little change in normal subjects.

The acid-secretion changes are striking. Pediatric patients studied overnight have had gastric secretion volumes between 600 to 2000 ml and corresponding basal acid secretion concentrations of 23 to 164 mEq/L. A BAO (basal acid output) exceeding 15 mEq/hr and an MAO (maximal acid output) above 100 mEq/hr are compatible with a gastrinoma. As the parietal cells are maximally stimulated to produce acid by gastrin released by the tumor, there is frequently an inappropriately small response to betazole (Histalog) or pentagastrin. A basal acid output greater than 60% of MAO or PAO (peak acid output) is suggestive of the diagnosis.

Treatment

Gastrinomas are generally small and often multiple. They cannot be localized by CT scan or ultrasound, and surgical exploration fails to find the tumor in most cases. There is no evidence to support the recommendation of attempts at primary resection of the gastrinoma without "chemical" or surgical total gastrectomy. The introduction of the H_2-receptor antagonist, cimetidine, has revolutionized the therapy of gastrinoma. It is the treatment of choice and may be associated with an anticholinergic agent taken at bedtime. If symptoms and gastric acid studies suggest failure of or escape from cimetidine, a vagotomy and pyloroplasty will further reduce acid secretion.

Total gastrectomy should be reserved for those with severe symptoms or with complications. Despite the fact that total excision of the tumor may be possible in only 10% of cases, surgical exploration is recommended after preparation of the patient with cimetidine. It should be noted that even after complete excision of gross tumor only 5% of patients have normal gastrin levels, the majority require lifetime cimetidine therapy. A recent adult series suggests a 5-year survival rate of 76% in patients where all gross tumor was removed compared to 21% when it was not possible. In cases where no tumor was seen, the survival rate was 100%.

CORROSIVE GASTRITIS

Acids, alkalis, and detergents affect the esophageal mucosa most severely, and in only a small number of cases is the stomach involved. After a rapid transit through the esophagus, the corrosive substance initiates pylorospasm and causes its maximum effect in the antrum. There are invariably superficial ulcerations and edema. Eventual scarring with an outlet obstruction is a distinct, long-term complication. Ferrous sulfate poisoning and calcium chloride are known to give rise to a severe form of chemical gastritis. Perforation of the stomach is reported from alkali ingestion in the form of Clinitest tablets. Liquid-Plumr (sodium hypochlorite and potassium hydroxide) has been associated with the presence of intramural bullous lesions in the stomach.

A recent report has attracted attention, albeit in adults, to a previously unsuspected high incidence of corrosive gastritis in the absence of lesions of the oropharynx and of the esophagus. This is more likely to occur with acids than with strong alkalis. Cautious fiberoptic endoscopy is advisable when there is a history of ingestion. The scope should not be advanced past esophageal lesions. However, when the esophagus appears intact, a thorough exploration of the stomach is indicated. The presence of diffuse gastritis with ulcerations, petechiae, and edema is an indication for conservative management. On the other hand, transmural necrosis, as evidenced by sheets of blackened mucosa, is an indication for an immediate laparotomy.

Abdominal pain, vomiting, and frank hematemesis closely follow the ingestion of corrosive agents. A soft rubber nasogastric tube should be inserted so that gastric lavage with antacids can dilute and neutralize the residual caustic. Subsequently, antacids are given hourly by mouth. Sedation, antibiotics, and parenteral fluids are administered while a close watch is kept for the development of signs and symptoms of peritonitis.

REFERENCES

Abe, K., Niikawa, N., and Sasaki, H.: Zollinger-Ellison syndrome with Marden-Walker syndrome, Am. J. Dis. Child. **133:**735-738, 1979.

Burmester, H.B.C., Hall, R., and Munainer, N.: The Zollinger-Ellison syndrome in a child, Gut **10:**800-803, 1969.

Drake, D.P., Maciver, A.G., and Atwell, J.D.: Zollinger-Ellison syndrome in a child: medical treatment with cimetidine, Arch. Dis. Child. **55:**226-238, 1980.

McCarthy, D.M.: Report of the U.S. experience with cimetidine in Zollinger-Ellison syndrome and other hypersecretory states, Gastroenterology **74:**453-458, 1978.

Roselund, M.L.: The Zollinger-Ellison syndrome in children: a review, Am. J. Med. Sci. **254:**884-892, 1967.

Roselund, M.L., Crean, G.P., Johnson, D.G., and others: The Zollinger-Ellison syndrome in a 10-year-old boy, J. Pediatr. **75:**443-448, 1969.

Schwartz, D.L., White, J.J., Saulsbury, F., and Haller, J.A.: Gastrin response to calcium infusion: an aid to the improved diagnosis of Zollinger-Ellison syndrome in children, Pediatrics **54:**599-602, 1974.

Regan, P.T., and Malagelada, J.R.: A reappraisal of clinical, roentgenographic and endoscopic features of the Zollinger-Ellison syndrome, Mayo Clin. Proc. **53:**19-23, 1978.

Wilson, S.D., Schulte, W.J., and Meade, R.C.: Longevity studies following total gastrectomy in children with the Zollinger-Ellison syndrome, Arch. Surg. **103:**108-115, 1971.

Zollinger, R.M., Ellison, E.C., Fabri, P.J., and others: Primary peptic ulcerations of the jejunum associated with islet cell tumors, Ann. Surg. **192:**422-427, 1980.

REFERENCES

Chong, G.C., Beahrs, O.H., and Payne, W.S.: Management of corrosive gastritis due to ingested acid, Mayo Clin. Proc. **49:**861-865, 1974.

Chung, R., and Den Besten, L.: Fibreoptic endoscopy in treatment of corrosive injury of the stomach, Arch. Surg. **110:**725-728, 1975.

Citron, B.P., Pincus, I.J., Geokas, M.C., and Haverback, B.J.: Chemical trauma of the esophagus and stomach, Surg. Clin. North Am. **48:**1303-1311, 1968.

GASTROINTESTINAL BLEEDING

Vomiting and rectal evacuation of blood constitute alarming symptoms that will promptly be brought to the physician's attention. Accurate diagnosis and proper management are often difficult. Lifesaving emergency treatment must be undertaken without delay in a number of cases in which the diagnosis is not immediately evident. In a small number, the precise origin of the bleeding cannot be found despite an extensive and prolonged diagnostic work-up.

The differential diagnosis of hematemesis and rectal bleeding in relationship with age and clinical features can be found in Part I of this book. Conditions that are more likely to affect each age group are listed in Fig. 7-12. The age range for each group of entities is the one associated with peak incidence but does not exclude their occurrence in other age groups. Over the past 5 years, there has been a decrease in the percentage of cases of severe upper gastrointestinal bleeding attributable to varices. We are now following a smaller number of children with extrahepatic portal hypertension. Another contributing factor has been the routine use of panendoscopy permitting identification of a bleeding site other than varices in a sizable proportion (20% to 30%) of children with portal hypertension. In a series of 68 pediatric patients, approximately 10% of upper gastrointestinal bleeds were caused by varices, whereas gastroduodenal ulcers accounted for close to 40%. Esophagitis and gastritis were responsible for close to 30%. The object of the following discussion is to provide an outline of the sequence of diagnostic and therapeutic measures that should be undertaken promptly in children with acute gastrointestinal bleeding.

Diagnosis

1. *Is it really blood and is it coming from the gastrointestinal tract?* Gastrointestinal bleeding in children can be acute and characterized by the vomiting of either fresh or altered blood or by the rectal evacuation of bright red blood or of melena. In other circumstances, when the bleeding is less severe or chronic, the diagnosis is more difficult and requires chemical detection. Since a number of substances may simulate hematochezia (food coloring, beets, Kool-Aid, gelatin desserts, ampicillin, and so on) or melena (iron preparations, bismuth, spinach, and so on), confirming the presence of blood with Hematest or Hemoc-cult on a stool specimen or on a finger-cot specimen should be done. Information related to antecedent epistaxis, significant coughing, or genitourinary problems may help identify the source of bleeding to a system other than the gastrointestinal tract.

2. *How much has the child bled, and what is the color and character of the blood?* A rough estimate of the quantity and a description of the color and character of the blood are important for the sorting out of diagnostic possibilities. Table 1-1 on p. 6 lists causes of gastrointestinal bleeding in relationship to the amount and appearance of blood in the stools. The following general guideline may assist the physician in localizing the source of the blood:

a. Bright red blood welling effortlessly out of the mouth usually indicates bleeding from esophageal varices.

b. Vomiting of bright red blood or of "coffee grounds" is usually associated with a lesion proximal to the ligament of Treitz.

c. Melena is indicative of a significant blood loss (over 50 to 100 ml per 24 hours) likely taking place proximal to the ligament of Treitz. In the event of massive bleeding from the upper tract, bright red rectal bleeding may occur.

d. Bright red or dark red blood in the stools is usually associated with a lesion originating in the ileum or colon.

e. Blood streaks on the outside of a stool localizes the lesion to the anal canal or rectal ampulla.

3. *Is the child acutely or chronically ill?* The most urgent part of the objective examination consists in evaluating the general condition of the child, with particular attention being given to the presence of signs of anemia or of shock. In this regard, pallor of the skin and mucous membranes is not so reliable as the loss of the normal red color in the creases of the extended hand. Pulse rate and blood pressure contribute to the assessment of the hemodynamic status of the patient. As a rule, a systolic blood pressure below 100 mm Hg or a pulse rate exceeding 100/min suggests that more than a 20% reduction of blood volume has occurred. A pulse rate increase of 20/min or a drop in systolic blood pressure greater than 10 mm Hg when the patient is made to sit up is a more sensitive index of a significant volume depletion.

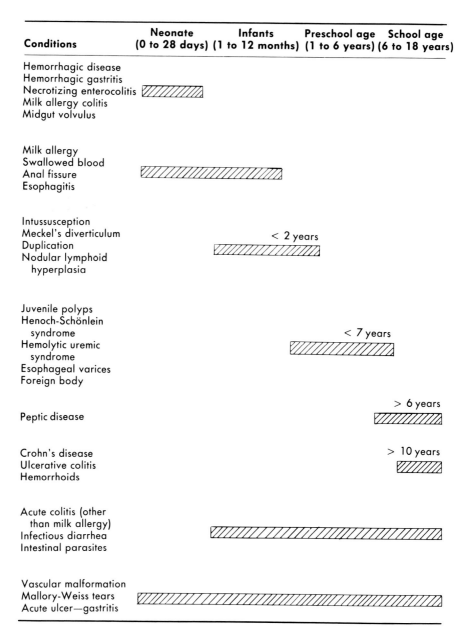

Fig. 7-12. Conditions associated with gastrointestinal bleeding in relation to age groups. (From Roy, C.C., et al.: Clin. Gastroenterol. 10:225, 1981.)

The physical examination should be thorough no matter how ill the patient is. Alertness to signs of portal hypertension or of intestinal obstruction and to the presence of icterus, ascites, abdominal distention or masses, spider nevi, petechiae, purpura, ecchymoses, angiomas, telangiectatic lesions, the mucosal pigmentation of Peutz-Jeghers, and the soft-tissue lesions or bone tumors of Gardner may rapidly lead to a diagnosis. The anus should be carefully inspected for fissures (before digital examination is done), the vagina for menstrual blood, and the nasal passages for signs of a recent epistaxis. Certain clinical points are particularly important to remember in children:

    a. Dizziness, pain, and loss of consciousness may be the only signs of bleeding.

    b. Physical evidence of liver disease may be minimal.

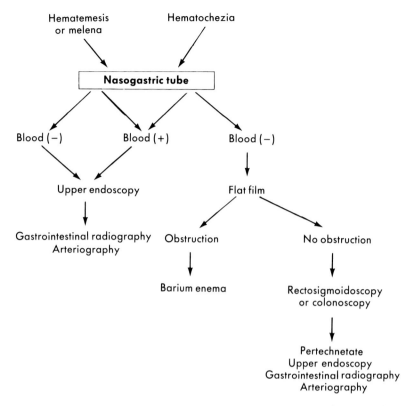

Fig. 7-13. Diagnostic approach to gastrointestinal bleeding. All cases with upper (hematemesis or melena) and lower (hematochezia) bleeding should have a nasogastric tube put in before further testing is carried out.

c. Family history is important in duodenal ulcers.

d. Retarded growth may be the only evidence of chronic inflammatory bowel disease.

e. Splenomegaly may be absent in extrahepatic portal hypertension.

f. Stress ulcers may occur days after trauma, burn, or the ingestion of drugs and are common with central nervous system problems.

4. Is the patient still bleeding, and from what site? The physiologic effects of gastrointestinal bleeding depend on both the amount of blood lost and the rapidity of the loss. Recording pulse, blood pressure, and respiratory rate every 15 minutes is essential to assess ongoing bleeding. Serial hemoglobin levels and hematocrit readings should be obtained hourly initially. Progressive decreases of both do not necessarily indicate active bleeding. The speed with which plasma expansion occurs varies from hours to days. Consequently, interpretation must also take into account clinical signs of active bleeding. A normal serum creatinine in the presence of a high BUN level indicates that a large amount of blood is in the small intestine. A progressive drop can be interpreted as an indication that active bleeding has stopped. In the presence of clinical and laboratory signs of active bleeding, bleeding time, prothrombin time, and platelet count are obtained to rule out a bleeding diathesis.

The most important diagnostic maneuver for serious upper or lower bleeding is nasogastric intubation (Fig. 7-13). In all cases of gastrointestinal bleeding, a small tube should be passed to sample gastric contents. Detection of blood in the gastric aspirate confirms a bleeding site proximal to the ligament of Treitz. However, the failure to find blood does not completely exclude the possibility that the duodenum may be the source of the blood.

If blood is recovered from the gastric aspirate, a large-bore tube should be placed in the stomach and gastric lavage with ice cold saline solution carried out until a clear or only a blood-tinged return is obtained. Esophagogastroduodenoscopy immediately follows ice-water lavage. A barium-contrast study of the esophagus, stomach, and upper intestine is carried out only in instances (10% to 15%) where a bleeding site is not found.

Panendoscopy is particularly well suited to help identify a bleeding site and lesions such as esophagitis, Mallory-Weiss tears, varices, stress ulcers, and gastritis unidentifiable roentgenologically. X rays cannot detect Mallory-Weiss tears. They also miss most cases of esophagitis, half of varices, and many gastric mucosal erosions, as well as a significant number of acute ulcers. There is no doubt that early endoscopy after stabilization of the patient's condition improves the accuracy of the diagnosis, but there is a study showing that it does not reduce the duration of the hospital stay, the outcome over the following year, and the mortality. However, there is a subgroup of patients with liver disease who may be benefited. There is still a case for a trial of medical therapy forgoing early endoscopy. Should bleeding recur or roentgenograms, done 24 to 48 hours after admission, fail to identify the source of bleeding, then endoscopy should be carried out. There is rarely (5% to 7%) a need for supplementary angiography. The major contribution of angiography is that the exact site of bleeding can be defined. Extravasation of contrast medium is observed but this is only possible if there is brisk active bleeding, 0.5 to 1.5ml/min, at the time of the study. If gastric or esophageal varices are the cause of hemorrhage, angiography will only rarely demonstrate extravasation. In esophagogastroduodenal lesions, celiac axis angiography is indicated. Superselective injection into the gastroduodenal and the left gastric arteries should be done if the information obtained is unsatisfactory. The arterial catheter can be used for therapy. Vasopressin is infused at a rate of 0.2 unit/min/1.73 m^2 for 24 hours and half that dose for a further 24 hours. Vasopressin (0.3 unit/min/1.73 m^2) is equally effective whether given intravenously or intra-arterially. Embolization of vessels is a promising form of intra-arterial therapy. We have successfully embolized a bleeding gastroduodenal artery in a 10-year-old child with portal hypertension and a large duodenal ulcer.

The *absence of blood from the gastric aspirates* essentially rules out an ongoing hemorrhage proximal to the ligament of Treitz and is most likely to be indicative of a distal lesion, though duodenal disease is still possible. Except for Meckel's diverticulum, most bleeding small bowel lesions also produce intestinal obstruction. A flat film of the abdomen and a barium enema should be done in such cases before an emergency laparotomy. If there is no obstruction and the bleeding seemingly comes from the colon or lower ileum, a rectosigmoidoscopy or preferably a colonoscopy should be carried out on an emergency basis before a barium enema. If a Meckel's diverticulum is suspected, it is best to forego roentgenographic studies and proceed with a ^{99m}Tc-pertechnetate scan (p. 137).

Detection of bleeding vascular tumors and lower intestinal mucosal lesions has been reported by use of in vivo ^{99m}Tc-pertechnetate red blood cells. Since acute hemorrhage from the small bowel or colon is rarely life threatening, except in cases of Meckel's diverticulum, extravasation can seldom be demonstrated by angiography. However, angiodysplastic hemangiomatous lesions and hereditary hemorrhagic telangiectasia (Osler's disease) can be diagnosed by angiography of the superior and inferior mesenteric arteries once arteriovenous connections are established. We have used vasopressin intra-arterially (by superior mesenteric artery) only once for the treatment of bleeding esophageal varices and have no experience with embolization of this arterial network.

Management

After blood is drawn out to rule out a hemorrhagic diathesis, vitamin K (5 to 10 mg) should be administered intravenously. Volume replacement should be done with a plasma expander until blood is available. Transfusion requirements can best be monitored by measurement of central venous pressure, with the physician remembering that children, particularly those with esophageal varices, tend to stop bleeding more rapidly when they are maintained in a state of relative hypovolemia.

The patient with upper gastrointestinal bleeding should be maintained in a semisitting position and in a calm environment. Sedation is used only exceptionally and reserved for severely anxious or agitated children. Special attention should be attuned to any signs of hepatic encephalopathy. If continued gastric lavage fails after an hour and the gastric tube still shows brisk ongoing bleeding requiring large amounts of blood, vasopressin is administered intravenously in a dose of 20 units/1.73 m^2 over a 20-minute period in 100 ml of 5% dextrose. If bleeding does not stop, a continuous infusion of vasopressin is started. A prospective randomized study has shown that there is no difference in the control of bleeding (56%) among patients receiving either intra-arterial or intravenous vasopressin. It is particularly effective in variceal bleeding. We therefore recommend vasopressin given intravenously at a rate of 0.3 to 0.4 unit/1.73 m²/min for 48 hours. The dosage can be decreased by half for the following 24-hour period. Patients receiving vasopressin need to be closely watched. Extreme pallor and severe limb arterial vasoconstriction leading to a disappearance of peripheral pulses are common. Moderate hypertension, water retention, and a worrisome hyponatremia are other side effects.

If angiography is done and demonstrates a bleeding point, intra-arterial vasopressin should be tried before one resorts to embolization with Gelfoam, the preferred method for the control of a bleeding gastroduodenal ulcer.

If maintenance of blood volume requires more than 10 to 15 ml/kg of blood every 4 hours in a child with varices, a pediatric Sengstaken-Blakemore tube should be used. This measure requires experience and constant nursing care, and we have employed it only four times in the past 5 years.

Most children with intact clotting mechanisms stop bleeding on bed rest, volume replacement, and gastric lavage. In children with stress ulcers, antacids given hourly (60 to 80 ml/1.73 m²/hour) to keep the pH above 7.0 may be helpful, but there are no reports of its efficacy as yet. Cimetidine (given intravenously at 1200 mg/1.73 m²/24 hours) has been tested and promotes a more rapid arrest of the bleeding than gastric lavage does alone. Vasopressin is particularly useful in variceal bleeding. The challenging patients are those with cirrhosis and a clotting defect unresponsive to repeated infusions of fresh frozen plasma (10 ml/kg).

Emergency sclerotherapy or a shunt operation should be considered when the above measures fail in variceal bleeding. Surgical treatment is warranted in peptic disease and stress ulcers if the bleeding is torrential or if it continues over several days despite aggressive medical management.

Because of the severity of the disease conditions associated with upper gastrointestinal bleeding secondary to stress-induced gastroduodenal mucosal erosions and ulcerations, prophylaxis has been advocated. Antacids and cimetidine seem to have a beneficial effect in patients at high risk for stress ulcers, that is, those with extensive burns, central nervous system trauma, and so on. A recent study has shown that Mylanta II at a dosage of 30 ml hourly was more efficacious than cimetidine.

REFERENCES

Athanasoulis, C.A.: Severe upper gastrointestinal bleeding. II. X-ray diagnosis and therapy, Clin. Gastroenterol. **10:**26-37, 1981.

Bauer, J.J., Kreel, I., and Kark, A.E.: The use of the Sengstaken-Blakemore tube for immediate control of bleeding esophageal varices, Ann. Surg. **179:**273-277, 1974.

Bernuau, J., Nouel, O., Belghiti, J., and Rueff, B.: Severe upper GI bleeding. III. Guidelines for treatment, Clin. Gastroenterol. **10:**38-59, 1981.

Boley, S.J., Brandt, L.J., and Frank, M.S.: Severe lower intestinal bleeding: diagnosis and treatment, Clin. Gastroenterol. **10:**65-91, 1981.

Conn, H.O.: Editorial: To scope or not to scope, N. Engl. J. Med. **304:**967-969, 1981.

Conn, H.O., Rameby, G.P., Storer, E.H., and others: Intra-arterial vasopressin in the treatment of upper gastrointestinal hemorrhage: a prospective, controlled clinical trial, Gastroenterology **8:**211-221, 1975.

Cox, K., and Ament, M.E.: Upper gastrointestinal bleeding in children and adolescents, Pediatrics **63:**408-413, 1979.

Fonkalsrud, E.W., Myer, N.A., and Robinson, M.J.: Management of extrahepatic portal hypertension in children, Ann. Surg. **180:**488-493, 1974.

Hastings, R.R., Skillman, J.J., Bushnell, L.S., and Silen, W.: Antacid titration in the prevention of acute gastrointestinal bleeding: a controlled randomized trial in 100 critically ill patients, N. Engl. J. Med. **298:**1041-1045, 1978.

Menguy, R.: Editorial: The prophylaxis of stress ulceration, N. Engl. J. Med. **302:**461-462, 1980.

Peterson, W.L., Barnett, C.C., Smith, H.J., and others: Routine early endoscopy in upper gastrointestinal tract bleeding: a randomized, controlled trial, N. Engl. J. Med. **304:**925-929, 1981.

Priebe, H.J., Skillman, J.J., Bushnell, L.S., and others: Antacid versus cimetidine in preventing acute gastrointestinal bleeding, N. Engl. J. Med. **302:**426-430, 1980.

Protell, R.L., Silverstein, F.E., Gilbert, D.A., and Feld, A.D.: Severe upper gastrointestinal bleeding. I. Causes, pathogenesis and methods of diagnosis, Clin. Gastroenterol. **10:**17-26, 1981.

Riff, E.J., Hayden, P.W., and Stevenson, J.K.: The detection of acute gastrointestinal bleeding using in vivo technetium 99m pertechnetate-labeled erythrocytes, J. Pediatr. **97:**956-958, 1980.

Roy, C.C., Morin, C.L., Weber, A.M.: Gastrointestinal emergency problems in paediatric practice, Clin. Gastroenterol. **10:**225-254, 1981.

Sunaryo, F.P., Boyle, J.T., Ziegler, M.M., and Heyman, S.: Primary nonspecific ileal ulceration as a cause of massive rectal bleeding, Pediatrics **68:**247-250, 1981.

Tedesco, F.J., Goldstein, P.D., Gleason, W.A., and Keating, J.P.: Upper gastrointestinal endoscopy in the pediatric patient, Gastroenterology **70:**492-494, 1976.

FOREIGN BODIES IN THE ALIMENTARY TRACT

The majority of children with gastrointestinal foreign bodies are 6 months to 4 years of age. As a general rule, any object that can be swallowed and reach the stomach will pass through the intestinal tract without difficulty in 90% of cases.

A foreign body that remains in the esophagus deserves immediate attention. Objects such as coins, buttons, and marbles can become lodged in the esophagus; however, the most dangerous ones are long and have sharp edges or angles that favor penetration of the mucosa. Foreign bodies of the esophagus are usually (70%) found at the level of the cricopharyngeal area, which corresponds to the fourth cervical vertebra. They may also be arrested in their progress in the middle and lower third of the esophagus. Children who have had surgery for a tracheoesophageal fistula are especially prone to impaction of the esophagus with partially chewed meat. Narrowing of the lumen at the level of the anastomosis is compounded by dysmotility of the distal part of the esophagus.

Symptoms of an esophageal foreign body are sometimes quite impressive and include gagging, attempts at vomiting, retrosternal pain, hypersalivation, and respiratory distress. If left in place, ulceration with bleeding and finally perforation with mediastinitis can occur. Under general anesthesia, removal should be done with an esophagoscope equipped with the appropriate forceps. Successful removal of smooth objects can be done by means of a Foley catheter (8 to 12 F), which is passed into the stomach, pulled back into the lower esophagus, inflated with 4 ml of meglumine diatrizoate (Gastrografin), and slowly pulled back under fluoroscopic guidance.

After reaching the stomach, a small percentage of foreign bodies may be arrested in their progress through the gastrointestinal tract at the level of the pylorus, the junction of the second and third duodenum, the ligament of Treitz, and the ileocecal region. Rarely, impaction of sharp objects is described in the anal canal.

Conservative management is in order for most foreign bodies that have reached the stomach. The progress of the foreign body can be followed by serial roentgenograms. In the case of coins, marbles, or toys that have no sharp edges, endoscopic or surgical removal should not be considered before 2 to 3 weeks have gone by without progress. An exception to this rule is the presence of objects containing lead or mercury, which could give rise to lead or mercury poisoning if immobilized in the stomach. Objects with sharp points such as straight pins, needles, open safety pins, thumb tacks, or small nails need to be watched clinically and roentgenographically daily. Parents are instructed to observe all stools and not to change the diet nor to give laxatives. Failure of progression over a period of a few days or any symptom that may relate to the presence of the foreign object is an indication for admission and treatment.

Long slender objects such as bobby pins, nails, and bolts, or even toothpicks, pose occasional problems because of their length, since they usually tumble end over end down the gastrointestinal tract. The critical length is probably over 5 cm in the younger child. They can pass through the stomach but then become lodged crosswise in the duodenum or in the intestine and lead to symptoms.

Complications of foreign objects distal to the esophagus include hemorrhage, especially in the case of glass objects, pressure necrosis (which leads to inflammation), obstruction, and perforation with peritonitis. In the case of foreign bodies trapped in the esophagus, perforation and mediastinitis can occur very rapidly after ingestion.

REFERENCES

Birkett, F.D.H., and Davies, C.J.: Safety-pin swallowers, Br. Med. J. **1:**504-527, 1971.

Brooks, J.W.: Foreign bodies in the air and food passages, Ann. Surg. **175:**720-732, 1972.

Brown, E.G., Hughes, J.P., and Koenig, H.M.: Removal of foreign bodies lodged in esophagus by a Foley catheter without endoscopy, Clin. Pediatr. **11:**468-471, 1972.

Carlson, D.H.: Removal of coins in the esophagus using a Foley catheter, Pediatrics **50:**475, 1972.

Chang, J.H.T., and Burrington, J.D.: Removal of coins from the esophagus: nothing new under the sun, Pediatrics **51:**313, 1973.

Hart, V.K.: Pins in the G.I. tract: some problems and their solutions and related clinical facts of pertinent interest, Eye Ear Nose Throat Mon. **47:**547-552, 1968.

Kassner, E.G., Rose, J.S., Kottmeier, P.K., and others: Retention of small foreign objects in the stomach and duodenum, Radiology **114:**683-686, 1975.

Larkworthy, W., Jones, R.T.B., Mahoney, M., and others: Removal of ingested coins utilizing fibre-endoscopy and special forceps, Br. J. Surg. **61:**750-752, 1974.

Norberg, H.P., and Reyes, H.M.: Complications of ornamental Christmas bulb ingestion, Arch. Surg. **110:**1494-1497, 1975.

Spitz, L.: Management of ingested foreign bodies in childhood, Br. Med. J. **4:**469-472, 1971.

BEZOARS
Trichobezoars and phytobezoars

The two main varieties of bezoars are trichobezoars and phytobezoars. Trichobezoars consist of large quantities of hair firmly matted together and assuming the shape of the stomach (Fig. 7-14) or the part of the small bowel in which they are occasionally located. Phytobezoars are composed of a variety of vegetable material forming a compact mass. Trichobezoars are far more common in the pediatric age group than phytobezoars and affect girls much more commonly than boys.

Symptoms of trichobezoars are vague and variable. They usually consist of vague upper abdominal pain with heaviness in the epigastrium, anorexia, intermittent vomiting, and weight loss. When the gastric trichobezoar has extended distally or has broken off, the symptoms may be those of a partial or complete intestinal obstruction. A similar mode of presentation is seen in children in whom the trichobezoar has formed in the small bowel without a gastric component.

Although a history of trichophagy is rarely volunteered, bald spots or sparse hair are not unusual in such children, who frequently suffer emotional disturbances. The association of trichophagy with iron-deficiency anemia has been recently suggested. In the course of a gastrostomy, the surgeon should carefully explore the small bowel for the presence of detached hairballs. Adequate psychotherapeutic measures are recommended in order to help the patient sort out his emotional problems, and, we hope, overcome trichophagy, the continuance of which may lead to a recurrence of the trichobezoar.

Lactobezoars and the "inspissated milk syndrome"

Lactobezoars may occur in infants as the result of feeding incorrectly prepared milk formula. In most cases, the gastric outlet obstruction is the result of using an inadequate amount of water to dilute a powdered formula. There are rare instances where it has occurred upon feeding a properly prepared 20 calories per ounce formula, but these infants were sick (diabetes insipidus, necrotizing enterocolitis). Both preterm and full-term infants fed formulas at a caloric density of 24 calories per ounce have been reported with the syndrome. However, in the past few years there has been a great increase in such cases in preterm babies. No single factor seems to be identified as

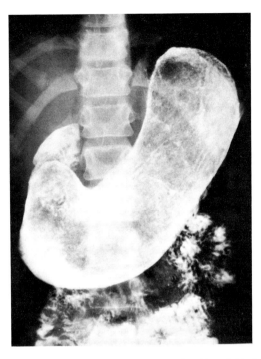

Fig. 7-14. Large trichobezoar. In this older child the only sign was an easily palpable abdominal mass. Some of these masses may extend through the pylorus to obstruct the duodenum. Fragments can break off and are usually passed wihtout incident. However, they can cause intestinal obstruction, particularly when they lodge at the ileocecal valve.

yet. The proliferation of cases coincides with the following changes in the nutritional management of infants born prematurely:

1. Trend to earlier feeding
2. Use of formulas with a higher caloric density
3. Advent of special premature formulas with a higher protein and calcium content and with a 40% concentration of medium-chain triglycerides
4. Increased utilization of the technique of continuous drip feeding

Continuous drip feeding seems to be the most important predisposing factor. From our own studies gastric emptying time does not seem to be decreased by the presence of 40% medium-chain triglycerides. Since the syndrome almost always develops within the first 2 weeks of life, it has been suggested that, during this period, intragastric drip feeding should not be done with a formula containing more than 20 kcal/30 ml.

The presenting symptoms include abdominal

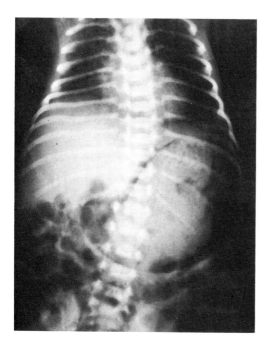

Fig. 7-15. Milk curd bezoar. The large mass of milk curd is outlined by gastric air.

distention, vomiting, an abdominal mass, and rarely diarrhea. Perforation of the stomach has been reported in four cases. The characteristic roentgenographic presentation of a lactobezoar consists of a well-formed intraluminal cast surrounded by air (Fig. 7-15). A routine screening method consisting in injection of 2 to 3 ml/kg of air through a nasogastric feeding tube before the use of a chest roentgenogram has been advocated. Withholding of feedings for 48 hours, gastric lavage with saline solution, and proper hydration bring about a resolution of symptoms. Relapses have never been reported upon resumption of feedings.

There have been reports of low intestinal obstruction secondary to milk curds. The "inspissated milk syndrome" occurs usually in premature infants who are being fed an artificial formula. It has also been described in full-term neonates. High-calorie feedings and recent surgery are commonly identified factors leading to the development of the syndrome. It has never been reported in breast-fed babies.

Classically, the affected neonate has passed meconium normally, followed by milk stools. At 5 to 15 days of age, vomiting and abdominal distention develop. On palpation "ropy" intestines and hard masses are felt in the right lower quadrant. Abdominal roentgenograms confirm a lower intestinal obstruction and reveal masses surrounded by gas within the lumen of the small bowel. Perforation rarely occurs.

Puttylike milk masses or copious amounts of firm, round yellowish pellets of milk curds are found in the lower ileum or in the colon. Necrotizing enterocolitis merits serious consideration when the syndrome occurs in premature infants. Hirschsprung's disease must also be considered. A contrast enema reveals a colon of normal caliber. Meglumine diatrizoate (Gastrografin) enemas have been used successfully in the treatment of this condition. Because of its enormous capacity to attract water, Gastrografin must not be administered without close attention being paid to the baby's hydration. Uneventful recoveries have also followed surgical removal.

Medication and food bezoars

Aluminum hydroxide, whether administered as a bolus or as a continuous drip, carries a risk for the formation of medication bezoars. Patients with renal failure, intestinal ileus, and borderline hydration are particularly vulnerable. Mixtures of magnesium and aluminum hydroxides are safer in this regard. There is one report of a gastric antacid bezoar in a newborn. Intestinal obstruction secondary to fecal impaction has been noted in three children receiving large doses of aluminum hydroxide after renal transplantation. Cholestyramine may also lead to intestinal obstruction. In patients with diseases such as Crohn's, bouts of intestinal obstruction have been described in association with medications administered in capsules.

Undigested pits, seeds, citrus rinds, and peanuts can obstruct the stomach and the lower ileum. Inadequate mastication is probably a contributory factor in young children. Rarely, excessive ingestion of strained carrots, used in the treatment of diarrhea, has resulted in small bowel obstruction.

REFERENCES

Bernstein, L.H., Gutstein, S., Efron, G., and others: Trichobezoar: an unusual cause of megaloblastic anemia and hypoproteinemia in childhood, Am. J. Dig. Dis. **18:**67-71, 1973.

Cremin, B.J., Smythe, P.M., and Cywer, S.: The radiological appearance of the "inspissated milk syndrome" as a cause of intestinal obstruction in infants, Br. J. Radiol. **43:**856-858, 1970.

DeBakey, M., and Ochsner, A.: Bezoars and concretions, Surgery **5:**132-160, 1939.

Duritz, G., and Oltorf, C.: Lactobezoar formation associated with high-density caloric formula, Pediatrics **63**:647-649, 1979.

Erenberg, A., Shaw, R.D., and Yousefzadeh, D.: Lactobezoar in the low-birth-weight infant, Pediatrics **63**:642-646, 1979.

Friedland, G.W., Rush, W.A., and Hill, A.J.: Smythe's "inspissated milk" syndrome, Radiology **103**:159-161, 1972.

Grosfeld, J.L., Schreiner, R.L., Franken, E.A., and others: The changing pattern of gastrointestinal bezoars in infants and children, Surgery **88**:425-431, 1980.

Portuguez-Malavasi, A., and Aranda, J.V.: Antacid bezoar in a newborn, Pediatrics **63**:679-680, 1979.

Rickham, P.P.: Intraluminal intestinal obstruction, Progr. Pediatr. Surg. **2**:73-82, 1971.

Schreiner, R.L., Lemons, J.A., and Gresham, E.L.: A new complication of nutritional management of the low-birth-weight infant, Pediatrics **63**:683-684, 1979.

Townsend, C.M., Remmers, A.R., Sarles, H.E., and others: Intestinal obstruction from medication bezoar in patients with renal failure, N. Engl. J. Med. **288**:1058-1059, 1973.

Zer, M., Tiqva, P., and Dintsman, M.: Intestinal obstruction in a young child due to impaction of undigested peanuts, J. Pediatr. Surg. **7**:439-441, 1972.

Ménétrier's disease

Hypertrophic gastritis is a common entity in adults. It is characterized by the presence of large rugal folds involving part or all of the stomach, upper abdominal pain, anorexia, vomiting hematemesis, and weight loss. It usually runs an unremitting, protracted course, and follow-up data suggest that gastric carcinoma may develop in a significant number of cases. The 17 children reported so far share with adult patients the same roentgenographic (Fig. 7-16), endoscopic, and biopsy findings. However, gastrointestinal symptoms are less conspicuous and are overshadowed by a clinically manifest protein-losing gastropathy present in only 25% of adults.

Vomiting and peripheral edema are invariably present. Abdominal pain is described in the majority. The differential diagnosis includes the nephrotic syndrome, entities responsible for a protein-losing enteropathy, and more specifically those associated with thick gastric folds such as peptic disease, Zollinger-Ellison syndrome, hamartomas of Peutz-Jeghers syndrome, juvenile polyposis of the stomach, lymphomas, and eosinophilic gastroenteritis. The last can mimic Ménétrier's dis-

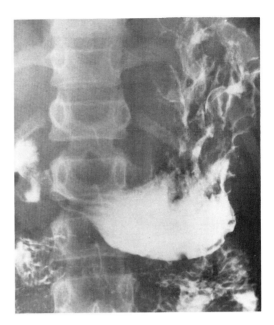

Fig. 7-16. This film taken from an 8½-year-old boy admitted for anasarca shows thickened and irregular mucosal folds in the upper part of the stomach. Gastric biopsy specimens showed hyperplastic pits with inflammation and cysts. Within 2 months, he recovered completely, and 4 months after the onset of symptoms, the histologic appearance of the stomach became normal.

ease clinically and roentgenologically, but biopsy results will establish the diagnosis.

Hypertrophic gastritis has also been called "thick gastric folds" in pediatric cases. In contrast to Ménétrier's disease in adults, the course of the disease is self-limited, transient, and benign. Complete recovery can be expected within a few months without treatment. The cause of the disorder is unknown in both adults and children. Of interest is the description of a few cases in which cytomegalovirus inclusion bodies have been found.

REFERENCES

Bloom, R.A., and Quaide, J.R.: Benign hypertrophic gastropathy, Clin. Pediatr. **19**:533-540, 1980.

Chouraqui, J.P., Roy, C.C., Brochu, P., and others: Ménétrier's disease in children: report of a patient and review of sixteen other cases, Gastroenterology **80**:1042-1047, 1981.

Scharschmidt, B.F.: The natural history of hypertrophic gastropathy (Ménétrier's disease), Am. J. Med. **63**:644-652, 1977.

8 *Diarrheal disorders*

PATHOGENESIS OF DIARRHEA

Diarrhea, defined as an increase in the number of stools or a decrease in their consistency, is the major clinical manifestation of alterations of water and electrolyte transport by the alimentary tract. It is the result of disorders involving digestive, absorptive, and secretory functions. A rational approach to diagnosis requires knowledge of normal water and electrolyte absorption and secretion by the physiologic unit made up of the small intestine and colon.

Each day, the adult human gut handles 7 liters of endogenous secretions (salivary, gastric, biliary, pancreatic, intestinal) and 2 liters of ingested fluids. Of this large volume, 3 to 5 liters are absorbed by the jejunum, 2 to 4 liters by the ileum, and 1 to 2 liters by the colon. Only 100 to 200 ml are lost in the stools. On a daily basis, the volume of fluid processed by the gut is equivalent to a major proportion of the extracellular fluid.

Transport of water and electrolytes

The transfer of water across the intestinal mucosa is a passive phenomenon that cannot occur without solute movement. When actively transported, substrates such as glucose and amino acids are absorbed, and the luminal solution becomes hypotonic relative to the interstitial fluid. As a result, water moves along this osmotic pressure gradient. It is likely that only a small proportion of water goes through the cells. Most of the water passes through the lateral intercellular spaces via the tight junctions, which are more permeable in the jejunum than they are in the ileum. Mucosal diseases (celiac disease) alter the size of the pores, distort the intercellular spaces, and consequently greatly affect the absorption of fluid and electrolytes. Water "pores" in the colon are less permeable than those in the small bowel.

Since the tight junctions through which water flows in the jejunum are large, sodium and potassium are swept in at the same time as water in response to the active absorption of water-soluble substrates. Solvent drag is not the only mechanism for sodium absorption, since it is also transported against an electrochemical gradient by an energy-requiring mechanism (Fig. 8-1). Glucose and sodium share a common carrier protein that transfers the pair into the cell much more efficiently than either alone. A more complete discussion of the coupling between glucose and sodium transport is presented in Chapter 9. Bicarbonate in bile and pancreatic juice is transported against a considerable gradient. It is removed from the lumen by the secretion of H^+, which, together with bicarbonate, generates H_2O and CO_2. It appears that bicarbonate can also stimulate Na^+ absorption; this is best explained by a Na^+/H^+ exchange process. The situation in the ileum is somewhat different from that in the jejunum. Na^+ is absorbed in exchange for H^+, but, in addition, there is another ion-exchange process that transports Cl^- in exchange for secreted HCO_3^- (Fig. 8-2). The colon has a lower permeability to ions and water and actively transports Na^+. Chloride is also absorbed actively, probably in exchange for bicarbonate, a situation analogous to that in the ileum. Potassium accumulates in the lumen by passive diffusion and also by active secretion in exchange for some absorbed sodium. It very efficiently dehydrates its contents. Aldosterone enhances colonic absorption of Na^+; in diarrheas with volume depletion and secondary hyperaldosteronism the effect of aldosterone may be clinically important.

Control of intestinal secretion

An accumulation of fluid and electrolytes, and its evacuation as diarrhea, can be the result of a decrease in the absorptive process and of an increase in the active secretory process as well. Increased luminal osmolarity, such as that which occurs in disaccharide intolerance, will increase the plasma to lumen flow. An increase of intravascular hydrostatic pressure and serosal pressure will have the same effect. The diarrhea associated with intravenous fluid overloading and the fluid accumulation resulting from intestinal obstruction with distention are best explained by this mechanism.

Cyclic AMP. Current information, albeit incomplete, suggests that absorptive processes are

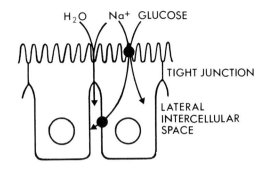

Fig. 8-1. Water and sodium absorption. Water flows into the lateral intercellular space because of the hypotonicity created by the active transport of glucose. Na^+ is dragged in the water stream (solvent drag), but it is also actively transported by sharing a common transport protein with glucose (Modified after Turnberg, L.A.: Water and electrolyte metabolism. In Sircus, W., and Smith, A.N., editors: Scientific foundations of gastroenterology, Philadelphia, 1979, W.B. Saunders Co.)

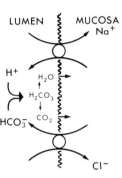

Fig. 8-2. Double ion–exchange process in the ileum. As H^+ is actively secreted, Na^+ is absorbed. With the secretion of HCO_3^-, Cl^- is absorbed. (Modified after Turnberg, L.A., et al.: J. Clin. Invest. **49**:548, 1970.)

confined to villous epithelial cells and that secretory processes take place in the crypt cells. Cyclic AMP inhibits absorption of NaCl in the villi and stimulates Cl^- secretion in the crypts. Acknowledged stimulators of mucosal cyclic AMP include vasoactive intestinal peptide (VIP), prostaglandins, deconjugated bile acids, and hydroxy fatty acids. Ricinoleic acid, the active principle of castor oil, also acts by stimulating colonic adenyl cyclase. Enterotoxins such as those of cholera and *Escherichia coli* and perhaps also the toxins of *Clostridium perfringens* and of *Staphylococcus aureus,* which are responsible for food poisoning, mediate diarrhea through cyclic AMP via adenyl cyclase (Fig. 8-3).

Non–cyclic AMP mediated secretion. Intestinal secretion can be enhanced by mechanisms other than cyclic AMP. In the case of the heat-stable enterotoxin of *E. coli,* it is through a stimulation of guanylate cyclase instead of adenylate cyclase. It subsequently leads to an increase of cyclic GMP. Many gastrointestinal hormones such as gastrin, cholecystokinin, glucagon, secretin, calcitonin, and serotonin are capable of stimulating secretion in man.

Effect of food on intestinal secretion. Gastrointestinal secretions are stimulated by food in-

take. Suppression of oral intake is a traditional approach to the early treatment of acute diarrheal disorders. It very effectively decreases the flow of water and electrolytes entering the intestinal lumen.

Fig. 8-4 shows the effect of fasting and food intake on the volume of intestinal secretions (upper panel) and the two individualized but usually concomitant mechanisms at play in the pathogenesis of diarrhea. Both increased secretion and decreased absorption lead to the accumulation of fluid and electrolyte in the lumen (upper panel).

Role of surface area and motility

Whereas a decrease in the surface area through a surgical resection or a mucosal disease has a profound effect on the enterosystemic cycle of water, the role of deranged motility is less clear. Although there are circumstances where hypermotility could play a primary role, in most instances a shortened transit time is secondary to net accumulation of water and electrolytes. Hypomotility is a more clearly defined etiologic factor for diarrhea. It leads to proliferation of the intestinal microflora in the upper small bowel, which is normally relatively sterile because it is responsible for the absorption of the bulk of nutrients,

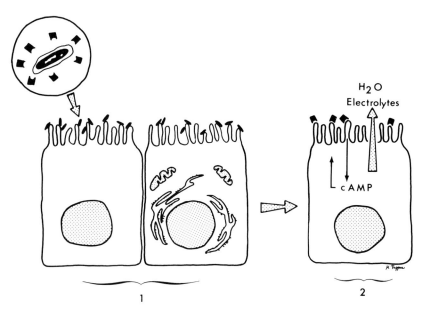

Fig. 8-3. Mechanism of secretory diarrhea. **1,** Enterotoxin-producing bacteria adhere to the brush border of enterocytes, where they release their exotoxin, which in turn binds to microvilli. The exotoxin stimulates adenyl cyclase production in the basal and lateral membranes of the cell. **2,** Adenyl cyclase leads to high intracellular concentration of cyclic AMP and active electrolyte and water secretion. (Courtesy G. Delage, microbiologist, Hôpital Sainte-Justine, Montreal.)

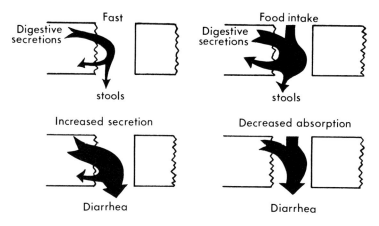

Fig. 8-4. Enterosystemic cycle of water. (From Desjeux, J., et al.: Colloques de l'Inserm **90:**39, 1979.)

as well as water and electrolytes. (Refer to the section on the contaminated small bowel syndrome.)

The following list summarizes the known mechanisms for the genesis of diarrhea. It is a pathophysiologic classification that, although helpful to the clinician, needs to be interpreted with the understanding that usually more than one mechanism must be invoked to explain the diarrhea.

Mechanisms of diarrhea

Osmotic factors
  Overfeeding
  Nonabsorbable solutes (lactulose, sorbitol, MgSO$_4$)
  Malabsorption of water-soluble nutrients
Diminished absorption or increased secretion of water and electrolytes
  Bacteria, viruses, and parasites
  Free bile acids (ileal resections, contaminated small bowel)
  Hydroxy fatty acids (ileal resections, contaminated small bowel)

Table 8-1. Etiologic classification of diarrhea

Type of disorder	Disease or etiologic agents
Infections	
Enteral	
Bacteria	Pathogenic *Escherichia coli,* shigellosis, salmonellosis, *Yersinia enterocolitica, Campylobacter, Staphylococcus aureus, Clostridium perfringens, Vibrio cholerae, Vibrio parahaemolyticus,* tuberculosis
Virus	Adenoviruses, rotavirus, parvovirus-like agents
Infestations	Amebiasis, giardiasis, ascariasis, coccidiosis
Parenteral	Urinary tract infections and otitis media
Inflammatory bowel disease	Crohn's, chronic ulcerative colitis, Whipple's disease, necrotizing enterocolitis of the newborn, nonspecific enterocolitis of infancy, pseudomembranous enterocolitis
Anatomic and mechanical causes	Short bowel syndrome, fistula, postgastrectomy effects, blind loop syndrome, partial small bowel obstruction, malrotation, Hirschsprung's disease, intestinal lymphangiectasis, chronic idiopathic intestinal pseudo-obstruction
Pancreatic and hepatic disorders	Cirrhosis, hepatitis, biliary atresia, chronic pancreatitis, pancreatic exocrine deficiency, cystic fibrosis of the pancreas, pancreatic hypoplasia
Biochemical causes	Celiac disease, disaccharidase deficiency, glucose-galactose malabsorption, abetalipoproteinemia, congenital chloridorrhea with alkalosis, acrodermatitis enteropathica
Neoplastic causes	Carcinoid, ganglioneuroma, neuroblastoma, Zollinger-Ellison syndrome, polyposis, lymphoma, adenocarcinoma, pancreatic islet cell tumor, medullary thyroid carcinoma
Immunity deficiencies	Acquired hypogammaglobulinemia, selective IgA deficiency, thymic hypoplasia, severe combined immunodeficiency syndrome
Endocrinopathies	Hyperthyroidism, congenital adrenal hyperplasia, hypoparathyroidism, Addison's disease
Malnutrition	Protein malnutrition (kwashiorkor), protein-calorie malnutrition (marasmus)
Dietary factors	Overfeeding, introduction of new foods
Food allergy	Milk colitis, allergic gastroenteropathy, milk and soy protein intolerance
Psychogenic or functional disorders	Irritable colon syndrome
Toxic diarrhea	Ingestion of heavy metals (arsenic, lead), organic phosphates, ferrous sulfate, antibiotics

Humoral factors (enterotoxins, vasoactive intestinal peptide, prostaglandins, serotonin, and so on)
Congenital chloridorrhea
Inflammatory and immune diseases
Mucosal disease (celiac disease)
Reduction in anatomic or functional surface area
Short bowel syndrome
Mucosal diseases
Altered motility
Hypomotility (malnutrition, scleroderma, chronic idiopathic intestinal pseudo-obstruction, glucagonoma)
Hypermotility (thyroid hormone, prostaglandins, serotonin)

What constitutes diarrhea is sometimes difficult to define in terms of number or consistency of stools because there are wide individual variations in colonic function. For example, one infant may have one firm stool every second or third day, whereas another passes from five to eight soft, small stools daily. A noticeable or sudden increase in the number of stools, a reduction in their consistency with an increase in their fluid content, and a tendency for stools to be green are more important features.

The physiologic consequences of diarrhea vary with its severity, its duration, associated symptoms, the age of the child, and his state of nutrition previous to its onset. Acutely, the loss of water and electrolytes leads to dehydration and electrolyte and acid-base disturbances. When diarrhea is protracted, chronic malnutrition may ensue.

Diarrhea is one of the symptoms most frequently encountered in pediatrics. It always should attract the physician's attention, particularly if the patient is younger than 2 years. Table 8-1 is a partial list of entities either presenting as diarrhea or giving rise to diarrhea as an associated symptom.

INFECTIOUS DIARRHEAS

When diarrhea is presumed or actually shown to be secondary to a virus, to a bacterial microorganism, or more rarely to a protozoan pathogen, the term "infectious gastroenteritis" is used. Acute transient attacks of diarrhea and vomiting are so common that they can almost be regarded as part of the normal way of life in all age groups. In the pediatric age group, infectious gastroenteritis is second only to upper respiratory tract infections as a cause of illness.

In developing countries, it remains the largest single cause of death because of rampant malnutrition, chronic parasitic infestation, and poor hygiene. Education, housing, hygiene, and climate significantly affect not only the incidence of infectious diarrheas but also their severity and outcome. With improvements in general health, nutrition, and hygiene, acute diarrheal disease in the first 2 years of life would no longer be one of the greatest health problems in the world.

Although in industrialized countries, infectious diarrheas are generally benign and self-limited, they are still a major pediatric problem and account for 3% to 5% of hospital admissions. At the Hôpital Ste-Justine and the Montreal Children's Hospital a recent survey has shown that less than 15% of the cases of acute gastroenteritis are of bacterial origin. *Salmonella* (4.4%), *Campylobacter* (4.3%), *Yersinia* (2.8%), and *Shigella* (1.1%) accounted for most. Enteropathogenic *Escherichia coli* was implicated in less than 1%. On the other hand, a viral cause (rotavirus) is found in more than 50% of cases. In the warmer climate of Houston and Mexico, rotavirus infections account for only 10% and 17% of enteropathogens, respectively. On the other hand, the incidence of *Shigella* (25%) and *Salmonella* (4%) is higher in Houston. Corresponding figures in Mexico are 14% and 12%. *Giardia lamblia* is often identified but is usually

associated with a subacute or chronic type of diarrhea rather than with the clinical picture of acute gastroenteritis. Although great progress has been made in the identification of new microorganisms responsible for acute gastroenteritis, there is still a large percentage (about 35%) of so-called acute nonspecific gastroenteritis. A number of organisms have at times been regarded as pathogenic. These include *Klebsiella, Enterobacter, Proteus, Citrobacter, and Pseudomonas*. The epidemiological evidence linking these bacteria with gastroenteritis in children should be interpreted with caution.

Pathophysiology of acute infectious gastroenteritis

Important information has emerged from studies on the pathogenesis and etiology of infectious diarrhea. In particular, a clearer delineation of clinical syndromes has come about through the description of the interaction of bacterial and viral pathogens with the intestinal mucosa (Table 8-2).

Interaction of bacterial pathogens with the intestinal mucosa

Enterotoxin production. Bacterial pathogens, such as *Vibrio cholerae* and certain strains of *E. coli,* do not invade the mucosal epithelium but produce disease through multiplication in the small intestine, followed by adhesion to the mucosa and release of an exotoxin that binds to the tips and crypts of small bowel villi. This binding can be blocked by neutralization of the toxin with antitoxin.

The interaction between the toxin and the epithelium activates adenyl cyclase in the cell membranes. This leads to an increase in cyclic adenosine monophosphate (AMP) from adenosine triphosphate (ATP). Cyclic AMP plays an important role in the intestinal secretion of fluid and electrolytes in the gut (Fig. 8-3). Both cholera and *E. coli* enterotoxin have the same effect as cyclic AMP on in vitro ileal preparations. Chloride secretion is stimulated and sodium absorption is inhibited. From a treatment standpoint, it is relevant to note that in cholera the addition of glucose, though it does not modify chloride secretion, will essentially restore sodium absorption and therefore passive water transport. However, this does not appear to be evident in *E. coli* infections.

Because these pathogens are noninvasive, histologic examination of the small bowel mucosa of infected individuals shows no morphologic changes.

Table 8-2. Pathogenesis and clinical syndromes associated with infectious gastroenteritis

Organisms	Localization	Pathogenesis	Clinical syndrome
Vibrio cholerae *Escherichia coli* *Shigella dysenteriae I* *Clostridium perfringens* A and D	Small bowel	Adherence and production of enterotoxin	Cholera-like diarrhea
Shigella *Escherichia coli* *Yersinia enterocolitica* *Campylobacter*	Colon mostly Colon Small and large bowel Small bowel mostly	Invasion with mucosal inflammation and destruction	Fever, diarrhea with blood and mucus
Viruses	Small bowel	Injury to microvilli, sometimes invasive and cytotoxic	Fever, diarrhea, rarely with blood
Salmonella	Small and large bowel	Penetration and systemic invasion	Mostly cholera-like; colitis is less frequent
Escherichia coli	Small and large bowel	Adherence without destruction of mucosa nor enterotoxin production?	Profuse diarrhea without blood or mucus

Clinically, fever is variable but generally low grade, and there may be significant abdominal distention.

Diarrhea is invariably watery and profuse, leading to dehydration and acidosis particularly in the first 2 years of life. *Clostridium perfringens* and *Shigella dysenteriae,* type 1, also produce enterotoxins.

Invasion and destruction of epithelial cells. *Shigella,* enteroinvasive *E. coli* (EIEC), *Yersinia enterocolitica, Campylobacter,* and certain species of viruses lead to illness through invasion of enterocytes, mucosal inflammation, and destruction. The infection may be limited to the small bowel or colon, but most invasive microorganisms involve both sites starting in the small bowel and soon leading to colitis with urgency, tenesmus, and bloody mucoid stools. Histologic examination reveals a friable mucosa with ulcerations. Bacterial organisms are seen within epithelial cells, where they multiply and cause superficial mucosal ulcerations.

Penetration of the lamina propria and systemic invasion. *Salmonella* organisms constitute the third important group of intestinal pathogens. This group invades the lamina propria, where it sets up an inflammatory reaction in the distal small bowel and in the colon. The epithelial lining usually shows mild changes. From the lamina propria, *Salmonella* organisms may reach the systemic circulation and lead to foci of infection elsewhere in the body.

Adherence without destruction of mucosa and without enterotoxin production. A recent report suggests a fourth interacting mechanism between microorganisms and enterocytes. Enteropathogenic *E. coli* (EPEC) penetrate the glycocalyx and adhere to the enterocyte surface. They do not invade, nor do they produce toxins, but disrupt the microvilli and modestly blunt the villi. More work needs to be done to confirm this.

Clinical aspects of acute infectious gastroenteritis (Table 8-3)

It is helpful for the physician to keep in mind the particular clinical patterns associated with the various microorganisms responsible for infectious gastroenteritis. In one study a bacterial origin was correctly predicted in 75% of cases. Microscopic examination of the stool for leukocytes has long been recognized as an important part of the diagnostic work-up. Stool specimens or rectal swabs are examined after a small fleck is placed on a glass slide and mixed with 2 drops

Table 8-3. Clinical features of acute infectious gastroenteritis

Clinical features	Rotavirus	Salmonella	Campylobacter	Yersinia	Shigella	*Escherichia coli* Enteropathogenic (EPEC)	Enterotoxigenic (ETEC)	Enteroinvasive (EIEC)
Age	Any age but more under 2 years	Any age	1 to 5 years mostly	Any age	Any age but more under 6 years	Under 1 year	All ages but more under 1 year	All ages
Diarrhea in contacts	30%	Variable	10%	<10%	>50%	—	—	—
Fever (>38.5° C)	Rare	Variable	Rare	About 50%	Frequent	Rare	Rare	Variable
Concomitant upper respiratory infection	Common	—	—	—	Common	—	—	—
Convulsions	—	Rare	—	—	Common	—	—	—
Vomiting	Invariable	Usual	About 30%	About 40%	Absent	Common	Common	Rare
Abdominal pain	Mild	Moderate	Severe	Crampy	Severe	—	—	—
Tenesmus	—	Rare	Frequent	—	Frequent	—	—	Frequent
Diarrhea	Watery	Loose and slimy	Mucoid and watery	Greenish	Mucoid and watery	Watery	Watery	Mucoid and watery
Blood	—	Rare	Usual	25%	>50%	—	—	Common
Fecal leukocytes	Unusual	Always	Always	Usual	Always	—	—	Usual

of methylene blue stain. A coverslip is then placed on the slide, and the examination is done a few minutes later. One can obtain a differential count by counting 200 cells when possible, but it is generally not helpful except in the case of typhoid fever and "allergic" diarrhea where the predominant cells are mononuclear instead of polymorphonuclear.

Value of stool cultures

The common practice of ordering "stool cultures ×3" has come under attack. Stool cultures are ordered needlessly when the probability of a positive culture is extremely low. The value of stool cultures could be increased when the clinical predictors described in Table 8-3 are used. A recent survey in adults has shown that a fever above 37.8° C with diarrhea for more than 24 hours with either blood (gross or occult) or nausea, vomiting, and abdominal pain are the best predictors of a positive stool culture. Foreign travel was also a factor that increased the chances of recovering a bacterial pathogen. An important finding is that there was little advantage in doing more than two cultures.

Bacteriology laboratories should be equipped to grow and isolate the bacterial pathogens, including *Campylobacter* and *Yersinia*. Serotyping is necessary for identification of *E. coli*, which is most commonly associated with acute diarrhea. Although there are many experimental systems to detect heat-labile and heat-stable toxin (LT and ST), none are suitable for use in routine clinical laboratories. Furthermore the detection of LT and ST is seldom indicated because enterotoxigenic *E. coli* is rarely found in acute gastroenteritis in North America.

Fungal and parasitic infection of the gastrointestinal tract

Fungi are normal inhabitants of the human small intestine. Overgrowth is common in association with long-term chronic debilitating illness, prolonged treatment with broad-spectrum antibiotics, the use of corticosteroids, and immunosuppressive therapy. Fungi seldom cause clinically significant disease in the gastrointestinal tract, but frequently they produce severe systemic disease. From time to time intestinal candidiasis is being resurrected as a cause of diarrhea in patients who are not on antibiotics and who are not immunosuppressed. The evidence is very tenuous because it

is strictly based on the recovery of *Candida* in the stools and on a prompt response to nystatin. Parasitic infections of the intestine are becoming more prevalent in our hemisphere because of increasing mobility and foreign travel. Giardiasis is one of the most frequent causes of chronic diarrhea, but it can also be implicated in epidemics of subacute diarrhea. The clinical response to *Giardia* infestation is variable, but children are more likely than adults to be acutely ill. A discussion of the more prevalent fungal and parasitic infections of the gastrointestinal tract can be found in Chapter 16.

REFERENCES

Binder, H.J.: Net fluid and electrolyte secretion: the pathophysiological basis of diarrhea, Viewpoints on Digestive Diseases, vol. 12, no. 2, March 1980.

Desjeux, J.-F., Heyman, M., and Mansour, R.B.: Water and ion movement in intestine, Les Colloques de l'Inserm **90:**39-52, 1979.

Dupont, H.L., and Hornick, R.B.: Clinical approach to infectious diarrheas, Medicine **52:**265-270, 1973.

Edelman, R., and Levine, M.M.: Acute diarrheal infections in infants. II. Bacterial and viral causes, Hosp. Pract. **15:**97-104, 1980.

Evans, N.: Pathogenic mechanisms in bacterial diarrhea, Clin. Gastroenterol. **8:**599-623, 1979.

Guerrant, R.L.: Editorial: Yet another pathogenic mechanism for *Escherichia coli* diarrhea?, N. Engl. J. Med. **302:**113-115, 1980.

Guerrant, R.L., Ganguly, W., Casper, A.G.T., and others: Effect of *Escherichia coli* on fluid transport across canine small bowel: mechanism and time-course with enterotoxin and whole bacterial cells, J. Clin. Invest. **52:**1707-1714, 1973.

Harris, J.C., Dupont, H.L., and Hornick, R.B.: Fecal leukocytes in diarrheal illness, Ann. Intern. Med. **76:**697-703, 1972.

Koplan, J.P., Fineberg, H.V., Benfari Ferraro, M.J., and Rosenberg, M.L.: Value of stool cultures, Lancet **2:**413-416, 1980.

Mark, M.I., Pai, C.H., Lafleur, L., and others: *Yersinia enterocolitica* gastroenteritis: a prospective study of clinical, bacteriologic and epidemiologic features, J. Pediatr. **96:**26-31, 1980.

Nelson, J.D., and Haltalin, K.C.: Accuracy of diagnosis of bacterial diarrheal disease by clinical features, J. Pediatr. **78:**519-522, 1971.

Pickering, L.K., Evans, D.J., Munoz, O., and others: Prospective study of enteropathogens in children with diarrhea in Houston and Mexico, J. Pediatr. **93:**383-388, 1978.

Plotkin, G.R., Kluge, R.M., and Waldman, R.H.: Gastroenteritis: etiology, pathophysiology and clinical manifestations, Medicine **58:**95-114, 1979.

Turnberg, L.A.: The pathophysiology of diarrhea, Clin. Gastroenterol. **8:**551-568, 1979.

Ulshen, M.H., and Rollo, J.L.: Pathogenesis of *Escherichia coli* gastroenteritis in man: another mechanism, N. Engl. J. Med. **302:**99-101, 1980.

Viral gastroenteritis

Community and family epidemics of so-called intestinal flu are well known to all physicians. These infections are typically very contagious, and most are presumably viral in origin. With application of improved virologic techniques, it has been shown that a number of viruses are indigenous to the gastrointestinal tract. However, there are at least two groups of viruses, parvovirus-like agents and rotaviruses, that have been clearly identified as causal agents of acute gastroenteritis in infants and children, as well as adults.

Etiologic agents

A number of viral infections may be associated with diarrhea, including measles, mumps, influenza, and infectious hepatitis. Enteroviruses are normal inhabitants of the human gastrointestinal tract, and polioviruses, coxsackieviruses, and echoviruses are rarely responsible for diarrheal disease. Other viral agents besides parvoviruses have also been etiologically implicated. These include astroviruses, picornaviruses, coronaviruses, and adenoviruses. They can be found in healthy persons, other viruses may be present with them, and the immune response is erratic. In contrast, parvovirus-like agents and rotaviruses are seldom encountered in healthy controls and they give rise to a good immune response. Nevertheless, epidemics of acute gastroenteritis have been reported with astroviruses and picornaviruses in infants and children. The role of corona-like viruses is more doubtful, but it is being closely examined because this group of agents is responsible for severe transmissible gastroenteritis in pigs and calves. Outbreaks of diarrheal disease secondary to adenoviruses have been described, and fatal cases have been reported.

Pathogenesis

There are now seven types of parvovirus-like agents, the most famous being the "Norwalk agent," which was held responsible for an epidemic of gastroenteritis in an elementary school in Norwalk, Ohio. These small 27 nm DNA viruses lead to jejunal abnormalities in symptomatic cases and within 24 to 48 hours in volunteers. The changes occur in both symptomatic and asymptomatic cases and are characterized by a blunting of villi and inflammatory changes in the lamina propria. On electron microscopy the microvillus pattern is distorted, brush-border enzymes are re-

duced, and a transient impairment of fat and D-xylose absorption may also occur. Histologic changes disappear within 2 weeks. The mechanism by which the Norwalk agent produces diarrhea is unknown, but it is not through stimulation of adenyl cyclase. Studies suggest that immunity to the Norwalk agent may be altogether absent after a challenge, may last for a variable period of time, or may be permanent. More work is necessary to understand this self-limited disease, which affects both children and adults and occurs in families, schools, and large communities.

As pointed out above, rotaviruses are the commonest cause of acute nonbacterial gastroenteritis in infancy and childhood; it can be a severe and even fatal disease as reported by the Toronto group. First described by a group from Melbourne, the rotaviruses are double-shelled particles with an average diameter of 70 nm (Fig. 8-5). Mucosal biopsy specimens show penetration and infection of the mature enterocyte population of the villi. The involvement is often patchy: the architecture may be severely distorted with an atrophic mucosa and severe inflammatory changes (Fig. 8-6) indistinguishable from those associated with celiac disease. The sloughed-off differentiated cells are replaced by immature cells, which cannot compensate for the absorptive defect. The D-xylose test is abnormal. The pathogenesis of the diarrhea remains unexplained and is different from that of cholera and ETEC. Adenyl cyclase and cyclic AMP are not increased.

Rotavirus infection is worldwide and has serious consequences in developing countries. Vaccination would be warranted because of the morbidity and mortality associated with such infections in view of their high incidence in a vulnerable age group. The vaccine would need to protect against several serotypes. The most serious problem is the difficulty of producing high yields of the human strains in cell cultures. Perhaps the problem could be solved by use of a bovine rotavirus, which can protect against infection by human strains.

Clinical findings

Norwalk agent. Epidemic nausea and vomiting secondary to infection with Norwalk agents occurs mostly in the winter. It affects all age groups and has an incubation period of 24 to 48 hours. Symptoms include fever, anorexia, vomiting, abdominal pain, diarrhea, and muscle pain. The at-

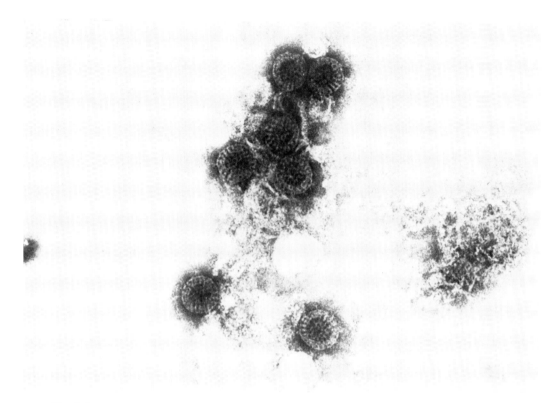

Fig. 8-5. Fecal rotaviruses show a sharply defined smooth rim (outer capsid) surrounding spoke-like subunits (inner capsid) that radiate outward from a hublike core. (Courtesy Dr. G. Delage, Hôpital Sainte-Justine, Montreal.)

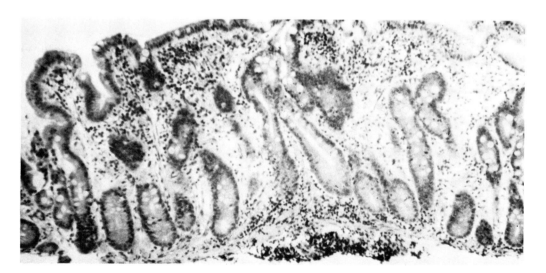

Fig. 8-6. Rotavirus gastroenteritis. These striking atrophic and inflammatory changes were observed in an 8-month-old infant with a 48-hour history of fever, diarrhea, and vomiting. (Courtesy J.R. Hamilton, Hospital for Sick Children, Toronto.)

tack rate within a home or a school can be as high as 30% or even 50%. The disease seldom lasts more than 3 days and is benign.

Rotavirus. Rotavirus infections are more severe. Their incidence is higher in the cooler months. During the winter, they may account for 80% of cases of acute gastroenteritis. Although all age groups are susceptible, the 6- to 24-month group is more vulnerable. There is no explanation why human neonates, though susceptible to infection, seldom become symptomatic, whereas newborn animals are more frequently and more severely affected during the first few weeks of life. Adult infections are mild and are usually associated with infection in the children of the household.

After an incubation period of 2 to 3 days, the illness starts abruptly with vomiting (almost 100%) and a fever of 38° C or above (10%). In most studies, 20% to 40% have an upper respiratory infection. Although fever and vomiting abate within 48 hours, diarrhea may persist for more than a week. Rectal biopsies are said to be normal though there is a report of rectal bleeding in 10% of cases. Dehydration, shock and death may occur. An unusually severe form of the disease in which death resulted from dehydration and hypernatremia has been reported from Toronto.

Differential diagnosis

Despite fever, vomiting, and diarrhea, affected children are not usually in a toxic condition. In most cases, except in the first few hours of the illness, patients will carry out their usual activities. One can rule out a bacterial infection by doing a stool culture when there is no evidence of a widespread community or family epidemic, especially if the patient is a young infant. Immunoelectron microscopy of a fecal filtrate can provide a diagnosis within 30 minutes. Solid-phase radioimmunoassay is more sensitive. Immune-adherence hemagglutination can be used to detect an immune response. The enzyme-linked immunosorbent assay (ELISA) is very sensitive, and the reagents are stable. It is the method of choice, particularly if there are large number of specimens to be examined.

Course and prognosis

Acute viral gastroenteritis is usually a self-limited disease running its course within a week. However, the histologic changes seen in most patients may persist for a week after disappearance of clinical symptoms. Carbohydrate intolerance to monosaccharides lasts until histologic repair. On the other hand, normal tolerance to disaccharides such as lactose may not return for several weeks, especially in infants younger than 6 months.

Although rotavirus gastroenteritis most often causes a relatively mild illness, dehydration requires intravenous therapy in a significant percentage of cases. It is on occasion a fatal disease.

Management

The most important part of the management is to decide whether the infant or child is ill and requires hospitalization. The mainstay of therapy consists of replacement of water and electrolyte losses through the oral administration of small amounts of clear fluids. If vomiting precludes use of the oral route, a period of fasting is indicated. Trimethobenzamide (Tigan), chlorpromazine, or sedatives should be used with caution and only when there is definite documentation of an epidemic or of a similar case in the family. In fact, these drugs may mask symptoms and render the clinical assessment of deterioration more difficult.

Similarly, the use of anticholinergic agents, of paregoric, or of antidiarrheal preparations has several disadvantages, particularly in relation to the younger child or the infant. They are not known to shorten the illness or to diminish the water and electrolyte losses, though the stools may be less frequent and less watery. In fact, one commonly used agent, a preparation of diphenoxylate hydrochloride and atropine (Lomotil), has been shown to be harmful in certain bacterial diarrheas. It is not known if this observation is also valid for viral diarrheas.

At the onset of intestinal symptoms such as vomiting, several hours of fasting are recommended. During that time, the infant or child should be kept quiet and closely observed. A teaspoonful or two of a cola drink may be first tried. Thereafter, oral fluids such as Pedialyte (Na^+ 30 mEq/L, K 20 mEq/L, and glucose 5%) or a home prepared solution containing 30 mEq/L of Na^+ and 18 mEq/L of K^+ is appropriate. The latter is prepared as follows: to 1 liter of fresh-frozen orange juice add 2.5 gm of table salt (½ teaspoon) and 1 liter of water. The risk of hyponatremia with this concentration of Na^+ is nil because the concentration of Na^+ in diarrheal stools is not as large as in cholera and ETEC infections. The risk of hypernatremia with the solution (Na^+ 90 and K^+ 20) recommended by the World Health

Organization is probably very small but nevertheless present. Clear soups or broth should not be used because their concentration of Na^+ may be very high (for example, Lipton's Chicken Noodle Soup Na^+ concentration is 238 mEq/L), and their concentration of K^+ is too low. Natural fruit juices are inappropriate because of their low Na^+ and K^+ content and their very high osmolalities. Apple juice and grape juice are over 700 and 1100 mOsm/kg of water, respectively. The same comments apply to fruit-flavored drinks and pop.

Recent studies have shown that glucose has no advantage over sucrose. In fact, sucrose has certain advantages because of its lower osmolality, ready availability, and lower cost. Attention is again drawn to the adverse effects of hyperosmolar solutions. A concentration of carbohydrates in excess of 5% is not recommended.

A teaspoonful should first be given, followed 15 minutes later by double that quantity. Thereafter an ounce or two of the same liquid should be given. Once vomiting has abated, more liberal amounts can be offered. Within a few days solids such as flavored gelatin desserts, soups, custards, bananas, applesauce, strained carrots, and toast with jelly can be given. The physician caring for the patient with viral gastroenteritis should be aware of the acquired monosaccharide intolerance during the acute phase of the illness. Checking for reducing substances may alert one to the need to reduce the carbohydrate content of clear fluids to 2.5% or to exclude them completely for a few days, especially since there is experimental evidence that in transmissible viral gastroenteritis (TGE) of young pigs glucose administration does not enhance sodium absorption in the infected pig. Reintroduction of lactose should be done progressively, after a waiting period of at least a week after the disappearance of all clinical symptoms. However, a recent study documents the fact that the length of the hospital stay of infants and children with mild acute gastroenteritis who are continued on their full-strength formula is not prolonged. Severe cases require hospitalization and intravenous rehydration.

REFERENCES

Adler, J.L., and Zickl, R.: Winter vomiting disease, J. Infect. Dis. **119**:668-673, 1969.

Banatvala, J.E.: The role of viruses in acute diarrhoeal disease, Clin. Gastroenterol. **8**:569-598, 1979.

Bishop, R.F., Davidson, G.P., Holmes, I.H., and others: Virus particles in epithelial cells of duodenal mucosa from children with acute nonbacterial gastroenteritis, Lancet **2**:1281-1283, 1973.

Chrystie, I.L., Totherdell, B.M., and Banatvala, J.E.: Asymptomatic endemic rotavirus infections in the newborn, Lancet **2**:1176-1178, 1978.

Davidson, G.P., and Barnes, G.L.: Duodenal changes with rotavirus gastroenteritis, Acta Paediatr. Scand. **68**:181-186, 1979.

Delage, G., McLaughlin, B., and Berthiaume, L.: A clinical study of rotavirus gastroenteritis, J. Pediatr. **93**:455-457, 1978.

Estes, M.K., and Graham, D.Y.: Epidemic viral gastroenteritis, Am. J. Med. **66**:1001-1007, 1979.

Finberg, L.: Oral electrolyte-glucose solutions for hydration, J. Pediatr. **96**:51-54, 1980.

Middleton, P.J., Abbott, G.D., Szymanski, M.T., and others: Orbivirus acute gastroenteritis of infancy, Lancet **1**:1241-1244, 1974.

Palmer, D.L., Koster, F.T., Rafiqui Islam, A.F.M., and others: Comparison of sucrose and glucose in the oral electrolyte therapy of cholera and other severe diarrheas, N. Engl. J. Med. **297**:1107-1110, 1977.

Portnoy, B.L., DuPont, H.L., Pruitt, D., and others: Antidiarrheal agents in the treatment of acute diarrhea in children, J.A.M.A. **236**:844-846, 1976.

Rees, L., and Brook, C.G.D.: Gradual reintroduction of full-strength milk after acute gastroenteritis in children, Lancet **1**:770-771, 1979.

Sack, D.A., Chowdhury, A.M.A.K., Eusol, A., and others: Oral hydration in rotavirus diarrhea: a double-blind comparison of sucrose with glucose electrolyte solution, Lancet **2**:280-283, 1978.

Steinhoff, M.C.: Medical Progress. Rotavirus: the first five years, J. Pediatr. **96**:611-622, 1980.

Tallet, S., MacKenzie, C., Middleton, P., and others: Clinical, laboratory and epidemiologic features of a viral gastroenteritis in infants and children, Pediatrics **60**:217-222, 1977.

Walker-Smith, J.: Gastroenteritis. In Diseases of the small intestine in childhood, ed. 2, Tumbridge Wells, Eng., 1979, Pitman Medical Pub. Co.

Wendland, B.E., and Arbus, G.S.: Oral fluid therapy: sodium and potassium content and osmolality of some commercial "clear" soups, juices and beverages, Can. Med. Assoc. J. **121**:564-569, 1979.

Wenman, W.M., Hinde, D., Feltham, S., and Gurwith, M.: Rotavirus infection in adults, N. Engl. J. Med. **301**:303-306, 1979.

Pathogenic *Escherichia coli* gastroenteritis

Since the early 1950s the concept has evolved that certain serotypes of *E. coli* are inherently enteric pathogens. Veterinary workers had recognized the association between *E. coli* and diarrhea before the turn of the century. The first study in man was reported in 1945. The classic enteropathogenic *E. coli* (EPEC) serotypes were described after the development of appropriate constituent monovalent serums and of the slide and tube agglutination methods. However, in the latter part of the 1950s evidence that put in question the inherent virulence of these serotypes, particu-

Table 8-4. Types and serotypes of *E. coli* associated with acute gastroenteritis

	Enteropathogenic (EPEC)	Enterotoxigenic (ETEC)	Enteroinvasive (EIEC)
Pathogenic mechanism	Probably a ''toxin''	Enterotoxin (ST, LT)	Epithelial cell invasion and multiplication
Age groups affected	Infants, but adults rarely	Infants and young children Adults (travelers)	All ages
Countries	Worldwide	Mainly developing, tropical countires	Worldwide
O groups associated (commonest)	26, 55, 86, 111, 114, 119, 126, 127, 128, 142	6, 8, 15, 25, 27, 63, 78, 148, 159	28ac, 112ac, 124, 136, 143, 144, 152, 164

As tabulated by B. Rowe: Clin. Gastroenterol. **8**:639, 1979.

larly in the sporadic cases of diarrheal disease, began to accrue. More than one EPEC strain could be found in patients with diarrhea. Furthermore, EPEC was identified with equal frequency in healthy persons.

After noting that only certain strains of *E. coli* 0111 caused secretory responses similar to those of cholera in a newly developed rabbit ileal-loop test, a group from India challenged the concept of serotyping to identify EPEC. This subsequently led to the identification of new serotypes, which produce heat-labile (LT) or heat stable (ST) toxin, or both enterotoxins. Investigations revealed that these enterotoxigenic *E. coli* (ETEC) could account for a significant proportion of travelers' diarrhea, for some community outbreaks of diarrhea, and also for a small number of cases of infantile gastroenteritis.

The first report that certain strains of *E. coli* could invade the mucosa and lead to a dysentery, shigella-like disease goes back to 1967. Most enteroinvasive *E. coli* (EIEC) serotypes are different from those of EPEC and ETEC (Table 8-4). Infections with EIEC can occur in all age groups and is worldwide.

Pathogenesis

E. coli attaches to the epithelial cells; EPEC and ETEC have a particular tropism for the upper small bowel (duodenum and jejunum), whereas EIEC mostly invade the large bowel, *E. coli* adherence studies suggest that it is mediated by the interaction of capsular antigens (K antigens) on brush-border receptors. After attachment, the EPEC and ETEC show no tendency to invade the host's tissues. Enterotoxins are known to be produced

by ETEC, whereas none have been identified for EPEC. However, it is likely that they also produce toxins, since EPEC infection reduces absorption and induces secretion of fluid and electrolytes. The presence of a cytotoxin has recently been suggested. There is intestinal distention, congestion, and minimal histologic changes; gross inflammation or ulceration of the mucosa is noticeably absent. However, in both rabbit and man, adherence to the mucosa and damage to the microvillous structure may be responsible for the net accumulation of fluid and electrolyte, as well as for digestive and absorptive defects.

Plasmids are extrachromosomal genetic elements that represent a regularly inherited, but dispensable, autonomously replicating gene pool. The ability of *E. coli* to produce enterotoxins is governcd by plasmids. The plasmid from ETEC produces either ST or both LT and ST. In contrast to ST, LT activates adenyl cyclase.

In rare cases in which the *E. coli* strain is invasive, it may set up widespread mucosal damage with acute inflammation. The organisms penetrate the cells of the intestinal epithelium and cause a syndrome similar to shigellosis. Infection with invasive *E. coli* gives rise to a dysentery-like picture characterized by fever, abdominal pain, tenesmus, urgency, blood, mucus and white cells in the diarrheal stools, and systemic toxemia. As in shigellosis, the colon seems to be a predominant site for multiplication of invasive *E. coli*.

The susceptibility of infants younger than age 6 months to certain strains of *E. coli* is related to the fact that maternal IgM is not transferred to the fetus because of its molecular weight (which is 900,000). It is known that antibodies against the

O antigen of gram-negative bacteria are mostly found in the IgM fraction of human immunoglobulins. Fully breast-fed babies are almost completely immune to pathogenic *E. coli* gastroenteritis. There is no doubt that colostrum and breast milk IgA prevents adhesion of bacteria to the intestinal mucosa and is truly an "antiseptic paint."

Epidemiology

In the past two decades, there has been a dramatic decrease in the incidence of epidemics of EPEC. Most outbreaks affected babies in hospital wards and in neonatal and day nurseries. There is no explanation for this change. It should be noted that from time to time there are still outbreaks reported with significant morbidity and even mortality. One such epidemic occurred in the winter of 1980 in Canada. It particularly affected North American Indian and Eskimo communities. The serotype 0111 K:58 H:2 identified in these cases was particularly virulent, leading to severe intractable diarrhea in a number of cases and exhibiting multiple antibiotic resistance. This is a reminder that although EPEC disease has undergone a sharp reduction, serious epidemic disease may still occur.

Screening for ETEC-associated LT and ST has been disappointing. Except for a few outbreaks in England and in the United States, it would seem that ETEC is not an important cause of infantile acute gastroenteritis as shown by reports from the United States, Sweden, and Canada. This may have to do with the unreliability and lack of standardization in the bioassays for the enterotoxins. However, there is no doubt that ETEC plays a major etiologic role in travelers' diarrhea. EIEC. infections are infrequent and in contrast to children and adults, neonates are not vulnerable to EIEC colitis. Water and food-borne epidemics of *E. coli* gastroenteritis have been well documented and are dealt with later in this section. An attack rate of 94% with *E. coli* 0124 was found in adults who had ingested contaminated imported French cheese.

Clinical findings

The onset may be gradual or abrupt. Cases with gradual onset tend to remain mild, whereas the most severe cases often begin abruptly.

Vomiting may be present from the onset and is associated with diarrhea that rapidly becomes explosive. The infant is toxic, and a fever is noted. Dehydration rapidly ensues. In some cases, vomiting precedes the diarrhea by a few days, abdominal distention is extreme, the fever is high, breathing is rapid and shallow, the fontanelle is depressed, the eyes are hollow, and there is persistence of the cutaneous fold. These physical signs may precede the diarrhea, since there is a paralytic ileus, and large fluid losses occur into the lumen of the gut.

The less severe cases present with diarrhea and a slight fever. The infant may be fretful or irritable. The stools are greenish and liquid, but there is no threat of dehydration. If treated symptomatically, the diarrhea may continue for weeks, thus leading to a significant loss of weight through gross malabsorption.

Since the clinical and histologic manifestations of EIEC infections are identical to those associated with *Shigella,* refer to that section.

Diagnosis

If there is evidence of epidemic, the diagnosis becomes obvious. However, the description of recent community epidemics in Canada is a reminder that enteropathogenic serotypes of *E. coli* can affect not only young infants but also children up to the age of 2 years. Nevertheless, one must be alert to signs of the disease, particularly in patients younger than 6 months old. The vomiting may be as projectile as that seen in pyloric stenosis, and diarrhea may be absent initially. Toxicity may be suggestive of sepsis and meningitis. In infants EPEC and ETEC gastroenteritis may be responsible for intractable diarrhea.

The isolation of pathogenic organisms should be attempted as early as possible. Despite its shortcomings, serotyping for EPEC should be carried out in cases of diarrhea in children below 2 years of age and also in older age groups if there is epidemiologic evidence of an outbreak. Identification of ETEC strains producing enterotoxin is beyond the expertise of standard clinical laboratories. Preliminary screening can be done by use of the available polyvalent and monovalent serums of EPEC. The majority of ETEC strains and EIEC strains will not be picked up by conventional serotyping. In the case of an outbreak, a few specimens should be sent to a reference laboratory equipped with diagnostic antiserums to cover all three ranges of diarrheogenic *E. coli:* EPEC, ETEC, and EIEC.

Prevention

Since neonates and low birth weight newborns are particularly susceptible to pathogenic *E. coli* gastroenteritis, breast feeding is undoubtedly the best preventive measure. The critical role of breast feeding in the prevention of gastroenteritis in developing countries has been amply demonstrated. Its value in the developed world is not fully appreciated despite numerous studies showing that pathogenic *E. coli* gastroenteritis is almost unheard of in the fully breast-fed infant.

Treatment

The essence of treatment is replacement of lost water and electrolytes. In milder cases, this can be done by mouth. It is important not to give solutions containing large amounts of sodium, since they may lead to hypernatremia. The amount of fluid to be given should be at least 150 ml/kg/24 hr. Tolerance for fluids is enhanced if small amounts are offered each time and if they are presented at room temperature rather than cold. There is both clinical and experimental evidence that in toxicogenic *E. coli* gastroenteritis, glucose may enhance the absorption of sodium and water and therefore reduce fecal losses. However, undiluted fruit juices are hypertonic and contain high concentrations of carbohydrates, which may lead to osmotic diarrhea.

Once vomiting has stopped and the stools become less frequent, milk feedings are resumed. Because of the evidence that after an *E. coli* gastroenteritis there is a temporary decrease in disaccharidase activity, affecting lactase particularly, it is recommended that a lactose-free formula be given after a severe bout. Very satisfactory results have been obtained with use of Nutramigen, or Pregestimil. These lactose-free formulas can be given for a few weeks after the acute illness.

Shock may be present within the first few hours after the onset. Since it is the result of a reduction in plasma volume secondary to loss of water and electrolytes, it should be corrected rapidly. This is followed by the provision of fluids to meet maintenance requirements and to repair deficits. Repair of deficit is calculated by estimation or documention of weight loss. A 5% loss corresponds to mild dehydration, 10% to moderate dehydration, and 15% to severe dehydration. One should evaluate continuing losses (Table 8-5) by weighing the patient daily and by monitoring losses.

Table 8-5. Electrolyte composition of stools (mEq/L)

	Na$^+$	K$^+$	Cl$^-$
Normal stools	22	54	21
Nonspecific diarrhea	54	33	47
Secretory diarrhea	120	40	94

Courtesy L. Chicoine, Hôpital Sainte-Justine, Montreal.

These losses are then added to maintenance and repair solutions.

When prompt resumption of oral feeding cannot be done within 4 or 5 days, it is advisable to meet energy and protein needs by peripheral parenteral nutrition (see section on intractable diarrhea).

Antibiotics

As J. Walker-Smith pointed out recently, antibiotics have little place in the management of children with gastroenteritis for the following reasons:

1. Bacterial pathogens are isolated in a minority (about 15%) of cases.
2. There is little evidence that they influence the natural history of the disease.
3. They may prolong the carrier state.
4. It is not certain that they eliminate the pathogenic bacteria from the gut.

Most infants with *E. coli* gastroenteritis recover uneventfully if water and electrolyte deficits are corrected promptly. By the time a bacteriological diagnosis is made, antibiotics are rarely needed. However, if the patient is still acutely ill when a bacteriologic diagnosis is made, neomycin is given at a dosage of 100 mg/kg/day in three divided doses for 5 days. Should testing show resistance of the implicated strain, colymycin (Colistin) is recommended and should be given at a dosage of 15 mg/kg/day in three divided does for 5 days. Because of the possible danger of sepsis and meningitis occurring during the first 6 months of life, a systemic antibiotic effective against *E. coli* should probably be given if there is clinical evidence that one is dealing with a dysentery-like syndrome indicative of an invasive strain. There is no indication for the use of parenteral or absorbable antibiotics in infants older than 3 months.

Complete eradication of the enteropathogenic *E. coli* is not the objective of antibiotic therapy unless the infant is going to an institution where, as a carrier, he could potentially be responsible for an epidemic. In that particular case, three consecutive negative cultures would be necessary before discharge.

The development of antibiotic resistance of *E. coli* is a problem that is better understood. When an antibiotic is given to an infant with *E. coli* gastroenteritis, the drug affects not only the bacterial strain responsible for the diarrhea but all the other microorganisms of the gastrointestinal tract. This normal flora may acquire drug resistance, which is then transferred by transmissible plasmids to pathogenic serotypes previously sensitive to the antibiotic in use.

Complications

It appears that the severity of *E. coli* gastroenteritis varies from time to time and from place to place. At the time of this writing, the disease in both the United States and England is usually mild in its endemic form. Recent epidemics in newborn nurseries have not been so severe as those reported in the early 1960s, when a mortality of 10% was not unusual. Infectious complications include sepsis and meningitis. Convulsions and brain damage secondary to shock and hypernatremia should prompt close monitoring of water and electrolyte needs.

REFERENCES

Boyer, K.M., Petersen, N.J., Farzaneh, I., and others: An outbreak of gastroenteritis due to *E. coli* 0142 in a neonatal nursery, J. Pediatr. **86:**919-927, 1975.

Gorbach, S.L., and Khurana, C.M.: Toxigenic *Escherichia coli:* a cause of infantile diarrhea in Chicago, N. Engl. J. Med. **287:**791-795, 1972.

Gross, R.J., Scotland, S.M., and Rowe, B.: Enterotoxin testing of *Escherichia coli* causing epidemic enteritis in the United Kingdom, Lancet **1:**629-630, 1976.

Gurwith, M.J., and Williams, T.B.: Gastroenteritis in children: a two-year review in Manitoba. I. Etiology, J. Infect. Dis. **136:**239-247, 1977.

Hirschhorn, N., McCarthy, B.J., Ranney, B., and others: Ad libitum oral glucose-electrolyte therapy for acute diarrhea in Apache children, J. Pediatr. **83:**562-571, 1973.

Ironside, A.G.: Gastroenteritis of infancy, Br. Med. J. **1:**284-286, 1973.

Levine, M.M., Bergquist, E.G., Nalin, D.R., and others: *Escherichia coli* strains that cause diarrhea but do not produce heat-labile or heat-stable enterotoxins and are non-invasive, Lancet **1:**1119-1121, 1978.

Marier, R., Wells, J.G., Swanson, R.C., and others: An outbreak of enteropathogenic *E. coli* food-borne disease traced to imported French cheese, Lancet **2:**1376-1378, 1973.

Nelson, J.D.: Duration of neomycin therapy for enteropathogenic *E. coli* diarrheal disease: a comparative study of 113 cases, Pediatrics **48:**248-258, 1971.

Nye, F.J.: Travellers' diarrhea, Clin. Gastroenterol. **8:**767-781, 1979.

Rodriguez-de-Curet, H., Lugo-de-Rivera, C., and Torres-Pinedo, R.: Studies on infant diarrhea, Gastroenterology **59:**396-404, 1970.

Rowe, B.: The role of *Escherichia coli* in gastroenteritis, Clin. Gastroenterol. **8:**625-644, 1979.

Rudoy, R.C., and Nelson, J.D.: Enteroinvasive and enterotoxigenic *Escherichia coli,* Am. J. Dis. Child. **129:**668-672, 1975.

Ryder, R.W., Wachsmuth, I.K., Buxton, A.E., and others: Infantile diarrhea produced by heat-stable enterotoxigenic *Escherichia coli,* N. Engl. J. Med. **295:**849-853, 1976.

Ste-Marie, M.T., Lee, E.M., and Brown, W.R.: Radioimmunologic measurements of naturally occurring antibodies. III. Antibodies reactive with *E. coli* and *Bacteroides fragilis* in breast fluids and sera of mothers and newborn infants, Pediatr. Res. **8:**815-819, 1974.

Salmonellosis

The incidence of typhoid fever has decreased within the past few decades. At the same time, the incidence of infections caused by salmonellas other than *Salmonella typhi* has increased. Salmonellas are often transmitted through food and food products such as meat, milk, eggs, and shellfish. In addition, these foods are subjected to complex manipulations during which one contaminated item can infect many other samples. More importantly, however, is the incidental contamination of food by food handlers in meat factories, poultry plants, and kitchens. In recent years, there has also been evidence of *Salmonella* infection of human beings occasioned by direct transmission from animals, particularly household pets such as cats, dogs, parakeets, and turtles. Water traps in resuscitators, cribs, tables, dust, and air have all been implicated.

Salmonellas invade the intestinal epithelium, but there is no extensive destruction. The precise mechanism whereby salmonellas evoke fluid secretion is unknown. Mucosal invasion appears essential for fluid loss to take place; perhaps a bacterial factor or property stimulates fluid secretion. Increased synthesis of prostaglandin has been shown, and there is one report of isolation of heat-stable and heat-labile enterotoxins closely related to those of ETEC. After a *Salmonella* infection, the epithelial lining is generally left intact, and the organisms reach the lamina propria, where they set up an inflammatory response. The nature of this inflammatory response determines the pathogenesis and resultant symptoms. In *S. typhi,* the inflammatory response is mononuclear, the organisms reach the circulation, and enteric fever with systemic symptoms and bacteremia results. When nontyphoid salmonellas are involved, the inflammatory response of the lamina propria is acute and involves the distal small bowel as well as the colonic mucosa. If the organisms are contained in the lamina propria, *Salmonella* gastroenteritis is the result. However, in a certain number of cases, particularly in young infants and in children with underlying debilitating diseases, *Salmonella* septicemia may occur, with foci of infection (pneumonia, meningitis) and abscess formation in diverse areas of the body.

Clinical findings

Gastroenteritis. The majority of cases of salmonellosis present with gastroenteritis. The rapid onset of diarrhea, vomiting, and fever 12 to 72 hours after the ingestion of contaminated food is suggestive of food poisoning. Severe abdominal pain with nausea and the absence of diarrhea may mimic acute appendicitis. However, in the average case, diarrhea is pronounced from the beginning. Since the stools are watery and may contain mucus, pus, and blood, the diagnosis can be clinically indistinguishable from shigellosis or other inflammatory bowel disease (Fig. 8-7).

In perhaps half of the cases, the temperature becomes normal within a few days and the diarrhea abates. In others, however, protracted diarrhea occurs but has little repercussion on the general well-being of the patients. In severe infections, dehydration and a shocklike picture are seen.

Septicemia. A small number of cases of salmonellosis, including all infections with *S. typhi,* present with septicemia. The incubation period is from 3 to 10 days. The fever is high, rising daily in a spiking fashion. No other symptoms may be observed at the onset, and the clinical picture may be that of fever of unknown origin. Nausea and vomiting are seen more commonly in the younger patients. Abdominal distention may develop. Diarrhea is present in some patients. On physical examination, an eruption resembling rose spots is occasionally seen. Meningism is occasionally present, and an enlarged spleen can be palpated in the patient with this form of salmonellosis. As a rule, symptons last a week, but the disease may take several weeks to run its course in the typical case of typhoid fever.

At Hôpital Sainte-Justine, Montreal, in 1971 to 1973, more than 40% of the cases of bacterial diarrhea were caused by a *Salmonella* infection.

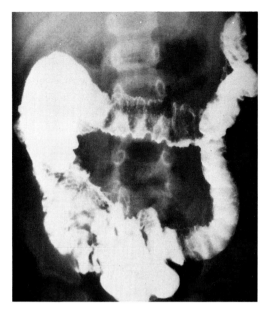

Fig. 8-7. Acute *Salmonella* enterocolitis with tenesmus, and pus and blood in stools. X-ray findings are indistinguishable from those of acute shigellosis. Mucosal irregularities are noted in the descending colon, and ulcerations are particularly well demonstrated in the transverse colon. Two weeks later, the barium enema was entirely normal.

Statistics for 1977-1978 at the same hospital combined with those of the Montreal Children's Hospital yield a much lower percentage (Table 8-6). This is attributable to the recognition of *Campylobacter* as an important pathogen and to an increasing percentage of bacterial diarrheas caused by *Yersinia* because the number of patients with salmonellosis has not changed. Close to half of the 503 cases were seen in patients in the first 2 years of life. In 15.5% of patients, a positive blood culture was obtained. The Montevideo and typhimurium serotypes accounted for close to 50% of the positive blood cultures. During that same period of time, there were only 4 cases of typhoid fever.

Diagnosis

Leukocytosis may or may not be present in the gastroenteric form, and a normal or low white blood cell count is seen in the septicemic form. Positive blood cultures indicate the diagnosis of systemic involvement and may also be found in the gastrointestinal type of clinical picture with which stool cultures are always positive and may remain positive for several weeks or months. Stool

Table 8-6. Relative frequency of isolation of *Salmonella* at Hôpital Sainte-Justine (HSJ) and at the Montreal Children's Hospital (MCH)

Year	Salmonella	Campylobacter	Yersinia	Shigella	Escherichia coli
HSJ					
(1971-1973)	40.5%	—	7.7%	4.5%	47.3%
HSJ and MCH					
(1977-1978)	29.3%	28.7%	18.7%	7.3%	6.7%

Table 8-7. Effect of treatment on convalescent phase of fecal excretion of *Salmonella*

	Number of Patients	Percent excreting same serotype			
		1 month	2 months	3 months	4 months
No treatment	57	62.5	29.4	33.3	25
Treatment	70	81.4	53.3	52.5	50

Data provided by G. Murray, R. Martineau, and G. Delage, Hôpital Sainte-Justine, Montreal.

smears characteristically show polymorphonuclear cells in *Salmonella* infections other than *S. typhi.* In the latter, mononuclear cells are noted.

Salmonella infections are diagnosed by isolation of the microorganism from the blood, stools, or urine. Direct rectal swabs are probably the most productive specimens. Indirect techniques of diagnosis rely on the rise of type-specific circulating antibodies for a given organism. Serologic testing may be useful 1 or 2 weeks after onset of typhoid fever, *Salmonella* sepsis, or the more severe cases of gastroenteritis, but it constitutes only second-best evidence.

Prognosis and complications

The prognosis is related to the age of the patient, the type of infecting microorganism, the extent of the infection, and the presence of complications. Intestinal hemorrhage and perforation occur rarely in children with typhoid fever. Disseminated intravascular coagulation occurs commonly and may become manifest as a hemolytic uremic syndrome. Immune complex glomerulonephritis has also been attributed to typhoid fever. Meningitis, pneumonia, osteomyelitis, and subacute bacterial endocarditis are serious ccomplications of *Salmonella* infections with bacteremia especially in young infants. Children with underlying immune defects such as chronic granulomatous disease are particularly vulnerable. A report of 11 fatal cases of necrotizing enterocolitis over a 10-week period in low birth weight newborns from whom *Salmo-*

nella was grown in six cases attracts attention to the lethal potential of the microorganism in newborn nurseries. The overall mortality probably is around 2% to 3%. In the series of 503 cases mentioned above, the mortality was 1.5%.

Treatment

Specific management. Although antibiotic therapy reduces the morbidity and mortality from typhoid fever and from bacteremia caused by other *Salmonella* serotypes, antibiotics have not proved similarly effective for the treatment of *Salmonella* gastroenteritis. In fact, recent studies have shown that administration of antibiotics may be associated with prolonged postconvalescent fecal excretion of *Salmonella* (Table 8-7). Furthermore, a certain percentage of these strains become resistant to antibiotics. Antibiotic therapy therefore increases the opportunity for person-to-person spread and for the dissemination of resistant organisms. Antibiotic therapy does not shorten or alter the course of the uncomplicated case of *Salmonella* gastroenteritis. Antibiotics appear to occasionally convert carrier states or cases of gastroenteritis to systemic disease with bactermia.

Despite these drawbacks, use of antibiotics is warranted in newborn infants, young infants, and children in a toxic condition. Their use is also indicated in salmonellosis associated with sickle-cell anemia, hemoglobinopathies, immune defects, and disseminated malignant diseases in which a septicemic form with its complications and metastatic infections is more likely to occur. Ampicillin, the antibiotic of choice, should be given at a dose of 100 mg/kg/24 hr for a week. In the case of enteric fever or of typhoid fever, antiobiotic treatment should be continued for 2 to 4 weeks or for at least a week after signs and symptoms have abated.

Studies from our hospital show that the serotypes typhimurium, Thompson, and Montevideo exhibit ampicillin resistance in percentages of 30%, 6%, and 3%, respectively; all the others are uniformly sensitive, including *S. typhi*. Chloramphenicol shows much less resistance and can be used if resistance to ampicillin is demonstrated. It should be noted, however, that resistance to chloramphenicol may, in certain areas, be higher than to ampicillin. For instance, it has been estimated that one third of *S. typhosa* strains in Los Angeles County are resistant to chloramphenicol. The dose is 100 mg/kg/24 hr until fever abates. It is then decreased to 50 mg and continued for 2 to 4 weeks. Prospective studies have shown that trimethoprim-sulfamethoxazole (TMS) at a dosage of 5 to 10 mg/25 to 50 mg/kg/day for a period of 7 days is a highly effective drug. It is essentially devoid of side effects, but resistance has been described. The combination of gentamicin and TMS has also been used.

General management. Salmonella gastroenteritis is usually a mild, self-limited illness. If careful attention is paid to fluid and electrolyte balance, recovery is generally uneventful. Bed rest is advocated for a few days. The patient should be carefully observed for signs of sepsis or other complications.

Because of the frequent incidence of cross infection in epidemics involving young children and particularly neonates, a careful search must be made for patients excreting salmonellas among all those admitted with diarrhea. Isolation of all such patients and discharge at the earliest possible time is recommended. Careful attention to general hygiene by hospital personnel having contact with patients is essential.

Contacts and carriers

Survey of household contacts is mandatory. Close to 50% are likely to be carrying the organism. The incidence of positive cultures is most frequent in younger members of the family, and a greater percentage of them are likely to show symptoms. Close observation of contacts carrying the organism is advocated. Asymptomatic carriers

of *S. typhi* should be treated with ampicillin for a few weeks.

About 40% to 60% of patients with salmonellosis are still excreting organisms 4 weeks after the acute phase of their illness. This frequency lessens sharply 2 months after the illness. After 1 year less than 3% are convalescent carriers and should not be treated unless they excrete *S. typhi* or paratyphoid B.

Immunization

Typhoid-paratyphoid immunization provides incomplete protection. Nevertheless, it is recommended for people at risk by exposure.

Protection is rapidly achieved when doses of 0.5 ml, 1 ml, and 1 ml intramuscularly at 1-week intervals are given. Fewer side effects and a slower immune response follow the subcutaneous administration of 0.5 ml, repeated after an interval of 4 weeks.

REFERENCES

Colon, A.R., Gross, D.R., and Tamer, M.A.: Typhoid fever in children, Pediatrics **56:**606-609, 1975.

Herzog, C.: Chemotherapy of typhoid fever: a review of literature, Infection **4:**166-173, 1976.

Kazemi, M., Gumpert, T.G., and Marks, M.I.: A controlled trial comparing sulfamethoxazoletrimethoprim, ampicillin, and no therapy in the treatment of *Salmonella* gastroenteritis in children, J. Pediatr. **83:**646-650, 1973.

Mandal, B.K.: Typhoid and paratyphoid fever, Clin. Gastroenterol. **8:**715-735, 1979.

Rosenstein, B.J.: Salmonellosis in infants and children: epidemiologic and therapeutic considerations, J. Pediatr. **70:**1-7, 1967.

Smith, E.R., and Badley, B.W.D.: Treatment of *Salmonella* enteritis and its effect on the carrier state, Can. Med. Assoc. J. **104:**1004-1006, 1971.

Stein, H., Beck, J., Solomon, A., and Schmaman, A.: Gastroenteritis with necrotizing enterocolitis in premature babies, Br. Med. J. **2:**616-619, 1972.

Shigellosis

Bacillary dysentery is an acute infection caused by various strains of *Shigella*. It is characterized by occurrence of diarrhea, fever, abdominal pain, tenesmus, and passage of stools that usually contain mucus, pus, and blood. There are four main groups of *Shigella* responsible for bacillary dysentery. Identification is established by culture properties and agglutination with standard typing sera. *S dysenteriae I* (Shiga bacillus) is alone associated with the production of an exotoxin. The toxin is heat labile and cytotoxic to intestinal cells, and its effect is not related to either inflammation or mucosal inury. Some strains of *S. dysenteriae* I lead to watery diarrhea without penetrating intestinal cells, whereas others are both invasive and toxigenic. Recently several strains of *S. flexneri* and *S. sonnei* have been shown to produce a cell-free toxin that causes secretion of intestinal fluid and electrolytes. This finding suggests that toxin may also be involved in the pathogenesis of infections caused by non-*dysenteriae* strains. *S. dysenteriae* is not seen in North America and is rare even in the tropics and in developing countries. The most recent large epidemic occurred in Bangladesh in 1974. *S. flexneri* and *S. sonnei* are usually implicated in Canada and in the United States, the latter being the most prevalent.

Dysentery is spread by the oral ingestion of microorganisms in contaminated food or drink. Flies can be the agent of transmission. The disease is more prevalent during the warm months, and its incidence is more frequent in tropic and subtropic areas. The severity of the illness is usually milder in areas in which it is more frequently seen.

The infection selectively affects the colon, the changes being more pronounced in the rectum and sigmoid colon. In milder cases, the colon is diffusely swollen and peppered with petechial hemorrhages. Usually, acute inflammatory exudates are seen in the mucosa and submucosa along with crypt abscesses. Shallow, irregular ulcerations follow the sloughing of patches of grayish membrane.

Clinical findings

Mild forms are most common and are clinically manifested by watery diarrhea with mild constitutional symptoms or without them. The more severe cases start abrupt with fever, abdominal pain, anorexia, and vomiting. Rapidly the symptoms are followed by diarrhea, crampy abdominal pain, and tenesmus. The stools are usually bloody and contain pus. The abdominal pain may be very severe and lead to a guarded abdomen in the absence of any other symptoms. Severe dehydration and peripheral collapse can affect patients of any age but particularly infants and young children. Fever commonly goes up to 40°s C. Meningism, delirium, and convulsions occur with some regularity in children. A concomitant upper respiratory infection and cough is often noted. A transient rose spot eruption, a morbilliform or petechial rash is also described. The acute symptoms may persist for a week or so. Gradually, the stools become less frequent and contain less blood. Convales-

cence may be prolonged for weeks with low-grade fever, intermittent diarrhea, and failure to thrive.

Diagnosis

The case of the typical ill patient presents no diagnostic problem. Mild cases exhibiting only watery diarrhea or severe cases presenting meningeal or appendiceal signs before emergence of diarrhea are harder to diagnose. That a fresh stool contains mucus, pus, and blood should alert the physician to consider this diagnosis. Sigmoidoscopic examination shows intense inflammation of the mucosa, which bleeds readily, along with pus and ulcerations. The diagnosis is established bacteriologically when *Shigella* is grown from the stools. The culture of specimens obtained when an ulcerated lesion is swabbed during endoscopy provides the most satisfactory approach. Culture plates should be inoculated as soon as possible. A significant, fourfold rise in agglutinins on paired serums establishes a retrospective diagnosis but is useful only in special epidemiologic studies.

The differential diagnosis includes other infectious diarrheas. On sigmoidoscopy, the findings are often indistinguishable from those of chronic ulcerative colitis, amebic dysentery, or invasive *E. coli* gastroenteritis. Meningeal and appendiceal signs are, at times, so prominent that meningitis and appendicitis need to be seriously considered.

Complications and prognosis

Sepsis and peritonitis are reported as rare complications of neonatal shigellosis. Disseminated intravascular coagulation, hemolytic-uremic syndrome with acute renal failure and pseudomembranous enterocolitis have been recorded in the course of epidemics. Most cases were caused by *S. dysenteriae* I. Keratoconjunctivitis, nonsuppurative arthritis, suppurative arthritis, and osteomyelitis rarely occur. The last is of particular concern in children with sickle-cell anemia.

Treatment

Shigellosis is a self-limited disease. Usually by the time the patient is seen he is symptomatically improved. The treatment, therefore, aims more at a bacterial cure than at a clinical cure. Most cases will not be clinically improved by use of antibiotics. However, it is recommended that all patients severely ill with shigellosis receive ampicillin for 5 days at a dose of 100 mg/kg. Bacteriologic cure rates after 48 hours of therapy are as great as 80% to 90%. Recent studies show that Lomotil or drugs that may slow intestinal motility are contraindicated because they may prolong the illness and may lead to toxic megacolon. A recent review concludes that when fever or dysentery (mucus, pus, blood in the stools, and tenesmus), or both, occur in the presence of acute diarrhea, an invasive pathogen should be suspected, and drugs that decrease gut motility are to be avoided. The proper replacement of water and electrolytes is of prime importance.

Proper control measures include the isolation of all cases of diarrhea until consecutive stool cultures are found negative for known bacterial pathogens such as *Shigella*. The patient with shigellosis should, of course, be strictly isolated, and discharged as promptly as possible.

In contrast to salmonellosis, in which antibiotic therapy tends to increase the percentage of convalescent carriers, there is evidence that ampicillin therapy decreases the percentage of convalescent patients excreting shigellas and reduces the risk of spread within a household. The ascendancy of *S. sonnei* as the predominant strain isolated from children with shigellosis is of importance because this subgroup is rapidly becoming ampicillin-resistant. The rising incidence of ampicillin resistance is occurring against a background of ever-increasing ampicillin usage. This is related to the fact that the *Shigella* organisms possess plasmids coding for transferable multiple antibiotic resistance.

At Hôpital Sainte-Justine in Montreal, only a small percentage of *S. sonnei* are ampicillin-resistant. There is a growing consensus that currently the drug of choice is trimethoprim-sulfamethoxazole (5 to 10 mg/25 to 50 mg/kg/day) in divided doses for 5 days. Forthcoming evidence may show that from a strictly epidemiologic standpoint all patients with shigellosis should be treated with antibiotics. Until such studies are made known, antibiotic therapy should be given to newborn infants, young infants, and sick children.

REFERENCES

Chang, M.J., Dunkle, L.M., Van Reken, D., and others: Trimethoprim-sulfamethoxazole compared to ampicillin in the treatment of shigellosis, Pediatrics **59**:726-729, 1977.

Davies, J.R., Farrant, W.N., and Uttley, A.H.C.: Antibiotic resistance of *Shigella sonnei*, Lancet **2**:1157-1159, 1970.

Haltalin, K.C.: Neonatal shigellosis, Am. J. Dis. Child. **114**:603-611, 1967.

Haltalin, K.C., Kusmiesz, H.T., Hinton, L.V., and others: Treatment of acute diarrhea in outpatients, Am. J. Dis. Child. **124**:555-561, 1972.

Keusch, G.T.: Shigella infections, Clin. Gastroenterol. **8**:645-662, 1979.

Koster, F., Levin, J., Walker, L., and others: Hemolytic-uremic syndrome after shigellosis: relation to endotoxemia and circulating immune complexes, N. Engl. J. Med. **298**:927-933, 1978.

Weissman, J.B., Gangarosa, E.J., Dupont, H.L., and others: Shigellosis. To treat or not to treat, J.A.M.A. **229**:1215-1216, 1974.

Yersinia infections of the gastrointestinal tract

Severe bacterial diarrhea has been associated primarily with infections due to salmonellas, shigellas, and enteropathogenic strains of *E. coli,* and these organisms still account for numerous cases of severe diarrheal diseases of childhood. A less common etiologic agent *Yersinia enterocolitica,* is being increasingly recognized, as borne out by Table 8-6. The incidence in Quebec and Ontario is so high as compared to the United States that a letter to the editor intimated that it could be a Canadian disease.

When an infection caused by *Y. enterocolitica* is suspected, the problem is not recovery of the organism from clinical material but rather its correct identification. It is a nonhemolytic aerobically growing gram-negative rod that resembles certain Enterobacteriaceae, particularly *Proteus* and other non–lactose fermenting Enterobacteriaceae. Appropriate bacteriologic diagnostic procedures are therefore necessary and appear to be particularly important since routine screening of stool specimens for *Y. enterocolitica* has disclosed the absence of *Yersinia* in children without gastrointestinal symptoms. Recovery of the organism should be regarded as indicative of actual or recent clinical disease.

A recent prospective study from the Montreal Children's Hospital and Hôpital Sainte-Justine has disclosed that infection assessed by culture or by the appearance of agglutination antibodies was commonly (greater than 20%) acquired by household contacts. However, symptoms were less likely to occur in adults than in children within a household.

Clinical findings

In our experience, the majority of infections with *Y. enterocolitica* occur in the first 3 years of life. Transmission by food and pets is known. An epidemic has been associated with contaminated

Table 8-8. Clinical picture associated with *Yersinia enterocolitica* serotype 0:3 gastroenteritis

Symptoms	Percentage	Duration in days
Diarrhea	98	14 (1 to 46)
Fever (>38.7° C)	68	3.9
Abdominal pain*	64.5	7.7
Vomiting	38.5	2.4
Bloody stools	26	—

Data tabulated from Marks, M.I., and others: J. Pediatr. **96**:26, 1980.

*In right lower quadrant in 13%.

chocolate milk. The incubation period is probably between 7 and 10 days.

The usual clinical picture is that of acute gastroenteritis (Table 8-8). On clinical grounds, one cannot draw up signs and symptoms more likely to occur with *Y. enterocolitica* than with other bacterial pathogens. However, severe persistent abdominal pain with fever, guarding, and vomiting may take precedence over diarrhea and suggest acute appendicitis. In this group, exploratory laparotomy may reveal acute terminal ileitis, acute appendicitis, acute mesenteric lymphadenitis, or all three. A more chronic granulomatous process has also been described. In such cases, diarrhea may be relapsing, and last several months. The disease process may be more diffuse and severe. There is sepsis with arthritis and a right lower guadrant pseudotumor formed by a mass of ileal loops with microabscesses and necrotic mesenteric lymph nodes. Seven children with thalassemia major and others with leukemia or aplastic anemia have been described with this form of the disease, which is fortunately rare.

Treatment

Yersinia is usually resistant to ampicillin and sensitive to aminoglycosides and trimethoprim-sulfathoxazole (TMS). It is rare that antibiotic treatment is warranted, since most cases are self-limited and the patients have already significantly improved by the time the diagnosis is made.

Course and prognosis

In most cases, the diarrhea lasts 1 to 2 weeks. The stools are watery, are often mucoid, and may contain blood (25%). Stools are commonly Hematest-positive. Recurrent chronic diarrhea

lasting for several months can also be seen. Gastrointestinal lesions can lead to peritonitis, massive gastrointestinal hemorrhage, sepsis, and death. We have not had any experience with such a severe form of the disease. Some authors have noted arthritic manifestations, myocarditis, and erythema nodosum as concomitants of *Y. enterocolitica,* gastroenteritis, and ileitis.

There is no evidence to show that acute terminal ileitis caused by *Yersinia* progresses to Crohn's disease. Patients followed for periods of 2 to 5 years after a bout of yersiniosis have not developed Crohn's disease, whereas 75% of those who had acute ileitis with negative cultures went on to develop Crohn's disease.

Yersinia pseudotuberculosis is a well-recognized cause of mesenteric lymphadenitis in Europe. Only rare cases have been reported from this hemisphere. The syndrome mimics acute appendicitis, but a normal appendix is found. The ileocecal lymph nodes are greatly enlarged, focal areas of necrosis are seen, and the sinusoids are filled with polymorphonuclear leukocytes. Direct culture of the lymph node and serologic testing will establish the diagnosis. The course of the illness is almost always benign and does not require antibiotics.

Campylobacter enteritis

It is only recently that *Campylobacter* organisms, well known for years in veterinary medicine, have been recognized as a cause of acute gastrointestinal infections in man. Campylobacters are thin, spirally curved, gram-negative rods with a single flagellum. Their morphologic similarity to *Vibrio cholerae* is quite striking. *Campylobacter fetus* subspecies *jejuni*, also known as "related vibrios," grow on blood agar but require reduced oxygen tension for growth. If campylobacters went undected for decades, the reason is that the techniques traditionally used in clinical laboratories did not suit their exacting growth requirements. Diagnostic human serology is useful. Paired serums usually show a fourfold or greater rise in antibody titer.

Systemic campylobacteriosis is reported, but it is rare. Five pediatric cases of sepsis and five of fatal neonatal meningitis have been reported. Although sepsis may occur in association with gastroenteritis, it is exceptional. The epidemiology of *Campylobacter* enteritis is not well understood as yet. Person-to-person transmission is most important with a secondary attack rate of about 10%. Food (butchered chicken) and water-borne infections are also known. The frequent early occurrence of profuse watery stools suggests a small bowel secretory component, but so far studies have failed to show the presence of enterotoxins or cytotoxins. The clinical picture is certainly suggestive of an invasive organism analogous to that seen in shigellosis. The principal site of infection is the jejunum and ileum. Extensive ulcerations and hemorrhagic ileitis may be the pathologic features, whereas in others there can be broadening and flattening of the jejunal mucosa. *Campylobacter*-caused colitis may be indistinguishable from other inflammatory causes of distal bowel disease.

Clinical findings

The incubation period is probably between 2 to 11 days. After the appearance of fever and abdominal pain, there is watery, profuse, and foul-smelling diarrhea. Most patients will develop blood-streaked stools shortly thereafter. The abdominal pain may be quite severe: it is crampy and generally periumbilical. Vomiting is infrequent. The illness generally lasts a week, but a longer course may occur. Relapsing diarrhea has also been reported.

At the Hôpital Sainte-Justine *Campylobacter* accounts for a significant percentage of the cases of bacterial gastroenteritis (Table 8-6). The largest experience reported in children is from Toronto where over a 6-month period *Campylobacter* was grown from nearly 23% of children with bacterial diarrheas. More than half were less than 3 years of age. Table 8-9 summarizes the clinical features in 37 cases.

Diagnosis

The diagnosis of *Campylobacter* enteritis should be entertained in children with fever, abdominal pain, and blood-streaked stools. Direct-phase microscopy is a fairly sensitive method for rapid diagnosis. Stool samples seem to give a higher yield of positive cultures than rectal swabs do. It is usually the sole enteric pathogen detected.

Abdominal pain may be severe enough to mimick an "acute abdomen." Acute appendicitis has been reported in the course of *Campylobacter* infections.

Treatment and prognosis

Most patients recover spontaneously, but erythromycin (20 to 40 mg/kg/day in four divided doses)

for 7 to 10 days is advocated. It has a low toxicity and is effective in speeding up the recovery and in shortening the duration of stool carriage. In the Toronto series, treated patients had a rapid resolution of their symptoms, and stools became negative within 48 hours of initiation of treatment. Two thirds of untreated children stopped having diarrhea within 1 week and 93% within 2 weeks. However, more than 50% still had a positive culture for *Campylobacter* after 3 weeks.

REFERENCES

Black, R.E., Jackson, R.J., Tsai, T., and others: Epidemic *Yersinia enterocolitica* infection due to contaminated chocolate milk, N. Engl. J. Med. **298:**76-79, 1978.

Bradford, W.D., Noce, P.S., and Gutman, L.T.: Pathologic features of enteric infection with *Yersinia enterocolitica*, Arch. Pathol. **98:**17-22, 1974.

Butzler, J.P., Alexander, M., Segers, A., and others: Enteritis, abscess and septicemia due to *Yersinia enterocolitica* in a child with thalassemia, J. Pediatr. **93:**619-621, 1978.

Butzler, J.P., and Skirrow, M.B.: *Campylobacter* enteritis, Clin. Gastroenterol. **8:**737-765, 1979.

Cadranel, S., Rodesch, P., Butzler, J.P., and Dekeyser, P.: Enteritis due to "related *Vibrio*" in children, Am. J. Dis. Child. **126:**152-158, 1973.

Delorme, J., Laverdière, M., Martineau, B., and Lafleur, L.: Yersiniosis in children, Can. Med. Assoc. J. **110:**281-284, 1974.

Gurry, J.F.: Acute terminal ileitis and *Yersinia* infection, Br. Med. J. **2:**264-266, 1974.

Gutman, L.T., Ottesen, E.A., Quan, T.J., and others: An inter-familial outbreak of *Yersinia enterocolitica* enteritis, N.Engl. J. Med. **288:**1372-1377, 1973.

Karmali, M.A., and Fleming, P.C.: *Campylobacter* enteritis in children, J. Pediatr. **94:**527-533, 1979.

Kohl, S., Jacobson, J.A., and Nahmias, A.: *Yersinia enterocolitica* infections in children, J. Pediatr. **89:**77-79, 1976.

Marks, M.I., Pai, C.H., Lafleur, L., and others: *Yersinia enterocolitica* gastroenteritis: a prospective study of clinical, bacteriologic and epidemiologic features, J. Pediatr. **96:**26-31, 1980.

Persson, S., Danielsson, D., Kjellander, J., and Wallensten, S.: Studies on Crohn's disease. 1. The relationship between *Yersinia enterocolitica* infection and terminal ileitis, Acta Chir. Scand. **142**(1):84-90, 1976.

Rettig, P.J.: Medical Progress. *Campylobacter* infections in human beings, J. Pediatr. **94:**855-864, 1979.

Saari, T.N., and Triplett, D.A.: *Yersinia pseudotuberculosis* mesenteric adenitis, J. Pediatr. **85:**656-659, 1974.

Waldschmidt, J.: *Yersinia enterocolitica* and *pseudotuberculosis* in children, Progr. Pediatr. Surg. **11:**97-105, 1978.

Food and water-borne infections and food poisoning

When acute diarrhea and vomiting rapidly occur after the ingestion of food contaminated with bacteria, containing their preformed toxin, or with a parasite, the diagnosis of food poisoning is made.

Table 8-9. Clinical features in 37 children with *Campylobacter* enteritis

Symptoms	Number of patients	Percentage
Diarrhea	35	95
Frank blood in stools	34	92
Fever	32	86
Abdominal pain	22	60
Vomiting	10	30

From Karmali, M.A., and others: J. Pediatr. **94:**527-533, 1979.

Table 8-10. Food poisoning and food-borne infection

Microorganism	Mechanism	Vehicle	Duration
Salmonella	Infection	Meat, poultry, dairy products	One week
Staphylococcus	Intoxication	Custards, pastries, meat, poultry	2 days
Clostridium perfringens	Infection, intoxication?	Meat, poultry, dairy products	2 days
Clostridium botulinum	Infection, intoxication?*	Honey?	Death, or recovery over several months
Vibrio parahaemolyticus	Infection	Seafood	1 week
Bacillus cereus	Intoxication	Boiled or fried rice	2 days
Campylobacter	Infection	Poultry, milk	1 week
Escherichia coli	Infection, intoxication?	Food	1 week
Shigella	Infection	Dairy products	1 week
Yersinia	Infection	Dairy products	1 week
Giardia	Infestation	?	Variable
Hepatitis virus	Infection	Shellfish	Variable

*In infant botulism, there is growth of the organism and local production of toxin.

Bacteriologic food poisoning agents can therefore be broadly classified within two categories.

1. True infections in which the bacteria once ingested multiply in the body.
2. Strictly intoxications in that the toxins are formed during growth of the microorganisms in the food before consumption.

Table 8-10 lists the principal pathogens, the type of food poisoning, the most common food vehicle, and the duration of the illness. Most foodborne outbreaks are caused by *Salmonella, Staphylococcus aureus,* and *Clostridium perfringens.* Despite all the drama and publicity given to botulism, this organism accounts for only a very small number of recorded food poisoning cases in the world.

Staphylococcal gastroenteritis (food poisoning)

All staphylococcal gastroenteritis results from ingestion of food that has been contaminated with staphylococci and that has not been either adequately cooked or refrigerated. Foods such as custards, mayonnaise, cream-filled pastries, and whipped cream constitute ideal culture media in which the staphylococcal enterotoxin is produced. The enterotoxin is heat-stable. Both coagulase-positive and coagulase-negative staphylococci are incriminated.

Clinical findings

The illness begins acutely within the first 4 to 6 hours after ingestion of the contaminated food.

Nausea, vomiting, severe abdominal cramps, and profuse diarrhea are regular features. Shock may occur in severe cases. Fever, if present, is mildly elevated. Improvement is already apparent within 24 hours.

Diagnosis

That there is an epidemic within a household and that the incubation period is short make the diagnosis evident.

Prognosis and treatment

The prognosis is excellent. The treatment is usually directed strictly to symptoms. Severe cases may require parenteral fluids.

Prevention

Prevention of staphylococcal food poisoning requires that a temperature of 150° F be maintained for at least 12 minutes, followed by refrigeration.

Staphylococcal enterocolitis

Staphylococcal enterocolitis is a rare and often fatal disease occurring more commonly in patients who have had surgery or have been treated with broad-spectrum antibiotics. It may give rise to ''pseudomembranous'' enterocolitis (p. 215 and Chapter 13). A diagnosis of staphylococcal enterocolitis should be made only when a pure culture of staphylococci is obtained from the stools. A Gram stain will readily identify them.

Botulism

This particular type of food poisoning results from the ingestion of toxin produced by *Clostridium botulinum,* of which there are six immunologically distinct strains. Types A, B, and E have been implicated in disease affecting man in the United States. Whereas spores of types A and B are widely distributed in soil, type E spores have been found on seashores and the sea bottom.

Botulinus toxins are the most potent poisons known; however, they are destroyed by boiling for 10 minutes or heating at 80° C for 30 minutes. Clinical botulism is produced when a food product is contaminated either with preformed toxin or with bacilli or spores. If spores are contaminating the food, they will germinate with time but only under certain conditions. Subsequently, when toxin is produced, the food product must not be heated if the toxin is to keep its pharmacologic action on cholinergic nerve transmission. Home-canned food, raw fish, and commercially processed fish products are known sources of botulism.

A particularly widely publicized form of food poisoning is the newly recognized entity "infant botulism." *Clostridium botulinum* is generally assumed to be unable to compete with the intestinal microflora. However in the more than 60 cases recorded there is evidence that in an infant less than 6 months of age, the organism can become established in the lower part of the bowel and produce toxin locally. Honey has been under strong suspicion as a source of spores, and a warning has been issued that it should not be given to babies less than 6 months of age.

Clinical features

Severity is related to host susceptibility and to the amount of toxin ingested. The disease may be so mild that consultation is not obtained; in other cases, it is fatal within a few hours. Within 12 hours to 3 days after ingestion of the contaminated food products, the individual suffers nausea, vomiting, and diarrhea. Central nervous system symptoms are related to the curare-like action on the motor end plate. The patient's mouth is dry, and he experiences dysphagia; vision is blurred, pupils are fixed, and diplopia occurs. Finally, the early signs of dizziness, weakness, and vertigo gradually lead to involvement of the respiratory muscles. When patients recover, improvement is apparent within a week of ingestion.

Diagnosis

The differential diagnosis must be made with Guillain-Barré syndrome and myasthenia gravis. The diagnosis can be confirmed when fresh serum is injected into mice with and without specific antiserum.

Treatment

Since respiratory failure is the real worry, tracheostomy should be done and positive-pressure respirators used early. Antitoxin should be given intravenously as early as possible after testing for sensitization. It is also advocated prophylactically in individuals who are known to have eaten contaminated food.

Prognosis

Once the patient has survived the paralytic phase, the outlook for complete recovery is excellent.

Mortality is as great as 65% in type A, 20% in type B, and 40% in type E.

Clostridial gastroenteritis (food poisoning)

Outbreaks of food poisoning in North America are more frequently associated with *Clostridium perfringens* than with staphylococci. The type A strains produce an enterotoxin that leads to a self-limited diarrheal illness 8 to 15 hours after the ingestion of contaminated food. All commercially available food can be at fault, but meat and poultry are more frequently involved.

Clostridial enteritis

Type C strains of *Clostridium perfringens* can cause necrotizing jejunitis and have been associated with the consumption of poorly cooked pork (pig feasting). It is especially frequent in children but has not been reported in North America.

Vibrio parahaemolyticus enterocolitis

Vibrio parahaemolyticus organisms are halophilic gram-negative rods responsible for an acute self-limited gastroenteritis bearing many similarities to *Salmonella* and *Shigella* infections. The incubation varies between 8 and 22 hours. Diarrhea, abdominal cramps, nausea, vomiting, and fever are the prominent symptoms. The dietary history invariably reports the ingestion of raw fish or uncooked shellfish.

REFERENCES

Arnon, S.S., Midura, T.F., Danus, K., and others: Honey and other environmental risk factors for infant botulism, J. Pediatr. **94:**331-336, 1978.

Black, R.E., Jackson, R.J., Tsai, T., and others: Epidemic *Yersinia enterocolitica* infection due to contaminated chocolate milk, N. Engl. J. Med. **298:**76-79, 1978.

Bolen, J.L., Zamiska, S.A., and Greenough, W.B.: Clinical features in enteritis due to *Vibrio parahaemolyticus,* Am. J. Med. **57:**638-641, 1974.

Breckinridge, J.C., and Bergdoll, M.S.: Outbreak of foodborne gastroenteritis due to a coagulase-negative enterotoxin-producing staphylococcus, N. Engl. J. Med. **284:**541-543, 1971.

Murrell, T.G.C., Roth, L., Egerton, J., and others: Pig-bel: enteritis necroticans: a study in diagnosis and management, Lancet **1:**217-222, 1966.

Turnbull, P.C.B.: Food poisoning with special reference to *Salmonella:* its epidemiology, pathogenesis and control, Clin. Gastroenterol. **8:**663-714, 1979.

DIARRHEA MISTAKEN FOR INFECTIOUS GASTROENTERITIS
Diarrhea related to use of antibiotics

The diarrheal complications of antibiotic usage are among the most frequent adverse drug reactions encountered in current-day practice. The diarrhea is usually profuse without blood or mucus and may have the color of the antibiotic suspension being administered. It does not contain fecal leukocytes. This type of nonspecific diarrhea will stop with discontinuation of the offending antibiotic, which is likely to be a broad-spectrum type. Occasionally it will take a few days to clear up and require a lactose-free diet or formula.

There is a considerable amount of information on antibiotic-induced malabsorption. Tetracyclines impair fat absorption in rats and iron absorption in both man and animals. Although kanamycin, bacitracin, polymyxin, and paromomycin are also known to produce malabsorption, its degree is milder than with neomycin. The latter causes striking fecal fat losses. It inhibits lipase hydrolysis of triglycerides; precipitates bile acids; interferes with protein, carbohydrate, sodium, calcium, iron, and vitamin B_{12} absorption; and causes mucosal cell damage with decreases in disaccharidase activity.

In rare patients, what seems to be a mild case of antibiotic-associated diarrhea is complicated by abdominal cramps, fever, and explosive stools with blood and mucus. This entity known as "pseudomembranous enterocolitis" may be caused by all antibiotics, but clindamycin and ampicillin have been more frequently implicated. It may occur as early as 4 days after initiation of antimicrobial treatment and as late as a few weeks after discontinuation. *Clostridium difficile* and its cytopathic toxin is the etiologic agent responsible for this severe affection, which may lead to toxic megacolon and perforation. A complete description can be found in Chapter 13.

Diarrhea associated with extraintestinal infections

The association between diarrhea and infections involving the urinary and the respiratory tract has long been known. The actual mechanism responsible for the presence of chronic diarrhea in young children with urinary tract infections is unknown. The diarrhea is often associated with evidence of failure to thrive, which is attributable to the infection and to anorexia (Fig. 8-8).

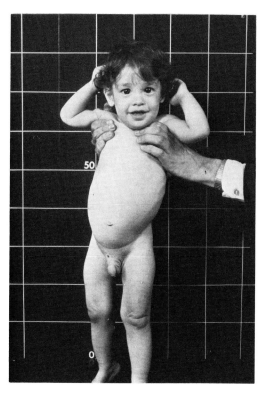

Fig. 8-8. Chronic diarrhea and urinary tract infection. This is a 15-month-old child with anemia, chronic diarrhea, and failure to thrive who was found to have hydronephrosis and infection secondary to congenital stenosis of the left ureteropelvic junction.

New epidemiologic information has become available on the relationship between respiratory infections and acute bouts of diarrhea. It is suspected that a concomitant infection of both the gastrointestinal and the respiratory tract is responsible, but as yet it remains unproved. A prospective study of 152 children with acute gastroenteritis has shown that 66% of the 74 with rotavirus in their stools had a respiratory infection, usually preceding the gastrointestinal symptoms. By comparison, evidence of respiratory infection was present in 26% of those with a bacterial enteritis and in 31% of the small number of children in whom other viruses were isolated from the stools. Of note is the observation that otitis was present in 27% of those with rotavirus gastroenteritis. It is disappointing that viral particles were not found in nine cases where electron microscopy of nasopharyngeal secretions was carried out.

Malnutrition and diarrhea

Malnourished children are more prone to suffer enteral infections. Depression in cell-mediated immunity and a decreased ability of the humoral system to respond to certain antigenic stimuli contribute to the propensity of malnourished children for infections. Malnutrition may lead to intestinal dysfunction characterized by an altered mucosal structure, defective disaccharidase activity, abnormal motility, and a changed intestinal bacterial flora. In countries in which protein malnutrition (kwashiorkor) or protein-calorie malnutrition (nutritional marasmus) affects the population, diarrhea occurs as part of the syndrome.

In the previously well-nourished infant who develops an acute bout of gastroenteritis, survival is more dependent on prompt and appropriate repair of water and electrolyte disturbances than on caloric needs. Little harm is done in well-nourished infants with diarrhea by starving them for a short period. On the other hand, in cases of malnutrition, survival may be limited not only by the disturbances in electrolyte and water balance but significantly by calorie deficit. It is now recognized that worsening of the diarrhea may be precipitated by ill-advised prolonged "resting of the alimentary canal" in children with diarrhea whose nutritional status is borderline and in whom one can assume that the integrity of the intestinal mucosa has been altered. It has been shown that the absorption of nutrients and electrolytes can be increased when the infant with diarrhea is fed. The stools, concomitantly, will be bulkier and more frequent, but there is at least tentative evidence that the duration of most diarrheal illnesses is not prolonged. However, the recommendation still stands that malnourished infants admitted with acute gastroenteritis should be offered a lactose-free formula. In addition to morphological changes of the brush border there are studies showing a reduction of pancreatic enzyme output, a decrease of conjugated bile acids, and alterations in intestinal function. A striking decrease in intestinal motility is a concomitant of protein-calorie malnutrition. This, in turn, leads to bacterial overgrowth in the upper bowel, further impairing micellar solubilization by deconjugating available conjugated bile acids and bringing about a decrease in disaccharidase content of the intestinal wall.

Over the years, we have been impressed with the number of young infants who, as a consequence of a prolonged or relapsing type of gastroenteritis, are admitted with iatrogenic malnutrition. Admittedly alterations in digestive functions manifested by diarrhea and malabsorption lead to multiple nutritional deficiencies. However, nutritional deficiencies of minerals, vitamins, proteins, and calories in infants with diarrhea are often in large part secondary to "starving" diets and contribute significantly to the morbidity and mortality associated with diarrheal diseases.

Treatment of the severely malnourished young infant with diarrhea is a challenge. The provision by the oral route of required nutrients and calories is usually impossible. Tolerance is greatly increased when one resorts to continuous nasogastric feeding of a 10 kcal/30 ml dilution of Pregestimil. Supplemental calories are given by peripheral parenteral nutrition. Because many infants with severe malnutrition and diarrhea suffer from "intractable diarrhea," the reader is directed to the discussion of that entity. Because of the readily established vicious circle of diarrhea → malnutrition → diarrhea in young infants, a plea is made for early repletion of protein and calorie deficits to reverse the gastrointestinal alterations associated with malnutrition.

Dietary diarrhea

The dietetic causes of diarrhea are numerous. Perhaps the most common factor responsible for dietary diarrhea in the infant is overfeeding. Most of the candidates for this type of diarrhea are babies who, in the first 3 months of life, are fussy and have colicky pain. Their cries will lead to their being fed excessively large amounts of formula. Gastric distention will stimulate the gastrocolic reflex shortening the transit time. The stage is then set for an osmotic type of diarrhea secondary to the incomplete digestion and absorption of osmotically active solutes.

A change in the composition of the infant's formula, a change in the added carbohydrates, a shift from breast feeding to a cow's milk formula, the introduction of new foods such as fruit juices, wheat cereal, egg yolk, vegetables, and so forth can all cause diarrhea. Usually, the infant looks well; more often than not, he may continue thriving despite the passage of loose, greenish stools containing mucus or undigested food particles. Careful history taking is usually sufficient to indicate the offending agent that should be excluded. In older children, ingestion of intestinal irritants such as spices and food high in fermentable roughage can lead to diarrhea.

In the acute and convalescent phases of acute diarrhea, when a milk-free diet is given, the osmotic load provided by large amounts of undiluted fruit juices (pineapple juice, 900 mOsm/L, and apple juice, 650 mOsm/L) may be responsible for continuing diarrhea. With an ever-increasing number of foods containing additives, it is likely that many more cases of chronic diarrhea will eventually be attributed to them.

Sorbitol, a sweet-tasting nonreducing polyalcohol sugar is used as a vehicle for oral medications, a substitute for sugar in candies and gums, an ingredient of some toothpastes, and a plasticizer of gelatin capsules. If consumed in large amounts, sorbitol will give rise to flatulence, abdominal distention, and an osmotic type of diarrhea.

Allergic diarrhea

Gastrointestinal allergy to dietary proteins is a frequently entertained diagnosis but a poorly documented clinical entity. Anaphylaxis is an immunologically mediated (reaginic) systemic reaction often of great severity and potentially life-threatening. Skin, respiratory, cardiovascular, and gastrointestinal manifestations can occur within minutes after exposure. Diarrhea may be a manifestation of anaphylaxis to foods such as eggs, soybeans, milk, nuts, fish and shellfish. Because of the present lack of an immunologic basis for most adverse reactions to foods and food additives, the term "food allergy" has been abandoned in favor of "food sensitivity." Because the laboratory is seldom useful, a rational clinical approach is necessary and includes:

A thorough history and physical examination

Reproduction of the adverse reaction by elimination followed by challenge with the suspected food

Objective confirmation by a double-blind challenge with the encapsulated food

In making a diagnosis of milk allergy, a positive family history, the presence of eczema, rhinitis, or asthma, and sensitivity to foods other than milk are helpful features. Prompt improvement of the diarrhea after milk withdrawal and recurrence of symptoms on readministration are supportive clinical observations. A peripheral eosinophilia, the presence of occult blood in the stools, and histologic and proctoscopic evidence of colitis may offer confirmatory evidence.

It is important to rule out other causes of diarrhea, particularly when the clinical entity and the laboratory findings do not overwhelmingly point toward allergy. When one's index of suspicion is high, a therapeutic trial with a cow's milk protein substitute formula is often warranted. It is important to remember that soy protein preparations give rise to diarrhea in a small number of normal infants but in a greater number of infants with milk allergy. Therefore, one should not rule out milk protein allergy if diarrhea continues in the infant receiving a soybean formula. On the other hand, a satisfactory response to soy formulas may be related not only to the elimination of bovine proteins but also to the exclusion of lactose. This difficult interpretation also applies when other lactose-free formulas such as Nutramigen are used as cow's milk substitutes. A description of allergic gastroenteropathy, milk-induced colitis, and milk allergy is found in Chapter 11.

REFERENCES

Bartlett, J.G.: Antibiotic-associated colitis, Clin. Gastroenterol. **8:**783-803, 1979.

Brunser, O.: Effects of malnutrition on intestinal structure and function in children, Clin. Gastroenterol. **6:**341-355 1977.

Charney, E.B., and Bodurtha, J.N.: Intractable diarrhea associated with the use of sorbitol, J. Pediatr. **98:**157-158, 1981.

Hirschhorn, N.: The treatment of acute diarrhea in children: an historical and physiological perspective, Am. J. Clin. Nutr. **33:**637-663, 1980.

Lewis, H.M., Parry, J.V., Davies, H.A., and others: A year's experience of the rotavirus syndrome and its association with respiratory illness, Arch. Dis. Child. **54:**339-346, 1979.

May, C.D., and Bock, S.A.: A modern approach to food hypersensitivity, Allergy **33**(4):166–88, 1978.

Rees, L., and Brook, C.G.D.: Gradual reintroduction of full-strength milk after acute gastroenteritis in children, Lancet **1:**770-771, 1979.

IRRITABLE COLON SYNDROME

Irritable colon syndrome is a clinical entity giving rise to a chronic nonspecific diarrhea in an otherwise well child. No organic disease is discoverable. For Davidson, who has carried out longitudinal observations, irritable colon syndrome masquerades under a variety of appellations. The newborn with colic the toddler with nonspecific diarrhea, and the older child with recurrent abdominal pain all represent instances of the irritable colon syndrome. In this context, the syndrome is a lifelong condition, symptoms of which may be manifested at any age.

Pathogenesis

The flow of small bowel contents in the colon is regulated by the ileocecal sphincter, which relaxes intermittently. With eating, ileal contents are discharged in the colon, which propels material with to-and-fro movements, permitting the absorption and secretion of water and electrolytes. Colonic motor activity is the result of the integration of segmental nonperistaltic contractions and of propulsive mass movements. Modulation of colonic segmentation is still poorly understood. It is essentially absent during sleep. Food is the main physiologic stimulus; HCl and gastrin do not seem to be involved. Cholecystokinin greatly stimulates segmental contractions; prostaglandins may also have an effect, but this is based on studies in inflammatory bowel disease. Mass movements are strong infrequent propulsive contractions, which occur three or four times a day, and usually start in the transverse colon. At the same time, haustral folds disappear ahead of the onward-moving contracting zone, permitting the rapid transit of material through the transverse and descending colon into the rectal ampulla. Mass movements are stimulated by the ingestion of foods and by an increased intake of dietary fiber.

There is evidence in the irritable colon syndrome that introduction of chilled foods or fluids may trigger mass movements. The role of the fat content of the diet has recently attracted attention because of a study showing that an increase in the percentage of calories ingested as fat leads to an amelioration or a disappearance of diarrhea in more than 80% of cases. A plausible explanation is that fat is a potent inhibitor of gastric emptying. On the other hand, it stimulates the release of cholecystokinin, which increases colonic motor activity. Motility studies carried out years ago by Almy and Davidson have shown an increased tone of the lower colonic segment. The area becomes virtually shut and unable to accept material for desiccation. During sleep, rectal spasm is lessened, and thereby desiccation is allowed to take place. This may be the reason that the head of the first morning stool in children with this disease is commonly of normal consistency. Much work remains to be done in the difficult area of colonic motility in response to stress and emotions.

The mouth-to-anus transit time of 14 ± 4.2

hours is shorter in children with the irritable colon syndrome than the values of 25.4 ± 7.6 hours obtained in age-matched controls. However, we have found no excessive losses of fat, nitrogen, or bile acids. Observations from work in adults suggest that a high-fiber diet (high-residue) "normalizes" both the short (diarrhea) and the prolonged (spastic constipation) transit time associated with the irritable colon syndrome. Preliminary information suggests that a high-fiber diet may also be helpful in children with chronic nonspecific diarrhea.

Clinical findings

The typical patient is described as a child between 8 months and 3 years of age who was a colicky baby and who gradually began having three to six loose stools per day. Most of the stools are passed early during the waking hours, and they are loose and contain undigested foods and mucus. There are no other symptoms present except for a diaper rash. The child is active, looks healthy, has a good appetite, and is growing normally. The diarrhea is made worse by a low-residue diet and by a low-fat and high-carbohydrate diet in relation to total calories. Bouts tend to be precipitated by stress or infection. Some children suffer only one brief episode lasting a few weeks or several months. In others, the functional diarrhea is recurrent or continuous. Regardless of the clinical pattern, there is, after a 2-year period of susceptibility, a gradual clearing of the symptoms. By 39 months of age, most patients are asymptomatic.

Differential diagnosis

Irritable colon syndrome is by far the most common cause of chronic diarrhea in the healthy child. In the majority of cases, a positive diagnosis can be made on the basis of the following clinical information:

1. Onset between 8 and 20 months of age
2. Normal growth and development
3. Loose stools, from three to six daily, with mucus and undigested foods
4. Family history of a functional bowel disorder

Despite the presence of the positive criteria listed, a stool culture, a search for *Giardia,* and testing of the stool pH should be carried out. An infectious type of diarrhea or a disaccharidase deficiency can thereby usually be ruled out. A de-

celeration of growth or a disparity between height and weight warrants testing for malabsorption. On rare occasions, *Giardia* infestation may mimic this clinical condition.

Most children with chronic nonspecific diarrhea are subjected to various restrictive diets in the course of their illness. Frequently the child is on a milk-free diet at the time of the initial consultation and compensates by drinking large amounts of chilled fruit juices, which tend to make things worse. Another qualitative dietary change reported, which not only perpetuates and worsens chronic nonspecific diarrhea but also precipitates it, is a diet deriving less than 30% of its calories from fat. Low-residue diets are also known to have an adverse effect on the symptoms. As a result of restricted diets over a period of several months, the caloric intake may have become insufficient to sustain growth. Therefore, flattening of the weight curve may be compatible with the diagnosis of chronic nonspecific diarrhea unless a thorough dietary history can otherwise document appropriate caloric intake. Needless extensive testing is often carried out because the physician overlooks the fact that the failure to thrive, which is occasionally found, is iatrogenic.

Treatment

Dietary management has dramatic results when the diet history shows a low fat intake in relation to normal amounts of calories (Table 8-11). The results are also impressive in those cases where the low fat intake is coupled with a low total caloric intake. The current advice is to give full-fat milk and to encourage foods with a high fat content such as cheese, butter, margarine, and peanut butter. Monitoring of compliance should be carried out to ensure that 30% to 50% of calories are derived from fat. Response to the diet may take 3 to 14 days. In some toddlers, we have been impressed with the dramatic response to the discontinuation of apple juice, which often is consumed in large amounts. Because it is normal for undigested fruits and vegetables to be recognized in the stools in those whose age group is prone to develop chronic nonspecific diarrhea, there is no indication to restrict them or to decrease other sources of fiber. Fiber is, in fact, helpful.

There is little if any place for drugs in this condition. In some cases Loperamide has been reported to be useful. There are also anecdotal reports on the beneficial use of Questran 2 to 4 gm

Table 8-11. Response of chronic nonspecific diarrhea to an increased intake of fat in relation to antecedent dietary history

Fat intake	Number	Percentage of responders
Adequate energy intake with low fat (<27%)	22	100%
Marginal energy intake with fat greater than 40%	7	85.7%
Adequate energy intake with normal fat (>28%)	15	53.3%

Adapted from Cohen, S.A. et al.: Pediatrics **64**(4):402, 1979, copyright American Academy of Pediatrics.

with breakfast. Finally, encouragement of early toilet training and reassurance that chronic nonspecific diarrhea is a benign self-limited condition are also important in the management.

REFERENCES

Cohen, S.A., Hendricks, K.M., Mattis, R.K., and others: Chronic nonspecific diarrhea: dietary relationships, Pediatrics **64**:402-407, 1979.
Cohen, S.A., Hendricks, K.M., Eastham, E.J., and others: Chronic nonspecific diarrhea: a complication of dietary fat restriction, Am. J. Dis. Child. **133**:490-492, 1979.
Davidson, M., and Wasserman, R.: The irritable colon of childhood, J. Pediatr. **69**:1027-1038, 1966.
Harvey, R.F., Pomare, E.W., and Heaton, K.W.: Effects of increased dietary fibre on intestinal transit, Lancet **1**:1278-1280, 1973.
Lloyd-Still, J.D.: Chronic diarrhea of childhood and the misuse of elimination diets, J. Pediatr. **95**:10-13, 1979.
Schneider, R.E., and Viteri, F.E.: Luminal events of lipid absorption in protein-calorie malnourished children: relationship with nutritional recovery and diarrhea, Am. J. Clin. Nutr. **27**:777-787, 788-796, 1974.
Thompson, G.R., Barrowman, J., Gutierez, L., and others: Action of neomycin on intraluminal phase of lipid absorption, J. Clin. Invest. **50**:319-323, 1971.
Viteri, F.E., and Schneider, R.E.: Gastrointestinal alterations in protein-calorie malnutrition, Med. Clin. North Am. **58**:1487-1505, 1974.
Walker-Smith, J.A.: Annotation. Toddler's diarrhea, Arch. Dis. Child. **55**:329-330, 1980.
Wender, E.H., Palmer, I.B., Herbst, J.J., and others: Behavioral characteristics of children with chronic nonspecific diarrhea, Am. J. Psychiatry **133**:20-25, 1976.

INTRACTABLE DIARRHEA OF INFANCY

Diarrhea in young infants is usually a self-limited disease responsive to supportive care. However, from time to time, the physician is confronted with an infant whose diarrhea is severe and refractory to standard treatment and rapidly leads to life-threatening fluid, electrolyte, protein, and caloric insufficiency. A wide variety of disorders are responsible for the intractable diarrhea syndrome. There are two forms of the syndrome, a primary form called nonspecific enterocolitis and a secondary form under which a number of disease entities are grouped, as follows:

Entities responsible for intractable diarrhea

Anatomical
    Hirschsprung's disease
    Short bowel syndrome
    Congenital or acquired stenosis
    Malrotation
    Contaminated small bowel syndrome
    Intestinal lymphangiectasia
Enteric infections and infestations
    Salmonella enteritis
    Escherichia coli enteritis
    Shigella enteritis
    Campylobacter enteritis
    Yersinia enteritis
    Staphylococcus enteritis
    Giardiasis
    Coccidiosis
    Candidal enteritis
Extraintestinal infection
    Urinary tract infection
    Sepsis
Acquired sugar intolerance
    Lactose intolerance
    Monosaccharide intolerance
Acquired protein intolerance
    Cow's milk protein intolerance
    Soybean protein intolerance
Cystic fibrosis
Selective inborn errors of absorption
    Sucrase-isomaltase deficiency

Glucose-galactose malabsorption
Congenital chloride diarrhea
Primary bile acid malabsorption
Congenital lactase deficiency
Inflammatory bowel disease
    Necrotizing enterocolitis
    Ulcerative colitis
    Granulomatous colitis
    Pseudomembranous enterocolitis
Tumors
    Neuroblastoma
    Ganglioneuroma
    VIP (vasoactive intestinal polypeptide)–secreting tumors
Endocrine disorders
    Adrenal insufficiency
    Adrenogenital syndrome
    Thyrotoxicosis
Miscellaneous
    Coeliac disease
    Abetalipoproteinemia
    Acrodermatitis enteropathica
    Enterokinase deficiency
    Defects of chylomicron formation and secretion
    Wolman's disease
    Immunodeficiency states

Nonspecific enterocolitis

Nonspecific enterocolitis is the most common cause of intractable diarrhea. Avery and his colleagues coined the affection and defined certain diagnostic criteria: diarrhea lasting more than 2 weeks during the first 3 months of life in the absence of any clinical, laboratory, or roentgenographic evidence of an identifiable disease entity. The pathophysiologic mechanisms responsible for the primary form of intractable diarrhea of early infancy are poorly understood. The primary event appears to involve damage to the mucosa of the small intestine, but the nature of the aggressor remains unknown. A workable hypothesis is that an undetected infection favors a hypersensitivity reaction to foreign proteins. Diarrhea rapidly becomes self-perpetuating through a combination of factors such as (1) loss of absorptive surface and diminution of brush-border enzymes, (2) injurious effect of undigested dietary antigens or of bacterial antigens on an inflamed mucosa that has lost its autodefense mechanisms, (3) bacterial overgrowth leading to invasion of the bowel wall, impaired monosaccharide transport, and bile salt deconjugation, and (4) pancreatic insufficiency and depressed local immune mechanisms, which are well known complications of starvation and malnutrition.

Clinical features

Although the average age of onset in most series is between 3 and 5 weeks, there are patients presenting as late as 4½ to 5 months. The initial phase can masquerade as a feeding problem. There is no fever and no signs of toxicity, and the diarrhea may appear to respond transiently after a formula change or a brief period of intravenous fluid therapy. In most cases, however, the symptoms are those of an infectious gastroenteritis.

The *diarrhea* is severe and profuse. It may respond favorably to a period of fasting or use of clear fluids orally, but it will begin again with the reintroduction of a formula. More often, the diarrhea is secretory and will continue unabated despite discontinuation of all oral intake. The number of stools may exceed 20 per day, and fecal losses may reach 100 ml/kg/day. Gross blood in the stool is rare but mucus is frequently noted.

Gastrointestinal symptoms other than diarrhea were initially considered relatively rare by our group. In retrospect, vomiting (70%) and abdominal distention (50%) are surprisingly common.

Systemic manifestations are most impressive. The clinical picture is dominated by dehydration, acidosis, and malnutrition. The majority of our own cases were below birth weight when first seen.

The *feeding history* is of interest in that invariably affected infants have been and are being formula-fed when the symptoms begin. We have yet to see a breast-fed baby with nonspecific enterocolitis.

Extraintestinal infections and administration of antibiotics can be documented by history in half the cases.

Laboratory, x-ray, and histologic findings

A constant finding is hypoalbuminemia. Air-fluid levels are especially evident in those infants with abdominal distention. Upper gastrointestinal and barium enema examinations are negative. Mild to severe inflammatory changes and mucosal alterations in the small bowel have been described. The histologic features of the upper small bowel do not correlate well with the severity of the symptoms or with the degree of malnutrition. However, a form of nonspecifc enterocolitis with a particularly bad prognosis is associated with small bowel biopsy specimens showing almost complete lack of recognizable mucosal architecture. They may be milder in the jejunum than in the ileum (Fig. 8-9). Inflammatory changes are also occa-

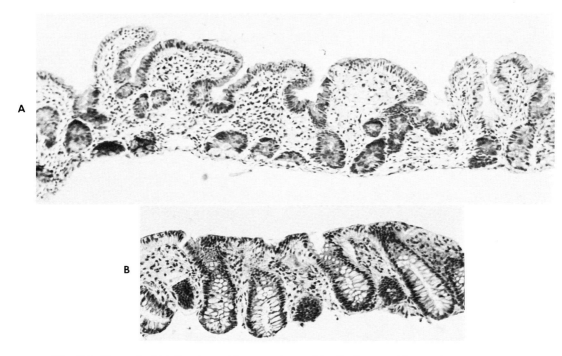

Fig. 8-9. Six-week-old infant boy with severe intractable diarrhea requiring total parenteral alimentation for a period of 3 months. **A,** Jejunal biopsy shows shortening and clubbing of villi. **B,** Changes are much more severe in the ileum, where there is total disappearance of normal architecture.

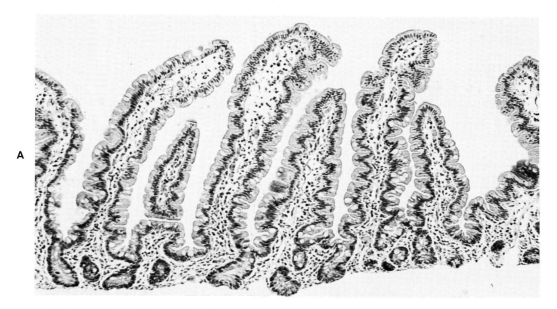

Fig. 8-10. Intractable diarrhea. **A,** This normal jejunal biopsy was taken from a 2-month-old infant with intractable diarrhea. The specimen was taken during the acute stage of the illness. **B,** In contrast, the rectal biopsy was abnormal. There were acute inflammatory changes. Polymorphonuclear cells are seen breaking through the epithelial lining of a crypt, giving rise to a typical crypt abscess.

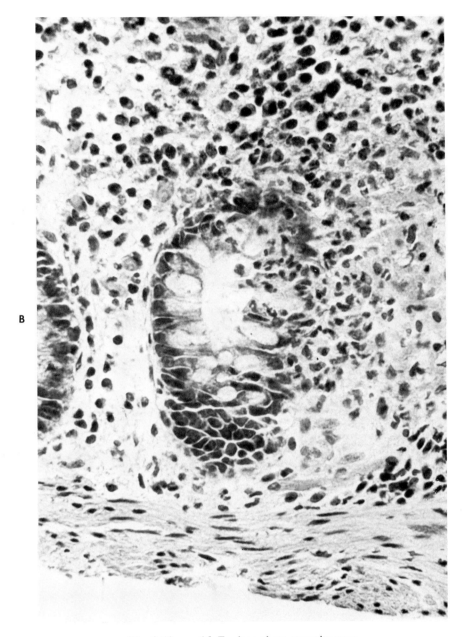

Fig. 8-10, cont'd. For legend see opposite page.

sionally noted in the colon; in certain instances, they may be more severe than in the jejunum (Fig. 8-10).

Secondary form of intractable diarrhea

In our experience, no specific diagnosis can be established in the majority of infants with intractable diarrhea. A discussion of each entity responsible for intractable diarrhea is found elsewhere in this book. The most frequently identifiable enti-

ties besides the short bowel syndrome are the following: Hirschsprung's disease, enteric infections, cow's milk protein intolerance, cystic fibrosis, and sucrase-isomaltase deficiency.

Diagnosis

The young infant with diarrhea that lasts for more than 2 weeks and shows continued loss of weight should be considered as having intractable diarrhea of infancy once results of stool examinations have indicated that pathogenic microorganisms (bacteria and viruses) are not present.

Stool pH and tests for reducing substances will permit detection of a primary or secondary disaccharidase deficiency. The physician should be aware, however, that finding a low pH and the presence of reducing substances is not unusual in diarrheal stools and is not necessarily indicative of the conditions for which the patient is being tested. Stools should also be checked for the presence of occult blood; milk colitis, allergic gastroenteropathy, and nonspecific enterocolitis may be seriously considered if stools are positive for blood.

A simple roentgenogram of the abdomen is rarely informative because air-fluid levels, so commonly present with an anatomic lesion such as a stenotic small or large bowel, are also seen in young infants with diarrhea from a variety of causes. A barium enema and an upper gastrointestinal examination are much more useful and should be done early in the investigation. A rectoscopic examination and rectal biopsy should be carried out, particularly if there is blood in the stools or if the clinical findings are compatible with Hirschsprung's disease. A small bowel biopsy is important for the diagnosis, especially since a few entities responsible for the secondary form of intractable diarrhea give rise to specific biopsy features. Because the duodenum is intubated for the small bowel biopsy, duodenal fluid can be collected through separate tubing for aerobic and anaerobic cultures for measurement of the percentage of free and secondary bile acids and quantitation of pancreatic enzymes.

Results of a sweat test and determination of stool chymotrypsin should help to rule out the possibility of cystic fibrosis, which stands high on the list of differential diagnoses. Remember that malnutrition readily brings about exocrine pancreatic insufficiency and that the associated hypoproteinemia and edema may give rise to falsely low sweat-chloride values. The serum electrolyte abnormalities seen in chloride diarrhea or the adrenogenital syndrome can be easily noted. Measurements of immunoglobulins and cellular immunity tests will rule out an immune defect.

Results of tests of carbohydrate absorption (glucose, D-xylose, disaccharides) are impossible to interpret in the infant suffering from diarrhea, and the tests are better put off until some degree of nutritional rehabilitation has been achieved. A

72-hour stool collection between two nonabsorbable markers will permit evaluation of stool volume and electrolyte concentrations. Bile acid excretion should be measured because primary bile acid malabsorption has been reported. Fat malabsorption is difficult to evaluate because these very sick infants do not ingest appropriate amounts of fat.

Catecholamine, vasoactive intestinal peptide (VIP), gastrin, and calcitonin assays will rule out tumors associated with diarrhea.

Treatment of nonspecific enterocolitis

Emergency therapy should be aimed at restoring blood volume and acid-base and electrolyte abnormalities. Because all these patients are severely malnourished, caloric deficits are high. Peripheral parenteral nutrition is initiated by use of Travasol 2.5 gm/kg, dextrose 10 gm/kg, Intralipid 2 gm/kg, and water 150 ml/kg of body weight. This provides 66 kcal/kg/day, which falls short of the usual needs but will slowly correct deficits during the initial period of observation and testing. A short period of bowel rest is recommended as part of the work-up, since it will provide the physician with an opportunity to see what effect it has on the stool output. Continuing severe diarrhea (more than 50 ml/kg/day) in the absence of any oral intake indicates a secretory type of intractable diarrhea, which will prove more difficult to control.

Experimental and clinical work has shown the importance of intraluminal nutrients to maintain the anatomic and functional integrity of the small bowel mucosa. This trophic effect is essentially absent when a monomeric diet (amino acids and dextrose is fed. We therefore attempt refeeding with Pregestimil (casein hydrolysate, long-chain and medium-chain triglycerides, and glucose polymer) given in small amounts at a concentration of 0.33 kcal/ml (10 kcal/30 ml). If tolerance is good, increasing quantities and concentrations are offered and the infant is discharged on this formula for the next few months.

In the absence of a satisfactory response, a low concentration and a small volume of the same formula is given continuously through a small nasogastric silicone rubber tube. During this period most of the calories are provided by the peripheral intravenous route. Enteral feedings are steadily increased in quantity and concentration. We agree with Ricour and colleagues in Paris that quantity

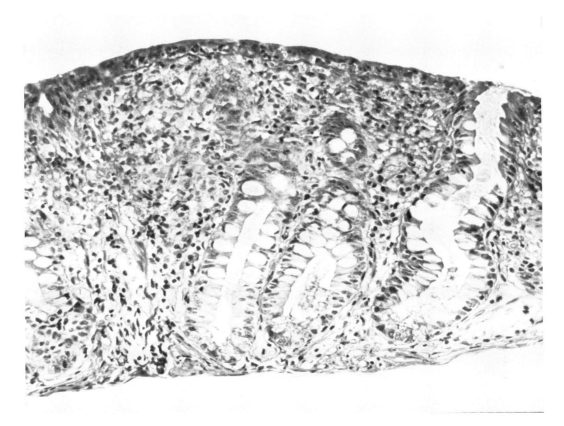

Fig. 8-11. Intractable diarrhea. This small bowel biopsy section taken after 7 months of total parenteral nutrition shows a totally atrophic mucosa with extensive epithelial changes and a dense inflammatory infiltrate.

can be increased in a stepwise fashion much more rapidly than concentration. Infants with intractable diarrhea are very sensitive to hyperosmolar solutions. Consequently, we suggest that solutions exceeding 285 mOsm/kg of water should not be given. On the other hand, the volume can often be pushed up to a range of 200 to 250 ml/kg/day. Tolerance is monitored by stool volume rather than by the number of evacuations. Stool pH and reducing substances are checked regularly as evidence of carbohydrate intolerance which is an indication to decrease the amounts fed or to change the composition of the formula. Attention has recently been drawn to difficulties with glucose polymers in a 7-week-old infant. Elemental diets are used by some groups; however, their high osmolality is a distinct disadvantage. Breast milk has also been used successfully.

Unfortunately, significant amounts of calories are poorly tolerated by a certain number of infants fed by either the intermittent oral or the continuous nasogastric route, and they have to be discontinued. These infants can be maintained on peripheral alimentation if they gain weight, but this is exceptional because the majority have high caloric needs (125 to 200 kcal/kg/day), which can only be met by a central catheter (see p. 874). A severe form of secretory diarrhea with 24-hour stool volumes of 100 to 300 ml/kg/day precludes enteral feedings. A central catheter is then necessary because total parenteral nutrition will need to be continued for a period of more than a month and sometimes for a period of more than a year. Attempts at reintroduction of oral feedings are made at monthly intervals.

Antibiotics have not been helpful. Corticosteroids have been used in some cases with severe atrophy and absence of signs of regeneration of the mucosa, however, they have not been shown to be effective. Antidiarrheal medications are useless and probably harmful. Cholestyramine is said to be effective in cases where large fecal bile acid losses are documented, yet we have had no success with this drug.

Prognosis

The outcome of this severe and challenging affection has changed dramatically with the advent of parenteral nutrition. The mortality has dropped from 75% to 10%. However, the morbidity is high and the course is often unpredictable. After the patient is discharged from a lengthy hospitalization, persisting diarrhea and failure to thrive are seen in a few patients whose small bowel histologic condition shows evidence of ongoing severe damage (Fig. 8-11). Fortunately, the majority of infants with nonspecific enterocolitis exhibit catch-up growth and follow normal developmental milestones.

REFERENCES

Avery, G.B., Villaviciencio, O., Lilly, J.R., and Randolph, J.G.: Intractable diarrhea in early infancy, Pediatrics **41:**712-722, 1968.

Balistreri, W.F., Partin, J.C., and Schubert, W.K.: Bile acid malabsorption: a consequence of terminal ileal dysfunction in protracted diarrhea of infancy, J. Pediatr. **89:**21-28, 1977.

Davidson, G.P., Cutz, E., Hamilton, J.R., and Gall, D.C.: Familial enteropathy: a syndrome of protracted diarrhea from birth, failure to thrive, and hypoplastic villus atrophy, Gastroenterology **75:**783-790, 1978.

Fisher, S.E., Leone, G., and Kelly, R.H.: Chronic protracted intolerance to dietary glucose polymers, Pediatrics **67:**271-273, 1981.

Greene, H.L., McCabe, D.R., and Merenstein, G.B.: Protracted diarrhea and malnutrition in infancy: changes in intestinal morphology and disaccharidase activities during treatment with total intravenous nutrition or oral elemental diets, J. Pediatr. **87:**695-704, 1975.

Gunn, T., Brown, R.S., Pencharz, P., and Colle, E.: Total parenteral nutrition in malnourished infants with intractable diarrhea, Can. Med. Assoc. J. **117:**357-360, 1977.

Heird, W.C., and Winters, R.W.: Total parenteral nutrition: the state of the art, J. Pediatr. **86:**2-17, 1975.

Heubi, J.E., Balistreri, W.F., Partin, J.C., and others: Refractory infantile diarrhea due to primary bile acid malabsorption, J. Pediatr. **94:**546-551, 1979.

Hyman, C.J., Reiter, J., Rodnan, J., and Drash, A.L.: Parenteral and oral alimentation in the treatment of the nonspecific protracted diarrheal syndrome of infancy, J. Pediatr. **78:**17-29, 1971.

Jonas, A., Avigad, S., Diver-Haber, A., and Katznelson, D.: Disturbed fat absorption following infectious gastroenteritis in children, J. Pediatr. **95:**366-372, 1979.

Keating, J.P., and Ternberg, J.L.: Amino-acid hypertonic glucose treatment for intractable diarrhea in infants, Am. J. Dis. Child. **122:**226-228, 1971.

Larcher, V.F., Shepherd, R., Francis, D.E.M., and Harries, J.T.: Protracted diarrhea in infancy: analysis of 82 cases with particular reference to diagnosis and management, Arch. Dis. Child. **52:**597-605, 1977.

Lloyd-Still, J.D., Shwachman, H., and Filler, R.M.: Protracted diarrhea of infancy treated by intravenous alimentation, Am. J. Dis. Child. **125:**358-364, 365-368, 1973.

MacLean, W.C., Lopez de Romana, G., Massa, E., and Graham, G.G.: Nutritional management of chronic diarrhea and malnutrition, primary reliance on oral feeding, J. Pediatr. **97:**316-323, 1980.

Sunshine, P., Sinatra, F.R., and Mitchell, C.H.: Intractable diarrhea of infancy, Clin. Gastroenterol. **6:**445-461, 1977.

Tamer, M.A., Santora, T.R., and Sandberg, D.H.: Cholestyramine therapy for intractable diarrhea, Pediatrics **53:**217-220, 1974.

ACRODERMATITIS ENTEROPATHICA

Acrodermatitis enteropathica is a rare autosomal recessive disorder of zinc absorption leading to chronic diarrhea and characteristic skin lesions. The term is also applied to any acquired zinc-deficiency state resulting in the same clinical picture.

Moynihan first recognized that plasma zinc was low and that recovery could be induced with zinc supplements. Early findings that human milk and diiodohydroxyquinolone were effective as therapy are now explained by an improved bioavailability of zinc. Although the zinc concentration of breast milk does not differ significantly from cow's milk, it contains low molecular weight zinc-binding ligands, which facilitate zinc absorption. Patients with this inborn disorder have a reduced accumulation of zinc in their mucosal biopsy specimens and are in negative balance when off therapy. In the face of low intraluminal zinc concentration provided by a normal diet, the absorption is defective. However, when higher amounts are provided, zinc absorption proceeds at a rate similar to that observed in normal subjects. Zinc is transported across the mucosal brush border by a mechanism that appears to require ATP. It then may be transported across the cell attached to an endogenous chelator. The inherited molecular defect in acrodermatitis enteropathica remains undetermined.

Acquired zinc-deficiency states occur when intake is inadequate, absorption is defective, or there are excessive losses. It is noted with some frequency in patients on total parenteral nutrition who are not provided with zinc and in disorders such as Crohn's and celiac diseases. Low zinc levels are reported in cystic fibrosis. Large losses are documented in some patients with an ileostomy. Urinary zinc excretion is also increased in various liver diseases.

Clinical features

The most consistent feature is a severe dermatitis over the peripheral aspects of the extremities and around the mouth, anus, and genitalia (Fig.

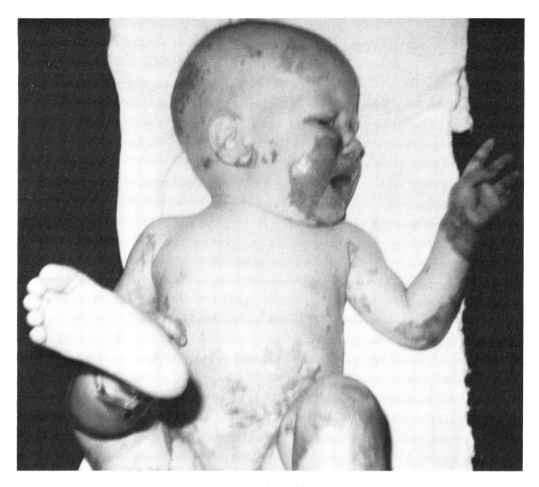

Fig. 8-12. Acrodermatitis enteropathica in an infant with alopecia and a widespread erythematous orificial acral rash. (Courtesy K.M. Hambidge and Spectrum Publications Inc., New York.)

8-12). It may become generalized. The lesions are erythematous, vesicobullous, pustular, or eczematoid, or of any combination. Severe nail dystrophy, alopecia, loss of eyebrows, conjunctivitis, photophobia, and corneal opacities are less constant. Chronic diarrhea is present in most patients, as well as hypogeusia, anorexia, and failure to thrive. Irritability, lethargy, and depression are well described neuropsychiatric manifestations. Increased susceptibility to infections is attributable to adverse effects of zinc deficiency on both cellular and humoral immunity. Hypogonadism is reported in adolescence.

Diagnosis

Because of the inconsistency of symptoms and signs, the clinician must have a high index of suspicion when faced with an anal and orificial rash in an infant who is formula-fed or who has been weaned a few months before the onset. Similarly, in conditions where zinc deficiency is known to occur, this diagnosis should be considered.

The most helpful laboratory determination to confirm the diagnosis is a plasma or serum zinc value below 6 μmol/liter. Only plastic ware should be used for sample collections, and rubber stoppers should be avoided. The few cases of acrodermatitis without hypozincemia are believed to result from sample contamination. The recent description of clinical features of the disease in a few premature breast-fed infants is the apparent result of an inability of some mothers to secrete zinc into their milk.

Treatment and prognosis

In the inborn disorder, oral zinc therapy has to be continued indefinitely. The quantity of zinc that is necessary varies between 30 and 45 mg regardless of age or size. It can be given as zinc sulfate or zinc acetate; 4.5 mg of the former and 3 mg of the latter is equivalent to 1 mg of elemental zinc. It is better absorbed if given between meals.

Oral zinc therapy results in rapid and complete clinical and biochemical remissions. The improvement is truly dramatic within a very short period of time after initiation of the treatment.

REFERENCES

Aggett, P.J., Atherton, D.J., Delves, H.T., and others: Studies in acrodermatitis enteropathica. In Kirchgeisner, M., editor: Proceedings of the Third International Symposium on trace element metabolism in man and animals, 1978, Technical University of Munich, Freising, pp. 210-215.

Cash, R., and Berger, C.K.: Acrodermatitis enteropathica: defective metabolism of unsaturated fatty acids, J. Pediatr. **74:**717-729, 1969.

Evans, G.W., and Johnson, P.E.: Zinc binding factor in acrodermatitis enteropathica, Lancet **1:**52, 1977.

Garrets, M., and Molokhia, M.: Acrodermatitis enteropathica without hypozincemia, J. Pediatr. **91:**492-494, 1977.

Hambidge, K.M., Walravens, P.A., and Neldner, K.H.: The role of zinc in the pathogenesis and treatment of acrodermatitis enteropathica. In zinc metabolism: current aspects in health and disease, New York, 1977, Alan R. Liss, Inc.

Kelly, P., Davidson, G.P., Townley, R.R.W., and Campbell, P.E.: Reversible intestinal mucosal abnormality in acrodermatitis enteropathica, Arch. Dis. Child. **51:**219-222, 1976.

Clinical approach to chronic diarrhea in infants and children

A considerable body of knowledge has developed concerning the structure, physiology, immunology, and developmental biochemistry of the gastrointestinal tract in children. The advent of sophisticated instrumentation and testing procedures has improved our capability to diagnose and manage certain specific entities responsible for diarrhea. However, there are still great gaps in our insight into a large number of infants and children with abnormal stools.

The clinician's dilemma is usually centered around deciding whether or not the child with persistent or recurrent diarrhea has an organic disease requiring investigation and treatment. The following discussion is a review of some aspects of the clinical assessment of the child with chronic diarrhea and an evaluaton of the usefulness of a certain number of clinical laboratory tests as well as of intestinal biopsies.

Chronic diarrhea: disease or symptom?

The differential diagnosis of chronic diarrhea in children is extensive and there is no substitute for a meticulous clinical assessment. It provides the clinician with the information required to sort out his patients into three different broad categories, as follows:

1. Those who only require watchful waiting
2. A certain proportion who should have a limited number of simple clinical laboratory tests
3. A small number who require extensive testing.

History

Because of the frequency and importance of congenital disorders, a thorough genetic history is essential. It should provide information on the health of relatives, consanguinity, and diseases and early deaths in siblings. A history of change in bowel habits is often more important than the number and consistency of stools. A precise record of the child's dietary and drug history should be obtained. Accurate information concerning the stooling pattern and the type of stools is important. Finally a description of associated symptoms and of the repercussions of the illness on the child's general health and growth should be sought.

We occasionally see children with an abnormal number and consistency of stools who turn out to have chronic constipation. A number of diseases of other systems or organs may secondarily affect gastrointestinal function and lead to diarrhea. In this regard, ear infections and urinary tract disease are well-known causes of chronic diarrhea, particularly in infants (Fig. 8-8). A secretory type of diarrhea may be associated with functional tumors. The majority are neuroblastomas (Fig. 8-13) or ganglioneuromas but vasoactive intestinal peptide–producing pancreatic tumors have also been reported. Although congenital structural anomalies of the gastrointestinal tract leading to diarrhea are usually associated with abdominal distention and vomiting, it may not always be the case (Fig. 8-14).

Because age is an important factor affecting the prevalence of certain conditions associated with chronic diarrhea, it provides helpful clues by limiting diagnostic hypotheses. However, there are pitfalls to a hermetic classification of chronic diarrhea on the basis of age; for example, chronic inflammatory bowel disease may start as early as the first 6 months of life. The timing of the diarrhea with respect to the dietary history is particularly important. Knowledge of the sequence of in-

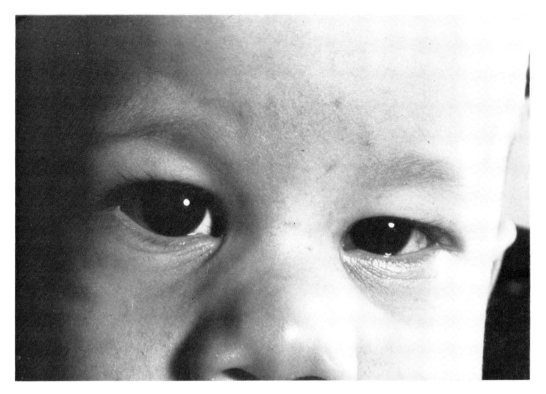

Fig. 8-13. Diarrhea associated with a neuroblastoma. This infant presented with profuse watery diarrhea, ptosis of the left upper eyelid, and meiosis (Horner's syndrome).

Fig. 8-14. Duplication of the ileum in an infant who presented with diarrhea and failure to thrive.

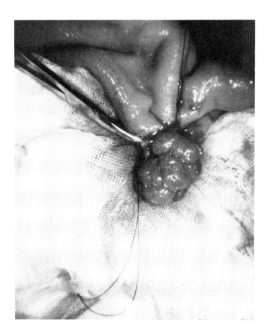

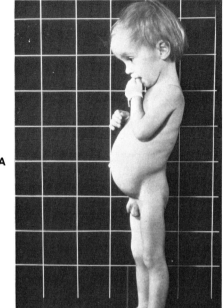

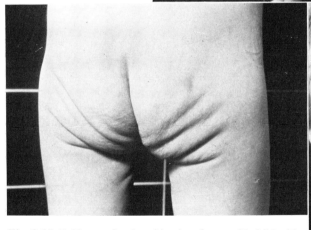

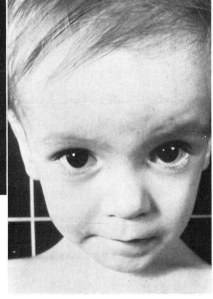

Fig. 8-15. Evidence of malnutrition in a 3-year-old child with celiac disease. Note, **A,** the distended lax abdomen with poor musculature, **B,** empty buttocks, and, **C,** sparse hair, large eyes, and thin face with a sad expression.

troduction of food products and their temporal relationship to diarrhea is essential. Since food additives and drugs can also be associated with diarrhea, this information should also be sought. In milk protein allergy, the dietary history is only helpful in those babies who are breast-fed and whose symptoms start at the time of weaning. The infant whose diarrhea starts shortly after the introduction of cereals and fruit is unlikely to be suffering from celiac disease but may have sucrase-isomaltase deficiency. Patients with gluten enteropathy become symptomatic several months after the introduction of gluten, but it may take years. The dietary history will also permit an estimate of total calories ingested and therefore of appetite. The good appetite of children with cystic fibrosis contrasts with the anorexia of those with celiac disease or with chronic inflammatory bowel disease.

Physical signs

A large number of physical signs have potential diagnostic value in the child with diarrhea. However, the most important information is often derived from the period of inspection during which the physician will come to grips with the following questions. Categorizing chronic diarrhea on the basis of its repercussions on the state of nutrition, growth, and pubertal changes is a most useful clinical tool. Clinical signs of malnutrition are at times evident (Fig. 8-15). It is surprising how often the clinician, rather than the parent, will be first to recognize failure to thrive. The subtle slowing of weight gain and statural growth is seldom appreciated in the close day-to-day relationship between mother and child. On the other hand, parents will readily recognize weight loss or lack of growth over a certain period of time. A decrease in the rate of weight gain out of proportion to that of height is usual in cases of chronic diarrhea with malabsorption or anorexia. Categorizing chronic diarrhea on the basis of its repercussions on nutrition and growth is not without occasional problems. Classically, sucrase-isomaltase deficiency is not associated with failure to thrive; however, this has not been our experience because more than 50% are below the third percentile in weight. Other entities known to have devastating effects on nutrition and growth may be missed if the clinician relies too heavily on the nutritional status of his patient. Celiac disease is occasionally associated with a reasonably normal state of nutrition, especially if the diagnosis is made early.

Iatrogenic failure to thrive is a frequent problem. Prolonged dietary restrictions for suspected food intolerance or for persistent diarrheal stools after a bout of gastroenteritis or as a component of maternal deprivation may lead to malnutrition. Failure to thrive is often wrongly attributed to chronic diarrhea and leads to considering a different category of entities unless the pediatrician recognizes that caloric intake has been drastically reduced. In order to have a balanced view of chronic diarrhea in the infant and toddler, it is important to remember that a large percentage of chronic diarrheas between the ages of 6 and 36 months can be attributed to the irritable bowel syndrome. A number of these children who are otherwise perfectly healthy undergo needless dietary restrictions, therapeutic interventions, and laboratory studies.

Laboratory tests

The clinician can go far in the differential diagnosis of chronic diarrhea by making a thorough clinical assessment of his patient. This can be supplemented by a few simple laboratory tests, which, to a large extent, can be performed in the office.

Stool

Stool examination. Examination of a stool is a valuable aid in the assessment of children with gastrointestinal disease. A microscopic examination of a small amount of feces emulsified with water and stained with methylene blue can lead to a diagnosis. Polymorphonuclear leukocytes are seen in acute bacterial enterocolitis, whereas lymphocytes may predominate in chronic inflammatory bowel disease. The presence of eosinophils suggests milk or soybean protein intolerance.

Fat. Neutral fat characterized by large globules, which will stain with Sudan red, suggests pancreatic insufficiency. Fatty acid diarrhea, such as seen in celiac disease, becomes manifest as refractile crystals under polarized light. These crystals do not stain with Sudan red.

Parasites. The main concern in the hunt for parasites is *Giardia*. One has to remember that 50% of patients with giardiasis will have a negative stool examination. A preparation for *Entamoeba histolytica* should also be examined.

pH and reducing substances. pH and reducing substances are useful tests for the diagnosis of sugar intolerance. Most newborns on breast milk and a significant number on formulas will have reducing substances in their stools. Assessment for reducing substances is especially important in the child who develops chronic watery diarrhea after a bout of acute enteritis. When the onset occurs shortly after birth, a diagnosis of primary lactose deficiency or of congenital glucose-galactose intolerance is probable. When a low pH and reducing substances are found shortly after the introduction of cereals or sucrose, sucrase-isomaltase deficiency should be suspected.

Blood. Testing stools for blood is an important office procedure in any child who has anemia, unexplained abdominal pain, or diarrhea. We still use Hematest tablets. Although such testing is not ideal, there are few false negatives and an acceptable number of false positives.

Cultures. In our experience, bacterial cultures are positive in less than 20% of children with acute enteritis and the yield of pathogens is very small in the case of chronic diarrhea, except for occasional cases of *Salmonella, Yersinia,* and *Campylobacter.*

Three-day stool collection

When one is confronted with an infant with chronic diarrhea and failure to thrive in the face of satisfactory caloric ingestions, fat malabsorption has to be suspected. A 3-day stool collection for fat and chymotrypsin is a practical technique to assess fat-absorptive function. Normal chymotrypsin values rule out a pancreatic cause but should be supplemented by a sweat test. In our lab, 3.5 gm of fat per 24 hours is the upper limit of normal during the first 2 years of life. Subsequently, 5 gm is the upper limit. We use carmine red markers for stool collection, which can be done at home. Close monitoring of fat intake is carried out only in children with questionable values or in those with a poor intake of fat.

Blood work and urine

Serum protein electrophoresis is a rough indicator of a child's state of nutrition or of the presence of a protein-losing enteropathy. Albumin synthesis is very sensitive to inadequate protein intake; however, it can keep up with a certain degree of protein-losing enteropathy (PLE). Consequently, serum protein electrophoresis may not pick up mild cases of protein-losing enteropathy. A study with chromium-labeled albumin may then be necessary. A complete blood count is a must, as well as a urine analysis and culture.

X-ray studies

Although the importance of a roentgenographic study of the gastrointestinal tract in infancy is undisputed, it is of limited value in the assessment of most children with chronic diarrhea or suspected malabsorption. Roentgenographic studies in the pediatric patient should never be considered a routine diagnostic procedure. Plain films of the abdomen, though of value under many circumstances, do not provide worthwhile information in most children with diarrhea. Exceptions are those infants in whom one suspects an anatomical lesion. Contrast films in children with chronic diarrhea and failure to thrive also have a very low diagnostic yield. One does not need an upper gastrointestinal series to diagnose cystic fibrosis or celiac disease, the two commonest disorders causing steatorrhea in infants. They should be reserved for cases in which an anatomic lesion is suspected.

D-Xylose

The 60-minute D-xylose absorption test is a very good measure of upper small bowel mucosal disease. We have yet to see a symptomatic case of celiac disease with a 60-minute D-xylose above 25 mg/dl. More recently, this test has also proved its value for the diagnosis of milk protein allergy. The normal D-xylose test obtained on a milk-restricted diet becomes abnormal within 5 days of a challenge with homogenized milk.

Small bowel biopsy

This procedure is associated with a very low risk. It is easily carried out and yields important information. Histologic changes are pathognomonic in a few disorders, they are of diagnostic value in many others. A diagnosis of celiac disease should never be made without a biopsy.

Rectoscopy and biopsy

A rectoscopy and biopsy should be carried out in all cases of chronic diarrhea with urgency, tenesmus, or night stooling, and if gross or occult blood is present. It is essential in all age groups where chronic inflammatory bowel disease is suspected.

Differential diagnosis

Chronic diarrhea may be secondary to a number of congenital and acquired disorders of the gastrointestinal tract of the liver and of the pancreas, but it can also reflect an underlying metabolic or endocrine problem, infections elsewhere, improper diet, or a drug reaction.

Although Table 8-12 may appear exhaustive, it only groups disease categories and entities in which chronic diarrhea may be an important feature. For instance, chronic liver disorders have not been listed because there are invariably other signs orienting the clinician. The table provides clues to the causes of chronic diarrhea based on age, type of diarrhea, salient anamnestic features, clinical signs, and repercussions on the patient's health and growth. The age shown refers to the usual age of onset of symptoms and does not exclude a later presentation. Table 8-12 makes no attempt at putting in proper perspective the relative frequency of this long list of entities. Probably over 95% of pediatric cases of chronic diarrhea can be attributed to half a dozen entities, which are irritable bowel syndrome, infections and infestations, chronic inflammatory bowel diseases, cystic fibrosis, celiac disease, and disaccharidase deficiencies.

Table 8-12. Guide to differential diagnosis of chronic diarrhea in infants and children

Disease category and entities	Age	Type of diarrhea	Associated clinical features	Repercussions on well-being and growth
Infections and infestations				
Salmonella, Yersinia	Any age	Watery, may contain mucus, pus, and blood	Pain, vomiting, fever	Chronic forms are unusual but may lead to significant weight loss
Giardia lamblia	Any age	Bulky, pale, malodorous, often nocturnal	Abdominal distention, flatulence, anorexia	Failure to thrive especially if associated immune defect
Parenteral infections				
Otitis media and urinary tract infection	< 2 years	Usually mild	Symptoms of underlying infection may be minimal	Vary with severity of infection
Postinfectious diarrhea				
(carbohydrate intolerance, fat malabsorption, malnutrition)	< 2 years	Can be severe if large carbohydrate intake or malnutrition	Clinical picture of carbohydrate intolerance, malabsorption, or marasmus	Malnutrition often iatrogenic, that is, secondary to ''starving'' diets
Dietary factors				
Overfeeding	< 6 months	Watery	Colicky baby	None, the baby is often fat
Milk protein allergy, soy protein allergy	< 2 months	Watery to fatty, at times mucus and blood	Vomiting, anemia; peripheral edema is rare	Mild (anemia) to severe (resembles celiac syndrome)
Intolerance to certain foods	< 6 months	Watery	Follows introduction of new foods	None
Acrodermatitis enteropathica	< 12 months	Severe	Alopecia, dermatitis, conjunctivitis, vomiting	Malnutrition

Continued.

Table 8-12. Guide to differential diagnosis of chronic diarrhea in infants and children—cont'd

Disease category and entities	Age	Type of diarrhea	Associated clinical features	Repercussions on well-being and growth
Irritable bowel syndrome	6 to 36 months	Watery, abundant mucus, undigested foods	None; often follows a bout of acute diarrhea and vomiting	None
Toxic diarrhea (Antibiotics, iron preparations, chemotherapy, radiation)	Any age	Loose, may contain modest amount of fat	Vomiting, anorexia	In the case of radiation enterocolitis, malnutrition may be severe
Functional tumors (Neuroblastoma, Zollinger-Ellison syndrome, carcinoid tumor, pancreatic cholera)	Any age	Severe, secretory diarrhea	Large spectrum of symptoms and signs; hypokalemia is common	Variable
Carbohydrate malabsorption Congenital Sucrose-isomaltose	< 6 months	Varies with sucrose intake	Abdominal distention, flatus, pain	Poor growth common if early onset
glucose-galactose	< 1 month	Watery, intractable	Dehydration, acidosis	Failure to thrive
Acquired lactose intolerance	4 to 8 years	Loose to watery	Abdominal pain, flatus	Normal growth
Secondary Lactose	Any age	Watery	Follows intestinal infections	Variable
Glucose-galactose	< 2 years	Severe watery	After surgery, infections, stagnant-look syndrome	Dehydration, acidosis
Pancreatic disorders Cystic fibrosis	< 6 months	Fatty	Repeated chest infections	Failure to thrive
Shwachman's disease	< 2 years	Fatty	Neutropenia, bone lesions	Variable degree of growth impairment
Chronic pancreatitis	Any age	Usually a late complication	Recurrent abdominal pain with vomiting	Variable degree of growth impairment
Celiac disease	< 2 years usually	Mild to severe	Vomiting, anorexia, abdominal distention	Failure to thrive
Intestinal lymphangiectasis	< 3 months	Mild to severe with fatty stools	Infections, vomiting, lymphedema	Failure to thrive

Table 8-12. Guide to differential diagnosis of chronic diarrhea in infants and children—cont'd

Disease category and entities	Age	Type of diarrhea	Associated clinical features	Repercussions on well-being and growth
Immune defects				
Acquired agammaglobulinemia and isolated IgA deficiency	Any age	Varying severity, often celiac syndrome	Recurrent sinopulmonary infections	Growth impairment
Defective cellular immunity and combined immune deficiency	< 2 years < 1 month	Severe with fat malabsorption	Feeding difficulties, skin rash, stomatitis, repeated infections	Desperately ill with severe failure to thrive
Inborn errors				
Familial chloride diarrhea	< 1 month	Profuse watery	Abdominal distention, alkalosis	Growth usually retarded
Abetalipoproteinemia and hypobetalipoproteinemia	< 3 months	Fatty	Abdominal distention, central nervous system disease	Failure to thrive
Wolman's disease	< 1 month	Severe fat	Vomiting, large liver	Severe malnutrition
Malabsorption of folic acid	< 1 month	Watery	Severe anemia, stomatitis, seizures	Failure to thrive and mental retardation
Galactosemia, tyrosinosis, fructose intolerance	< 3 months	Not invariably present	Vomiting, large liver, icterus, seizures	Failure to thrive
Primary bile acid malabsorption	< 1 month	Intractable diarrhea with carbohydrate intolerance and fat malabsorption	Dehydration, wasting	Failure to thrive
Anatomic abnormalities				
Congenital				
Malrotation, partial small or large bowel obstruction, short bowel	< 3 months	Intractable diarrhea, may be like celiac syndrome	Vomiting, abdominal distention	Failure to thrive
Acquired				
Blind or stagnant loop syndrome	Any age	Severe with carbohydrate and lipid malabsorption	History of surgery, vomiting, distended abdomen	Significant stunting of growth and malnutrition
Chronic intestinal pseudo-obstruction	Usually > 4 years	Bouts of obstipation with chronic diarrhea	Recurrent bouts of intestinal obstruction	Progressive weight loss and growth impairment
Lymphosarcoma	> 4 years	—	Crampy pain, intussusception	Weight loss and anemia
Familial polyposis	Teen-agers	Watery with blood	Abdominal pain, anemia	None unless malignancy

Continued.

Table 8-12. Guide to differential diagnosis of chronic diarrhea in infants and children—cont'd

Disease category and entities	Age	Type of diarrhea	Associated clinical features	Repercussions on well-being and growth
Inflammatory bowel disease				
Crohn's disease	Usually > 10 years	Loose stools, often nocturnal	Pain more severe in Crohn's disease	Severe growth retardation in Crohn's disease; less pronounced in chronic ulcerative colitis; delayed puberty
Chronic ulcerative colitis	Usually > 10 years	Diarrhea with blood, nocturnal	Tenesmus in chronic ulcerative colitis Anorexia, fever; extraintestinal manifestations often predominant in Crohn's disease	
Intractable diarrhea of early infancy (nonspecific enterocolitis)	< 3 months	Explosive watery diarrhea	Vomiting and fever common at onset	Cachexia
Hirschsprung's enterocolitis	< 1 year	Pea soup and putrid	Abdominal distention, vomiting, fever, and periods of obstipation	Toxic, failure to thrive
Eosinophilic gastroenteritis	Any age	Watery and at times severe	Vomiting; eczema and asthma are common	Failure to thrive common in infants
Malnutrition and maternal deprivation	< 1 year	Loose stools	Apathy, lethargy, abnormal affect, signs of battering	Retarded growth and neuromotor development
Endocrinopathies				
Hyperthyroidism	Any age	Watery	Signs of hyperthyroidism	
Congenital adrenal hyperplasia	< 1 month	Watery	Vomiting usually predominates	Failure to thrive

9 *Carbohydrate intolerance*

Carbohydrates comprise a substantial proportion of the diet of man. In the Western world, an adult ingests about 350 gm of carbohydrates daily; starch accounts for 60% of this intake, sucrose 30%, and lactose 10%. Other oligosaccharides such as trehalose (young mushrooms) and stachyose (lentils, kidney, and navy beans) are ingested in small amounts and only intermittently. Milk is the only food containing lactose, and man is the only mammal drinking milk throughout its lifetime and sustaining a high intestinal lactase activity throughout life. Carbohydrate intolerance may involve monosacharides disaccharides, or polysaccharides. Some of the conditions are secondary to an underlying intestinal disease, whereas others are primary. In this latter group, a certain number are permanent, with the rest being temporary and attributable to a developmental lag. Table 9-1 summarizes the conditions of clinical significance.

NORMAL INTRALUMINAL CARBOHYDRATE DIGESTION

Starch is a polysaccharide of molecular weight ranging from 100,000 to 1 million. It is made up of two glucose polymers, amylose and amylopectin (Table 9-2), and is extensively digested by hydrolytic enzymes within the intestinal luminal fluid. *Amylose* is made up of a straight chain of glucose molecules linked by α-1,4 oxygen bridges. Salivary and pancreatic alpha-amylases attack the interior α-1,4 junctions but cannot hydrolyze the outermost links, and therefore maltose (two glucose units), maltotriose (three glucose units), and other oligosaccharides (5%), containing four to nine glucose molecules, are the final products. Intestinal mucosal maltases (glucoamylase) hydrolyze these oligosaccharides to yield glucose molecules. *Amylopectin* makes up 80% of ingested starch. It has a more complex structure than amylose. In addition to the straight α-1,4 chain of glucose molecules, it possesses α-1,6 branching points every 25 glucose units along the chain with continuation as an α-1,4 straight chain. The salivary and pancreatic alpha-amylases selectively attack the interior α-1,4 glucose-glucose links but cannot hydrolyze either the exterior ones or the ones ad-

Table 9-1. Carbohydrate malabsorption in neonates and children

Type	Reduced brush-border enzyme activity	Impaired monosaccharide transport
Primary	Congenital sucrase-isomaltase deficiency	Glucose-galactose malabsorption
	Congenital lactase deficiency	
	Late-onset lactase deficiency	
	Temporary lactose malabsorption in newborns	
Secondary	Lactase deficiency	Acquired monosaccharide malabsorption
	Lactose, sucrose, and oligosaccharide malabsorption if extensive brush-border damage	

jacent to branching points. Thus the end products of intraluminal digestion of starch are maltose, small amounts of oligosaccharides, and alpha-dextrins (Fig. 9-1). The latter are hydrolyzed to glucose molecules by mucosal alpha-dextrinase (isomaltase).

INTESTINAL OLIGOSACCHARIDASE AND DISACCHARIDASE ENZYMES

The products of salivary and pancreatic alpha-amylases, as well as the dietary disaccharides sucrose and lactose, are hydrolyzed by enzymes located in the brush-border membrane of intestinal villus cells. Hydrolysis occurs on the outside of the intestinal membrane at a site exterior to the permeability barrier. Recent studies provide evidence that disaccharidases are topographically located (Fig. 9-2) so that they can bind disaccharides and very efficiently deliver their products of hydrolysis to the monosaccharide transport systems of the cell. (See Chapter 10.) It has been

Table 9-2. Intraluminal and mucosal digestion of carbohydrates

Diet (percentage of carbohydrate intake)	Luminal enzymes	Oligosaccharides and disaccharides presented to mucosa	Mucosal enzymes	End products
Starch (60%)				
Amylopectin	Salivary and pancreatic alpha-amylases →	Maltose, maltotriose, and other oligosaccharides α-1,4 linkage)	Glucoamylase (maltase) →	Glucose
		Alpha-dextrins (α-1,6 linkage)	Alpha-dextrinase (isomaltase) →	Glucose
Amylose	Salivary and pancreatic alpha-amylases →	Maltose, maltotriose, and other oligosaccharides	Glucoamylase (maltase) →	Glucose
Sucrose (30%)	→	Sucrose	Sucrase →	Glucose and fructose
Lactose (10%)	→	Lactose	Lactase →	Glucose and galactose
Trehalose	→	Trehalose	Trehalase →	Glucose

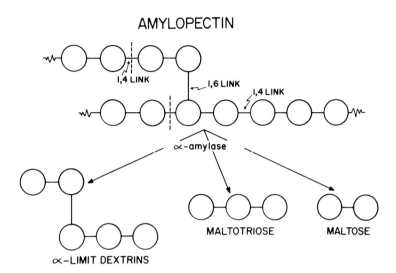

Fig. 9-1. Action of salivary and pancreatic alpha amylases on branched starch (amylopectin). The hydrolytic products maltose and maltotriose also originate from the digestion of straight-chain amylose, whereas alpha-limit dextrins are unique to digested amylopectin. (From Gray G.M.: N. Engl. J. Med. **292:**1225, 1975.)

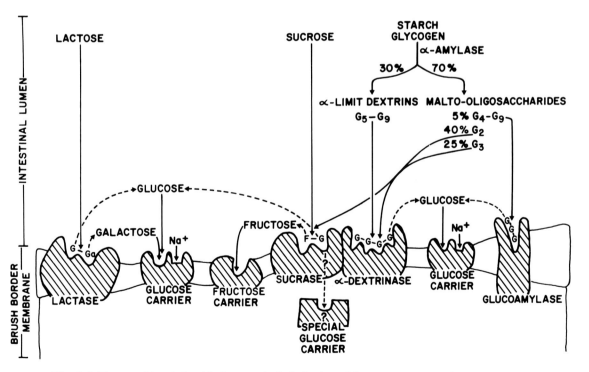

Fig. 9-2. Topographic relationship between hydrolytic sites of lactose, sucrose, and starch at the brush border and the carriers for the resultant monosaccharides. (From Gray, G.M.: N. Engl. J. Med. **292:**1225, 1975.)

shown that glucose is absorbed more rapidly if it is administered as a disaccharide.

Factors affecting hydrolytic activity

Distribution in gastrointestinal tract and cell cycle. Oligosaccharidase and disaccharidase activity is higher in the jejunum and proximal ileum than in the duodenum and distal ileum. As shown in Fig. 9-3, the basic functional unit of the small intestine consists of a crypt and villus. Epithelial cells originate at the base of the crypt where DNA and protein synthesis are very active. These cells are immature and do not have a microvillous structure. As they migrate up the villus, they acquire the machinery for the hydrolysis and transport of carbohydrates. The appearance of oligosaccharidase and disaccharidase activity is therefore dependent on the presence of mature, well-differentiated epithelial cells. The half-life of carbohydrate hydrolytic enzymes is said to be limited to a few hours. Separation of brush-border membrane proteins now permits the correlation of enzyme activity with a specific protein band. Results so far suggest that the band is present, albeit reduced, even in cases where enzyme activity is completely absent.

Effect of age, diet, and drugs. Unlike many other mammals, the full-term infant is born with a full complement of carbohydrate hydrolytic enzymes. However, the activity of lactase, in contrast to those of sucrase and maltase, which are already high in the 10-week-old fetus, develops late in gestation. Lactase is a nonadaptable enzyme; neither a lactose-free nor a lactose-rich diet influences its activity. This is in contrast to sucrase and maltase, which increase on feeding of fructose, sucrose, and maltose. Corticosteroids stimulate the precocious development of sucrase and alpha-dextrinase activity in immature animals.

Starch intolerance

Salivary amylase is detectable during the last half of gestation. The digestion of starch begins in the mouth and will continue in the stomach if the pH is high. Pancreatic alpha-amylase is the principal enzyme for the digestion of starch but shows little or no activity in the first 4 to 6 months of life. On the other hand, intestinal glucoamylase levels in 1-month-old infants are comparable to those of 5-year-old children. Glucoamylase, though more active on oligosaccharides of 5 to 9 glucose units, may also contribute to the hydrolysis of starch.

Although not a clinical problem of recognized significance, limitations in the capacity of newborns and young infants to digest starch have been

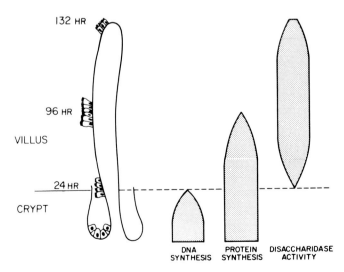

Fig. 9-3. Life cycle of epithelial cells on the crypt-villus unit as a function of oligosaccharidase and disaccharidase activity. Hydrolytic activity begins as the cell emerges from the crypt, increases as it migrates up the villus, and decreases as it becomes senescent before being extruded. (From Gray, G.M.: N. Engl. J. Med. **292:**1225, 1975.)

found. Amylopectin hydrolysis is particularly affected. Iatrogenic diarrhea can be caused by large amounts of cereals offered to neonates and young infants in a "thickened feeding" regimen to reduce gastroesophageal reflux. A recent study shows that glucoamylase activity decreases with increasing severity of villus atrophy but that the degree of depression tends to parallel maltase rather than the more severe decreases in lactase, sucrase, and alpha-dextrinase. Thus, a relative degree of starch intolerance may be seen in three circumstances. First, in young babies because of the normal developmental delay in pancreatic alpha-amylase activity and, second, in any age group when there is severe mucosal damage. Finally, starch intolerance may be found in infants with sucrase-isomaltase deficiency.

Disaccharide intolerance

Normally hydrolyzed disaccharides disappear from the intestinal lumen in the proximal part of the small intestine, and their constituent monosaccharides are rapidly absorbed. Inadequate disaccharidase levels, on either a congenital or an acquired basis, constitute the first cause of disaccharide intolerance. A second important reason is inadequate exposure of disaccharides to enzyme hydrolysis, which may result from a shortening of the small intestine or an increased rate of transit through the small bowel. Because lactase activity is low compared to other disaccharidases, a number of clinical entities can be associated with lactose intolerance despite normal lactase levels in jejunal homogenates.

Symptoms associated with disaccharide intolerance include a watery type of diarrhea, bloating, distention, borborygmi, flatulence, and cramps. Recurrent severe abdominal pain and nausea may also occur. The pathophysiologic action of unabsorbed disaccharides on intestinal function has been well studied. The osmotic action of the offending disaccharide causes a large increase in intestinal fluid secretion, which in turn stimulates intestinal motility and shortens the transit time. When the disaccharide reaches the distal intestine and colon where the microflora is luxuriant, enteric bacteria ferment the sugar to hydrogen, carbon dioxide, and organic acids, especially lactic acid, which further raise the osmolarity, lower the pH, and interfere with the reabsorption of fluid. In a 24-hour stool sample there are only trace amounts of lactic acid (under 50 mg); the amount goes up to more than 1 gm in the stools of patients with disaccharide intolerance, and accordingly the pH drops below 5.5. Unabsorbed carbohydrates fermented by the microflora can also be detected in expired air as hydrogen. Carbohydrates that have escaped hydrolysis and fermentation can be found in stools as reducing substances, with more than 0.5% being significant.

Disaccharidase deficiencies are either primary or secondary. In the primary, or genetically determined, form, the enzyme deficit is usually isolated, the disaccharide intolerance theoretically should persist throughout life, and the intestinal tissue structure is normal.

The acquired form of disaccharidase deficiency is usually transient. It involves a quantitative decrease of all disaccharidase enzymes, though, clinically, lactose intolerance is by far the most common. Histologic studies will often reveal the small bowel mucosal changes of the underlying disorder. A general diagnostic approach to children suspected of disaccharide intolerance is summarized below. Symptoms are caused by unabsorbed sugars; therefore great importance should be attached to the triggering and the amelioration of symptoms shortly after the introduction and withdrawal of the suspected carbohydrate. Detection of the unabsorbed carbohydrate by stool pH, reducing substances, and breath hydrogen excretion constitute confirmatory evidence. Oral lactose and sucrose absorption tests have been abandoned because there is no correlation between the maximum rise in glucose and diarrhea. Measurement of disaccharidase activity on a biopsy specimen does not fare better except in situations where one is trying to document if the carbohydrate intolerance is primary and involves a single enzyme (lactase or sucrase-isomaltase) or if it is secondary to brush-border damage and involves all disaccharidase enzymes.

Diagnosis of disaccharidase deficiency

1. History
2. Breath hydrogen (H_2) test after ingestion of lactose or sucrose
3. Examination of stools
   a. pH in watery supernatant
   b. Reducing substances
4. Oral mucosal biopsy
   a. Histologic studies
   b. Enzyme assay
5. Clinical response to removal of suspected sugar from diet

PRIMARY (CONGENITAL) DISACCHARIDASE DEFICIENCIES
Sucrase and isomaltase deficiency

Among the primary forms of enzymatic deficiency, sucrase and isomaltase deficiency is by far the most common. It is inherited according to an autosomal mode of transmission. The incidence of this disorder is very high and may reach up to 10% among Greenland Eskimos. The combined defect always coexists in the same patient.

Sucrase-isomaltase is an integral brush-border protein built up of two distinct polypeptides having either sucrase or isomaltase (alpha-dextrinase) activity. Although some studies indicate that the enzymatic activity is caused by an absent protein, others suggest the presence of an inactive enzyme. A recent report has shown the presence of free isomaltase in brush-border membrane proteins of one patient and suggests that although the majority lack both the sucrase and the isomaltase polypeptides some may retain active isomaltase polypeptide.

Clinical findings

Diarrhea is the main symptom. It usually appears when sucrose, Dextri-Maltose, and starch are fed to the baby. In breast-fed babies, feeding of solid foods, especially fruits, triggers the symptom. The stools are liquid and frothy and have a sour smell. They commonly cause a diaper rash quite resistant to local measures.

A long history of crampy abdominal pain and chronic diarrhea in association with abdominal distention, flatulence, borborygmi, and toilet-training difficulties is common. Infants tend to be quite sick with this disorder, some may present with intractable diarrhea, others with repeated attacks of explosive diarrhea requiring hospital admissions. Failure to thrive is usually seen in such cases and may be quite severe. A summary of findings associated with sucrase-isomaltase deficiency in infants is found in the following list:

Clinical findings in infants with sucrase-isomaltase deficiency

Age of onset
  Shortly after birth if a sucrose-containing formula is given or upon introduction of solid foods
Symptoms and signs
  Stools invariably watery
  Bouts of dehydration frequent
  Vomiting reported in almost half of cases
  A distended tympanitic abdomen usual
  Colicky pain and borborygmi common

Laboratory tests
  Stool pH < 5.5
  Reducing substances in stools
  Abnormal breath H_2 test after a sucrose load
  Undetectable sucrase activity in jejunal biopsy specimens
  Steatorrhea and hypoproteinemia in more than half of infants
Repercussions on growth
  There is commonly failure to thrive and evidence of malnutrition

Diagnosis

Unhydrolyzed disaccharides cause considerable movement of electrolytes and water into the lumen of the proximal intestinal tract and therefore give rise to an osmotic type of diarrhea. Consequently, sucrose is commonly found in the stools. This can be documented by paper chromatography or, more easily, by the following bedside or office determination. To 5 drops of the liquid part of a stool add 10 drops of 1 N HCl and boil for a few seconds. Add a Clinitest tablet.

Unabsorbed sucrose and alpha-dextrins are hydrolyzed more or less completely into monosaccharides by the colonic flora. Fermentation yields hydrogen, which can be monitored in expired air after the ingestion of a standard dose (2 gm/kg to a maximum of 50 gm/kg) of sucrose. Discrimination between sucrose-tolerant and -intolerant children with the interval breath hydrogen collection is best obtained at 90 minutes. The pH of loose stools evacuated within 6 to 8 hours of a sucrose load is generally below 5.5. A physician should be in attendance when the test is done in infants and young children because explosive stools and shock may occur.

The intestinal mucosa is invariably normal. Quantitative determination of sucrase-isomaltase activity in jejunal mucosal homogenates shows very low levels or total absence of sucrase activity. Maltase is moderately decreased, whereas lactase is usually in the upper range of normal.

Treatment

Rigid exclusion of sucrose from the diet constitutes a valid therapeutic test. Within a few days, children with chronic diarrhea since birth may become constipated.

Subsequently, the diet can be somewhat liberalized under the dietitian's supervision. The average patient will be able to tolerate a diet excluding only foods with a sucrose content of more than 2% (Chapter 28).

It is important to remember that some infants will have diarrhea when receiving proprietary formulas containing Dextri-Maltose, a carbohydrate formula modifier. Similarly, a starch-rich diet will lower the stool pH and produce diarrhea. If impairment of starch digestion is present, it is limited to the first year of life.

The prognosis is good, but the amount of sucrose tolerated by each patient varies. Patients tend to know their own limit of tolerance. Ingestion of significant amounts of sucrose is invariably followed by bloating, gas pain, flatus, and diarrhea. The tolerance for sucrose improves somewhat with age, but enzyme levels remain permanently very low. It has been suggested that the homozygote for this mutant gene has symptoms all his life and that the heterozygote may be either symptomatic only in childhood or never be affected.

Congenital lactase deficiency

Congenital lactase deficiency is a very rare condition, since only a few patients appear to satisfy the following diagnostic criteria:
1. Severe diarrhea from birth
2. Very low levels of lactase activity in conjunction with normal activity of other disaccharidases
3. Normal small bowel histologic condition
4. Permanent defect of lactase activity with no improvement of symptoms upon subsequent milk ingestion.

Separation of brush-border membrane proteins reveals a reduction of the protein band rather than its absence. This pattern observed in three patients with congenital lactase deficiency corresponds to that seen in the late onset type of lactase deficiency. This suggests that congenital lactase deficiency results from a defect in a regulatory gene rather than in a structural gene. Investigators in another study, however, could not find residual brush-border lactase activity in four patients and suggest that congenital lactase deficiency is the result of a structural mutation leading to the inability to synthesize the enzyme protein.

Clinical findings

Theoretically, diarrhea should start when the first feedings of a lactose-containing formula or of breast milk are given. Vomiting is not uncommon along with colicky pain and abdominal distention. Explosive, watery, acid diarrhea constitutes the most constant clinical finding. Malnutrition may supervene if the diagnosis is not promptly made. Steatorrhea is rare but has been described.

Diagnosis

The stool pH can be as low as 3.8. Reducing substances are usually present in the stools. Instances of lactosuria, aminoaciduria, proteinuria, acidosis, and an elevated blood urea nitrogen (BUN) level have been described in infants. An oral lactose absorption test in an infant believed to have the disease, and from whose diet lactose has been withdrawn, is likely to precipitate symptoms of intolerance within 8 hours.

Since explosive diarrhea and shock may ensue, a physician should be in attendance when the test is performed. The breath hydrogen test will be positive, and high concentrations (more than 0.5%) of reducing substances will be found in the stools.

It is necessary to establish that there is no mucosal damage, which may be responsible for secondary lactase deficiency, by use of a small bowel biopsy, which also permits direct estimation of the disaccharidase level. However, the absence of histologic abnormalities in jejunal mucosa with little or no lactase activity does not establish with certainty a diagnosis of primary lactase deficiency, since it is known that in the aftermath of acute small bowel mucosal disease, lactase activity may not return for periods of up to 6 months.

The presence of reducing substances in the stools of neonates, whether breast-fed or formula-fed, is normal and tends to be more severe and prolonged in prematures. However, the absence of reducing substances would militate against the diagnosis. It is important to remember that most neonates who are intolerant to formulas have milk protein sensitivity rather than lactose intolerance.

Treatment

A lactose-free formula should be ordered as soon as the diagnosis is suspected.

SECONDARY (ACQUIRED) DISACCHARIDASE DEFICIENCIES
Late-onset lactase deficiency

Inherited delayed-onset lactase deficiency affects the majority of humans, but there are striking ethnic differences in its prevalence (10% to 90%). Family studies from various ethnic groups have established that the condition is transmitted by an autosomal recessive gene. The residual 10% or less of lactase activity is derived from the same protein band found in the brush border of individuals who have normal lactase activity. Therefore, the mutation that affects the capacity for lactose digestion in adulthood probably affects a regulatory gene rather than a structural gene.

At the time of weaning, all land mammals have a striking drop in lactase activity. The decrease found in 5% to 12% of adult whites and in 70% of adult blacks in the United States is generally present by the age of 3 to 6, but it may occasionally be delayed until the teens. The hypothesis that lactase is an adaptable enzyme is no longer tenable. The geographic hypothesis proposes that lactose digestion in adulthood is characteristic of only a minority of the world's peoples, those whose ancestors inhabited the dairying zones of the Old World. Individuals with the mutant gene had a selective advantage in terms of fertility because they had access to a food of high nutritional value, which also protected them against metabolic bone disease through its high calcium content.

There is poor correlation between clinical symptoms of milk intolerance and the results of lactose-tolerance tests as well as of lactase-activity determinations in biopsy specimens. Recent studies have pointed out that although most lactose malabsorbers will experience symptoms when given 50 gm of lactose (equivalent to lactose in a liter of milk) the majority will tolerate 12 to 18 gm (lactose content of 1 to 1½ glass of milk). The need for double-blind studies in determining the true frequency and clinical significance of a suspected food intolerance such as lactose has been emphasized by a study showing that only 16% of lactose malabsorbers (glucose rise of less than 26 mg/dl) reported symptoms after the ingestion of 25 gm of lactose.

The usual clinical manifestations of diarrhea, bloating, flatulence, and crampy abdominal pain occur within 8 hours of ingestion of an amount of lactose ranging from 2 to a maximum of 50 gm/kg. These findings have led to the investigation of the role of lactose in the pathogenesis of common gastrointestinal conditions such as the irritable colon syndrome and recurrent abdominal pain (RAP) in children. One study showing that close to 30% of those with recurrent abdominal pain may have lactose intolerance on the basis of an abnormal lactose-tolerance test and of improvement on an elimination diet could not be confirmed. Another report using the breath hydrogen test, a more reliable measurement of lactose malabsorption, indicated that 40% of 80 children with recurrent ab-

dominal pain were lactose malabsorbers and that 20 of 28 responded favorably to a milk-free diet. This report must be interpreted with caution because (1) it was not a blinded study, (2) patients with recurrent abdominal pain who absorb lactose were not tried on the diet, and (3) no measure of lactose consumption was made during the lactose-containing diet periods.

Most individuals with low lactase levels can consume a certain amount of lactose. They can tolerate lactose in its fermented forms, such as cheese or yogurt, but may have to limit themselves to milk that is added to beverages or foods. In young children, who should consume significant amounts of milk, a commercially available yeast lactase enzyme has been found to be useful. Five to 10 drops of Lact-Aid (Sugar-Lo Company, Atlantic City, N.J.) is added to a liter of milk, which is then placed in the refrigerator. Twenty-four hours later 70% to 100% of the lactose is hydrolyzed to glucose and galactose and the milk can be tolerated by most children with late-onset lactase deficiency.

Temporary lactose malabsorption in newborns

Both term and premature newborns have a limited capacity to absorb lactose when it is tested by the lactose-tolerance test. This ''physiologic'' malabsorption is said to be more frequent in breast-fed babies because of its higher lactose content. Unabsorbed lactose probably plays a role in the predominance of the bifidobacilli flora in breast-fed babies.

Lactose is of nutritional importance, since it accounts for almost 40% of calories provided by breast milk. The degree of lactose sequestration in the colon is particularly impressive in prematures. It has been estimated to correspond to 64% of intake by lactose breath hydrogen tests. According to reports the results of these tests are positive in 75% of prematures during the first 2 weeks. In contrast to what was expected, the percentage increased to 100% by the end of the third week. Stool-reducing substances can be detected in up to half of formula-fed as well as breast-fed newborns, but the concentration rarely exceeds 0.5% when tested by Clinitest tablet.

Although lactase activity is low until the last 2 months of gestation, there are undoubtedly other factors, such as jejunal hurry, that compound the digestive defect. Lactose malabsorption in newborns is not associated with symptoms unless lactose concentration is increased above 10%. Therefore, the presence of reducing substances and a positive breath test does not warrant replacement of lactose by other dietary carbohydrates.

In the past few years, attention has been drawn to the possibility that phototherapy-associated diarrhea could be attributable to low lactase levels. However, lactose intolerance has not been confirmed by others. Unconjugated bilirubin, present in significant concentrations in the intestinal lumen of light-treated neonates, appears responsible for the increased fecal water loss and shortened transit time because it is a powerful inducer of intestinal secretion.

Secondary lactase deficiency

Since the disaccharidases are found in the brush border, they are likely to be affected in any disorder in which the intestinal mucosa is damaged. Lactase deficiency is the most important type of secondary disaccharidase deficiency for the following reasons:

1. Lactase does not reach optimal activity until the very end of gestation and it is present in concentrations lower than those of sucrase-isomaltase.
2. It cannot be induced by lactose feeding.
3. A lag of several months may be seen between histologic repair and the return of normal activity.

Following is a list of some of the conditions associated with secondary lactase deficiency:

Celiac disease
Tropical sprue
Cystic fibrosis
Severe malnutrition
Crohn's disease
Postoperative intestinal surgery in infants
Blind loop syndrome
Abetalipoproteinemia
Giardiasis
Intractable diarrhea
Viral or bacterial gastroenteritis
Immune defects
Chronic ulcerative colitis
Neomycin administration

A significant number of children with cystic fibrosis have been found to have low lactase levels. Hypolactasia is of no clinical significance because children with cystic fibrosis tolerate milk nor-

mally. In untreated celiac disease, lactase activity may be extremely low but surprisingly the tolerance for milk is generally quite good. Most cases of clinically significant secondary lactase deficiency are found in infants recovering from viral and bacterial gastroenteritis.

Secondary sucrase deficiency

Intestinal mucosal damage tends to lower the levels of all disaccharidases. Signs of sucrose intolerance are usually masked by the more striking symptoms related to lactose intolerance. Infectious diarrhea is the more commonly observed disease leading to secondary sucrose intolerance.

DIARRHEA FROM "SUGAR-FREE" GUM AND CANDIES

Sorbitol, mannitol, and xylitol are the alcohol derivatives of the natural sugars glucose, mannose, and xylose, respectively. Because they are not absorbed to any significant extent, they may cause diarrhea if taken in excess.

REFERENCES

AAP Committee on Nutrition: The practical significance of lactose intolerance in children, Pediatrics **62:**240-245, 1978.

Ament, M.E., Perera, D.R., and Esther, L.: Sucrase-isomaltase deficiency: a frequently misdiagnosed disease, J. Pediatr. **83:**721-727, 1973.

Antonowicz, I., Lebenthal, E., and Schwachman, H.: Disaccharidase activities in small intestinal mucosa in patients with cystic fibrosis, J. Pediatr. **92:**214-219, 1978.

Auricchio, S., Ciccimarra, F., Moauro, L., and others: Intraluminal and mucosal starch digestion in congenital deficiency of intestinal sucrase and isomaltase activities, Pediatr. Res. **6:**832-839, 1972.

Bakken, A.F.: Temporary intestinal lactase deficiency in light-treated jaundiced infants, Acta Paediatr. Scand. **66:**91-96, 1977.

Barr, R.G., Levine, M.D., and Watkins, J.B.: Lactose intolerance and recurrent abdominal pain in childhood, N. Engl. J. Med. **300:**1449-1452, 1979.

Christensen, M.F.: Prevalence of lactose intolerance in children with recurrent abdominal pain, Pediatrics **65:**680, 1980.

Ebbesen, F., Edelsten, D., and Hertel, J.: Gut transit time and lactose malabsorption during phototherapy. I. A study using lactose free human mature milk; II. A study using raw milk from the mothers of the infants, Acta Paediatr. Scand. **69:**65-68, 69-71, 1980.

Freiburghaus, A.U., Schmitz, J., Schindler, M., and others: Protein patterns of brush-border fragments in congenital lactose malabsorption and in specific hypolactasia of the adult, N. Engl. J. Med. **294:**1030-1032, 1976.

Gilat, T., Dolizky, F., Gelman-Malachi, E., and Tamir, I.: Lactase in childhood—a nonadaptable enzyme, Scand. J. Gastroenterol. **9:**395-398, 1974.

Gracey, M., and Burke, V.: Sugar-induced diarrhea in children, Arch. Dis. Child. **48:**331-336, 1973.

Gray, G.M.: Carbohydrate digestion and absorption, N. Engl. J. Med. **293:**1225-1230, 1975.

Gudmand-Höyer, E., and Krasilnikoff, P.A.: The effect of sucrose malabsorption on the growth pattern in children, Scand. J. Gastroenterol. **12:**103-107, 1977.

Harrison, M., and Walker-Smith, J.A.: Reinvestigation of lactose intolerant children: lack of correlation between continuing lactose intolerance and small intestinal morphology, disaccharidase activity, and lactose tolerance tests, Gut **18:**48-52, 1977.

Kilby, A., Burgess, E.A., Wigglesworth, S., and Walker-Smith, J.A.: Sucrase-isomaltase: a follow-up report, Arch. Dis. Child. **53:**677-679, 1979.

Kwon, P.H., Rorich, M.H., and Scrimshaw, N.S.: Comparative tolerance of adolescents of differing ethnic backgrounds to lactose containing and lactose free dairy drinks. I. Initial experience with a double blind procedure; II. Improvement of a double blind test, Am. J. Clin. Nutr. **33:**17-21, 22-26, 1980.

Lebenthal, E., and Lee, P.C.: Gluocoamylase and disaccharidase activities in normal subjects and in patients with mucosal injury of the small intestina, J. Pediatr. **97:**389-393, 1980.

Lebenthal, E., Rossi, T.M., Nord, K., and others: Recurrent abdominal pain and lactose absorption in children, Pediatrics **67:**828-832, 1981.

Lebenthal, E., Sunshine, P., and Kretchmeer, N.: Effect of carbohydrate and corticosteroids on activity of α-glucosidases in intestine of the infant rat, J. Clin. Invest. **51:**1244-1250, 1972.

Liebman, W.M.: Recurrent abdominal pain in children: lactose and sucrose intolerance, a prospective study, Pediatrics **64:**43-45, 1979.

Lifshitz, F.: Carbohydrate problems in paediatric gastroenterology, Clin. Gastroenterol. **6:**415-429, 1977.

Lisker, R., and Aguilar, L.: Double blind study of milk lactose intolerance, Gastroenterology **74:**1283-1285, 1978.

MacLean, W.C., and Fink, B.B.: Lactose malabsorption by premature infants: magnitude and clinical significance, J. Pediatr. **97:**383-388, 1980.

Perman, J.A., Barr, R.G., and Watkins, J.B.: Sucrose malabsorption in children: noninvasive diagnosis by interval breath hydrogen determination, J. Pediatr. **93:**17-22, 1978.

Rosensweig, N.S.: Editorial on lactose-hydrolyzed milk, Am. J. Clin. Nutr. **32:**1979, 1979.

Simoons, F.J.: The geographic hypothesis and lactose malabsorption: a weighing of the evidence, Am. J. Dig. Dis. **23:**963-980, 1978.

Skovbjerg, H., and Krasilnikoff, P.A.: Immunoelectrophoretic studies on human small intestinal brush border proteins: the residual isomaltase in sucrose intolerant patients, Pediatr. Res. **15:**214-218, 1981.

Whitington, P.F.: Effect of jaundice phototherapy on intestinal mucosal bilirubin concentration and lactase activity in the congenitally jaundiced Gunn rat, Pediatr. Res. **15:**345-349, 1981.

MONOSACCHARIDE MALABSORPTION
Absorption of monosaccharides

Glucose, galactose, and fructose are the end products of intraluminal (salivary and pancreatic amylase) and membrane (disaccharidase) digestion of dietary carbohydrates. The specific transport mechanism for glucose and galactose involves several steps (Fig. 9-4). Mucosal entry re-

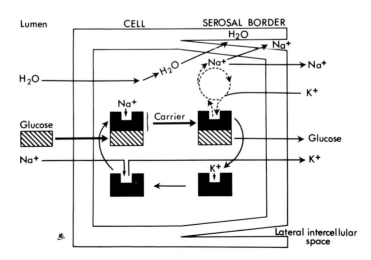

Fig. 9-4. Carrier-mediated glucose transport. The various steps of glucose transport in and out of the cell are described in the text. The pumping out of Na^+ in the lateral intracellular space and across the serosal-cell border provides an osmotic gradient that brings about the passive diffusion of water into the cell and out in the lateral intercellular space. (Modified from Singer, I., and Rotenberg, D.: N. Engl. J. Med. **289:**257, 1973.)

quires interaction of the substrate with a carrier molecule to form a complex that depends on Na^+ to maintain the proper carrier-sugar relation. This complex made up of carrier, sugar, and Na^+, diffuses to the serosal border of the cell, where a cation pump pushes Na^+ off the carrier and out of the cell. K^+ then replaces Na^+ on the carrier. This exchange greatly reduces the affinity of the carrier for the sugar, so that the monosaccharide can leave the cell by diffusion. The carrier then diffuses back to the mucosal side of the cell, where Na^+ from the lumen replaces K^+ on the carrier. This active process is energy dependent and permits absorption against a lumen-to-cell concentration gradient. Fructose entry into the cell is also carrier mediated; however, it is largely energy independent. Most of the data available suggest that it cannot be transported against a concentration gradient.

Two types of *monosaccharide malabsorption* have been described: (1) the primary, familial, autosomal-recessive, inherited disorder known as glucose-galactose malabsorption (see Chapter 17), and (2) the secondary, acquired, temporary type that involves not only glucose and galactose but also fructose and D-xylose.

Acquired monosaccharide malabsorption
Clinical findings

The clinical features associated with acquired monosaccharide malabsorption are essentially the same as those seen with disaccharidase deficiency states described in the previous section. The main symptom is diarrhea, the stool pH is below 5.5, and reducing substances can be identified in excessive amounts. After a glucose tolerance test, explosive diarrhea may occur. A Clinistix (glucose oxidase) test will be strongly positive if glu-

cose is fed. The disease is mainly seen in the perinatal period and in young infants. It is described with many conditions (Table 9-3). Disaccharides and monosaccharides alike are malabsorbed. Unlike patients with primary or secondary disaccharidase deficiency, these infants continue to have diarrhea when fed formulas containing the monosaccharides glucose, galactose, and fructose. Metabolic acidosis and hypoglycemia are threatening complications.

Pathogenesis

The pathogenesis in some cases remains obscure. Mucosal biopsy specimens may show essentially no histologic changes and normal disaccharidase activity. In protein-calorie malnutrition and in cases developing after surgery of the gastrointestinal tract, the contaminated small bowel syndrome has been documented (p. 381). Free bile acids, identified in the upper gastrointestinal tract of these infants, are known to interfere with intestinal transport of monosaccharides.

In most cases with intractable diarrhea of early infancy, the inability to absorb monosaccharides is caused by a severe decrease in effective absorptive surface. A recent report has shown that the surface area can be reduced to as little as 10% of normal during the acute stage of the disease. There was a linear relationship between structure and function assessed by jejunal biopsies and perfusion studies. On follow-up study, it appeared that microvilli recovered much more slowly than villi.

Treatment

An awareness of the clinical conditions favoring the development of this temporary entity is extremely important. Intravenous feeding is usually needed initially. A carbohydrate-free soy-based formula (RCF, Ross Laboratories, Columbus, Ohio) or else a casein hydrolysate (2.5%) with medium-chain triglyceride oil (2.5%) or vegetable fat (3%) can be used. Intravenous carbohydrates should be discontinued very slowly as small concentrations of oral glucose or Dextri-Maltose are introduced, being started at 1% and worked up to 5% over a period of weeks; otherwise hypoglycemia may occur. A prolonged period of parenteral alimentation is usually necessary in cases of intractable diarrhea because malnutrition is invariably present and may contribute to the impairment of monosaccharide absorption. Sequential

Table 9-3. Acquired monosaccharide malabsorption

First few months of life	Infants
Necrotizing enterocolitis	Gastroenteritis
Contaminated small bowel	(rotavirus
syndrome	particularly)
Acute gastroenteritis	Protein-calorie
Intractable diarrhea of early	malnutrition
infancy (primary type)	
Neonatal surgery of gas-	
trointestinal tract	

intestinal biopsy specimens are particularly useful for assessment of the response of the mucosa and for planning of the therapeutic regimen.

REFERENCES

Akesode, F., Lifshitz, F., and Hoffman, K.M.: Transient monosaccharide intolerance in a newborn infant, Pediatrics **51:**891-897, 1973.

Gracey, M., and Burke, V.: Sugar-induced diarrhea in children, Arch. Dis. Child. **48:**331-336, 1973.

Heyman, M., Desjeux, J.-F., Grasset, E., and others: Relationship between transport of D-xylose and other monosaccharides in jejunal mucosa of children, Gastroenterology **80:**758-762, 1980.

Howat, J.M., and Aaronson, I.: Sugar intolerance in neonatal surgery, J. Pediatr. Surg. **6:**719-723, 1971.

Klish, W.J., Udall, J.N., Rodriguez, J.T., and others: Intestinal surface area in infants with acquired monosaccharide intolerance, J. Pediatr. **92:**566-571, 1978.

Lifshitz, F., and Coello-Ramirez, P.: Monosaccharide intolerance and hypoglycemia in infants with diarrhea, J. Pediatr. **77:**595-603, 1970.

Viteri, F.E., and Schneider, R.E.: Gastrointestinal alterations in protein-caloric malnutrition, Med. Clin. North Am. **58:**1487-1505, 1974.

10 *Malabsorption syndrome*

Intestinal malabsorption may be defined as any state in which there is a disturbance of the digestive-absorptive sequence of any dietary constituent across the intestinal mucosa. The two basic requirements of the process of digestion and absorption are as follows:

1. Chemical modifications of substrates in the lumen, on the surface, or in the enterocyte so that they can be absorbed.
2. The transport of fat-soluble substances through the aqueous environment of the lumen and of water-soluble substrates across the protein-lipid membrane.

Absorption is largely dependent on normal digestion; therefore diseases interfering with pancreatic exocrine function and with the production and flow of biliary secretions readily give rise to malabsorption.

The majority of diseases related to an absorptive defect are diseases of the small intestine or conditions that affect its normal function. Not only should the small bowel be of sufficient length, but the mucosal surface area available for absorption must not be decreased beyond a certain extent. A disturbed anatomy or motility not only will interfere with normal propulsive movements and mixing of food with pancreatic and biliary secretions but can lead to an altered bacterial flora, which can also be responsible for malabsorption. Impairment of portal venous return, anoxia and lymphatic abnormalities are well-described causes of malabsorption.

There are now a number of biochemical abnormalities, most of which fit the category of inborn errors of metabolism, known to block either the hydrolysis (disaccharidase deficiency) or the uptake (glucose-galactose malabsorption) of nutrients by the intestinal epithelium, or the movement of absorbed substrates from the cell to the extracellular compartment (abetalipoproteinemia). Malnutrition, endocrine conditions, immunity deficiencies, and emotional factors (maternal deprivation) are well-described conditions leading to malabsorption but for which a specific mechanism has not been pinpointed in most cases.

DIGESTION AND ABSORPTION OF DIETARY CONSTITUENTS (Fig. 10-1)
Fat

The dietary lipids are water insoluble. They require the detergent action of bile to maintain them in the aqueous phase in the gut lumen, but the protein-lipid membrane of the enterocyte offers little resistance to their translocation. Ninety percent are in the form of long-chain triglycerides made up of three long-chain fatty acids on a glycerol backbone. Other sources of dietary lipids are phospholipids, cholesterol, plant sterols, and fat-soluble vitamins.

Lipolytic phase

The degree of emulsification and hydrolysis of fat taking place in the stomach seems to contribute little to normal triglyceride digestion. However, gastric lipolytic activity against milk triglycerides is quite high (Table 10-1). Gastric lipolysis is of importance in the first few months of life and perhaps also later in life when pancreatic insufficiency is present.

Pancreatic juice has lipolytic activity against the major dietary esterified lipids. Three enzymes have been isolated: lipase (and colipase), esterase, and phospholipase. Triglycerides undergo extensive hydrolysis in the proximal small intestine and yield two fatty acids and a beta-monoglyceride (fatty acid combined with glycerol in beta position) through the action of lipase. The efficiency of lipase digestion is profoundly influenced by particle-size distribution of the fat emulsion and the surface area of the oil-water interface.

Most dietary triglycerides are probably presented for intestinal digestion as emulsions covered by proteins or phospholipids, or both. In order for lipolysis to take place, pancreatic lipase must adsorb to the lipid-water interface of the triglyceride droplet. However, in the presence of bile salts, this binding does not take place unless colipase is bound to lipase. Colipase provides an anchor for the binding of lipase to the interface provided that the latter is "desorbed" of its proteins by bile salts and of phospholipids through their

249

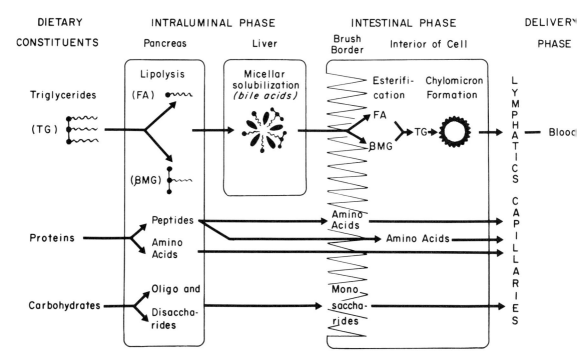

Fig. 10-1. Digestion and absorption of triglycerides, proteins, and carbohydrates.

Table 10-1. Gastric lipolysis of a feeding

Feeding	Subjects	Time after meal (minutes)	Triglyceride hydrolysis (%)
Human milk*	Pyloric stenosis	10	20
Human milk†	Low birth weight	60	15
Cream (10%)‡	Adults	4	3
Isomil§	Low birth weight	7	15.6

*Olivecrona and others: Acta. Paediatr. Scand. **62**:520, 1973.
†Frederickson and others: Acta Paediatr. Scand. **66**:479, 1977.
‡Hamosh and others: J. Clin. Invest. **55**:908, 1975.
§Hamosh and others: J. Pediatr. **93**:674, 1978.

hydrolysis by phospholipase (Fig. 10-2). Some insoluble lipids, such as cholesterol, are not altered chemically during digestion, but rather micellar solubilization is required for their absorption. In contrast, lipids such as medium-chain triglycerides require only chemical hydrolysis, since the digestive products are water soluble.

Micellar solubilization

Bile acids, synthesized in the liver from cholesterol, are conjugated with either glycine or taurine

in a ratio of 2.5:1, secreted into the bile by a special transport mechanism, and stored in the gallbladder. When food is taken, bile acids enter the duodenum in high concentration, where they form micelles with the products of pancreatic lipolysis (Fig. 10-3).

Micellar solubilization is a property of all detergents. Bile acids, when present at a sufficient intraluminal concentration (critical micellar concentration), form macromolecular aggregates with the more polar products of lipolysis. In turn, these mixed micelles can then incorporate into their molecular structure (and therefore solubilize) nonpolar dietary constituents such as cholesterol. Micelles serve as carriers. They are broken up and deliver their constituent molecules to the intestinal surface. Since bile acids are poorly absorbed from the jejunum, where fat is almost completely taken up, they serve for the formation of other micelles before moving downstream.

An efficient absorption of bile acids takes place in the ileum, so that only a small amount is lost in the feces (Fig. 10-4). Bile acids return to the liver in the portal vein, thus completing their enterohepatic circulation. The bile acid pool circulates approximately six times in 24 hours (twice with each meal); it is maintained constant by the

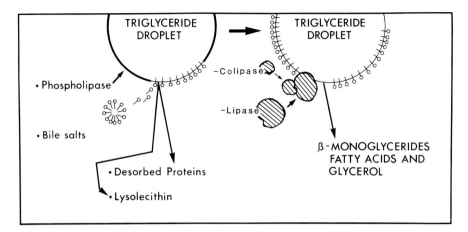

Fig. 10-2. Luminal events leading to the hydrolysis of triglycerides. Lecithin adsorbed to the surface of the triglyceride droplet is hydrolyzed to lysolecithin through the action of phospholipase A_2 while bile salts remove proteins. Lipase and colipase form a complex to ensure its binding to the droplet and subsequent hydrolysis of the latter.

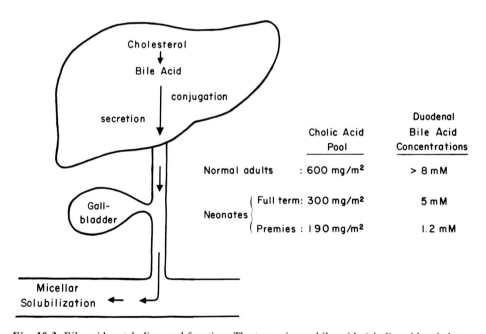

	Cholic Acid Pool	Duodenal Bile Acid Concentrations
Normal adults	: 600 mg/m²	> 8 mM
Neonates { Full term:	300 mg/m²	5 mM
Premies :	190 mg/m²	1.2 mM

Fig. 10-3. Bile acid metabolism and function. The two primary bile acids (cholic acid and cheno-deoxycholic acid) are synthesized by the liver. The third bile acid component of bile is deoxycholic acid. It is the product of bacterial dehydroxylation of cholic acid in the lower ileum and colon and accounts for 20% of total duodenal bile acid concentration in adults. It is largely absent during the first year of life. Bile acid synthesis is reduced in neonates, particularly in low birth weight babies. Reduced bile acid concentrations are believed to be largely responsible for the fat malabsorption of the newborn period (p. 301). (Modified after Watkins, J.B., et al.: N. Engl. J. Med. **288:**431, 1973.)

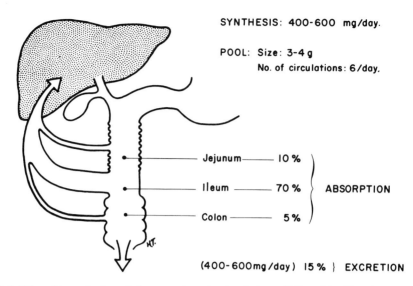

SYNTHESIS: 400-600 mg/day.

POOL: Size: 3-4 g
No. of circulations: 6/day.

Jejunum——— 10 %
Ileum ———— 70 % } ABSORPTION
Colon ———— 5 %

(400-600mg/day) 15 % } EXCRETION

Fig. 10-4. Bile acid synthesis and the enterohepatic circulation of bile acids. The chances of a bile salt's being absorbed are affected by its polarity and solubility, by the presence of food residue, and by the intestinal transit time. Bile acids are passively absorbed in the jejunum and colon, and they are actively transported in the ileum. Resection or disease involving the ileum is associated with an increased fecal sequestration of bile acids and a compensatory increase of synthesis by the liver.

daily hepatic synthesis of the amount sequestered in the stool (Fig. 10-4). Micellar solubilization is defective, and fat malabsorption occurs when duodenal concentrations of bile acids are too low (under 3 mM). This can be the result of defective synthesis by the liver (hepatocellular damage, prematurity), intrahepatic and extrahepatic cholestasis or excessive losses in the stools (short bowel syndrome). In this regard, it is interesting to note in Fig. 10-3 the small cholic acid pools and the low duodenal concentrations of bile acids in neonates and particularly in low birth weight newborns in whom fat malabsorption is invariably found.

Fat uptake

As seen previously, the intraluminal phase of digestion and absorption is an open system in which digestion products are continuously generated and removed. The uptake is a passive process that proceeds down a potential gradient against two major resistances: a diffusion barrier caused by an unstirred water layer on the luminal side of the brush border, and a resistance to translocation through the membrane lipid.

In discussing fat uptake from the lumen, we need to recognize five individual steps (Fig. 10-5).

Diffusion through unstirred water layer. In any situation in which a biologic membrane or cell sulface is immersed in a solution there exist concentric layers of water extending out from the aqueous lipid interface. Since the effective surface area of the unstirred water layer in the small bowel is small in relationship to the greater surface area of the underlying villi and microvilli, the unstirred water layer constitutes an important diffusion barrier. In fact, the diffusional resistance of the unstirred water layer to total absorption is greater than that of the protein-lipid membrane because of the poor aqueous diffusibility of lipolytic products. Shorter chain length and the presence of one or more double bonds in the individual fatty acids exhibit greater aqueous diffusibility. Although products of triglyceride lipolysis (monoglycerides and fatty acids) can be absorbed to some extent from an oil phase where they are present as emulsified droplets, they are much more readily absorbed from the aqueous phase as a monomolecular solution or as micelles.

Diffusion of short- and medium-chain fatty acids through the unstirred water layer would not be facilitated by micellar formation because of their high solubility and low molecular weight. The situation is different with long-chain fatty acids. The

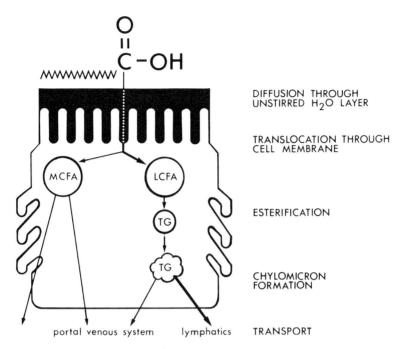

Fig. 10-5. Uptake of long-chain (LCFA) and medium-chain fatty acids (MCFA). Five well-individualized steps are recognized for LCFA. The two intracellular events esterification and chylomicron formation are bypassed by MCFA. After extrusion from the enterocyte LCFA are transported mainly through the lymphatics, whereas that of MCFA occurs through the portal venous system. (From Roy, C.C.: In Lebenthal, E., editor: Textbook of gastroenterology and nutrition in infancy, New York, 1981, Raven Press.)

flux of fatty acids in micelles through the unstirred layer may be 25 to 100 times greater than the corresponding flux of fatty acids in solution. Micelles therefore constitute an ideal shuttle between the bulk water phase and the water-microvillus interface (Fig. 10-6). The major physiologic function of the bile acid micelle is to overcome unstirred water layer resistance. Fatty acids of medium chain length are absorbed nearly as well in the absence as in the presence of bile acid micelles. As the chain length is increased, the fatty acids become progressively more dependent on the presence of bile acid micelles. In the case of a very hydrophobic compound such as cholesterol, no absorption occurs in the absence of bile acids.

Dietary phospholipids and the quantitatively more important biliary phospholipids (1:5 ratio) need to be hydrolyzed before being absorbed. Pancreatic phospholipase A_2 specifically frees the fatty acid in position 2 of the molecule of lecithin to yield lysolecithin. Hydrolysis of lecithin reduces the load of micellar solutes and therefore the size of micellar aggregates because lysolecithin is a soluble

amphiphil (to water and fat) that readily leaves micelles to enter a monomolecular solution. The greater size of lecithin-containing micelles increases the resistance to diffusion across the unstirred water layer and may account for studies showing that lecithin inhibits the absorption of linoleic acid, taurocholate, and cholesterol.

Translocation through cell membrane. Penetration of lipid molecules does not occur through aqueous channels but by diffusion through the structured protein-lipid membrane as monomers. Micellar aggregates break up at the surface, the component molecules partition between the unstirred aqueous layer and the cell membrane, and then diffusion takes place. There is evidence that a protein in the cytosol of the enterocyte may facilitate the transport of fatty acids to the endoplasmic reticulum and thereby reduce the resistance to translocation. Of interest is the observation that a diet high in unsaturated fat increases the fatty acid–binding protein (FABP) in the distal small bowel, which constitutes a reserve area for absorption in situations such as in the newborn

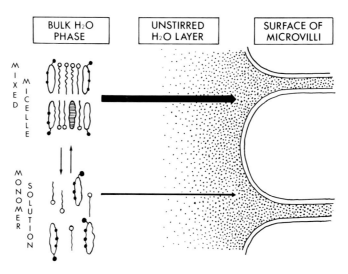

Fig. 10-6. Bile acid–lipid–water interactions and transport across the unstirred layer. There is no sharp boundary between the bulk water phase and the unstirred water layer; the transition is gradual. As monomer concentration of bile salts increase, bile salt micelles are formed. They take up cholesterol and nonionized long-chain fatty acids from oil droplets (not shown) and products of lipolysis (lysolecithin, monoglycerides, ionized fatty acids), as well as some lecithin present in the bulk water phase as a monomolecular solution. Component molecules of the micelle are continuously entering and leaving it. The heavier arrow through the unstirred water layer indicates that diffusion of lipolytic products and their delivery to the membrane is much more effective when they form micelles with bile salts than when they are monomer solutions. (From Roy, C.C.: In Lebenthal, E., editor: Textbook of gastroenterology and nutrition in infancy, New York, 1981, Raven Press.)

period during which fat intake is considerable and the digestive phase is impaired. Values after medium-chain triglyceride (MCT) feeding suggests that the fatty acid–binding protein is not involved in the transport of MCT in the cell cytosol.

Esterification. Fatty acids and monoglycerides are largely resynthesized to triglycerides after having been taken up by the enterocytes. Activation of fatty acids by the microsomal fatty acid CoA lipase is an essential step before esterification. The levels of both activating and esterification enzymes are higher in the jejunum than in the ileum. Jejunal and ileal esterification reach their peak during weaning and adulthood, respectively. Luminal contents (oral intake and pancreaticobiliary secretions) appear to be important in the development and maintenance of intestinal fatty acid esterification. Although it is difficult to extrapolate animal data to humans, the information currently available suggests that the process of fatty acid activation and esterification does not appear to be a limiting step in the process of fat absorption, even in unfavorable situations such as the newborn period.

Chylomicron formation. The intracellular event that follows the resynthesis of triglycerides is the formation of intestinal chylomicrons (Fig. 10-7). The bulk of dietary lipids (triglycerides and cholesterol) are transported as chylomicrons. Very low density lipoproteins (VLDL) are also formed postprandially but play only a minor role. In the fasting state, VLDL predominate and are responsible for the transport of endogenous lipids (intestinal and biliary). Nascent high-density lipoproteins (N-HDL) are also synthesized by the intestine. They mainly transport cholesterol but also long-chain fatty acids, and in contrast to chylomicrons and VLDL, they are released not only in lymph but also in the portal venous system.

There are still few studies on the efficiency of chylomicron formation in the newborn period. Chylomicrons are not observed postprandially during the first week of life. Of interest is the fact that gestational age does not seem to influence the appearance of chylomicrons, or their size or number. These data do not necessarily suggest that poor formation of chylomicrons may be a limiting step in the overall scheme of fat uptake by the entero-

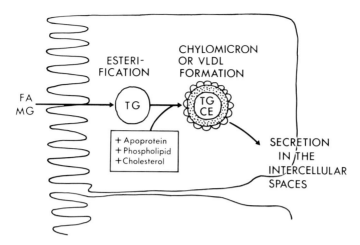

Fig. 10-7. Formation of chylomicrons and very low density lipoproteins. The core of these particles is composed of resynthesized triglycerides (TG) and esterified cholesterol (CE). Samll amounts of free cholesterol and phospholipids are added to a surface coat of apoproteins. Assembly takes place in the endoplasmic reticulum. They then move to the Golgi apparatus where additional sugars are added to apoproteins and form vesicles. The Golgi vesicles migrate to the lateral basal aspect of the cell, fuse with the plasma membrane, and release their contents by reverse pinocytosis into the interstitial space and lymphatics.

cyte. It is possible that a high turnover rate of absorbed lipids could explain these results. In circumstances where the absorptive capacity of the small bowel is challenged by large fat loads, the distal segments have been shown to accumulate more fat than the proximal segments do. This has been attributed ot the limited capacity of the ileum for chylomicron synthesis or secretion. Since the lower bowel is called upon as a reserve area for absorption in the newborn period where the fat load is considerable in the face of a digestive phase defect, it is possible that a limited ability to synthesize chylomicrons could contribute to fat malabsorption.

Transport in lymphatics or portal venous system. The final step in the uptake of fat from the lumen is its transport within the cell and its exocytosis. Although the bulk of long-chain fatty acids are exported in the lymphatics, a certain amount is transported in the portal venous system (Fig. 10-5). They can be bound to albumin and get into the systemic circulation as monomers or else enter into the formation of nascent high-density lipoproteins. The proportion of long-chain fatty acids transported in the portal vein varies with the amount of fat presented to the absorptive appartus and the solubility of the perfused fatty acids. The importance of this finding in the context of the better coefficient of fat absorption associated with unsat-

urated long-chain fatty acid feeding of infants remains unknown. Medium-chain fatty acid absorption in lymph is negligible and occurs almost entirely in the portal vein in their nonesterified form and bound to albumin.

Proteins

Protein accounts for 11% to 14% of total calories. It is essential to maintain an appropriate nutritional status and to ensure growth and development. It plays an important role for the release of gastrointestinal hormones such as cholecystokinin-pancreozymin and secretin, which influence not only the secretion of pancreaticobiliary secretions but also perhaps the growth of the pancreas.

Digestion of proteins starts in the stomach by the action of pepsin. However, the bulk of dietary protein is hydrolyzed in the duodenum and upper jejunal lumen by pancreatic proteolytic enzymes screted in an inactive form. Trypsinogen is catalyzed into active trypsin by the enzyme enterokinase present in the brush border of the upper small bowel. Trypsin then activates autocatalytically the bulk of trypsinogen and the other zymogens, chymotrypsinogen, proelastase, and procarboxypeptidase (p. 841). The products of pancreatic proteolysis are small peptides and amino acids. The former either undergo further hydrolysis by brush border peptidases or else are taken up by the enterocytes, in which specific intracellular peptidases are responsible for their final breakdown into amino acids.

In the jejunum, intracellular peptidases are mainly responsible for mucosal hydrolysis, whereas in the ileum both brush border and cytosolic peptidases are important. Of interest is the observation that after a high-protein meal, peptides are still present in the ileum. A recent study showing differences in the absorption of two different protein hydrolysates confirms the presence of specific peptide-transport systems for dipeptides and tripeptides. Experimental data suggest that administration of peptides has significant advantages over free amino acid mixtures in children with a reduced absorptive surface area. Furthermore, the intact peptide-transfer mechanism is age-dependent in that the influx of certain dipeptides is greater in young animals than in adults.

Amino acids are taken into and transported across the intestinal cell by an active sodium-dependent process similar to the one described below for glucose.

Although the bulk of proteins to be digested and absorbed are dietary, endogenous protein is also important for nitrogen balance through failure of absorption or loss in the lumen, that is, protein-losing enteropathy (Chapter 11).

On perfusion of human volunteers with amino acids, branched-chain amino acids (leucine, isoleucine, and valine) display the highest rate of absorption and glutamic acid and aspartic acid the lowest. Because small peptides made up of either dicarboxylic amino acids (glutamic acid and aspartic acid) or imino acids (proline, hydroxyproline) and glycine undergo little hydrolysis at the brush border and are preferentially taken up as peptides, the transport mechanisms for these two classes of amino acids may not have the same physiologic importance as for the other amino acids.

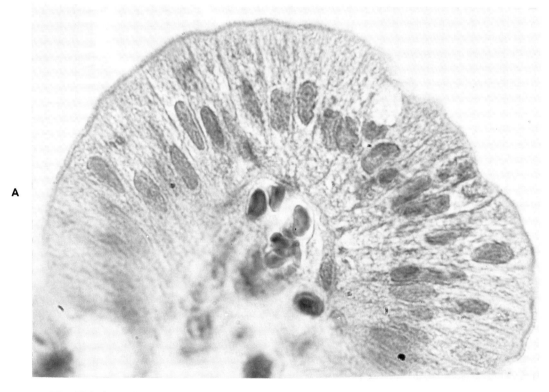

A

Fig. 10-8. **A,** Under the light microscope with oil immersion the microvillous pattern can already be appreciated. **B,** However the electron microscope permits an evaluation of the size, shape, and distribution of microvilli. Note the presence of the ''fuzzy coat'' that covers the surface of these fingerlike projections; it probably plays an important role in absorptive function and defense mechanism.

It has long been known that the immature intestinal cell of the newborn can absorb unhydrolyzed protein for several months. Work in this area suggests that transport of macromolecules may continue throughout life. It never occurs in sufficient quantities to be of nutritional importance but may have far-reaching consequences in the pathogenesis of a number of intestinal and systemic disease states because of the potential obsorption of bacteria, toxins, enzymes, and ingested food antigens.

Carbohydrates

The type of carbohydrates in the diet and their intraluminal and bursh-border digestion are discussed in Chapter 9. Glucose and galactose are actively transported across the intestine by a process requiring energy and Na^+, whereas the absorption of fructose occurs by facilitated fiffusion using a carrier mechanism independent of Na^+ and of the glucose-galactose transport mechanism.

Mucosal entry requires interaction of the substrate with a protein carrier molecule in the brush border to form a complex that will move across the lipoprotein membrane barrier along with sodium. The presence of Na^+ is necessary to maintain the proper carrier-sugar relationship because glucose and Na^+ share a common carrier. Reciprocally, glucose is known to stimulate the absorption of sodium. Once taken into the cell, the actively transported sugar can be metabolized locally and provides energy for the active pumping of Na^+ out at the base and lateral sides of the enterocyte. The transported sugar moves out of the enterocyte as it reaches concentrations exceeding those in blood (downhill transport). Through this mechanism, sodium moves into the cell down a concentration gradient, since intracellular Na^+ is kept low (10 mEq/L) by a sodium pump that requires energy. Actively transported sugars, on

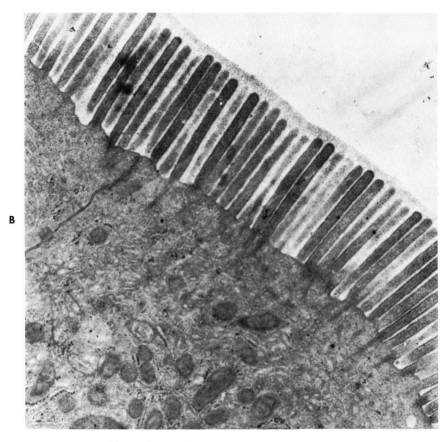

Fig. 10-8, cont'd. **B,** For legend see opposite page.

the other hand, can make their way into the cell even when their concentration is much lower than that of the absorptive cells (uphill transport). This is usually the case in the small bowel distal to the first foot or so of jejunum.

It has long been known that glucose is more efficiently absorbed when offered to the mucosal surface as a disaccharide. The accepted explanation is that brush-border disaccharidase enzymes are topographically distributed so that carrier molecules can complex with the monosaccharides more readily. Recent evidence suggests that glucose released from sucrose, maltose, and isomaltose may be transported into the enterocyte in the absence of Na^+. The hypothesis is that brush-border disaccharidases may serve as vectors that transport the products of their enzymatic activity across the membrane.

The efficiency of carbohydrate uptake depends to some extent on the relative sterility of the small bowel as well as on its motility, which, if reduced, may increase the thickness of the unstirred water layer and retard diffusion of carbohydrates to the surface of microvilli. However, the most critical factor is the structural and functional integrity of the enterocyte and of its brush border. The most distinctive feature of the enterocyte is its apical brush border composed of a row of closely packed microvilli (Fig. 10-8). External to these is the glycocalyx, which is rich in carbohydrate material. It may play a role in digestion and protects the microvillus surface by acting as a molecular sieve. Mucosal injury and inherited defects lead to a list of brush-border membrane diseases, most of them affecting carbohydrate hydrolysis and uptake (Table 10-2).

Vitamin B_{12}

The major source of dietary vitamin B_{12} is animal protein and B_{12} producing microorganisms.

Vitamin B_{12} is attached to dietary protein from which it is freed by gastric pepsin. This step is not rate limiting since absorption of protein-bound vitamin B_{12} may also take place. Free vitamin B_{12} binds to two molecules of intrinsic factor, a glycoprotein secreted by gastric parietal cells. The complex preserves vitamin B_{12} from utilization by bacteria and from the formation of unabsorbable macromolecular aggregates during transport in the small bowel. In the ileum, the complex binds to receptor sites, and intrinsic factor remains

Table 10-2. Brush-border membrane diseases

Enzyme defect
Congenital lactose maldigestion
Adult lactose maldigestion
Sucrose-isomaltose maldigestion
Trehalose maldigestion
Enterokinase deficiency
Carrier protein defect
Glucose-galactose malabsorption
Neutral amino acid malabsorption
Basic amino acid malabsorption
Amino acid–glycine malabsorption
Folate malabsorption

From Crane, R.K., and others: Membranes and diseases, New York, 1976, Raven Press.

attached to the receptor after facilitating B_{12} entry into the enterocyte. Surface-bound intrinsic factor may then promote the uptake of more vitamin B_{12}.

The four basic mechanisms of vitamin B_{12} deficiency associated with malabsorption are as follows:

1. Deficiency of intrinsic factor secondary to gastric disorders
2. Utilization or adsorption of vitamin B_{12} by parasites or bacteria
3. Malabsorption of vitamin B_{12} in disease or resection of the ileum
4. Malabsorption of vitamin B_{12} in chronic pancreatic insufficiency

Folic acid

Normal metabolism in man necessitates certain derivatives of folic (pteroylglutamic) acid, and there is no biosynthesis of these substances within the body. They or their precursors must be obtained from the diet by absorption in the small intestine. The normal absorption of folate compounds is therefore of great importance in the maintenance of normal metabolism. Hematologic and neurologic repercussions of folate deficiency are well known.

Folates are widely distributed in plant and animal tissues, and 75% of the daily folate intake of 700 μg is in the form of pteroylpolyglutamates. Folic acid is rapidly absorbed from the duodenum and jejunum. Dietary pteroylpolyglutamates are hydrolyzed at the intestinal brush-border surface by a specific peptidase to yield monoglutamates and diglutamates. These products are then hydrolyzed by enterocyte lysosomes before being methylated.

Drugs associated with folate malabsorption include phenytoin, sulfasalazine, para-aminosalicylates, and oral contraceptives. The folate deficiency of alcoholics and of cirrhotics is believed to reflect nutritional deprivation and associated intestinal or metabolic abnormalities rather than folate malabsorption. Controversy exists as to whether the transport process of folates is active or passive. Recent evidence suggests that it is passive and cannot take place against a concentration gradient. It is absorbed primarily from the upper third of the small intestine. However, all disorders of the small intestine can be associated with reduced absorption. Chronic vomiting can lead to folate deficiency.

Vitamin D and calcium

Orally administered vitamin D is primarily absorbed in the jejunum in a process similar to that described for fat. After absorption, the vitamin enters the lymphatic system as a constituent of chylomicrons. The vitamin then enters the liver, where it is converted into its 25-hydroxy derivative, which in turn is transformed by the kidney mitochondria into the final metabolically active form of vitamin D, the 1,25-hydroxy derivative. Because this product is synthesized in the kidney and has its function in intestine and bone, it clearly fits the prerequisites for a hormone. Dihydroxy D_3 is 100 and 1000 times more potent than 25-OH D_3 and vitamin D, respectively, in promoting calcium mobilization from bone and absorption from the intestine. Its rate of synthesis is regulated by dietary calcium and ultimately by the serum calcium concentration.

The transfer of calcium with phosphate as the normal accompanying anion against an electrochemical gradient requires oxidative metabolism and is therefore an active transport process. Current information is that there is a bidirectional flux of calcium at both the luminal and serosal side of the enterocyte throughout the small intestine. Net absorption (insorption-exsorption) is maximal in the duodenum. The effect of vitamin D on calcium absorption is mediated by an increase in the permeability of the intestinal cell membrane and by the promotion of the synthesis of a calcium-binding protein that carries the absorbed calcium

to the base of the intestinal cell. Calcium absorption is impaired when absorption of the fat-soluble vitamin D or its conversion into active metabolites is defective. Calcium becomes unavailable for absorption in the presence of large amounts of fatty acids by forming insoluble calcium soaps, which are then excreted in the feces.

Fat-soluble vitamins A, D, E, and K

The fat-soluble vitamins are found associated with dietary lipids and share the same sequence of events for their digestion and absorption. Consequently, disease conditions associated with severe fat malabsorption usually lead to simultaneous malabsorption of the fat-soluble vitamins A, D, E, and K.

Iron

The diet should provide 1 mg/kg/day of iron, which is the recommended daily allowance. Dietary iron is unavailable to the body unless the foodstuff is first digested and the freed iron is rendered soluble.

Under normal circumstances, iron is absorbed in the duodenum and upper small bowel. Hemoglobin iron is the most efficiently absorbed and is not bound like inorganic iron (ferrous and ferric) by carbonates, phytates, and oxalates into unabsorbable forms. At the acid pH of the stomach and duodenum, ferrous and ferric iron are rendered soluble by chelation with ascorbic acid, carbohydrates, or amino acids. Approximately 5% to 10% of dietary iron is absorbed, and this corresponds closely with daily losses through the gut, skin, and urine. The quantities absorbed in a given individual are closely geared to the body's requirements, since processes for enhancing iron excretion are quite limited.

The absorbing capacity of mucosal cells is strongly influenced not only by intraluminal events and the anatomic and functional integrity of enterocytes but also more importantly by the size of iron stores, which regulates the enterocyte transport protein. The processes of mucosal uptake and serosal transfer are both tightly regulated by mucosal cell transferrin, which is a close reflection of the total iron body stores. Absorption of iron is carrier mediated because transferrin binds iron in the lumen of the gut and transports it across the brush border.

Magnesium and zinc

The two elements magnesium and zinc have considerable importance in normal body functions are are commonly deficient in conditions giving rise to the malabsorption syndrome. Magnesium is absorbed equally well in the jejunum and ileum. Calcium and magnesium transport systems are separate, but both are influenced by vitamin D. As is the case for calcium, magnesium forms complexes with phosphate, citrate, and sulfate and is bound to proteins. Chronic diarrhea, muscular cramps, and tetany are the important manifestations of hypomagnesemia.

Average zinc absorption has been estimated to be 20% to 30% of that ingested. A zinc-binding ligand transports zinc across the mucosal cell to receptors on the serosal surface. Absorbed zinc is transported in the portal system bound to albumin and to a lesser extent to transferrin. In the presence of steatorrhea, zinc forms insoluble complexes with fat. High concentrations of zinc are found in ostomy fluids and zinc deficiency is a well known complication of Crohn's disease and celiac disease. Anorexia, hypogeusia, delayed wound healing, skin lesions, and diarrhea are common manifestations. A more complete discussion of zinc deficiency states can be found in Chapter 17.

Water and electrolytes

See Chapter 8.

PATHOPHYSIOLOGIC CLASSIFICATION

Assimilation of nutrients is dependent on their proper digestion and absorption, which take place in the lumen of the small intestine (luminal phase), on the surface, and within the enterocytes (intestinal phase), and is also dependent on their removal from the cells and delivery to the body (delivery phase). The sequence of events for the three major dietary constituents shown in Fig. 10-1 serves as the framework for the classification of malabsorptive conditions. A pathophysiologic grouping of disease conditions is helpful to the clinician in his differential diagnostic approach to the patient.

Intraluminal phase abnormalities

Acid hypersecretion—Zollinger-Ellison syndrome
Gastric resection
Inadequate lipolysis and proteolysis
Cystic fibrosis
Chronic pancreatitis

Pancreatic pseudocysts
Shwachman's syndrome
Enterokinase deficiency
Lipase deficiency
Malnutrition
Decreased conjugated bile acids
  Liver production and excretion
    Neonatal hepatitis
    Biliary atresia: intrahepatic and extrahepatic
    Acute and chronic active hepatitis
    Disease of the biliary tract
    Cirrhosis
    Fat malabsorption in the premature infant
  Intestinal factors
    Short bowel syndrome
    Bacterial overgrowth
      Blind loop
      Fistula
      Strictures—regional enteritis
      Scleroderma, intestinal pseudo-obstruction

Abnormalities of the intestinal phase

Mucosal diseases
  Infection, bacterial or viral
  Infestations
    Giardia lamblia
    Fish tapeworm
    Hookworm
  Malnutrition
    Marasmus
    Kwashiorkor
  Dermatitis herpetiformis
  Folic acid deficiency
  Drugs: methotrexate, antibiotics
  Crohn's disease
  Chronic ulcerative colitis
  Cow's milk intolerance and soy protein
    intolerance
  Secondary disaccharidase deficiency
  Hirschsprung's disease with enterocolitis
  Tropical sprue
  Celiac disease
  Radiation enteritis
  Lymphoma
  Eosinophilic gastroenteritis
Circulatory disturbances
  Cirrhosis
  Congestive heart failure
Abnormal structural makeup of gastrointestinal tract
  Dumping syndrome after gastrectomy
  Malrotation
  Stenosis of jejunum or ileum
  Small bowel resection—short bowel syndrome
  Polyposis
Selective inborn absorptive defects
  Congenital malabsorption of folic acid

Selective malabsorption of vitamin B_{12}
Cystinuria, methionine malabsorption
Hartnup's disease, blue diaper syndrome
Glucose-galactose malabsorption
Primary disaccharidase deficiency
Acrodermatitis enteropathica
Abetalipoproteinemia
Congenital chloridorrhea (chloride diarrhea)
Primary hypomagnesemia
Hereditary fructose intolerance
Familial hypophosphatemic rickets
Endocrine diseases
Diabetes
Addison's disease
Hyperthyroidism
Hypoparathyroidism, pseudohypoparathyroidism
Neuroblastoma, ganglioneuroma

Defective delivery phase

Whipple's disease
Intestinal lymphangiectasis
Congestive heart failure
Regional enteritis with lymphangiectasis
Lymphoma
Abetalipoproteinemia

Miscellaneous

Renal insufficiency
Carcinoid, mastocytosis
Immunity defects
Familial dysautonomia
Maternal deprivation?
Collagen diseases
Wolman's disease
Histiocytosis X
Intractable diarrhea of early infancy

REFERENCES

Adibi, S.A.: Intestinal phase of protein assimilation in man, Am. J. Clin. Nutr. **29:**205-215, 1976.

Ammon, H.V., Thomas, P.J., and Phillips, S.F.: Effect of lecithin on jejunal absorption of micellar lipids in man and on their monomer activity in vitro, Lipids **14:**395-400, 1979.

Bläckberg, L., Hernell, O., Bengtsson, G., and Olivecrona, T.: Colipase enhances hydrolysis of dietary triglycerides in the absence of bile salts, J. Clin. Invest. **64:**1303-1308, 1979.

Borgström, B.: Importance of phospholipids, pancreatic phospholipase A_2 and fatty acid for the digestion of dietary fat, Gastroenterology **78:**954-962, 1980.

Crane, R.K., Menard, D., Preiser, H., and Cerda, J.: Brush border membrane. In Bolis, L., Hoffman, J.F., and Leaf, A., editors: Membranes and diseases, New York, 1976, Raven Press.

Dallman, P.R.: New approaches to screening for iron deficiency, J. Pediatr. **90:**678-681, 1977.

Fairclough, P.D., Hegarty, J.E., Silk, D.B.A., and Clark, M.L.: Comparison of the absorption of two protein hydrol-

ysates and their effects on water and electrolyte movements in the human jejunum, Gut **21:**829-834, 1980.

Friedman, H.A., and Nylund, B.: Intestinal digestion, absorption and transport, Am. J. Clin. Nutr. **33:**1108-1139, 1980.

Gray, G.M.: Carbohydrate digestion and absorption, N. Engl. J. Med. **292:**1225-1230, 1975.

Hambidge, M.: Trace element deficiencies in childhood. In Suskind, R.M., editor: Textbook of pediatric nutrition, New York, 1980, Raven Press.

Hamosh, M.: A review. Fat digestion in the newborn: role of lingual lipase and preduodenal digestion, Pediatr. Res. **13:**615-622, 1979.

Himukai, M., Konno, T., and Hoshi, T.: Age-dependent change in intestinal absorption of dipeptides and their constituent amino acids in the guinea pig, Pediatr. Res. **14:**1272-1275, 1980.

Hofmann, A.F.: Lipase, colipase, amphipathic dietary proteins, and bile acids: new interactions at and old interface, Gastroenterology **75:**530-532, 1978.

Jeejeebhoy, K.N., Chu, R.C., Marliss, E.B., and others: Chromium deficiency, glucose intolerance, and neuropathy reversed by chromium supplementation, in a patient receiving long-term total parenteral nutrition, Am. J. Clin. Nutr. **30:**531-538, 1977.

Koldovsky, O.: Digestion and absorption. In Stave, U., editor: Perinatal physiology, ed. 2, London, 1978, Plenum Publishing Co.

Mansbach, C.M.: Conditions affecting the biosynthesis of lipids in the small intestine, Am. J. Clin. Nutr. **29:**295-301, 1976.

Matthews, D.M., and Adibi, S.A.: Peptide absorption, Gastroenterology **71:**151-161, 1976.

Mertz, W., Toepfer, E.W., Roginski, E.E., and Polansky, M.M.: Present knowledge of the role of chromium, Fed. Proc. **33:**2275-2280, 1974.

Ockner, R.K., and Manning, J.A.: Fatty acid binding protein in small intestine: identification, isolation and evidence for its role in cellular fatty acid transport, J. Clin. Invest. **54:**326-328, 1974.

Rosenberg, I.H.: Absorption and malabsorption of folates, Clin. Haematol. **5:**589-618, 1979.

Roulet, M., Weber, A.M., Paradis, Y., and others: Gastric emptying and lingual lipase activity in cystic fibrosis, Pediatr. Res. **14:**1360-1363, 1980.

Sabesin, S.M., and Frase, S.: Electron microscopic studies of the assembly, intracellular transport, and secretion of chylomicrons by rat intestine, J. Lipid Res. **18:**496-511, 1977.

Shiau, Y.F., Umstetter, C., Kendall, K., and Koldovsky, O.: Development of fatty acid esterification mechanisms in rat small intestine, Am. J. Physiol. **237:**E399-403, 1979.

Silk, D.B.A., Chung, Y.C., Kim, Y.S., and others: Comparison of oral feeding of peptide and amino acid meals to normal human subjects, Gastroenterology **70:**A79/937, 1976.

Simmonds, W.J.: Uptake of fatty acid and monoglyceride. In Rommel, K., Goebell, H., and Böhmer, R., editors: Lipid absorption: biochemical and clinical aspects, Lancaster, Eng., 1976, MTP Press, Ltd., p. 51.

Sleisenger, M.H., and Kim, Y.S.: Protein digestion and absorption, N. Engl. J. Med. **300:**659-663, 1979.

Surawica, C.M., Sillery, J., Saunders, D.R., and Rubin, C.E.: Human jejunal absorption of long-chain fatty acid (LCFA) without chylomicron formation, Gastroenterology **76:**1256, 1979 (Abstract).

Tso, P., Balint, J.A., and Simmonds, W.J.: Role of biliary lecithin in lymphatic transport of fat, Gastroenterology **73:**1362-1367, 1977.

Westergaard, H., and Dietschy, J.M.: The mechanism whereby bile acid micelles increase the rate of fatty acid and cholesterol uptake into the intestinal mucosa cell, J. Clin. Invest. **58:**97-108, 1976.

Woodward, J.C., Webster, P.D., and Carr, A.A.: Primary hypomagnesemia with secondary hypocalcemia, diarrhea and insensitivity to parathyroid hormone, Am. J. Dig. Dis. **17:**612-618, 1972.

CLINICAL FINDINGS
History

The general approach to a patient believed to be affected with malabsorption should include recording a detailed and accurate history. The following points are particularly important to consider:

1. The chronologic sequence of events is of primary importance in determination of the onset of and the relationship between symptoms and the introduction of various nutrients, as in milk protein intolerance, disaccharidase deficiency, celiac disease, or the administration of drugs.
2. An accurate dietary history in terms of quantity and quality is essential, since many children present with malnutrition, which may be secondary to restricted diets enforced to control symptoms.
3. A thorough subjective examination may uncover extraintestinal constitutional disorders that are associated with malabsorption.
4. That the patient has undergone previous abdominal surgery may lead one to consider the anatomic causes of malabsorption.
5. That he suffered repeated infections orients the diagnosis toward cystic fibrosis or immunity defects.
6. The knowledge of visits to tropical countries or to areas where certain infestations are endemic is important.
7. In some cases, the complaints may not refer to the gastrointestinal tract alone. Failure to thrive, weight loss, peripheral edema, unexplained fever, anorexia, and fatigue may be the first signs of chronic liver disease or of Crohn's disease.

Physical examination

During the examination, particular attention should be given to the nutritional status and to certain physical signs.

The severity of symptoms or their chronicity will evidently take on added significance if the examiner can show that the underlying illness is interfering with normal growth. Plotting the child's height and weight on a growth chart will, at a glance, demonstrate in most cases of generalized malabsorption a discrepancy between height and weight. Stunting is particularly severe in cystic fibrosis, celiac disease, and chronic inflammatory bowel diseases such as chronic ulcerative colitis and regional enteritis. Delayed development of secondary sexual characteristics is regularly seen in these conditions.

Recent loss of weight is usually confirmed by appreciation of the thickness of subcutaneous tissue and by the abnormal elasticity of the skin. Muscle wasting should also be looked for and is best demonstrated in the buttocks, thighs, and arms.

Inspection of the extremities may show peripheral edema in those malabsorptive states accompanied by a protein-losing enteropathy or by severe malnutrition. Color and texture of hair are usually altered in protein-deficiency states. Clubbing of fingers, frequently associated with chronic liver or bowel disease, is also a common feature in cystic fibrosis with severe lung disease.

Examination of the abdomen should be particularly directed to the estimation of enlargement, distention, and the presence of generalized discomfort or of localized painful areas and masses.

Deficiencies in fat-soluble vitamins can be indicated by the presence of skin bruises (vitamin K) and by evidence of rickets (vitamin D). Anemia is commonly associated with malabsorption syndromes. Acute dermatitis may be a manifestation of zinc deficiency.

Locomotor and nervous system examination can demonstrate muscle weakness, arthralgia or arthritis, and the muscle cramps associated with the tetany of celiac disease. Patients with a malabsorption syndrome are often depressed, irritable, uncooperative, and difficult to approach.

LABORATORY DIAGNOSIS

It is difficult to plan an easy and rational approach to the investigation of malabsorption. The tests that may be employed in any individual patient depend greatly on the initial clinical presentation, the physical findings, and the repercussions that the disease has had on the nutritional status and on growth. When clinical findings are equivocal, the following work-up is recommended:

Examination of stools and stool assessment
  Cultures
  Microscopic studies for ova, cysts, and parasites
  Microscopic examination for neutral fat and fatty acids
  Test for occult blood
  Determination of stool pH and presence of reducing substances
  Quantification of stool fat in a 3-day sample collected between nonabsorbable markers
Urine—analysis and culture
Hematologic evaluation
  Complete blood cell count
  Reticulocyte count
  Platelet count
  Erythrocyte sedimentation rate
  Prothrombin time
Biochemical evaluation
  Protein and immunoglobulin electrophoresis
  Determination of sodium, potassium, chloride, carbon dioxide
  Determination of calcium, phosphorus, alkaline phosphatase, folic acid, and vitamin B_{12}
  D-Xylose absorption test
  Sweat test
X-ray study
  Assessment of bone age
  Survey of the chest
  Barium meal and small bowel follow-through
  Barium enema

Perhaps the most important feature in the diagnosis of generalized malabsorption is steatorrhea. Accurate measurement of fecal fat is the most valuable diagnostic aid. Screening tests such as serum carotene and vitamin A are unreliable.

Additional testing is necessary to establish the site of the digestive-absorptive defect and to determine the extent of the malabsorption. The following list is a compilation of the diagnostic determinations that we have found most helpful in infants and children with a presumptive diagnosis of malabsorption. A discussion of their place and value in the work-up of the child with malabsorption can also be found in Part III.

Fat absorption
  Determination of 72-hour fecal fat excretion and preferably of the coefficient of fat absorption
Protein absorption and loss
  Serum protein electrophoresis
  Determination of fecal excretion of ^{51}Cr-albumin
Carbohydrate absorption
  D-Xylose absorption test
  Determination of stool pH and reducing substances
  Breath hydrogen excretion after lactose or sucrose

Absorption of fat-soluble vitamins
  Determination of prothrombin time before and 24 hours after administration of parenteral vitamin K (5 mg)
  Determination of calcium, phosphorus, and alkaline phosphatase
Absorption of folic acid and vitamin B_{12}
  Schilling test
  Determination of serum levels of folic acid and vitamin B_{12}
  Bone marrow examination
Absorption of iron
  Determination of iron levels in serum
  Assessment of total iron-binding capacity
Bacterial infection and parasitic infestation
  Stool and jejunal cultures
  Examination of duodenal juice and of impression smear of jejunal mucosa for *Giardia lamblia*
  Bile acid breath hydrogen test
X-ray studies
  Upper gastrointestinal series with small bowel study
  Barium enema
  Roentgenographic assessment of bone age
Pancreatic exocrine function
  Sweat chlorides (iontophoresis)
  Determination of fecal chymotrypsin in a 72-hour stool collection
  Examination of duodenal aspirate for volume, viscosity, pH, bicarbonate, trypsin, lipase, and amylase activity before and after intravenous administration of secretin and pancreozymin
Liver function
  Bilirubin, SGOT, alkaline phosphatase
  Sulfobromophthalein test (BSP)
  Serum bile acids
Structural and enzymatic integrity of peroral small bowel
  Mucosal biopsy
  Examination of specimen with the dissecting, light, and electron microscopes
  Disaccharidase determination
Structural integrity of large intestine
  Rectosigmoidoscopy and rectal biopsy
Miscellaneous
  Immunoglobulin levels, lipoprotein electrophoresis, catecholamines, 5-hydroxyindole acetic acid, gastrin, vasoactive intestinal peptide, calcitonin, cortisol, and thyroid function

Small bowel x-ray examination

Plain films of the abdomen may show gas patterns suggestive of ileus or obstruction or the calcification associated with neuroblastomas, ganglioneuromas, chronic pancreatitis, gallstones, antecedent meconium peritonitis, and duplications.

Barium sulfate contrast studies of the stomach

and entire small bowel are useful in defining gross anatomic defects of these organs or of closely related neighboring structures and viscus. However, they can also be of great value for identification of diffuse lesions of the small intestine and can orient the clinician toward a specific diagnosis.

The roentgenographic classification that follows is based on small intestinal diameter and mucosal fold thickness. This grouping of malabsorptive conditions under roentgenologic patterns should, of course, be correlated with clinical, laboratory, and histologic findings to maximize its value on the diagnostic process required for the child suspected of having a digestive-absorptive defect.

*Roentgenographic classification of malabsorptive conditions**

Pattern I. Normal small intestine pattern
  Pancreatic insufficiency other than cystic fibrosis
  Drug-induced malabsorption: antibiotics, methotrexate, para-aminosalicylic acid
  Disaccharidase deficiency with a normal biopsy
Pattern II. Dilated small intestine with normal folds
  Obstruction and ileus
  Celiac disease
  Collagen diseases: systemic lupus erythematosus, dermatomyositis, scleroderma
  Chronic idiopathic pseudo-obstruction
Pattern III. Thickened regular folds with or without dilation
  Celiac disease
  Hypoproteinemia
  Edema
  Lymphangiectasia
  Amyloidosis
  Lymphoma
Pattern IV. Thickened irregular or nodular folds with or without dilatation
  Cystic fibrosis
  Crohn's disease
  Lymphoid nodular hyperplasia
  Whipple's disease
  Mastocytosis
  Eosinophilic gastroenteritis
  Abetalipoproteinemia
  Zollinger-Ellison syndrome
  Lymphoma

*Modified from Tully, T.E., and Feinberg, S.B.: A roentgenographic classification of diffuse diseases of the small intestine with malabsorption, Am. J. Roentgenol. Radium Ther. Nucl. Med. **121**:283-290, 1974.

Small intestinal biopsy

Suction biopsy of the small intestine is a safe procedure even in neonates. The description of the instrument and of the technique used can be found in Chapter 31. Over the past few years, we have carried out intestinal biopsies much earlier in the course of investigating children with suspected malabsorption, short-cutting a significant number of tests found to be of poor value in localizing and characterizing a digestive-absorptive defect. The information provided by a peroral biopsy of the small intestine is not limited to histologic features. Enzymatic, metabolic, immunologic, and microbiologic studies are useful. Future developments in this area are very promising.

Histology

The diagnostic value of a small bowel biopsy varies with the distribution, specificity, and constancy of the histologic changes associated with various entities. Biopsy specimens for most diagnostic purposes are taken from the duodenojejunal junction at the ligament of Treitz, since this area is invariably involved in the diffuse diseases of the small bowel. Serial biopsy specimens from other areas are reserved for cases in which changes may be patchy. The amount and reliability of the information provided by a biopsy at the ligament of Treitz can be categorized as follows*:

Biopsy at ligament of Treitz

Diagnostic biopsy
  Celiac disease
  Whipple's disease
  Abetalipoproteinemia
  Combined immunodeficiency disease
  Acquired agammaglobulinemia
Diagnostic or nondiagnostic biopsy
  Intestinal lymphangiectasia
  Eosinophilic gastroenteritis
  Giardiasis
  Crohn's disease of proximal jejunum
  Isolated IgA deficiency
  Dysgammaglobulinemia
  Mastocytosis
  Lymphoma
Nonspecific changes
  Milk or soy protein intolerance
  Malnutrition

*Modified from Trier, J.S.: Diagnosis value of peroral biopsy of the proximal small intestine. N. Engl. J. Med. **285**:1470-1473, 1971.

Intractable diarrhea of early infancy
Antibiotic- or methotrexate-induced malabsorption
Tropical sprue
Contaminated small bowel syndrome
Radiation enteritis

Studies other than histology

Enzymatic studies. The routine determination of disaccharidase activity should be carried out and is of diagnostic value in isolated lactase deficiency, in congenital sucrase-isomaltase deficiency, and in cases of general decrease of disaccharidase activity associated with various mucosal disorders. Enterokinase determinations will identify rare cases of congenital enterokinase deficiency.

Metabolic studies. In vitro transport of labeled substrates such as glucose and amino acids can be done in cases of inborn errors with selective defects of absorption.

Immunologic studies. Immunofluorescent studies with immunoglobulin and complement fraction antibodies can be done in suspected immunity defects.

Microbiologic studies. Direct isolation and culture or immunofluorescent identification can be done for bacteria, viruses, and parasites.

Culture of explants. This remains a research tool.

REFERENCES

Anderson, C.M.: Malabsorption in children, Clin. Gastroenterol. **6:**355-375, 1977.

Berg, N.O., Borulf, S., Jakobsson, I., and Lindberg, T.: How to approach the child suspected of malabsorption, Acta Paediatr. Scand. **67:**403-411, 1978.

Russell, R.I., and Lee, F.D.: Tests of small intestinal function: digestion, absorption, secretion, Clin. Gastroenterol. **7:**277-315, 1978.

Walker-Smith, J.: Diseases of the small intestine in childhood, ed. 2, Bath, Engl., 1979, Pitman Medical Publishing Co., Ltd.

SPECIFIC ENTITIES
Celiac disease (gluten enteropathy)

Together with cystic fibrosis, celiac disease is the most common cause of malabsorption in infants and children. It is a disease in which the mucosa of the small bowel of susceptible patients is damaged by gluten-containing foods. Clinical symptoms and histological changes remit on gluten withdrawal, and histologic relapse occurs within

Table 10-3. Incidence of celiac disease

	1971-1975	1976-1980
St. James's Hospital* (Leeds)	32	9
Hôpital Sainte-Justine (Montreal)	31	12

*Courtesy J.M. Littlewood, Leeds, England.

2 years of reintroducing gluten in the diet. This definition implies that gluten intolerance is permanent. However, recent reports suggest that a small percentage (5%) of patients will not relapse after 2 years of gluten challenge and may suffer only from temporary gluten intolerance. The present evidence indicates that the gluten intolerance is persistent; long-term studies are needed to prove it to be permanent.

The relative importance of heredity and environmental factors in the origin of gluten enteropathy remains unsettled. It is still unknown what the respective role of genetics and environmental factors is. The relationship between the incidence of the disease, infant-feeding practices, and the age of introduction of gluten-containing foods has yet to be defined. The incidence is higher in Europe and in Canada than in the United States. Recent reports suggest that the incidence of celiac disease is decreasing (Table 10-3). This has been attributed to the fact that a large proportion of infants with chronic diarrhea are placed on a milk-free, egg-free, and gluten-free diet before being referred. Others suggest that a change in recent feeding practices, particularly the delayed introduction of solid foods, is the important factor.

The highest incidence of celiac disease presenting in children has been found to be 1 in 597 in the west of Ireland. It is uncommon in blacks and Asians, but it has been described in Asian Indians. Celiac disease often occurs in several members of one family; in fact, intestinal biopsy specimens have shown mucosal abnormalities in 5% to 10% of first-degree relatives. An important link between genetic factors and sensitivity to gluten is the finding of a highly significant increase in the incidence of certain histocompatibility antigens. HLA-B8 is found in 60% to 90% of patient with celiac disease, a fourfold increase over its incidence in a normal population.

Pathogenesis

In the 1950s, it was established that the intestinal malabsorption of celiac disease was related to a factor present in wheat, rye, barley, and oats. A clinical relapse occurred when children with the disease were fed gluten (wheat protein) and gliadin (ethanolic extract of gluten). Subsequent studies showed that the clinical toxicity of gliadin was not altered by peptic-tryptic digestion or by further hydrolysis with pancreatin. The peptide structure is essential for toxicity; gliadin hydrolyzed to its constituent amino acids is harmless to a gluten-sensitive mucosa. Chromatography of gliadin digests has permitted the identification of acidic peptides, which are highly toxic (fraction 9, alpha-gliadin).

Two theories have been proposed to explain the susceptibility of certain individuals to develop the intestinal lesions of celiac disease on exposure to the toxic peptides of gluten.

Metabolic defect. One theory holds that celiac disease may be the result of the lack of an intestinal enzyme for the ultimate detoxification of gluten. This results in the accumulation of material toxic to the susceptible mucosa. When subfractions of fraction 9 obtained from a peptic-tryptic-pancreatic digest of wheat gliadin are incubated with mucosal homogenates, a higher amount of residual peptides are detected in digestion experiments conducted with histologically normal celiac mucosal homogenates than with controls. This lends some support to the hypothesis of an enzyme deficiency. However, most of the evidence indicates that peptidase deficiencies are secondary to mucosal damage. Since no biochemical or physiologic abnormalities can be found in the healed celiac mucosa, the peptidase deficiency appears to be reversible by dietary treatment and is therefore considered a consequence of the disease rather than its primary cause. A cell surface membrane defect that would allow gluten to act as a lectin and bind to the cell surface remains hypothetical.

Immunologic disorder. The immunologic theory has gained increasing support. It holds that celiac disease, through an interplay of genetic and environmental factors, is primarily attributable to an immunologic dysfunction of the intestinal mucosa. Gliadin plays the role of an antigen that evokes an injurious immune response.

1. The rapid development of "gliadin shock" in a few celiac children shortly after the reintroduction of gluten suggests an anaphylactic reaction. However, a delayed Arthus type of reaction has been noted after intradermal testing of celiac patients with gluten fractions. The prompt improvement of celiac disease after corticosteroid treatment and suppression of the toxic effect of gluten on addition of corticosteroids to cultured biopsy specimens favor an immunologic reaction.

2. High titers of antibodies to dietary antigens, especially to gluten, gliadin, and its fractions, have been found in serum and intestinal contests of celiac patients. However, many normal children have antibodies to gluten and also seem to have been immunized by gluten. The finding of complement-fixing antibodies to gliadin that belong to the IgM class has been found only in celiac patients.

3. A rise in serum IgA is a common finding during the active phase of the disease. High levels of serum secretory IgA have also been found. More pertinent, perhaps, are the reports of increased synthesis of IgA and IgM by the intestinal mucosa. A substantial portion of these immunoglobulin have been identified as antigluten antibodies.

4. Circulating immune complexes have been detected in celiac patients. Because immune complexes containing IgM and IgG activate the classic complement pathway, the metabolism of C_3 has been examined. Only a modest lowering has been reported. More interesting is an increased fractional catabolic rate suggesting perhaps activation by immune complexes in the intestinal mucosa.

5. As an alternative to a possible antibody-mediated response to gluten, cell-mediated responses have been sought. The production of macrophage-inhibition factor (MIF) by lymphocytes exposed to gluten has permitted the identification of 90% of patients. The production of macrophage-inhibition factor by cultured celiac mucosa further supports the role of a cellular immune reaction mediated by a lymphocyte population sensitized to gluten.

6. Organ cultures of intestinal biopsies taken from celiac patients in exacerbation and incubated with gliadin responded differently from those taken from patients in remission. Since tissues from patients in remission are not affected by the presence of gluten, it is suggested that gluten protein is not directly toxic to the epithelial cells. Proof that an endogenous effector mechanism, such as humoral substances or sensitized cells, must first trigger the cytotoxic effect was obtained when co-

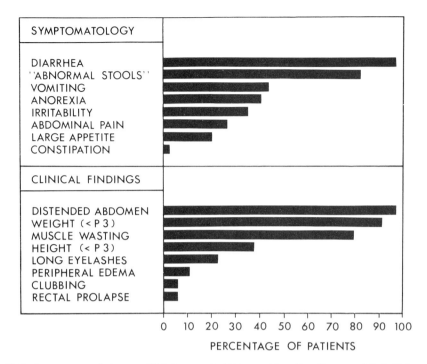

Fig. 10-9. Symptoms and signs in 39 infants and children with celiac disease. $< P\ 3$, Below the third percentile. (From Buts, J.P., et al.: Union Med. Can. **105:**1660, 1976.)

culture of ''remission'' biopsy material with ''exacerbation'' biopsy material in the presence of gluten rendered the former susceptible to the toxic effect of gluten. Although the precise mechanism by which gluten produces cell damage is not known, it is likely to be mediated by either T-cells or B-cells. Histocompatibility antigens such as HLA-B8 could facilitate binding of gluten fractions to epithelial cells. This hypothesis is now supported by the observation that biopsy specimens obtained from patients with HLA-B8 celiac disease are much more susceptible to gluten injury than specimens from those who do not carry this histocompatibility antigen.

Clinical findings (Fig. 10-9)

The so-called textbook picture of the disease is seen in an 18-month-old infant with a history of diarrhea starting between 6 and 12 months of age. His height is stunted and is well below the third percentile for weight. Wasting of the limbs contrasts with a relatively round face and a strikingly distended abdomen (Fig. 10-10). He is described as anorexic and irritable.

Unfortunately, the age and mode of presentation are extremely variable and require elaboration.

Age of onset. Gluten enteropathy usually has its onset between 8 and 24 months. The youngest patient we have seen with the disease is a 3-month-old infant who presented with intractable diarrhea. Although its is unusual for the disease to present for the first time in the teen-age years because of a natural tendency for gluten enteropathy to undergo clinical remission during that period, there are occasional cases in that age group. In England, the commonest age of presentation is between 9 and 12 months of age.

Mode of presentation. In reviewing the modes of presentation, it is important to remember that many patients with celiac disease may never seek medical attention. The study of relatives has, in fact, yielded a number of asymptomatic cases. In general, the mode of onset tends to be more acute in the younger age group, but even then the clinical manifestations are protean.

Diarrhea. Initially, the diarrhea may be intermittent and somehow related to upper respiratory infections or repeated attacks of infectious gastroenteritis. Subsequently, the diarrhea becomes more chronic. In only half the cases, the typical, pale, foul, greasy, bulky stools are reported by parents. A small number of infants may be desperately ill with a profuse diarrhea leading to de-

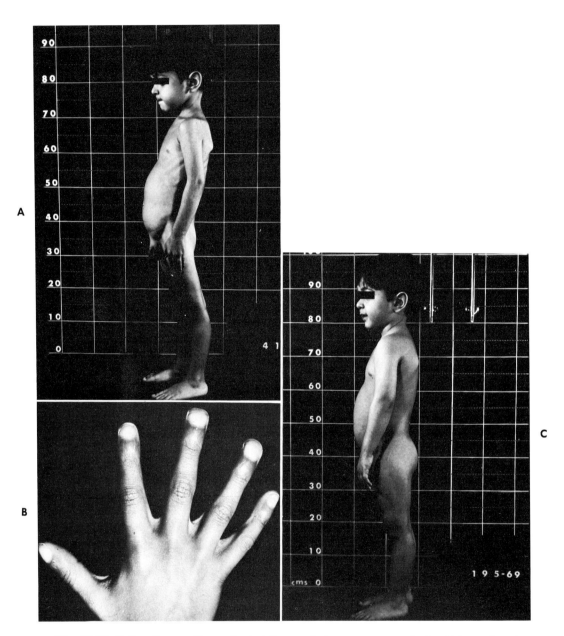

Fig. 10-10. Celiac disease. These physical features before treatment and after 7½ months of receiving a gluten-free diet were present in a 4-year-old child with a 1-year history of passing voluminous, pale, greasy, offensive stools. The following physical features are noted in **A:** stunting (fiftieth percentile for 2 years), wasting, flat buttocks, prominent abdomen, relatively fat face. Clubbing of the fingers is better seen in **B. C,** After 7½ months of receiving a gluten-free diet, the habitus has changed remarkably. The child has gained a significant amount of weight and has grown 9 cm; the buttocks have filled out. Musculature has improved remarkably, particularly in the extremities. The abdomen remains protuberant.

hydration, acidosis, and shock (celiac crisis). Although diarrhea is, with failure to thrive, the most common symptom, diarrhea is often absent (10% to 25%). However, the absence of diarrhea is more likely to occur in older children.

Constipation, vomiting, and abdominal pain. In one series, constipation was found in 10%. Fecal impaction can be quite severe and be secondary to reduced intestinal motility. We have been impressed with the frequency of vomiting, which can actually dominate the picture. Constipation, vomiting, and abdominal pain will sometimes lead to a clinical diagnosis of intestinal obstruction, especially intussusception.

Anorexia and abnormal behavior. Poor appetite is believed to be invariably present, though, by history, it is sometimes difficult to document. A large appetite is sometimes documented. The abnormalities of behavior associated with celiac disease have been well described. Patients are usually fretful, irritable, uncooperative, and difficult to handle, but they can be apathetic. A dramatic personality change is rapidly noted on withdrawal of dietary gluten.

Failure to thrive and wasting. A decreased caloric intake compounds the caloric fecal loss and rapidly brings about a deceleration of growth illustrated by plotting height and weight curves. As expected in malnutrition secondary to poor intake and malabsorption, weight is comparatively more affected than height. However, in older children, especially in those with few symptoms, such a discrepancy is less likely to be found. Short stature may be the only presenting clinical feature. It has recently been suggested that a small bowel biopsy should be part of the work-up in children with short stature and a 4-year delay in bone age especially if serum folate and iron are abnormal.

In established cases, not only is there growth arrest, but loss of weight can be documented. Muscle wasting seems to affect with particular predilection the proximal limbs and the buttocks (Fig. 10-10, *A*). Concomitantly, the abdomen becomes progressively more distended because of poor musculature, altered peristaltic activity, and accumulation of intestinal secretions and gas. Dilated loops of bowel are often easily identified through the thin abdominal wall.

Peripheral edema and other physical signs. Usually confined to the lower extremities, peripheral edema secondary to hypoproteinemia may be intermittent at first and is found in close to one

third of young patients. Clubbing of fingers (Fig. 10-10, *B*), smooth tongue, long eyelashes, and delayed dentition and motor development are other features.

Anemia and signs of vitamin deficiencies. Anemia is usually present and most often secondary to iron deficiency. Serum iron levels are usually low, as are serum folate levels. Serial estimation of the latter is believed to be a useful means for assessment of the compliance of patients with the gluten-free diet.

Deficiencies in fat-soluble vitamins are common. Hypoprothrombinemia can be severe and is responsible for epistaxis, ecchymoses, and sometimes intestinal hemorrhage. Correction with vitamin K should precede intestinal biopsy. Since there is growth arrest, malabsorption of vitamin D leads more often to osteomalacia than to rickets. Osteomalacia has been reported as a mode of presentation in young adults. Tetany with low calcium and magnesium levels occurs in a small number of cases of severe celiac disease beginning at an early age.

Laboratory investigations

Fecal fat excretion. Since steatorrhea is absent in 10% to 25% of children with celiac disease, and its degree is more closely related to the extent of the mucosal lesion in the small bowel than to its severity, a normal fecal fat output does not rule out gluten enteropathy.

A 3-day stool collection is easily carried out at home. It is essential, especially in the child who passes stools irregularly or who does not have diarrhea, to collect the feces between nonabsorbable markers. Because celiac patients are anorexic, it is best to calculate fat intake during the collection. Expressed as a percentage of intake, the untreated celiac patient usually excretes between 15% and 35% of his fat intake. Normal values are less than 10%. In infants and children, a fat excretion exceeding 3.5 gm/24 hr and 4.5 gm/24 hr, respectively, is considered abnormal in our laboratory. In 35 patients with celiac disease with a mean age of 25.4 months at the time of diagnosis, the average ($X \pm$ standard deviation) 24-hour fat excretion was 8.2 ± 4.2 gm. These data from the Hôpital Sainte-Justine point to the fact that the steatorrhea associated with celiac disease is less severe than that with cystic fibrosis where corresponding values recorded in 43 patients was 17.0 ± 10.5 gm.

D-Xylose absorption. The D-xylose absorption test is now considered the most sensitive screening test for celiac disease. An oral dose of 5 gm, followed by a 60-minute blood level determination, leads to the complete separation of untreated celiacs from controls, with 20 mg/dl being used as the minimal normal rise. The discriminant value of D-xylose after a dose of 14.5 gm/m^2 given as a 10% aqueous solution is better than the 5 gm dose, which may be too small for older children. We consider a result of 25 mg/dl or less at 60 minutes as an indication for a small bowel biopsy.

Protein metabolism. Almost half the children with active disease have decreased total serum proteins with albumin levels below 3.5 gm/dl. The hypoalbuminemia is usually secondary to abnormal exudation of proteins and is best demonstrated by the fecal clearance of ^{51}Cr-albumin. The protein-losing enteropathy may at times dominate the clinical picture and be as severe as that seen in intestinal lymphangiectasia. Abnormal nitrogen losses in the stools are seen in 50% of cases and tend to follow quite closely the degree of steatorrhea. They are secondary to increased cell exfoliation and protein-losing enteropathy and to decreased amino acid uptake in the atrophic mucosa.

Pancreatic function. Since cystic fibrosis and celiac disease are the most common entities responsible for the malabsorption syndrome in children, a sweat test should always be carried out. Furthermore, there are now a small number of cases in which celiac disease and cystic fibrosis are present in the same patient. A relative degree of pancreatic insufficiency is described in adults with gluten enteropathy. This is related to an inadequate relase of cholecystokinin despite hyperplasia of the small intestinal mucosal cells containing cholecystokinin. More recently a few cases of celiac disease with severe pancreatic insufficiency attributable to protein malnutrition and requiring pancreatic enzymes have been described.

Bile acid metabolism. Impaired cholecystokinin release leads to gallbladder inertia, low concentration of bile salts in the duodenum, and a decreased enterohepatic circulation of an enlarged bile acid pool in adults. In children, we have found normal fecal bile acid excretion, which seems to confirm the finding of normal bile acid turnover in adults. Liver function tests are usually normal.

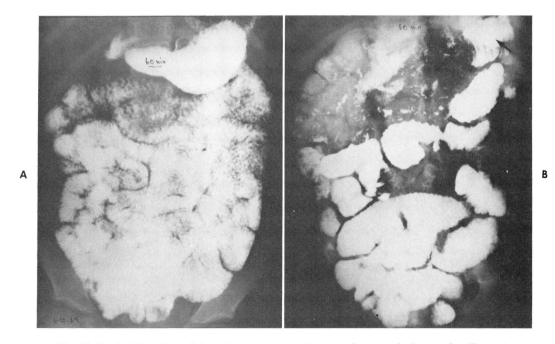

Fig. 10-11. A, Normal small bowel shows a smooth mucosal pattern in loops of uniform size that are well filled with a continuous column of barium. **B,** In contrast, the celiac picture is characterized by dilatation of the loops, segmentation of the barium, hypersecretion, and nonobstructive intussusception, *arrow.*

Hematology studies. Red blood cell smears usually show hypochromia. Serum iron and folate are low. If there is ileal involvement, serum vitamin B_{12} may also be decreased. Hypoprothrombinemia is often found.

Immune correlates. Because of the relatively frequent association between immune defects and celiac disease, immunoglobulin determinations should be done. Increased IgA levels are commonly found in the acute stage of the disease.

After a challenge with gluten, increased synthesis of IgA, and IgM as well, can be demonstrated in biopsy specimens. Various investigators have shown that patients have a high ratio of circulating antibodies to gluten and to various other foods. However, the diagnostic relevance of this finding is in doubt since these antibodies can also be found in controls. Various attempts have been made to find a satisfactory skin test for celiac disease. A positive Arthus type of reaction is reported after the intradermal testing with subfraction B_2 of gluten. After a challenge with gluten, jejunal biopsy specimens show an increased number of IgA and IgM-secreting cells in the lamina propria and of lymphocytes in the surface epithelium.

X-ray studies

Bone age. Celiac patients, especially those who have not received treatment for a long-standing illness giving rise to few intestinal symptoms, exhibit significant retardation of bone age. In assessment of the effect of treatment, it is important to document restoration of a normal growth pattern.

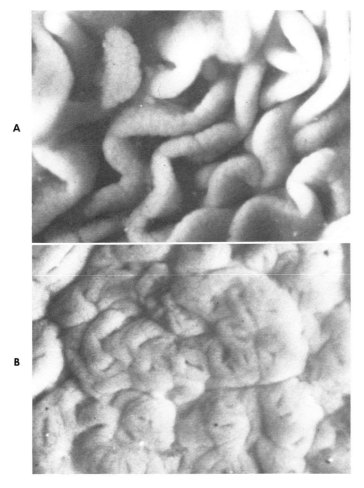

Fig. 10-12. Under the dissection microscope, **A,** the normal pattern of the small bowel is easily recognizable, and contrasts, **B,** with the severe atrophy noted in active celiac disease. (Courtesy Dr. Ramón Tormo, Clínica Infantil de la Seguridad Social, Barcelona.)

Bones. Roentgenograms of the bones reveal diffuse demineralization with reduction in cortical thickness. Osteomalacia and osteoporosis are common. Frank rickets is uncommon.

Small intestine. The roentgenographic pattern of malabsorption commonly associated with celiac disease varies with the patient's age and the duration and severity of the disease. Generally, by barium meal most patients have demonstrable changes in the small intestine characterized by dilatation, segmentation, fragmentation, and hypersecretion (Fig. 10-11, *B*).

Dilatation. The dilated loops are long and have flaccid and pliable walls. Dilatation is more striking in the jejunum and tends to be more pronounced in severe cases.

Segmentation. Within dilated loops, large masses of barium are seen; between these segmented clumps of barium, wormlike or stringlike strands of barium are noted. In a number of cases, there is a so-called moulage of the segmentally dilated loop through masking of the valvulae conniventes by fluid accumulation.

Hypersecretion. A coarse, granular appearance of the barium with areas of flocculation is indicative of hypersecretion. Accessory signs include diffuse thickening of the mucosal folds. The signs may be indicative of hypoproteinemia and is

therefore nonspecific. It also has been reported as the result of significant hypersecretion. Nonobstructive intussusception is rarer (Fig. 10-11, *B*). Transit time is particularly slow in severe cases with significant alteration of the dynamic state of the bowel and hypersecretion. The clinical picture may be that of an intestinal obstruction.

Barium studies of the small intestine are also necessary for ruling out anatomic abnormalities such as malrotation, the stenotic segments of regional enteritis, scleroderma, ileal stenosis, and ileocolic fistulas, which are well-known causes of malabsorption.

Peroral jejunal biopsy. The definitive diagnostic procedure is the peroral small bowel biopsy. Inspection of the biopsy specimen with a dissection microscope will usually reveal severe shunting or complete absence of intestinal villi (Fig. 10-12). As a result of gluten sensitivity, the mucosal architecture, surface epithelium, and cell population of the lamina propria are greatly altered.

Mucosal architecture and surface epithelium (Table 10-4). The initial event is an increased rate of shedding of enterocytes. This, in turn, leads to compensatory enlargement of the proliferative compartment in the crypts. The disappearance of the normal mucosal pattern occurs when entero-

Table 10-4. Comparative features of jejunal mucosa in normal state and in celiac disease

	Normal	Celiac disease
	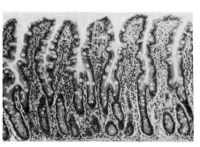	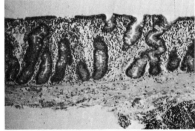
Shape of villi	Long fingerlike villi	Subtotal or total atrophy of villi
Villous epithelium	Tall columnar cells with basally oriented oval nuclei (Fig. 10-8, *A*)	Cells short and cuboid in shape; nuclei have lost their basal polarity. (Fig. 10-15)
Crypts	Short crypts in relation to length of villi (villus-to-crypt ratio: > 2:1)	Elongated deep crypts (Fig. 10-14) in relation to villi (villus-to-crypt ratio: < 2:1)
Cellularity of lamina propria	Moderate	Increased (Fig. 10-16)

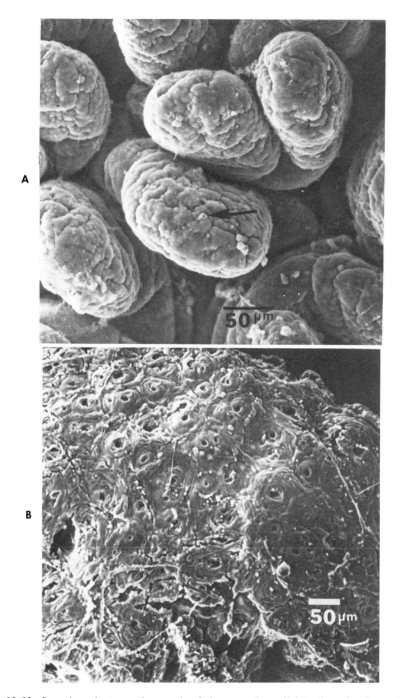

Fig. 10-13. Scanning electron micrograph of the normal small intestine, **A,** shows the three-dimensional contours of fingerlike villi with their circumferential grooves and discrete openings of crypts, *arrow*. The moonlike landscape of the celiac mucosa is featureless except for the large openings of the crypts, **B.** (Courtesy Harry L. Greene, Vanderbilt University Hospital, Nashville, Tenn.)

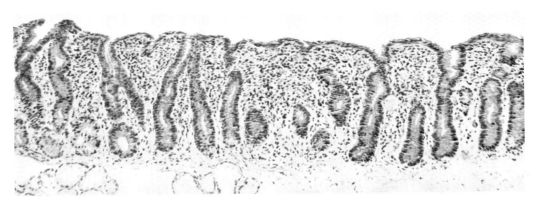

Fig. 10-14. Subtotal atrophy of villi, with deep and often tortuous bifid crypts.

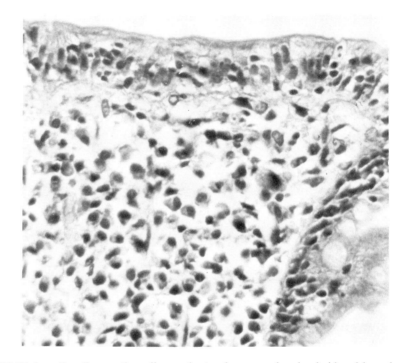

Fig. 10-15. In celiac disease, the cells are shorter than normal and cuboid and have basophilic cytoplasm. The nuclei are round but have irregular shapes and have lost their basal polarity.

blastic hyperplasia incompletely compensates for the shortened enterocytic life-span of the enterocytes of the mucosa. In children, villous atrophy is usually more complete than in adults; the presence of leaflike villi or of ridges giving rise to mild clubbing or to partial villous atrophy is not satisfactory evidence for celiac disease. The villi are totally or almost totally absent, with only a suggestion of villous stumps, which in fact represent areas between adjacent crypts. Scanning electron microscopy shows wide openings of crypts, which open into a flat absorptive surface (Fig. 10-13). The crypts are elongated, increased in diameter, and often bifid and tortuous (Fig. 10-14). These architectural changes greatly decrease the effective absorptive surface. Because the epithelial cells are always abnormal (Fig. 10-15), whatever is left of the absorptive surface is severely compromised.

Lamina propria. There is usually a heavy cellular infiltration consisting predominantly of plasma cells. Lymphocytes are also increased and are seen

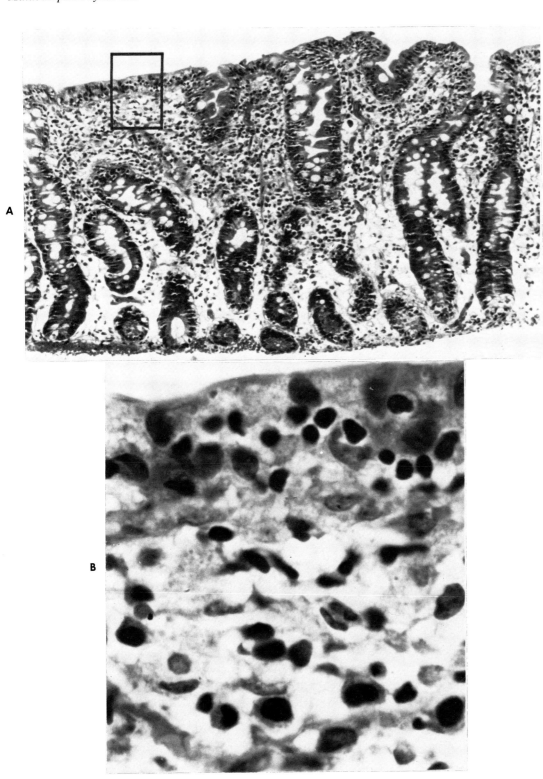

Fig. 10-16. These photomicrographs show typical changes of celiac disease. Particular attention is attracted to, **A,** a dense, chronic inflammatory reaction in the lamina propria and to, **B,** epithelial cell changes and infiltration of the epithelium with a large number of lymphocytes (theliolymphocytes).

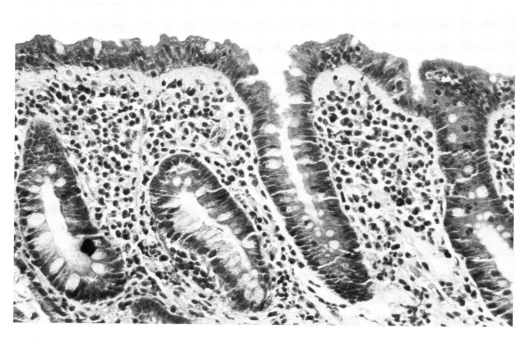

Fig. 10-17. Thin strip of collagen separates the epithelium from the lamina propria in this biopsy section from an infant with severe gluten enteropathy.

between the enterocytes (Fig. 10-16). An increased amount of collagen in the subepithelial portion of the lamina propria is occasionally seen (Fig. 10-17). Its relationship with "collagenous sprue," which presumably fails to respond to gluten withdrawal, remains unclear.

Although the lesion of celiac disease is characteristic, it is not totally specific. "Collagenous sprue" (if it does constitute a separate entity), protein-calorie malnutrition, intestinal lymphoma, infectious gastroenteritis, giardiasis, tropical sprue, immune defects, and cow's milk and soy protein intolerance can produce jejunal changes closely resembling those in biopsy specimens from patients with celiac disease.

Although celiac disease is primarily a mucosal disease involving the proximal jejunum, there is evidence that 40% of children also have morphologic changes in their ileum. There is a good correlation between the severity of symptoms and the length of the small bowel involved.

Diagnosis

Celiac disease can only be truly excluded by demonstration of the presence of a normal jejunal mucosa in a child known to have a normal gluten intake. To establish the diagnosis definitively, one needs to obtain an initial biopsy with typical findings, a second one after strict adherence to a gluten-free diet, and one after a gluten challenge to show return of the disease.

We are still faced with referrals of patients who have been diagnosed on the basis of clinical history and response to gluten withdrawal. At least two thirds of these children are subsequently proved by biopsy not to have celiac disease after 6 months on a normal diet. Therefore a therapeutic trial on a gluten-free diet without a prior biopsy is a poor practice that should be abandoned.

It is important to know that celiac disease has been described in association with cystic fibrosis, diabetes mellitus, cow's milk intolerance, immune defects, and dermatitis herpetiformis.

The majority of patients with dermatitis herpetiformis are HLA-B8 positive and have at least a mild mucosal lesions consistent with celiac disease. However, it is only the rare patient with gluten enteropathy who will develop lesions of dermatitis herpetiformis. The therapeutic response of the skin lesions to sulfone and of the intestinal lesion to a gluten-free diet are independent of each other. The recent findings of defective Fc-receptor function in patients with dermatitis herpetiformis and in HLA-B8–positive controls strengthens the case for the hypothesis that celiac disease is the result of an aberrant immunologic response to gluten.

Complications

Celiac crisis. The grave life-threatening complication of celiac crisis is fortunately quite rare. It may be precipitated by an intercurrent infection, a prolonged fast, or anticholinergic medication. It is characterized by dehydration and acidosis secondary to severe intractable diarrhea and vomiting. The abdomen is usually severely distended. There may be evidence of intestinal obstruction and shock.

Malignancy. In adults with celiac disease the risk for the development of malignant lymphoma of the small bowel and for carcinomas of the gastrointestinal tract, particularly of the esophagus and the stomach, is increased. The risk is also higher in their relatives. At present, there is no evidence in adults that a gluten-free diet provides protection. However, the possibility that the risk of malignancy can be decreased has not been totally excluded, since a population with celiac disease continuously maintained on a gluten-free diet since early childhood has not been studied.

Miscellaneous. Malnutrition may lead to permanent stunting of growth in long-standing cases. Anemia from iron and folic acid deficiency, rickets, osteomalacia, pathologic fractures, tetany, muscle weakness, and·peripheral neuropathy constitute some of the extraintestinal manifestations and complications. Ulceration and stricture of the small intestine is a rare local complication but is not reported in children.

Treatment

Celiac crisis. A nasogastric tube should be placed on intermittent suction and intravenous fluids started. Potassium deficits can be large. Calcium gluconate and magnesium can be given if there is tetany. Salt-poor human albumin infusions can be used as a volume expander if shock or a significant degree of hypoproteinemia is present. Intravenous hydrocortisone (10 mg/kg/24 hr) usually leads to a rapid improvement, and within a few days it can be discontinued in favor of prednisone (1.5 mg/kg/24 hr) with progressive resumption of oral intake. Progressive weaning of the corticosteroids should be carried out after a few weeks of treatment and the patients maintained on a strict gluten-free diet with supplemented vitamins.

Prompt histologic recovery with corticosteroids suggests that short-term administration of prednisone may also be used in severely ill infants in whom anorexia and malabsorption do not rapidly respond to the gluten-free diet.

Gluten-free diet. Although sensitivity to oats is variable, it is best to eliminate oats along with the more toxic wheat, rye, and barley cereal grains. Prescribing a gluten-free diet does not settle the malabsorption and malnutrition problem of a significant number of children who are anorexic and whose diarrhea is exacerbated when appropriate calories are given. The intake at first may have to be quite limited. In cases with significant malnutrition, a short-term period of peripheral parenteral alimentation with amino acids, glucose, and Intralipid may be very helpful.

The clinical response to withdrawal of gluten is often dramatic. Within a few days or weeks, the child's appearance and disposition changes. The stools become more formed and less frequent. The appetite improves. Rapid restoration of normal weight is seen within a few months, along with a slower, progressive catch-up pattern for height. Within 6 months, normal mucosal architecture can be documented (Fig. 10-18). The diet of the infant or child who fails to respond within a few weeks should be carefully reviewed, for its is likely that he is inadvertently being fed small amounts of gluten.

Much experience has confirmed the toxic effects of gluten in the pathogenesis of celiac disease and the efficacy of the gluten-free diet. Although failure to adhere strictly to the diet is the most common cause of this occurrence, one must keep in mind the absence of response of patients with hypogammaglobulinemia, diffuse lymphoma of the small intestine, collagenous sprue, or "unclassified sprue." A few reports suggest that occasional patients who fail to respond to a gluten-free diet should be studied for evidence of sensitivity to other proteins.

Necessary duration of diet. Because no series of patients have been followed and reexamined throughout life, permanence of gluten intolerance has not been proved. However, only a small number of patients show no evidence of relapse after 2 years of reintroduction of gluten.

Current information is that most will have a relapse of their disease and the rest will exhibit growth retardation, anemia, or osteomalacia after 8 to 19 years of follow-up. Although only one

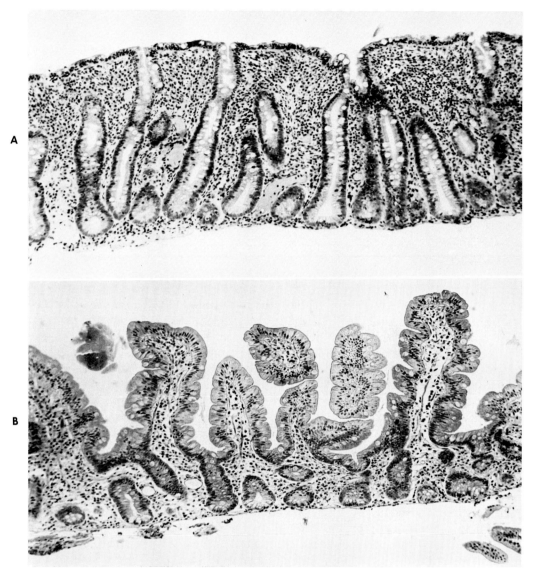

Fig. 10-18. **A,** Initial biopsy of a 2-year-old child showed total villous atrophy. **B,** Repeat biopsy section 6 months later shows a normal mucosa.

third have become symptomatic on a slice of bread a day for a period of a year after 2½ years of strict adherence to the diet, all have been found to eventually develop typical mucosal lesions. It becomes apparent that there is a relationship between age, duration of symptoms, and response to the diet. Adults often do not respond so readily and completely as children. There is a theoretical possibility that the celiac child who clinically tolerates gluten after a few years on the diet may have a relapse as a young adult and not respond to withdrawal of gluten.

We have much difficulty in convincing parents that permanent dietary restriction is necessary for their child, who seems to be perfectly healthy on a full diet even though there is evidence of histologic relapse. Parents need considerable help initially. Despite few signs of ill health, the invariable improvement of growth parameters, disposition, and appetite that follows gluten withdrawal is usually quite impressive and needs to be stressed during follow-up visits. The increased availability of gluten-free products makes the diet less of a burden than it was a few years ago.

Indications for the reintroduction of gluten in the diet. If the diagnosis of celiac disease has been made on clinical grounds alone without confirmation by biopsy, it is mandatory that gluten be introduced progressively into the diet. A biopsy should be performed as soon as symptoms occur or after 3 to 6 months if the patient remains asymptomatic.

In well-documented cases who show satisfactory clinical improvement on a gluten-free diet, it is recommended to control the laboratory tests, which were initially abnormal, and to repeat the peroral biopsy 3 to 6 months after the diagnosis is made. Reintroduction of a normal diet to test for the permanence of gluten intolerance is suggested after 2 years of dietary treatment. A biopsy should be performed 3 to 6 months later or as soon as symptoms recur. If the biopsy is still normal after 2 years on a normal diet, one can conclude that the gluten intolerance was temporary. It would appear more likely to occur in patients in whom the diagnosis is made before the age of 1 year. Temporary gluten intolerance has been reported in infants with milk protein intolerance. Initial reports of this entity by Finnish workers were confirmed by other groups in Europe. From an in vitro study of rat-fetus small intestine it has been shown that gliadin and its peptides have toxic effects that disappear with maturation. The speculation is that with injury (infection, milk protein intolerance) normal detoxifying mechanisms could regress. A recent European survey shows that less than 5% of patients with celiac disease fall into this category though in one report the figure reaches 20% after 6½ years of a gluten challenge. Young infants with milk protein intolerance may also respond adversely to gluten. This gluten intolerance is reported to be of a temporary nature and a secondary phenomenon. A challenge is especially important in such cases.

It is mandatory to challenge the patients in whom either the mucosal lesions were not so characteristic as one usually sees or the response to gluten withdrawal in terms of symptoms or growth was not so good as expected.

At least one group of workers has elected to maintain those patients who have a histologic relapse on a normal diet as long as they remain symptom-free and grow normally. Of interest is their report of three patients who relapsed histologically on a normal diet and healed their lesion in their midteens even though they had continued to ingest gluten. The recent description of gluten-sensitive diarrhea without any histologic signs and only discrete signs of celiac disease suggests a form of gluten intolerance different from celiac disease and from temporary gluten intolerance. The evidence so far points to a small subset of patients with a form of food-induced diarrhea associated with gluten.

Disaccharide-free diet. Because the disaccharidases of the small intestinal mucosa are located in the microvilli of the epithelial absorptive cells, the disaccharidase activity is greatly depressed where the jejunal mucosa is diffusely damaged as in celiac disease. Maltase and sucrase activity are less significantly affected than lactase is. Their corresponding substrates, maltose and sucrose, need not be restricted. It is advisable to remove milk and lactose-containing products for a few weeks after the diagnosis only if intolerance is clinically manifest.

REFERENCES

Anderson, C.M., Gracey, M., and Burke, V.: Celiac disease: some still controversial aspects, Arch. Dis. Child. **47:**292-298, 1972.

Baker, A.L., and Rosenberg, I.H.: Refractory sprue: recovery after removal of nongluten dietary proteins, Ann. Intern. Med. **89:**505-508, 1978.

Congdon, P., Mason, M.K., Smith, S., and others: Small bowel mucosa in asymptomatic children with celiac disease, Am. J. Dis. Child. **135:**118-121, 1981.

Cooper, B.T., Holmes, G.K.T., Ferguson, R., and Cooke, W.T.: Celiac disease and malignancy, Medicine **59:**249-261, 1980.

Cooper, B.T., Holmes, G.K.T., Ferguson, R.A., and others: Gluten-sensitive diarrhea without evidence of celiac disease, Gastroenterology **79:**801-806, 1980.

De Ritis, G., Occorsio, P., Auricchio, S., and others: Toxicity of wheat flour proteins and protein derived peptides for in vitro developing intestine from rat fetus, Pediatr. Res. **13:**1255-1261, 1979.

Falchuk, Z.M., Gebhard, R.L., Sessoms, C., and Strober, W.: An in vitro model of gluten-sensitive enteropathy: effect of gliadin on intestinal epithelial cells of patients with gluten-sensitive enteropathy in organ culture, J. Clin. Invest. **53:**487-500, 1974.

Falchuk, Z.M., Nelson, D.L., Katz, A.J., and others: Gluten-sensitive enteropathy: influence of histocompatibility type on gluten sensitiveity in vitro, J. Clin. Invest. **66:**227-233, 1980.

Groll, A., Candy, D.C.A., Preece, M.A., and others: Short stature as the primary manifestation of coeliac disease, Lancet **2:**1097-1099, 1980.

Hamilton, J.R., and McNeill, L.K.: Childhood celiac disease: response of treated patients to a small uniform daily dose of wheat gluten, J. Pediatr. **81:**885-893, 1972.

Lawley, T.J., Hall, R.P., Fauci, A.S., and others: Defective Fc-receptor functions associated with the HLA-B$_8$/DRW$_3$ haplotype, N. Engl. J. Med. **304:**185-192, 1981.

Lebenthal, E., and Branski, D.: Childhood celiac disease: a reappraisal, J. Pediatr. **98**:681-690, 1981.

Lloyd-Still, J.D., Grand, R.J., Khaw, K.T., and Shwachman, H.: The use of corticosteroids in celiac crisis, J. Pediatr. **81**:1074-1081, 1972.

Low-Beer, T.S., Heaton, K.W., Pomare, E.W., and Read, A.E.: The effect of celiac disease upon bile salts, Gut **14**:204-208, 1973.

McNeish, A.S., and Anderson, C.M.: The disorder in childhood, Clin. Gastroenterol. **3**:127-144, 1974.

Mylotte, M., Egan-Mitchell, B., Fottrell, P.F., and others: Family studies in coeliac disease, Q. J. Med. **43**:359-369, 1974.

Nusslé, D., Mégevand, A., Delèze, G., and others: Non coeliac gluten intolerance without associated milk protein allergy, Acta Paediatr. Belg. **29**:261, 1976 (Abstract).

Packer, S.M., Charlton, V., Keeling, J.W., and others: Gluten challenge in treated coeliac disease, Arch. Dis. Child. **53**:449-453, 1978.

Regan, P.T., and DiMagno, E.P.: Exocrine pancreatic insufficiency in celiac sprue: a cause of treatment failure, Gastroenterology **78**:484-487, 1980.

Robinson, D.C., Watson, A.J., Wyatt, E.H., and others: Incidence of small-intestinal mucosal abnormalities and of clinical celiac disease in the relatives of children with celiac disease, Gut **12**:789-793, 1971.

Rolles, C.J., Nutter, S., Kendall, M.J., and Anderson, C.M.: One-hour blood-xylose screening test for celiac disease in infants and young children, Lancet **2**:1043-1045, 1973.

Schmitz, J., Jos, J., and Rey, J.: Transient mucosal atrophy in confirmed coeliac disease. In McNicholl, B., McCarthy, C.F., and Fottrell, P.F., editors: Perspectives in coeliac disease, Lancaster, Eng., 1978, MTP Press.

Shmerling, D.H.: Questionnaire of the European Society for Paediatric Gastroenterology and Nutrition on coeliac disease. In McNicholl, B., McCarthy, C.F., Fottrell, P.F., editors: Perspectives in coeliac disease, Lancaster, 1978, MTP Press, Ltd.

Walker-Smith, J.: Celiac disease. In Diseases of the small intestine in childhood, ed. 2, Kent, Eng., 1979, Pitman Medical Publishing Co., Ltd.

Weir, D.G., and Hourihane, D.O'B.: Celiac disease during the teenage period: the value of serial serum folate estimations, Gut **15**:450-457, 1974.

Weiser, M.M., and Douglas, A.P.: An alternative mechanism for gluten toxicity in coeliac disease, Lancet **1**:567-569, 1976.

Young, W.F., and Pringle, E.M.: 110 children with celiac disease, Arch. Dis. Child. **46**:421-436, 1971.

Tropical sprue

Tropical sprue is a common cause of chronic diarrhea and malabsorption in people from tropical areas. It has a peculiar geographic distribution and occurs both in epidemic and endemic form. All age groups are affected, though the attack rate is significantly higher in adults. In the event of an epidemic, younger age groups usually become symptomatic later than adults.

The pathogenesis of the disease is still unknown. Three factors have been invoked:

1. Nutritional deficiency
2. Dietary antigen
3. Transmissible infectious organism

There is no evidence to support the suggestion that it may be a nutritional deficiency disease. Malnutrition is the result rather than the cause. The possibility that a dietary antigen is responsible has not been substantiated. No causal agent—bacterial, viral or parasitic—has ever been identified. Epidemiologic studies show that some patients develop the disease within days of entering an endemic area whereas others become ill years after leaving it.

The intestinal microflora of people living in tropical and subtropical countries is abnormal by Western standards. Although abnormal bacterial colonization is present in some patients, it is not so extensive as in the contaminated small bowel syndrome and there is no consistent pattern. However, the success of antibiotic treatment maintains one's interest in the role of bacteria.

Clinical findings

In a series of pediatric patients the youngest age at onset of symptoms was 7 months. The most regularly found symptoms include weight loss or failure to grow, anorexia, weakness, chronic diarrhea, and pallor. On physical examination, most patients are well below the third percentile in weight. Glossitis is usually mild and is rarely accompanied by burning. Abdominal distention and pain may be present.

Laboratory findings

Patients may have macrocytosis and megaloblastosis. The majority are anemic and have low levels of iron, serum folate, and vitamin B_{12}. D-Xylose absorption and fecal fat excretion are often abnormal. The prothrombin time may be prolonged, and hypoproteinemia is common. Small bowel roentgenograms can show a malabsorption pattern, and the breath hydrogen test may confirm the presence of bacterial contamination of the upper small intestine.

Biopsy findings

Morphologic changes do not correlate well with the severity of the absorptive abnormalities and are gnerally less severe than in celiac disease. Shortening and elongation of crypts can be impressive, but the surface epithelium is relatively well preserved. The disease involves the entire small bowel, though the proximal lesions are more severe than those in the ileum.

The significance and specificity of these lesions are now seriously doubted since identical changes have been described in asymptomatic individuals living in the same areas.

Diagnosis

The diagnosis should be suspected in areas where the disease is endemic in any child with chronic diarrhea, malnutrition, or megaloblastic anemia. A history of having visited areas where the disease is present is necessary before one entertains the possibility of tropical sprue. It should be noted that the length of the stay can be as short as a week. Other possibilities that should be considered include amebiasis, strongyloidiasis, capillariasis, bacterial infections, and celiac disease.

Therapy

Treatment is aimed at correction of the nutritional deficiencies after initial care of the acute water, electrolyte, and acid-base problems, which may be associated with severe diarrhea. No dietary restrictions are recommended. Vitamin B_{12} and folic acid administration is associated with a rapid amelioration of the patient's general condition and in some cases with normalization of the intestinal lesion.

The most effective drug at the moment is tetracycline, administered for a period of a few weeks. Long-term treatment (6 months) appears effective for the prevention of frequently encountered relapses.

Prognosis

The prognosis is generally good. Many patients appear to recover spontaneously, whereas in others there is a high rate of relapse.

REFERENCES

Cook, G.C.: Breath hydrogen after oral xylose in tropical malabsorption, Am. J. Clin. Nutr. **31**:555-560, 1980.

Guerra, R., Wheby, M.S., and Bayless, T.M.: Long-term antibiotic therapy in tropical sprue, Ann. Intern. Med. **63**:619-634, 1965.

Kapadia, C.R., Bhat, P., Jacob, E., and Baker, S.J.: Vitamin B_{12} absorption: a study of intraluminal events in control subjects and patients with tropical sprue, Gut **16**:988-993, 1975.

Klipstein, F.A., and Baker, S.J.: Regarding the definition of tropical sprue, Gastroenterology **58**:717-721, 1970.

Mathan, M., Mathan, V.I., and Baker, S.J.: An electron microscopic study of jejunal macrosal morphology in control subjects and in patients with tropical sprue in southern India, Gastroenterology **68**:17-32, 1975.

Santiago-Borrero, P.J., Maldonado, M., and Horta, E.: Tropical sprue in children, J. Pediatr. **76**:470-479, 1970.

Tomkins, A.M., Drasar, B.S., and James, W.P.T.: Bacterial colonization of jejunal mucosa in acute tropical sprue, Lancet **1**:59-62, 1975.

Contaminated small bowel syndrome

Since an abnormal intestinal bacterial flora may become established in the absence of an intestinal "blind loop" or "stagnant loop," the term "contaminated small bowel syndrome" is now used to define a clinical condition characterized by a malabsorptive syndrome associated with the proliferation of excessive numbers of chiefly anaerobic bacteria in the small intestine. The term "blind loop" refers to a special type of bacterial overgrowth syndrome that occurs in an intestinal loop disconnected from the main stream.

Etiology

Contaminated small bowel syndrome is a heterogeneous disorder and has numerous causes. The list of diseases associated with contamination of the small bowel grows increasingly large. In certain diseases, bacterial overgrowth may be a non-specific finding, whereas in others listed below, it appears to be responsible for significant symptoms and absorptive defects.

Conditions associated with the contaminated small bowel syndrome in infants and children

Postoperative phase of intestinal surgery in young infants

Protracted diarrhea after a bout of acute gastroenteritis

Blind loop by an end-to-side anastomosis

Continent ileostomy

Congenital or acquired strictures, stenotic areas, fistulas, diaphragms

Crohn's disease

Intestinal scleroderma and chronic idiopathic intestinal pseudo-obstruction

Protein-calorie malnutrition and tropical sprue

Intestinal microflora

Population. The proximal and mid-small bowel of healthy human beings is sparsely populated with bacteria, consisting predominantly of facultatively aerobic bacteria (under 10^4/ml), together with small numbers of Enterobacteriaceae and *Bacteroides*.

The upper intestinal flora of people living in tropical countries is more profuse. The distal ileum represents a transition zone between the upper small bowel and colon; it harbors a sparse microbial flora in approximately one fifth of normal subjects. Despite the presence of a variety of aerobic and anaerobic *(Bacteroides)* organisms in most normal adults, bacterial counts are still modest in the ileum (10^5 to 10^8) in comparison with the colon and feces (10^{11}/ml). Across the ileocecal valve, the flora is dominated by the nonsporeforming anaerobic organisms, principally *Bacteroides fragilis* (46%), and other *Bacteroides* species along with *Bifidobacterium, Eubacterium,* and *Propionobacterium.* These outnumber facultative anaerobic bacteria such as *Streptococcus faecalis, Escherichia coli,* and lactobacilli by a factor of 1000.

Colonization in the newborn. The alimentary canal is sterile at birth. Within a few hours, there is very quick colonization of the gastrointestinal tract. Under the influence of breast feeding, a stable microflora is developed in the colon and feces within 3 or 4 days. More than 99% of the cultivable flora consists of the anaerobic *Lactobacillus bifidus.* There is a paucity of putrefactive bacteria such as the gram-negative anaerobes *(Bacteroides, Clostridium,* and *Proteus).* This accounts for the low pH (4.5 to 5.1) of stools from breast-fed infants.

Formula feeding does not prevent the growth of gram-negative anaerobes. *Lactobacillus bifidus* still is an important part of the flora, but it is often surpassed by the putrefactive ''*Bacteroides* group,'' which render the stools ''more alkaline'' (pH 5.5 to 8.3). Differences in enteric flora among bottle-fed babies, older children, and adults are not very pronounced.

Stability of the flora. Although the bacterial population of the gut may vary considerably from one individual to another, the flora in a given individual remains remarkably stable.

The anatomic and structural integrity of the gastrointestinal tract is essential to limit bacterial proliferation and to keep the colonic flora in its place. Disorders leading to partial obstruction or associated with defective peristalsis are therefore important factors limiting the ability of the portion of the gut responsible for digestion and absorption to remain relatively bacteria-free. The stomach with its gastric acid contents and the ileocecal valve constitute other important components. Bile acids exhibit antibacterial activity.

Physiologic concentrations of free bile acids (cholic and deoxycholic acid) readily inhibit anaerobic human intestinal bacteria in vitro but have little effect on aerobic organisms. Conjugated bile acids (taurocholic and glycocholic acid) have few or no bacteriostatic properties. The well-documented contaminated small bowel associated with hepatic cirrhosis or the one that occurs after extensive intestinal resections may be explained by decreases in the intestinal concentrations of bile acids and particularly deoxycholic acid. There are a number of other factors that are probably important, such as mucus, lysozyme, and fatty acids, in the complex system that maintains the balance between host and flora. Immunologic mechanisms probably do not play a determinant role though secretory IgA has been shown to prevent the adhesion of pathogenic organisms to the mucosa. As stated elsewhere, hypogammaglobulinemic patients do not suffer from a bacterial overgrowth syndrome.

Dietary changes, even when drastic, bring about only minor changes. Addition of cellulose sometimes causes reduction in the anaerobic colonic flora. The consumption of up to 1 kg of yogurt or the ingestion of up to 20 capsules a day of *Lactobacillus acidophilus* (10^{12}) does not significantly change the fecal flora. Lactulose (D-fructofuranose) is a nonabsorbed disaccharide that is useful in treating hepatic encephalopathy. One of its postulated modes of action was that it reduced urea-splitting bacteria in the colon. Recent evidence suggests that the small reductions seen are related to its laxative effect and that the same changes can be observed with osmotic agents such as mannitol or sorbitol. We have recently examined the fecal flora of patients on elemental diets for a period of 3 weeks and have failed to identify significant changes.

Mucosal flora. The luminal flora, because of its accessibility, has attracted much more attention than the adherent mucosal flora. Part of the intestinal microflora is carried downstream, but large numbers of bacteria adhere to epithelial cells and establish a close mucosa-microbe relationship of much greater importance that the luminal flora. The involvement of this flora in pathologic processes through their potential to cause injury, to secrete toxins, to modify mucus secretion, to trigger an immune response, or to protect the mucosa from potentially pathogenic bacteria are largely unknown.

Effects on morphology and function (Table 10-5). Indigenous microorganisms influence alimentary physiology in many ways, not only because of their presence in the lumen, but also because of their close association with the epithelium through their embedment in the "fuzzy coat," or glycocalyx. Studies in germ-free animals contaminated with intestinal microorganisms show a rapid acceleration of intestinal cell turnover. Crypts become deeper, and the mucosa is thickened. Simultaneously, there are important changes in bile acid metabolism and in absorptive function. This does not deter from the fact that the intestinal flora plays a critical role. The numerous studies on the contaminated small bowel syndrome are particularly convincing in this respect.

Bile acid metabolism. The primary bile acids synthesized by the liver (cholic and chenodeoxycholic acid) are conjugated with taurine or glycine. In the lower small bowel and colon they are largely deconjugated and dehydroxylated (to deoxycholic and lithocholic acid). Further transformations include oxidation to form keto bile acids and reduction to either alpha or beta hydroxyl groups. In the contaminated small bowel syndrome, bacterial transformation of bile acids takes place in the upper gut (Fig. 10-19). This greatly impairs fat absorption because free and dehydroxylated bile acids cannot form micelles with the products of lipolysis and because, in contrast to conjugated bile acids, which are absorbed in large part in the ileum, they can be passively transported in the upper bowel. As a result, bile acid concentrations may be too low to ensure micellar solubilization.

Fat absorption. Fat malabsorption is not only secondary to a diminution of the micellar solubilization of fat but could also relate to the inhibition of uptake and reesterification of fatty acids by free and secondary bile acids. Unabsorbed fatty acids may be metabolized by intestinal bacteria to produce long-chain hydroxy acids, some of which are structurally similar to a well-known cathartic, ricinoleic acid. Hydroxy fatty acids impair net water and sodium transport and induce water secretion. They are in part responsible for the watery diarrhea associated with the contaminated small bowel syndrome.

Absorption of water-soluble substrates. Enteric microorganisms metabolize carbohydrates and transform them into organic acids and hydrogen. A further defect may be related to the inhibition of monosaccharide transport by deconjugated bile acids. The inhibition is reversible and leads to monosaccharide malabsorption after small intestinal surgery in the neonatal period, during the course of infectious gastroenteritis, and in the other causes of the contaminated small bowel syndrome. It is more likely the result of mucosal disfunction.

Table 10-5. Pathophysiology of contaminated small bowel syndrome

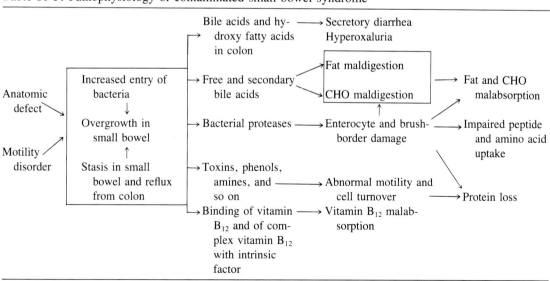

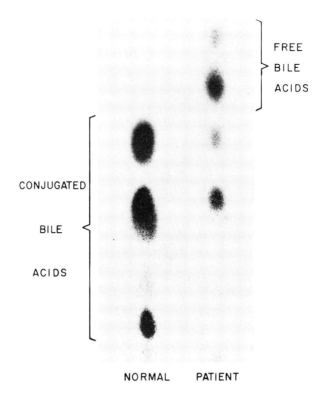

FREE
BILE
ACIDS

CONJUGATED

BILE

ACIDS

NORMAL   PATIENT

Fig. 10-19. Free bile acids in the contaminated small bowel syndrome. This thin-layer chromatographic plate shows large amounts of free bile acids in the upper jejunum of a patient with chronic idiopathic intestinal pseudo-obstruction (p. 123).

Hypoproteinemia is repeatedly found in the "blind loop" syndrome. Studies with ^{51}Cr-albumin do show an excessive loss, but the increased fecal excretion is still small in relation to the hypoalbuminemia. Bacteria can use amino acids. The resulting end products can be absorbed and excreted in the urine. This is the basis for the use of indicanuria as a marker of excess bacterial metabolism of tryptophan. Bacterial injury to the brush border leads to decreased levels of enterokinase and peptidase activities. In addition, dipeptide and amino acid uptake may be inhibited by deconjugated bile acids. Thus there are four mechanisms involved:

1. Increased protein loss in lumen
2. Utilization of amino acids by bacteria
3. Impaired digestion of proteins
4. Decreased transport of peptides and amino acids

Vitamin B$_{12}$ deficiency. The available evidence suggests that the ileal receptor for the vitamin B$_{12}$–intrinsic factor complex is intact. Certain bacteria can bind vitamin B$_{12}$ and compete with intrinsic factor. It is also probable that they can bind the vitamin B$_{12}$–intrinsic factor complex and thereby prevent its attachment to ileal receptors. Anaerobes, particularly *Bacteroides,* appear to play a major role in vitamin B$_{12}$ malabsorption. In contrast to aerobic bacteria, intrinsic factor does not protect against extensive binding of the vitamin by anaerobes.

Hyperoxaluria. The hyperoxaluria documented in the short bowel syndrome is also seen in the contaminated small bowel syndrome and may lead to nephrolithiasis. The mechanism responsible for the increased excretion of oxalates in the urine has been a subject of controversy. It now seems that normal amounts of oxalate are produced in the intestinal lumen and negligible amounts from the glycine moiety of conjugated bile acids. However, because of the presence of unabsorbed fatty acids, luminal calcium is used up to form calcium soaps and is not available to prevent the intestinal absorption of dietary oxalate by forming insoluble calcium oxalate. In addition, fatty acids and bile acids unabsorbed in the small bowel increase colonic mucosal permeability to dietary oxalate.

Structural changes. It has been widely accepted

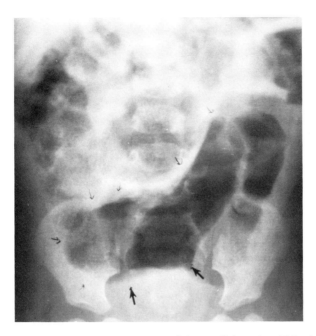

Fig. 10-20. Blind loop with bacterial overgrowth of the small intestine. This simple film of the abdomen shows a widely dilated small bowel loop, *arrows,* proximal to an end-to-side ileal anastomosis performed after a neonatal resection for volvulus. Malabsorption and malnutrition were severe. Antibiotics produced dramatic results. The patient was reoperated on after a period of peripheral parenteral alimentation.

that bacterial contamination of the upper gut is not accompanied by changes in villous architure or epithelial cell structure, though infiltration of the underlying lamina propria by inflammatory cells is usual. Reports suggest histologic abnormalities that may be of functional importance to explain the absorptive defects described previously. Ultra-structural changss are much more impressive and include damage to microvilli, mitochondria, and the Golgi apparatus. Disaccharidase deficiency has been documented and appears to be the result of brush-border damage by *Bacteroides*-secreted proteases.

Clinical findings

The patient with the contaminated small bowel syndrome usually has symptoms of malabsorption and demonstrates more or less profound nutritional consequences. Significant growth retardation may be seen if symptoms are long-standing. The history can be that of a primary intestinal disease such as Crohn's disease with strictures or chronic idiopathic intestinal pseudo-obstruction with pronounced alterations in the motility of the small bowel (Chapter 4). That the patient underwent surgery during the neonatal period (Fig. 10-20) or

later in life with bypassing or resection of segments of the small intestine is very important information in the subjective examination of the patient with malabsorption. It is not unusual for the contaminated small bowel syndrome to start years after such a surgical procedure.

Congenital anomalies are particularly important in the etiology of the contaminated small bowel syndrome in children. A number of these anomalies give rise to partial obstruction and do not lead to early surgical intervention. They may first become manifest later in life when they may mimic celiac disease. Entities such as intestinal malrotation and congenital kinking, stenosis, or diaphragms are particularly important.

More specific clinical findings orienting the diagnosis toward the syndrome include repeated attacks of abdominal pain that are colicky in nature and associated with abdominal distention. Anorexia, nausea, vomiting, the passage of pale, malodorous stools floating in water, and megaloblastic anemia are also seen. It is well to remember that the typical picture is hardly constant. Consequently, the diagnosis of contaminated small bowel syndrome should be considered in all patients with malabsorption.

Children with the contaminated small bowel syndrome often have severe watery diarrhea with water, electrolyte, and acid-base balance problems. Hypoproteinemia, hypocalcemia, hypomagnesemia, hypoprothrombinemia constitute other biologic correlates. The watery diarrhea is particularly impressive in neonates during the first month or two after surgery.

Diagnosis

The diagnosis rests first on proving that there is malabsorption and defining its consequence on the patients' growth and nutritional state. Second, certain criteria must be satisfied before one attributes malabsorption to intraluminal bacteria.

1. Available methods for investigation of intestinal bacterial populations fall short of the ideal. Intubations of the small bowel are carried out in our institution with an open tube. The specimens are obtained under anaerobic conditions and transported in a GasPak jar. They are serially diluted and cultured on several selective media.

2. Since one of the most striking consequences of massive proliferation of bacteria in the small intestine is malabsorption of vitamin B_{12}, an abnormal Schilling test carried out with intrinsic factor constitutes important evidence favoring the diagnosis.

3. The absorption of D-xylose may be abnormal. This does not necessarily imply that absorption is defective, since bacteria can utilize D-xylose and account for falsely low values in the plasma. Evidence of intraluminal bacterial catabolism of D-xylose can be documented in adults by measurement of $^{14}CO_2$ after a 1 gm dose of ^{14}C-xylose or in children by monitoring of breath hydrogen (H_2) after a standard dose (0.5 gm/kg) of D-xylose. Lactulose is a β-galactoside and is therefore not absorbable. It has been used as a substrate for a hydrogen breath test in adults.

4. The major diagnostic problem is to determine whether bacterial overgrowth in the small intestine is responsible for the absorptive defects. Since most of the available evidence indicates that the steatorrhea is tied with alterations of bile acid metabolism, tests are currently available to detect bile acid deconjugation by the overgrowth of bacteria. One can demonstrate precipitation of free bile acids by showing that a major portion of the bile acids in intestinal contents are not in the aqueous phase after centrifugation. The presence of a significant percentage of free bile acids not

normally present in the jejunum can be established by thin-layer chromatography (Fig. 10-19). Large fecal losses of bile acids can be documented in the absence of an intestinal resection (See Chapter 4 on the subject of intestinal pseudo-obstruction). Bacterial overgrowth can be established indirectly by the bile acid deconjugation breath test. The cholyl-^{14}C-glycine breath test can be considered the most useful and the most sensitive test to detect bacterial degradation of bile acids. Under normal conditions, almost all the ingested labeled bile acid is absorbed intact and recirculated to the liver. In contrast, whenever the glycine-conjugated bile acid is exposed to large quantities of bacteria before being absorbed, deconjugation and metabolism of ^{14}C-glycine produces large amounts of $^{14}CO_2$ excreted by the lungs. Measurements are usually carried out over 6 hours. Because the labeled bile acid is mixed with the bile acid pool, the test reflects the fractional deconjugation rate and not the total amount of bile acid undergoing deconjugation. Because false-positive results may result from increased concentrations of bile acids spilling into the colon, the fecal excretion of the label should also be measured. The availability of stable isotopes will undoubtedly contribute to the wider use of this test in pediatrics.

5. The roentgenologic demonstration of abnormal anatomy and peristalsis is particularly important (Fig. 10-20). One should recall, however, that the absence of a stenotic area with proximal dilatation does not rule out the diagnosis. Poor propulsive action in a hypertrophied segment proximal to the site of a patent anastomosis may be sufficient evidence.

6. Small bowel mucosa from patients with the contaminated small bowel syndrome is commonly reported as being normal. Electron microscopy may be helpful, as demonstrated in a few patients.

7. Response to antibiotic therapy constitutes an additional diagnostic feature, but treatment failure does not rule out diagnosis.

Treatment

The aims of treatment are threefold: correction of the nutrition problem, elimination of the bacterial overgrowth, and, when feasible, restoration of the small bowel's anatomic and functional integrity.

The initial efforts should be directed at correction of the acute and chronic nutritional deficiencies with appropriate administration of nutrients and vitamins. Steatorrhea and diarrhea can be helped by a low-fat diet (10 to 20 gm of long-chain triglycerides) supplemented with medium-chain triglycerides (Pregestimil, Portagen, medium-chain triglyceride oil). Parenteral alimentation may have to be used for short periods. The sugar content of the formula is carefully monitored in young infants who are recovering from intestinal surgery and who so frequently have gross monosaccharide malabsorption. If a concentration of 2.5% is poorly tolerated, sugar is completely restricted and given intravenously. Cholestyramine appears helpful in adults and is aimed at controlling watery diarrhea secondary to the presence of free bile acids. Unfortunately it is seldom effective in children.

Reduction or elimination of the bacterial overgrowth can be attempted by the administration of tetracycline, lincomycin, clindamycin, or metronidazole. These antibiotics are particularly effective against the anaerobes that are largely responsible for the spectrum of associated absorptive defects. Little data exist in respect to what is appropriate long-term antibiotic therapy, but the antibiotics need close follow-up study, especially during the first few weeks in view of the problems associated with their administration in some patients (Chapter 13). Intermittent therapy, one week out of every two, and a change of antimicrobial agent from time to time are recommended.

Surgical correction of the abnormality causing small bowel stasis is clearly the ultimate aim. All children should be considered potential candidates for surgery, except those with scleroderma or intestinal pseudo-obstruction.

REFERENCES

Ament, M.E., Shimoda, S., Saunders, D.R., and Rubin, C.E.: The pathogenesis of steatorrhea in three cases of small intestinal stasis syndrome, Gastroenterology **63:**728-747, 1972.

Bayes, B.J., and Hamilton, J.R.: Blind-loop syndrome in children, Arch. Dis. Child. **44:**76-81, 1969.

Borriello, P., Hudson, M., and Hill, M.: Investigation of the gastrointestinal bacterial flora, Clin. Gastroenterol. **7:**329-349, 1978.

Brunser, O.: Effects of malnutrition on intestinal structure and function in children, Clin. Gastroineterol. **6:**341-353, 1977.

Caspary, W.F.: Breath tests, Clin. Gastroenterol. **7:**362-364, 1978.

Challacombe, D.N., Richardson, J.M., Rowe, B., and Anderson, C.M.: Bacterial microflora of the upper gastrointestinal tract in infants with protracted diarrhea, Arch. Dis. Child. **49:**270-277, 1974.

Drude, R.B., and Hines, C.: The pathophysiology of intestinal bacterial overgrowth syndromes, Arch. Intern. Med. **140:**1349-1352, 1980.

Isaacs, P.T., and Kim, Y.S.: The contaminated small bowel syndrome, Am. J. Med. **67:**1049-1057, 1979.

Jonas, A., Krishnan, C., and Forstner, G.: Pathogenesis of mucosal injury in the blind loop syndrome, Gastroenterology **75:**791-795, 1978.

Kern, L.: Bacterial contamination syndrome of the small bowel, Clin. Gastroenterol. **8:**397-401, 1979.

Kilby, A.M., Dolby, J.M., Honour, P., and Walker-Smith, J.A.: Duodenal bacterial flora in early stages of transient monosaccharide intolerance in infants, Arch. Dis. Child. **52:**228-234, 1977.

King, C.E., and Toskes, P.P.: Small intestine bacterial overgrowth, Gastroenterology **76:**1035-1055, 1979.

Mallory, A., Kern, F., Smith, J., and Savage, D.: Patterns of bile acids and microflora in the human small intestine, Gastroenterology **64:**26-33, 34-42, 1973.

Northfield, T.C., Drasar, B.S., and Wright, J.T.: Value of small intestinal bile acid analysis in the diagnosis of the stagnant loop syndrome, Gut **14:**341-347, 1971.

Riepe, S., Goldstein, J., and Alpers, D.H.: Effect of secreted *Bacteroides* proteases on human intestinal brush border hydrolases, J. Clin. Invest. **66:**314-322, 1980.

Roy, C.C., and Weber, A.: Clinical implications of bile acids in paediatrics, Clin. Gastroenterol. **6:**377-395, 1977.

Schoeller, D.A., Schneider, J.F., Solomons, N.W., and others: Clinical diagnosis with the stable isotope ^{13}C in CO_2 breath tests, J. Lab. Clin. Med. **90:**412-421, 1977.

Wanitschke, R., and Ammon, H.V.: Effects of dihydroxy bile acids and hydroxy fatty acids on the absorption of oleic acid in the human jejunum, J. Clin. Invest. **61:**178-186, 1978.

Welkos, S.L., Toskes, P.P., Baer, H., and Smith, G.W.: Importance of anaerobic bacteria in the cobalamin malabsorption of the experimental rat blind loop syndrome, Gastroenterology **80:**313-320, 1981.

Short bowel syndrome

The short bowel syndrome is the result of alterations of gastrointestinal motility, secretion, digestion, and absorption that occur after an extensive small bowel resection. The most common clinical conditions that require the removal of significant lengths of the small intestine occur in the neonatal period.

Short bowel syndrome in neonate

Intestinal malrotation with volvulus and bands
Jejunoileal atresias
Meconium ileus
Omphalocele and gastroschisis with volvulus
Duplications and other abdominal tumors
Internal hernias
Congenitally short small bowel

In older infants and in children, intussusception with gangrenous small bowel and Crohn's disease are the two entities that most commonly lead to the short bowel syndrome.

Differences between the jejunum and ileum

A brief recall of the structural and functional differences between the jejunum and ileum is essential to understand the physiopathology of the short bowel syndrome.

Anatomic differences. The small intestine of the neonate measures about 250 cm. There is no specific anatomic structure that marks the end of the jejunum and the beginning of the ileum. The proximal two fifths is the jejunum, and the rest is the ileum. However, the structural and functional differences between the two are important and significantly modify the severity, treatment, and prognosis of the short bowel syndrome. The diameter of the proximal jejunum is twice that of the distal ileum; its surface area is greatly increased by the circular folds (plicae circulares), which are sparser and smaller in the ileum. These folds are covered by mucosa that, throughout the small intestine, is composed of villi, crypts, lamina propria, and muscularis mucosae. A further anatomic advantage of the jejunum over the ileum

in terms of surface area relates to the fact that villi are taller.

Functional differences. The inner layer of the mucosa consists of a continuous sheet of a single layer of columnar epithelial cells lining both the crypts and the villi. Crypt epithelium is largely made up of undifferentiated cells that will acquire absorptive properties as they travel up the villi to replace senescent enterocytes coming off the tip of the villi. The luminal surface of each absorptive cell (mature enterocyte) is increased thirtyfold by great numbers of microvilli that in turn are covered by a surface coat of glycoprotein (Fig. 10-8, *B*). The microvilli not only are responsible for absorption but also participate in the digestion of carbohydrates and proteins because they are the site of several enzymes hydrolyzing these substrates. Microvilli are also endowed with specific receptor sites that play an important role in the absorption of vitamin B_{12}–intrinsic factor complex, calcium, iron, and perhaps also conjugated bile acids. The surface-coat glycoprotein ("fuzz") provides a unique microenvironment where dietary constituent molecules are trapped and may come into contact with adsorbed pancreatic en-

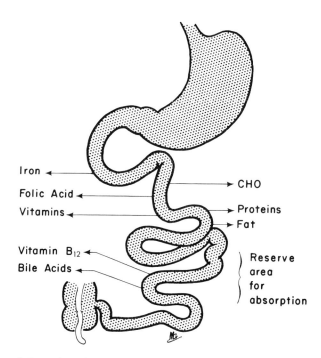

Fig. 10-21. Sites of absorption of dietary nutrients. The duodenum and jejunum are responsible for the absorption of all substrates except vitamin B_{12} and bile acids. The ileum does absorb small amounts in the normal situation and can, to a certain extent and after a variable adaptation period, take over for the diseased or resected jejunum.

zymes and with the apical plasma membranes of microvilli. As shown on Fig. 10-21, the duodenum and jejunum are responsible for the absorption of most dietary constituents except vitamin B_{12} and bile acids. With regard to fat absorption, experimental studies suggest that the capacity of the ileum to form chylomicrons is limited when compared to that of the jejunum.

Capacity of adaptation of the small intestine. The ileum compensates for its smaller surface area by a slower transit. It has a very effective functional reserve capable of taking over for the resected jejunum. The latter has a limited capacity to adapt to and compensate for the absorptive function of the ileum. This is attributable partly to the more rapid transit through the jejunum and partly to the lack of specific receptors for vitamin B_{12} and conjugated bile acids on the microvillous membrane of the jejunum.

Adaptation of the remaining small bowel plays an important role in the prognosis, but there have been few measurements of the residual small bowel in man. Roentgenographic studies invariably show dilatation of remaining small bowel loops and eventually elongation over a certain period of time. Examination of biopsy specimens show a true increase in villous size, the result of expansion of the proliferative zone (crypt size). As a result of this adaptive hyperplasia, which takes place over a period of several months, there is an increased surface area available for absorption and a corresponding improvement in absorption.

Intestinal growth is controlled by a feedback mechanism that is governed by exogenous (diet) and a number of endogenous agents. From animal studies, several mechanisms have been suggested to mediate adaptation after small bowel resection (Fig. 10-22).

Luminal contents. Animals maintained on total parenteral nutrition after intestinal resection do not undergo adaptation. Gastric infusion of a polymeric diet is more effective than a monomeric diet. Fat, with the exception of medium-chain triglycerides, appears to be the most effective dietary

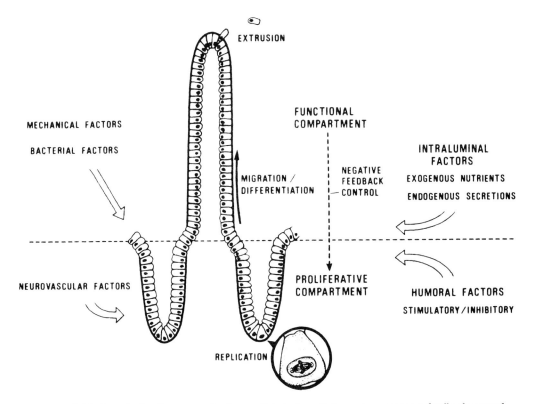

Fig. 10-22. Intestinal cell turnover in the small intestine. Enterocytes possess a feedback control whereby cell division in the proliferative compartment (the crypts) is regulated by the number of cells in the functional compartment. Exogenous and endogenous factors listed are discussed in the text. (From Williamson, R.C.N.: N. Engl. J. Med. **298:**1445, 1978.)

component to stimulate adaptation. It is not yet clear whether the effect of these nutrients is direct or is mediated by bile and pancreatic secretions, which, even in the absence of chyme, have been shown to stimulate mucosal growth in the ileum.

Gastrointestinal hormones. Because luminal nutrients are critical for adaptation to take place, it was logical to examine the possibility that hormones secreted in response to enteric feeding could be involved. Pentagastrin is ineffective except in the duodenum. Secretin and cholecystokinin may have an effect, but it is probably mediated by their effect on pancreaticobiliary secretions. Enteroglucagon does seem to have a trophic effect. Mineralocorticoids have also been shown to promote structural and functional adaptation in rat small bowel.

Dilatation and stasis of the remaining gut may enhance functional adaptation. Neurovascular changes that occur after a resection may contribute to adaptive hyperplasia though evidence in this regard is still fragmentary.

Physiopathology

Gastrointestinal motility. Factors that lead to alterations in gastrointestinal motility include the following:

1. Gastric hypersecretion has been documented in 50% of adults with extensive small bowel resection. It is usually transitory. Gastrin levels are normal in children. However, supranormal maximal gastric hydrochloric acid output is reported in 4 of 12 infants studied.

2. The extent of the decrease in surface area available for absorption is a critical factor. The absorptive capacity of the remaining bowel is influenced by the presence or absence of the ileocecal valve as well as of the colon. Diarrhea is less of a problem in patients in whom the ileocecal is preserved. Furthermore, conservation of the valve plays a significant role in prevention of the development of the contaminated small bowel syndrome. Outcome is also more favorable if the colon has not been resected. The absorptive capacity of the colon should not be underestimated, since it has considerable potential for water, electrolyte, and short-chain fatty acid transport.

3. Bacterial contamination of the upper bowel is almost always present in the early phase after a wide resection. Through the production of phenols and amines bacterial overgrowth may affect motility.

4. Deconjugated (free) and dehydroxylated (secondary) bile acids, as well as hydroxylated fatty acids, are potent cathartics.

Impairment of digestion. Factors leading to impairment of digestion include the following:

1. Pancreatic function is impaired whenever malnutrition is present. Even in normal newborns, a relative degree of exocrine pancreatic insufficiency is described. Gastric hypersecretion and a shortened transit time can decrease the transformation of zymogens into active proteolytic enzymes and the hydrolysis of fat by lipase.

2. Micellar solubilization is defective because of a decrease in conjugated bile acids. Newborn and premature infants constitute the majority of pediatric patients with the short bowel syndrome, and they already have a significant degree of fat malabsorption during the first month of life because of low intraduodenal concentrations of conjugated bile acids (see discussion of malabsorption in the first month of life, in this chapter). After an ileal resection, losses in the feces (Fig. 10-23) often exceed the capacity of the liver to maintain critical micellar concentrations. Even in cases where concentrations found in the duodenum are theoretically sufficient to form micelles, it is likely that micellar solubilization is defective. There is invariably a very high predominance of glycine over taurine conjugated bile acids (G/T) ratio) as a result of large fecal losses. Because of their low pK_a, glycoconjugates may be precipitated if the duodenum is acidic and therefore may not be available for solubilization of fat. Furthermore, in the common situation in which the small bowel is contaminated, the bile acids are deconjugated and therefore cannot form micelles with the products of lipolytic digestion.

3. Digestion of disaccharides and peptides is reduced because of accelerated transit and brushborder changes through bacterial contamination. Impairment of disaccharide and peptide digestion also occurs in the event that a wide resection of the jejunum has been done, since it is at that level that disaccharidase and peptidase activities are largely concentrated.

Absorptive defects. All nutrients, including water, electrolytes, fat, protein, carbohydrate, and all vitamins, are absorbed subnormally after massive resection of the small intestine. The degree of malabsorption varies with the type of resection. Large extents of mid–small bowel can be resected without many problems. However, when much

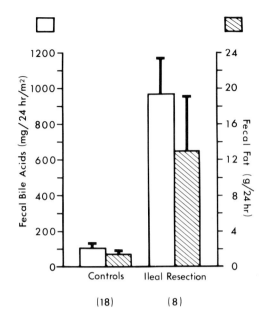

Fig. 10-23. Fecal sequestration of bile acids (mg/24 hr/ m²) in 8 young infants with the short bowel syndrome, after an ileal resection, represents more than an eight-fold increase above control values. In these patients, pool size and intraduodenal concentrations of bile acids are commonly decreased, since compensatory synthesis is often exceeded. The reserve capacity of the liver for bile acid production is variable but appears generally limited to a sevenfold to tenfold increase.

smaller segments of the proximal or distal small intestine are removed, severe symptoms can develop. Removal of a considerable length of distal small bowel can be tolerated if the ileocecal valve is left in place, since its absence predisposes the remaining small intestine to bacterial contamination and perhaps also accelerates transit time.

Clinical findings

The clinical picture produced by massive small bowel resection is one of starvation and diarrhea. Appetite is invariably voracious unless there is a significant degree of abdominal distention. The latter is an indication that the continuity of the bowel or its motility is compromised or, more frequently, that unabsorbed nutrients are undergoing bacterial breakdown in the colon, thus producing large amounts of gas. Vomiting suggests stenosis or stricture at the anastomotic site or the formation of a stagnant loop.

The diarrhea is often intractable but tends to improve as compensatory changes take place. In fact, it has been clinically demonstrated that there

is an increase in the absorptive surface of the remaining small intestine by increases in diameter and thickness of the wall and concomitant widening of villi with increased arborizations. Furthermore, there is a gradual decrease in the gastric hypersecretion and in the motility of the stomach and small bowel with a corresponding increased absorptive capcity for fat, proteins, and carbohydrates. These adaptive changes may gradually modify the clinical picture, but they occur more frequently in the ileum after proximal resection than in the jejunum when the distal small bowel has been removed.

There is usually a rapid weight loss with muscle wasting and decreased body fat. Excessive water and electrolyte losses lead to dehydration and a strong craving for salt. Anorexia and vomiting may occur when there is a significant degree of metabolic acidosis.

Anemia and hypoproteinemia are constant features. Manifestations of impaired protein absorption are low levels of serum proteins and hypoalbuminemia. Low serum carotene and cholesterol values associated with steatorrhea reflect the diminished absorption of fat. As a consequence of fat malabsorption, there is commonly evidence of vitamin D deficiency and malabsorption of calcium. Hypocalcemia is more likely to develop when the ileocecal valve has been resected. Magnesium balance tends to parallel that of calcium. Tetany may occur during the early phase, and osteomalacia in long-standing cases. Iron deficiency is likely to develop if the upper bowel has been removed, and vitamin B_{12} deficiency if the ileum was resected. Purpura and generalized bleeding reflects impaired coagulation caused by malabsorption of vitamin K.

Laboratory and x-ray findings

The transit time from mouth to anus measured with a nonabsorbable marker such as carmine red can be as short as 12 minutes. Roentgenographic studies should be done for assessment of the length of the remaining bowel, and for making sure that it is of reasonably normal caliber throughout and is emptying itself of its contents.

Cultures of small bowel contents for aerobic and anaerobic microorganisms are essential if there is a poor therapeutic response or if roentgenographic findings show dilatation proximal to the anastomotic site.

The biologic nutritional profile is characteristic

of starvation. Absorption studies may be useful in assessment of absorptive function of the remaining bowel and compensatory changes that will eventually occur.

Carbohydrates. Intolerance to monosaccharides and disaccharides is almost always present initially and can be evaluated by D-xylose and lactose absorption tests. Reducing substances in acidic stools (pH less than 5.5) are usually found. Unconjugated bile acids are responsible for the malabsorption of monosaccharides; they indicate bacterial contamination of the upper bowel, but it is usually temporary unless there is a structural problem (stenosis) or a functional problem (side-to-side anastomosis with stagnant loop) at the anastomotic site. Disaccharidase activity may be normal in the jejunum, but disaccharides are poorly tolerated because of jejunal hurry; this tends to decrease with time. In the rare cases of jejunal resections, the normally low disaccharidase activity in the ileum will gradually increase.

Fat and proteins. Fat and nitrogen balance studies should be done to help plan dietary management. The coefficient of fat and nitrogen absorption is always abnormal. Sequential measurements are useful in planning dietary manipulations. Hypoalbuminemia is particularly severe when the short bowel syndrome is complicated by a stagnant loop.

Vitamins, iron, bile acids, and oxalate. Vitamin B_{12} malabsorption (Schilling test with intrinsic factor) improves with time even in the event that the entire ileum has been removed. All fat-soluble vitamins are poorly absorbed. Calcium absorption will be significantly improved when fat malabsorption is under control (low-fat diet and medium-chain triglycerides). Serum iron is usually normal if the duodenum and jejunum are left in place. Bile acid concentrations are expected to be below 3 mM in 50% of infants. The G/T ratio may reach figures in excess of 10/1 (normal: 2/1). Should the contaminated small bowel syndrome be present, a significant proportion of duodenal bile acids may be free or secondary. The combined solvent effects of bile acids and lecithin maintain the solubility of cholesterol in bile and prevent the formation of gallstones. The severe bile acid loss and the depleted bile acid pool that follow wide ileal resections lead to an increase in cholesterol and the development of cholelithiasis, a complication seen occasionally in infants. Fecal bile acid measurements are useful in ileal resec-

tions because the documentation of a massive loss of bile acids is an indication that a ''cholerrheic enteropathy'' may exist and respond to cholestyramine. Hyperoxaluria (p. 284) and its complication, nephrolithiasis, are common in adults with the short bowel syndrome. Urinary oxalate excretion is also increased in most infants who have had an extensive intestinal resection. We have seen an infant with complete renal shutdown from oxalate stones.

Management

The infant with a massive small bowel resection presents a challenging management problem. It is impossible to plan for proper care unless the clinician establishes close contact with the surgeon to determine the area and length of small bowel resected, the presence or absence of the ileocecal valve, the type of anastomosis, the presence or absence of adhesions or peritonitis, and, most important, the percentage and apperance of the remaining small bowel.

Diet. Small amounts of (10 ml/kg) of a dilute formula (0.33 kcal/ml) adminstered every 3 hours should be started promptly. Protein hydrolysates have an osmotic advantage over amino acids. A mixture of monosaccharides and polysaccharides is preferable to disaccharides. Long-chain triglycerides (LCT) are poorly tolerated and should be partially replaced by medium-chain triglycerides (MCT). We favor Pregestimil, and we gradually increase the volume before increasing the caloric density to 0.50 kcal/ml and eventually to full strength, which is 0.67 kcal/ml. An increased stool output with the appearance of fecal reducing substances is an indication that tolerance limits have been exceeded. A 24- to 48-hour period of fasting is then indicated before resumption of the formula at a lower caloric density.

There is now considerable experience on both sides of the Atlantic with the use of continuous enteral feeding. It represents a significant advantage. A larger number of calories (up to 180 cal/kg/day), water (up to 275 ml/kg/day), and electrolytes can be provided while low-osmolality feedings are used. Although elemental diets have theoretical disadvantages (amino acids, monosaccharides, absence of fat, high osmolality) in terms of tolerance and capacity to induce adaptive changes in the remaining bowel, they are used with success by some groups. The largest experience is that of Ricour, who uses a formulation with an osmolality of about 300 mOsm/kg, which provides the patient with the following:

Monosaccharides, disaccharides, and polysaccharides	18 to 24 gm/kg
Protein hydrolysate	3 to 4 gm/kg
Medium-chain triglycerides	3 to 5 gm/kg

Formula should be started very cautiously. In a significant number of cases, steatorrhea and diarrhea will continue for a period of months and become chronic. Nutrient needs are therefore higher in resected individuals. Frequent small meals are always in order, and the single most effective dietary manipulation to control symptoms and assure growth on a long-term basis is a low-fat diet supplemented with MCT (Portagen and MCT oil).

Vitamins, iron, and trace elements. Intravenous or intramuscular administration is in order at least in the early phase.

Parenteral alimentation. The degree of panmalabsorption is usually severe, and parenteral alimentation is necessary to supplement insufficient oral calories. Peripheral vein alimentation regimens described for infants in Chapter 28 can provide 66 to 96 kcal/kg/day and are well tolerated. Even if oral calories are practically negligible, the oral route should be maintained, since experimental evidence suggests that maintenance of a normal mucosa and adaptation are dependent to some extent on luminal nutrition. In the event that oral intake is totally impossible because of excessively large water and electrolyte losses, or there is less than 80 cm of bowel left, a central catheter is used. Total parenteral nutrition may be necessary for extended periods. A more complete discussion of parenteral alimentation can be found in Chapter 28.

Therapy of specific problems

1. Antidiarrheal agents such as anticholinergic agents or opiates are contraindicated. They readily bring about abdominal distention.

2. Antacids are used in adults in an effort to reduce the consequences of gastric hypersecretion on motility, fat digestion, and mucosal damage. Cimetidine and antacids have not been helpful in children.

3. Cholestyramine (2 to 4 gm four times a day) can be useful in treating the explosive watery diarrhea associated with large losses of bile acids (chloerrheic enteropathy). Our own experience with small infants has not been rewarding in this regard. They seem to behave more like adults with very extensive resections (over 100 cm) who have a hydroxy fatty acid diarrhea (p. 283). A fat-free or low-fat diet with MCT is more beneficial, and cholestyramine seldom does any good.

4. Antibiotics should be used if, after the first few weeks, a contaminated small bowel can be documented. However, it is only a temporary measure. Surgery is the only treatment if roentgenographic studies suggest a stagnant loop.

As discussed before, oxalic acid is more extensively absorbed because of the presence of fatty acids and bile acids in the colon. A low-fat diet protects against hyperoxaluria.

6. The leading cause of death in infants with short-gut syndrome receiving total parenteral nutrition is sepsis. A high index of suspicion should be maintained and a complete septic work-up is called for in the presence of poor weight gain despite appropriate calories, fever of undetermined cause, and obstructive jaundice. Removal of the central catheter and systemic antibiotics are indicated in such circumstances.

The outcome after a wide intestinal resection is mainly dependent on the following:

1. Extent of resection
2. Area of small bowel (jejunal or ileum) resected
3. Function of remaining bowel
4. Preservation of ileocecal valve
5. Ability of shortened intestine to adapt

In a survey of 50 infants who had an extensive resection before the age of 2 months, less than 5% of cases with 38 to 75 cm of remaining small bowel died. The mortality was 50% in those who had between 15 and 38 cm of small bowel left. The presence of the ileocecal valve was quite critical. There were no survivors in 11 patients who were left with 40 cm or less of small intestine and in whom the ileocecal valve had been resected.

The presence of associated anomalies or of extreme prematurity adds to the risk. Significant as a poor prognostic factor is the appearance of distention, anorexia, or vomiting, since chances are that a further resection will be necessary. Parenteral nutrition has remarkably improved the prognosis of the short bowel syndrome by ensuring survival while compensatory changes occur in the remaining small bowel. Since there are isolated cases of survival in infants who had less than 15 to 20 cm of remaining small bowel after surgery, the physician cannot "close the door" on young infants with massive resections.

As more young infants survive the immediate postoperative period, a few reports are now giving accounts of the long-term course of these patients in terms of growth and development. Most patients by 2 or 3 years of age can consume a reasonably normal diet except for a moderate reduction of fat. They may grow well despite persisting defects in absorption. Developmental delays are quite common, but most seem unrelated to the short-gut syndrome. The presence of associated anomalies, extreme prematurity, or central nervous system complications add to the risk.

REFERENCES

Bohane, T.D., Haka-Ikse, K., Biggar, W.D., and others: A clinical study of young infants after small intestinal resection, J. Pediatr. **94:**552-558, 1979.

Buts, J.P., Morin, C.L., and Ling, V.: Influence of dietary components on intestinal adaptation after small bowel resection in rats, Clin. Invest. Med. **2:**59-66, 1979.

Compston, J.E., and Creamer, B.: The consequences of small intestinal resection, Q. J. Med. **46:**485-497, 1977.

Gracey, M., Burke, V., Oshin, A., and others: Bacteria, bile salts and intestinal monosaccharide malabsorption, Gut **12:**683-692, 1971.

Greenberger, N.J.: The management of the patient with short bowel syndrome, Am. J. Gastroenterol. **70:**528-540, 1978.

Hofmann, A.F., and Poley, J.R.: Role of bile acid malabsorption in pathogenesis of diarrhea and steatorrhea in patients with ileal resection. I. Response to cholestyramine or replacement of dietary long-chain triglyceride by medium-chain triglyceride, Gastroenterology **62:**918-934, 1972.

Krejs, G.J.: The small bowel. I. Intestinal resection, Clin. in Gastroenterol. **8:**373-386, 1979.

Malangoni, M.A., Cakmak, O., and Grosfeld, J.L.: Adverse effects of endotoxin following massive distal bowel resection, J. Pediatr. Surg. **14:**708-711, 1979.

Morin, C.L., and Ling, V.: Adaptation of the small bowel after resection in response to intraluminal lipid, Gastroenterology **74:**1070, 1978 (Abstract).

Ricour, C., Duhamel, J.F., and Nihoul-Fekete: Nutrition entérale à début constant chez l'enfant, Arch. Franc. Pédiatr. **34**(2):154-170, 1977.

Rickham, P.P.: Subtotal intestinal resection in the newborn, Ann. Chir. Infant. **18:**173-182, 1977.

Tefas, J.J., MacLean, W.C., Kolbach, S., and Shermeta, D.W.: Total management of short gut secondary to midgut volvulus without prolonged total parenteral alimentation, J. Pediatr. Surg. **13:**622-626, 1979.

Valman, H.B.: Growth and fat absorption after resection of ileum in childhood, J. Pediatr. **88:**41-45, 1976.

Valman, H.B., Oberholzer, V.G., and Palmer, T.: Hyperoxaluria after resection of ileum in childhood, Arch. Dis. Child. **49:**171-173, 1974.

Weser, E.: Intestinal adaptation after small bowel resection, Viewpoints on Digestive Diseases **10:**(2):1-4, 1978.

Williamson, R.C.N.: Intestinal adaptation, N. Engl. J. Med. **298:**1393-1402, 1443-1450, 1978.

Wilmore, D.W.: Factors correlating with a successful outcome following extensive intestinal resection in newborn infants, J. Pediatr. **80:**88-95, 1972.

DISORDERS OF LIPID TRANSPORT THROUGH FAILURE OF CHYLOMICRON FORMATION AND SECRETION

The intestine synthesizes chylomicrons after the uptake of the lipolytic products of intraluminal long-chain triglyceride digestion. Chylomicrons provide a means of transporting large quantities of triglycerides. The sequence of assembly, intracellular transport, and secretion of chylomicrons is still incompletely elucidated. Apoproteins B, A-I, A-II, A-IV, and C-II are synthesized by ribosomes on the rough endoplasmic reticulum, whereas triglycerides, cholesterol, and phospholipids are located in the smooth endoplasmic reticulum. The triglyceride core is coated with cholesterol ester, phospholipids, and apoproteins. These nascent chylomicrons are then transported to the Golgi apparatus where concentration and glycosylation occur. After being released into the intercellular space, the chylomicrons must traverse the basal membrane of the enterocyte and then diffuse between the immunocyte population of the lamina propria before entering lymphatics through gaps between endothelial cells of the lymphatic channels.

Abetalipoproteinemia and hypobetalipoproteinemia

Abetalipoproteinemia is a rare autosomal recessive disease that was described 25 years ago by Bassen and Kornzweig. It is characterized by the association of a severe malabsorption syndrome with a slowly progressive neuromuscular disorder resembling Friedreich's ataxia, retinitis pigmentosa, and acanthocytes. These patients cannot synthesize apoprotein B and therefore cannot form chylomicrons, nor can they secrete very low density lipoproteins (VLDL), which are eventually converted into low-density lipoproteins (LDL). As a result, chylomicrons, VLDL, and LDL are undetectable. The high ratio of free cholesterol to phospholipids and deficiencies of vitamins E and A and of essential fatty acids probably account for the red blood cell changes and for the retinal and neurologic disorder.

Clinical findings

Affected children become symptomatic within the first year of life. Failure to thrive is a common initial complaint. Diarrhea and abdominal distention are invariably present. Later there is progressive ataxia, loss of muscle strength, and nystagmus.

The gastrointestinal symptoms are indistinguishable from those of other causes of the malabsorption syndrome, like celiac disease and cystic fibrosis. Whereas the gastrointestinal problems tend to improve, the neural and ophthalmic ones become worse with age. The child is described as clumsy for the first few years. This progresses to frank ataxia with loss of deep tendon reflexes and loss of vibratory sense and position. Retinal changes seldom appear before adolescence. Cirrhosis has been reported.

Milder forms of the disease have been reported with hypobetalipoproteinemia.

Laboratory findings

The amount of plasma cholesterol is less than 60 mg/dl, and triglyceride levels are very low (less than 20 mg/dl). The electrophoretic pattern of lipoproteins shows the total absence of, or a striking decrease in, beta-lipoproteins and the absence of apoprotein B. Plasma concentration of carotene and of vitamins A and E is very low. Steatorrhea is invariably present. A snow-white duodenum may be seen on endoscopy. A small bowel biopsy specimen shows a normal pattern of villi, but the epithelial cells are engorged with lipid droplets identified as triglycerides (Fig. 10-24). Acanthocytes are best detected by wet smear. Lipid content of red blood cells can be measured.

Diagnosis

The differential diagnosis includes the various causes of the malabsorption syndrome in the first few years of life. Later, the symptoms are predominantly neurologic and may mimic Friedreich's ataxia.

Treatment

There are now a few reports on the successful use of a large dose of vitamin E (100 mg/kg per day) as well as of vitamin A (7500 to 25,000 IU per day). They may be effective in delaying the development or progression of the neurologic and retinal lesions. A low-fat diet supplemented with

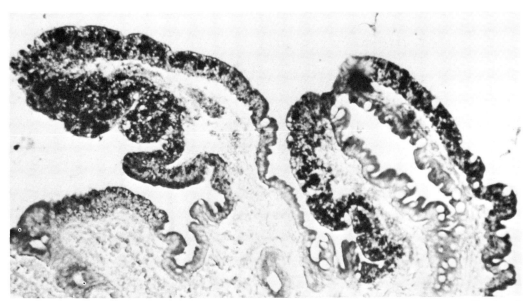

Continued.

Fig. 10-24. Abetalipoproteinemia. A 3-month-old infant with diarrhea, steatorrhea, and failure to thrive since birth. This oil-red-O stain of a peroral small bowel biopsy section shows vacuolation of enterocytes by neutral lipids. Total cholesterol was 50 mg/dl and triglycerides were 15 mg/dl. Beta lipoproteins could not be identified by electrophoresis. Low density lipoprotein apo B was not measurable, and no chylomicrons could be detected after a fatty meal of 50 gm/1.73 m^2.

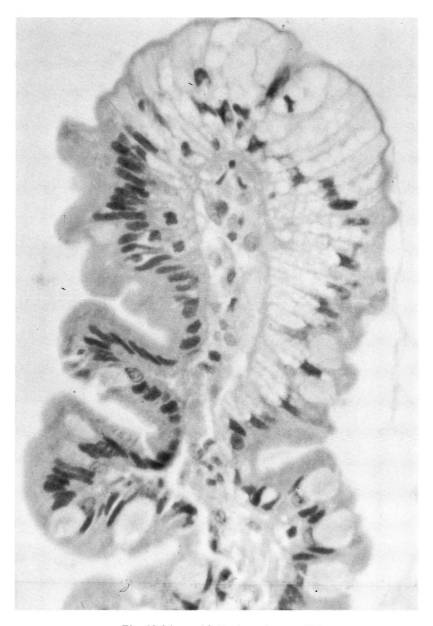

Fig. 10-24, cont'd. For legend see p. 295.

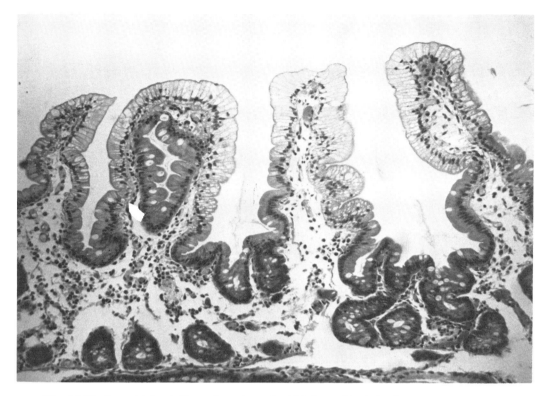

Fig. 10-25. Peroral jejunal biopsy in a 4-month-old infant with chylomicron retention disease. Despite 12 hours of fasting, the epithelial layer covering the upper two thirds of each villus is distended by fat. The cytoplasm of enterocytes is fenestrated by fat droplets, which cannot be exported into the lymphatics because of failure of chylomicron formation.

medium-chain triglycerides very effectively corrects the malabsorption syndrome.

The maintenance of high plasma levels of beta-lipoproteins in a patient has been ineffective in improving triglyceride transport. It is thus believed that the defects associated with this disease are not simply the result of the lack of circulating beta-lipoproteins.

Defect of chylomicron formation or secretion with normal apoprotein B (chylomicron retention disease)

Over the past few years we have seen seven children with this new syndrome. They developed a celiac-like syndrome during the first 3 months of life. A low 1-hour D-xylose level was noted in the majority along with hypoalbuminemia. Steatorrhea was uniformly present and amounted to about 12 gm/day. Low levels of carotene, vitamin A, and vitamin E and hypoprothrombinemia were documented. The jejunal biopsy changes (Fig. 10-25) are indistinguishable from those seen in abetalipoproteinemia and hypobetalipoproteinemia. Hypocholesterolemia was noted. Fasting triglycerides were normal but failed to respond to a fatty meal, and no chylomicrons were seen.

Of interest is the observation that these patients have normal serum apoprotein B (apo B) and only a small decrease in apo A-I and apo A-IV. Increased amounts of apo B are present in their intestinal mucosa. Electron microscopy (Fig. 10-26) suggests that chylomicrons are formed, since uniform-sized particles are membrane bound. Perhaps the final packaging of chylomicrons is defective, but it is more likely a defect in secretion.

The importance of this disorder stems from the fact that 3 of 8 patients have neurologic manifestations and 5 of 8 have abnormal ophthalmic findings. At present all these patients are on the following treatment regimen:

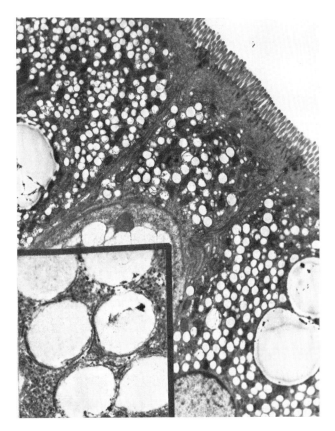

Fig. 10-26. Chylomicron retention disease. This electron micrograph (×4500) after a 12-hour fast shows small vacuoles of uniform size in addition to a few large ones. Part of a goblet cell nucleus is seen above the inset. *Inset* (×30,000) shows small vacuoles that are widely distributed in the cytoplasm of the enterocytes. They are membrane wrapped and have the morphologic features of chylomicrons.

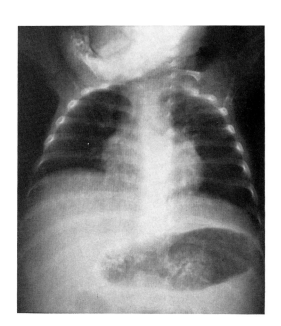

Fig. 10-27. Wolman's disease. Extensive calcification of both adrenal glands was seen in a 3 month old with diarrhea since birth and massive hepatomegaly.

Low-fat, medium chain triglyceride–supplemented
  diet
Vitamin K, 5 mg daily
Vitamin A, 15,000 units/m^2 daily
Vitamin E, 100 mg/kg daily

WOLMAN'S DISEASE

This rare autosomal recessive storage disease is
secondary to deficiency of lysosomal acid esterase. Consequently, cholesterol esters and triglycerides accumulate in all organs. Patients present
with diarrhea, hepatomegaly, and severe failure to
thrive within the first few months of life. Adrenal
glands are calcified (Fig. 10-27), the bone marrow shows fat-laden macrophages, the villous pattern of the small bowel is grossly distorted by a
lamina propria swollen by sheets of foamy macrophages (Fig. 10-28). Most patients have a rapidly downhill course and die before 1 year of age.
There is no treatment available.

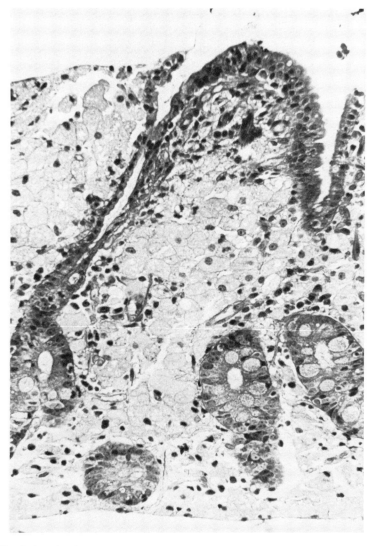

Fig. 10-28. Wolman's disease. The villous architecture is distorted by massive infiltration of the
lamina propria by fat-laden macrophages. The latter were also abundant in a rectal biopsy specimen.

REFERENCES

Azibi, E., Zaidman, J.L., Eschar, J., and Szeinberg, A.: Abetalipoproteinemia treated with parenteral and oral vitamins A and E and with medium chain triglycerides, Acta Paediatr. Scand. **67**:797-801, 1978.

Cottrill, C., Glueck, C.J., Leuba, V., and others: Familial homozygous hypobetalipoproteinemia, Metabolism **23**:779-791, 1974.

Fosbrooke, A., Choksey, S., and Wharton, B.: Familial hypo-β-lipoproteinemia, Arch. Dis. Child. **48**:729-732, 1973.

Lees, R.S., and Ahrens, E.H.: Fat transport in abetalipoproteinemia, N. Engl. Med. **280**:1261-1266, 1969.

Mars, H., Lewis, L.A., Robertson, A.L., and others: Familial hypo-β-lipoproteinemia, Am. J. Med. **46**:886-900, 1969.

Muller, D.P.R., Lloyd, J.K., and Bird, A.C.: Long-term management of abetalipoproteinemia, Arch. Dis. Child. **52**:209-214, 1977.

Partin, J.S., Partin, J.C., Schubert, W.K., and McAdams, J.: Liver ultrastructure in abetalipoproteinemia: evolution of micronodular cirrhosis, Gastroenterology **67**:107-118, 1974.

Patrick, A.D., and Lake, B.D.: Wolman's disease. In Hers, H.G., and Van Hoof, F., editors: Lysosomes and storage disease, New York, 1977, Academic Press, Inc.

Robinson, W.G., Kuwabara, T., and Bieri, J.G.: Vitamin E deficiency and the retina: photoreceptor and pigment epithelial changes, Invest. Ophthalmol. Visual Sci. **18**:683-690, 1979.

Roy, C.C., Sniderman, A., Deckelbaum, R., and others: Normal concentrations of serum and increased intestinal apo B with failure of chylomicron secretion: a new disorder of lipid transport, Pediatr. Res. **16**:175A, 1982 (Abstract).

Sabesin, S.M., and Frase, S.: Electron microscopic studies of the assembly, intracellular transport and secretion of chylomicrons by rat intestine, J. Lipid Res. **18**:496-511, 1977.

Scott, B.B., Miller, J.P., and Losowsky, M.S.: Hypobetalipoproteinemia: a variant of the Bassen-Kornzweig syndrome, Gut **20**:163-168, 1979.

MALABSORPTION IN THE FIRST MONTH OF LIFE

The functional immaturity of the intestinal tract, liver, and pancreas during the first few weeks of life has important clinical implications because of the short-term and long-term repercussions of malnutrition on growth and development. The greater vulnerability of the infant with a low birth weight is related to the following factors:

1. Greater caloric needs in relationship with surface area
2. Metabolic immaturity, which limits the extent of possible dietary manipulations
3. Fecal sequestration of ingested calories, which is more extensive and compounded by a restricted gastric capacity and the frequent occurrence of an incompetent gastroesophageal sphincter

Carbohydrates

Intestinal maltase and sucrase reach mature values by the sixth to eighth month of intrauterine life, whereas lactase reaches normal values only close to term. Reducing substances are commonly found in the stools of newborns and breath hydrogen excretion confirm that some degree of lactose malabsorption is present even in full-term neonates. Most formulas contain lactose as the sole carbohydrate source so as to simulate human milk. Recently formulas have been introduced for low birth weight infants in which 50% of carbohydrate is in the form of glucose polymer. Since salivary amylase and brush-border glucoamylase are present at birth, it is assumed that hydrolysis of the polymer is unlikely to be a problem despite the absence of pancreatic amylase. It should be noted however that transport of glucose is not so effective during the first few months of life (Fig. 10-29) as it is later. The rate of jejunal transport of glucose does not go beyond 4.5 gm/hr, whereas in adults it is 30 gm/hr. This difference is not strictly related to the surface area available for absorption since the K_m (the affinity of glucose for its carrier) is three times lower than it is in adults. In this context, the finding of reducing substances in the stools of neonates is not surprising. It may be of clinical significance in situations where the concentration of carbohydrates in a formula exceeds 10 gm/dl.

Proteins

In the period of life during which anabolic activity is at its highest level, providing the proper amount of high-quality proteins is critical for the accretion and synthesis of proteins.

The proteolytic activity of gastric pepsin is less in preterm than in full-term infants. Enterokinase, essential for the conversion of trypsinogen into trypsin, is only measurable at the end of gestation, whereas brush-border peptidase activity is already high during the third trimester.

Pancreatic proteases are found in substantial quantities in newborns. However, the functional response of the pancreas in the early postnatal period to secretagogues is absent up to 1 month of age. After 1 month, only chymotrypsin output increases significantly after cholecystokinin and secretin. Despite these limitations there is no evidence that a digestive-phase defect constitutes a significant handicap for the absorption of proteins. There are indications from analysis of il-

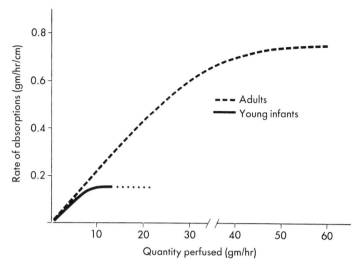

Fig. 10-29. Kinetics of glucose absorption in infants and adults from various studies analyzed by Younoszai. (From Younoszai, M.K.: J. Pediatr. **85**:446, 1974.)

eocecal contents that breast milk proteins are more completely hydrolyzed than cow's milk proteins.

It is possible that the transport defect documented for monosaccharides also applies to amino acids. This has not yet been studied, but even if some degree of limitation were present, it would not constitute a significant handicap because the major proportion of substrates made available for the synthesis of proteins are absorbed as dipeptides and tripeptides and not as amino acids. As is the case for disaccharides and glucose polymers, the lower osmolality of peptides presents a distinct advantage. The substitution of whole proteins for a hydrolysate is only indicated if a digestive-phase defect or if protein intolerance is present.

Extent of fat malabsorption and pathogenesis

Only the normal full-term neonate on breast milk can achieve a normal (greater than 95%) coefficient of fat absorption. In the low birth weight newborn, figures of 75% to 85% on breast milk drop significantly (45% to 60%) when cow's milk is given. Substituting vegetable oils (soya, olive, corn) for butterfat leads to a significant improvement in the coefficient of fat absorption (70% to 85%) achieved by formula-fed low birth weight newborns. Correction of fat malabsorption can be effected by a formula in which 40% to 80% of the lipid source is medium-chain triglycerides.

As borne out by the preceding paragraph, long-chain saturated fatty acids (except when breast milk is their source) are poorly tolerated by neonates. Significant improvement occurs with unsaturated fatty acids and complete correction with medium-chain fatty acids. Positional arrangement of fatty acids within the triglyceride molecule constitutes an important determinant affecting neonatal fat absorption. In this regard, the great advantage of human milk fat has to do with the fact that palmitic acid is predominantly esterified at position 2 (beta position). In butterfat, this long-chain saturated fatty acid is equally distributed among all three positions of the triglyceride. Absorbability of palmitic acid is greater as a beta-monoglyceride than as a free fatty acid. It is not known at this point whether immaturity of small bowel mucosal function could contribute to the fat malabsorption of the neonate.

The digestive phase of fat absorption is abnormal in the newborn period. Duodenal fluid contains inadequate amounts of pancreatic lipase and there is no response to cholecystokinin-pancreozymin. The presence of triglycerides in the stools confirms the presence of a lipolytic-phase defect. The physical events leading to the micellar dispersion of lipolytic products are altered in view of significant abnormalities of bile salt metabolism. The intraluminal concentration of bile salts is commonly below the one required to solubilize the products of lipolysis. This is attributable to the following:

1. Large fecal loss secondary to a defective ileal transport.

2. Contraction of pool size related to an inadequate compensatory synthesis

As a result, micellar solubilization of lipids is poor and fat transport through the unstirred water layer to the water-microvillus interface is hampered. There is little or no data in neonates suggesting that translocation, esterification, chylomicron formation, or transport of lipids out of the enterocyte are defective.

The coefficient of fat absorption in breast-fed babies is higher. This is of particular importance in low birth weight neonates who may sequester more than 30% of ingested fat in their stools or regular formulas. The presence of lipoprotein lipase and of bile salt–stimulated lipase in breast milk leads to partial hydrolysis of lipids, which, once in the stomach, are more susceptible to enzymatic attack by lingual lipase than unsaturated long-chain triglycerides present in formulas.

The observation that fat absorption in breast-fed neonates is higher relative to the intraluminal bile salt concentrations is also explained by the triglyceride configuration of breast milk lipids. As discussed on the preceding page, a large percentage (55%) of palmitic acid, a poorly saturated long-chain fatty acid, is in the beta position of breast milk triglycerides. Therefore after lipolysis, palmitate will be delivered to the unstirred water layer as the more soluble and more diffusible beta-monoglyceride. There is experimental evidence that the mucosal uptake of fat is inhibited by the binding of fatty acids to casein, albumin, and soy protein. The significance of this finding in infants has not been examined. Perhaps the lower concentration of breast milk proteins and their more extensive digestion could contribute to the more complete absorption of breast milk fat.

Management

Undernutrition is probably the most pernicious problem that besets the low birth weight infant. Concern over the impossibility of providing appropriate calories and nutrients by mouth and by intermittent gavage has led to continuous nasogastric or nasoduodenal feeding. Although short circuiting the stomach offers some measure of protection against vomiting and aspiration pneumonia, it decreases the coefficient of fat absorption because it bypasses the gastric phase of fat lipolysis. Furthermore it has been associated with intestinal perforation, intussusception, and necrotizing enterocolitis. Despite these drawbacks, there is still a place for transpyloric feeding in special circumstances such as severe esophageal chalasia or perhaps in cases where gastric distention is unassociated with any other contraindication to oral alimentation. Parenteral alimentation as the sole source of nutrition or as a supplement to oral feedings represents a significant advance, but it is not without risk.

Recent evidence indicates that the milk of mothers giving birth prematurely is suited to their infant's requirements in terms of increased protein and mineral content. There are still conflicting views as to the appropriate composition of formula for the low birth weight infant. Protein should be supplied as a 60 to 40 ratio of whey protein to casein at a concentration of 2.5 to 4 gm/100 kcal. Soy protein formulas should not be used. The carbohydrate source should probably be a mixture of lactose and glucose polymers. With regard to fat, which constitutes the predominant source of energy, formulas that contain 40% to 50% of their fat as medium-chain triglycerides have distinct advantages in terms of fat absorption, nitrogen retention, and early growth.

REFERENCES

Auricchio, S., Rubins, A., and Murset, G.: Intestinal glycosidase activities in the human embryo, fetus and newborn, Pediatrics 35:944-954, 1965.

Borgström, B., Lindquist, B., and Lundh, G.: Enzyme concentration and absorption of protein and glucose in duodenum of premature infants, Am. J. Dis. Child. 99:338-343, 1960.

Chiles, C., Watkins, J.B., Barr, R., and others: Lactose utilization in the newborn: role of colonic flora, Pediatr. Res. 14:356, 1980 (Abstract).

De Belle, R.C., Vaupshas, V., Vitullo, B.B., and others: Intestinal absorption of bile salts: immature development in the neonate, J. Pediatr. 94:472-476, 1979.

Fomon, S.J.: Infant nutrition, ed. 2, Philadelphia, 1974, W.B. Saunders Co.

Ghadimi, H., Anulanantham, K., and Rathi, M.: Evaluation and nutritional management of the low birth weight newborn, Am. J. Clin. Nutr. 26:473-476, 1973.

Grand, R.J., Watkins, J.B., and Torti, F.M.: Development of the human gastrointestinal tract: a review, Gastroenterology 70:790-810, 1976.

Katz, L., and Hamilton, J.R.: Fat absorption in infants of birth weight less than 1,300 gm, J. Pediatr. 85:608-614, 1974.

Lebenthal, E., and Lee, P.C.: Development of functional response in human exocrine pancreas, Pediatrics 66:556-560, 1980.

Nutrition Committee, Canadian Pediatric Society: Feeding the low–birth weight infant, Can. Med. Assoc. 124:1301-1311, 1981.

Pereira, G.R., and Lemons, J.A.: Controlled study of transpyloric and intermittent gavage feeding in the small preterm infant, Pediatrics 67:68-72, 1981.

Roy, C.C., Ste-Marie, M., Chartrand, L., and others: Correction of the malabsorption of the preterm infant with a medium-chain triglyceride formula, J. Pediatr. **86:**446-450, 1974.

Signer, E., Murphy, G.M., Edkins, S., and others: The role of bile salts in the fat malabsorption of premature infants, Arch. Dis. Child. **49:**174-180, 1974.

Valman, H.B., Aikens, R., David-Reed, Z., and Garrow, J.S.: Retention of nitrogen, fat and calories in infants of low birth weight on conventional and high-volume feeds, Br. Med. J. **3:**319-210, 1974.

Watkins, J.B., Bliss, C.M., Donaldson, R.M., and Lester, R.: Characterization of newborn fecal lipid, Pediatrics **53:**511-515, 1974.

Watkins, J.B., Szczepanik, P., Gould, J.B., and others: Bile salt metabolism in the human premature infant, Gastroenterology **69:**706-713, 1975.

Younoszai, M.K.: Jejunal absorption of hexose in infants and children, J. Pediatr. **85:**446-448, 1974.

Zoppi, G., Andreotti, G., Pajno-Ferra, F., and others: Exocrine pancreatic function in premature and full-term neonates, Pediatr. Res. **6:**880-886, 1972.

Protein-losing enteropathy

Excessive loss of plasma proteins into the gastrointestinal tract occurs with a number of well-defined disorders. Protein-losing enteropathy has been described with at least 85 different diseases, most of which, except for gastric polyps and gastric carcinoma, have been observed in the pediatric population. Some causes of abnormal enteric protein loss are as follows:

Disorders associated with protein-losing enteropathy

Heart
    Congestive heart failure
    Constrictive pericarditis
    Atrial septal defect
    Primary myocardial disease
Stomach and esophagus
    Reflux esophagitis
    Ménétrier's disease
    Allergic gastroenteritis
    Multiple gastric ulcers
Small intestine
    Celiac disease
    Cystic fibrosis
    Cow milk intolerance or soy protein intolerance
    Intestinal lymphangiectasis
    Tropical sprue
    Crohn's disease
    Lymphosarcoma
    Gastrointestinal infections and infestations
    Giardiasis
    Allergic gastroenteritis
    Contaminated small bowel syndrome
    Radiation enteritis
    Abetalipoproteinemia
    Chronic volvulus, malrotation, or stenosis
    Dermatitis herpetiformis
    Chronic intestinal pseudo-obstruction
    Ulcerative jejunoileitis
Colon
    Ulcerative colitis
    Hirschsprung's disease
    Polyposis
Immune deficiency states
    Agammaglobulinemia
    Wiskott-Aldrich syndrome

ALBUMIN METABOLISM

Hypoalbuminemia constitutes a good index of a protein-losing enteropathy. However, it occurs in a variety of circumstances, and its clinical significance can be appreciated only if it is realized that albumin level is the complex end result of a number of interrelated factors regulating its synthesis, degradation, and distribution. Normal values for albumin metabolism are shown in Table 11-1.

Role of structure

Albumin is the major protein synthesized by the liver and exported into plasma. The polypeptide chain of molecular weight (69,000 to 70,000) is folded in such a way that nine double loops are formed and held in place by disulfide bridges. Albumin serves in the plasma to maintain osmotic pressure and to carry metals, ions, fatty acids, amino acids, metabolites, bilirubin, enzymes, drugs, and hormones. The polyribosomes bound to the endoplasmic reticulum of the liver cell synthesize albumin. Experimental work shows that the process takes 20 minutes and that probably only a third of the liver cell population is active in the synthesis of albumin. Newly synthesized molecules are released directly into hepatic sinusoids, with hepatic lymph normally playing only a small and insignificant role. However, when sinusoids are distorted or when there is postsinusoidal portal hypertension, as occurs in cirrhosis of the liver, as much as 87% of newly synthesized albumin bypasses the vascular compartment of the liver, as well as hepatic lymphatics, and may be lost directly into ascites.

Distribution

Serum albumin is widely distributed in an intravascular and an extravascular pool. After the intravenous injection of labeled albumin, equilibrium within the vascular pool occurs within minutes. However, distribution equilibrium between the intravascular and extravascular pools requires 7 to 10 days. The intravascular space contains 35% of the albumin mass, and the extravascular space, 65%. Close to 50% of the available extravascular albumin is found in the skin. Within 2 days of leaving the vascular system, 80% of the albumin is returned to the plasma, mainly by the thoracic

Table 11-1. Normal albumin metabolism*

Subject of study	Serum albumin level (gm/dl)	Albumin synthesis (mg/kg/24 hr)	Albumin degradation (% plasma albumin pool/ 24 hr)	Exchangeable albumin pool (gm/kg)	Intravascular albumin (%)
Adults					
Male	3.5-4.5	120-200	6-10	4.0-5.0	38-45
Female	3.5-4.5	120-150	6-10	3.5-4.5	38-45
Children					
13 days to 14 months	3.3-4.3	180-300	10-11	6.0-8.0	33-43
3 to 8 years	4.2-5.0	130-170	6-9	3.0-4.0	46-51

*From Rothschild, M.A., Oratz, M., and Schreiber, S.S.: N. Engl. J. Med. 286:748-755, 1972.

duct. The extravascular exchangeable pool of albumin can be rapidly mobilized into the plasma in response to hemorrhage, massive proteinuria, protein-losing enteropathies, or starvation.

Factors influencing synthesis and degradation

Amino acids. The most important factor regulating albumin synthesis is nutrition, or more specifically, the supply of amino acids at the site of synthesis. Studies have shown that the effect of altered protein intake on albumin synthesis is much more pronounced than on total liver protein production. Albumin synthesis decreases by 50% within 24 hours of a total fast or shortly after initiation of a protein-deficient diet. On refeeding proteins to protein-depleted animals, albumin synthesis increases much more than total liver protein synthesis. The reduction in albumin synthesis in starvation occurs despite an endogenous supply of amino acids through the recycling of liver proteins. With excessive degradation of liver proteins the rate of synthesis falls. This leads to a drop in plasma concentration, which in turn brings about a decrease in catabolic rate. It has been shown in postoperative patients intravenously infused with glucose that the muscle and hepatic catabolic pools of amino acids are insufficient and that an exogenous supply is necessary to achieve a high rate of albumin synthesis. All amino acids are not effective. Tryptophan is the least abundant amino acid in liver proteins and may be rate limiting during starvation or protein deprivation. Arginine, lysine, phenylalanine, glutamine, alanine, threonine, proline, and ornithine are also known to be particularly effective. The observation that all the amino acids known to stimulate albumin production also stimulate urea production has led to the concept that the urea cycle may play an important role in the regulation of protein synthesis.

Hormones. Cortisone, thyroid growth hormone, and insulin are known to stimulate albumin synthesis. However, it has overall antianabolic effects because of enhanced gluconeogenesis, which leads to a decrease in the availability of amino acids to the synthetic machinery. Insulin and glucagon also play a role. Glucose, by eliciting a rise in insulin and a fall in glucagon, improves the utilization of infused amino acids for synthesis and decreases the degradation of proteins.

Hepatic milieu intérieur. The hepatic interstitial fluid contains only low concentrations of albumin and is probably a very sensitive system influencing albumin synthesis. A decrease in the colloid content at or near the site of albumin turns on synthesis. A rise in plasma albumin in response to salt-poor albumin infusions could turn off synthesis if the hepatic interstitial fluid oncotic pressure is increased as a result of the infusions.

Catabolism. The factors regulating the degradation of albumin are poorly understood. Degradation affects new and old albumin molecules alike; 3% to 4% of exchangeable albumin is degraded daily. The mechanisms involved are mass dependent and are equally affected by the intravascular mass of albumin and by the total pool of exchangeable albumin. Accordingly, hypoalbuminemia should be associated with a drop in catabolic rate. In practice, this relationship does not always hold. Induced hyperalbuminemia leads to an increase in catabolic rate; however, there is little change in synthetic rate. Therefore, degradation and synthesis are not independent in that situation.

The normal kidney plays a minor role in albumin degradation. The liver and the gastrointestinal tract are probably responsible for 10% each of the total mass of albumin lost and degraded daily. Plasma proteins of all classes are present in low concentrations, in saliva and gastrointestinal secretions and on the mucosal surface of the gastrointestinal tract. It is likely that this leakage, which accounts for 10% of the total quantity of albumin catabolized daily, occurs as a result of the loss of lymph from the lamina propria at the apex of the intestinal villi with desquamating cells. After hydrolysis, the constituent amino acids of albumin and of other proteins lost in the lumen are reabsorbed and reutilized.

A number of hepatic and gastrointestinal diseases are associated with continued loss of albumin. Of importance in cirrhotics is the report that in most patients the albumin synthetic rate is not depressed. The hypoalbuminemia is more related to catabolism through sequestration in ascitic fluid. In protein-losing enteropathies, the synthetic rate cannot keep up with losses. Depressed rates of synthesis have been noted even when malnutrition is not a problem and also in situations where the leakage of proteins is taking place high in the gastrointestinal tract, permitting the reabsorption of amino acids. The lack of response of the synthetic mechanism to the stimulus of an increased degradation rate remains frequently unexplained.

PATHOGENESIS

An excessive loss of enteric proteins may be associated with a variety of diseases involving any segment of the gastrointestinal tract. These disorders can be grouped under two basic pathologic processes. One mechanism is a blockage of lymphatics, and the second is an abnormal mucosal permeability to protein.

Pathogenesis of protein-losing enteropathy

Blockage of lymphatics
  Intestinal lymphangiectasis
  Crohn's disease
  Intestinal malrotation or volvulus with lymphovenous
    obstruction
  Whipple's disease (only one poorly documented case
    in children)
  Compression of lymphatics or thoracic duct by a tumor
  Cirrhosis of the liver
  Constrictive pericarditis, congestive heart failure

Increased mucosal permeability to proteins
  Celiac disease
  Tropical sprue
  Contaminated small bowel syndrome
  Gastrointestinal infections and infestations
  Ulcerative colitis, radiation enteritis
  Polyps
  Ménétrier's disease

Hypoalbuminemia occurs if the hepatic synthetic mechanism is not able to compensate because of the severity of the protein-losing enteropathy. It may also occur with a modest degree of enteric protein loss if the synthetic mechanism cannot be increased on account of malnutrition, malabsorption of amino acids, or chronic infection. It is clear that in most diffuse diseases of the gastrointestinal tract associated with a protein-losing enteropathy, malnutrition and malabsorption compound the problem by decreasing the ability of the liver for compensatory synthesis. The diagnosis of a protein-losing enteropathy cannot invariably be made on the basis of serum albumin level, since the synthesis rate can in some cases compensate for the loss. It should be assessed by a direct measurement of enteric protein loss.

CLINICAL FINDINGS

The spectrum of clinical signs and symptoms identified with protein-losing enteropathy is very large. Some patients may have no symptoms referable to the gastrointestinal tract and have only the signs of a chronic illness with lowered plasma osmotic pressure manifested as edema. The edema may be localized; occasionally it is nonpitting and asymmetric (intestinal lymphangiectasis). Anasarca is not uncommon, and chylous ascites may occur. Weight gain is invariably poor, and height is often stunted. Evidence of fat-soluble vitamin deficiencies is common. The anemia present is often hypochromic, though not uncommonly megaloblastic. The latter form can be related to vitamin B_{12} or folic acid malabsorption. In severe cases, it can be related to extremely low levels of circulating proteins. Most patients present severe, longstanding gastrointestinal symptoms. Although there is nonselective "bulk loss" of a number of plasma proteins into the enteric lumen, albumin is usually the most depressed of the plasma proteins.

Quantitation of enteric protein loss

Although the estimation of fecal nitrogen may be helpful in certain circumstances, it should be

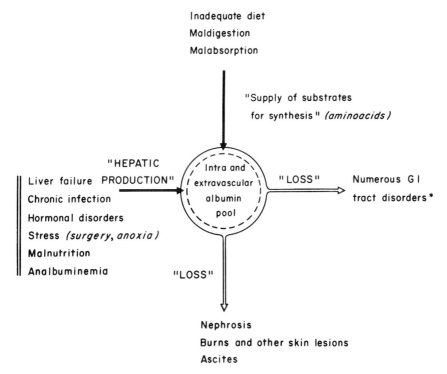

Fig. 11-1. Etiology of hypoalbuminemia. *Listed on first page of Chapter 11.

remembered that in most cases of protein-losing enteropathy the stool nitrogen level is not abnormally elevated, since the amino acids derived from the hydrolysis of exuded plasma proteins can be reabsorbed.

Quantitation of intestinal losses of albumin is best carried out by use of ^{51}Cr-albumin. In normal subjects the ^{51}Cr label is neither significantly absorbed from nor secreted into the gastrointestinal tract; it is therefore perfectly suited for the quantitation of intestinal losses of albumin. The 4-day stool collection after an intravenous injection of ^{51}Cr-albumin never contains more than 0.7% of the injected radioactivity in normal subjects. This figure in most patients with protein-losing enteropathy is greater than 3% and may be as great as 60%.

Differential diagnosis

The diagnosis of protein-losing enteropathy can be considered when one is assured that the dietary intake is adequate and that malnutrition does not account for the hypoproteinemia. Also, since hypoalbuminemia can be related to either a lowered production or an increased catabolic rate, it is important that the physician rule out hepatic disease

and make certain that no significant proteinuria is present (Fig. 11-1).

Treatment

Once the diagnosis of protein-losing enteropathy is made, an extensive search must be made of the cardiovascular system and gastrointestinal tract for a treatable lesion. Temporary benefits can be derived from albumin infusions and diuretics when there is severe plasma contraction and anasarca. The dietary approach and specific treatments are discussed with each entity.

REFERENCES

Greenberg, G.R., Marliss, E.B., Anderson, G.H., and others: Protein-sparing therapy in postoperative patients: effects of added hypocaloric glucose or lipid, N. Engl. J. Med. **294:**1411-1416, 1976.

Rosenoer, V.M., Skillman, J.J., Hasting, P.R., and others: Albumin synthesis and nitrogen balance in postoperative patients, Surgery **87:**305-312, 1980.

Rothschild, M.A., Oratz, M., and Schreiber, S.S.: Editorial. Extravascular albumin, N. Engl. J. Med. **301:**497-498, 1979.

Rothschild, M.A., Oratz, M., and Schreiber, S.S.: Albumin synthesis. In Javitt, N.B., editor: Liver and biliary tract physiology. I. International review of physiology, vol. 21, Baltimore, 1980, University Park Press.

Rothschild, M.A., Oratz, M., and Schreiber, S.S.: Albumin synthesis, N. Engl. J. Med. **286:**748-756, 816-821, 1972.

SPECIFIC ENTITIES
Intestinal lymphangiectasis
Lymph circulation

The intestinal mucosal lacteals represent a very important component of the absorptive apparatus. They follow the arcuate pattern of small blood vessels. They are lined by very thin endothelial cells with overlapping cytoplasmic protrusions between which chylomicrons, water and electrolytes penetrate. Mucosal lacteals are terminal lymphatics and empty into collecting lymphatic channels, which, in contrast to lacteals, are capable of contraction and dilatation through their myogenic activity. Furthermore, they are equipped with valves, which regulate lymph flow. In the mesentery and omentum, the outstanding feature is the presence of large saccular structures, which are 5 to 10 times larger than collecting lymphatic channels. A drop in blood volume or in colloid pressure impairs the capacity of lacteals to drain the interstitium. Blind ending, distortion, or increased pressure in the lymphatic channels will result in leakage of lymph.

Etiology

Intestinal lymphangiectasis is a primary or secondary disorder of the gastrointestinal tract associated with lymphatic dysfunction, bulk loss of lymph into the bowel lumen, and protein-losing enteropathy.

Etiologic classification of intestinal lymphangiectasis

Primary form
   Limited to the lamina propria
   Intact lamina propria with involvement of the submucosa, subserosa, mesentery, and omentum
   Generalized lymphangiomatosis
Secondary form
   Functional
      Malrotation with lymphovenous compression
      Congestive heart failure
      Constrictive pericarditis
      Cirrhosis
   Blockage of lymph flow
      Crohn's disease
      Intestinal scleroderma
      Whipple's disease
      Panniculitis of the mesentery (Weber-Christian)
      Retroperitoneal tumors
      Lymphomas

The primary form is the result of a congenital disorder of the lymphatic system. Support for this concept comes from the frequent incidence of associated lymphatic aberrations in the limbs and in many other anatomic locations. The occurrence of intestinal lymphangiectasis in patients with Turner's syndrome and Noonan's syndrome has been described. The secondary form is the result of lymph stasis, which may be functional as in malrotation with lymphovenous compression, congestive heart failure, constrictive pericarditis, and cirrhosis. Blockage of lymph flow may be associated with inflammatory and infiltrative disorders of the intestine and its mesentery. These diseases include Crohn's disease, panniculitis of the mesentery, Whipple's disease, intestinal scleroderma, retroperitoneal tumors, and lymphomas. A subset of patients have variable signs of inflammatory disease and a secondary form of lymphangiectasis that responds to corticosteroids.

As a result of protein leakage in the lumen of the bowel, protein loss is large, and although reabsorption of amino acids occurs, synthesis by the liver may not keep up with the loss, leading to hypoalbuminemia and edema. Fat malabsorption is usually present and its extent is variable. Since most thoracic duct lymphocytes belong to a pool of thymus-dependent cells that recirculate from blood to lymph, the bulk loss of lymph may lead to a depression of both humoral and cellular immunity. There is hypogammaglobulinemia, lymphocytopenia (less than 1500 mm^3), cutaneous anergy, depressed in vitro lymphocyte reponses to a variety of stimuli, and an increased incidence of neoplasia.

Clinical features

Peripheral edema is the most common complaint. Failure to thrive, diarrhea, abdominal distention (Fig. 11-2), lymphedematous limbs (Fig. 11-2), repeated infections, or tetany are the outstanding features. Gastrointestinal symptoms, usually mild but possibly severe, include diarrhea, intermittent vomiting, and abdominal pain. Ascites and pleural and pericardial effusions may be secondary to hypoalbuminemia, or they may be chylous in nature and be the result of lymphatic anomalies in these areas (Fig. 11-3). Careful attention to the cardiac examination is needed to rule out constrictive pericarditis.

The major laboratory findings are a low level of serum albumin, decreased immunoglobulin levels, and lymphopenia. Anemia may also be found. Serum calcium is frequently depressed, and stool fat content is usually elevated. Lymphocytes may be seen in large numbers on a stool smear.

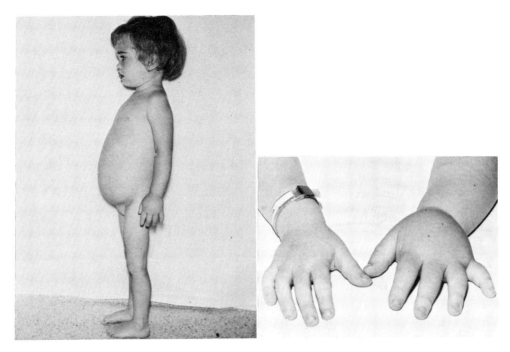

Fig. 11-2. Intestinal lymphangiectasis. This 2-year-old girl had chronic diarrhea, failure to thrive, abdominal distention, peripheral edema, and a lymphedematous left arm and hand. A low-fat diet supplemented with medium-chain triglycerides led only to mild improvement of her protein-losing enteropathy.

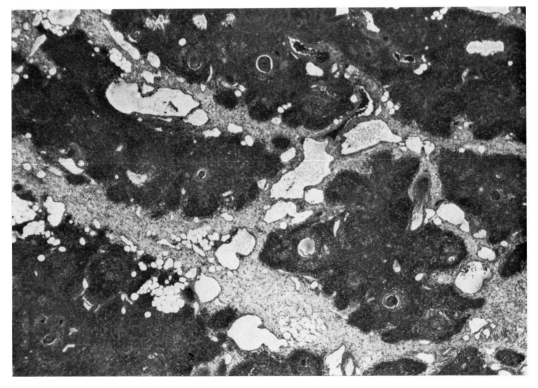

Fig. 11-3. This photomicrograph shows a thymus riddled with dilated lymphatics. The patient was a 6 year old with extensive lymphatic anomalies and no gastrointestinal manifestations.

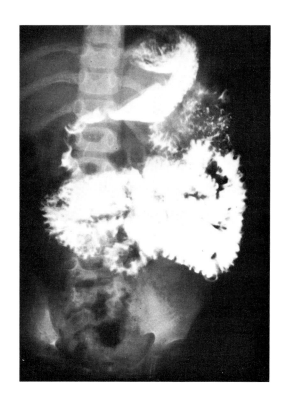

Fig. 11-4. Lymphangiectasis of the small bowel. A grossly coarsened mucosal pattern such as this is beyond the limits of normal variation. Several diagnoses are possible, including parasitic infestation, particularly *Giardia,* and involvement of the bowel with lymphoma. The presence of peripheral lymphedema in this patient made the true diagnosis easy.

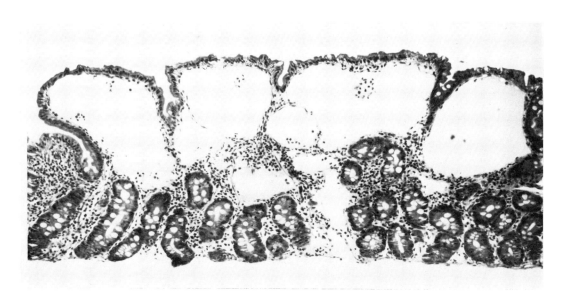

Fig. 11-5. Histologic changes associated with intestinal lymphangiectasis. The normal architecture of these jejunal villi are distorted. The core of the villi are fenestrated by large, dilated lacteals. In one villus (second from the left) the lacteal is actually seen bursting through the surface of the epithelium.

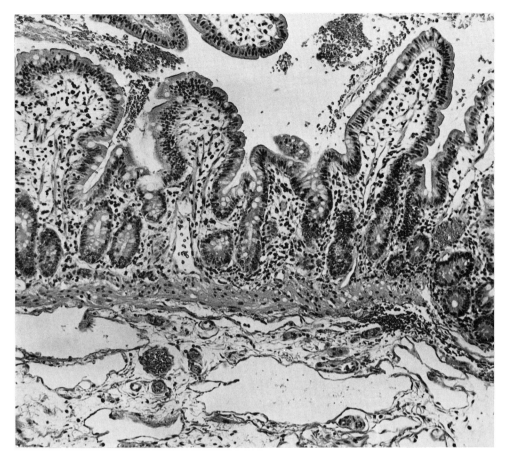

Fig. 11-6. Submucosal form of lymphangiectasis in an 11-year-old girl with profuse diarrhea and hypoproteinemia. A suction biopsy specimen of the jejunum had proved to be normal, but a segmental resection was carried out after a peroperative lymphangiogram. There has been a substantial improvement of gastrointestinal symptoms, but hypoalbuminemia persists, since there is also significant involvement of the pleura and lungs.

Results of studies of albumin loss, metabolism, and synthesis will confirm the gastrointestinal protein loss. Gastrointestinal protein loss may be modest to absent in cases where the lamina propria is not involved. The hypoalbuminemia in such patients is the result of trapping of albumin in telangiectatic areas and local catabolism. Appearance of the small bowel on roentgenograms can be normal in as many as 20% of patients. The abnormal characteristics (Fig. 11-4) include (1) dilution of the barium column distally and (2) absent or minimal dilatation of the bowel. Results of a small bowel biopsy confirm the diagnosis by revealing dilated lacteals in the villi (Fig. 11-5). In other cases, the mucosal biopsy may be normal because the lymphangiectasis affects the submucosa (Fig. 11-6) and the serosa leaving the villous

architecture intact. Lymphangiography is difficult to perform on pediatric patients, but it may demonstrate the generalized nature of this entity. A peripheral lymphangiogram may reveal stasis and reflux into the abdominal and mesenteric lymphatics with extravasation of contrast material or dye into the proximal small intestine. More commonly the examination will show diffuse hypoplasia of peripheral lymphatics, hypoplasis of periaortic lymph nodes with a variable degree of hypoplasia (Fig. 11-7), or else the total absence of the thoracic duct.

Differential diagnosis

All the entities that lead to protein-losing enteropathies must be considered when hypoalbuminemia is found. In the hypoalbuminemic patient

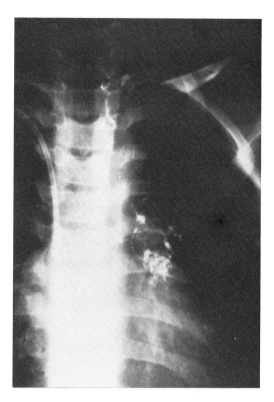

Fig. 11-7. This lymphangiogram shows to the left of T6 and T7 a network of varicose lymphatic vessels that are closely associated with the pericardium. The patient was a 6-year-old boy with chylothorax, chylopericardium, and a congenital anomaly of the thoracic duct.

without liver, kidney, or heart disase, intestinal lymphangiectasia should be seriously considered. The dilated lacteals associated with Crohn's disease are easily distinguished from those of congenital lymphangiectasis, since chronic inflammatory changes are present (Fig. 11-8). The finding of lymphedematous limbs, ascites, or a pleural effusion in association with the clinical features mentioned before stongly indicates a congenital type of intestinal lymphangiectasis.

Complications and sequelae

Failure to thrive, episodes of tetany, and increased numbers of infections are the frequent complications of this disease. Lymphedema of the limbs may be disfiguring because it leads to increased bone growth and hemihypertrophy.

Treatment

Specific surgical therapy is indicated in rare cases when the lesion is localized to a small area of the bowel (identified by means of mesenteric lymphography). Surgery is also indicated for situ-

ations when the pleura and the pericardium are involved. Surgical attempts in intractable cases have included peritoneal anastomosis of a saphenous vein.

Medical management is directed toward reduction of the intestinal lymphatic pressure by elimination of long-chain fats from the diet. Substitution diets utilizing medium-chain triglycerides offer the best form of treatment. They are consistently successful only in patients where lymphangiectasis is limited to the lamina propria. Water-soluble vitamins and calcium supplements are needed. Gamma globulin injections may be indicated if levels are extremely low. Antibiotics are used for specific infections. Albumin infusions with diuretics provide symptomatic relief.

Prognosis

Exacerbations and remissions sometimes occur. Dietary manipulations may bring about dramatic results in some cases; in others, use of medium-chain triglycerides has little effect in modifying the disease.

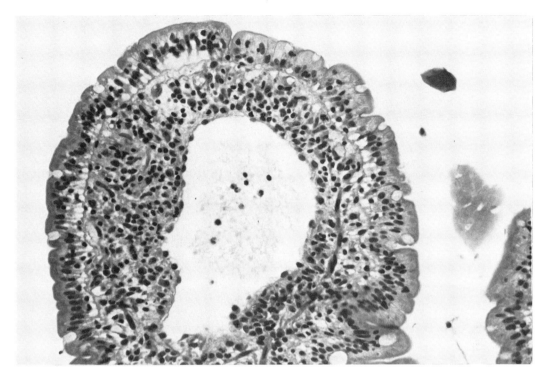

Fig. 11-8. Dilated lacteal surrounded by a dense chronic inflammatory infiltrate in a jejunal villus from a 15-year-old girl with Crohn's disease. She presented with peripheral edema and chronic abdominal pain.

REFERENCES

Fleisher, T.A., Strober, S., Muchmore, A.V., and others: Corticosteroid-responsive intestinal lymphangiectasia secondary to an inflammatory process, N. Engl. J. Med. **300:**605-606, 1979.

Herbst, J.J., Johnson, D.G., and Oliveros, M.A.: Gastroesophageal reflux with protein-losing enteropathy and finger clubbing, Am. J. Dis. Child. **130:**1256-1258, 1976.

Kinmonth, J.B., and Cox, S.J.: Protein-losing enteropathy in primary lymphoedema: mesenteric lymphography and gut resection, Br. J. Surg. **61:**589-593, 1974.

Nelson, D.L., Blaese, R.M., Strober, W., and others: Constrictive pericarditis, intestinal lymphangiectasia and reversible immunologic deficiency, J. Pediatr. **86:**548-554, 1975.

Parsons, H.G., and Pencharz, P.B.: Intestinal lymphangiectasia and colonic polyps: surgical intervention, J. Pediatr. Surg. **14:**530-532, 1980.

Schussheim, A.: Protein-losing enteropathies in children, Am. J. Gastroenterol. **58:**124-132, 1972.

Shimkin, P.M., Waldmann, T.A., and Krugman, R.L.: Intestinal lymphangiectasia, Am. J. Roentgenol. Radium Ther. Nucl. Med. **110:**827-841, 1970.

Vardy, P.A., Lebenthal, E., and Shwachman, H.: Intestinal lymphangiectasis: a reappraisal, Pediatrics **55:**842-851, 1975.

Chylous ascites

Chylous ascites results from effusion of mesenteric, cisternal, or lower thoracic duct lymphatic fluid into the peritoneal cavity. The condition is secondary to a lymphatic obstruction, the likely result of a congenital malformation, trauma, a chronic inflammatory process, peritoneal bands, or tumors. However, in the neonate, the cause is unknown.

Clinical findings

In the congenital form, a history of a rapidly enlarging abdomen, diarrhea, and failure to thrive are the only manifestations. The abdomen is often distended; a fluid wave and shifting dullness are demonstrable. Unilateral or generalized peripheral lymphedema may be present.

In older children, the history is most important in that trauma, infection, tumor, and previous surgery may play a major role. The signs and symptoms are otherwise similar to those observed in the congenital form.

When chylous ascites becomes massive, scrotal edema, inguinal and umbilical hernias, breathing difficulties and edema of the lower extremities may occur.

Since the leak of lymphatic fluid takes place

somewhere between the intestinal walls and the thoracic duct, its contents include the nutrients absorbed through the lacteals and the proteins from the extracellular fluid that are passed in the lymphatic system. Paracentesis yields milky fluid with a high lipid content and 3% proteins if the patient has been fed. Chylous ascites may be observed in newborn infants even preceding the institution of any feeding; in such cases, the fluid is clear and is indistinguishable from ascites secondary to liver disease, an obstructive uropathy, or multicystic kidneys. Laboratory findings include hypoalbuminemia, hypogammaglobulinemia, and lymphopenia.

Complications

Severe chylous ascites may be fatal. Chronic loss of albumin and immunoglobulins may lead to severe malnutrition. The often observed lymphopenia potentiates the risk of infection.

Treatment

Surgical measures are helpful when a specific cause can be found. When a congenital abnormality such as hypoplasia, aplasia, or ectasia of the lymphatics exists, injection of chemical irritants, lymphatic ligation, or a peritoneovenous shunt can be helpful. Attempts to relieve the ascites by bringing the saphenous vein into the peritoneal cavity have been tried, with partial success. General measures include institution of a fat-free diet, or, better, a fat-free diet supplemented with medium-chain triglycerides to decrease the formation of chylous ascitic fluid. The congenital form of chylous ascites often disappears after paracentesis and the use of a medium-chain triglyceride diet. No reasonable explanation has been offered for the phenomenon. Repeated paracentesis is to be condemned as a form of treatment. Parenteral alimentation, by keeping lymph flow to a minimum, may permit sealing of the chyle leak and is currently the most effective form of treatment (Chapter 28).

Prognosis

Prognosis is guarded, though a number of spontaneous cures have been reported. The disease is often chronic in nature and reflects only one aspect of a more generalized lymphatic abnormality. Generalized lymphangiomatosis is associated with a high mortality, particularly in those cases with involvement of the lungs, bones, and other viscera such as the spleen.

REFERENCES

Chang, J.H.T., Newkirk, J., Carlton, G., and others: Generalized lymphangiomatosis with chylous ascites: treatment by peritoneo-venous shunting, J. Pediatr. Surg. **15**:748-750, 1980.

Sanchez, R.E., Machour, G.H., Brennan, L.P., and Woolley, M.M.: Chylous ascites in children, Surgery **69**:183-188, 1971.

Viswanathan, U., and Putnam, T.C.: Therapeutic I.V. alimentation in traumatic chylous ascites in a child, J. Pediatr. Surg. **9**:405-410, 1974.

Warwick, W.J., Holman, R.T., Quie, P.G., and Good, R.A.: Chylous ascites and lymphedema, Am. J. Dis. Child. **98**:317-329, 1959.

Chylothorax

Chylous pleural effusions in the neonatal period, though rare, represent the most common form of pleural fluid accumulation in early life. In most cases, the cause is unknown. It may be unilateral or bilateral and may be associated with generalized lymphangiomatosis. Recently it has been reported as a complication of parenteral nutrition through a central catheter in four low birth weight infants. Thrombosis of the superior vena cava and of the left innominate vein near the point at which the thoracic duct empties was responsible for the bilateral chylothorax. In older infants and children, it may be associated with thoracic surgery, trauma, or a tumor. Repeated paracenteses are contraindicated. Respiratory distress and infections are noteworthy. Medium-chain triglycerides (MCT) are useful in decreasing chyle flow. However, complete cessation of oral intake and parenteral alimentation is usually necessary along with the chest tube drainage. In the absence of successful drying up of the effusion poudrage, chemical irritants, and eventually pleurectomy are in order.

REFERENCES

Brodman, R.F., Zavelson, T.M., and Scheibler, G.L.: Treatment of congenital chylothorax, J. Pediatr. **85**:816-817, 1974.

Curci, M.R., and Dibbins, A.W.: Bilateral chylothorax in a newborn, J. Pediatr. Surg. **15**:663-665, 1980.

Gershanik, J.J., Jonsson, H.T., Riopel, D.A., and Packer, R.M.: Dietary management of neonatal chylothorax, Pediatrics **53**:400-403, 1974.

Vain, N.E., Swarner, O.W., and Cha, C.C.: Neonatal chylothorax: a report and discussion of nine consecutive cases, J. Pediatr. Surg. **15**:261-265, 1980.

Cow milk protein intolerance

Adverse reactions to cow milk and to milk-base formulas can be manifestations of lactose intolerance (p. 243), glucose-galactose malabsorption, and galactosemia, but much more frequently intolerance to the protein component is the responsible factor. Intolerance to cow milk proteins has been the subject of much study over the past several years. It is no longer the catchall for a wide spectrum of respiratory, dermal, and gastrointestinal disorders that appear to be improved after elimination of milk from the diet.

The better definition, stricter application of diagnostic criteria, and critical evaluation of certain immunologic correlates have significantly contributed to a better understanding and a greater awareness of the entity.

Pathogenesis

Different immunologic mechanisms have been shown to be abnormal, but it is still not clear whether they cause the symptoms or are secondary phenomena. So, despite increasing evidence that a hypersensitivity reaction mediates the clinical manifestations and the tissue injury, it is still more prudent to term the entity "cow milk protein intolerance."

Metabolic abnormality. On the basis of a series of studies with ^{51}Cr-labeled red cells and ^{121}I-albumin, a loss of blood and albumin in stools was shown to be substantially greater when susceptible infants ingest homogenized milk instead of a heat-processed formula. A heat-labile toxic protein has been suggested to explain these findings. The possibility that whole proteins or large peptides could exert a direct toxic effect on a genetically predisposed intestinal mucosa or one that is an immature or injured (by gastroenteritis) is likewise a plausible explanation. Perhaps the mucosa is vulnerable because of a congenital, developmental, or acquired failure of a normal detoxifying mechanism.

Hypersensitivity reaction. Cow's milk contains at least 20 antigenic protein components. Beta-lactoglobulin, absent from breast milk, is the one with the greatest antigenicity; lactalbumin, casein, and bovine serum albumin are less potent. Intestinal transport of macromolecules is especially important during the early months of life when the immune system cannot as effectively prevent the absorption of antigens and neutralize the ones gaining access to the circulation (Fig. 11-9). Besides the qualitative properties and the size of the antigen load, three other factors may enhance the absorption of macromolecules:

1. Decreased intraluminal proteolytic activity, a frequent complication of malnutrition

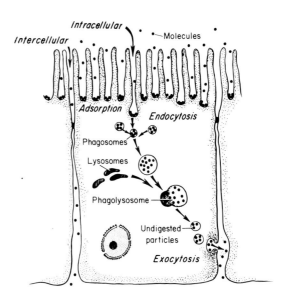

Fig. 11-9. Absorbed antigens penetrate the microvillous membrane by endocytosis. The macromolecules stored in small vacuoles (phagosomes) fuse with lysosomes and are hydrolyzed. Undigested macromolecules migrate to the basal surface of the cell and are released by exocytosis through the basolateral membrane. (From Report of the 72nd Ross Conference on Pediatric Research, 1977; with permission of Dr. Allan Walker and Ross Laboratories, Columbus, Ohio.)

2. Defective mucosal barrier secondary to immaturity or injury
3. Relative deficiency of secretory IgA from decreased synthesis in the neonate

Response of humoral immunity to milk proteins. Antibodies to ingested proteins found in the serum (circulating antibodies) and in intestinal secretions (coproantibodies) are of doubtful significance, since there is a wide overlap with normal controls. A recent study shows that all infants given either milk-based or soy-based formulas develop a prompt rise in hemagglutinins, in contrast to those fed a casein hydrolysate formula. Low titers also reported in breast-fed infants suggest that proteins vary in their antigenic potential.

Since IgG and IgM antibodies to milk are present, they would be expected to react in the presence of an antigen excess and lead to complement activation. One study showing a decrease in complement on oral challenge could not be confirmed by another group. The case is therefore very weak for an Arthus type of delayed reaction in milk hypersensitivity.

The immunologic basis for an immediate hypersensitivity reaction is not more securely established though clinically anaphylactic reactions are well known. The role of reaginic IgE antibodies is supported by the presence of IgE milk antibodies and by the observation that symptoms can be prevented by disodium cromoglycate (cromolyn sodium). However, there is no objective proof that IgE antibodies are fixed to mast cells and induce the release of mediators. By use of the RAST technique, titers of IgE antibodies have been found to be higher in milk sensitive children and increased mucosal IgE cells have been found after a challenge with milk. However, the RAST test to milk proteins may also be positive in atopic patients. Increased IgE plasma cells have been found in conditions such as celiac disease and gastroenteritis.

Is cell-mediated immunity involved? The only indication that cell-mediated immunity could be involved comes from the observation that lymphocytes from patients with milk intolerance may undergo blast transformation when cultured in the presence of cow milk antigens. There are currently several groups examining the in vitro response of mucosal explants to milk antigens in terms of release of chemical mediators that induce inflammatory changes. Preliminary results are encouraging.

Incidence

Cow milk protein intolerance is overdiagnosed when the diagnosis rests only on the symptomatic improvement of digestive disturbances after removal of milk from the diet. Even reliance on the strict criteria of Goldman may not be appropriate to determine the incidence. The three recommended clinical remissions and exacerbations do not necessarily occur within 48 hours of elimination and reintroduction of milk. A conservative figure for the incidence of milk protein intolerance can probably be set at 0.5% with a predominance in males.

The incidence is greatly increased in children from families having allergies (asthma, rhinitis, urticaria, atopic dermatitis). Atopy is found in 47% to 80% of families of affected infants. It is said to be more frequent in cases of selective IgA deficiency. A few studies indicate that breast feeding may protect infants born to atopic families from eczema and asthma, but this will require confirmation. There are no data on the protective effect of exclusive breast feeding during the first 4 to 6 months against the development of cow

milk protein intolerance. We believe that breast feeding during the first 2 to 3 months is not protective.

Clinical features

A wide range of symptoms and signs affecting the gastrointestinal tract, the respiratory system, and the skin are described.

Clinical manifestations associated with cow milk protein intolerance

Acute forms of the disease
  Anaphylactic reaction
  Gastroenteritis
  Intractable diarrhea
  Necrotizing enterocolitis
  Acute colitis
Chronic syndromes
  Wilson-Heiner-Lahey syndrome
  Allergic gastroenteritis
  Celiac-like syndrome
  Infantile colic?

Acute manifestations. The disease may be acute and manifest itself as an anaphylactic reaction. Its role in the sudden infant death syndrome has been suggested. In other cases, the onset is characterized by a bout of gastroenteritis from which the infant fails to convalesce. Whether such patients who can go on to "intractable diarrhea" (Fig. 11-10), represent complications of infectious gastroenteritis remains to be determined. Necrotizing enterocolitis (NEC) could be an acute and catastrophic manifestation of cow milk and soy protein intolerance. It has been described in several low birth weight infants, but cow milk protein intolerance may be a complication of necrotizing enterocolitis rather than its cause. Acute cow milk- or soy protein–induced colitis is an occasional mode of presentation. It occurs within the first week or two. Clinical, roentgenographic, endoscopic and histologic findings (Fig. 11-11) do not differ from those of an infectious colitis or a chronic ulcerative colitis. Prompt remission usually occurs after elimination of milk- or soy-based formulas.

Wilson-Heiner-Lahey syndrome. Chronic intestinal blood loss is common in cow milk protein intolerances. It is usually occult, will go unnoticed for long periods, and may result in profound iron-deficiency anemia through the loss of 0.6 to 10.3 ml of blood per day, which varies with the amount of milk ingested and decreases if heat treatment is carried out instead of pasteurization.

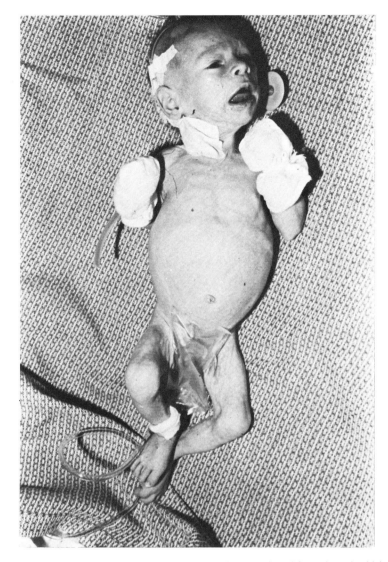

Fig. 11-10. Intractable diarrhea with severe malnutrition developed in a 5-week-old infant who was fed homogenized milk from birth.

The syndrome occurs mainly between 3 and 12 months of age and resolves by 2 years.

Allergic gastroenteritis. An abnormal response of the gastrointestinal tract to cow milk often leads to significant losses of proteins. The syndrome was originally described as "allergic gastroenteropathy." It involves infants with eosinophilia and varying degrees of eczema, asthma, or allergic rhinitis and who, on milk ingestion, develop vomiting, diarrhea, peripheral edema with hypoalbuminemia, occult blood in the stools with hypochromic anemia, and failure to thrive. Steatorrhea and jejunal mucosal changes are not features of this condition. Further characterization of this syndrome reveals striking gastric mucosal changes (Fig. 11-12) and only modest patchy jejunal histologic anomalies. Only one of these six recently reported cases responded to milk withdrawal. The others required intermittent cortocosteroid therapy and therefore behaved more like patients with eosinophilic gastroenteritis (p. 323). A satisfactory response to milk withdrawal has been obtained in the two patients we have seen with this syndrome.

Celiac-like syndrome. This clinical entity consists of chronic diarrhea with some vomiting and a variable degree of fat malabsorption. The symptoms may go unnoticed until failure to thrive and eventual malnutrition attracts attention. D-Xylose

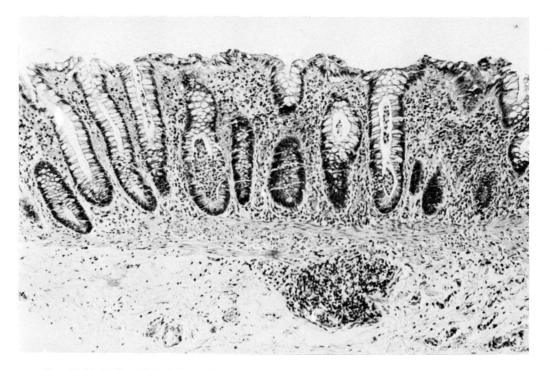

Fig. 11-11. Milk colitis. This suction rectal biopsy was taken from a 1-week-old infant with bloody diarrhea. Acute inflammatory changes are prominent, and three crypts contain collections of polymorphonuclear cells. There is actual breakdown of the wall of one crypt (crypt abscess). Within a week after discontinuation of the milk-based formula, there was complete healing of this lesion.

is invariably abnormal and the intestinal biopsy shows an enteropathy of variable severity. The lesion may be indistinguishable from the one seen in celiac disease, but generally the atrophy is less severe and is patchy. Disaccharidase activity correlates well with the severity of the histologic changes.

Infantile colic. Generally speaking, paroxysmal fussing is not helped by dietary manipulations and it occurs as frequently on breast milk as on milk-based formulas. A recent paper showing that elmination of cow milk from the diet of lactating mothers had a favorable effect on infantile colics awaits confirmation.

Diagnosis

Close attention to the dietary history is essential, especially in infants who, for variable periods, have been breast fed. The feeding of supplements is important to document along with a detailed sequence of the introduction of weaning foods. In the infant who has been breast fed for an extended period of time, gluten and cow milk are often introduced within a short interval of time.

Adverse reactions to cow milk proteins usually occur within a few days after their introduction. The symptom-free interval tends to last a few months when gluten is the culprit.

Until recently the diagnosis of cow milk protein intolerance was based on clinical criteria described by Goldman:

1. Remission of symptoms after elimination of cow milk from the diet
2. Relapse within 48 hours of beginning a milk challenge
3. Positive reactions to three such challenges, each with a similar onset, duration, and clinical features

Health professionals and parents are reluctant to risk a serious reaction after the first positive challenge. A second drawback mentioned earlier is the fact that in our hands symptoms triggered by cow milk proteins may take much longer than 48 hours before being apparent. The delay can be as long as 1 month.

Although there is solid clinical evidence of a cause-and-effect relationship between the ingestion of milk proteins and the symptoms described

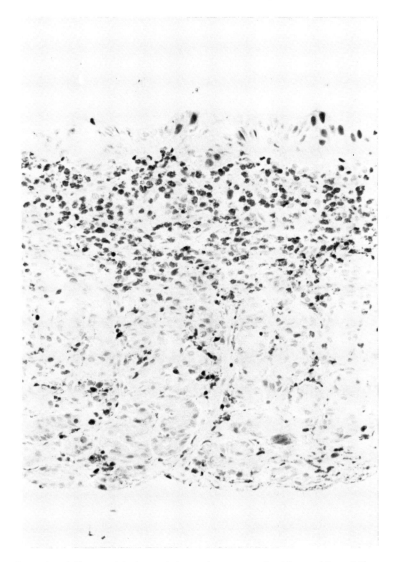

Fig. 11-12. Eosinophilic gastritis in an infant who presented with vomiting, failure to thrive, peripheral edema, and eosinophilia (29%). This Luna stain of a gastric biopsy section shows minimal epithelial necrosis. Below the epithelium there is a dense infiltrate of eosinophils. The small bowel biopsy specimen was normal. There was a prompt resolution of symptoms and of biopsy changes within a period of 2 months after withdrawal of a milk-based formula.

above, the immunologic correlates are weak and cannot be used to confirm or rule out the diagnosis. Some workers have suggested that routine histological examination of small intestinal biopsy specimens before and after a cow milk challenge is useful (Fig. 11-13). Others suggest that jejunal biopsies are not necessary because symptomatic children invariably have histologic changes.

The 1-hour blood-xylose test is a reliable index of small bowel mucosal function (Chapter 10) and

has proved to be a valuable means of validating the diagnosis, particularly in children who do not develop symptoms or who have an equivocal response during the few days after a milk challenge. The diagnosis can be validated safely and noninvasively by the following approach worked out by Dr. Morin at the Hôpital Sainte-Justine:

1. History and symptoms compatible with the diagnosis while the child is on a milk-based formula

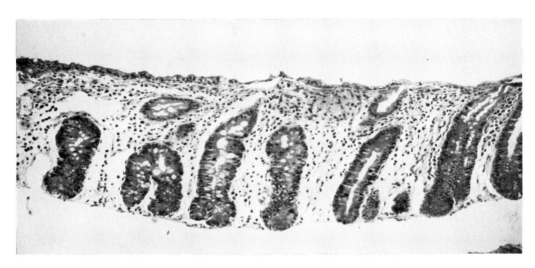

Fig. 11-13. Severe jejunal changes associated with reintroduction of milk in an infant. There is total villous atrophy, deep crypts, and a very abnormal epithelium. The changes are indistinguishable from those seen in celiac disease.

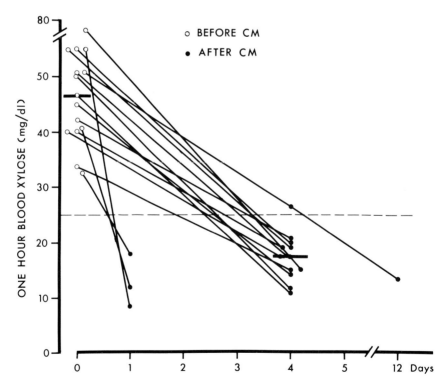

Fig. 11-14. One-hour blood xylose levels before and after a cow-milk challenge (CM) in 15 infants with cow-milk protein intolerance. *Dotted line,* Lower limit of normal in 126 controls. In three patients, the D-xylose test had to be carried out 24 hours after cow milk was given because the severity of symptoms precluded continuation of the challenge. Of the 12 others, seven had mild to moderately severe symptoms and five remained asymptomatic. (From Morin, C.L., et al.: Lancet **2:**1102-1104, 1979.)

2. Good clinical progress on a milk-free diet
3. Normal 1-hour blood-xylose level 4 to 10 weeks after clinical recovery
4. Significant drop of the 1-hour blood-xylose level with or without symptoms 4 days after reintroduction of cow milk proteins (Fig. 11-14)

The milk challenge should preferably be carried out in a hospital setting though close surveillance for a severe reaction is generally not necessary beyond the first 36 hours. An intravenous is started before 5 ml of cow milk is given; the same amount is repeated 4 hours later. If no severe reaction is noted, cow milk is offered ad libitum over the next 4 days. In those patients who develop no symptoms and whose blood-xylose level does not drop, a milk-based formula is resumed and it is concluded that either they never had cow milk protein intolerance or else that they have regained their tolerance.

Treatment

In most cases, milk elimination results in a rapid amelioration of symptoms and nutritional rehabilitation.

In long-standing cases with malnutrition and mucosal damage, improvement may take longer and require parenteral nutrition followed by continuous nasogastric alimentation.

Nutramigen is a casein hydrolysate formula that can be used as a milk substitute. In some cases, it appears to be poorly tolerated on the basis of persisting allergenicity (large peptides) or of its acidogenic properties, particularly in malnourished infants.

Pregestimil is a formula that we have found very helpful; its protein source is casein hydrolysate. In unusual cases with extreme milk protein sensitivity, symptoms may persist on Pregestimil. A good response will be obtained by use of Vivonex, an elemental product comprised of amino acids and no peptides.

Intolerance to soy is present or develops in 30% to 40% of infants with cow milk protein intolerance. Soy formulas are therefore contraindicated during the first few weeks in view of the fact that response to the initial period of milk withdrawal is crucial for confirmation of the diagnosis. The cost acceptability of casein hydrolysate formulas warrant the use of a soy formula on a long-term basis.

Therapeutic failures are commonly seen in older infants who are exposed to foods containing dairy products or bovine proteins. Transient gluten intolerance is a separate entity (p. 279), but it can develop in conjunction with cow milk protein intolerance. In certain instances, patients will develop symptoms while receiving a milk protein substitute a short time after introduction of gluten. In patients with long-standing and severe symptoms who have never been exposed to gluten, it is our policy to postpone the introduction of gluten for a few months. Reintroduction of cow milk and bovine proteins is best carried out in the context of a carefully monitored challenge after the age of 12 months.

The use of corticosteroids has been advocated in the early stages of treatment of the atopic infant with allergic gastroenteritis. The ones who strictly have the gastrointestinal symptoms generally respond favorably to milk restriction.

Prevention

Breast feeding is strongly advocated as the sole article of nutrition for the first 6 months, especially in infants with a family history of atopy. A casein hydrolysate formula would appear to have some benefits in terms of milk hemagglutinins, but there is no information on the protection it may confer against intestinal manifestations of cow milk protein intolerance. A recent paper suggests that breast feeding offers no protection against the development of extraintestinal manifestations such as atopic dermatitis and asthma.

The presence of cow milk proteins in breast milk and of antibodies to cow milk in cord blood warrants the recommendation that women with a family history of allergy not assume large quantities of milk during pregnancy and lactation.

Prognosis

Death resulting from anaphylactic shock is rare and there is no proof that sudden infant death syndrome is related to it. Intractable diarrhea has a morbidity but is presently associated with a low mortality.

Generally speaking, once management with a milk-free diet has been initiated, the prognosis is excellent. The disease is limited in time because most infants tolerate milk by the age of 12 to 18 months though intolerance may persist until 3 to 5 years of age.

Because of the potential danger of a severe reaction on reintroduction of milk at 1 year of age, it is advisable to carry out a milk challenge under close medical supervision. Because anaphylactic reactions are bound to occur early after the first few milliliters, 8 hours with an intravenous tube in place is probably sufficient.

Soy protein intolerance

Soy formulas account for 10% of commercial formula sales. They are recommended for a wide variety of infantile gastrointestinal disorders such as paroxysmal fussing, regurgitation, vomiting, diarrhea, galactosemia, lactose, and cow milk protein intolerance.

Although the antigenicity of present-day heat-processed soy protein–isolate formulas is less than soy flour, there are still concerns with regard to the high incidence (about 30%) of milk-sensitive infants who are intolerant for soy protein. Although most infants with soy protein intolerance have concomitant cow milk intolerance, there are some cases where soy protein sensitivity appears to be primary and not facilitated by a preceding injury to the mucosal barrier.

The following is a list of disorders associated with soy protein intolerance along with references of initial reports:

Anaphylactic reaction (Fries, J.: J. Asthma. Res. **3**:209, 1966)
Necrotizing enterocolitis (Powell, G.K.: J. Pediatr. **88**:840, 1976)
Colitis (Halpin, T.C., and others: J. Pediatr. **91**:404, 1977)
Enterocolitis with a flat mucosa (Ament, M.E., and others: Gastroenterology **62**:227, 1972)

Breast feeding constitutes the most appropriate preventive measure against the development of allergic manifestations in infants born to atopic families. Along with restriction of bovine products, eggs, and wheat for a period of 9 months, a soy formula has been found to be beneficial. This advantage of soybean over cow milk protein could not be confirmed in a laboratory study showing that in terms of circulating antibodies both are equally antigenic.

REFERENCES

Bhana, S.L., and Heiner, D.S.: Cow's milk allergy: pathogenesis, manifestations, diagnosis and management Adv. Pediatr. **25**:1-37, 1978.

Delèze, G., and Nusslé, D.: L'intolérance aux protéines du lait de vache chez l'enfant, Helv. Paediat. Acta **30**:135-149, 1975.

Eastham, E.J., and Walker, W.A.: Effect of cow's milk on the gastrointestinal tract: a persistent dilemma for the pediatrician, Pediatrics **60**:477-481, 1977.

Eastham, E.J., Lichauco, T., Grady, M.I., and Walker, W.A.: Antigenicity of infant formulas: role of immature intestine on protein permeability, J. Pediatr. **93**:561-564, 1978.

Gerrard, J.W., MacKinzie, J.W.A., Goluboff, N., and others: Cow's milk allergy: prevalence and manifestations in an unselected series of newborns, Acta Paediatr. Scand. (Suppl.) **234**:1-21, 1973.

Goldman, A.S., Anderson, D.W., Sellers, W.A., and others: Milk allergy: oral challenge with milk and isolated milk proteins in allergic children, Pediatrics **32**:425-443, 1963.

Gruskay, F.L.: Prophylaxis of allergic disease. Does milk-free diet help? A prospective study, Tenth International Congress of Allergology, Jerusalem, Nov. 1979.

Halpin, T.C., Byrne, W.J., and Ament, M.E.: Colitis, persistent diarrhea and soy protein intolerance, J. Pediatr. **91**:404-407, 1977.

Iyngkaran, N., Abdin, Z., Davis, K., and others: Acquired carbohydrate intolerance and cow milk protein sensitive enteropathy in young infants, J. Pediatr. **95**:373-378, 1979.

Iyngkaran, N., Yadav, M., Balabaskaran, S., and Sumithran, E.: In vitro diagnosis of cow's milk protein sensitive enteropathy by organ culture method, Gut **22**:199-202, 1980.

Jakobsson, I., and Lingberg, T.: Cow's milk as a cause of infantile colic in breast-fed infants, Lancet **1**:437-439, 1978.

Katz, A.J., Goldman, H., and Grand, R.J.: Gastric mucosal biopsy in eosinophilic (allergic) gastroenteritis, Gastroenterology **73**:705-709, 1977.

Kjellman, N.M., and Johansson, S.G.O.: Soy versus cow's milk in infants with a biparental history of atopic disease: development of atopic disease and immunoglobulins from birth to 4 years of age, Clin. Allergy **9**:347-358, 1979.

Kleinman, R.E., and Walker, W.A.: The enteromammary immune system: an important new concept in breast milk host defense, Dig. Dis. Sci. **24**:876-882, 1979.

Kramer, M., and Moroz, B.: Do breast-feeding and delayed introduction of solid foods protect against subsequent atopic eczema?, J. Pediatr. **98**:546-550, 1981.

Kuituven, P., Rapola, J., Savilahti, E., and Visakorpi, J.K.: Response of the jejunal mucosa to cow's milk in the malabsorption syndrome with cow's milk intolerance, Acta Paediatr. Scand. **62**:585-595, 1973.

Morin, C.L., Buts, J.P., Weber, A., and others: One-hour blood xylose test in diagnosis of cow's milk protein intolerance, Lancet **1**:1102-1104, 1979.

Nusslé, D., Bozic, C., Cox, J., and others: Non celiac gluten intolerance in infancy. In McNicholl, B., McCarthy, C.F., and Fottrell, P.F., editors: Perspectives in coeliac disease, Lancaster, 1978, MTP Press, Ltd.

Powell, G.K.: Enterocolitis in low birth weight infants associated with milk and soy protein intolerance, J. Pediatr. **88**:840-844, 1976.

Savilahti, E.: Immunochemical study of the malabsorption syndrome with cow's milk intolerance, Gut **14**:491-501, 1973.

Seban, A., Konijn, A.M., and Freier, S.: Chemical and immunological properties of a protein hydrolysate formula, Am. J. Clin. Nutr. **30**:840-846, 1977.

Sumithran, E., and Iyngkaran, N.: Is jejunal biopsy really necessary in cow's milk protein intolerance?, Lancet **2**:1122-1123, 1977.

Waldman, T.A., Wochner, R.D., Laster, L., and Gordon, R.S.: Allergic gastroenteropathy, N. Engl. J. Med. **276:**761-769, 1967.

Walker-Smith, J.: Dietary protein intolerance. In Diseases of the small intestine in childhood, ed. 2, Kent, Eng., 1979, Pitman Medical Publishing Co., Ltd.

Whitington, P.F., and Gibson, R.: Soy protein intolerance: four patients with concomitant cow's milk intolerance, Pediatrics **59:**730-732, 1977.

Woodruff, C.W., and Clarke, J.L.: The role of fresh cow's milk in iron deficiency. I. Albumin turnover in infants with iron deficiency anemia. II. Comparison of fresh cow's milk with a prepared formula, Am J. Dis. Child. **124:**18-30, 1972.

Eosinophilic gastroenteritis

A rare condition of unknown cause, eosinophilic gastroenteritis is characterized by a variety of polypoid or infiltrative lesions in the stomach or small bowel that have in common a chronic inflammatory reaction with many eosinophils, peripheral eosinophilia, and abnormal symptoms after ingestion of specific foods. There are still only a few cases reported in the pediatric age group.

Two clinical forms of the disease are recognized. In the mucosal form, intermittent vomiting, diarrhea, abdominal pain and failure to thrive or to gain weight are the most important symptoms. Other manifestations of allergy, such as atopic dermatitis, allergic rhinitis, and asthma, are commonly found in the patient's past or present history. Peripheral eosinophilia, hypoalbuminemia with increased enteric loss of proteins, mild or absent steatorrhea, increased levels of IgE, iron-deficiency anemia with occult blood in the stools, and a flat D-xylose absorption tests may be found. The small bowel roentgenographic examination shows a malabsorption pattern with edematous folds. A peroral biopsy of the stomach and proximal small bowel reveals mild to severe eosinophilic infiltration with varying degrees of mucosal changes and epithelial abnormalities. Villous structural changes in the jejunum are often patchy.

Elimination diets (milk, gluten, eggs, pork and beef) are indicated. However, symptoms and signs are often intermittent, and flare-ups may occur without an identifiable precipitating cause. Intermittent corticosteroid therapy is helpful. Initial results with cromolyn sodium have been disappointing.

In the second form of allergic gastroenteritis, the lesions are more deeply infiltrative and give rise to considerable thickening and rigidity, mostly in the stomach but also in the small bowel, appendix, large bowel, and mesentery leading to eosinophilic ascites in some cases. The symptoms may be ulcerlike and associated with pyloric outlet obstruction. In other cases, the lesions are focal and form distinct tumor masses that are eosinophilic granulomas. One such eosinophilic granuloma gave rise to an ileoileal intussusception in a 3-year-old child. The deeply infiltrative and polypoid form of the disease is rarely associated with eosinophilia and an allergic history is infrequent. They are not associated with the ingestion of specific foods. Corticosteroids are believed to be effective.

REFERENCES

Campbell, W.L., Green, W.M., and Seaman, W.B.: Inflammatory pseudotumor of the small intestine, Am. J. Roentgenol. Radium Ther. Nucl. Med. **121:**305-311, 1974.

Cello, J.P.: Eosinophilic gastroenteritis: a complex disease entity, Am. J. Med. **67:**1097-1104, 1979.

Greenberger, N., and Gryboski, J.D.: Allergic disorders of the intestine and eosinophilic gastroenteritis. In Sleisenger, M.H., and Fordtran, J.S., editors: Gastrointestinal disease, ed. 2, Philadelphia, 1978, W.B. Saunders Co.

Jona, J.Z., Belin, R.P., and Burke, J.A.: Eosinophilic infiltration of the gastrointestinal tract in children, Am. J. Dis. Child. **130:**1136-1139, 1976.

Katz, A.J., Goldman, H., and Grand, R.J.: Gastric mucosal biopsy in eosinophilic (allergic) gastroenteritis, Gastroenterology **73:**705-709, 1979.

Persoff, M.M., and Arterburn, J.G.: Eosinophilic granuloma causing intussusception in a 3-year-old child, Am. J. Surg. **124:**676-678, 1972.

12 *Immune homeostasis and the gut*

The gut occupies a unique role in the development and maintenance of immune homeostasis. The intestinal mucosa is a lymphoid organ at the interface between man and his environment. Only a monolayer of epithelial cells separates the *milieu intérieur* from a wide variety of potential antigens made up of products of digestion, drugs, and microorganisms. Well-recognized immune deficiency states frequently give rise to gastrointestinal manifestations, and many gastrointestinal disorders may lead to secondary immune deficiency or be associated with abnormal immune responses of the gut.

OVERVIEW OF IMMUNE SYSTEM
Ontogeny of immune response (Fig. 12-1)

The thymus, spleen, lymph nodes, and Peyer's patches of the lower small bowel are largely responsible for the development and the proliferation of cells involved in immune responses. Their main cellular component is the lymphocyte, which, like megakaryocytes, red cells, granulocytes, and monocytes, originates from stem cells in the bone narrow. Lymphocytes have the capacity to recognize antigens by means of special receptors on their surface. One population of lymphocytes (T cells) differentiates by contact with the epithelial component (Hassall's corpuscles) and with humoral factors (such as thymosin) of the thymus. The members of a second lymphocyte population (B cells) are responsible for antibody production and evolve from the bone marrow without the influence of the thymus, In the chicken, the central lymphoid organ responsible for the differentiation of stem cells into B lymphocytes corresponds to the bursa of Fabricius, a small lymphoid organ located at the end of the gastrointestinal tract. In mammals, gut-associated lymphoid tissue such as the appendix and Peyer's patches have been examined but do not appear to represent bursal equivalents.

T and B lymphocytes

Lymphocytes share a unique capacity to recognize all antigens likely to be met in a lifetime by surface receptors, but the two populations differ in their response. On contact with antigens, some T cells differentiate into large lymphocytes and release lymphokines, which attract macrophages and lymphocytes and induce an inflammatory response. They act directly (cell-mediated immunity) and play a major role in transplant and tumor rejection and in hypersensitivity reactions. They provide the resistance against viral, bacterial, and fungal infections, particularly against intracellular microorganisms. There are two other subpopulations of T cells: helper cells, which by their interaction with B cells amplify antibody production, and suppressor cells, which regulate both the cell-mediated and the humoral immune response.

Role of macrophages

B cells are stimulated to make antibody not only by the help of T cells (helper T cells), which presumably have come into contact with the same antigen, but also by antigen that has been previously processed by macrophages derived from monocytes. Macrophage-processed antigen is essential for T-cell activation. Therefore phagocytosis and processing of antigens by macrophages constitute essential steps before the development of specific immune responses involving T and B cells.

Mononuclear monocytes may not only present antigen in a highly immunogenic form to lymphocytes but they can also destroy antigens. However, their killing power for pathogenic organisms is not comparable to that of granulocytes.

Complement function

The complement system is an interrelated complex of serum proteins that is closely associated with the humoral antibody system. The reaction sequence of the 12 proteins is initiated by antigen-antibody complexes involving IgM and most classes of IgG. The major role of complement is to modulate and regulate the immune response. Its various activation units share a vast range of biologic activity. They mediate chemotaxis, histamine release, smooth muscle contraction, capillary permeability, yeast opsonization, cell-membrane damage, release of antigen-antibody complexes,

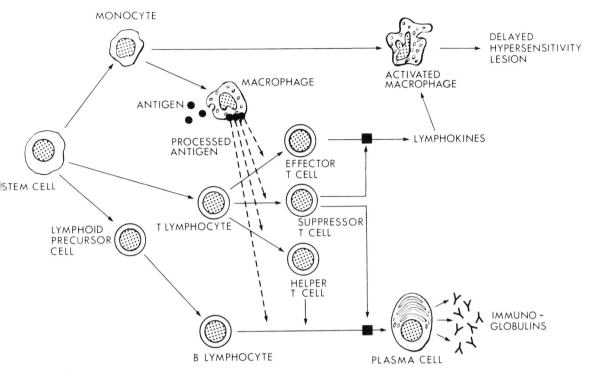

Fig. 12-1. Ontogeny of the immune response. (Modified after Rose, N.R.: Sci. Am. **224:**80-103, 1981.)

and perhaps also the production of certain antibodies.

Structure and function of gastrointestinal immune system

The gut serves as one of the largest peripheral depositories for cells differentiated along the lines of small lymphocytes or plasma cells. In this environment, the gut-associated lymphoid tissue proliferates and responds immunologically to various antigenic stimuli. Most gut-associated immunocompetent cells are located in the mucosal surface and therefore constitute the first line of defense against infection and aggression by a host of antigens.

Peyer's patches, tonsils, and the appendix are the principal nodular lymphoid tissues though lymphoid nodules can also be seen elsewhere from the pharynx to the anus. The size and structure of lymphoid nodules are influenced by the degree of antigenic stimulation. Peyer's patches extend through the lamina propria and submucosa of the small intestine. Their epithelium is flattened and essentially devoid of crypts and villi. It consists of M cells specialized for antigen absorption by means of pinocytosis.

A distinguishing morphologic feature of B and T cells is their preferential localization in different areas of peripheral lymphoid tissues. B cells are found in the superficial cortical areas of lymph nodes, where they participate in the formation of primary and secondary follicles and in the medullary cords. T cells are found primarily in the deep cortical areas of lymph nodes around the germinal centers. The anatomic juxtaposition of B and T cells has a functional counterpart. There are, in fact, numerous examples of cooperative interactions between both types of cells. The humoral response to certain antigens by B cells shows a strong dependency on the presence of T cells despite the fact that the two cell types are different in terms of bearing specific recognition units for antigen.

There are substantial numbers of individual lymphoid cells, plasma cells, and monocytes dispersed within the lamina propria of the entire gastrointestinal tract, along with eosinophils, other polymorphonuclear lymphocytes, and mast cells.

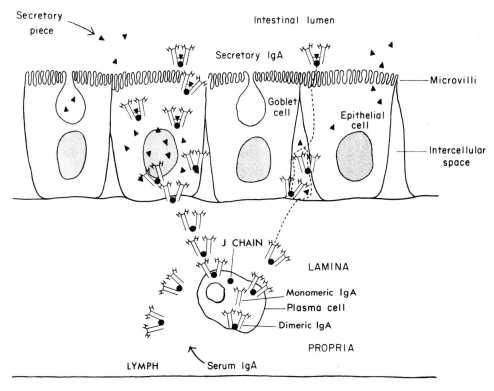

Fig. 12-2. Synthesis of secretory IgA. (Modified from Tourville, D.R., Alder, R.H., Bienenstock, J., and Tomasi, T.B.: J. Exp. Med. **129:**411-429, 1969.)

Intraepithelial lymphocytes also constitute an important component of the nonaggregated lymphoid tissue. These cells occupy intercellular positions and are usually located between the nucleus and the basement membrane of enterocytes. The prevailing opinion is that intraepithelial lymphocytes are T cells, whereas the lamina propria population is mostly made up of B cells, the majority of which contain, synthesize, and secrete IgA.

Both T and B lymphocytes have the capacity to return "home" to the aggregated lymphoid tissue, such as Peyer's patches and the appendix. They enter through interfollicular venules, populate the nodular lymphoid tissue, and come into contact with antigens. They then start differentiating before entering efferent lymphatic mesenteric lymph nodes, the thoracic duct, and the general circulation, after which they migrate back to the intestine. During this "maturation journey" the 2% of IgA-carrying B cells identified in Peyer's patches increase to 90% by the time they return to the lamina propria.

It is now the consensus that the aggregated lymphoid tissues initiate immune responses. Because of size, structure, and ability to trap antigens, the chances of an encounter between an antigen and lymphocytes with the appropriate receptor are greatly increased in nodular lymphoid tissues. The immunocyte population in the lamina propria and in the epithelial layer are effector cells; they both carry out immune responses.

The majority of plasma cells in the gastrointestinal tract mucosa contain IgA. Approximate proportions of IgA, IgM, and IgG cells are 82%, 16% and 2%, respectively. Secretory IgA is the predominant class of immunoglobulins involved in the defense of the intestinal mucosa and is the only quantitatively important immunoglobulin in the secretions of the gut. Secretory IgA differs in several respects from serum IgA. The latter exists in either a monomer or dimer form with sedimentation coefficients of 7S and 11S, respectively. Stabilization of the dimeric serum IgA is effected by the presence of a J chain originating from plasma cells. The physicochemical differences between the 11S serum IgA and secretory IgA are the result of the presence in secretory IgA of a glycoprotein referred to as a secretory component. In man, the primary site of synthesis of the IgA portion of the secretory molecule is the plasma cells of the lamina propria (Fig. 12-2). The secretory component, on the other hand, is synthesized in the epithelial cells and attached to a dimeric form of IgA either in the basement membrane or within the cytoplasm of specialized epithelial cells in the crypts. Secretory components can also combine with polymeric 19S IgM.

There is normally little dimeric IgA in the serum because 80% to 90% of IgA is in the monomeric form. Levels of IgA in bile are 10 times higher than in serum, whereas IgG concentrations are 30% to 50% lower than those of serum. The liver plays an important role in the delivery of dimeric IgA from the circulation to the biliary tract. During this transport, the secretory component presumably synthesized within the biliary tract is attached to form SIgA (secretory IgA). High concentrations of SIgA have been reported in obstructive jaundice and can be helpful in the differentiation of various categories of obstructive jaundice in infancy. Biliary SIgA is thus another route, distinct from local secretion across the epithelial layer, to make SIgA available to the gut lumen. It is likely that dimeric IgA synthesized in lamina propria cells could reach the liver through the general circulation and lymphatics.

The biologic role of secretory IgA in the normal body defense mechanisms and in various diseases remains unclear. The normal flora is certainly a major stimulus for the gut-associated plasma cells, as shown by studies in germ-free mice. It seems likely that secretory IgA, despite the fact that it does not fix complement, plays an important role in the resistance of mucous membranes to pathologic microorganisms and dietary antigens. Secretory IgA has antibody activity against bacteria, viruses, autoantigens, toxins, and a variety of food antigens. More important perhaps is the finding that it is resistant to proteolytic degradation, strongly adheres to epithelial surfaces through interaction with mucin, blocks bacterial adherence to mucosal surfaces, and prevents absorption of potentially antigenic macromolecules.

Development and maintenance of immune competence

The third-trimester fetus already has developed a competent immune system. This is of importance for survival, since the gastrointestinal tract

situated at the interface between the internal and external environments is exposed to abundant sources of antigen. In the fetus, the intestine is devoid of plasma cells, and their appearance and subsequent role in immunoglobulin synthesis is probably a result of antigen stimulation (by microorganisms and food) from the intestinal lumen. The second repository for the intestinal "immunocyte complex," the aggregated lymphoid nodules known as Peyer's patches and found in the lamina propria and in the submucosa, is poorly developed at birth and continues to increase in size and number for the first 10 years of life. Its growth is also a result of stimulation from the external environment. Studies in animals show that the bacterial flora has a key role in this regard.

The newborn has significant immunologic defects. The newness of his T lymphocytes, slow to respond to antigenic stimuli because of the absence of previous contact, constitutes a serious handicap. B cells are also affected since T helper cells will not drive B cells to differentiation and antibody production. The intrinsic capacity of B cells to form antibodies is also handicapped. The newborn has a complement of IgG, which he acquired transplacentally, and he readily produces IgM and IgG. However, his serum level of IgA remains low for months; he is therefore dependent on an exogenous source.

Breast milk provides large quantities of secretory IgA and confers passive mucosal immunity by giving the gastrointestinal tract additional resistance to invasion by food antigens and microorganisms (viruses and bacteria) until the infant's own mucosal immune system has matured. Breast milk is a source of macrophages, B cells, and T cells, which are immunologically similar to lymphocytes present in the gastrointestinal tract. The T cells exhibit the full range of T-cell activities in vitro and respond to a number of antigenic stimuli, particularly those encountered in the intestine. It has been suggested that colostral lymphocytes could implant themselves in the lamina propria of the newborn intestinal tract. In addition, human milk provides specific antibodies produced by the mother against her enteric flora. Thus maternal milk provides a specific immunity against potentially harmful enteric antigens by an enteromammary secretory immune system, which appears to involve cells and immunoglobulins (Fig. 12-3).

It is well known that breast feeding protects against intestinal infection. The degree of protection it confers against necrotizing enterocolitis is

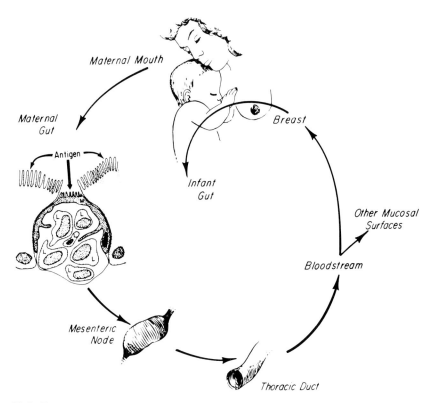

Fig. 12-3. Enteromammary immune system. Antigens in the lumen are processed by M cells. The antigens then trigger the production of specific IgA by lymphoblasts that migrate to the systemic circulation, populate the breast, and produce secretory IgA, which is ingested by the infant. (From Kleinman, A., and Walker, A.: Dig. Dis. Sci. **24:**876-882, 1979.)

still controversial. However, we have yet to see a fully breast-fed baby with intractable diarrhea of early infancy. Recent reports emphasize the fact that the overall risk even of extraintestinal infections is decreased, even in our own affluent society. Breast milk is said to have significant long-term advantages in infants from atopic families with regard to systemic manifestations of allergy such as rhinitis, asthma, and eczema. However a recent report has not been able to confirm this. Finally, the tentative identification of defects in the immunologic apparatus of the intestine in celiac disease and in chronic inflammatory bowel disease should serve to reinforce the idea that particular attention should be paid to optimizing the conditions under which the immune system is developing during the early months of life.

REFERENCES

Abrahamson, D.R., Powers, A., and Rodewald, R.: Intestinal absorption of immune complexes by neonatal rats: a route of antigen transfer from mother to young, Science **206:**567-569, 1979.

Bullen, C.L., Tearle, P.V., and Stewart, M.G.: The effect of ''humanised'' milks and supplemented breast feeding on the fecal flora of infants, J. Med. Microbiol. **10:**403-413, 1977.

Cunningham-Rundles, C., Brandeis, W.E., Good, R.A., and Day, N.K.: Milk precipitins, circulating immune complexes and IgA deficiency, Proc. Natl. Acad. Sci. USA **75:**3387-3389, 1978.

Goldblum, R.M., Ahlstedt, S., Carlsson, B., and others: Antibody forming cells in human colostrum after oral immunization, Nature **257:**797-798, 1975.

Goldblum, R.M., Powell, G.K., and Van Sickle, G.: Secretory IgA in the serum of infants with obstructive jaundice, J. Pediatr. **97:**33-36, 1980.

Katz, A.J., and Rosen, F.S.: Gastrointestinal complications of immunodeficiency syndromes. In Immunology of the gut, Ciba Foundation Symposium **46:**243-261, 1977.

Kleinman, R.E., and Walker, W.A.: The enteromammary immune system: an important new concept in breast milk host defense, Dig. Dis. Sci. **24:**876-882, 1979.

McFarlin, D.E., Strober, W., and Waldman, D.: Ataxia-telangiectasia, Medicine **51:**281-314, 1972.

Ogra, S.S., and Ogra, P.L.: Immunologic aspects of human colostrum and milk, J. Pediatr. **92:**550-555, 1978.

Orlans, E., Peppard, J., and Hall, J.: Rapid active transport of immunoglobulin A from blood to bile, J. Exp. Med. **147:**588-592, 1978.

Parrott, D.M.V.: The gut as a lymphoid organ, Clin. Gastroenterol. **5**:211-228, 1976.

Schlesinger, J.J., and Covelli, H.D.: Evidence for transmission of lymphocyte responses to tuberculin by breast-feeding, Lancet **2**:529-533, 1977.

Tomasi, T.B., Larson, L., Challacombe, S., and McNabb, P.: Mucosal immunity: the origin and migration patterns of cells in the secretory system, J. Allergy Clin. Immunol. **65**:12-19, 1980.

Walker, W.A.: Antigen absorption from the small intestine and gastrointestinal disease, Pediatr. Clin. North Am. **22**:731-746, 1976.

GASTROINTESTINAL DISEASES WITH IMMUNOLOGIC COMPONENTS

The three main functions of the lymphoid system are (1) antibody and immunoglobulin production, (2) graft-versus-host reactivity, cell-mediated graft rejection, and delayed hypersensitivity, and (3) chyle transport and lymphocyte circulation. It is clear that the abundant gut-associated lymphoid tissue, the lacteals of the intestinal villi, and the lymphatic channels of the bowel wall and mesentery are anatomic structures of major importance for the maintenance of immune homeostasis. Therefore, it is not surprising that certain primary diseases of the gastrointestinal tract result in a secondary humoral and cellular immunodeficiency. These conditions are discussed in Chapter 11, which is devoted to protein-losing enteropathies.

Immunocompetence is adversely affected by malnutrition. The clinician should keep in mind the fact that the sick child with failure to thrive and evidence of severe malnutrition has involuted central (thymus) as well as peripheral lymphoid tissues and impaired cell-mediated immunity. Rosette-forming T lymphocytes are decreased, and there may be a failure of response to antigens used to test delayed hypersensitivity. In contrast, B lymphocytes are present in normal numbers and immunoglobulin levels are commonly high though there are reports showing that secretory IgA may be low. Complement proteins are also decreased in concentration and affect chemotaxis, opsonization, and microbial lysis. Finally, the bactericidal capacity of granulocytes may be impaired. With correction of the nutritional status, there is rapid recovery of normal immunologic function.

The large number of immunologically competent cells and their location within the gastrointestinal tract may be of pathophysiologic importance in certain gastrointestinal disorders. The gut may be the location of abnormal immune responses to normal or abnormal antigenic stimuli. Abnormal immune responses may result in the formation of autoantibodies or of sensitized lymphocytes. These may be cytotoxic to the host and therefore of etiologic significance, or they may be merely a result of antigen release and therefore represent only a concomitant response. The sections devoted to pernicious anemia, celiac disease, milk allergy, and inflammatory bowel disease describe several alterations in immunologic mechanisms; however, as the reader will discover, none of these entities can be clearly shown to be of immune or of autoimmune etiology.

INTESTINAL DISEASE IN CHILDREN WITH PRIMARY IMMUNE DEFICIENCIES

Respiratory infection is the most common illness associated with immunodeficiency syndromes. However, gastrointestinal abnormalities are frequent and may be the initial complaint leading to a diagnosis of a primary immune deficiency (Table 12-1).

Congenital sex-linked agammaglobulinemia (Bruton)

This well-known hereditary condition occurring only in males usually becomes manifest during the first year of life. It is characterized by deficient serum and secretory immunoglobulins, but cellular immunity is intact. Gastrointestinal symptoms are infrequently reported in these patients. In our experience, diarrhea is usually mild and intermittent; it tends to improve with age. Chronic rotavirus infection has been reported. Giardiasis may be present and may lead to variable degrees of jejunal changes and to isolated lactase deficiency in a certain number. Of note is the recent description of multiple crypt abscesses in patients who had no symptoms of colitis.

Idiopathic acquired agammaglobulinemia and dysgammaglobulinemia

Described in both sexes, the defect in humoral immunity is usually not so severe as in the congenital form. Symptoms begin later in life, but gastrointestinal manifestations are present in the majority (60%) (Fig. 12-4). *Giardia lamblia* infestation is common in this group, and it is reported that 50% of children with acquired agammaglobulinemia have chronic gastrointestinal symptoms. Steatorrhea, partial atrophy of villi,

Table 12-1. Immune disorders associated with gastrointestinal manifestations

Disorder	Frequency of disease
Deficiency in antibody production	
Sex-linked agammaglobulinemia	+
Acquired idiopathic agammaglobulinemia	+ + +
Isolated deficiency of IgA	+
Dysgammaglobulinemia	+ +
Deficiency in cell-mediated immunity with or without deficiency in antibody production (T cell and T-B cell deficiency)	
Chronic mucocutaneous candidiasis	+ + +
Nezelof's syndrome	+ +
Severe combined immunodeficiency disease	
No enzyme defect	+ + +
Adenosine deaminase	+ + +
Nucleoside phosphorylase	+ + +
Wiskott-Aldrich syndrome	+ *
Disorders of phagocytosis, chemotaxis, and complement function	
Chronic granulomatous disease	+ + +
Acrodermatitis enteropathica	+ + +

*Gastrointestinal bleeding from thrombocytopenia.

nodular lymphoid hyperplasia, and a generalized decrease in disaccharidase activity is common. Aerobic and anaerobic cultures of the upper intestinal tract may show excessive numbers of anaerobes. However, the correlation between symptoms and lesions is poor. When giardiasis is present, the intestinal lesion may respond to treatment with metronidazole. A gluten-free diet generally fails when there is no improvement after eradication of *Giardia* trophozoites. Gamma globulin injections have no effect in the majority of cases. The presence of crypt abscesses has been noted in a small proportion of patients with acquired agammaglobulinemia in the absence of signs and symptoms of colitis. There are reports of chronic inflammatory bowel disease with this form of immune deficiency.

Diarrhea, steatorrhea, and generalized malabsorption have also been associated with the primary immune deficit in which IgA and IgG are low but IgM is normal or high (dysgammaglobulinemia). Giardiasis has been found and nodular lymphoid hyperplasia described (Fig. 12-5).

Isolated IgA deficiency

Isolated IgA deficiency is by far the most prevalent form of primary immune deficiency. It is said to be present in 1 of 700 patients. These patients have an increased incidence of autoimmune disease, autoimmune phenomena, recurrent sinopulmonary infections, pernicious anemia, cirrhosis, and malignancies. Most patients are asymptomatic, and the incidence of gastrointestinal manifestations is low. Gastrointestinal diseases associated with isolated IgA deficiency include gastric atrophy with pernicious anemia, ulcerative colitis, regional enteritis, lactase deficiency, nodular lymphoid hyperplasia, disaccharidase deficiency, giardiasis, and celiac disease. The last is indistinguishable from the classic gluten enteropathy, and there is a good response to a gluten-free diet (Fig. 12-6). Some patients cases fail to respond to all forms of treatment and die with intractable diarrhea and malabsorption.

Patients who lack IgA are known to have high titers of antibodies to foods and have an increased incidence of cow milk protein intolerance.

T-cell and T-B cell deficiency

Infants with isolated T-cell and combined T- and B-cell deficiency almost invariably have severe gastrointestinal manifestations with oral candidiasis and failure to thrive. However, in DiGeorge's syndrome, intestinal symptoms may be absent. In the other disorders where both immunoglobulin production and cell-mediated immunity are defec-

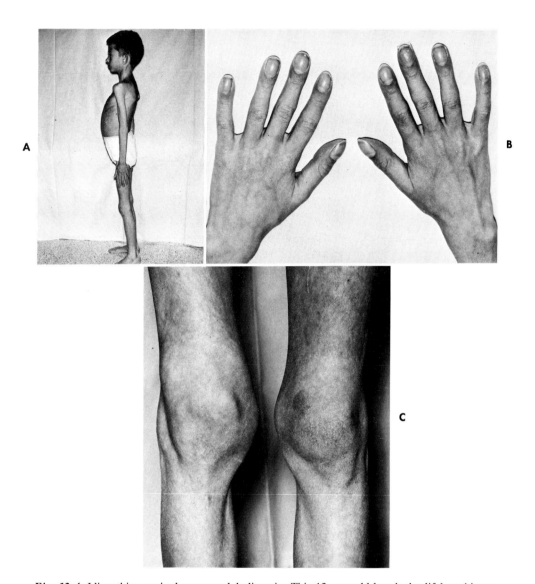

Fig. 12-4. Idiopathic acquired agammaglobulinemia. This 12-year-old boy had a lifelong history of repeated infections and failure to thrive. He has chronic pulmonary disease and severe malabsorption with wasting and stunting. A solitary rheumatoid right knee has been documented over the years. There is abdominal distention, winging of the scapulae (**A**), clubbing of the fingers (**B**), and a deformed right knee (**C**). The small bowel biopsy showed partial atrophy of villi. Stool fat was in excess of 20 gm daily. There was no response to a gluten-free diet.

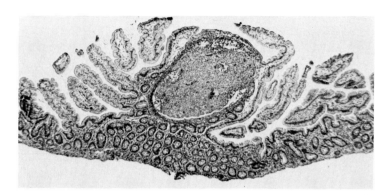

Fig. 12-5. Nodular lymphoid hyperplasia in type I dysgammaglobulinemia. This biopsy of the upper jejunum shows a normal villous pattern except for the presence of a large lymphoid follicle. The patient was an 11-year-old without any symptoms referable to the gastrointestinal tract.

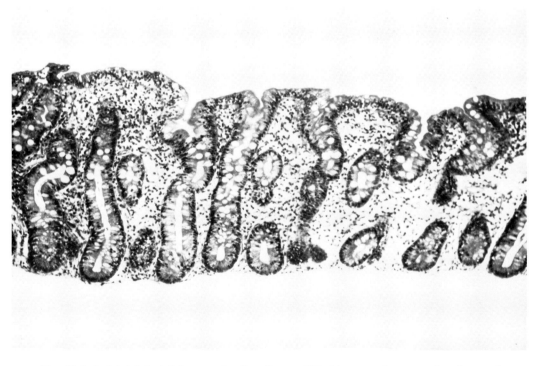

Fig. 12-6. Isolated IgA deficiency and celiac disease. This biopsy section was taken from a 5 year old whose atrophic mucosa failed to improve after metronidazole treatment of giardiasis. He responded to a gluten-free diet.

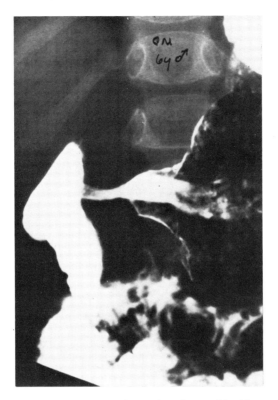

Fig. 12-7. Chronic granulomatous disease in a 6 year old with antral stenosis.

tive, diarrhea is intractable. It may be bloody and associated with evidence of colitis. Malabsorption of fat and carbohydrate and deficiency of disaccharidase have been described. The small bowel biopsy tissue may be normal, except for a decrease in the immunocyte population of the lamina propria. In others, there may be villous atrophy and PAS-positive foamy macrophages close to the tips of the villi.

Chronic mucocutaneous candidiasis

The majority of children have symptoms referable to oral and esophageal candidiasis. Chronic ulcerations in the mouth and esophagus may lead to scarring and severe strictures. Chronic diarrhea and severe fat malabsorption are complications that may be seen when chronic mucocutaneous candidiasis is associated with hypoparathyroidism and Addison's disease.

Chronic granulomatous disease

In chronic granulomatous disease, which usually becomes manifest before the age of 1 year, there is inability to kill bacteria despite normal phagocytosis. Persistent infections, eczematoid

dermatitis, recurrent lymphadenopathy, suppuration, draining granulomatous lesions, and osteomyelitis are usually the main problems.

The most consistent gastrointestinal manifestation is hepatosplenomegaly. Ulcerative stomatitis and esophagitis, chronic enteritis, colitis, and perirectal abscess are common. Of particular interest is the recent report of gastric antral narrowing by granulomas (Fig. 12-7). Gastric involvement leads to recurrent vomiting, and in some patients it may be the first manifestation of the disease.

Histologic studies of the stomach and of the small and large bowel reveal the presence of granulomas with multinucleated giant cells and foamy macrophages (Fig. 12-8). Villous atrophy may be present.

General findings

Although there are still comparatively few clinical studies describing the gastrointestinal manifestations in children presenting with primary immune deficiencies, previously discussed, current information can be summarized as follows:

1. Diarrhea is more or less constant and often

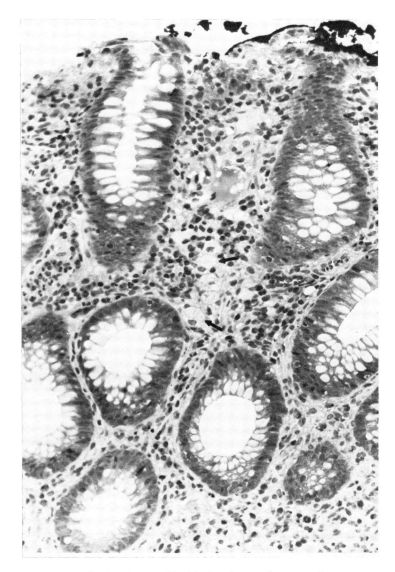

Fig. 12-8. Rectal biopsy from a 12 year old with chronic granulomatous disease. *Arrows,* Cluster of foamy pigment-laden macrophages.

severe in patients with defective cellular immunity.

2. Gastrointestinal disease is mild and quite rare in sex-linked agammaglobulinemia when compared to the acquired idiopathic form and to dysgammaglobulinemia.

3. Most patients with isolated IgA deficiency are free of gastrointestinal problems.

4. Recent studies point to the importance of one searching thoroughly for *Giardia lamblia,* remembering that it may account for the diarrhea, malabsorption, and small bowel changes.

5. Despite the finding of excessive numbers of microorganisms in the upper intestine, antibiotics are rarely helpful, and therefore it is unlikely that patients with primary immune deficiencies have a "contaminated small bowel syndrome" of clinical importance. In a significant number, a decrease in disaccharidase activity has been documented.

6. Despite the fact that a history of milk intolerance cannot be elicited in most, a trial on a milk-free diet is warranted.

7. In contrast to the respiratory problems, the gastrointestinal disease associated with pri-

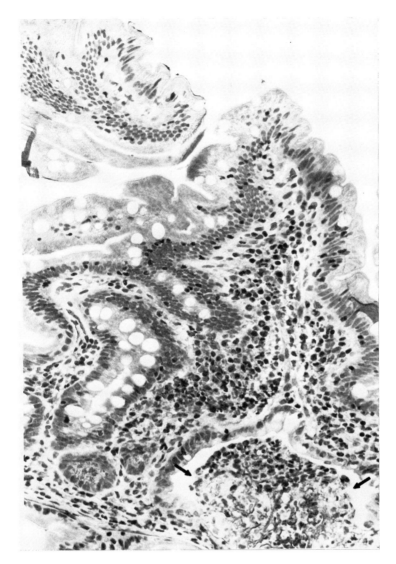

Fig. 12-9. Crypt abscess in a 5 year old with acquired idiopathic agammaglobulinemia (common variable immunodeficiency). *Arrows,* Crypt filled with inflammatory cells. The rest of the mucosa is relatively intact.

mary immune defects usually does not respond to plasma or globulin injections.

8. Patients with immunoglobulin deficiencies frequently have histologic evidence of colitis (Fig. 12-9), despite the absence of symptoms and of rectosigmoidoscopic findings.

9. Children with immunodeficiency disorders are at risk for a variety of autoimmune disorders such as chronic active hepatitis and thyroiditis, and long-standing cases may develop malignancies and particularly lymphomas.

REFERENCES

Ament, M.E., and Ochs, H.D.: Gastrointestinal manifestations of chronic granulomatous disease, N. Engl. J. Med. **288:**382-387, 1973.

Ament, M.E., Ochs, H.D., and Davis S.D.: Structure and function of the gastrointestinal tract in primary immunodeficiency syndromes: a study of 39 patients, Medicine **52:**227-248, 1973.

Amman, A.J.: T cell and T-B cell immunodeficiency disorders, Pediatr. Clin. North Am. **24:**293-313, 1977.

Brown, W.R., Butterfield, D., Savage, D., and Tada, T.: Clinical, microbiological and immunological studies in patients with immunoglobulin deficiencies and gastrointestinal disorders, Gut **13:**441-449, 1972.

Carroll, J.E., and Silverman, A., and Isobe, Y.: Inflammatory myopathy, IgA deficiency and intestinal malabsorption, J. Pediatr. **89:**216-219, 1976.

Chandra, R.K.: Interactions of nutrition, infection and immune response, Acta Paediatr. Scand. **68:**137-144, 1979.

Chandra, R.K.: Acrodermatitis enteropathica: zinc levels and cell-mediated immunity, Pediatrics **66:**789-791, 1980.

Dubois, R.S., Roy, C.C., Fulginiti, V.A., and others: Disaccharidase deficiency in children with immunologic deficits, J. Pediatr. **76:**377-385, 1970.

Goldman, A.S., and Goldblum, R.M.: Primary deficiencies in humoral immunity, Pediatr. Clin. North Am. **24:**277-293, 1977.

Hermans, P.E., Diaz-Buxo, J.A., and Stobo, J.D.: Idiopathic late-onset immunoglobulin deficiency: clinical observations in 50 patients, Am. J. Med. **61:**221-237, 1977.

Horowitz, S., Lorenzsonn, V.W., Olsen, W.A., and others: Small intestinal disease in T cell deficiency, J. Pediatr. **85:**457-462, 1974.

Johnston, R.B., and Newman, S.L.: Chronic granulomatous disease, Pediatr. Clin. North Am. **24:**365-377, 1977.

Perry, G.S., Spector, B.D., Schuman, L.M., and others: The Wiskott-Aldrich syndrome in the United States and Canada, J. Pediatr. **97:**72-78, 1980.

Savilahti, E., Pelkonen, P., and Visakorpi, J.K.: IgA deficiency in children: a clinical study with special reference to intestinal findings, Arch. Dis. Child. **46:**665-670, 1971.

Webster, A.D.B.: The gut and immunodeficiency disorders, Clin. Gastroenterol. **5:**323-340, 1976.

13 *Inflammatory bowel diseases*

ACUTE DISEASES
Appendicitis

An increase in the incidence of appendicitis in the Western world was noticed in 1920 and has its parallel today in many developing countries where there have been significant dietary changes in terms of a decrease in cellulose and an increase in sugar consumption. Intestinal transit time, particularly through the colon, is closely related to the bulk of bowel content. A cellulose-depleted diet not only slows transit but also results in firmer stools and increased intraluminal pressures favoring obstruction and infection.

The pathogenesis of appendicitis is poorly understood, but it appears that bacterial invasion of the appendix is greatly favored by obstructive phenomena. Fecaliths, parasites, and lymphoid hyperplasia are probably important predisposing factors. Fecaliths are found in close to 25% of cases; pinworms, on the other hand, are found in less than 10%, and their role remains problematic. Appendicitis has occurred in association with enteric infections. Similarly, preceding extraintestinal infections (particularly those of the upper respiratory tract) could also possibly trigger an acute inflammatory process in the appendix. In 1% of cases of acute appendicitis, pneumonia is also present.

Acute appendicitis is the condition most commonly requiring abdominal surgery during childhood, and it affects all age groups. There are now more than 100 cases reported in the neonatal period but less than 10% of cases occur below the age of 5. A third of the cases are in the 5 to 10-year-old group. The highest incidence is in the 10- to 15-year-old group.

Clinical findings

The triad of abdominal pain, fever, and localized abdominal tenderness indicates appendicitis until proved otherwise. The most important finding is right lower quadrant pain, which has often been preceded by diffuse or periumbilical pain. Vomiting occurs in most patients. Fever is commonly low grade (38° or 38.5° C); however, temperatures can become hyperpyretic (to 40° C) if the patient has peritonitis.

Below two years of age, the child is unable to explain his symptoms and a third party is always involved. Recognition of the distress depends on perceptiveness of the parent or guardian. It is then the physician's difficult task to decide if the pain is intra-abdominal in origin. Establishing with some accuracy the time of onset and making a prompt decision are especially important in infants and young children, since perforation occurs rapidly after pain begins.

Periumbilical pain in the initial stage of the disease is attributable to stretch receptors embedded in the small blood vessels of the appendix. They transmit the first signs of inflammation along the mesenteric nerves and then to the spinal nerve (T10) which supplies the dermatome at the level of the umbilicus. After a few hours, vomiting will occur and rapidly the pain will shift to the right lower quadrant because the inflamed appendix will exude small amounts of inflammatory fluid on the parietal peritoneum. In cases of retrocecal appendicitis, pain does not shift from the periumbilical area after perforation. This relative *accalmie* (momentary calmness) contrasts with a concomitant deterioration of the child's general condition. Vomiting becomes more frequent, the fever rapidly increases, and the respiration is rapid with a short inspiratory phase and grunting.

A careful examination of the abdomen is essential in any child with abdominal pain, since the clinical picture of appendicitis is often atypical, particularly in infants and young children. For instance, diarrhea may substitute for constipation, and the abdominal pain may never localize to the right lower quadrant. Palpation of the abdomen of the young child should be done with the fingers, not with the hand, beginning in nonsensitive areas. The child is asked to identify the quadrant in which pain on palpation is felt. If pain is intense, it leads to voluntary contraction of the abdominal musculature. Guarding is often difficult to elicit. The hand should press down slowly as the examiner attempts to distract the child. It should be maintained a few seconds in the same position when the abdominal wall is sufficiently depressed before quick removal of the hand. In cases where the appendix is already perforated, there is involuntary rigidity through spasm of the rectus muscle. It is often difficult to distinguish spasm from voluntary contraction. Sequential examinations over several hours by the same physician are invaluable. However, even in cases of peritonitis, involuntary contraction of the abdominal musculature can be absent in young infants. Peristalsis is difficult to assess; total absence or increase with high-pitched sounds constitutes additional evidence. A rectal examination should always be done, even though its interpretation is particularly difficult in the young child.

Appendicitis in the neonatal period is especially difficult to diagnose. More than 100 cases have been reported. It is more frequent in boys than in girls. It may masquerade as necrotizing enterocolitis, and its association with Hirschsprung's disease has been previously described. The mortality (80%) is extraordinarily high, and a number of factors such as a thin-walled appendix, a small omentum, and impaired defense mechanisms are contributory, but perhaps the most important is the failure to consider the diagnosis in the sick neonate who will be treated conservatively until perforation and sepsis occur.

Laboratory and x-ray findings

The white blood cell count (WBC) is seldom higher than 15,000. As a general rule a WBC of 20,000 or more without signs of appendiceal perforation invalidates the diagnosis of appendicitis. A low WBC with a striking preponderance of bands can be seen with the presence of an abscess or with generalized peritonitis.

Roentgenographic findings parallel the pathologic stage. In children, appendicitis frequently is the result of obstruction of the appendiceal lumen by a fecalith, which is often visible on a plain film of the abdomen (Fig. 13-1). The presence of a roengenographically detectable fecalith in a child with clinical findings suggestive of appendicitis is associated with a perforation in 75% of cases below the age of 6, and in 33% of those over 6 years of age in 96 cases reported from Hôpital Sainte-Justine. One or two air-filled small bowel loops in the right lower quadrant indicate localized ileus (sentinel loops) and early localized inflammation, as does a fluid level in the cecum.

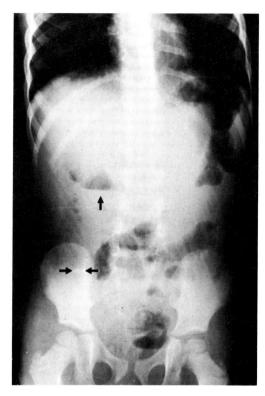

Fig. 13-1. Perforated appendix. A 3-year-old child had a 24-hour history of vomiting and abdominal pain. Generalized abdominal guarding was present on admission, and the white blood cell count was 14,200 with 23% bands. Film shows a few hydroaeric levels in the vicinity of the right lower quadrant, *arrow*. It is impossible to delimit the inferior margin of the liver, and there is slight scoliosis secondary to abdominal muscle spasm. A fecalith is present, *arrows*.

Scoliosis and abdominal wall edema are other valuable roentgenographic signs. In the case of peritonitis, transient hydroureter and hydronephrosis may be seen. A soft-tissue mass in the right lower quadrant may be a localized abscess. Multiple bowel loops throughout the abdomen, particularly with some free peritoneal fluid, are likely findings in generalized peritonitis. However, free peritoneal air is seldom seen with ruptured appendix. A calcified fecalith, shown on an abdominal film in a patient who has no acute symptoms, is regarded as potentially dangerous and constitutes an indication for elective appendectomy.

A barium enema examination of the unprepared colon is a safe procedure. It may be helpful in cases where the diagnosis is uncertain. Although failure of the appendix to fill has no value, extrinsic compression of the tip or medial wall of the

Table 13-1. Stages of appendicitis

Parameter	Inflamed (<24 hr)	Infected (24-48 hr)	Complicated (>48 hr)
Temperature	<38° C	38°-39° C	>39° C
Pulse	<100/min	100-110/min	>110/min
White blood cell count	Normal	Raised	Raised
Neutrophils	Raised	Raised	Raised
Erythrocyte sedimentation rate	Normal	Raised	Riased
Pus cells in appendix	None to few	Moderate	Numerous

From Doraiswamy, N.V.: Br. J. Surg. **65:**877, 1978.

cecum, an abrupt cutoff of the barium, or a distortion in shape or caliber provides useful information. Attention is drawn to the fact that since the length of the appendix is unknown, a "normally filled" appendix does not exclude distal obstruction and perforation.

Differential diagnosis

According to a recent report, the disease progresses in three stages, each lasting 24 hours. Close attention to the sequence inflamed-infected-complicated may help the diagnosis because 92% of the 100 children reported satisfied at least four criteria for the three stages of development shown in Table 13-1.

Since atypical cases are common, intrathoracic infection and urinary tract infection need to be ruled out in all cases of acute abdominal pain. Particular attention should be paid to the general appearance of the patient, his breathing rate, the presence of grunting, a limp, difficulty in climbing onto the examining table, or the scoliosis associated with abdominal muscle spasm.

Because physical findings are often inconclusive, a great many diagnostic errors can be prevented if one sequentially examines the abdomen over a period of a few hours and follows closely the evolution of the presenting symptoms.

A long list of conditions (Table 13-2) giving rise to "acute abdomen" in the pediatric age group should be kept in mind.

Should a history of chronic constipation be elicited, the presence of a large mass of hard stools in the rectum warrants the administration of enemas, which will promptly bring relief of the pain. The early phase of gastroenteritis can mimic acute appendicitis. In this regard salmonellosis and shigellosis are particularly important to consider. Food poisoning is another important consideration and the history of cases in the family is a critical diagnostic clue. In girls, particular attention should be paid to *mittelschmerz* and to pelvic inflammatory disease. The presence of pneumonia on roentgenograms does not rule out acute appendicitis; a pleural effusion is commonly seen when a subphrenic abscess is present.

Complications

Perforated appendix. The incidence of perforation is very high and seems to be increasing. A figure of 40% was obtained in recent surveys from the Children's Hospital of Los Angeles and from the Children's Hospital of Columbus. Age is a critical factor. Below 2 years of age 93% were perforated, the figures for the age groups 3 to 5, 6 to 10, and over 10 were 71%, 40%, and 33% respectively in the Columbus study. Optimizing communications with parents and obtaining a more thorough history are obviously important, but more critical is a precise physical examination coupled with appropriate interpretation of physical findings, which may help to decrease the delay in diagnosis, as seen in 30% to 50% of patients. Finally, no patient with acute abdominal pain and fever should be sent home without appropriate laboratory and roentgenographic examination and reevaluation over several hours.

Most perforated appendices are associated with voluntary guarding, rebound tenderness, and tenderness upon rectal examination. A rectal mass and rigidity of the abdominal wall can be expected in 20% of such cases.

Table 13-2. Etiologic classification of "acute abdomen" in pediatric age group

Mechanical obstruction		Inflammatory diseases and infections			
		Gastrointestinal disease	Paralytic ileus	Blunt trauma	Miscellaneous
Intraluminal	Extraluminal				
Foreign body	Hernia	Appendicitis	Sepsis	Accident	Lead poisoning
Bezoar	Intussusception	Crohn's disease	Pneumonia	Battered-child	Sickle-cell crisis
Fecalith	Volvulus	Ulcerative colitis	Pyelonephritis	syndrome	Familial Medi-
Gallstone	Duplication	Henoch-Schönlein	Peritonitis		terranean
Ascariasis	Stenosis	purpura and	Pancreatitis		fever
Meconium ileus	Tumor	other causes of	Cholecystitis		Porphyria
equivalent	Mesenteric	vasculitis	Renal and		Diabetic aci-
Tumor	cyst	Peptic ulcer	gallbladder		dosis
Fecaloma	Superior mes-	Meckel's diverticu-	stone		Addisonian
	enteric ar-	litis	Pelvic inflam-		crisis
	tery syn-	Acute gastroenteri-	matory dis-		Torsion of testis
	drome	tis	ease		Torsion of ovar-
		Food poisoning	Mittelschmerz		ian pedicle
		Pseudomembranous			Hydronephrosis
		enterocolitis			Rheumatic fever
					Streptococcal
					infection
					Nodular lym-
					phoid hyper-
					plasia

From Roy, C.C., Morin, C.L., and Weber, A.M.: Clin. Gastroenterol. **10**:225, 1981.

Peritonitis. Perforation, which may occur as early as a few hours after the onset of symptoms, provides a short-lived relief from the severity of the abdominal pain. The development of peritonitis is accompanied by signs of toxicity: tachycardia, a high temperature (39° or 40° C), and pallor. The child lies quietly, breathing superficially and rapidly. The abdomen is diffusely tender and is usually rigid.

Intra-abdominal abscess. Perforation of the appendix may cause an intra-abdominal abscess, which may localize in the pelvic area and eventually fistulize in the rectum or vagina. Subphrenic abscess, a rare complication of the perforated appendix, may provide a few localizing physical signs, but frequently is associated with a pleural effusion. A fever typical of sepsis develops. Splinting of the diaphragm provokes respiratory difficulties and shoulder pain; a pleural effusion is not uncommon.

An appendiceal abscess may at times be difficult to diagnose because of the intermittence of symptoms after the initial walling-off process. A mass, a tendency for pain to become localized, and the appearance of edema or redness of the abdominal wall are useful diagnostic features.

Pylephlebitis. Septic thrombosis of the appendiceal vessels can lead to an extensive inflammation of the portal system and multiple liver abscesses. This complication has been practically nonexistent since the advent of antibiotics.

Mucocele of the appendix. Obstruction of the lumen of the appendix by a foreign body or an inflammatory process may sometimes lead to a great accumulation of mucus that distends the lumen, resulting in a so-called mucocele of the appendix.

Treatment

Since virtually all reported deaths occur in children with a perforated appendix, conservative management dictates an appendectomy when the diagnosis cannot be ruled out after a period of close observation. If, at laparotomy, the appendix is normal, conditions such as torsion of an ovarian cyst, regional enteritis, or Meckel's diverticulum should be looked for.

For the extremely ill child with a perforated appendix, operation should be delayed. Oxygen therapy, rehydration, correction of blood volume with albumin or plasma, systemic antibiotics (ampicillin, gentamicin, and clindamycin), nasogastric suction, and a high Fowler's position (to facilitate drainage in the pelvic area) are all essential measures. After 4 to 12 hours, the temperature and pulse rate will have dropped somewhat, and surgery should be carried out. It is not rare for the child with a perforated appendix to experience a prolonged period of ileus postoperatively. This should be treated conservatively. Conservative management is also advocated when a mechanical obstruction develops within 10 days after excision of a perforated appendix with generalized peritonitis. Parenteral hyperalimentation may be useful in such cases. To diminish the incidence of postoperative complications, one should routinely drain the peritoneal cavity if either a localized abscess or diffuse peritonitis is present. In those cases with peritonitis, peritoneal lavage with saline solution is recommended.

Prognosis

For the fortunate patients in whom the diagnosis is made before perforation occurs and for whom early operation is performed, the mortality is negligible. When delay in diagnosis results in perforation, numerous complications occur, resulting in prolonged hospitalizations and a mortality of 0.1% to 0.5%.

"Appendiceal colic": an entity requiring surgery?

A recent paper suggests that an elective appendectomy is curative for a certain percentage of children with chronic recurrent abdominal pain (RAP). The criteria for "appendiceal colic" warranting surgery were as follows:

1. Invalidating pain
2. Tenderness on deep palpation of the right lower quadrant
3. A filling defect or distention of the appendix best seen on a film taken 24 hours after a barium swallow with small bowel follow-through

An 86% correlation was found between the roentgenographic findings and inspissated fecal material. The appendices were normal except for lymphoid hyperplasia (37%), which, by narrowing the appendiceal lumen, was believed to contribute to the entrapment of fecal material and to its subsequent inspissation. The high prevalence of inspissated fecal material (72.8%) in the appendices removed from the 70 children with "appendiceal colic" contrasts with the low figures of 8.2% and of 33.8% documented in appendices removed during the course of another operation and in cases of acute appendicitis, respectively. Less than 5% of these children experienced return of their abdominal pain during a follow-up period of 2 months to 11 years. Since other studies have shown a recurrence rate of 30% to 50% in series where the criterion for surgery was the severity and the frequency of the bouts of pain, confirmation of these findings by others is anxiously waited. The only indication for an elective appendectomy in cases of recurrent abdominal pain is in those who have a fecalith on a plain film.

REFERENCES

Ackerman, N.B.: The continuing problems of perforated appendicitis, Surg. Gynecol. Obstet. **139:**29-32, 1974.

Doraiswamy, N.V.: Progress of acute appendicitis: a study in children, Br. J. Surg. **65:**877-879, 1978.

Fee, H.J., Jones, P.C., Kadell, B., and O'Connell, T.X.: Radiologic diagnosis of appendicitis, Arch. Surg. **112:**742-744, 1977.

Folkman, M.J.: Appendicitis. In Ravitch, M.M., Welch, K.J., and Benson, C.D., editors: Pediatric surgery, ed. 3, Chicago, 1979, Year Book Medical Publishers, Inc.

Grosfeld, J.L., Weinberger, M, and Clatworthy, H.W.: Acute appendicitis in the first 2 years of life, J. Pediatr. Surg. **8:**285-293, 1973.

Holgersen, L.A., and Stanley-Brown, E.G.: Acute appendicitis with perforation, Am. J. Dis. Child. **122:**288-293, 1971.

Kwong, M.S., and Dinner, M.: Neonatal appendicitis masquerading as necrotizing enterocloitis, J. Pediatr. **96:**917-918, 1980.

Liebman, W.M., and St. Geme, J.W., Jr.: Enteroviral pseudoappendicitis, Am. J. Dis. Child. **120:**77-78, 1970.

Marchildon, M.B., and Dudgeon, D.L.: Perforated appendicitis: current experience in a children's hospital, Ann. Surg. **185:**84-87, 1977.

Parsons, J.M., Miscall, B.G., and McSherry, C.K.: Appendicitis in the newborn infant, Surgery **67:**841-843, 1970.

Savrin, R.A., and Clatworthy, H.W.: Appendiceal rupture: a continuing diagnostic problem, Pediatrics **63:**37-43, 1969.

Schisgall, R.M.: Appendiceal colic in childhood: the role of inspissated caste of stool within the appendix, Ann. Surg. **192:**687-693, 1980.

Shandling, B., Ein, S.H., Simpson, J.S., and others: Perforating appendicitis with antibiotics, J. Pediatr. Surg. **9:**79-83, 1974.

Pseudomembranous enterocolitis (antibiotic-associated colitis)

Pseudomembranous enterocolitis is a distinctive form of inflammatory bowel disease. It is usually associated with antibiotic therapy and is etiologically related to the cytotoxin of *Clostridium difficile.* Thirty-five cases have been reported in the pediatric age group. All children had been treated with antimicrobials either as single agents or in combination. Ampicillin and amoxicillin have been

Table 13-3. Clinical and laboratory findings in seven cases of pseudomembranous enterocolitis

Case	Age (years)	Fever (° C)	Stools/ day	White blood cell count	Proteins (gm/dl)	Antibiotic therapy	
						Type*	Time (days)
1	5⁵/₁₂	40	8	30,700	4.3	P, A	13
2	6	38	43	68,000	4.5	A	1
3	6	37.5	23	32,000	3.1	A	4
4	9	40	13	27,000	4.6	C	8
5	12	39.5	10	18,000	6.4	P	15
6	5½	39	7	26,300	6.3	P	7
7	6	39	22	45,100	4.5	P, A	10

*A, ampicillin; P, penicillin G or V; C, clindamycin.

most commonly (16 cases) implicated followed by clindamycin and lincomycin (7 cases) and penicillin G or penicillin V (6 cases). Cephalosporins and sulfonamides have been associated with the disease in adults; at least one case has occurred in a patient or trimethoprim and sulfamethoxazole. Pseudomembranous enterocolitis has been reported in four normal adults without a history of concomitant or antecedent antibiotic therapy. A provocative study has shown that *Clostridium difficile* organisms and toxin were found in 9 of 15 patients with chronic ulcerative colitis and Crohn's disease who had a severe relapse of their disease. Because the microbe is normally found in the vagina and rapidly disappears from the stools after the first few months of life, it is likely that transmission from the vaginal flora accounts for the high rate (50%) of isolation from the stools of healthy neonates.

Stools from patients with pseudomembranous enterocolitis contain the heat-labile cytotoxin of *Clostridium difficile.* Because the cytopathic changes observed after the addition of the ultrafiltrate of stools from patients is neutralized by the antitoxin of *Clostridium sordelli,* it was originally believed that the latter organism was implicated. This tissue culture assay also allows the measurement of titers. Colonization by *Clostridium difficile* is facilitated by the fact that antibiotics decrease the population of other components of the competing colonic flora. It constitutes the most rapid, simple, and sensitive method to prove the cause of the disease, especially in cases where the clinical diagnosis is in doubt.

Clinical findings

There is a range of clinical severity. Some patients may only have diarrhea, some will develop frank colitis, and others will have the full-blown clinical picture. Symptoms usually begin 4 to 10 days after initiation of antimicrobials, but they may start as early as during the first day of administration or as late as 3 weeks after discontinuation. Diarrhea is uniformly present and is generally severe (Table 13-3). Dehydration, fever, vomiting, crampy abdominal pain, tenesmus, and abdominal distention are common. Toxic megacolon and perforation are complications.

Laboratory, X-ray, and endoscopic findings

Hypoproteinemia is usual, and leukocytosis is impressive. The flat film of the abdomen (Fig. 13-2) is of some diagnostic help and the barium enema is contraindicated because the risk of perforation is high. Endoscopy should be carried out as soon as the diagnosis is suspected. The classic proctoscopic findings of raised yellowish white plaques are diagnostic (Fig. 13-2). Histologic examination confirms the presence of necrosis and pseudomembranes, which may be extensive, or focal and more superficial (Fig. 13-3). In milder forms of the disease the colon may be normal and show only evidence of erythema or more commonly show "nonspecific colitis." The cytotoxin is said to be present in only 20% of such cases.

Although the colon is the usual site of the disease (Fig. 13-4), we believe that the term "enterocolitis" is still warranted. We have documented small bowel involvement (Fig. 13-5) in two cases. In one of them the diagnosis was made by a small bowel biopsy (Fig. 13-6) and the rectoscopic findings were totally nonspecific. The absence of membranes at sigmoidoscopy does not rule out the disease as coloscopy is sometimes necessary for identification of the pathognomonic features.

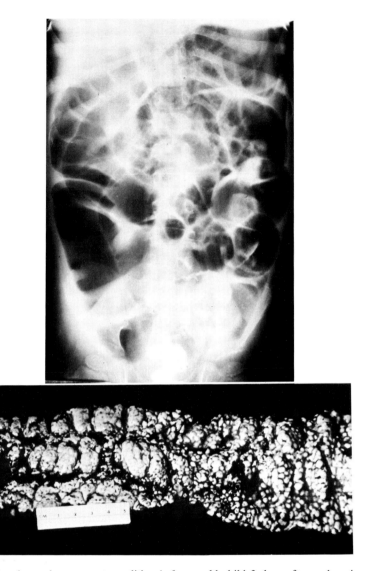

Fig. 13-2. Pseudomembranous enterocolitis. A 6-year-old child 3 days after undergoing a mastoidectomy suffered diarrhea, vomiting, abdominal distention, dehydration, hypoproteinemia, and shock. The flat film of the abdomen shows greatly distended colonic and small bowel loops characteristic of an ileus. The patient's condition worsened, and he died despite a colostomy. Postmortem examination showed extensive involvement of the ileum and entire colon in an ulceronecrotic process, with formation of yellow-gray, greatly adherent membranes that could not be scraped off.

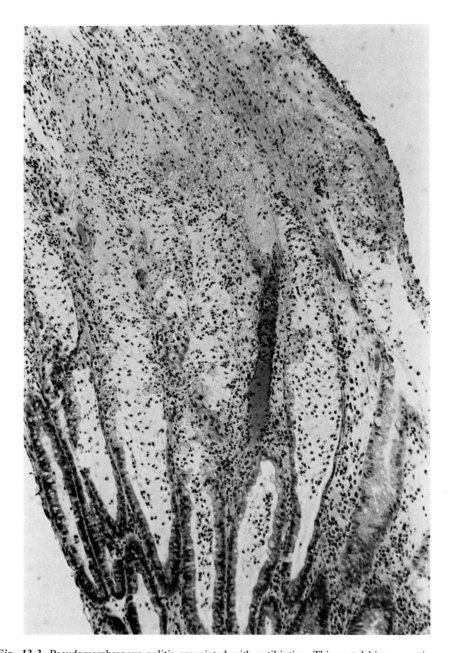

Fig. 13-3. Pseudomembranous colitis associated with antibiotics. This rectal biopsy section was taken from a 10-year-old boy who developed profuse diarrhea and severe abdominal pain 2 days after completing a 3-week course of penicillin for otitis media. On endoscopy, the mucosal surface was studded with raised yellow membranous plaques that, in some areas, became confluent. There is extensive necrosis of the crypts and complete disappearance of the superficial epithelium. The membrane is made up of fibrin, mucus, and inflammatory cells. The patient made an uneventful recovery.

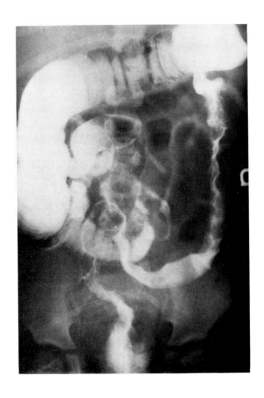

Fig. 13-4. Pseudomembranous colitis associated with the hemolytic-uremic syndrome. This barium enema shows extensive large nodular contour defects in the left colon and in the rectosigmoid. On endoscopy, the changes were typical of pseudomembranous colitis. Initial symptoms were those of fever, abdominal distention, vomiting, and bloody diarrhea. The patient, a 6-year-old boy, died 3 days after admission.

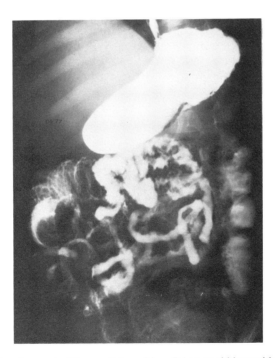

Fig. 13-5. Striking involvement of the small bowel in a 5½-year-old boy with pseudomembranous enterocolitis.

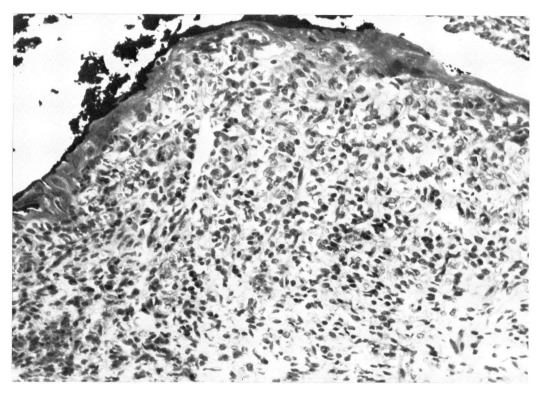

Fig. 13-6. Suction biopsy section of the small bowel in a child with pseudomembranous enterocolitis. Note the necrotic epithelium with fibrin exudate. There is total disappearance of the usual histologic features. A dense inflammatory infiltrate is present.

Differential diagnosis

The disease may mimic infections, gastroenteritis, inflammatory bowel disease, or even intestinal obstruction. The following conditions can lead to pseudomembranous enterocolitis, but it is uncertain if antibiotics are additional risk factors for the development of the disease.

Necrotizing enterocolitis (p. 87)
Hirschsprung's enterocolitis (p. 69)
Congenital heart disease with ischemia or severe heart failure
Uremic colitis
Hemolytic-uremic syndrome (p. 347)

Management

A high index of suspicion is necessary if the disease is to be diagnosed early. Profuse diarrhea in a child on antibiotics warrants an endoscopic examination, prompt discontinuation of antimicrobials if possible, a stool culture for anaerobes, and a specimen for detection of the *Clostridium difficile* toxin. Any patient with severe diarrhea, cramps, fever, leukocytosis, and abdominal dis-

tention needs to be closely screened for the possibility that antibiotic exposure has taken place during the preceding 3 weeks.

Immediate supportive therapy includes rehydration electrolyte replacement and salt-poor albumin. Many patients respond dramatically to discontinuation of the antibiotic. When antibiotic therapy is considered indispensable, a different, less frequently implicated agent should be given, and vancomycin should be started orally. Vancomycin, 125 to 500 mg/1.73 m^2 four times a day, is also advocated in all cases where the onset of the disease occurs some time after antimicrobials have been stopped. In such cases, the disease tends to be more severe and prolonged and parenteral alimentation may be indicated.

Oral vanocomycin has dramatic effects. Within 2 to 3 days an amelioration is usually noted. Therapy should be continued for at least 1 week. Of note is the report of symptomatic relapses in 14% occurring 4 to 21 days after completion of the first course of vancomycin. Repeated courses of vancomycin have been necessary in selected patients. Oral bacitracin is also effective. A less favorable experience has been reported with cholestyramine, which binds the cytotoxin.

As pointed out recently, the disease could have been prevented in many reported pediatric patients, since the indications for antimicrobial therapy could be questioned in most.

Prognosis

The mortality in 25 children reported before the use of vancomycin was 28%. In a more recent series of 10 children a favorable outcome is reported though one suffered two relapses and required three courses of vancomycin to eradicate the disease.

REFERENCES

Bartlett, J.G.: Antibiotic-associated colitis, Clin. Gastroenterol. **8:**783-801, 1979.

Bartlett, J.G., Tedesco, F.J., Shull, S., and others: Symptomatic relapse after oral vancomycin therapy and antibiotic-associated pseudomembranous colitis, Gastroenterology **78:**431-434, 1980.

Buts, J.P., Weber, A.M., Roy, C.C., and Morin, C.L.: Pseudomembranous enterocolitis in childhood, Gastroenterology **73:**823-827, 1977.

Devroede, G., Poisson, J., Madarnas, P., and others: Lincomycin-clindamycin colitis is not an entity, Can. J. Surg. **20:**326-335, 1977.

Fekety, R., Kim, K., Brown, D., and others: Epidemiology of antibiotic-associated colitis, Am. J. Med. **70:**906-908, 1981.

Larson, H.E., and Price, A.B.: Pseudomembranous colitis: presence of clostridial toxin, Lancet **2:**1312-1314, 1977.

Sutphen, J.S., and Grand, R.J.: New identification of *Clostridium difficile* as a cause of chronic diarrhea without classic signs of colitis, Pediatr. Res. **15:**622, 1981 (Abstract).

Tedesco, F., Markham, R., Gurwith, M., and others: Oral vancomycin for antibiotic-associated pseudomembranous colitis, Lancet **1:**226-228, 1978.

Trnka, Y.M., and LaMont, J.T.: Association of *Clostridium difficile* toxin with symptomatic relapse of chronic inflammatory bowel disease, Gastroenterology **80:**693-696, 1981.

Viscidi, R., Willey, S., and Bartlett, J.G.: Isolation rates and toxigenic potential of *Clostridium difficile* isolates from various patient populations, Gastroenterology **81:**5-9, 1981.

Wald, A., Mendelow, H., and Bartlett, J.G.: Non-antibiotic associated pseudomembranous colitis due to toxin-producing clostridia, Ann. Intern. Med. **92:**798-799, 1980.

Colitis of hemolytic-uremic syndrome

The hemolytic-uremic syndrome is characterized by acute renal failure, hemolytic anemia, and thrombocytopenia. Intestinal manifestations are present early, and the most common are abdominal pain and diarrhea. Later in the disease there is bloody diarrhea and evidence of colitis with frank ulcerations, focal areas of necrosis, submucosal hemorrhage (Fig. 13-7), fibrinoid necrosis of small arterioles, and extensive thromboses. The colitis can progress to pseudomembranous enterocolitis and toxic megacolon. We have several patients with rectal prolapse, and this has also been described by others.

Sigmoidoscopy and biopsy are indicated in all patients with severe gastrointestinal symptoms. Close monitoring is also recommended during the course of the illness. Toxic megacolon and evidence of perforation are indications for surgery, but the prognosis is extremely grave though segmental resection of gangrenous colon may be life saving. After the acute phase of the disease, long-term follow-up study of the colitis is necessary because strictures requiring surgery may occur.

REFERENCES

Berman, W., Jr.: The hemolytic-uremic syndrome: initial clinical presentation mimicking ulcerative colitis, J. Pediatr. **81:**275-278, 1972.

Koster, F., Levin, J., Walker, L., and others: Hemolytic-uremic syndrome after shigellosis: relation to endotoxemia and circulating immune complexes, N. Engl. J. Med. **298:**927-933, 1978.

Lieberman, E.: Hemolytic-uremic syndrome, J. Pediatr. **80:**1-16, 1972.

Sawaf, H., Sharp, M.J., Youn, K.J., and others: Ischemic colitis and stricture after hemolytic-uremic syndrome, Pediatrics **61:**315-317, 1978.

Schwartz, D.L., Becker, J.M., So, H.B., and Schneider, K.M.: Segmental colonic gangrene: a surgical emergency in the hemolytic-uremic syndrome, Pediatrics **62:**54-56, 1978.

Tochen, M.L., and Campbell, J.R.: Colitis in children with the hemolytic-uremic syndrome, J. Pediatr. Surg. **12:**213-219, 1977.

Intestinal manifestations of Henoch-Schönlein purpura

Anaphylactoid purpura is a common illness that is well described in pediatric texts. The gastrointestinal manifestations can precede the skin purpura and are commonly severe.

Any part of the gastrointestinal tract can be involved, with the possible exception of the esophagus. Hemorrhage occurs into the intestinal wall, with edema of the mucosa and submucosa. Extensive scalloping and thumbprinting may be seen on roentgenograms (Fig. 13-8). Local ulceration of the mucosa associated with a diffuse arteriolitis and fibrinoid necrosis may occur, though most accounts limit their findings to localized submucosal hemorrhage and intussusception.

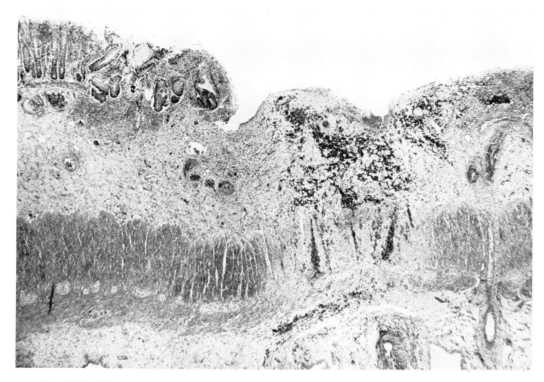

Fig. 13-7. This segment of large bowel was taken from a 21-month-old boy with hemolytic uremic syndrome who died with multiple large bowel perforations. Transmural necrosis is present with extensive venous thromboses.

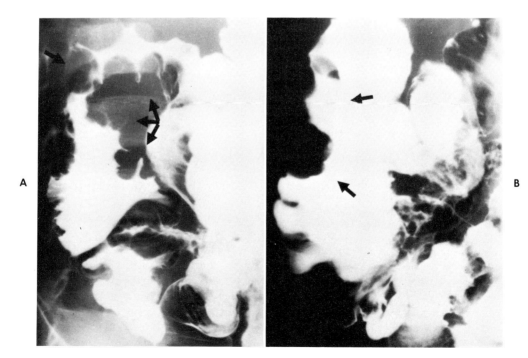

Fig. 13-8. Intramural colonic hematoma. During the course of Henoch-Schönlein purpura, this 4-year-old child developed abdominal pain, vomiting, and mild distention. **A,** Barium enema shows a well-circumscribed lesion at the splenic flexure, *arrows*. **B,** Note the extensive thumbprinting, *arrows,* suggestive of blood accumulating between the mucosa and the deeper layers of the colonic wall.

Clinical findings

Abdominal pain, which is present in close to two thirds of patients, is colicky and can be very severe. Exploratory laparotomy, in one series, has been carried out in 10% of cases. Hematest-positive stools and melena are described in 50% and 30%, respectively. Intussusception is said to occur in 3%, and massive intestinal hemorrhage in 5% to 10%. It is interesting to note that gastrointestinal manifestations tend to be more frequent and severe in older children than in toddlers and preschoolers.

Diagnosis

The differential diagnosis includes the medical and surgical conditions responsible for an "acute abdomen."

Treatment

There is no satisfactory treatment for the common manifestations of anaphylactoid purpura. Corticosteroid therapy, however, has been shown to be very useful in patients with acute gastrointestinal manifestations. Usually within a few hours after hydrocortisone is started intravenously, the patient's pain decreases. Recurrence of severe pain may be seen on weaning of the patient from corticosteroid therapy.

REFERENCES

Goldman, L.P., and Lindenberg, R.L.: Henoch-Schönlein purpura: gastrointestinal manifestations with endoscopic correlation, Am. J. Gastroenterol. **75:**357-360, 1981.
Rodriguez-Erdmann, F., and Levitan, R.: Gastrointestinal and roentgenological manifestations of Henoch-Schönlein purpura, Gastroenterology **54:**260, 1968.
Smith, H.J.: Spontaneous perforation in Schönlein-Henoch purpura, South. Med. J. **73:**603-606, 1980.

Radiation enterocolitis

Gastrointestinal symptoms frequently occur during the first or second week of radiation therapy. Nausea, vomiting, diarrhea, and rectal bleeding are common. In children, pelvic irradiation is rare; therefore the endarteritis is more likely to involve the small bowel and occurs some months after completion of radiation therapy. The small bowel biopsy shows a shortening of villi with edema and inflammatory cells in the lamina propria. Signs and symptoms of malabsorption with protein-losing enteropathy may be present. Elemental diets are helpful, but parenteral alimentation is necessary in severe cases.

REFERENCES

De Poerck, A.F., Engelholm, L., De Toeuf, J., and others: Radiation enteritis of small intestine, J. Belg. Radiol. **63:**573-579, 1980.
Tankel, H.I., Clark, D., and Lee, F.D.: Radiation enteritis with malabsorption, Gut **6:**560-569, 1965.

INFLAMMATORY BOWEL DISEASE

The term "inflammatory bowel disease" is used to designate two chronic intestinal disorders: chronic ulcerative colitis and Crohn's disease. They are grouped together because of the many similarities in their epidemiologic, immunologic, and clinical features.

Inflammatory bowel disease (IBD) constitutes an increasingly larger proportion of chronic intestinal disease in the pediatric age group. The chronicity of ulcerative colitis and of Crohn's disease, the severity of their complications, and the management problems have led to much research into pathogenetic mechanisms.

Etiology: current lines of research

The answer is not available yet, but there are a number of important leads suggesting that inflammatory bowel disease is the result of a genetically conditioned susceptibility to one or more environmental influences.

Immune factors

Humoral immunity. Anticolon antibodies directed against colonic epithelial cell antigens and cross-reacting with antigens from *Escherichia coli* have been demonstrated in both blood and colon. However they are nonspecific, since comparable titers are present in many other diseases. Furthermore they do not cause cell damage to tissue cultures in vitro. The deposition of antigen-antibody complexes has been suggested as a possible cause. Complement and gamma globulin deposition has been demonstrated, and there is some evidence for the presence of circulating immune complexes. This could be a consequence of the inflammation rather than the cause, especially since complement aberrations in patients are modest, at best, and inconsistent. Relatively recent reports on the efficacy of cromoglycate have not been confirmed and therefore have largely defused the idea that an immediate hypersensitivity reaction could cause degranulation of mast cells in the bowel wall. Current evidence linking antibody-mediated reactions to the pathogenesis of inflammatory bowel disease is weakened by reports of that disease in patients with acquired hypogammaglobulinemia and with selective IgA deficiency.

Cell-mediated immunity. Although a number of studies have shown that patients with inflammatory bowel disease have T cells, which are coated with processed colon and bacterial antigens, both in their circulation and in the lamina propria of their intestine, there is no evidence that this is specific to these patients and that these sensitized T cells have a cytotoxic effect against intestinal cells. There is a stronger case, however, that lymphocytes with an Fc receptor (null cell) may attach to the Fc portion of an antibody coating the target colon epithelial cell and exert direct cytotoxicity. This has been shown by incubation of lymphocytes from patients with inflammatory bowel disease with colon epithelial cell cultures. The case for the role of an antibody-dependent cell-mediated cytotoxicity is weakened by the observation that within a few days after resection of the diseased bowel, this special class of lymphocytes lose their cytotoxicity toward colon cells.

A large volume of work has identified impairment of cellular immunity in patients with inflammatory bowel disease. It is more common in Crohn's disease than in ulcerative colitis, with cutaneous anergy noted in 70% of the former and in 48% of the latter. Our own experience suggests that in patients with Crohn's disease, cellular immunity is significantly correlated with the severity of the disease particularly with malnutrition. Although anergy disappears after proctocolectomy in ulcerative colitis, it tends to persist in Crohn's disease after surgery. As yet there is no explanation for this observation, but the case for a primary defect in cellular immunity is still weak. The evidence suggests that it is a secondary phenomenon, especially since an increased incidence of cutaneous anergy in siblings and parents of patients has not been demonstrated.

Histocompatibility antigens. Because ankylosing spondylitis, a disease associated with the presence of HLA-B27, is considerably more frequent in patients with inflammatory bowel disease, it was logical to examine HLA antigenemia profiles. The search has not been fruitful, except for the observation of concordance of HLA haplotypes in 4 of 5 sibling pairs with Crohn's disease. This suggests a genetic predisposition but does not provide us with a specific HLA haplotype that could help us understand the pathogenesis by identification of individuals at risk for inflammatory bowel disease.

Infectious agents

Bacteria. Mice, rats, guinea pigs, and rabbits have been used in the past decade in attempts to reproduce granulomas after inoculation of these animals with Crohn's disease tissue homogenates. However, granulomas have also appeared after injections with ulcerative colitis and normal colonic tissue. Thus the formation of granulomas from transmission experiments appears to be a nonspecific tissue reaction.

Because of clinical observations and of studies showing a cross-reactivity of *Escherichia coli* and colon antigenic determinants for colon antibodies, the microflora has been examined. Perhaps the complexity of the flora and the crudeness of currently available techniques explain in part the failure to identify a specific organism or an enterobacterial antigen. Two recent reports suggesting that *Clostridium difficile* is grown with some regularity in patients with inflammatory bowel disease experiencing a severe relapse is of interest. Should this be confirmed, it would provide a treatable and perhaps preventable etiologic factor for relapses.

Also of great interest are studies examining the possibility that cell wall–deficient bacteria might be involved. The most provocative results have documented the presence of a cell wall–defective *Pseudomonas* and high antibody titers to this bacterium in patients with Crohn's disease. Tissues and blood obtained from patients with ulcerative colitis and with other diseases were normal.

Viruses. Extensive screening for viruses was initiated 20 years ago and has continued over the years. Cytomegalovirus has been implicated in ulcerative colitis but this has not been confirmed. When ultrafiltrates of diseased bowel from patients with inflammatory bowel disease is added to tissue culture, a cytopathic effect is observed and is neutralized by guinea pig antiserum to Crohn's disease and ulcerative colitis tissue culture fluid. A few reports have shown viruslike particles on electron microscopy, but others have not detected their presence.

Psychogenic factors

In the past decade the pendulum has swung away from the possibility that psychologic influences could play a pivotal role in the pathogenesis of inflammatory bowel disease. The frequency of emotional disturbances in patients with ulcerative colitis and their important relationship to exacerbations has frequently been stressed. Children with this disease are described as emotionally fragile, vulnerable to stressful situations, and overly dependent on domineering, overprotective, and self-centered mothers. However, the prevailing opinion is that patients with inflammatory bowel disease do not have a higher incidence of personality problems or of psychiatric illness than children or adolescents suffering from other chronic diseases. Undoubtedly chronic invalidism, the threat of a severe relapse or of surgery, and anxiety concerning schooling and career constitute stressful situations that a number of adolescents are ill equipped to face, especially if family and physician fail to provide appropriate support. Psychologic problems do not play a role in the pathogenesis of the disease but may accentuate symptoms and the severity of a relapse.

Dietary and other environmental factors

In view of the increasing incidence of Crohn's disease and of the greater vulnerability of urban dwellers, the eventual role of foods, food additives, and environmental pollutants is under scrutiny. Although exposure to carrageenan (an emulsion stabilizer) and to environmental mercury, an insufficient intake of fiber, and an increased consumption of refined sugars and of cornflakes have all been implicated as potential factors, the evidence so far is anecdotal. More investigation and epidemiologic surveys will be necessary before preventive nutrition and environmental measures can be suggested.

REFERENCES

Auer, I.O., Buschmann, C., and Ziemer, E.: Immune status in Crohn's disease. 2. Originally unimpaired primary cell mediated immunity in vitro, Gut **19**:618-626, 1978.

Cave, D.R., Mitchell, D.N., and Brooke, B.N.: Experimental animal studies of the etiology and pathogenesis of Crohn's disease, Gastroenterology **69**:618-624, 1975.

Clancy, R.: Isolation and kinetic characteristics of mucosal lymphocytes in Crohn's disease, Gastroenterology **70**:177-180, 1978.

Dvorak, A.M., Dickersin, G.R., Osage, J.L., and Monahan, R.A.: Absence of virus structures in Crohn's disease tissues studied by electron microscopy, Lancet **1**:328, 1978.

Gitnick, G.L., Rosen, V.J., Arthur, M.S., and Hertweck, S.A.: Evidence for the isolation of a new virus from ulcerative colitis patients: comparison with virus derived from Crohn's disease, Dig. Dis. Sci. **24**:609-619, 1979.

Gitnick, G.L.: Etiology of inflammatory bowel diseases: are we making progress? Gastroenterology **78**:1089-1091, 1980.

Meyers, S., Sachar, D.B., Taub, R.N., and Janowitz, H.D.: Significance of anergy to dinitrochlorobenzene in inflammatory bowel disease: family and postoperative studies, Gut **19**:249-252, 1978.

Parent, K., and Mitchell, P.: Cell wall–defective variants of *Pseudomonas*-like (group Va) bacteria in Crohn's disease, Gastroenterology **75**:368-372, 1978.

Rabin, B.S., and Rogers, S.J.: A cell-mediated immune model of inflammatory bowel disease in the rabbit, Gastroenterology **75**:29-33, 1978.

Rawcliffe, D.M., and Truelove, S.C.: Breakfast and Crohn's disease, Br. Med. J. **2**:539-540, 1978.

Sachar, D.B., Auslander, M.O., and Walfish, J.S.: Aetiological theories of inflammatory bowel disease, Clin. Gastroenterol. **9**:231-257, 1980.

Soltis, R.D., Hasz, D., Morris, M.J., and Wilson, I.D.: Evidence against the presence of circulating immune complexes in chronic inflammatory bowel disease, Gastroenterology **76**:1380-1385, 1979.

Trnka, Y.M., and LaMont, J.T.: Association of *Clostridium difficile* toxin with symptomatic relapse of chronic inflammatory bowel disease, Gastroenterology **80**:693-696, 1981.

Epidemiology and genetics of inflammatory bowel disease

Epidemiologic surveys directed at the incidence and prevalence of inflammatory bowel disease have reported figures that are very variable. Although diagnostic criteria and methodology (inpatients versus outpatients) may explain some of these differences, there are undoubtedly geographic, eth-

Table 13-4. Epidemiologic survey of inflammatory bowel disease

Health organization	Period of survey	Inflammatory bowel disease	
		Total number	Crohn's disease to ulcerative colitis
CHMC (Boston)	1967-1976	139	1.53:1
HSJ (Montreal)	1969-1979	138	1.82:1
Cleveland Clinic	1965-1974	482	2.27:1
HSC (Toronto)	1969-1976	148	1:1.42

No. of patients

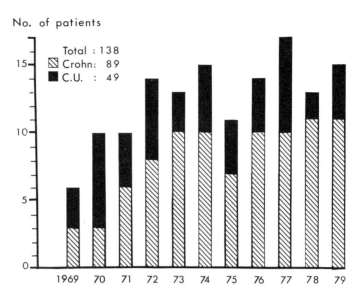

Fig. 13-9. Chronic inflammatory bowel diseases. Comparative incidence of Crohn's disease and chronic ulcerative colitis over a period of 11 years at the Hôpital Sainte-Justine, Montreal, 1969-1979.

nic, and racial factors affecting susceptibility. Males and females are equally affected. Inflammatory bowel disease is less frequent in blacks, Orientals, and Israeli Jews. Jews living in Europe and North America seem to be at higher risk. Inflammatory bowel disease is more common in non-Latin Western European countries than in France, Italy, and Spain. All studies have shown that urban populations are at higher risk than rural dwellers.

The annual incidence rate of ulcerative colitis varies between 3.7 to 7.3 per 100,000 with a prevalence of 37.4 to 100. These rates have not changed over the past 2 decades, whereas those for Crohn's disease show a rapid increase over the same period. The early (1960 to 1963) survey of Crohn's disease in the Baltimore area recorded an incidence of 1.8, but in the more recent one (1973) it doubled to 3.7. A study conducted in 1978 by the Research Committee of the Organisation Mondiale de Gastro-entérologie established the ratio of Crohn's disease to ulcerative colitis at 1 to 1.24.

The proportion of cases of inflammatory bowel disease becoming symptomatic during childhood and adolescence varies between 15% and 30%. A somewhat lower figure is reported for ulcerative colitis than for Crohn's disease. A higher incidence of Crohn's disease is apparent at the Children's Hospital Medical Center, the Hôpital Sainte-Justine, and the Cleveland Clinic, but this has not

been the case over essentially the same period of time at the Hospital for Sick Children in Toronto (Table 13-4).

A yearly breakdown of our own cases (Fig. 13-9) shows that for the 5-year period 1969 to 1974 less than 60% of our patients with inflammatory bowel disease were suffering from Crohn's disease. During the 1975 to 1979 period, Crohn's disease accounted for more than 70%. This increase in Crohn's disease is unlikely to be fortuitous, since over the past 2 years we have still been seeing more than 2.3 patients with Crohn's disease for each one with ulcerative colitis. Furthermore, most of these patients are reevaluated and followed regularly by the gastrointestinal clinic so that the same diagnostic criteria have been applied over the years. This trend was confirmed at the Cleveland Clinic: in the 1960s a little more than 60% of their 431 cases below 20 years of age had Crohn's disease, whereas for the first half of the 1970s the percentage had gone up to 70%.

Familial aggregation of inflammatory bowel disease has been known for about 20 years. Usually only one disease is seen in the same sibship. However, parents of index cases as well as their children are often discordant for the same disease. In monozygotic twins, concordance is higher in Crohn's disease (7 of 8) than in ulcerative colitis (5 of 11). A large family study has been recently conducted in 838 pediatric cases collated over a

Table 13-5. Results of family study in 838 pediatric cases of inflammatory bowel disease (IBD)

IBD	Number	Percentage with IBD in first-degree relatives	Rate of occurrence in first-degree relatives (%)	
			Siblings	Parents
Ulcerative colitis	316	15.8	4	6
Crohn's disease	522	16.6	6	8

Data from Farmer, R.G., Michener, W.M., and Mortimer, E.A.: Clin. Gastroenterol. **9:**271-278, 1980.

period of 20 years (1955 to 1974) (Table 13-5).

In our own survey about 13% of children with Crohn's disease had first-degree relatives with inflammatory bowel disease, and the incidence was 6.5% in those with ulcerative colitis. These figures contrast with those from Toronto where the familial incidence was higher in the cases with ulcerative colitis (15%) than in those with Crohn's disease (8.2%).

When the authors of the study in Table 13-5 included grandparents, aunts, uncles, and cousins, one third of all patients had abnormal family histories. However, the inheritance of inflammatory bowel disease does not follow mendelian principles unless a very low penetrance is postulated.

The role of the environment is difficult to define but certainly appears minimal when compared to the genetic background. There are few examples of inflammatory bowel disease in people sharing the same immediate environment such as spouses, adopted children, and even half-siblings. This weakens the case for environmental influences unique to living in the same household and emphasizes the key role of genetic susceptibility.

REFERENCES

Aiges, H., Portnoy, J., Silverberg, M., and others: Families of adolescents with inflammatory bowel disease: demographic analysis, Pediatr. Res. **12:**364, 1978 (Abstract).

Brahme, F., Lindström, C., and Wenckert, A.: Crohn's disease in a defined population, Gastroenterology **69:**342-351, 1975.

Farmer, R.G., Michener, W.M., and Mortimer, E.A.: Studies of family history among patients with inflammatory bowel disease, Clin. Gastroenterol. **9:**271-278, 1980.

Kirsner, J.B.: Genetic aspects of inflammatory bowel disease, Clin. Gastroenterol. **2:**557-575, 1973.

Lewkonia, R.M., and McConnell, R.B.: Familial inflammatory disease: heredity or environment? Gut **17:**235-243, 1976.

Mendeloff, A.I.: The epidemiology of inflammatory bowel disease, Clin. Gastroenterol. **9:**259-270, 1980.

Rosen, P., Zonis, J., Yekutiel, P., and others: Crohn's disease in the Jewish population of Tel-Aviv–Yafo, Gastroenterology **76:**25-30, 1979.

Singer, H.C., Anderson, J.G.D., Frischer, H., and others: Familial aspects of inflammatory bowel disease, Gastroenterology **61:**423-430, 1971.

• • •

Much attention has been focused on the relationship of ulcerative colitis to Crohn's disease. Under this impetus, certain clinical, roentgenographic, and pathologic features have provided sound bases for distinguishing the two conditions. However, there are still some cases for which differentiation is not possible. In the absence of any clue to the cause of either, it is impossible to determine whether they represent two distinct entities, a different tissue reaction to the same etiologic agent, or different stages of the same disease. Accordingly, some authors have questioned the sharp distinction classically drawn between ulcerative and granulomatous colitis. Despite these drawbacks and before we proceed with a detailed description of both entities, a list of clues that may help in the differential diagnosis of ulcerative colitis and Crohn's disease is provided in Table 13-6.

Ulcerative colitis

Ulcerative colitis is an acute inflammatory disease of the mucosa of the colon and rectum. It affects both sexes equally, usually runs a chronic course interspersed with acute exacerbations, and occurs in all pediatric age groups. Although occasionally seen in infants during the first year of life, the mean age at diagnosis is around 11. As a rule, until the onset of ulcerative colitis the children have enjoyed good health and normal devel-

Table 13-6. Differential diagnosis between ulcerative colitis and Crohn's disease

Feature	Ulcerative colitis	Crohn's disease
Relative incidence of symptoms		
Rectal bleeding (gross)	Common	Rare
Diarrhea	Often severe	Moderate or even absent
Pain	Less frequent	Almost always
Anorexia	Mild or moderate	Can be severe
Weight loss	Moderate	Severe
Growth retardation	Usually mild	Often pronounced
Extraintestinal manifestations	Common	Common
Involvement		
Small bowel		
Extensive	—	10%
Lower ileum	5% to 10%	90%
Colon	100%	75%
Rectum	95%	50%
Anus	5%	85%
Distribution of lesions	Continuous	Segmental
Roentgenologic features	Superficial ulcers, loss of haustration, no skip areas, shortening	Serpiginous ulcers, thumbprinting, skip areas, string sign
Pathologic changes	Diffuse mucosal disease	Focal transmural disease granulomas
Response to treatment		
Steroids and sulfasalazine	75%	25% to 50%
Parenteral nutrition and elemental diets	Poor	Very good to induce a remission
Azathioprine and 6-mercaptopurine	Good in selected cases	Good in selected cases
Surgery	Excellent	Fair or poor
Course		
Remissions	Common	Difficult to define
Relapse after surgery	Common if rectum not removed	35% to 100%
Cancer risk	High in pancolitis	Slight

opment. Even though symptoms are usually acute, the interval of time between onset of symptoms and diagnosis is often quite long. However, a greater awareness of the disease has decreased this interval from 14 months to less than 4 months in our own experience.

Intestinal manifestations (Fig. 13-10)

Bloody diarrhea. Frequent passage of loose or watery stools containing small amounts of feces with variable quantities of pus, mucus, and blood is almost always present at the time of diagnosis. However, at the onset of symptoms only two thirds have diarrhea and less than one third have gross blood in their stools. Nocturnal diarrhea is present in the majority. Nocturnal bowel movements are a sign of severe involvement. Urgency with incontinence can be documented in 25% to 30% of cases. The painless passage of red blood mistaken for a benign anal abnormality can be the first sign.

Abdominal pain and tenesmus. The abdominal pain of ulcerative colitis, not so severe as that seen in Crohn's disease, is probably related to the failure of peristaltic waves to progress normally through diseased areas, leading to colonic distention. The pain is usually colicky; it can be made worse by the ingestion of food and is somewhat relieved by defecation.

The typical crampy lower abdominal pain of ulcerative colitis is accompanied by a sensation of urgency of defecation. In fact, tenesmus may be virtually constant, forcing the patient to make repeated futile attempts at defecation resulting in the passage of only small collections of mucus or blood.

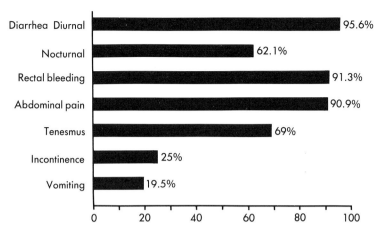

Fig. 13-10. Intestinal symptoms associated with 46 cases of chronic ulcerative colitis in children with a mean age of 11.4 ± 3.9 years.

Anorexia, nausea, and vomiting. Severe anorexia is usual in the acute stage of the illness. Later on, a lack of appetite can be the result of severe depression, or it may be secondary to exacerbation of abdominal pain brought about by ingestion of food. Nausea and vomiting, worrisome symptoms, are indicative of severe progressive disease. Associated with severe abdominal distention, nausea and vomiting may be indicative of toxic megacolon or of an impending local complication such as a free colonic perforation.

Extraintestinal manifestations

Many extraintestinal clinical features may precede by months or years the intestinal symptoms. Extraintestinal manifestations are present in most children.

Dehydration, weight loss, and retarded maturation. Acute depletion of body water and electrolytes occurs only in severe attacks. In young children, particularly, potassium deficits may be considerable. Weight loss is a constant feature of the acute disease but is not so frequent or severe as in Crohn's disease.

The time lag between the onset of symptoms and the diagnosis and the extent of the disease affect the incidence and the severity of growth retardation. Somewhat less than a third of children stand below the third percentile for weight and 10% below the third for height. Minimal gastrointestinal symptoms can sometimes be overshadowed by a strikingly stunted growth. Delayed puberty is reported in 20% of cases.

Nonspecific signs of inflammatory disease. A low-grade fever peaking in the evening can be documented for prolonged periods of time. Chills, fever, and leukocytosis are likely in the initial stage of the disease.

Mucocutaneous lesions. Erythema multiforme or erythema nodosum can be seen during the acute stage of the disease. Pyoderma gangrenosum is described as the more typical skin lesion associated with ulcerative colitis in adults but is rare in children (Fig. 13-11). Aphthous stomatitis extending to the palate and pharynx is more common in Crohn's disease but is seen in more than 10% of cases.

Musculoskeletal and ocular involvement. There appears to be a close association of skin, joint, and ocular involvement. Episodes of arthralgia or arthritis often coexist with colonic symptoms and are described in 10% to 20% of children with ulcerative colitis. Ankylosing spondylitis has not been reported in children. Conjunctivitis is frequently recorded, with uveitis being much rarer. Finger clubbing is likely in long-standing cases.

Liver disease. Fatty infiltration of the liver is the most common hepatic lesions and is probably related to chronic malnutrition. Chronic active hepatitis is the second most common form of liver disease in children with ulcerative colitis. We have seen four cases of chronic active hepatitis associated with ulcerative colitis, an incidence of more than 8%. Pericholangitis is the dominant lesion in adults. The presence of liver disease cannot be positively correlated with the extent, duration, or activity of the colitis.

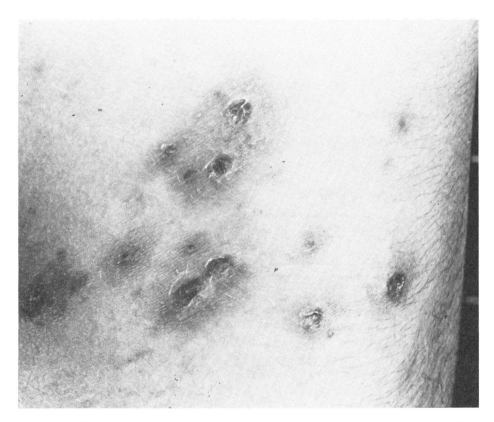

Fig. 13-11. Typical lesions of pyoderma gangrenosum in an adolescent with pancolitis. These irregularly shaped ulcers with rolled-out margins are characterized by a heavy infiltration of chronic inflammatory cells and occasional giant cells. There is perivascular hyalinization and fibrin deposition.

Liver function of all patients with ulcerative colitis should be tested. A liver biopsy should be done if there is hepatomegaly, consistently abnormal results of liver function tests, or symptoms such as jaundice or pruritus.

Laboratory findings

Hypochromic anemia, mainly attributable to chronic blood loss, develops in most patients. Half the patients can be expected to have a hemoglobin below 11 gm, an elevated erythrocyte sedimentation rate, and hypoalbuminemia (<3.5 gm/dl). The last constitutes a good index of relapse and is indicative of protein-losing enteropathy.

Fat malabsorption associated with ulcerative colitis is rare. The occasional malabsorption of vitamin B_{12} does not seem to correlate positively with the presence of so-called backwash ileitis. Disturbed colonic motility promotes ileocecal valve incompetence and brings about an abnormal bacterial colonization of the lower small bowel, explaining vitamin B_{12} malabsorption.

X-ray studies

In the very sick child with ulcerative colitis, plain films of the abdomen and proctoscopy should be done rather than a barium enema. Contrast studies may be dangerous in severe acute colitis. There are numerous reports of toxic megacolon within 48 hours of a barium study. We have the impression that it can at least exacerbate symptoms and prefer to wait until cooling down of the colitis has occurred. On the other hand, if symptoms are moderate, an air-contrast study is more likely to yield information than an ordinary barium enema.

Early roentgenographic changes in ulcerative colitis are nonspecific and may be totally absent. This has occurred in a third of our cases. However, there is usually loss of haustration and mucosal mottling. Later, the roentgenograms show superficial ulcerations (Fig. 13-12) and thickening of the bowel wall. At the time of diagnosis 25% of patients show involvement of their entire colon (Fig. 13-13); it is limited to the left and transverse

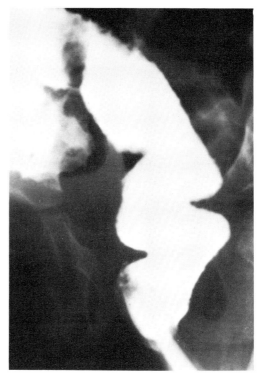

Fig. 13-12. Ulcerative colitis. A 15-year-old girl was admitted to hospital for rectal bleeding and anemia. Proctoscopic examination showed a superficial inflammatory and ulcerative process limited to the first 10 cm proximal to the anal margin. A barium enema shows fine spicules indicative of superficial ulcerations, which are also seen in cases of bacterial or amebic colitis.

A 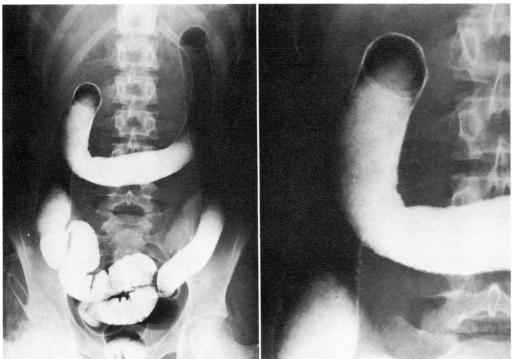 B

Fig. 13-13. Ulcerative colitis. A, There is total colonic involvement characterized by complete loss of haustration and by the presence of fine spicules indicative of superficial ulcerations. The abnormal mucosal pattern is better appreciated on the enlarged spot film of the hepatic flexure, B. The thin barium mixture shows multiple tiny collections of more concentrated medium in the myriad of superficial ulcers. This patient had the disease for 1 year and already presents with severe, advanced roentgenologic evidence of ulcerative colitis.

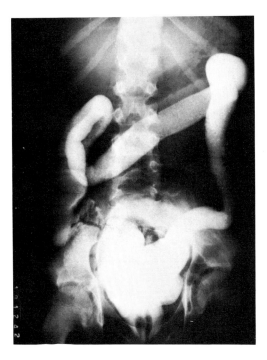

Fig. 13-14. Ulcerative colitis with "backwash" ileitis. The colon wall is stiff, straight, and smooth. At this advanced stage, there is total loss of normal haustration throughout the colon except for the region of the cecum. In this patient the terminal ileum is also involved.

colon in 50%. In 15% to 25% the disease does not go beyond the rectosigmoid and the left colon. "Backwash ileitis" is noted in the last few centimeters of the ileum in 10% of patients with pancolitis (Fig. 13-14).

A remarkable characteristic of roentgenographic features associated with ulcerative colitis is the speed and the extent with which severe changes can come and go. This is, of course, related to the superficial nature of the inflammatory process. However, in long-standing cases where the disease has extended to the submucosa and has run a chronic course, the "burnt-out" colon is present. It is characterized by the complete disappearance of haustral markings, shortening of the colon, and uniform reduction in its caliber (lead-pipe colon). Recently described segmental strictures may occur and mimic carcinomatosis; however, they appear to be reversible.

Endoscopic findings

In our experience general anesthesia is never necessary for a rectosigmoidoscopic examination and sedation is not routinely used except for in-

fants, preschoolers, and older children who are particularly anxious or who are in severe pain.

Endoscopic features are extremely variable and several features are shared by ulcerative colitis and Crohn's disease. A third of the patients with ulcerative colitis may at the onset have essentially normal findings. Mild disease is characterized by erythema, edema, and loss of vascular pattern. The next stage leads to granularity and friability, which is best elicited when the mucosa is swabbed vigorously with a cotton applicator. Frank ulcerations, when present, represent more severe disease and invariably are surrounded by a mucosa that is greatly hyperemic, edematous, and friable. Although there are no truly pathognomonic features in Crohn's colitis, certain features such as aphthous or frank ulcerations widely dispersed in a normal mucosa, bumpy indurations, and linear longitudineal ulcers are quite distinctive.

Coloscopy is now an accepted procedure in pediatric patients and is proving to be a useful tool in these ways: (1) a significant number of adult patients reported by roentgenography to have a left-sided form of ulcerative colitis have been shown to have disease extending proximally, (2) direct access to a stricture or polypoid lesion permits identification of its nature (inflammatory, fibrotic, or cancerous), (3) it is invaluable in the follow-up study of long-standing cases so that one may document the presence of dysplastic changes, which identifies patients at greatest risk for carcinoma.

Rectosigmoidoscopic examination is essential for the clinical diagnosis of colitis and in the followup care of patients. It is remarkable how rapidly after disease onset severe changes appear and yet can be reversed when the disease is under control. Rectosigmoidoscopic examination may be more difficult in more chronic cases, because the colonic walls are much less flexible and the colonic lumen is reduced.

Biopsy features

Even if there are no significant roentgenographic or rectosigmoidoscopic findings, mucosal biopsies or a full-thickness biopsy from a rectal valve should be done. Normal endoscopic findings do not rule out the diagnosis of ulcerative colitis.

Although there are no specific features in the histology of ulcerative colitis, there are patterns of inflammation that are characteristic for the different clinical phases of the disease. In the acute

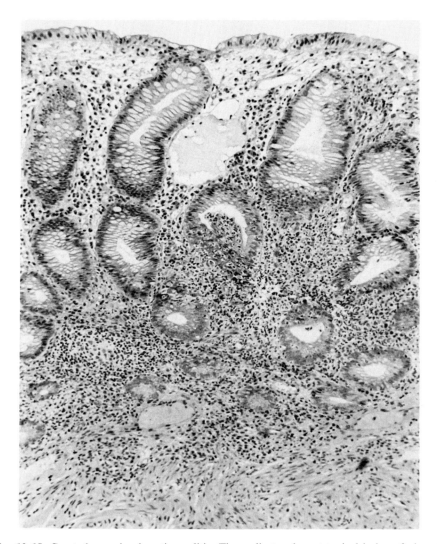

Fig. 13-15. Crypt abscess in ulcerative colitis. The earliest and most typical lesion of ulcerative colitis is a crypt abscess, an accumulation of polymorphonuclear cells in a crypt of Lieberkühn with breakdown of its wall. The superficial epithelial layer is well preserved in this case.

stage, mucosal inflammation is severe, with an increase in the lymphocyte and plasma cell content of the lamina propria and focal polymorphonuclear infiltration. The presence of crypt abscesses (Fig. 13-15) is compatible with ulcerative colitis. Acute bacterial *(Salmonella, Shigella, Yersinia, Campylobacter)* colitis may give rise to the same findings. Furthermore crypt abscesses are described in Crohn's disease. If there is severe mucosal destruction and the formation of ulcers, the superficial tela submucosa may be infiltrated with inflammatory cells. The mucosal epithelium shows varying degrees of destruction; often it appears to be melting away, and goblet cells are notably absent.

The inflammatory process may at times invade the submucosa and muscular layers. The resulting deeper ulcerations coalesce and form deep furrows in the long axis of the colon (Fig. 13-16). In certain cases, the mucosal inflammatory response is totally nonspecific: vasculitis is characterized by thickening of vessel walls and thrombi.

In a matter of a few weeks, the mucosal inflammation may subside dramatically and the goblet cell population return. There may be atrophy with diminution in the number and size of the glands as well as branching of the crypts and thickening of the lamina muscularis mucosae in patients who have had repeated bouts of colitis. There are also some patients in whom the inflammation is a more

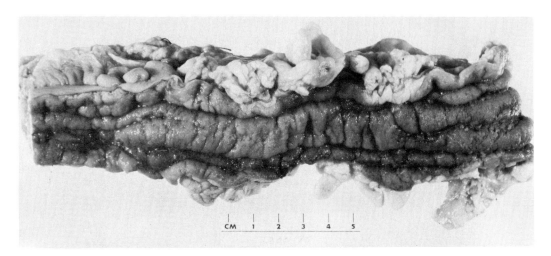

Fig. 13-16. Ulcerative colitis is primarily a mucosal disease with infrequent initial involvement of the other layers. However, in long-standing cases, the adjacent submucosa often participates in the process. This specimen shows pronounced thickening of the colon and deep linear ulcerations undermining the mucosa and extending into the submucosa.

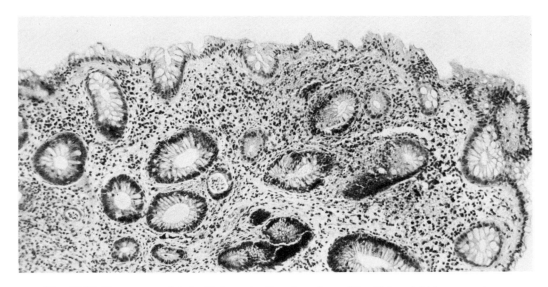

Fig. 13-17. Changes associated with long-standing ulcerative colitis. This rectal biopsy specimen shows a loss of the normal parallelism of the crypts. Several are atrophic, and there are foci of acute inflammatory cells. The specimen was taken from an asymptomatic 15-year-old girl who has had ulcerative colitis for 6 years. Roentgenograms and endoscopy were negative at the time this biopsy section was obtained.

continuous process of low-grade activity in which the salient features of acute disease are muted. Serial biopsies can be profitable when one is monitoring the response to therapy (Fig. 13-17) and have been used in adults to identify signs of severe epithelial dysplasia that may represent a precancerous lesion.

Now accepted is the concept that carcinoma does not arise from morphologically normal mucosa but from a precarcinomatous lesion, which can be identified. It occurs almost exclusively in patients with long-standing pancolitis and may be present in flat mucosa and hyperplastic mucosa and in polypoid mucosal lesions. The crypt architecture shows branching and may assume a villous configuration. The cells lining the crypts are crowded together; they show hyperchromatic nuclei and numerous mitoses in the upper portion of the crypts. The pathologist may have difficulty separating dysplasia from the epithelial hyperplasia caused by regeneration, since in the latter there is invariably acute inflammation.

Clinical course

Ulcerative colitis is a disease that is highly variable in severity, clinical course, and ultimate prognosis. The initial as well as subsequent exacerbations may be insidious or abrupt. Neither the severity of the initial attack nor the paucity of early symptoms has any prognostic value in children. However, it is said that adults with severe or fulminant ulcerative colitis commonly remain more refractory to medical therapy.

Basically, ulcerative colitis is defined as an acute or chronic recurrent disease. Clinical observation and long-term follow-up studies in children permit the identification of two distinct patterns of the disease, which are as follows.

Remitting colitis. The most commonly seen form of ulcerative colitis is the remitting type. The patient has remissions and exacerbations that are likely to be severe and frequent during the first few years of this disease. After this initial stage, a permanent remission may occur, or the pattern continues in a manner seen in the chronic, continuous type. It has been reported that in the remitting type of disease the risk of carcinomatosis is lower, but this remains controversial.

Chronic, continuous colitis. Patients with chronic, continuous colitis are never very sick, but neither are they ever well. A complete remission can never be documented. Intestinal symptoms may be minimal. Chronic malnutrition and anemia are common, but diarrhea is mild, and rectal bleeding may be completely absent. In contrast to the children with the remitting type of ulcerative colitis, the ones with the chronic, continuous clinical course respond poorly to medical therapy.

Pancolitis versus ulcerative proctitis and left-sided colitis. The extent of the disease has very important clinical implications with regard to the severity of symptoms, the response to treatment, the need for hospitalization and for surgery, the degree of invalidism, and most importantly the risk for carcinomatosis.

Pancolitis. The majority (80%) of children with ulcerative colitis have universal involvement of their colon 5 years after onset, whereas the corresponding figure in adults probably does not exceed 50%. When the diagnosis is first made, roentgenographic findings identify lesions proximal to the splenic flexure in 50% of our patients, and at rectosigmoidoscopy there are no identifiable limits to them. These patients have a higher incidence of extraintestinal manifestations, with hypoalbuminemia and anemia being invariably present and toxic megacolon a threat. Recurrences tend to be severe during the first few years, and response to therapy can be a problem. Surgery has to be carried out within the first few years in 20% to 30%. After the first few years, a certain number become relatively asymptomatic (chronic continuous colitis) and are handicapped by a burnt-out colitis. They run a high-risk of carcinomatosis, especially since a proctocolectomy is difficult to sell to patients who are not severely handicapped by their disease.

Ulcerative proctitis and left-sided colitis. Only a small percentage (20%) of children have ulcerative colitis limited to the rectum, the sigmoid, and the descending colon. If one relies on roentgenographic findings at diagnosis, as many as 50% do not have lesions in the ascending colon and in the transverse colon, but in the majority roentgenographic evidence of pancolitis will become apparent over the next 5 years. A large-scale adult study has shown that 30% of cases in whom roentgenographic changes were limited to the left colon can be expected to develop more extensive disease in a 5-year-period.

Ulcerative proctitis is an inflammatory process limited to the rectum or rectosigmoid junction. The symptoms consist of rectal bleeding, mild diarrhea, abdominal cramping, and tenesmus. Extracolonic manifestations are rare, and the disease only has minimal repercussions on the patient's general state of health. The response to treatment is good, but relapses occur. Surgery is rarely necessary. In such cases microscopic examination reveals that the disease process also involved the descending colon. In 10% of adult cases, the disease becomes more extensive. On the other hand, spontaneous remissions also occur. Experience with this form of ulcerative colitis is very limited in children. Most of the cases we have seen have extended to the left colon as compared to a 30% chance in adults.

Left-sided colitis is associated with a more severe form of disease. Extraintestinal manifestations and recurrences are more frequent and severe, and surgery may be necessary. In adults, the chance of extension of the disease proximal to the splenic flexure within 5 years after the original diagnosis has been estimated to be 21% by roentgenographic study but only 10% by a colonoscopic study. In our experience, a serious relapse of left-sided colitis in children often indicates the development of universal colitis.

Diagnosis

A number of conditions may, at times, mimic the clinical, proctoscopic, histologic, or roentgenographic findings, with the entity most difficult to dislodge from this group being granulomatous colitis. Infections, infestations with amebas, connective tissue diseases, pseudomembranous colitis, allergic gastroenteropathy, and the irritable colon syndrome are the entities that also need to be ruled out.

The diagnosis of ulcerative colitis in the typical patient is not difficult. However, an alert clinician can also suspect this diagnosis in children who merely have a change in bowel habits, experience an acute nonspecific gastroenteritis, or pass a few drops of blood painlessly in a normal stool. Hemorrhoids are rare in children, and anal fissures are invariably seen in children with the history of the painful defecation of constipated stools. When there is reasonable doubt about the possibility of ulcerative colitis, proctoscopy, rectal biopsy, and barium enema should be carried out.

Endoscopic findings do not invariably permit the establishment of a positive diagnosis of ulcerative colitis, but certain conditions can be ruled out when one is aware of their distinguishing features:

Infectious colitis
  Intense mucosal hyperemia with much sticky mucus.
  Mucosa is generally not so fragile as in ulcerative colitis.
Amebic colitis
  Ulcers are deep and "punched out." They are invariably surrounded by a rim of intense erythema.
Pseudomembranous colitis
  Yellowish plaques small and widely disseminated or large and confluent on a mucosa that is not very friable.
Crohn's colitis
  Rectosigmoidoscopy and rectal biopsy specimens are normal in more than two thirds of children with Crohn's disease. If colitis is present, patchy lesions of mucosal erythema with a moderate degree of friability and ulcerations may be seen. The presence of tiny aphthous ulcerations in a normal-looking mucosa is an early and reliable sign of granulomatous colitis.

Complications

The many, varied complications of ulcerative colitis are likely to occur at any time during the course of the disease. They can be classified as local and systemic. Because of the special concern for the risk of carcinoma, it is discussed separately.

Local complications

Hemorrhoids. Hemorrhoids are a complication more frequently encountered in ulcerative colitis than in Crohn's disease. It is rare in children and mentioned only because hemorrhoids are easily confused with skin tags, a very frequent finding in Crohn's disease.

Fissures. Anal fissures are less frequently seen in ulcerative colitis than in granulomatous disease. The patient with a fissure who has no consistent history of constipation, and especially if he

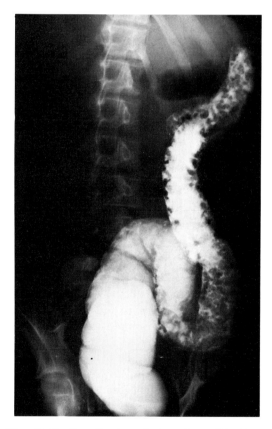

Fig. 13-18. Complication of ulcerative colitis. Pseudopolypoid formation is dramatically illustrated. The pseudopolyps are more likely to occur in severe cases and are the result of accumulated normal mucosa separated by deep ulcerations.

has experienced some rectal bleeding, should be suspected of having ulcerative colitis. On the other hand, anorectal fistulas and perirectal disease are rare in ulcerative colitis and common in Crohn's disease.

Perforations and fistulas. With progression of the disease, ulcers within the mucosa may extend to outer layers of the bowel wall, leading to perforations, which are occasionally free. They commonly evolve slowly, thereby creating internal fistulas with other loops of bowel or with an extraintestinal organ. Perforations occur more rapidly in a patient with toxic megacolon.

Strictures. The chronic course interspersed by acute exacerbations leads to strictures mostly in the rectosigmoid and less frequently in the transverse colon. These strictures are the apparent result of hypertrophy of the tunica muscularis mucosae and are potentially reversible.

Pseudopolyps. This is a very common complication of long-standing disease. Pseudopolyps represent islands of inflamed mucosa surrounded by ravaged atrophic mucosa. With time, pseudopolyps will grow and project into the lumen (Fig. 13-18). Some remain sessile; others become pedunculated. Bleeding from these inflammatory polyps (Fig. 13-19) is rare, but their presence indicates severe disease. Giant inflammatory polyps are described in adults, in whom they may be mistaken for a carcinoma and may lead to obstruction, particularly in burnt-out colitis, when the colon is narrowed by chronic changes.

Toxic megacolon. Although in fulminating cases colonic dilatation is occasionally noted, toxic

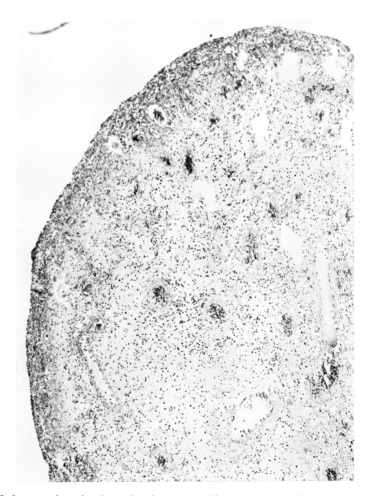

Fig. 13-19. Large pedunculated pseudopolyp removed from a 14-year-old girl with pancolitis who had protracted rectal bleeding.

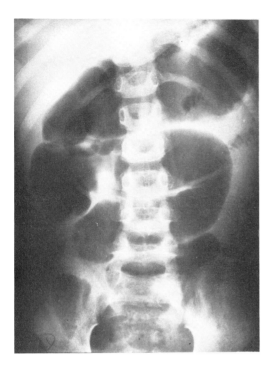

Fig. 13-20. Toxic megacolon in an 18-year-old child who had been treated medically. Despite conservative management of this dramatic complication, surgery had to be performed.

megacolon is infrequent in children. Early warning signs include a steadily progressive inflammatory process and a relentlessly deteriorating course. The temperature rises, the bowel sounds and diarrhea diminish, and the abdomen becomes more distended, tender, and tympanitic.

Toxic megacolon may occur in 5 to 10% of patients with inflammatory bowel disease; it is more frequent in ulcerative colitis than in Crohn's colitis. It usually is indicative of pancolitis with intense inflammation and deeply penetrating ulcerations. This then produces ileus and dilatation. The role of antidiarrheal agents (opiates and anticholinergics) and an antecedent barium enema examination has been underscored by many studies. Plain films (Fig. 13-20) will show segmental or universal dilatation of the colon. There is an absence of the haustral pattern and pneumatosis may be seen.

The patient is toxic and often tends to go into shock. Hypoalbuminemia and electrolyte disturbances are invariably present. Gram-negative sepsis, massive hemorrhage, and perforation are life-threatening complications. Nasogastric suction, intravenous fluid, albumin, whole blood, antibiot-

ics, and corticosteroids should be promptly started, and a surgeon should be on the alert for a complication or a clinical condition that fails to improve over a 72-hour period.

Massive hemorrhage. This rare complication may occur as the opening symptom, but it occurs more frequently in the course of an exacerbation in patients with the remitting type of colitis.

Systemic complications

Growth retardation and delayed puberty. Profound retardation of physical growth and sexual development can be one of the most devastating of all systemic complications of ulcerative colitis and may be a compelling indication for colectomy. However, it is much less commonly seen than in Crohn's disease.

Ankylosing spondylitis. Spndylitis and colitis tend to cluster in families. In contrast to the arthropathy that is an extraintestinal manifestation of ulcerative colitis and parallels the activity of the bowel disease, spondylitis may precede or follow the onset of colitis and progresses more or less independently of the primary disease. Although more frequently associated with ulcerative colitis, it may also occur in Crohn's disease. We have not seen ankylosing spondylitis in children with colitis. Because of the association between spondylitis and uveitis, the teenager with uveitis should be screened for the possibility of spondylitic colitis. It is of interest that both conditions have been found to be associated with the histocompatibility antigen HLA-B27.

Nephrolithiasis. Five percent of adults with inflammatory disease of the bowel eventually develop renal stones. In those patients who have had a proctocolectomy and ileostomy, calcium oxalate stones are frequently described (Chapter 10).

Hepatic lesions. Over the years, it has become evident that there is a high correlation between hepatic dysfunction and ulcerative colitis, and this is particularly true if the latter is of long standing. Chronic active hepatitis is commonly an associated disease rather than a complication. Pericholangitis is a complication of the colitis and may progress to cirrhosis.

Thrombophlebitis. Rarely described in the pediatric age group, thrombophlebitis can be a disastrous complication. We have seen a 16-year-old who had chronic continuous colitis and suffered a deep ileofemoral thrombophlebitis.

Carcinoma. The association of cancer of the large intestine and ulcerative colitis is well known.

The risk is believed to be high in patients whose disease starts in childhood and during adolescence, but this belief has been recently challenged. Susceptibility to neoplastic degeneration increases with the duration of ulcerative colitis. Most of the patients who develop carcinoma of the colon have had their disease for 10 years or longer. Although there have been no reports of cancer developing before 7 years, our own experience with one patient with pancolitis treated for 2 years and in whom the onset of the disease could be traced back for only 5 years is of some concern. The cumulative cancer risk is only 5% at 10 years; it then rises to 25% at 20 years. After 20 years, the chances for the development of carcinoma of the colon are 50%. Other studies were carried out in adults and show a 3.5% risk at 10 years, with a yearly increase of 1% subsequently.

Patients with total colonic involvement are particularly at risk. The risk is very small in those with proctitis (rectosigmoiditis) and with left-sided colitis. In one study the incidence of cancer was 5% and the median duration of the disease was 32 years. Corresponding figures in a group with universal colitis were 13% and 20 years. More optimistic are the views expressed by another group stating that the risk of carcinomatosis in left-sided colitis is slightly if at all greater than that of the normal population. The severity of the disease influences very little the risk of carcinomatosis. The patient with the chronic continuous type of colitis is more at risk because it is unlikely that a proctocolectomy will be done on the basis of a relatively mild disease. In fact, studies show that 55% of patients with cancer had mild disease with no extraintestinal manifestations and little in the way of systemic and local complications.

It is important to remember that the carcinomas of ulcerative colitis are poorly differentiated and metastasize early. The prognosis for a 5-year survival is about 25%. Even the most conscientious efforts may fail to detect a carcinoma in time. Carcinomas complicating ulcerative colitis differ from spontaneously occurring lesions in that they have less predilection for the rectosigmoid area. They tend to be multiple, flat, and intramural with rapid spread, and they are intrinsically more malignant than other carcinomas. Conventional roentgenographic examination is unsatisfactory. Dysplasia is a precarcinomatous lesion that can be detected by endoscopy. Since dysplasia is a focal lesion, multiple biopsies should be done, particu-

larly in areas where there are suspicious changes such as polypoid and nodular formations and also plaque-like areas. The yield appears just as good with rectosogmoidoscopy as with colonoscopy. The latter is theoretically better and should be repeated every third year, whereas proctoscopy can be done yearly and has the advantage of providing deeper biopsies. The detection of dysplasia should lead to elective surgery. Of concern is the presence of carcinoma in a sizable proportion of colons removed electively.

Treatment

The management of ulcerative colitis requires a great deal of attention because it is directed to the care of the patient rather than to the disease process. The patient must be seen frequently, particularly during the acute stage of the disease. Subtle symptoms should be looked for, especially since overt symptoms may be absent in the presence of ongoing, smoldering disease. The disorder is life long and invalidating physically and psychologically. Children need to be told that treatment has improved over the past decade and that their disease can be medically controlled or surgically cured so that they can enjoy a normal life style and life expectancy.

Diet and activity. Although a high-protein, high-carbohydrate, normal-fat, high-vitamin diet is recommended, it is difficult for the sick child to take. The main concern should be serving meals that the child will eat. It is sometimes better to allow the patient to choose his own diet, espcially in the acute stages of the disease, when anorexia can be quite a problem. The frequent incidence (40%) of decreased lactase activity during the first few months of the disease may warrant trial of a milk-free diet, espcially if symptoms are slow to respond to other measures.

No blanket policy exists for controlling the activity of these children. One should individualize the amount of physical activity permitted according to the clinical condition of the patient. Similarly, early resumption of schoolwork should be advised on the condition that the patient is not pushing himself beyond his physical capabilities.

Hospitalization. A change of environment is often strikingly beneficial for the patient. Furthermore, it permits the physician sustained contact with the patient and his family. Such contact is essential not only for a complete diagnostic evaluation but also for the thorough indoctrination of the parents in the nature and outlook of the disease as well as for planning the therapeutic approach and long-term care.

In severe attacks of chronic ulcerative colitis, especially in those children with abdominal distention and dehydration, hospitalization is mandatory. Adequate fluid replacement, repair of plasma or blood volume contraction, and use of hydrocortisone or ACTH and a broad-spectrum antibiotic may all be needed on admission. Signs of toxicity or vomiting warrants nasogastric suction. Parenteral alimentation may sometimes be used for a few weeks (pp. 368 and 874).

Antidiarrheal agents. Opiates are useful for ameliorating pain but should be used with caution in the acute severe stages of the disease. Anticholinergic agents reduce rectal spasm and can be effective when used continuously. Diphenoxylate (Lomotil) has been disappointing in pediatric patients, and we have abandoned its use. Imodium has been totally ineffective.

Sulfasalazine (salicylazosulfapyridine). It is well known that salicylazosulfapyridine (now officially sulfasalazine) is of therapeutic benefit in the management of ulcerative colitis. This medication combines in the same molecule a salicylate and a sulfonamide moiety. It is split in the colon by the microflora, and the sulfapyridine is absorbed, transformed in the liver, and excreted in the urine. The 5-aminosalicylic acid, on the other hand, is largely unabsorbed and is believed to be the active anti-inflammatory agent, though the possibility that sulfapyridine during its passage through the colonic mucosa may also be effective has not been ruled out.

Side reactions to this drug are frequent and are related to serum sulfapyridine levels, which tend to be significantly affected not only by the dosage used but also by the capacity of the liver to acetylate (slow and fast acetylator phenotypes). The serious side effects need to be anticipated and recognized early. A serum sickness–like reaction can be serious, with fever, arthritis, and erythema multiforme. More common is a Heinz body hemolytic anemia, which should also force discontinuation. We have not seen the peculiar "cyanosis" complication, nor have we documented agranulocytosis. Anemia may not only be attributable to hemolysis but also to interference with folic acid absorption (Chapter 10). Attention has been recently drawn to bloody diarrhea, vomiting, and fever are a triad of symptoms attributable to the

drug rather than to a flare-up of the disease, We have seen two patients who had explosive diarrhea repeatedly triggered by sufasalazine. Since exacerbations of ulcerative colitis have been reported in association with the presence of *Clostridium difficile,* it is of interest to speculate that the growth of this organism could be facilitated by the drugs.

Because of the extremely common side effects of anorexia, nausea, and headache, the drug should be introduced gradually and taken with food. We recommend either the enteric-coated or the non–enteric coated tablets at a dose of 500 mg. If the drug is well tolerated, the dose is increased gradually to 3 to 4 gm daily over a period of 1 week. Because the therapeutic efficacy of the drug is entirely dependent on the bacterial azo-splitting of the molecule in the colon, antibiotics should not be used concomitantly by the oral route. Weekly checks on the white blood cell count and on a red blood cell smear and hematocrit reading are essential during the first month or two of therapy or at any time when the dosage is increased. Over the past few years, there has been a net tendency to decrease the total dosage administered. There is no indication that a dosage exceeding 3 to 4 gm/24 hr is advantageous from a therapeutic point of view, and the evidence clearly shows that side effects are more frequent with a larger dosage.

Sulfasalazine is used alone in mild cases of ulcerative colitis, in combinaton with corticosteroid enemas in left-sided colitis, and in association with oral prednisone in patients who are severely ill and have extraintestinal manifestations. Sulfasalazine suppositories and enemas are reportedly effective when the disease process is limited to the rectum and rectosigmoid junction. There is now strong evidence that a dosage of 500 mg administered four times a day should be continued indefinitely to prevent recurrences unless it is contraindicated by side effects.

ACTH and corticosteroids. In severe attacks of ulcerative colitis, ACTH or hydrocortisone, given intravenously, are indicated. Some authors prefer ACTH 80 units/1.73 m^2; we use hydrocortisone 10 mg/kg/day over a period of 7 to 10 days. With clinical improvement, intravenous therapy is discontinued in favor of oral prednisone 1 to 2 mg/kg with a maximum of 60 mg/day to be continued for a period of 6 to 8 weeks. Gradual weaning should then take place over a period of several weeks with special attention being paid to symptoms likely because of an exacerbation or a relapse.

Long-term morbidity and mortality studies of ulcerative colitis in the eras before and since the use of steroids show a reduction of mortality by one half. Nevertheless, continuous steroid treatment should not be undertaken lightly, especially in children. Maintenance steroids (prednisone), 7.5 to 15 mg/24 hr, should be reserved for cases in which more conservative measures fail. Unfortunately, some children with ulcerative colitis will require prolonged treatment with corticosteroids. There is no good study on the value of long-term prednisone treatment of the chronic continuous type of ulcerative colitis compared to that of a placebo. However, clinical experience dictates that it is a sound approach in a certain percentage of patients, since stopping of steroid therapy in such patients results in a flare-up of the disease. The physician must choose between colectomy and the long-term use of a larger dose of prednisone with the associated complications (growth failure, iatrogenic hyperadrenocorticism, osteoporosis with vertebral collapse).

Administration of prednisone, 10 to 15 mg in a single dose on alternate days, has been found to be effective once control of the acute symptoms has been achieved by full daily dosage. Alternate-day therapy is instituted in the following manner. Once the patient is under satisfactory control with prednisone 20 mg/day, the even-day dosage is decreased weekly by 2.5 to 5 mg, and the dosage of 20 mg is maintained on uneven days. Subsequently, the odd-day dose of 20 mg should be reduced to 10 to 15 mg if possible. With this regimen, patients can remain essentially free of symptoms and side effects. It is often difficult to disentangle the respective role of corticosteroid therapy from that of ongoing smoldering disease giving rise to a few symptoms. A dosage of 10 mg/day of prednisone is believed to be sufficient to impair growth; therefore alternate-day therapy has significant advantages in this respect. Remember, however, that maintenance prednisone (15 mg/day) has not been shown to prevent recurrences in adults in remission from their disease. Therefore attempts at weaning children completely from prednisone should be made under close supervision before one decides that maintanance therapy on a daily or alternate-day basis is necessary.

Corticosteroid retention enemas are particularly useful in cases of proctosigmoiditis and left-sided colitis. A recent study has shown that most patients who fail to respond had, by colonoscopy, a form of disease that extended beyond the left colon. Moderate absorption of the prednisolone occurs and may give rise to some degree of adrenal suppression. This form of therapy has no place in the treatment of pancolitis though it may serve as an adjunt to sulfasalazine in cases where rectal disease is particularly severe. We recommend Cortenema or methylprednisolone acetate (Depo-Medrol) 20 to 40 mg in 100 ml of saline solution on a twice-a-day basis initially. With abatement of symptoms, this can be reduced to a once-a-day administration at bedtime. The knee-chest position is preferable during the administration, and then the child is asked to stay in bed for an hour or so. The Cortifoam preparation should be reserved for cases where the proctitis is limited to the distal part of the rectum though this form of disease is very rare in children.

Immunosuppressive drugs. Azathioprine (Imuran) has been used both acutely and chronically. None of the few clinical trials offer convincing evidence that azathioprine (Imuran) is effective in the treatment of an acute attack of ulcerative colitis when added to corticosteroids. There is a suggestion, however, that it may have a role in the maintenance treatment of the disease. Azathioprine has an anti-inflammatory effect and does permit, in certain instances, a significant reduction of steroid dosage, particularly in those patients who require large maintenance dosage of corticosteroids to remain clinically well. There is no clear-cut evidence to indicate that clinical improvement is related directly to any effect that azathioprine may have on the immune response. Potential side effects and hazards such as risk of infection, bone marrow depression, and risk of pancreatitis should be taken into consideration. Concern for the risk of malignancy, particularly since ulcerative colitis is in itself carcinogenic, has largely disappeared, since azathioprine-associated malignancies have been reported only in transplant patients. Treatment whould be started in the hospital, and the patient needs to be followed closely. The dosage we have been using is 2 mg/kg/24 hr. We have seen relapses on withdrawal of immunosupressive therapy.

Other drugs. We have had no experience with disodium cromoglycate, a mast cell membrane stabilizer. Most studies do not report that this drug is effective except, perhaps, in the treatment of proctitis, a rare disease in children that responds to other forms of treatment. Metronidazole has also been used in chronic proctitis, but it has not proved to be effective.

Hyperalimentation. Although there is good experimental evidence from a research team in our unit that parenteral nutrition or enteral alimentation with an elemental diet induces dramatic atrophic changes in the colon, results in ulcerative colitis have been disappointing. Total bowel rest is highly effective in Crohn's disease (see next section), but it has not been useful in inducing remissions in ulcerative colitis. However, total parenteral nutrition is a precious adjunct for nutritional rehabilitation of the severely malnourished and for meeting the nutritional needs of children with severe colitis (Chapter 29).

Surgery

Fulminant colitis. Emergency surgery is lifesaving in the case of fulminant disease with toxic megacolon. These patients should be identified early, and as soon as toxic megacolon is suspected, a surgeon should be consulted. If after 72 hours of nasogastric suction, appropriate replacement of fluid, electrolytes, colloids, and red blood cell mass deficits and administration of parenteral antibiotics and corticosteroids there is little improvement, a subtotal colectomy and ileostomy should be done. Evidence of perforation or peritonitis is an indication for immediate surgery. There are no data in children, but in adults about two thirds of cases with toxic megacolon require surgery.

Severe attacks of fulminant colitis may not necessarily be associated with a large amount of air in the colon, but the patient may be just as toxic. Gram-negative sepsis and massive hemorrhage may complicate the clinical picture. We believe that these patients deserve surgery if there is little or no response to aggressive medical treatment and parenteral alimentation over a period of 1 to 2 weeks. This approach appears to be warranted, especially since the pediatric experience for this category of patients is that within 2 years 40% will require surgery because of intractability of the disease and serious complications.

Long-standing colitis. Recent series suggest that 20% to 30% of children and adolescents with ulcerative colitis require surgery within 5 years of the onset of their disease. The following are indications for elective surgery:

Invalidating disease with chronic ongoing colitis despite 2 years of adequate medical therapy

Severe growth retardation before epiphyseal closure

Serious side effects in patients who require a high dosage of steroids

Pancolitis of a duration of more than 7 years with evidence of a dysplastic mucosa

Type of operation. In contrast to Crohn's disease, ulcerative colitis is surgically curable. Proctocolectomy in one or two stages has been the most commonly practiced and accepted operation. Children adapt quite readily to an ileostomy. Although life with an ileostomy has serious drawbacks, most patients accept this handicap as a significant improvement over the disability of a serious disease. Results are truly dramatic and a normal life expectancy is at hand after a proctocolectomy. For the small number of patients who do not adjust satisfactorily to an ileostomy, a continent ileostomy can be suggested. Kock's procedure consists in constructing an ileal reservoir and a flush skin-level stoma. The patient empties the pouch several times a day with a tube and keeps a gauze pad on the stoma.

Colectomy and ileorectal anastomosis has been favored by many groups, particularly in England and in France. It is believed that the diseased rectum tends to heal after the procedure. The operation is contraindicated when rectal disease is severe. In other cases, an initial colectomy and ileostomy is followed later by an ileorectal anastomosis. If rectal involvement is mild, colectomy and ileorectal anastomosis are done in one stage. Meticulous supervision of the preserved rectum is mandatory. Persistent rectal disease is of significant concern; in only 30% of pediatric patients was an acceptable result obtained. The rectum had to be removed in more than 50%. Others suggest a figure of 75% for proctectomy within 5 years.

In the past few years, there have been several reports of a successful ileoanal-endorectal anastomosis after a total colectomy and a mucosal proctectomy. The rectal mucosa is stripped from the muscular wall of the rectum, and the ileum is sutured to the ileal mucosa. The chances for a successful operation are said to be enhanced by a 4- to 6-week period of parenteral alimentation and rectal steroids to facilitate dissection of the mucosa.

Psychotherapy. The need for a formal psychiatric referral is individualized. The physician responsible for the total care of the patient has a

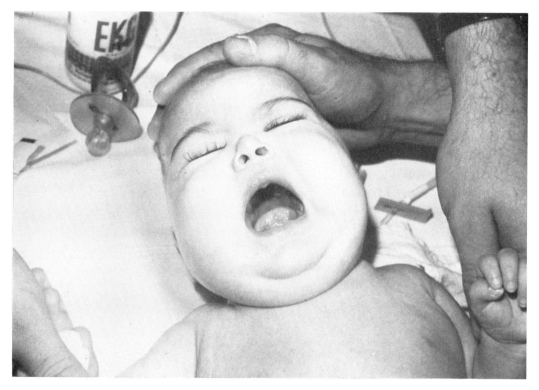

Fig. 13-21. Severe side effects of prednisone therapy in an infant with ulcerative colitis. The disease proved resistant to large doses that led to a number of complications. Surgery had to be performed when the infant was 10 months of age.

dual role in the emotional health of children with ulcerative colitis: (1) he must try to modify the patient's environment by reducing stressful situations, and (2) he must work at increasing the patient's tolerance for a chronic illness attended by complications.

The child with this disease should be seen regularly in the office and given a chance to openly discuss his illness. The physician must be supportive and understanding without fostering self-pity and invalidism. It is wise to utilize a multidisciplinary approach as long as the pediatrician remains at the hub and can call on the services of his surgical and psychiatric colleagues as the need arises.

Prognosis

It is practically impossible to make a long-term prognosis for the individual patient recovering from his first attack of ulcerative colitis. However, the extent of the initial disease and the severity of the first attack provide useful indicators. In patients who are very sick (30% to 50%), anemic, and hypoalbuminemic, the response to medical management is usually satisfactory at first, but a significant number will require surgery within a few years. A few fail to go into a remission and cannot be weaned from a large dose of steroids. This has been particularly true in infants. (Fig. 13-21).

The long-term use of sulfasalazine has significant protective value against exacerbations, but the degree of protection is variable. Exacerbations may follow respiratory infections, emotional upsets, infectious gastroenteritis, or perhaps a control barium enema. In most cases, exacerbations occur without apparent provocation and may be fulminant especially during the first few years. The mortality from a severe initial attack or a fulminant exacerbation is very low.

The chances of a complete and permanent remission after the first bout are much less than the 10% recorded for adults. Most patients have relapses that are mild to moderately severe. A remarkable feature of ulcerative colitis is the speed with which the patient and his colon recover from exacerbations. Most pediatric patients initially diagnosed as having proctitis will have an extension of their disease shortly after the first attack. Perhaps 30% of our patients have left-sided colitis. The disease is better controlled with drugs, and exacerbations are less frequent and severe. Total colonic involvement affects the majority, and relapses tend to be worse during the first few years.

More than 50% of children do well on medical therapy and have a normal life style. The disease is smoldering but gives rise to few symptoms except during acute bouts. In others, the inflammatory process is continuously active and is inadequately controlled by drugs. This chronic continuous type of clinical course is disabling, and elective surgery is required for 20% of patients so affected within 5 years.

The present concern is for children with pancolitis who are doing reasonably well on medical therapy and who run a high risk of carcinomatosis. A surveillance program is in order to detect mucosal dysplasia. Surgical advances permitting removal of the colon and of the diseased mucosa with intestinal continuity and the rectum being preserved will, we hope, improve the quality of life and assure a normal life expectancy to children with ulcerative colitis.

REFERENCES

Alexander-Williams, J., and Buchmann, P.: Criteria of assessment for suitability and results of ileorectal anastomosis, Clin. Gastroenterol. **9**:409-417, 1980.

Ament, M.E.: Immunodeficiency syndromes and gastrointestinal disease, Pediatr. Clin. North Am. **22**:807-825, 1975.

Baker, W.N.W., Glass, R.E., Ritchie, J.K., and others: Cancer of the rectum following colectomy and ileorectal anastomosis for ulcerative colitis, Br. J. Surg. **65**:862-868, 1978.

Blackstone, M.W., Riddell, R.H., Rogers, B.H.G., and others: Dysplasia-associated lesion or mass detected by colonoscopy in long-standing ulcerative colitis: an indication for colectomy, Gastroenterology **80**:366-374, 1981.

Das, K.M., Morecki, R., Nair, P., and Berkowitz, J.M.: Idiopathic proctitis. I. The morphology of proximal colonic mucosa and its clinical significance, Dig. Dis. Sci. **22**:524-528, 1977.

Devroede, G.J., and Taylor, W.F.: On calculating cancer risk and survival of ulcerative patients with the life table method, Gastroenterology **71**:505-509, 1976.

Farmer, R.G., Whelan, G., and Sivak, M.V.: Colonoscopy in distal colon ulcerative colitis, Clin. Gastroenterol. **9**:297-306, 1980.

Fonkalsrud, E.W., Ament, M.E., and Byrne, W.J.: Clinical experience with total colectomy and endorectal mucosal resection for inflammatory bowel disease, Gastroenterology **77**:156-160, 1979.

Greenstein, A.J., Sachar, D.B., Smith, A., and others: Cancer in universal and left-sided ulcerative colitis: clinical and pathologic features, Mount Sinai J. Med. **46**:25-32, 1979.

Hamilton, J.R., Bruce, G.A., Abdourhaman, M., and Gall, D.G.: Inflammatory bowel disease in children and adolescents, Adv. Pediatr. **26**:311-341, 1979.

Karjoo, M., and McCarthy, B.: Toxic megacolon of ulcerative colitis in infancy, Pediatrics **57**:962-965, 1976.

Lennard-Jones, J.E., Morson, B.C., Ritchie, J., and others: Cancer in colitis: assessment of individual risk by clinical and histologic criteria, Gastroenterology **73**:1280-1289, 1977.

Lindham, S., and Lagercrantz, R.: Ulcerative colitis in childhood: should the rectum be preserved at surgery? Scand. J. Gastroenterol **15**:123-127, 1980.

Martin, L.W., and Le Coultre, C.: Technical considerations in performing total colectomy and Soave endorectal anastomosis for ulcerative colitis, J. Pediatr. Surg. **13**(6D):762-764, 1978.

Meyers, S., and Janowitz, H.D.: The place of steroids in the therapy of toxic megacolon, Gastroenterology **75**:729-731, 1978.

Nugent, F.W., and Haggit, R.C.: Long-term follow-up, including cancer surveillance for patients with ulcerative colitis, Clin. Gastroenterol. **9**:459-476, 1980.

Powell-Tuck, J., Ritchie, J.K., and Lennard-Jones, J.E.: Prognosis of idiopathic proctitis, Scand. J. Gastroenterology **12**:727-732, 1977.

Ritchie, J.K., Powell-Tuck, J., and Lennard-Jones, J.E.: Clinical outcome of the first ten years of ulcerative colitis and proctitis, Lancet **1**:1140-1143, 1978.

Ruddell, W.S.J., Dickinson, R.J., Dixon, M.F., and Axon, A.T.R.: Treatment of distal ulcerative colitis (proctosigmoiditis) in relapse: comparison of hydrocortisone enemas with rectal hydrocortisone foam, Gut **21**:885-889, 1980.

Strauss, R.G., Gwishan, F., Mitros, F., and others: Rectosigmoidal colitis in common variable immunodeficiency disease, Dig. Dis. Sci. **25**:798-801, 1980.

Truelove, S.C., Willoughby, C.P., Lee, E.G., and Kettlewell, M.G.W.: Further experience in the treatment of severe attacks of ulcerative colitis, Lancet **2**:1086-1088, 1978.

Werlin, S.L., and Grand, R.J.: Bloody diarrhea—a new complication of sulfasalazine, J. Pediatr. **92**:450-453, 1978.

Werlin, S.L., and Grand, R.J.: Severe colitis in children and adolescents: diagnosis, course and treatment, Gastroenterology **73**:828-832, 1977.

Crohn's disease

When first described by Crohn, Ginsburg, and Oppenheimer in 1932, the disease was called "regional ileitis." This chronic inflammatory disorder affects any part of the gastrointestinal tract from mouth to anus, and in a small number of patients there is no evidence of ileitis. The term "Crohn's disease" is therefore more appropriate. It has a distinctive pattern of clinical and pathological features (Table 13-6) but none of them taken individually is essential for establishing the diagnosis. When Crohn's disease is limited to the colon, the overlap in the clinical and pathologic feratures with ulcerative colitis is such that in 20% of adults with colitis a precise diagnosis cannot be made.

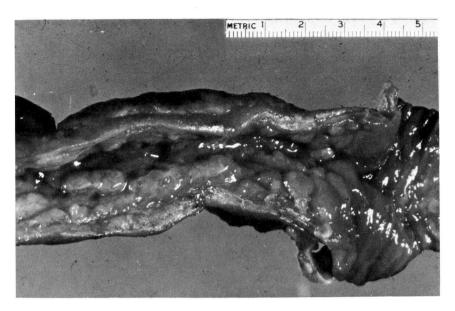

Fig. 13-22. Crohn's disease of the ileum. The bowel wall is greatly thickened. Its mucosal surface is distorted by polypoid masses of heaped mucosa separated by multiple deep, linear ulcerations.

Pathologic condition

The same focal and transmural changes may be observed in this disease no matter which part of the gastrointestinal tract is involved (Fig. 13-22). The bowel wall is thickened; narrowing of the lumen can lead to complete obstruction. The classic hose-pipe stricture is characterized by a rigid, edematous, fibrotic bowel wall. In other cases, longitudinal and transverse deep ulcerations predominate. Mucosa collected between intercommunicating crevices or fissures gives a cobblestone appearance to the involved bowel. Lesions are often discontinuous along the length of the bowel, giving rise to so-called skip areas.

Intestine that lies adjacent to or between diseased segments looks perfectly normal except for a dilated appearance immediately proximal to narrowed or stenotic areas. The surgeon will usually find a greatly thickened, fatty, and edematous mesentery. Fingerlike projections of thick mesentery characteristically extend over the serosal surface toward the antimesenteric border of the bowel (creeping fat). Mesenteric nodes are enlarged, firm, and matted together to form an irregular mass. The indurated mesentery, thickened mesenteric fat, and enlarged lymph nodes commonly lead to deformities of the cecum and ascending colon, which may be mistaken for intrinsic involvement of the colon. Because the serosa and mesentery are regularly inflamed, a characteristic feature is the tendency for involved bowel loops to be firmly matted together by fibrotic peritoneal and mesenteric bands. This adhesive process, in conjunction with the transmural involvement, is responsible for another characteristic phenomenon, the tendency for fistula formation. A fistulous tract may join together diseased bowel loops, but more often it will establish communication between a diseased segment of bowel and a healthy one. Although a fistula may establish a communicating tract with other intra-abdominal organs (bladder, vagina) and structures (perineum, abdominal wall), most often it will end blindly and form an intraperitoneal or retroperitoneal abscess.

Microscopically, a chronic granulomatous inflammatory reaction with edema and fibrosis involves all layers of the intestinal wall. The most useful diagnostic feature is the presence of noncaseating granulomas containing multinucleated giant cells and epithelioid cells (Fig. 13-23). These focal granulomas are found in 60% of resected bowel and in 25% of regional lymph nodes. In the absence of granulomas, the presence of broad ulcerations extending deep into the submucosa (Fig. 13-24) and the muscular layers is suggestive, particularly if submucosal inflammation appears intense and if there are large numbers of lymphoid aggregates. In cases of proximal involvement of

Fig. 13-23. Granuloma and giant cells of Crohn's disease. **A,** The granuloma represented here was found in a rectal biopsy specimen. The lesion, roughly nodular, is composed of epithelial cells with multinucleated giant cells; a dense chronic inflammatory reaction is seen peripherally. **B,** Giant cells are present in a jejunal villus in the absence of other obvious inflammatory changes.

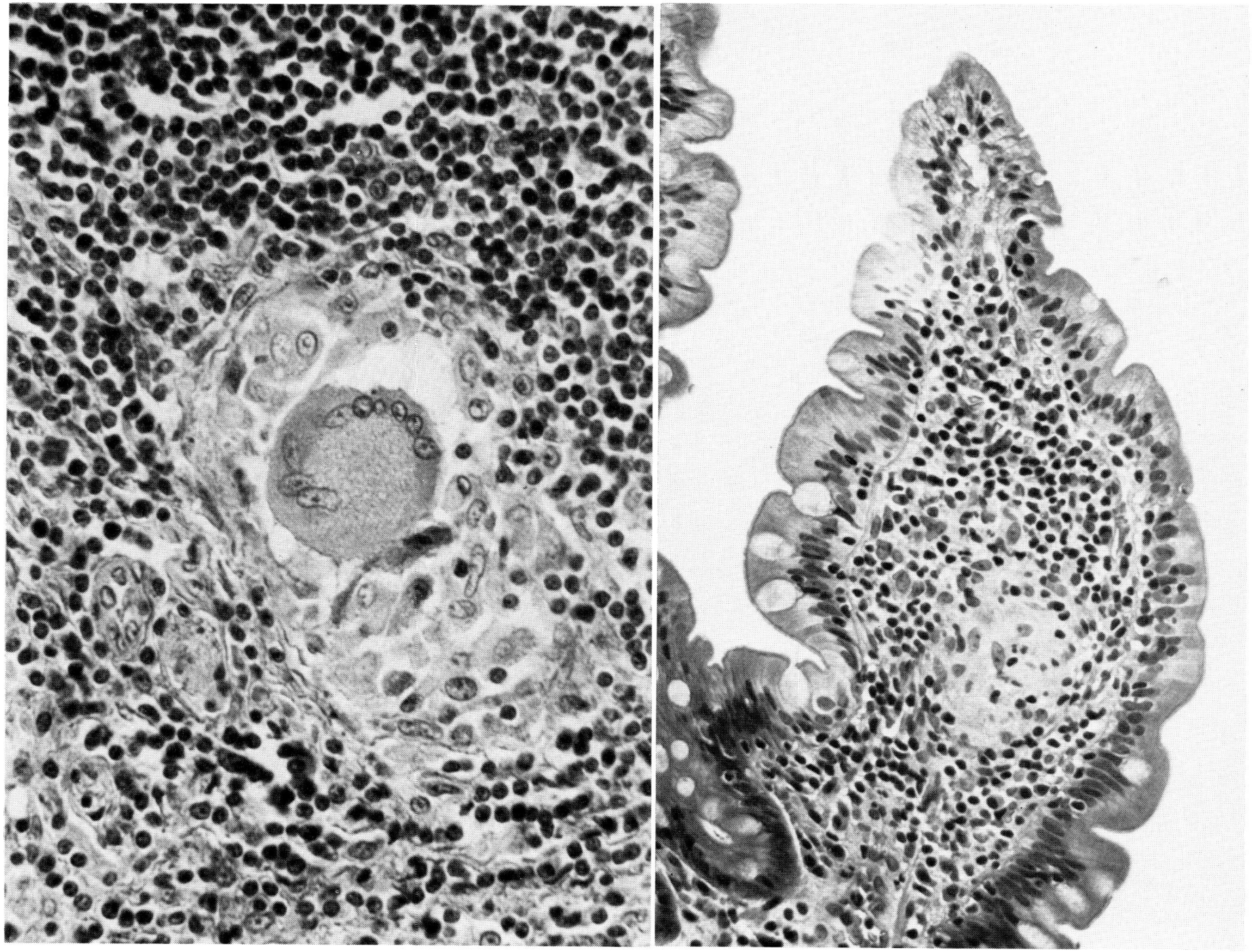

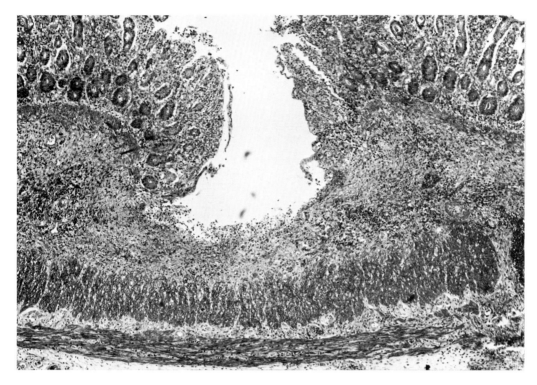

Fig. 13-24. Submucosal ulceration in Crohn's disease. An irregular, somewhat flask-shaped ulceration extending into the tela submucosa through a thickened lamina muscularis mucosae is seen. Nerve tissue is prominent between the two muscular layers. Note the nodular aggregates of lymphoid cells in the submucosa.

the small bowel, a peroral biopsy specimen may be diagnostic if multinucleated cells can be identified in the lamina propria (Fig. 13-23).

Rectal biopsy is an important technique for the differentiation of Crohn's disease from ulcerative colitis (Fig. 13-23). The detection of granulomas is pathognomonic and may be found in the mucosa or submuscosa. Granulomas are commonly found in anal lesions; therefore, if the diagnosis is in doubt, they can be biopsied. The absence of endoscopic findings usually indicates that useful information is unlikely to be found on the biopsy material. Granulomas are not essential to support a clinical diagnosis. An intact mucosa beneath which there is submucosal inflammation is rather typical. Patchy lesions are unusual in ulcerative colitis and more likely in Crohn's disease (Fig. 13-25). In contrast to ulcerative colitis, where ulcerations are disseminated in a diffusely abnormal mucosa, the rectal mucosa early in the course of Crohn's colitis may only show a few small aphthous ulcerations. Later on, the mucosa may be diffusely erythematous but less friable than in

ulcerative colitis and may show cobblestoning, as well as linear and confluent ulcers. Crypt abcesses are not exceptional in Crohn's colitis and should not be considered pathognomonic of ulcerative colitis.

Clinical features

In adult patients the disease will be limited to the ileum in somewhat less than 30% of cases. It involves both the colon and the ileum in 40% and the colon alone in 25%. Diffuse disease (stomach, jejunum, ileum, and often colon) is present in 5% of cases. Finally, a small number may have only anorectal area. Large pediatric series have reported a comparable anatomic distribution, but our experience has been different. The pure colonic form is less frequent, and extensive proximal small bowel involvement is more common (Table 13-7). More than a year usually elapses between onset of symptoms and diagnosis. This interval of time is more than doubled in those who have extensive small bowel disease probably because a smaller number of these patients have

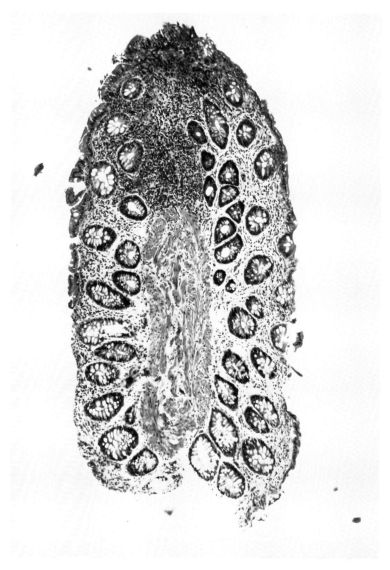

Fig. 13-25. This biopsy specimen of a rectal valve in a patient who had minimal endoscopic changes shows superficial ulceration and disappearance of glands in a focal area of inflammation that reaches beyond the lamina muscularis mucosae.

Table 13-7. Site of disease and duration of symptoms in 93 children with Crohn's disease at Hôpital Sainte-Justine

Site	Percentage	Duration of symptoms (months)
Ileum and colon	61	13 ± 3
Terminal ileum	26	9 ± 2
Extensive small bowel disease	10	31 ± 10
Colon	3	13 ± 7

diarrhea (Fig. 13-26). Anal lesions are said to be less common in children than in adults. However, most children with colonic involvement will have some anorectal abnormality at some time during the course of their disease. When first seen, more than 37% of our patients had either a fissure or a fistula.

The clinical features of Crohn's disease depend to some extent on the part and extent of the gut affected. We have come to consider typical the child with a history of recurrent, ill-localized ab-

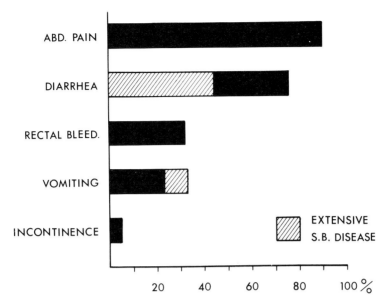

Fig. 13-26. Relative incidence of gastrointestinal symptoms in 93 cases of Crohn's disease in children. Diarrhea is less frequent and vomiting is more common when extensive small bowel disease is present. (Data from LeLuyer, B., et al.: Hôpital Sainte-Justine, Montreal, 1981.)

dominal pain, late afternoon and evening low-grade fever, lassitude, anorexia, and weight loss of several months' duration. However, some of the other modes of presentation listed are also common and explain the long interval between onset of symptoms and diagnosis.

Modes of presentation of Crohn's disease

Fever of undetermined origin
Arthritis (rheumatic fever or rheumatoid arthritis)
Anorexia nervosa
Dwarfism with osteoporosis
Acute appendicitis
Relapsing gastroenteritis
Recurrent mouth sores
Anal fissure, abcess, or fistula

Intestinal manifestations

Abdominal pain. Crampy abdominal pain often triggered by eating is usually the predominant symptom. Defecation does bring about some relief when the colon is involved; in these cases, tenesmus may also be present.

There is no doubt that the abdominal pain of Crohn's disease is much more severe than in ulcerative colitis. In most instances, it is periumbilical, but the pain tends to localize in the right lower quadrant. In adults, one third of the patients may initially have an acute condition of the abdomen mimicking an attack of appendicitis. A similar

mode of presentation does occur in children. In patients in whom the upper gastrointestinal tract is involved, the pain can be epigastric and mimic peptic disease (Fig. 13-27).

Anorexia, nausea, and vomiting. Commonly, appetite progressively decreases during the inital stage of the disease and during acute exacerbations. Many children will decrease their food intake to avoid the abdominal pain that occurs after eating. Nausea and vomiting indicate that the patient is acutely ill or has long-standing disease with partial or complete intestinal obstruction. The anorexia may be severe enough to be mistaken for anorexia nervosa.

Diarrhea. Loose, frequent stools may be the initial complaint. A small number of patients may have the initial clinical picture of a gastroenteritis. When the disease is confined to the small bowel, diarrhea is less frequent and severe than when the colon is involved. Movements may be watery but are more often soft and loose. Urgency of defecation and nocturnal diarrhea are generally present only if the colon is involved. Tenesmus and incontinence indicate that the disease process is present in the rectum. Although consistently bloody bowel movements are more likely to occur in ulcerative colitis, a massive rectal hemorrhage may be the presenting feature in Crohn's disease. The diarrhea of Crohn's disease seldom contains the

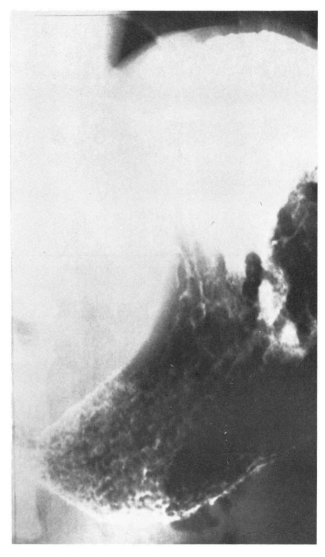

Fig. 13-27. Crohn's gastritis in a 10½-year-old boy who had extensive small bowel involvement. Symptoms were remindful of peptic disease. There is pronounced thickening of central folds, mucosal nodularity, and "cobblestoning."

mucopurulent material seen in ulcerative colitis unless there is acute and severe involvement of the rectosigmoid.

Extraintestinal manifestations. Stomatitis (Fig. 13-28), arthralgia, arthritis, erythema nodosum, pyoderma gangrenosum, conjunctivitis, and uveitis may predominate over the intestinal symptoms. In our experience, a third of patients have joint symptoms and 10% have erythema nodosum. The most frequently encountered extraintestinal manifestation is growth retardation. The majority are below the third percentile for weight, and a third of affected children stand below the third percentile for height by the time a diagnosis is made. Fever (70%) is generally intermittent and, in the absence of complications, rarely exceeds 39° C. A fever of unknown origin should attract attention to the possibility of Crohn's disease.

Physical examination

Most children with Crohn's disease suffer stunted growth by the time the diagnosis is made. Mal-

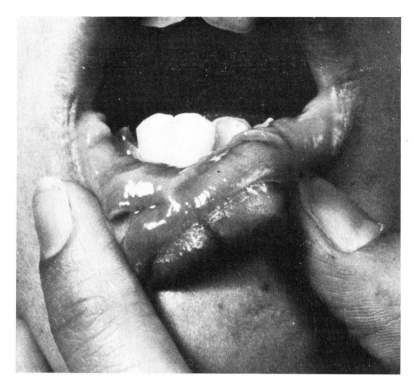

Fig. 13-28. Crohn's stomatitis. The most common type is aphthous stomatitis with superficial and painful ulcerations on the gums and mucosae. This is a rare form with deep fissure-like ulcerations.

nutrition is more or less constant. Children with the disease look chronically ill and debilitated, have recently lost weight, and show evidence of muscle wasting. Peripheral edema and clubbing of the fingers and toes (20%) are common findings (Fig. 13-29). Occasionally, a youngster will present with an "acute abdomen" and is very toxic, but invariably telltale signs of protracted chronic illness are apparent.

The abdomen should be examined with great care. The patient will often pinpoint a precise area of tenderness at palpation. Short of an abdominal mass, in the right lower quadrant the careful examiner may find an area in which there is mild guarding or at least a decrease in the natural softness and mobility of the abdominal contents. Rectal examination may demonstrate an indolent, long-standing anal fissure, ulceration, abscess, fistula, or skin tag, which may precede the abdominal symptoms. In long-standing cases, perirectal disease can become so severe that rectal examination is impossible.

Laboratory findings

In the presence of active disease, the sedimentation rate is usually increased, and an iron-deficiency anemia is documented. Interpretation of other laboratory tests needs to take into consideration the fact that the nutritional problems of children with Crohn's disease result in large part from a grossly inadequate food intake in the face of increased requirements and losses through the diseased intestinal tract.

In our hands, mild to pronounced hypoalbuminemia is present in 60% of cases; the albumin level may drop below 2 gm/dl in patients with extensive small bowel disease. A normal Schilling test does not rule out severe ileal disease, but the test is abnormal in close to 40% of our cases. Steatorrhea, an abnormal D-xylose absorption test, and low serum folate levels are invariably present with proximal small bowel disease. Approximately 25% of children with Crohn's disease have a moderate degree of steatorrhea and increased fecal losses of bile acids. The presence of a stricture

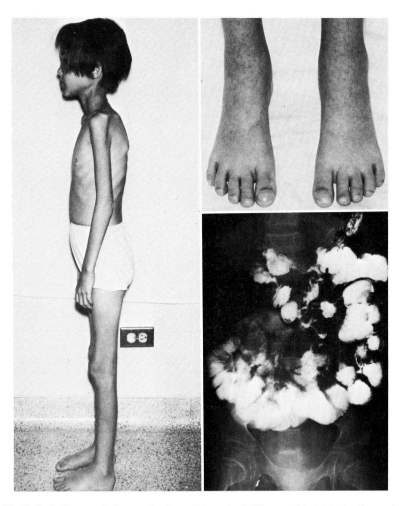

Fig. 13-29. Crohn's disease of the proximal small bowel. A 10-year-old girl had a 3-year history of anorexia, weight loss, arthralgia, anemia, and fever in the evenings. On physical examination, there was considerable wasting, peripheral edema, and clubbing of the fingers and toes. Malabsorption, hypochromic anemia, and hypoproteinemia were documented. The jejunum shows extensive changes, with the ileum relatively normal. During a follow-up period of 4 years, there was no extension of her disease but very little amelioration of her clinical malnutrition. Intermittent courses of antibiotics were temporarily beneficial, but symptoms of partial intestinal obstruction led eventually to a partial resection of the jejunum.

Fig. 13-30. Crohn's ileocolitis. A 4 cm area around the ileocecal valve shows an irregular constriction that extends into the terminal ileum. The remainder of the colon is entirely normal. Ileocecal valve involvement predisposes to bacterial colonization of the small intestine.

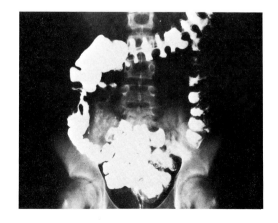

or of a stenotic area of small bowel commonly leads to the contaminated small bowel syndrome (Fig. 13-30) with the malabsorption syndrome described in Chapter 10.

X-ray features

Roentgenographic examination should include both a complete upper gastrointestinal series with small bowel follow-through and a barium enema. Early changes may be limited to peristaltic abnormalities in involved areas. The most common signs are a thickened mucosa with fine irregularities and ulcerations, pseudopolypoid formation with cobblestone appearance, areas of dilatation proximal to stenotic zones with rigid walls, diffuse narrowing of the terminal ileum (Figs. 13-31 and 13-32), longitudinal ulcerations with transverse fissures, and wide separation between small bowel loops. When the colon is involved, there is loss of haustration, ulceration, extensive thumbprinting, and finally, shortening of the colon. Skip areas and a widened space between the rectum and the sacrum are helpful roentgenographic features of Crohn's disease of the large bowel.

Although in most cases of extensive small bowel disease the ileum is involved, there are instances where it is free of disease. Duodenal and jejunal disease is characterized roentgenographically by the presence of stenotic segments and strictures with dilatation of proximal loops. Spasm and irritability of the duodenum are described when jejunitis is present and must be distinguished from the roentgen findings of Crohn's duodenitis. Crohn's gastritis never occurs without coexisting extragastric disease (Fig. 13-27)

In patients who have had surgery, evidence of recurrence or recrudescence should be looked for at the level of the anastomosis or proximal to it. Finally, although clinical remissions are usually associated with the persistence of roentgenographic signs, there are instances of remarkable healing of lesions initially considered to be irreversible. Edema and spasm in diseased areas of

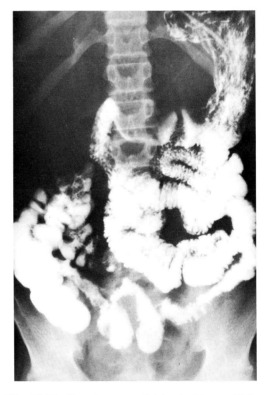

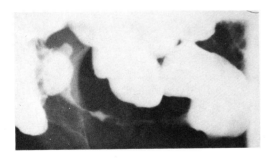

Fig. 13-31. Crohn's disease of the terminal ileum. There is severe thickening of the lumen of the terminal ileum. This patient was first admitted to the hospital with a history of anorexia nervosa. Growth failure in the absence of gastrointestinal symptomats prompted endocrine studies and psychiatric referral. Two years after the diagnosis of Crohn's disease was made, she was readmitted with signs of partial intestinal obstruction confirmed by the presence of a so-called string sign in a rigid, fibrotic terminal ileum. An intestinal resection was carried out, but 18 months later there was evidence of colonic and rectal involvement.

Fig. 13-32. Granulomatous ileitis. A 12-year-old boy had a 2-year history of abdominal cramps and arthralgia. Three weeks before admission to the hospital, he began suffering severe diarrhea, weight loss, erythema nodosum, aphthous ulcers, and fever. There is extensive involvement of the terminal ileum, a cobblestone appearance being particularly prominent. On fluoroscopy, normal peristalsis was absent; on palpation, the right lower quadrant was rigid and painful.

bowel largely account for such observations.

In view of the findings in the National Cooperative Crohn's Disease Study, which showed that the pattern of roentgenographic features and its extent do not correlate with clinical symptoms or response to drug therapy, the need for ''ritual'' roentgenograms in the follow-up study appears questionable except in the following circumstances: (1) severe clinical exacerbation if a stricture or a fistula is suspected, (2) preoperative evaluation to guide the surgeon, and (3) postoperative evaluation of the patient who experiences a clinical recrudescence or recurrence.

Endoscopic features

Every patient suspected of having Crohn's disease should have a rectosigmoidoscopic examination. Normal findings can be expected in half the cases; erythema, edema, increased friability, and aphthous ulcerations in 25%; and pathognomonic noncaseating granulomas can be identified in as many as 25%. Colonoscopic examination has a place in the initial work-up if the proctoscopy shows normal tissue and if the barium enema cannot rule out colonic disease. Colonoscopy is useful preoperatively to determine the extent of colonic involvement.

Upper gastrointestinal endoscopy is indicated in patients with known Crohn's disease who have an abnormal upper small bowel series. In these children the differential diagnosis is usually between peptic disease and Crohn's disease. If a peptic ulcer is seen in a patient already on prednisone, its treatment will be different from that of a lesion representing an extension of Crohn's disease. The gastroscopic picture of Crohn's disease of the stomach is remarkable and remindful of granulomatous colitis. We have seen two patients with a cobblestone pattern and large deep longitudinal ulcers. The histologic changes are commonly those of pronounced inflammation of the mucosa (Fig. 13-33) with submucosal fibrous and transmural involvement. Giant cells can sometimes be identified in the ulcerated mucosa.

Complications

In contrast to ulcerative colitis, acute fulminating episodes are rare. Generally speaking, patients with Crohn's disease follow a more chronic and unremitting course. Acute exacerbations intercalated with periods of relative quiescence is the usual course of the disease, particularly during the early years. Most of the complications are related to the transmural inflammation leading to intestinal obstruction (25%), a stagnant loop syndrome, internal fistulization (Fig. 13-34), and abscess formation (50%). A massive hemorrhage is an occasional event.

Toxic megacolon. This complication is less frequent (less than 5%) than in ulcerative colitis but needs to be recognized promptly. The transverse colon and splenic flexure are the sites of maximal dilatation, but there is air throughout the colon in contrast to mechanical obstruction. Air fluid levels are present; pneumatosis and free air should be looked for. The patient is very toxic; the abdomen is distended and tender. Guarding, rebound tendernss, and shoulder pain indicate a free perforation. Hypoalbuminemia is invariably present. Gram-negative sepsis and shock are ominous complications of toxic megacolon.

Carcinoma. There are more than 30 cases of carcinoma of the small bowel reported in Crohn's disease. Most carcinomas have been found in the distal ileum of patients who have had the disease for more than 10 years. It is of interest to note that 12 have occurred in loops that had been short circuited by bypass surgery. Although the incidence of carcinoma of the colon is low when compared to ulcerative colitis, it is believed to be increased twentyfold. We are not aware of its occurrence during the adolescent years.

Perianal and perineal lesions. Perianal fissures, abscesses, or fistulas may occasionally precede intestinal involvement or constitute the sole manifestation of the disease. However, perianal and perineal lesions usually evolve together with more proximal disease and constitute a serious and disabling complication. The more distal the intestinal lesion, the higher is the incidence of perianal disease. A recently published series documents a figure of 12% when the disease is limited to the small bowel, 15% in ileocolic forms, 41% with large bowel involvement with rectal sparing, and 92% when the rectum is affected. The experience in pediatric patients is somewhat different. Our observation is that close to 4 of every 10 children and adolescents with Crohn's disease has either skin tags, fissures, or fistulas. In the largest group of pediatric patients ever reported, perianal disease was seen in 26%, 36%, and 19% of cases with disease affecting the small bowel, both the small and the large bowel, and the colon, respectively. Chronic indurated rectal fissures and fistu-

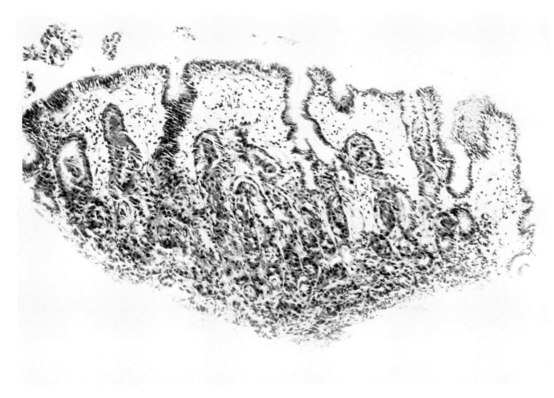

Fig. 13-33. Crohn's gastritis. Biopsy specimen of the fundus shows infiltration of the mucosa by a dense chronic inflammatory process. No giant cells could be identified.

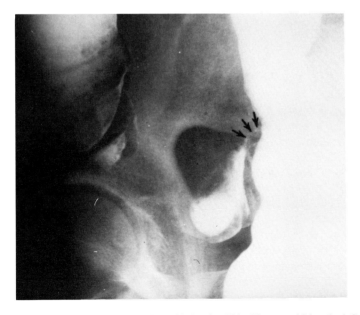

Fig. 13-34. Crohn's disease with an ileosigmoid fistula. This 18 year old has had Crohn's ileocolitis for 4 years. Four months after a 1-week bout of fever, abdominal pain, and diarrhea, the barium enema shows a fistulous tract between the rectosigmoid and the ileum, *arrows*. The patient is currently asymptomatic on prednisone and sulfasalazine.

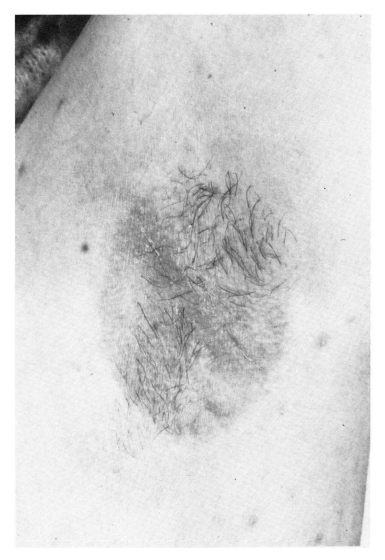

Fig. 13-35. Axillary lesions in a 17 year old with an ileostomy occurring after an ileocolectomy for Crohn's disease. Within 7 weeks of oral treatment with zinc sulfate, there was complete clearing of the oozing and crusty dermatitis. Identical lesions were seen in the inguinal creases.

las are associated with perirectal abscesses, perineal sepsis, rectovaginal fistulas, and varying degrees of destruction of the rectal sphincters.

Urinary tract complications. The ureter and bladder may be involved. Hydronephrosis may be secondary to compression of the ureters. Oxalate and uric acid stones are not uncommon. An enterovesical fistula is a serious complication. Frequency, dysuria, and pneumaturia are the usual symptoms.

Liver disease. The spectrum of liver complications is the same as in ulcerative colitis except that chronic hepatitis is rare. The incidence of he-

patic problems is higher with extensive colonic disease. We have not had any patients with abnormal liver function tests.

Impaired growth and delayed sexual maturation. Growth retardation may precede clinical symptoms by years and may be unrelated to the severity of disease. Impaired linear growth is a frequent and serious complication that is already present in 20% to 30% at the time of diagnosis. Despite appropriate medical therapy, 50% of those who are initially below the third percentile for height remain stunted, and 25% of those who at the time of diagnosis stand above the third per-

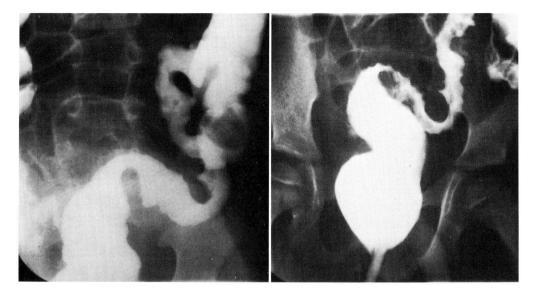

Fig. 13-36. Granulomatous colitis versus ulcerative colitis. The onset seemed to indicate ulcerative colitis, with vomiting, high fever, and abdominal distention; furthermore, the disease was limited to the sigmoid colon. The x-ray pattern of deep ulcerations and cobblestone appearance was more compatible with granulomatous colitis. Histologic diagnosis was that of nonspecific chronic inflammation.

centile for height will fall below this percentile. As pointed out by others, appropriate medical, nutritional, and surgical interventions are likely to be effective in terms of catch-up'' growth only if they are initiated well before puberty.

Deficiencies of specific nutrients. In addition to calorie-protein malnutrition, patients may present deficiencies of vitamins (A, D, C, folic acid, and B_{12}), minerals (Ca, Mg), or trace elements (Zn, Cu). A recent study has shown that 30% to 40% have a low serum zinc concentration. This may contribute to growth retardation, anorexia, abnormalities in taste, hypogonadism, and skin lesions. The skin lesions may be confused with recurrent herpes because of circumoral involvement. The crusting lesions are also found on the genitalia and extremities (Fig. 13-35). They rapidly respond to zinc sulfate.

Diagnosis

If the inflammatory process involves both the small and the large intestines, there is little doubt that one is dealing with Crohn's disease, though ulcerative colitis with backwash ileitis needs to be ruled out. However, when the colon alone is involved (Fig. 13-36), one has to rely on biopsy findings or on the presence of skip lesions, which are never described with ulcerative colitis.

The differential diagnosis of Crohn's disease of the small bowel includes other granulomatous processes such as tuberculosis, histoplasmosis, amebiasis, and sarcoidosis, which are very rare conditions during childhood. Lymphomas, adenocarcinomas, and intestinal scleroderma may also mimic Crohn's disease. Patients with chronic granulomatous disease, acquired hypogammaglobulinemia, and selective IgA deficiency have been described with gastrointestinal involvement sharing many of the characteristics of Crohn's disease.

As noted previously, extraintestinal manifestations such as fever of unknown origin, arthralgia, mouth sores, and erythema nodosum should alert one to the possibility of Crohn's disease. All children with perianal disease should be suspected of Crohn's disease. Since a significant percentage of normal children experience recurrent abdominal pain, further information should be sought as to location of pain (in the right lower quadrant) and the presence of associated symptoms (such as fever or diarrhea) and signs (malnutrition) compatible with Crohn's disease. It is important to note that a low percentage (10% to 18%) of children with Crohn's disease present as acute appendicitis but, in retrospect, a history of diarrhea and recent weight loss can be elicited in most cases.

Management

Since Crohn's disease is a chronic, potentially lifelong, and invalidating affection of unknown cause, there is no single medication, therapeutic regimen, or surgical procedure that can be advocated. The management depends on the individual patient's condition and his tolerance for the disease.

Once the diagnosis is made, the physician's role goes far beyond the writing of orders or of prescriptions. It is his responsibility to establish a sound relationship with patient and parents and to provide information concerning the nature of the illness and the challenges that lie ahead. The message should clearly indicate that there is no cure for the disease. However an optimistic outlook is necessary. An important point is that significant advances have been made with regard to the control of symptoms and the prevention of complications. Patients should be told that with proper guidance, good compliance, and self-discipline they can enjoy an essentially normal life style with a minimum of incapacitation and have long intervals without any symptoms.

A complete assessment of the patient's condition, of the extent and severity of the disease, and of the presence or imminence of complication, is essential for short-term and long-term planning of an appropriate management regimen. It is very useful to assess the repercussions of the disease in order to be able to evaluate the effectiveness of treatment. The Crohn's disease activity index (CDAI) is a very useful tool (Table 13-8). Its interpretation is shown in Table 13-9. After completion of roentgenological, endoscopic, histologic, and biochemical studies, a calorie count using a 3- to 7-day dietary recall and anthropometric measurements (height, weight, and subscapular and triceps skinfolds) should be done.

At the onset, or during an acute relapse, patients should have bed rest, and most do better as inpatients. In those patients with vomiting and signs of partial intestinal obstruction, continuous nasogastric suction is indicated. This will generally allow the edema and spasm to subside. Intravenous rehydration and nutritional rehabilitation are necessary during this acute phase. A surgical consultation should be obtained early so that one can plan surgery if medical management fails to reverse the intestinal obstruction.

Dietary care. Dietary management should center around (1) the design of a balanced, nutritious

Table 13-8. Calculation of Crohn's disease activity index (CDAI)

	Calculation
Total number of diarrheal stools for each of previous 7 days	×2 . . . .
Abdominal pain for each of previous 7 days	×5 . . . . . .
None = 0	
Mild = 1	
Moderate = 2	
Severe = 3	
General well-being for each of previous 7 days	×7 . . . . . .
Well = 0	
Below par = 1	
Poor = 2	
Very poor = 3	
Terrible = 4	
Clinical signs during the 7 days	×20 . . . . . .
Arthritis or arthralgia = 1	
Skin or mouth lesions = 1	
Iritis or uveitis = 1	
Anorectal lesion = 1	
Other fistulas = 1	
Fever over 38° C during the week = 1	
Lomotil and opiates for diarrhea	×30 . . . . . .
No = 0 Yes = 1	
Adominal mass	×10 . . . . . .
None = 0	
Questionable = 2	
Definite = 3	
Hematocrit	×6 . . . .
For boys, 47 − Hematocrit	
For girls, 42 − Hematocrit	
Body weight	×1 . . . .
$\left(1 - \dfrac{\text{Body weight}}{\text{Standard weight}}\right) \times 100$	
Total	

Table 13-9. Interpretation of CDAI values

Quiescent disease	<150
Relatively well	150-300
Sick patient	300-400
Dangerously ill	>400

Table 13-10. Continuous enteral alimentation as primary therapy

Protocol (10 patients 14.1 ± 3.4 years of age)
  Nasogastric Vivonex for 3 weeks
  Gradual weaning over a 10-day period and progression from a polymeric liquid formula to a low-residue and a normal diet
  Prednisone, 0.35 mg/kg/day, started upon discontinuation of nasogastric Vivonex

Results	*Before*	*At 3 weeks*	*At 3 months*
Caloric intake (kcal/kg)	39 ± 9	81 ± 17	—
Weight (kg)	36 ± 15	40 ± 16	43 ± 16
CDAI (Table 13-8)	307 ± 75	69 ± 36	99 ± 83

From Morin, C.L., and others: Pediatr. Res. **13**:405, 1979.

high-protein and high-caloric diet with supplemental vitamin B_{12}, folate, iron, trace elements, and multivitamins, and (2) the acceptance and tolerance of this diet by an anorexic and often nauseated child or teen-ager who, for months, has been eating fewer than half the calories he requires.

As no specific dietary constituent has been implicated in the pathogenesis of the disease, it is best to have the patient design his own diet using his preferences and aversions as guidelines. In the presence of severe postprandial abdominal pain, it is best to restrict residues as much as possible and to suggest small frequent meals. Liquid polymeric formulas provide a very acceptable, though expensive source of extra calories and nutrients for the ambulatory patient. Children can increase their energy intake by 1000 to 12000 calories in this way and achieve a positive caloric balance.

A relapse can be successfully managed by adherence to a diet where most calories are provided by a liquid formula. A number of children in relapse are not only anorexic, but also restrict their food intake because eating leads to severe postprandial abdominal pain. We find liquid formulas very useful in such circumstances.

Elemental and polymeric diets. If a thorough assessment has revealed that a significant degree of malnutrition is present and oral intake of appropriate calories is an unrealistic goal, continuous enteral alimentation with an elemental diet should be seriously considered. A large experience with inpatients shows that "putting the bowel to rest" brings about a dramatic relief of intestinal and extraintestinal symptoms most often in the absence of other medications. Table 13-10 summarizes this regimen and the results achieved in 10 patients. Recently, however, we have come to better define its indications and limitations. It should be used with caution in patients who have

a CDAI above 400. Continuous enteral alimentation with an elemental diet has further applications. A relatively short course followed by a normal diet and a small dose of prednisone (0.35 mg/kg/day) leads to a resumption of normal growth, which continues for a period of about 3 months after termination of the 6-week period of elemental diet. Preliminary data suggest that 4- to 6-week courses repeated every 3 to 4 months with prednisone 0.35 mg/kg/day can maintain patients in remission and allow them to grow satisfactorily.

Judicious flavoring of elemental diets can enhance palatability and permit adequate oral intake in selected adolescents, but total caloric intake is lower. Therefore oral elemental and polymeric diets are ineffective when severe malnutrition and growth failure are present.

Elemental diets are successfully used for the treatment of complications such as fistulas and perianal disease. High-output fistulas are unlikely to respond, but one can expect good results for the ileal fistulas. Successful closure of enterovesical, enterocutaneous, and enteroperitoneal fistulas with abscess formation has been achieved. We have also had gratifying results in perianal Crohn's disease with severe fistulous disease that had failed to respond to steroids, Flagyl, and azathioprine.

Parenteral nutrition. This approach is very valuable in severely ill patients with Crohn's disease and in those in whom enteral alimentation attempts have failed. Studies in adults show that a remission can be induced in 80% and persist for more than 3 months in 60%. If a fistula is present, closure can be expected in more than 40%. A dramatic reversal of malnutrition and a change in growth velocity can be expected in all children on parenteral nutrition. Home total parenteral nutrition has been a successful approach in select patients. The attendant risks and costs of total parenteral nutrition are such that indications are restricted to those children in whom the oral route is precluded. Some patients should be started on total parenteral nutrition and then gradually weaned to continuous enteral alimentation.

Antidiarrheal and analgesic agents. In children with watery diarrhea, certain specific measures may be helpful. Because a small number have bile acid or hydroxy fatty acid diarrhea even before having undergone an ileal resection, a low-fat diet supplemented with medium-chain triglycerides (Portagen and MCT oil) may be helpful in conjunction with cholestyramine. Since disaccharidase activity may be reduced even in the absence of significant jejunal involvement, a lactose-free diet may provide some relief.

We are totally unhappy with diphenoxylate (Lomotil) and do not administer opiates. Anticholinergic agents such as propantheline bromide (Pro-Banthine) may relieve cramps but should be used with caution. Darvon and acetaminophen may be used as analgesics. Aspirin products are avoided.

Sulfasalazine (salicylazosulfapyridine). The drug should be considered "initial" therapy for mild and moderate disease activity without significant extraintestinal manifestations and malnutrition. Perhaps 10% of children with Crohn's disease fit into this category. If it seems to be effective in achieving a remission, it should be continued indefinitely. Theoretically it should only be effective in patients with Crohn's colitis or with an ileocolic form of the disease, but we certainly have had some success in a few patients with disease limited to the distal ileum. The National Cooperative Crohn's Disease Study has shown that it is effective for the treatment of active symptomatic disease. It is not superior to prednisone alone or when given in combination with prednisone. Finally, sulfasalazine is not considered an effective drug to prevent relapses once a remission has been obtained.

It is difficult to decide to discontinue the drug when the child has improved roentgenographic findings, is asymptomatic, and is growing well. The question of prophylaxis after surgical resection must also be raised. Recurrences occur in both medically and surgically induced "remissions" despite steroids or sulfasalazine, or both. The problem is that a clinically and roentgenologically quiescent disease does not necessarily mean that there is a remission. Physicians who advocate

continuous therapy believe that Crohn's disease is always active and that symptoms need to be controlled. There is certainly no place for the drug after an ileostomy and after surgery when the anastomosed margins are free of disease.

Side effects are said to occur in 15% of adults on 35 mg/kg/day of sulfasalazine. The advocated dosage in pediatric patients is 50 mg/kg/day up to a maximum of 4 gm/day in the acute phase. Maintenance dosage is 2 gm/day. The schedule recommended for the introduction of the drug in ulcerative colitis applies also to Crohn's disease.

Steroids. Hydrocortisone, given intravenously, and prednisone, given orally, result in dramatic remissions. Fever, malaise, and diarrhea decrease, the appetite returns, and extraintestinal manifestations vanish along with the fullness or mass in the right lower quadrant. Upon stopping of the steroids, symptoms generally recur because, in most cases, the disease process is chronic and smoldering. Controlled studies have shown that prednisone is effective in the acute stage, but it has not been proved to be useful in preventing relapses.

The recommended dosage of prednisone is 1 to 2 mg/kg/day (maximum dose 60 mg/day) for 6 to 8 weeks with gradual weaning according to the recommendations made in the section on ulcerative colitis. The majority (80%) of our patients are steroid dependent. A large proportion of those are under good control with alternate-day therapy (12.5 to 20 mg). The rest require a daily dose (12.5 to 20 mg) given at breakfast.

As previously mentioned, the steroid dosage necessary to bring about a dramatic resolution of symptoms is much smaller if an enteral alimentation regimen is also prescribed in the acute phase of the disease. Topical steroids have no place in the treatment of Crohn's disease.

Immunosuppressive agents. Immunosuppressive therapy has been tried in Crohn's disease since 1965. Ineffective in a dose of 1 mg/kg/day, azathioprine can maintain a patient in clinical remission if the dosage is doubled to 2 mg/kg/day. It controls symptoms at a lower dosage of prednisone and allows reduction of corticosteroid dosage in cases in which a large daily maintenance dose (more than 15 mg) is necessary. Withdrawal of the drug substantially increases the risk of relapse. A 4.4% incidence of pancreatitis is reported within a month of starting azathioprine (Imuran). We have seen a few patients on the combination of prednisone and Imuran who developed zoster lesions. Hepatic and hematologic complications are also reported.

A recent study has shown convincingly that 6-mercaptopurine (6-MP) (1.5 mg/kg/day) is effective. Response to therapy may take as long as 3 to 6 months. It is reasonably safe and can be administered for prolonged periods of time. Patients with colitis and ileocolitis fare better on the drug than in cases where the disease is limited to the small bowel. The main indication appears to be in cases where sulfasalazine does not prevent relapse and where steroids cannot be reduced or stopped. From the studies available, 6-MP appears to be more effective than azathioprine. Perhaps this is related to the fact that only 50% of azathioprine is metabolized to 6-MP.

Antibiotics. Wide-spectrum antibiotics can lead to some improvement when there is evidence of a stricture and the contaminated small bowel syndrome. They should be used in the presence of an overt abdominal abscess or an acute abdominal or toxic megacolon. In such cases the parenteral administration of ampicillin and gentamicin is recommended. Antibiotics are not generally effective in the treatment of perianal abscesses and fistulas; however, encouraging results have been reported with metronidazole (Flagyl) 1 to 1.5 gm/day over a period of a few months.

Surgery. Crohn's disease is neither a medically nor a surgically curable condition. One should speak of surgical management instead of treatment since operative procedures should be reserved for acute and chronic complications.

Emergency surgery in the pediatric age group is likely to be done in the initial stage of the disease when the patient presents with severe abdominal pain mimicking acute appendicitis. A certain percentage of these will turn out to have acute ileitis and 90% will recover completely (see p. 389). However, the majority presenting acutely will turn out to have Crohn's disease and run a chronic course. It is now considered safe to do an appendectomy even if the cecum is involved; the risk of a fistula is very low. Other indications for emergency surgery include a massive hemorrhage, a free perforation, and a toxic megacolon that continues to deteriorate despite aggressive medical treatment.

Indications for elective surgery include severe growth failure, intractability of the disease, repeated bouts of intestinal obstruction, and an abscess that fails to respond to conservative measures. Enteroenteric fistulas are generally left alone unless the fistula short-circuits the absorptive apparatus or drains poorly. An enterovesical fistula is an absolute indication for surgery. Extensive small bowel disease with gastric and duodenal involvement poses a special problem. Vagotomy and a posterior gastrojejunostomy has been proposed, but we have no experience with this operation in the few children we have with duodenal Crohn's disease. In other situations, resection rather than bypass is currently the preferred procedure. In an attempt to rid the patient of disease and prevent or lessen the chance of recurrence, many surgeons resect a wide margin of grossly normal bowel on either end of the involved bowel. A recent study shows that there is only a small, nonsignificant increase in the incidence of recurrence of the disease at the suture line requiring surgery in cases where margins of anastomosis were histologically involved. Conservative resection is therefore recommended. Perianal disease also calls for a conservative approach. Abscesses should be drained and fistulas laid flat when possible. Perianal wounds will heal by themselves, but they generally follow fairly well the evolution of the disease elsewhere. When rectal involvement is contiguous to the anal disease, the situation is more complex and often requires a proctocolectomy.

A large percentage of pediatric patients will require surgery. The Cleveland series shows that during a follow-up period of 7.7 years almost 70% of 522 children and adolescents had to be operated on. In our own series of 93 children and adolescents more than 1 out of 3 had surgery within 3 years. Of interest is the fact that in more than 25% of those who had elective surgery, growth failure, and disease intractability were the indications for a resection. Surgery generally has a favorable impact on growth in prepubertal children and will buy time. Relative freedom from symptoms and resumption of growth can be expected, but the likelihood of a recurrence is very high and it may occur very early after the initial resection. Rough figures for recurrences after an operation is 20% after 2 years and 40% after 3½ years.

The Los Angeles group reports that the risk of recurrence over 5 years is much higher in ileocolic disease (64%) than in ileal disease (25%). There are no figures for the rate of recurrence in pediatric patients after a proctocolectomy for disease confined to the colon. The figure in a large adult series is 20% after 5 years.

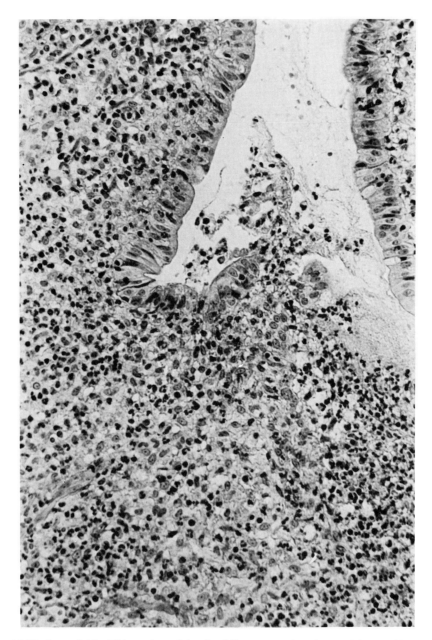

Fig. 13-37. Acute ileitis. This section of the distal ileum was taken from a 15-year-old boy who presented with signs of acute appendicitis. In contrast to biopsy findings in Crohn's disease, the infiltrate is acute, and an ulceration is clearly visible on the right. The patient made an uneventful recovery and has been asymptomatic for the past decade.

The best operation for extensive Crohn's colitis is a proctocolectomy, but the price to pay is an ileostomy. Ileorectal anastomosis should be offered to pediatric patients. If the rectum is moderately involved, a temporary ileostomy may be done in the hope that diversion of the feces will allow the rectum to heal. However, this has not been a good approach. It is now believed that if the rectum appears worth saving, an ileorectal anastomosis should be carried out after medical attempts at improving the rectal involvement. Perianal disease, unless there is destruction of sphincters and incontinence, is not an absolute contraindication. Proctocolectomy and ileostomy will be eventually necessary in a significant number of youngsters with an ileorectal anastomosis, but it is worth the risk.

Prognosis

The disease in the young remains very active over several years. A percentage of patients may go into a permanent "remission," but most have a smoldering disease that can be controlled medically but acute exacerbations occur from time to time and cannot be predicted or prevented. Ileocolic forms are more disabling and postsurgical recurrence is very high when compared to that of the ileal variety. Although surgery is not curative, a median relapse time of 16 months after medical therapy and of 48 months after surgery has been reported in a pediatric series from England.

About 20% have a severe disabling disease, whereas 20% have few symptoms and describe themselves as perfectly healthy. The majority therefore do experience symptoms that impose some limits on their quality of life.

Acute ileitis

In a small percentage of children who present acute appendicitis, the surgeon will find a thickened and inflamed terminal ileum. The past history is totally negative for telltale symptoms and signs of a chronic smoldering disease such as Crohn's. Careful inspection will reveal that the cecum is uninvolved. The inflammatory process is acute, it is not transmural, and the mesentery is intact. Cultures and serologic study may confirm the presence of a *Yersinia* infection. Few patients (10% to 20%) initially diagnosed as having acute ileitis on the basis of histologic features (Fig. 13-37) progress to typical Crohn's disease with its previously described course and complications.

REFERENCES

Alexander-Williams, J., and Buchmann, P.: Criteria of assessment for suitability and results of ileorectal anastomosis, Clin. Gastroenterol. **9:**409-417, 1980.

Allan, R., Steinberg, D.M., Williams, J.A., and others: Crohn's disease involving the colon: an audit of clinical management, Gastroenterology **73:**723-732, 1977.

Ament, M.D.: Inflammatory disease of the colon: ulcerative colitis and Crohn's colitis, J. Pediatr. **86:**322-334, 1975.

Block, G.E.: Surgical management of Crohn's colitis, N. Engl. J. Med. **302:**1068-1070, 1980.

Burbige, E.J., Huang, S.S., Bayless, T.M.: Clinical manifestations of Crohn's disease in children and adolescents, Pediatrics **55:**866-872, 1975.

Calam, J., Crooks, P.E., and Walker, R.J.: Elemental diets in the management of Crohn's perianal fistulae, J.P.E.N. **4:**4-8, 1980.

Cavell, B., Hildebrand, H., Meeuwisse, G.W., and Lindquist, B.: Chronic inflammatory bowel disease, Clin. Gastroenterol. **6:**481-497, 1977.

Farmer, R.G., and Michener, W.M.: Prognosis of Crohn's disease with onset in childhood or adolescence, Dig. Dis. Sci. **24:**752-757, 1979.

Fillit, H., Bernstein, L., Davidson, M., and others: Primary acquired hypogammaglobulinemia and regional enteritis, Arch. Intern. Med. **137:**1252-1254, 1977.

Fonkalsrud, E.W., Ament, M.E., Fleisher, D., and others: Surgical management of Crohn's disease in children, Am. J. Surg. **138:**15-21, 1979.

Gryboski, J.D., and Spiro, H.M.: Prognosis in children with Crohn's disease, Gastroenterology **74:**807-817, 1978.

Hamilton, J.R., Bruce, G.A., Abdourhaman, H., and others: Inflammatory bowel disease in children and adolescents, Adv. Pediatr. **26:**311-341, 1979.

Holter, A., and Fisher, J.E.: Adenocarcinoma of the small bowel associated with Crohn's disease, Arch. Surg. **113:**991-993, 1978.

Homer, D.R., Grand, R.J., and Colodney, A.H.: Growth, course and prognosis after surgery for Crohn's disease in children and adolescents, Pediatrics **59:**717-725, 1977.

Kaufman, S., Chalmer, B., Heilman, R., and others: A prospective study of the course of Crohn's disease, Dig. Dis. Sci. **24:**269-276, 1979.

Kelts, D.G., Grand, R.J., Shen, G., and others: Nutritional basis of growth failure in children and adolescents with Crohn's disease, Gastroenterology **76:**720-727, 1979.

Kirschner, B.S., Voinchet, O., and Rosenberg, I.H.: Growth retardation in inflammatory bowel disease, Gastroenterology **75:**504-511, 1978.

Kirschner, B.S., Klich, J.R., Kalman, S.S., and others: Reversal of growth retardation in Crohn's disease with therapy emphasizing oral nutritional restitution, Gastroenterology **80:**10-15, 1981.

McClain, C., Soutor, C., and Zieve, L.: Zinc deficiency: a complication of Crohn's disease, Gastroenterology **78:**272-279, 1980.

Morin, C.L., Roulet, M., Roy, C.C., and others: Continuous elemental enteral alimentation in children with Crohn's disease and growth failure, Gastroenterology **79:**1205-1210, 1980.

O'Donoghue, D.P., and Dawson, A.M.: Crohn's disease in childhood, Arch. Dis. Child. **52:**627-632, 1977.

O'Donoghue, D.P., Dawson, A.M., Powell-Tuck, J., and others: Double blind withdrawal trial of azathioprine as maintenance treatment for Crohn's disease, Lancet **2:**955-957, 1978.

Present, D.H., Korelitz, B.I., Wisch, N., and others: Treatment of Crohn's disease with 6-mercaptopurine, N. Engl. J. Med. **302:**981-987, 1980.

Sohn, N., Korelitz, B.I., and Weinstein, M.A.: Anorectal Crohn's disease: definitive surgery for fistulas and recurrent abscesses, Am. J. Surg. **139:**394-397, 1980.

Strauss, R.G., Ghishan, F., Mitros, F., and others: Rectosigmoidal colitis in common variable immunodeficiency disease, Dig. Dis. Sci. **24:**798-801, 1980.

Summers, R.W., Switz, D.M., Sessions, J.T., and others: National cooperative Crohn's disease study: results of drug treatment, Gastroenterology **77:**847-869, 1979.

Watts, J.M., and Hughes, E.S.R.: Ulcerative colitis and Crohn's disease: results after colectomy and ileorectal anastomosis, Br. J. Surg. **64:**77-83, 1977.

Whittington, P.F., Baunes, H.V., and Bayless, T.M.: Medical management of Crohn's disease in adolescence, Gastroenterology **72:**1338-1344, 1977.

Winship, D.H., Summers, R.W., Singleton, J.W., and others: National Cooperative Crohn's Disease Study: study design and conduct of the study, Gastroenterology **77:**829-842, 1979.

14 *Constipation, fecal incontinence, and proctologic conditions*

PHYSIOLOGY OF DEFECATION AND CONTINENCE
Colonic motility

The intrinsic innervation of the colon consists of excitatory (cholinergic and noncholinergic) and inhibitory (adrenergic and nonadrenergic) nerves. The relative importance of the four types of innervation is not entirely clear, but the gross abnomalies of colonic function in conditions such as Hirschsprung's disease point to the importance of an intact myenteric plexus in maintaining integrated colonic motility.

The colon exhibits several types of contractile activity, the main kind being segmentation of the lumen by stationary, narrow contraction rings that form the well-known haustra, the result of structural and functional properties of the colon. Segmentation is present in the sigmoid colon about half the time and less than that in the other parts of the colon. Such contractile activity produces slow to-and-fro internal circulation of the feces but no propulsion. After kneading the fecal mass for several hours, the segmenting contractions stop, and a "mass movement" advances the stool to a more distal section of the colon before segmenting contractions start again. The stool is thus delivered to the rectum after three or four stops and starts over a period of one to several days. Segmentation, which increases resistance to net flow, is depressed in diarrheal states. "Mass movements" occur three to four times a day, usually within an hour after eating, and are not present during sleep in the normal colon.

Cholinergic drugs, such as prostigmine, augment segmentation, whereas anticholinergic or atropine-like drugs inhibit it. Glucagon is a potent inhibitor of electrical and pressure changes in the colon. Recent interest in prostaglandins stems from work showing increased synthesis and release in inflammatory bowel disease. Sulfasalazine and corticosteroids respectively inhibit synthesis and release of prostaglandins. Morphine, codeine, diphenoxylate, and loperamide increase segmentation activity in both the large and small bowel, and it in this way that they are effective antidiarrheal agents. Motor activity of the large bowel is affected by the fiber content of the diet, by drugs, and by the use of laxatives. Excessive colonic contractions may play a part in the pathogenesis of certain types of abdominal pain.

Instruments of continence

The rectum normally contains little or no material. Before defecation, it fills with feces propelled by the sigmoid colon. Sphincters of the rectum and anus are controlled both consciously and unconsciously in order to be entirely effective at all times of the day and night. The receptors that provide knowledge of the content of the anal canal lie in the bowel wall and the surrounding pelvic and perineal muscles. The muscles that govern the flow of flatus, feces, and mucus are the internal and external sphincters and the levator ani muscles. The second, third, and fourth sacral segments of the spinal cord link the sensory and motor sides of the nervous arc with the higher centers of the central nervous system. The levator musculature very closely wraps the part of the anal canal that is cranial to the pectinate line. By its pull, it maintains an 80-degree angle between the axis of the rectum and the anal canal. The part of the anal canal that is distal to the pectinate line is clothed by the encircling internal and external sphincters (Fig. 14-17).

Although the anal canal caudal to the pectinate line is endowed with sensory receptors for pain, touch, cold, pressure, and friction, the part cranial to the pectinate line and lined by rectal mucosa is endowed only with distention sensory receptors. Most authors believe that rectal distention, acutely sensed by the rectal mucosa, leads to relaxation of the internal sphincter. The relaxed internal sphincter allows the contents to contact the very sensitive and effective anal canal receptors, inducing external sphincter contraction. Others believe that the initiating signal of rectal distention may be picked up not only by the rectal mucosa, but also by the levator ani muscle complex. In congenital anorectal malformations, both the internal and external sphincters may be rudimentary, and yet a high degree of continence can be achieved if the sleeve and sling complex is in-

391

tact. Gas, liquid, or solid moving into the sleeve and sling zone provides a stretch that is immediately and keenly appreciated. Since reconstruction of an anal canal devoid of sphincters (internal and external) but endowed with the sleeve and sling sphincter leads to satisfactory continence, it seems reasonable to believe that the sleeve and sling complex has an important sensory function.

In the normal resting state, the lumen of the anal canal is occluded by the sleeve and sling sphincter and by the resting tone of the external and internal sphincters. The first warning of gas, liquid, or solid in the part of the anal canal cranial to the pectinate line is picked up by the stretch receptors of the sleeve and sling complex. If the peristaltic wave is weak, the contraction of the complex will barely reach consciousness. A stronger peristaltic drive creates tension in the sleeve and sling, which calls for more urgent contraction, occluding the anal canal with the help of the external sphincter under voluntary control. As the calls become more insistent, colic appears. The sleeve and sling can perceive the difference between impending passage of flatus, solid, and fluid and has the ability to permit one to escape with or without the other.

Pathophysiology of incontinence

Rectal continence can be achieved when the capacity to resist the urge to defecate is physiologically possible and has been acquired. This presupposes the integrity of muscular and sensory structures. The internal sphincter, a smooth muscle in continuity with the rectal musculature, is in a state of relative contraction until distended by gas or fecal material, which brings about its relaxation. The external sphincter and the levator ani complex are voluntary muscles completing the group of structures essential for continence in normal human beings.

In infants up to 8 to 12 months of age and in patients with spinal cord injury proximal to the second and third sacral nerves, defecation is entirely by reflex, since relaxation of the internal sphincter, in the absence of the conscious urge to defecate, leads to automatic defecation. When continence is achieved, relaxation of the internal sphincter increases pressure on the external sphincter and levator ani muscles, which, under voluntary control, are either contracted to prevent defecation or relaxed to allow defecation with the assistance of abdominal muscles, the diaphragm, and the levator ani complex.

In chronic constipation, the sleeve and sling, easily tired by impacting feces, become relaxed and permit shortening of the anal canal to the length only of the skin-lined anus. It is then found that the short passage, though encircled by external and internal sphincters, is barely sphincteric, permitting constant leakage that is momentarily arrested only at the time of conscious (15 to 60 seconds) muscular contractions of the external sphincter surrounding the skin-lined anus.

The constant fecal soiling associated with constipation (encopresis) should not be confused with incontinence caused by incompetent sphincter mechanisms. Neurologic lesions, congenital or acquired, lead to severe incontinence problems through denervation of the external sphincter and of the sleeve and sling complex. There is loss of the mechanosensory receptors, bringing about an absence of sensation of rectal fullness and of the presence of stools in the anal canal, as well as a loss of sphincteric function.

In congenital anorectal malformations requiring reconstruction of the anal canal, both the internal and external sphincters may be functionally or anatomically absent. If no damage has been done to the puborectalis sling and the levator ani muscles, the sensory and motor functions of this complex are sufficient to ensure continence.

SIMPLE CONSTIPATION
Definition and pathophysiology

Constipation defined as a condition in which bowel movements are infrequent leads to much overtreatment. The frequency of defecation is influenced by social and dietary customs, and it is only recently that a normal pattern of defecation has been agreed on, albeit in adults. Older children and adolescents who have fewer than three bowel movements a week can be considered as outside the normal range but do not, on this basis alone, require treatment any more than does the breast-fed infant who passes a soft stool every 3 or 4 days. Constipation refers to the character of the stool rather than to the frequency of defecation and to associated symptoms such as difficulty in expulsion of the stools, blood-streaked bowel movements, and abdominal discomfort. The neonate or the infant brought to the office because he is fussy, cries, turns red, and draws up his legs on passing a soft stool is not constipated, and neither is the 12-month-old infant who acts as though he is having great difficulty in evacuating a normal stool when, in fact, he is attempting to withhold a stool. Constipation may represent the regular passage of firm or hard stools or else of small, hard masses at extremely long intervals (obstipation). In its most severe form, constipation may be accompanied by fecal soiling (encopresis).

Familial, cultural, and social factors influence the genesis, development, and course of constipation to varying degrees. A few babies are constipated during the neonatal period and, despite a variety of formula changes, persist in having constipation. Studies of colonic motility indicate differences in the motility pattern between control subjects and patients with constipation. Anterior location of the anus should be looked for. Psychologic factors, methods involved in toilet training, diet (particularly excessive milk intake), and misuse or abuse of laxatives and enemas may influence the development of toilet habits. Well-designed physiologic studies suggest that the increased rate of water and electrolyte absorption in the colon of constipated adults is totally accounted for by a slower transit brought about by an element of anorectal obstruction. Whether these findings also apply to infants and children remains unknown.

Clinical findings

A multitude of symptoms, such as fever, convulsions, nervousness, school failure, and bad breath, have been attributed to constipation. It is extremely unlikely that failure to have a bowel movement results in any of these.

The neonate or the infant often appears to be having a great deal of difficulty passing a stool. His face may turn red, and he draws up his legs on the abdomen even when the stool passed is quite soft. This pattern erroneously may be considered an indication of constipation. In a similar vein, the infant from 6 to 12 months of age may become flushed, draw up his legs, and act as though he is having a great deal of difficulty in having a bowel movement. Frequently, quite the contrary is true—he may be attempting to withhold a stool. The ability and the recognition of the ability to withhold a stool frequently become apparent to the child at this time. Failure to appreciate this normal development pattern may lead to the unwise use of laxatives or enemas.

As the child becomes ambulatory, far too many new and exciting activities arise to detract from the ''call to stool,'' much to the distress of all but the child. He may pass enough stool to relieve the pressure while continuing to play, and gradually

he develops an effective capacity to ignore the rectal fullness. In the older child, school, games, social events, and the hurried pace of life's activities may all complicate the development of any pattern of regularity. Many teen-age girls, for example, may become constipated because of reluctance to use toilet facilities other than at home.

Differential diagnosis

Constipation is a symptom associated with many gastrointestinal disorders and systemic diseases; therefore the following differential diagnosis is considerable:

Etiologic classification of constipation

Idiopathic or constitutional causes
Dietary causes
    Undernutrition
    Protracted vomiting
    Excessive intake of cow's milk
    Lack of bulk
Drugs and abuse of cathartics
Structural defects of gastrointestinal tract
    Anus and rectum
        Anal fissure, hemorrhoids, abscess
        Congenital anal and rectal stenosis
        Presacral teratoma
        Rectal prolapse
    Small bowel and colon
        Tumor
        Stricture
        Chronic volvulus
        Intussusception
        Internal hernia
Smooth muscle diseases affecting gastrointestinal tract
    Scleroderma and dermatomyositis
    Systemic lupus erythematosus
    Primary chronic intestinal pseudo-obstruction
Abnormalities of myenteric ganglion cells
    Hirschsprung's disease
    Hypoganglionosis and hyperganglionosis
    von Recklinghausen's disease
    Multiple endocrine neoplasia type 2B
Absence of abdominal musculature
Spinal cord defects
    Spina bifida
    Myelomeningocele
    Meningocele
    Diastematomyelia
    Paraplegia
    Cauda equina tumor
Metabolic and endocrine disorders
    Hypothyroidism
    Hypoparathyroidism
    Renal tubular acidosis
    Diabetes insipidus
    Vitamin D intoxication

Idiopathic hypercalcemia
Hypokalemia
Neurologic and psychiatric conditions
   Myotonic dystrophy
   Amyotonia congenita
   Brain tumors
   Mental retardation
   Psychosis

A careful history should document the age of onset, its relationship to changes in the diet or in the child's environment, and its response to various therapeutic measures. The presence of associated symptoms such as vomiting, abdominal distention, or pain, and evidence of growth failure point to an organic cause requiring further investigation. Iron preparations, psychotropic agents, anticonvulsants, diuretics, antacids, and anticholinergic agents can give rise to constipation. A thorough physical examination is in order to rule out findings compatible with the large differential diagnosis, particularly if the change in bowel habits has occurred for no reason. A rectal examination is mandatory but should never be done before close inspection of the anus, the perirectal tissues, and the lower spine.

Anterior location of the anus is a recognized clinical entity. Although more commonly seen in females, it also has been described in males. The anus is displaced anteriorly and well forward of the midpoint between the vaginal fourchette and the tip of the coccyx (Fig. 14-1). In males no such landmark is available and the diagnosis is more difficult to make. Rectal examination demonstrates a normal sphincter. Beyond the sphincter, there is usually a posterior shelf, which is found when one hooks the index finger on the back lip of the anus (Fig. 14-2). This shelf may be obstructive and may require anoplasty if conservative management, described below, fails.

Short-segment Hirschsprung's disease may present a clinical picture similar to that of chronic constipation. Rectal biopsy at 3 cm from the anal margin may be helpful, since ganglion cells are absent. A manometric study will confirm the diagnosis. One should remember, however, that in long-standing constipation, with or without encopresis, reflex relaxation of the internal sphincter may be blunted (Fig. 14-3).

Treatment

Dietary corrective measures include attempts to increase the intake of fluids, high-residue foods (bran, whole wheat, fruit, and vegetables), prune juice, prunes, and plums. In infants, the use of a

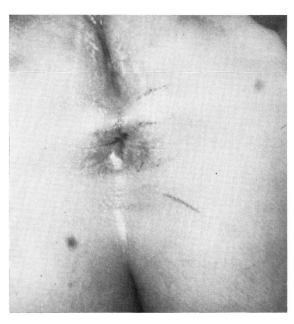

Fig. 14-1. Normally the anus is situated at a midpoint between the fornix and the tip of the coccyx. In this case there is significant anterior displacement of the anus. (Courtesy Dr. A. Bensoussan, Hôpital Sainte-Juustine, Montreal.)

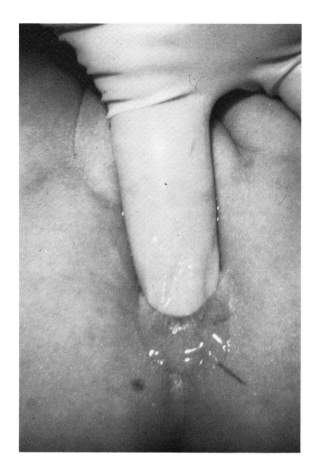

Fig. 14-2. In this case of anterior displacement of the anus a posterior shelf is easily demonstrated. Surgical correction is sometimes necessary. (Courtesy Dr. A. Bensoussan, Hôpital Sainte-Justine, Montreal.)

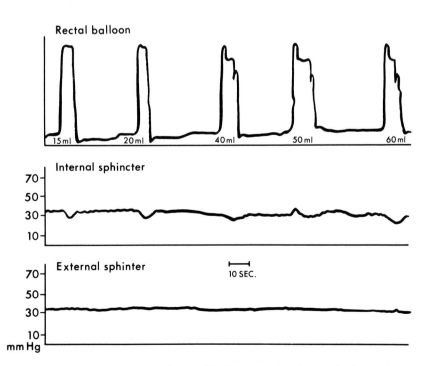

Fig. 14-3. This tracing taken from a 6-year-old child with chronic constipation and encopresis shows normal relaxation of the internal sphincter and no contraction of the external sphincter in response to considerable distention of the rectal ampulla. (Courtesy Dr. A. Bensoussan, Hôpital Sainte-Justine, Montreal.)

barley malt extract such as Maltsupex is most gratifying. Adding 1 or 2 tsp to feedings two or three times a day is usually sufficient.

Stool softeners such as dioctyl sodium sulfosuccinate (Colace), 5 to 10 mg/kg/24 hr, can be prescribed alone or in combination with other agents. This substance prevents excessive drying of the stool and may be safely administered for prolonged periods of time. However, it is completely ineffective when stool retention is voluntary.

Cathartics are not recommended because they rapidly lead to dependence and often give rise to abdominal cramps. In patients with neurologic disorders we use Dulcolax suppositories along with enemas, oral lactulose (5 to 10 ml twice a day), or Colace. Mineral oil taken by mouth or through the rectum is discussed in the following section.

CONSTIPATION WITH ENCOPRESIS (PSYCHOGENIC CONSTIPATION)

The dividing line between simple and psychogenic constipation is arbitrary. However, the constant or intermittent involuntary seepage of feces is characteristic of psychogenic constipation, in which there is usually a huge mass of feces in the rectal ampulla and sigmoid colon. In large outpatient series of children treated for constipation, two thirds of the patients present with soiling. Children affected by psychogenic constipation suffer from emotional disturbances that almost invariably disappear with relief of the constipation. There is no doubt, however, that in a certain number of cases, the emotional problems may lead to the symptom complex described or to the uncommon situation (5%) where there is encopresis without constipation.

Pathogenesis

Psychogenic factors. Most mothers know only too well how often their infant passes feces, and they are quick to seek a remedy for any disturbance of traditional normality. The overconcern of many mothers for a regularly functioning gastrointestinal tract is gradually overtaken by that for achievement of rectal continence. Gradually the young child becomes aware of the taboo against indiscriminate defecation, and voluntarily control is usually learned before the age of 3 years. During the period of toilet training (9 months to 3 years), the automatic, involuntary process of def-

ecation becomes a voluntary act associated with morality and taboos at a time when the speed of emotional and intellectual development is near its height and patterns of behavior are labile and easily distorted. Functional, habit, or "psychogenic" megacolon can be defined as a state of voluntary fecal retention to such as degree that impaction, encopresis, and megacolon result. The cause of "holding back" may relate to attempts to accomplish toilet training at an inappropriately early age, coercive attitudes toward rectal continence, or placement of a high love premium on a perfect daily performance. According to some authors, the "potting couple" (mother and child) is not at fault but rather the child's own neurodevelopment. In these children, there is not only poor response to rectal distention, but also other signs of neurodevelopmental dysfunction, such as hyperactivity, distractibility, poor motor coordination, or disabilities in the process of learning. Painful defecation and resulting habit constipation, with or without fecal soiling, is most often the cause of psychogenic problems related to bowel dysfunction.

Constitutional factors. In cases of idiopathic constipation there is a delayed transit time and an increased absorption of water in the colon that appears to be secondary to the slow transit time and to the increase in colonic volume. An element of anorectal obstruction or segmental colonic inertia could explain these findings. In children with chronic constipation and encopresis, the colon propels feces normally and effectively to the rectum, in which a large mass gathers. There may be primary rectal inertia; in these cases, the history of constipation goes back to the first few months of life. In others, rectal inertia may be precipitated by an acute episode of constipation or by a painful condition of the anus such as a fissure. Distention and pressure build up in the rectal lumen, stimulating the rectal mucosa and the sleeve and sling muscle complex and bringing about relaxation of the internal sphincter. Attempts to defecate are painful, and "holding back" ensues. Failure to evacuate results in a megarectum, and the sleeve and sling become relaxed and permit shortening of the anal canal to the length only of the skin-lined anus. The short passage, though encircled by the external sphincter, is barely sphincteric and permits constant leakage.

Recent studies in both adults and children with chronic constipation have strengthened the hypothesis that most cases are attributable to an outlet obstruction. The pattern of transit of radiopaque markers through the colon suggests that outlet obstruction is more common than colonic inertia. Manometric studies show that most children with constipation have one abnormality or a combination of the following:

A higher-than-normal intrarectal pressure necessary to elicit relaxation of internal sphincter (Fig. 14-3)

Increased anal resting pressure

Blunted subjective perception of urge to defecate

A few years ago, a small number of constipated children with encopresis were shown to have ganglion cells and absence of relaxation of their internal sphincter. The term "anal achalasia" was coined for this small subset of patients who are believed to have a form of Hirschsprung's disease. In such cases medical treatment may be associated with a progressive decrease in the intrarectal pressure necessary to bring about relaxation of the internal sphincter. In others the treatment advocated for ultrashort-segment (less than 5 cm) Hirschsprung's disease is recommended.

Clinical findings

Regardless of the cause of constipation at the onset, the child holds back, a habit that results in his horrendous problem, since the accumulation of feces makes defecation even more difficult and painful. Soon he begins to soil himself, and if he is attending school, he becomes isolated and an outcast. At home, he is in no better favor.

The cardinal feature of encopresis, withholding of stools, is often not recognized by the parents. They commonly give a history of the child's making valiant efforts at defecation, whereas in fact he is holding back. Another mode of presentation is chronic diarrhea that is caused by the flow of fluid intestinal contents around a large fecal impaction and subsequent leakage through an external sphincter that has lost its competence.

Constipation with encopresis rarely starts before the age of 3 years. Boys are much more frequently (6 to 1) affected than girls. Failure to thrive is very uncommon and requires that another diagnosis be considered. Although stools are more likely to be evacuated in the daytime and outside the schoolroom, nighttime soiling occurs in about half the patients. A recent series has shown that 40% were never toilet trained. In close to half of those who had achieved continence before becoming encopretic a "disruptive" event seemed to play a role.

Colicky abdominal pain is often documented and leads to the evacuation of a large, impacted stool mass that can block the toilet plumbing. Although the child may be retaining large amounts of fecal material easily palpated through the abdominal wall, the abdomen is moderately distended because gas escapes normally. Enuresis is an associated complaint in 30%, and the incidence of urinary tract infections is increased.

On examination, the child is usually withdrawn and depressed and will not volunteer any information about his problem. On rectal examination, the anal canal is noticeably shortened and barely sphincteric. The rectal ampulla is large and filled with a mass of fecal material.

Differential diagnosis

It is most important to recognize that fecal incontinence may occur with or without constipation. The physiologic and psychologic mechanisms associated with incontinence in the constipated child represent a specific entity distinct from incontinence in the child who does not have constipation. Fecal soiling is a condition in which children who, at an age when most others are out of diapers, continue to defecate into their diapers or underclothes. Neurologic abnormalities (Fig. 14-4), progressive degenerative diseases, and mental retardation should be ruled out.

At times, symptoms of Hirschsprung's disease are not prominent in infancy and may become typical only in early or even late childhood. The relationship between the length of the aganglionic segment and the severity or age of onset of the symptoms is poor except in short or ultrashort segment aganglionosis. In these cases, symptoms are likely to start in early childhood. It is important to remember that a small proportion may have soiling. Care should be taken not to confuse them with cases of idiopathic megacolon.

In a recent report, 10% of children resistant to medical management of constipation that had started either at birth or during the first year were identified as having ultrashort segment (less than 5 cm from the anal margin) Hirschsprung's disease (Table 14-1).

Encopresis in the child who has no history of constipation does not yield to the regimen described below. In such cases, there is either persistence of, or reversion to, the infantile pattern

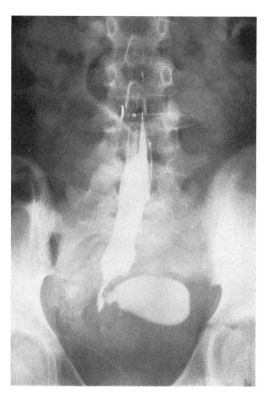

Fig. 14-4. Chronic constipation in a 10 year old with agenesis of the right hemisacrum and an anterior lipidomeningocele demonstrated by myelography.

Table 14-1. Clinical features in ultrashort segment Hirschsprung's disease

	Constipation (85)	Hirschsprung's disease (10)
Onset from in- fancy	49	9
Stooling at more than 10-day interval	15	4
Abdominal dis- tention	27	8
Soiling	51	4
Neonatal ob- struction	3	4
Family history	25	0
Psychologic problem	20	2

From Clayden, G.S., and Lawson, J.O.N.: Arch. Dis. Child. **51:**918-923, 1976.

of uninhibited defecation. Attention should also be paid to the possibility of an underlying systemic or gastrointestinal disease when constipation is of recent onset and is particularly severe. Abdominal pain persisting after removal of an impaction is a cause for concern.

All cases of long-standing, protracted, severe constipation, particularly if failure to thrive and abdominal distention are present, call for investigation of the possibility of Hirschsprung's disease. With recent reports of encopresis associated with short segment aganglionosis and with segmental dilatation of the colon, roentgenographic investigation of all cases of "idiopathic megacolon" is recommended. The next step is to take successive suction biopsy specimens at 3, 4, and 5 cm from the anal margin. However, ultrashort segment Hirschsprung's disease may be missed by a biopsy and may only show failure of the internal sphincter to relax on distention of the rectum.

In psychogenic constipation, a simple roentgenograph of the abdomen shows a colon dilated with stool and indistinguishable from the scout films

seen in congenital aganglionic megacolon. Barium enema, on the other hand, shows in the former entity a dilated colon extending to the anus. Oblique views must be made to avoid covering a spastic segment by a dilated portion. The functional megacolon usually evacuates barium readily, whereas in aganglionosis, evacuation is poor. If the initial barium enema was performed without previous cleansing enemas (best to detect a spastic segment), a repeat roentgenographic study should be done within 1 to 2 weeks, or sooner if symptoms occur.

Treatment

Removal of the fecal impaction is the first step. This can be accomplished by the administration of 3 ml/kg of hypertonic phosphate enemas (pediatric Fleet enemas); giving two at a 1-hour interval is highly effective. One must remember, however, that hypertonic dehydration, hyperphosphatemia, and hypocalcemic tetany have been reported. To prevent this complication when the first hypertonic phosphate enema is ineffective, one should follow it with an isotonic saline enema, remembering, however, that shock has also been reported after instillation of large amounts of saline solution.

Once the fecaloma has been evacuated, daily normal saline enemas are given for a week. If the fecaloma is particularly hard, it is best to use rectal instillation of 120 ml of mineral oil, followed, a few hours later, by a saline enema. This may have to be repeated twice a day for a few days. The second phase of the management consists in giving increasing amounts of mineral oil sufficiently large to result in three or four loose bowel movements that the child cannot ''hold back.'' A good starting dose is 30 ml/10 kg in divided dosage morning and evening. Potting the child for a short period twice a day after breakfast and dinner is recommended, so that, over a period of 3 months, regular bowel habits are developed. Doses of oil are gradually reduced during the ensuing 2 to 3 months. Prevention of a relapse is important, particularly in patients with a history of constipation since birth. Leakage of oil may be a sign that a new impaction has formed and that the amounts of oil recommended were insufficient. Attention to dietary factors is important. A multivitamin preparation is best administered a few hours before mineral oil.

After this initial phase, the use of a stool softener (Colace, 5 to 10 mg/kg/24 hr) may be necessary on a chronic basis, but it should not be used until regular habits have been acquired and until the child has no longer any desire to withhold. Psychiatric help is indicated for patients with recurring symptoms and for those with overt severe emotional disturbances.

In the past few years submucosal resection of a thin strip of muscle, including the full thickness of the internal sphincter and both layers of the rectal musculature, has been carried out in both adults and children with ultrashort segment Hirschsprung's disease, as well as in those with idiopathic megacolon. Results in the latter condition are not satisfactory in adults if colon inertia is present. In 11 children, two were cured, six were improved, and two were unchanged. Anal dilatation under general anesthesia should be attempted before a sphincterotomy is done. A cure can be expected in close to 50%, but relapses have been reported.

Behavior-modification techniques and biofeedback training are noninvasive and associated with promising results. Of 40 patients with functional constipation, 24 had no soiling and 14 had only minor soiling after two to five sessions during which the child is asked to duplicate and reinforce the sphincter pressure responses observed on the oscilloscope as a result of inflation of a rectal balloon. A home program of exercise for anal muscle contraction and regular toileting are the other components of this exciting approach to a difficult problem.

REFERENCES

Bentley, J.F.R.: Constipation in infants and children, Gut **12:**85-90, 1971.

Christensen, J.: The controls of gastrointestinal movements: some old and new views, N. Engl. J. Med. **285:**85-97, 1971.

Clayden, G.S., and Lawson, J.O.N.: Investigation and management of long-standing chronic constipation in childhood, Arch. Dis. Child. **51:**918-923, 1976.

Davidson, M., and Bauer, C.H.: Studies of distal colonic motility in children. IV. Achalasia of the distal rectal segment despite presence of ganglia in the myenteric plexuses of this area, Pediatrics **21:**746-761, 1958.

Davidson, M., Kugler, M.M., and Bauer, C.H.: Diagnosis and management in children with severe and protracted constipation and obstipation, J. Pediatr. **62:**261-275, 1963.

Devroede, G.: Constipation: mechanisms and management. In Sleisenger, M.H., and Fordtran, J.S., editors: Gastrointestinal disease, ed. 2, Philadelphia, 1978, W.B. Saunders Co.

Fitzgerald, J.F.: Difficulties with defecation and elimination in children, Clin. Gastroenterol. **6:**283-297, 1977.

Hata, Y., Duhamel, M., Pages, R., and others: Mégarectum de l'enfant, Ann. Chir. Infantile **15:**65-75, 1974.

Hendren W.H.: Constipation caused by anterior location of the anus and its surgical correction, J. Pediatr. Surg. **13:**505-512, 1978.

Leape, L.L., and Ramenofsky, M.L.: Anterior ectopic anus: a common cause of constipation in children, J. Pediatr. Surg. **13:**627-630, 1978.

Levine, M.D.: Children with encopresis: a descriptive analysis, Pediatrics **56:**412-416, 1975.

Martelli, H., Devroede, G., Arhan, P., and Duguay, C.: Mechanisms of idiopathic constipation: outlet obstruction, Gastroenterology **75:**623-631, 1978.

Meunier, P., Marechal, J.M., and Jaubert de Beaujeu, M.: Rectoanal pressures and rectal sensitivity studies in chronic childhood constipation, Gastroenterology **77:**330-336, 1979.

Olness, K., McParland, F.A., and Piper, J.: Biofeedback: a new modality in the management of children with fecal soiling, J. Pediatr. **96:**505-509, 1980.

Scobie, W.G., Kirwan, W.O., and Smith, A.N.: Colonic motility in children with constipation, Dis. Col. Rect. **20:**672-676, 1977.

Shandling, B., and Desjardins, J.G.: Anal myomectomy for constipation, J. Pediatr. Surg. **4:**115-118, 1969.

Taichert, L.C.: Childhood encopresis: a neurodevelopmental-family approach to management, Calif. Med. **115:**11-18, 1971.

CONGENITAL AGANGLIONIC MEGACOLON (HIRSCHSPRUNG'S DISEASE)

Congenital aganglionic megacolon was decribed more than a hundred years ago, but the pathogenesis has been known for only a little more than 25 years. The incidence of the disease is 1 in 5000 live births. It is rare (2.6%) in low birth weight infants and there is no known racial predilection. Although classically known as a disease of the very young, older children, adolescents, and adults may suffer from this condition. Hirschsprung's disease accounts for 20% to 25% of cases of neonatal intestinal obstruction. Its frequent association with Down's syndrome is worth remembering. The disease is four times more common in boys than in girls. However, in cases where the aganglionosis extends beyond the sigmoid colon (long segment disease) the ratio drops below 3 to 1. A familial pattern is described in 7% of all patients, but it increases to 21% if one examines only cases of total colonic aganglionosis with or without small bowel involvement. Of interest also in the 1979 survey of the members of the surgical section of the American Academy of Pediatrics is the observation that the percentage of girls with a positive family history is somewhat greater, but a 3 to 1 preponderance of boys is still present. The risk of the disease developing in siblings is variable. It runs from 0.6% for sisters of boys with a short segment to 18% in brothers of girls with a long segment.

Pathogenesis

The primary defect in Hirschsprung's disease is regarded as the total absence of the intramural ganglion cells of the submucosal and myenteric plexuses. Studies of human embryos and fetuses suggest that this is the result of a defective migration of ganglion cell precursors of the neural crest into the hindgut. Hirschsprung's is therefore a neural crest disease and is one of a growth of neurocrestopathies such as pheochromocytoma, neuroblastoma, and medullary carcinoma of the thyroid, which are all associated with intestinal hyperganglionosis and bouts of intestinal obstruction. Von Recklinghausen's disease is another neurocrestopathy; it can be associated with obstruction through intestinal neurofibromas. Intestinal muscular activity is regulated by cholinergic excitatory sympathetic and parasympathetic fibers and by adrenergic inhibitory fibers. The autonomic innervation also includes noncholinergic excitatory and nonadrenergic inhibitory fibers. The distal rectum, the internal sphincter, and the anal canal are normally in a state of near continuous activity. The current hypothesis is that the neurons of the nonadrenergic inhibitory system are in the myenteric plexus. If inhibitory nerves synapse in ganglion cells, in the absence of ganglion cells coordinated relaxation cannot take place. As a result the aganglionic segment, the internal sphincter, and the anal canal in Hirschsprung's disease are in a state of constant contraction. Acetylcho-

line concentrations in aganglionic segments are threefold lower than in ganglionic segments. Muscle strips from patients with Hirschsprung's disease are much less responsive to the excitatory effect of acetylcholine than those from controls. Recent studies suggest that muscarinic cholinergic receptors are normal. Thus, the information is still fragmentary but the evidence points to a defective inhibitory activity rather than to an increased cholinergic excitatory activity.

Over the past few years, failure of relaxation of the internal sphincter on rectal distention has been recognized as pathognomonic of the disease and as an important determinant of clinical manifestations. At the level of the internal sphincter and for a distance of 3 cm inside the anal canal, there is a very poor correlation between structure (ganglion cells) and function (relaxation of the sphincter). As is the case with denervation of smooth muscle, the internal sphincter remains in a state of constant contraction and prevents evacuation not only of solids but also of liquids and gas. It is likely that the degree of internal sphincter dysfunction assumes an important role in the genesis of symptoms. Achalasia of the internal sphincter may be the only abnormality remaining after surgery and may account for persistence of symptoms.

The recent description in both humans and animals of hypoganglionosis, segmental absence, degenerative changes, or immaturity of ganglion cells is forcing the idea that the presence of ganglion cells in no way assures normal colonic function. Perhaps perinatal and postnatal environmental factors also play a role in the pathogenesis of Hirschsprung's disease.

Pathologic findings

Classic Hirschsprung's disease. Agenesis of ganglion cells between the mucosa and the submucosa (Meissner's plexus) and between the muscular layers (Auerbach's plexus) is usually associated with hyperplastic nerve fibers characterized by a striking proliferation of Schwann's cells (Fig. 14-5). This finding can be of great help in the diagnosis of Hirschsprung's disease in infants and children.

Meissner's plexus has very little influence on colonic motility, but it participates in the abnormal developmental pattern of Auerbach's plexus. The easy accessibility of Meissner's plexus (Fig. 14-6) through a suction biopsy is somewhat coun-

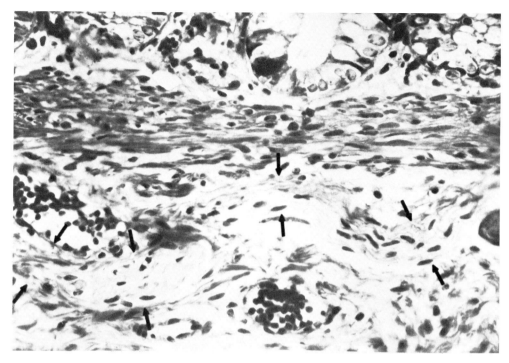

Fig. 14-5. Meissner's plexus in Hirschsprung's disease. This suction biopsy specimen of the rectum taken at 5 cm from the anal verge shows, in the submucosa, hyperplastic nonmyelinated nerve fibers and the complete absence of ganglion cells, *arrows*.

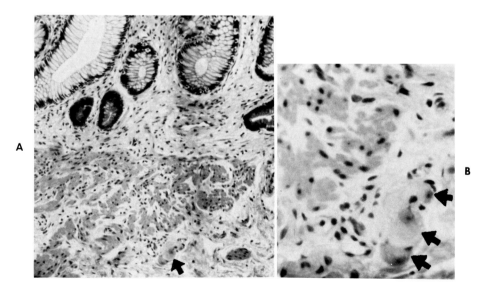

Fig. 14-6. *A,* Ganglion cells in the submucosa, *arrow*. Although ganglion cells are usually smaller in size in Meissner's plexus (submucosal) than in Auerbach's plexus (myenteric), they can be readily identified. **B,** Three of them are present in this rectal suction biopsy specimen, *arrows*.

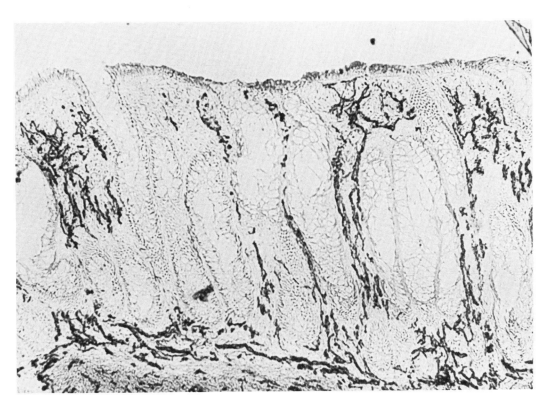

Fig. 14-7. Acetyl cholinesterase stain of a rectal suction biopsy specimen. This technique is an important adjunct to the diagnosis. Normally, staining is essentially absent in the mucosa. In this biopsy section taken from a young infant, staining is pronounced and indicates that hyperplastic and hypertrophic nerve fibers extend all the way up to the periphery of the mucosa.

terbalanced by the fact that its ganglion cells are more sparsely distributed and generally smaller. For some authors failure to identify submucosal ganglion cells or the presence of proliferated nerve fibers, or both, in a patient for whom the clinical diagnosis is in doubt calls for a punch biopsy of a rectal valve. A further important point is that ganglion cell density varies greatly from one area of the colon to another. Ganglion cells are particularly sparse in the transverse colon though plentiful at both the hepatic and splenic flexures and in the lower rectum. Ganglion cells are rarely seen within the first 2.5 to 3 cm of the rectum. Furthermore, small ganglion cells are described in the internal sphincter of patients with authenticated cases of congenital megacolon. Consequently, biopsy specimens should not be relied on for the diagnosis unless they are taken proximal to the internal sphincter.

Incoming autonomic nerve fibers synapse in the submucosal (Meissner's) and in the intermuscular (Auerbach's) plexus. Postganglionic fibers are then distributed to all layers from the mucosa to the serosa. In the absence of ganglion cells, there is a remarkable hyperplasia and hypertrophy of the myenteric plexus along with a proliferation of nerve fibers throughout the mucosa. These proliferated mucosal nerve fibers are readily identified by a special stain for acetylcholine esterase (Fig. 14-7) and constitute an important addition to the work-up of the patient with Hirschsprung's disease. Acetylcholine esterase is an enzyme essential for the hydrolysis of acetylcholine. Its activity measured chemically in biopsy specimens shows a mean sixfold increase in Hirschsprung's disease.

The aganglionic segment remains persistently contracted, whereas the proximal segment above retains its peristaltic function. As a result, there is work hypertrophy, eventual dilatation (megacolon), and sometimes perforation of the normally innervated colon.

Pseudo-Hirschsprung's disease and related disorders. The recent description of a number of patients with essentially the same clinical and

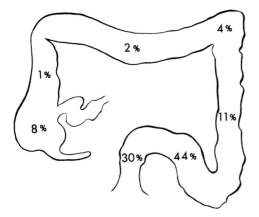

Fig. 14-8. Length of aganglionic segment in 998 cases of Hirschsprung's disease. (Drawn from data by Kleinhaus, S., et al.: J. Pediatr. Surg. **14:**588-600, 1979.)

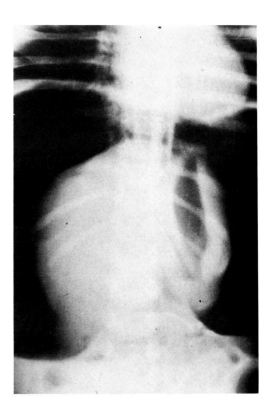

Fig. 14-9. Neonatal intestinal perforation with Hirschsprung's disease. The diagnosis of Hirschsprung's disease must be ruled out in all cases of neonatal intestinal obstruction or perforation. There is generalized free pneumoperitoneum in this 2-week-old infant with constipation since birth, abdominal distention, and bilious vomiting.

roentgenographic picture as in Hirschsprung's disease but in whom no histologic abnormalities have been found is forcing reappraisal of the pathogenesis of the disease. It is also hard to understand why Hirschsprung's disease can be well tolerated for years, or decades, and then can finally give rise to the classic picture of congenital megacolon or to intestinal obstruction. The frequent disparity between the length of the aganglionic segment and its clinical repercussions suggests that there may be relative degrees of functional impairment of colonic evacuation. Finally, there are indications that achalasia of the internal sphincter may play a significant role in the overall picture.

Length of bowel involved and associated anomalies. The extent of the aganglionosis varies enormously. It may involve only the area close to the internal sphincter, or it may affect the entire colon and small bowel, giving rise to clinical signs of a congenital duodenal obstruction. Fig. 14-8 summarizes the relative distribution of cases in terms of length of involvement. It can be seen that in most cases (75%) the aganglionic segment is limited to the rectosigmoid colon. Only 15% extend beyond the splenic flexure, and 8% involve the entire colon alone or the colon with various lengths of the small bowel.

The frequency of associated anomalies in Hirschsprung's disease is small compared to other anomalies of the digestive tract. However, there is a striking increase in Down's syndrome (3.2% in the series of Swenson and colleagues). Megaloureters are noted in 2.5%.

Clinical findings

It is surprising to note in the American Academy of Pediatrics survey that during the period of 1971 to 1975, only 15% of cases were diagnosed during the first 30 days of life whereas close to two thirds were identified by 3 months of age. A very small proportion are diagnosed beyond 5 years of age, and they usually have a short (rectosigmoid) or more often an ultrashort (less than 5 cm) segment.

Since the symptoms and signs vary to some extent according to the age of the patient with Hirschsprung's disease, it is important to describe the aggregation of clinical findings seen at different ages.

First week of life. The newborn infant, usually of average weight, will fail to pass meconium; this is rapidly followed by reluctance to eat, bilious vomiting, and abdominal distention, which may provoke rapid breathing and grunting. The classic picture of acute intestinal obstruction secondary to Hirschsprung's disease may be impossible to distinguish from that secondary to other conditions such as meconium ileus, ileal atresia, or large bowel obstruction. Obstruction may lead to an ileal, appendiceal, or colonic perforation (Fig. 14-9).

In other cases, there is delay in passing meconium within the first 24 to 48 hours. This is followed by obstipation associated almost invariably with varying degrees of abdominal distention. If the degree of partial intestinal obstruction is severe enough, vomiting is noted. The neonate usually has a worried or frowning appearance, which, combined with thin features, makes the baby look like a little old man. Often the baby is irritable, feeds poorly, and fails to thrive.

Infancy. The infants whose initial symptoms are not correctly interpreted and are merely treated with digital rectal dilatations and enemas may have a temporary remission of a few weeks' duration, but the majority respond poorly and may develop severe diarrhea in addition to the triad of failure to thrive, abdominal distention, and vomiting (Fig. 14-10). The presence of diarrhea is an ominous sign because it usually is indicative of enterocolitis associated with a high mortality in the first few months of life. It is characterized by explosive, liquid stools, fever, and severe prostration. Enterocolitis is essentially never seen beyond 2 years of age: two thirds occur in infants diagnosed within the first 3 months. Of great interest is the recent observation that its incidence is relatively low (10%) during the first month of life but climbs to 30% and 33% at 2 and 3 months.

One must remember that enterocolitis may exist even in the absence of diarrhea. Unexplained fever and poor feeding may be the earliest symptoms of enterocolitis. The pathologic lesion shows acute inflammatory and ischemic changes; perforation and sepsis are common.

Childhood. If symptoms during early infancy are not prominent, the affected child suffers from obstinate constipation, the stools are offensive and ribbonlike, the abdomen is enlarged, the veins are prominent, peristaltic patterns are readily visible, and fecal masses are easily palpated (Fig. 14-11). Intermittent bouts of intestinal obstruction from fecal impaction, hypochromic anemia, hypoproteinemia, and failure to thrive are added features. Encopresis is rare in Hirschsprung's disease but may occur when the disease is limited to an ultrashort segment (less than 5 cm). Table 14-1 shows

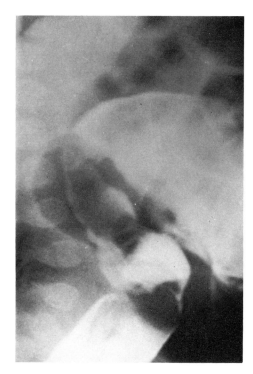

Fig. 14-10. Hirschsprung's disease with a short aganglionic segment. A 1-month-old infant suffered obstipation since birth. There was a significant degree of abdominal distention. The barium injected under low pressure shows a spastic segment leading into a colonic lumen dilated by air, fluid, and feces.

comparative clinical findings between ultrashort segment Hirschsprung's disease and idiopathic megacolon.

Diagnosis

Rectal examination. On digital examination of the rectum, the anal canal and rectum are devoid of fecal material and may feel narrow and grip the finger. As the finger is withdrawn, there may be a forcible gush of flatus and liquid, offensive, pale stools. The presence of fecal colonic impaction associated with an empty rectum is most suggestive of the disease.

Roentgenographic studies. A plain roentgenograph of the abdomen with the patient in the prone position with a vertical beam may show a severe degree of gaseous distention and, more importantly, how far into the colon and rectum the gaseous distention extends. In a neonate, the absence of gas in the pelvis is suggestive of Hirschsprung's disease. However, in infants, it is difficult to distinguish between dilated small intestine

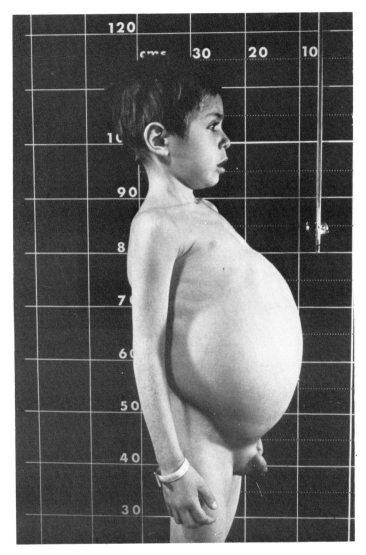

Fig. 14-11. Hirschsprung's disease in a 6-year-old boy. This youngster suffered from chronic constipation from birth. The symptoms were controlled by medication, and growth was satisfactory until a few weeks before admission when he developed intestinal obstruction.

and dilated large bowel; therefore no etiologic diagnosis can be made.

A barium enema should be done by introduction of a small amount of radiopaque material through a catheter, with the tip inserted barely beyond the anal sphincter. The most reliable roentgenographic finding of Hirschsprung's disease is a clear-cut zone of transition between the aganglionic distal segment, which is narrow or of normal caliber, and the dilated proximal with normal ganglion cells (Fig. 14-12). Such a clear-cut zone often is not present at birth. When colonic involvement is total or when the zone of transition cannot be identified, one has to rely on late films taken 12 to 48 hours after evacuation. Barium retained after 24 hours is uniformly distributed throughout the colon (Fig. 14-13). In the normal child or one with chronic constipation, the retained barium is usually collected as a bolus in the rectum and sigmoid. This sign can be lost if a water-soluble contrast enema is used. Of interest is the observation that the widest rectal diameter is usually smaller than that of the widest rectal diameter of the sigmoid loop, even in the absence of a roentgenographically definite transition segment.

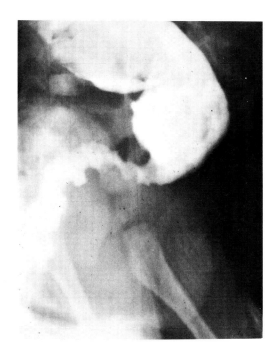

Fig. 14-12. Aganglionic megacolon. The irregular spastic segment is clearly differentiated from the dilated portion above. Oblique or lateral projections are practically always necessary to demonstrate a short segment such as this, since in the anteroposterior projection a dilated part lies over it.

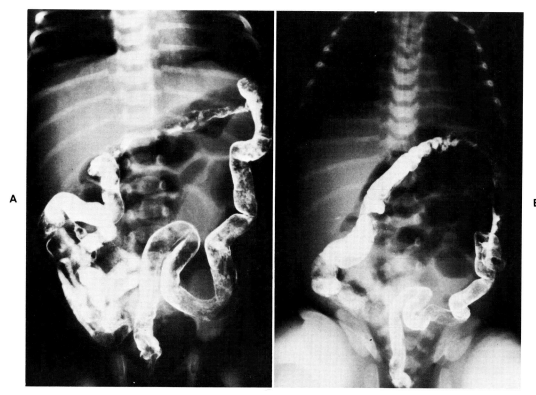

Fig. 14-13. Total aganglionosis. A 2-day-old neonate failed to pass meconium and suffered abdominal distention and vomiting. **A,** Barium enema shows a colon of reduced caliber and outlines the distal ileum. **B,** Twenty-four hours later, hardly any barium has been evacuated and it is uniformly distributed throughout the colon. A rectal suction biopsy showed absence of ganglion cells. An ileostomy was performed. The postoperative course was complicated by malnutrition and enteritis, which required parenteral hyperalimentation.

Rectal biopsy. Besides a number of false negative or equivocal roentgenographic patterns, false positives are also reported. Rectal biopsy is the most reliable method of diagnosis and should be performed in all cases, since the diagnosis rests on histologic evidence of aganglionosis.

The simplicity and safety of rectal suction biopsies make this the procedure of choice. The presence of ganglia in the submucosa is reassuring and rules out the diagnosis. However, the absence of ganglia is more difficult to interpret because ganglion cells in young infants may be small and monopolar. The presence of large nonmyelinated nerve trunks in the submucosa adds considerable weight to the diagnostic value of absent ganglion cells. These conglomerations of nerve fibers are particularly prominent near the transition zone. Acetylcholine esterase histochemistry is invaluable because it not only permits the specific staining of the neuroma-like conglomerations of nerve fibers but also shows the fine network of nerves extending in the mucosa (Fig. 14-7). We are impressed with the reliability of suction biopsy specimens examined for ganglion cells and for high acetylcholine esterase activity. We no longer find it necessary to do a full-thickness biopsy of the lower rectal valve. The only indication for a full-thickness biopsy is determination of the length of aganglionic segments at surgery. Our policy has been to take successive biopsies at 3, 4, and 5 cm from the anal margin and to cut the entire blocks.

Manometric study. Pressure recordings are obtained from the internal and external sphincters in response to transient balloon distention of the rectum. Anorectal manometry should be available for the routine investigation of all infants and children in whom the diagnosis of Hirschsprung's disease is entertained. The rectoanal inhibitory reflex, that is, internal sphincter relaxation in response to a transient rectal distention, is absent in Hirschsprung's disease (Fig. 14-14). The presence of the reflex rules out the disease, but there are false negative results associated with longstanding cases of constipation (anal achalasia) with or without encopresis. Tracings in newborns pose particular problems though it is in this age group that accuracy of the manometric diagnosis is particularly important.

In a study of 45 full-term infants, manometric recordings have revealed that in 11% internal sphincter relaxation was present at birth, in 50% on the third day, and in all of them by the twelfth day. With special refinements in technique, it has been demonstrated that a normal anorectal reflex can be recorded in 95% of prematures with a mean birth weight of 1600 gm and at a mean age of 11.7 days.

A delayed maturation of the intramural nerve plexuses can be caused by hypoxia, respiratory distress syndrome, and prematurity. The associated functional intestinal obstruction is the result of a high barrier of anorectal resting pressure and an absent internal sphincter relaxation reflex.

Differential diagnosis

As alluded previously, the various causes of intestinal obstruction need to be ruled out. Since neonatal, cecal, appendiceal, or colonic perforation has been associated with congenital megacolon, the disease should be ruled out in all cases of intestinal perforation. Delayed passage of meconium is an indication for a rectal biopsy and a manometric study. Meconium plug syndrome may be the mode of presentation of Hirschsprung's disease (Fig. 14-15). The megacystis–microcolon–intestinal hypoperistalsis syndrome has to be kept in mind, but it occurs only in girls. The small left colon syndrome may give rise to a pseudo-transitional zone at the splenic flexure. Sepsis, respiratory distress syndrome, central nervous system problems, and extreme prematurity are some of the entities responsible for functional intestinal obstruction in the newborn (Chapter 3).

Functional or psychogenic megacolon has many distinguishing features. Our attitude has been to do manometric studies and biopsies if there is a reasonable doubt.

Acquired megacolon may be secondary to an anal stricture; it is also seen in cretinism, mental retardation, and the so-called pseudo-Hirschsprung's disease. The few patients suffering this latter disease have the same clinical and roentgenographic characteristics as those with bona fide Hirschsprung's disease. However, the dilated bowel does not have the commonly noted muscular hypertrophy, and ganglion cells are present in the rectum. Hypoganglionosis and immaturity of ganglion cells remain hypothetical explanations for this disorder.

Zonal colonic aganglionosis has been well documented, and its mode of presentation does not differ from the usual form of the disease, though symptoms tend to be less severe. An ultrashort distal rectal segment (less than 5 cm from the anal

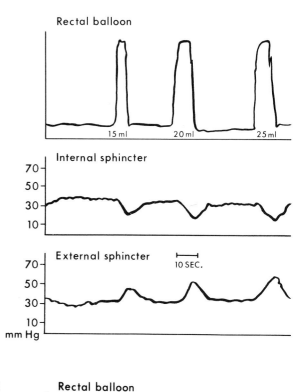

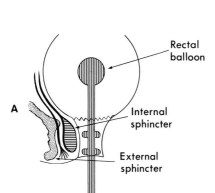

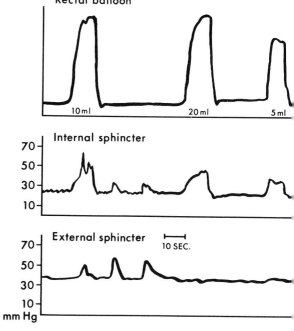

Fig. 14-14. Diagrammatic representation of the rectal probe to show relationship of the balloon system with the rectal ampulla and with both the internal and external sphincters, **A.** When the rectal balloon is distended by use of 15 ml of water, the internal sphincter relaxes and the external sphincter contracts, **B.** In contrast to this normal response, the other tracing demonstrates failure of relaxation and enhanced rhythmical activity of the internal sphincter, **C.** (Courtesy Dr. A. Bensoussan, Hôpital Sainte-Justine, Montreal.)

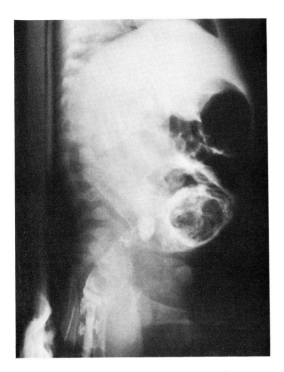

Fig. 14-15. Hirschsprung's disease presented as meconium plug syndrome. This 1-month-old infant failed to develop normal colonic function after having been relieved of obstructing meconium plugs by barium enema. There is a distal spastic segment, and the colonic portion is distended by air, fluid, and feces.

margin) may give rise to atypical symptoms more suggestive of idiopathic megacolon and to normal roentgenographic and biopsy findings if the tissue is removed from a rectal valve. Suction biopsy can miss only the rare patients with ultrashort segments. In such cases a manometric study is the only means of making a diagnosis. Segmental dilatation of the colon is characterized by severe constipation from birth. A variable segment of the colon (sigmoid, transverse, or the entire colon except for the rectosigmoid) may be dilated. The muscular wall of the involved segment is hypertrophic. Ganglion cells are present throughout.

Because of the frequent occurrence of enterocolitis during the first few months of life, intractable diarrhea or a severe bout of gastroenteritis should force close scrutiny of the patient for a history of delay in passing meconium and chronic constipation. The disease may also be mistaken for celiac disease because of the striking abdominal distention and failure to thrive.

Complications

Intestinal perforation is rare, but it has been described as the first sign of Hirschsprung's disease; appendiceal perforation appears to be a common site for perforation in the newborn infant. Perforations are also described all along the dilated proximal colon. Perforations of the ileum are described when aganglionosis of the colon is total.

Enterocolitis is a hazardous complication and the major cause of death in infants with Hirschsprung's disease. The survey conducted by the pediatric surgeons of the American Academy of Pediatrics shows that the mortality (30%) of patients with enterocolitis at the time of diagnosis (15%) has not changed during the last 20 years. Its incidence is very low after the age of 2 and most occur during the first 3 months. Enterocolitis is more common with long segment aganglionosis, but it does occur even in cases where the disease is limited to the rectum. Its postoperative occurrence is high, particularly after a Swenson or a Soave procedure.

The mode of presentation is variable; it may run a chronic course characterized by foul-smelling diarrhea, abdominal distention, and failure to thrive. In other instances, it is a fulminating disease characterized by hyperthermia, hypovolemic shock, vomiting, explosive stools, and rectal bleeding. Repeated bouts of enterocolitis separated by intervals of relative good health is the pattern seen from time to time after surgery. Pneumatosis may be present, and a barium enema will be that of ulcerative colitis. The histologic picture is that of a severe type of colitis characterized by extensive ulceronecrotic changes in the mucosa.

Induction of water intoxication from tapwater enemas was reported a few years ago; more recently, shock and hypertonic dehydration have resulted from the use of saline and hypertonic phosphate enema solutions.

Chronic malnutrition, failure to thrive, anemia, a protein-losing enteropathy, and repeated episodes of intestinal obstruction are well-described complications in patients whose difficulty goes undiagnosed and untreated.

Treatment

The goals of surgery are to permit normal defecation and to ensure continence and normal sex-

Table 14-2. Surgical results (%) in 1009 patients

	Swenson (390)	Duhamel (339)	Soave (93)	Boley (187)
Mortality	2.5	1.8	3.2	1.1
Complications	48	45.1	54.4	39.6
Enterocolitis	15.6	5.9	15.0	2.1
Incontinence	3.2	1.1	2.1	1.1
Anal stenosis	9.5	5.5	15.1	9.4
Obstruction	9.0	7.1	3.2	1.6
Fecal fistula	6.2	2.9	1.1	1.1
Disrupted anastomosis	11.2	2.4	1.1	5.8

Data from Kleinhaus, S., and others: J. Pediatr. Surg. **14:**588-600, 1979.

ual function by a procedure associated with little morbidity and no mortality.

Decompression surgery should be carried out on an emergency basis. Beforehand it is essential to deflate the abdomen with repeated rectal irrigations of normal saline solution through a carefully inserted rectal rubber cannula. Irrigations should be carried out two to four times daily until clear returns are obtained. This is a lifesaving procedure in young infants with enterocolitis. The fever drops and the infant's general condition improves almost miraculously. Close attention should be given to preoperative rehydration and to the correction of shock and hypoalbuminemia, which is almost uniformly present. The colostomy should be performed in an area of the colon in which ganglion cells are present by frozen section. When the entire colon is involved, an ileostomy is carried out.

In healthy patients with a short segment, a colostomy is usually not necessary and daily rectal irrigations can be carried out until definitive surgery. However, Nixon's recommendation is that "no baby suspected of Hirschsprung's disease should leave the hospital before diagnosis and no confirmed case should leave without an operation of either colostomy or definitive surgery. Otherwise, fatalities from supervening enterocolitis will continue to occur."

Definitive surgery is better postponed until the infant is 10 to 14 months of age. In cases diagnosed later, the colostomy is left in place for a period of 3 months before the final surgical procedure. Four basic procedures are available: the rectosigmoidectomy of Swenson, the retrorectal transanal pull-through of Duhamel, the endorectal pull-through either without primary anastomosis (Soave) or with primary anastomosis (Boley). Description of these techniques is beyond the scope of this discussion. More important is close examination of the results (Table 14-2), which attract attention to the fact that complications follow 45% to 60% of operations and that we should theoretically favor the procedure associated with the lowest percentage of ileocolitis. Resection of the aganglionic segment is delayed until the infant is at least 6 months of age.

Hirschsprung's disease has postoperatively recurred in some cases, probably because of the dropping out of ganglion cells secondary to vascular impairment in some, and in others because of chronic inflammatory changes leading to stenosis.

Posterior sphincterotomy of the internal sphincter produces excellent results when abnormal spasticity of the internal sphincter, or the so-called ultrashort aganglionic segment, is present either as the initial diagnosis or in the postoperative phase when signs of obstruction or, more importantly, of enterocolitis are present.

Prognosis

In the neonatal period, mortality reaches 25% to 35%. Enterocolitis before or after surgery is an ominous complication that accounts for 30% of the deaths in young infants. A plea is made for a high index of suspicion, a complete work up, and aggressive treatment because this is the only means of reducing mortality. Of note is the fact that only 10% of infants have enterocolitis during their first month, this percentage trebles during the second and third months of life.

REFERENCES

Aldridge, R.T., and Campbell, P.E.: Ganglion cell distribution in the normal rectum and anal canal, J. Pediatr. Surg. **3:**475-490, 1968.

Bentley, J.F.R., Nixon, H.H., and Ehrenpreis, T.: Seminar on pseudo-Hirschsprung's disease and related disorders, Arch. Dis. Child. **41:**143-154, 1966.

Campbell, P.E., and Noblet, H.R.: Experience with rectal suction biopsy in the diagnosis of Hirschsprung's disease, J. Pediatr. Surg. **4:**410-415, 1969.

De Lorimier, A.A., Benzian, S.R., and Gooding, C.A.: Segmental dilatation of the colon, Radiology **112:**100-104, 1971.

Deodhar, M., Sieber, W.K., and Kiesewetter, W.B.: A critical look at the Soave procedure for Hirschsprung's disease, J. Pediatr. Surg. **8:**249-254, 1973.

Kleinhaus, S., Boley, S.J., Sheran, M., and Sieber, W.K.: Hirschsprung's disease: a survey of the members of the surgical section of the American Academy of Pediatrics, J. Pediatr. Surg. **14:**588-600, 1979.

MacIver, A.G., and Whitehead, R.: Zonal colonic aganglionosis, a variant of Hirschsprung's disease, Arch. Dis. Child. **47:**233-237, 1972.

Martin, L.W., Buchino, J.J., LeCoultre, C., and others: Hirschsprung's disease with skip area, J. Pediatr. Surg. **14:**686-687, 1979.

Meier-Ruge, W., Lutterbeck, P.M., Herzog, B., and others: Acetylcholinesterase activity in suction biopsies of the rectum in the diagnosis of disease, J. Pediatr. Surg. **7:**11-17, 1972.

Meunier, P., Marechal, J.M., and Mollard, P.: Accuracy of the manometric diagnosis of Hirschsprung's disease, J. Pediatr. Surg. **13:**411-415, 1978.

Morikawa, Y., Donahoe, P.K., and Hendren, W.H.: Manometry and histochemistry in the diagnosis of Hirschsprung's disease, Pediatrics **63:**865-871, 1979.

Nissan, S., and Bar-Moar, J.A.: Changing trends in presentation and management of Hirschsprung's disease, J. Pediatr. Surg. **6:**10-15, 1971.

Prévot, J., Bodart, N., Babut, J.M., and others: Hirschsprung's disease with total colonic involvement, Progr. Pediatr. Surg. **4:**63-89, 1971.

Sane, S.M., and Girdany, B.P.: Total aganglionosis coli, Radiology **107:**397-404, 1973.

Siber, W.K.: Hirschsprung's disease. In Ravitch, M.M., Welch, K.J., Benson, C.D., Aberdeen, E., and Randolph, J.G., editors: Pediatric survey, ed. 3, Chicago, 1979, Year Book Medical Publishers, Inc.

Suzuki, H., White, J.J., Shafie, M.E., and others: Nonoperative diagnosis of Hirschsprung's disease in neonates, Pediatrics **51:**188-191, 1973.

Swenson, O., Sherman, J.O., and Fisher, J.H.: Diagnosis of congenital megacolon: an analysis of 501 patients, J. Pediatr. Surg. **8:**587-594, 1973.

Torone, B.H., Stocker, J.T., Thompson, H.E., and Chang, J.H.T.: Acquired aganglionosis, J. Pediatr. Surg. **14:**688-690, 1979.

FECAL INCONTINENCE

The control of defecation is the result of complex sensory, motor, and psychologic factors (see discussion on physiology of defecation and continence and on pathophysiology of incontinence). One of the most difficult problems faced by the pediatrician is fecal incontinence in a child. In this section, discussion refers to patients who have a neurogenic type of incontinence because of a congenital malformation of the central nervous system (myelomeningocele), an acquired peripheral neurologic deficit (spinal cord trauma), or a deficit after operations for imperforate anus and Hirschsprung's disease. Fecal incontinence is tolerable for many years and is handled by diapering. However, when the child reaches school age, parents and the medical team start looking frantically for a solution, on which school enrollment is contingent.

Clinical findings

The history should document the severity of the incontinence. Can the patient defecate voluntarily at times? Is the incontinence selective for liquids and gas? Does it occur only when the stools are loose? The information concerning the circumstances surrounding the onset of symptoms and their progress is essential. If the age of the patient permits, the interviewer should find out if the lack of sensation of rectal fullness and of passage of stools is complete or not, and if it is constant or intermittent.

A neurogenic bladder, paresis of the lower extremities, hydrocephalus, spinal deformities, and rectal prolapse are common findings associated with myelomeningoceles. A lipoma, hemangioma, localized hair growth, or a midline sinus or dimple in the lumbosacral area should attract attention to a spina bifida with or without extrusions of the contents of the vertebral canal and associated myelodysplasia.

On rectal examination, an impaction may be discovered. There is usually little or no perianal cutaneous sensation, the anal canal usually offers little resistance ot the examining finger, and voluntary contractions on the finger are either weak or totally absent. Stimulation of the perianal skin does not lead to reflex "puckering" of the anus.

Some of these children are more or less constantly soiled and require constant diapering (fecal soiling). Others may have a sudden evacuation but

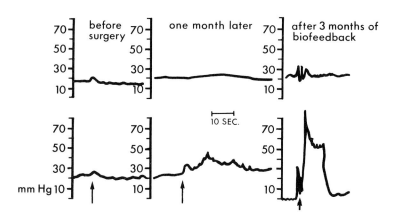

Fig. 14-16. Manometric tracings in a case of imperforate anus before transplantation of the gracilis muscle and after surgery and biofeedback training. *Two panels on left,* Absence of sphincteric activity on voluntary contractions. Some activity is present 1 month after surgery, *center panels,* and increased remarkably after postoperative stimulation with Continaid during the day. (Courtesy Dr. A. Bensoussan, Hôpital Sainte-Justine, Montreal.)

can be relatively clean except for mild staining of their underpants (fecal staining).

Manometry

A manometric study is useful even though the correlation between clinical findings and manometric assessment of sphincters in response to rectal distention is often poor.

In general, the patients with neurologic lesions, except those with spina bifida occulta, have an internal sphincter that relaxes normally but no external sphincter contraction. Various attempts have been made to obtain objective measurements of factors related to continence in patients with congenital imperforate anus who have fecal incontinence. Manometric investigation shows that poor clinical results after reconstructive surgery for a high lesion are associated with a grossly abnormal function of the anorectal structure. The rectoanal inhibitory reflex is usually absent, there is a low resting pressure in the upper anal canal, and pressure developed during voluntary contraction of the external sphincter is reduced. However, the correlation between continence and sphincteric abnormalities is not very good, since one study showed that 50% of continent patients after operation for a high type of anomaly and 30% after a low type had normal continence despite significant sphincteric abnormalities on manometry.

Management

Most children with the neurologic problems just discussed have an internal sphincter that relaxes normally on distention of the rectum, but they fail to feel the stools in contact with the anal canal and cannot prevent defecation. In others, the absence of perception for feces in the rectum leads to constipation and impaction instead of incontinence. The rectum can be emptied regularly before it fills and causes reflex relaxation of the internal sphincter. This can be achieved with a bisacodyl (Dulcolax) suppository once a day, or a saline enema. If this technique is to give optimal results, the parents must assume responsibility to decide the time of day and the best method to achieve bowel evacuation. The incontinent patient can be tried on dietary measures to produce constipated stools that can be evacuated by straining of abdominal muscles and manual pressure over the abdomen at regular intervals. In other children, the urge to defecate may be perceived if stools are rendered bulkier with Metamucil. When conservative measures fail, an abdominal colostomy should be seriously considered.

The child with an imperforate anus of the low type can be expected to develop continence because in addition to an intact puborectalis sling of the levator ani he has sensation in his anal canal and an internal sphincter that functions normally. On the other hand, the patient with a supralevator type of imperforate anus such as rectal agenesis may be slow to achieve continence. He relies solely on sensory receptors in his puborectalis sling and has no internal sphincter and little or no striated external sphincteric musculature. However, as noted previously, the striated muscle that is most important in continence is the puborectalis sling and not the external sphincter. Toilet training should be delayed. With time, what is left of the sphincteric musculature will be stronger and the child will become motivated to achieve continence.

Favorable results have been obtained by biofeedback in 10 patients 4 to 18 years of age who had been incontinent after repair of a supralevator type of imperforate anus despite enemas, laxatives, behavior modification, and psychotherapy. Transplantation of the gracilis muscle offers an opportunity to achieve continence in children with a high-lying imperforate anus (Fig. 14-16). It is a last "resort" approach after surgical attempts upon the levator sling and after medical management.

REFERENCES

Arhan, P., Faverdin, C., Devroede, D., and others: Manometric assessment of continence after surgery for imperforate anus, J. Pediatr. Surg. **11**:157-166, 1976.

Eisner, M.: Functional examination of rectum and anus in normals, in disturbances of continence and defecation and in congenital malformation, Scand. J. Gastroenterol. **7**:305-308, 1972.

Haberkorn, H., Chrispin, A., and Nixon, H.H.: Assessment of fecal incontinence by manometric and radiological techniques, J. Pediatr. Surg. **9**:43-49, 1974.

Holschneider, A.M., Kellner, E., Streibl, P., and Sippell, W.G.: The development of anorectal continence and its significance in the diagnosis of Hirschsprung's disease, J. Pediatr. Surg. **11**:151-156, 1976.

Olness, K., McParland, F.A., and Piper, J.: Biofeedback: a new modality in the management of children with fecal soiling, J. Pediatr. **96**:505-509, 1980.

Raffensperger, J.: The gracilis sling for fecal incontinence, J. Pediatr. Surg. **14**:794-797, 1979.

Schnaufer, L., Mahesh Kumar, A.P., and White, J.J.: Differentiation and management of incontinence and constipation problems in children, Surg. Clin. North Am. **50**:895-905, 1970.

White, J.J., Suzuki, H., El Shafie, M., and others: A physiologic rationale for the management of neurologic rectal incontinence in children, Pediatrics **49**:888-893, 1972.

PROCTOLOGIC DISORDERS

An anorectal examination should be part of every physical examination of the neonate, infant, and child. Anorectal disease in pediatric patients may go unrecognized and be dismissed under such diagnoses as infantile colic, constipation, emotional problems, or pinworms.

The main cause of anorectal disease in infants or children is the trauma produced by the mechanical abrasion of the anal canal by hard stools or by the irritating effect of diarrheal stools. Once the normal mucosal barrier has been crossed, bacteria gain access to the perianal structures (Fig. 14-17).

Anal fissures

Anal fissures are the most common proctologic disorder during infancy and childhood. The slit-like tear in the anal canal is usually caused by the passage of hard, large, scybalous fecal masses. In older children, a crypt abscess that has broken down leads to the laying down of scar tissue easily torn by hard stools. Explosive diarrhea can also be a contributing factor.

Clinical findings

The infant or child cries at defecation and often will try to hold back his stools. Irritability, tenesmus, and colic may be associated. Bright red blood in sparse amounts follows defecation. The anal canal to the mucocutaneous junction can be seen if the patient is held in a knee-chest position and the buttocks are spread apart. A digital or proctoscopic examination need not be done if the superficial tear is easily identified. Anterior, lateral, and multiple fissures are most common in infants and young children. Those of posterior location affect older children. A rectal examination will elicit sphincter spasm especially in the older children.

Differential diagnosis

When a fissure cannot be identified beyond a reasonable doubt, it is essential to rule out other causes of rectal bleeding such as polyposis, ulcerative colitis, and so forth. That an anal fissure is resistant to therapy might indicate the presence of a burrowing cryptitis or of chronic inflammatory bowel disease (Crohn's disease or ulcerative colitis).

Treatment

Anal fissures should be treated promptly and vigorously, especially in infants, to break the constipation-fissure-constipation cycle. We recommend the use of dioctyl sodium sulfosuccinate, 5 to 10 mg/kg/24 hr, given with feedings.

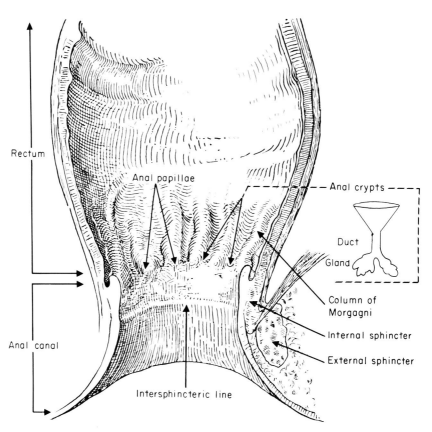

Fig. 14-17. Anatomic landmarks of the anorectum. The internal sphincter, a continuation of the circular smooth muscle layer, extends to within 0.5 to 1 cm of the anal orifice in children. The external sphincter encircles the anal canal, and its fibers are closely associated with those of the levator ani muscle, which takes off at a 45-degree angle. The intersphincteric line can usually be palpated; it is somewhat grooved and paler in color. The columns of Morgagni are longitudinal folds of rectal mucosa whose distal ends or papillae are epithelial tags of somewhat polypoid appearance. Between the papillae are the rectal sinuses, which extend distally as anal crypts. The anal crypts fill up with stools and may become infected and lead to obstruction and infection of the anal ducts and glands.

If this does not prove sufficient, 1 ounce of either mineral oil or olive oil is injected rectally with an ear syringe at bedtime. Proctosedyl, a cream containing neomycin B (Soframycin), hydrocortisone, and dibucaine hydrochloride (Cinchocaine) is very useful and can be applied after defecation and sitz baths. If painful defecation persists, warm baths three or four times a day, and twice-a-day anal dilatation with a generously lubricated finger cot can be added to the regimen.

Surgery is indicated if a fissure fails to heal after 2 to 3 months of treatment, is indurated, and is associated with a skin tag distally and with a hypertrophied anal papilla proximally.

Cryptitis

Cryptitis is a common proctologic condition that may be caused by constipation or diarrhea. The symptoms include burning of the anal area, painful defecation, and tenesmus; there is also usually spasm of the internal sphincter. Rectoscopic examination shows deepening of the crypts, hypertrophy of the papillae, and venous congestive changes. The inflammatory changes may be localized (abscess) or more diffuse. Cryptitis is usually self-limited unless infection, after spreading to the anal ducts and glands, invades perianal and perirectal tissues (anal abscess and fistula). Treatment is essentially the same as in anal fissures, since it is aimed at quickly alleviating the constipation.

Anal abscess and fistula

Infection of the perianal ducts and glands taking off from the bottom of the crypts of Morgagni (cryptitis) generates this proctologic condition. An abscess is formed in the poorly draining duct. Infection then spreads within, through, or outside the sphincteric zone to finally invade the subcutaneous tissue. An abnormal communication (fistula) is finally established between the rectum and the skin of the perianal area. Alternatively, the abscess may extend upward through the puborectalis musculature into the deeper tissues and form an ischiorectal abscess.

Recent series have stressed a striking preponderance of the condition in boys (80%), which is particulary evident in infants. The majority of affected children are less than 3 years of age. More than half the cases occur during the first 6 months of life. Triggering events are hard to determine, though sometimes the patient has chronic constipation or a history of gastroenteritis. Fever and an area of lumpy perianal redness with induration or with an intermittent discharge giving rise to painful defecation is the usual mode of presentation. In contrast to adult series where 75% grow gramnegative organisms, *Staphylococcus aureus* is present in more than half the cases. Incision and drainage is the recommended treatment if there is fluctuation or no improvement with warm soaks and antibiotics after a few days. Vigorous treatment is especially warranted in patients with compromised immunity. A fistula in ano is a complication in 25% to 30%. It requires fistulotomy and excision of the tract. The differential diagnosis should include cellulitis with beta-hemolytic streptococci and furuncles. The presence of an anal fistula in an older child who is not otherwise perfectly well should make one entertain the diagnosis of Crohn's disease.

The fistula should be incised and drained as soon as the diagnosis is made. The internal opening of the fistula is usually located 1 to 2 cm from the mucocutaneous junction. Fistulectomy is necessary to prevent recurrences.

Perianal cellulitis caused by beta-hemolytic streptococci of group A

Perianal cellulitis is a rare entity characterized by perianal erythema, edema, and tenderness to palpation. The lesion involves an area about 2 inches around the anal orifice and renders defecation painful. The history of a preceding streptococcal pharyngitis, perianal cultures positive for the same organisms, and complete resolution with penicillin substantiate the evidence for this unusual manifestation of streptococcal infections.

Hemorrhoids

Hemorrhoids are rare in children, and they are all external. Internal hemorrhoids almost never exist and do not account for rectal bleeding in the pediatric population. External hemorrhoids can be the result of anal infections (cryptitis) spreading to the hemorrhoidal veins or the result of anorectal disease associated with granulomatous ileocolitis. In portal hypertension, portal blood is commonly diverted from the inferior mesenteric vein to the systemic circulation through the venous plexus of the anal canal. Although hemorrhoidal venous pressure can become very high in such a situation, the incidence of hemorrhoids in extrahepatic or intrahepatic portal hypertension is infrequent.

Conservative management includes regulation of bowel habits, and use of sitz baths, dibucaine ointment, or rectal astringent suppositories. In cases of thrombosed hemorrhoids resistant to medical treatment, removal of the hematoma is in order.

Chronic fissure, skin tag, and anal stenosis

More than 40% of children with Crohn's disease have anal disease, which usually remains asymptomatic. In most patients with anal symptoms there is an associated abscess, a poorly draining fistula, or a tight anal stenosis preventing normal defecation. Stenosis of the anal canal usually extends proximally to the lower rectum. There is a combination of linear ulceration, edema, and fibrosis. Treatment should be conservative. Dilatation is best carried out under general anesthesia and is then continued daily by the patient who is advised to keep his stools soft with mineral oil, Colace, or Metamucil. A complete discussion of Crohn's disease is found in Chapter 13 and of congenital anal stenosis in Chapter 3.

Prolapse of the rectum

Telescoping of the rectum and the anus is a physiologic phenomenon associated with defecation. Prolapse of the rectum refers to the abnormal descent or protrusion of one of more coats of rectum through the anus.

Predisposing factors in childhood include (1) a flat sacrum and coccyx, (2) an abnormal mobility

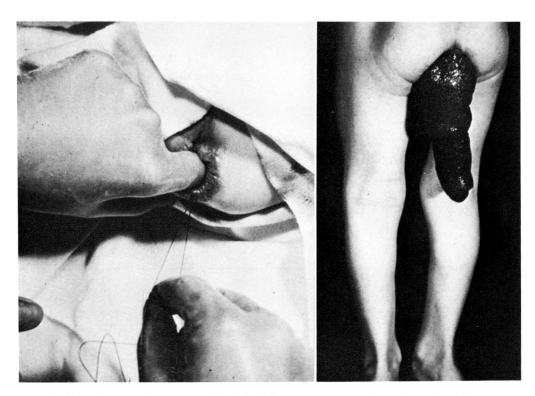

Fig. 14-18. Prolapse of the rectum. The full thickness of the rectum has prolapsed (procidentia). Visible folds are absent and the mucosa is edematous and dark red. The prolapse had become chronic in a child with a myelomeningocele and poor anal sphincter tone. Surgery was carried out.

of the sigmoid colon, (3) poor development of supporting muscular structures, and (4) rectal mucosa loosely attached to the underlying tunica muscularis.

Clinical findings

The condition usually affects infants less than 1 year old, but it is frequent up to 2 years of age. The mother will notice a 1 to 2 cm red protrusion from the anus at the time of defecation. The mucosal pattern cannot be recognized. When, less commonly, the full thickness of the rectum prolapses (procidentia), the mucosal folds are concentric and readily identified.

Constipation, long sessions at stool, coughing as in whooping cough, malnutrition, and an increase in intra-abdominal pressure (ascites) are precipitating factors. Its association with myelomeningocele, mental retardation, celiac disease, the Ehler-Danlos syndrome, and particularly cystic fibrosis is important to remember.

At first the prolapsed rectum is normal in color. As the protrusion becomes chronic, the mucosa is edematous, dark red, and dull (Fig. 14-18). Stools commonly contain much mucus and small amounts of blood. Tenesmus is common.

Treatment

Reduction can be easily carried out by the mother. Attention should be directed toward treatment of constipation, which is the most common predisposing factor. The disease is usually self-limited. If, despite these measures, the prolapse becomes chronic, strapping of the buttocks has been advocated.

Manual reduction can at times be unsuccessful. In such instances, intussusception is likely. There is rapid onset of edema, purplish discoloration of the intussusception head, and intestinal obstruction.

In chronic troublesome cases continuing beyond 2 years of age, injection of a sclerosing agent into the rectal submucosa can be rewarding. A report shows satisfactory results in 91 of 100 cases with the use of 10 ml of almond oil in 5% phenol injected in four or five sites circumferentially. Of the 100 cases reported, four had mental retardation, two had cystic fibrosis, one had celiac disease, and two others had Ehler-Danlos syndrome. All of those with an underlying disease required a second injection.

Surgery should be reserved for the rare patients in whom conservative measures and time fail to correct this self-limited condition or for those who have sigmoidorectal intussusception.

REFERENCES

Arminski, T.C., and McLean, D.W.: Proctologic problems in children, J.A.M.A. **194:**1195-1197, 1965.

Craff, A.R., and Alexander-Williams, J.: Fissure-in-ano and anal stenosis, Clin. Gastroenterol. **4:**619-634, 1975.

Duhamel, J.: Anal fistulae in childhood, Am. J. Proctol. **26:**40-43, 1975.

Emberg, R.N., Cox, R.H., and Burry, V.F.: Perirectal abscess in children, Am. J. Dis. Child. **128:**360-361, 1974.

Hirschfeld, A.J.: Two family outbreaks of perianal cellulitis associated with group A beta-hemolytic streptococci, Pediatrics **46:**799-802, 1970.

Krieger, R.W., and Chusid, M.J.: Perirectal abscess in childhood, Am. J. Dis. Child. **133:**411-412, 1979.

Mentzer, C.G.: Anorectal disease, Pediatr. Clin. North Am., pp. 113-125, 1956.

Rowe, R.J.: Symposium on the management of hemorrhoidal disease, Dis. Colon Rectum **11:**127-136, 1968.

Wyllie, G.G.: The injection treatment of rectal prolapse, J. Pediatr. Surg. **14:**62-64, 1979.

15 *Psychophysiologic recurrent abdominal pain*

Any pediatric caregiver must soon become impressed by the number of children who have either acute or recurrent abdominal pain as a major symptom. Psychophysiologic recurrent abdominal pain is a distinct pediatric entity characterized by at least three attacks of pain, severe enough to affect routine activity and occurring over a period of time longer than 3 months. The pain episodes occur in the *absence* of demonstrable organic disease but in the presence of identifiable psychophysiologic determinants. In fact, less than 5% of all children with recurrent abdominal pain have an organic disease that can account for their symptoms.

Several surveys of unselected school children found the frequency of this syndrome to be between 10% to 15%. The large number of cases further compounds the already difficult problem of diagnosis and treatment of any individual case of recurrent abdominal pain. Frequently, coping with a physical complaint of emotional origin is not an easy task for most physicians trained in diagnosis and treatment of organic disease. Too often the pediatric caregiver assigns the cause of the abdominal pain to an ill-defined organic condition such as "stomach flu," "intestinal virus," or "excess stomach acid," which temporarily satisfies the parent seeking a simple but not serious medical explanation. Unfortunately, this approach serves only to compound the emotional confusion already existing in the anxious child. Despite passage of sufficient time to allow for resolution of the considered diagnoses, including the use of a variety of medications (antacids, anticholinergics), worsening of symptoms both in frequency and severity is reported rather than improvement. The problem now assumes the more formidable challenge in size and scope once the physician realizes that he is dealing with a recurrent physical disability that is functional in nature. Since the child's behavior can often be regarded as a barometer of the family emotional climate, the presence of psychophysiologic recurrent abdominal pain usually signifies not only a disorder of the whole child, but a disturbance of some aspects of the family unit as well.

Once established, the clinical features of this condition seldom vary in expression, and deviations from such a pattern may signify an intercurrent organic condition. It is worth remembering that emotionally triggered illnesses do not immunize against organic disease. Consequently, both the physician and the parents must exercise particular caution while considering each episode of pain, especially if the rare organic cause is to be recognized.

Etiology

The etiology of this syndrome is not completely understood though many interrelated factors are probably responsible for its evolution (Fig. 15-1). The concept that psychogenic factors are triggering events in the production of physical pain is generally accepted. Emotional events may usher in the pain syndrome. The development of pain syndromes as a response to threatened, fantasized, or actual loss (separation-anxiety states) is extremely common in children. The chronic pain may come into play after an illness that unmasks the specific vulnerability of the child. This latter phenomenon is frequently seen after gastrointestinal viral illness or other diseases that commonly refer pain to the abdomen. It would appear that both a genetic and an acquired susceptibility probably play a role in the evolution of this condition in most children.

Psychophysiologic disorders are largely dependent on the autonomic nervous system, and this integrated dependency requires both learned and conditioned responses. It is clear that complex interrelationships exist between cortex and hypothalamic preganglionic nerve cells that are capable of producing pain by this pathway. Although the gastrointestinal tract seems to be the dominant target organ receiving the brunt of emotionally triggered autonomic discharges, a generalized disturbance, or imbalance between excitatory and inhibitory aspects of autonomic nervous system function, may also exist.

The group "at risk," being most likely to develop somatic manifestations to repeated stresses, are those children with a high arousal state. They

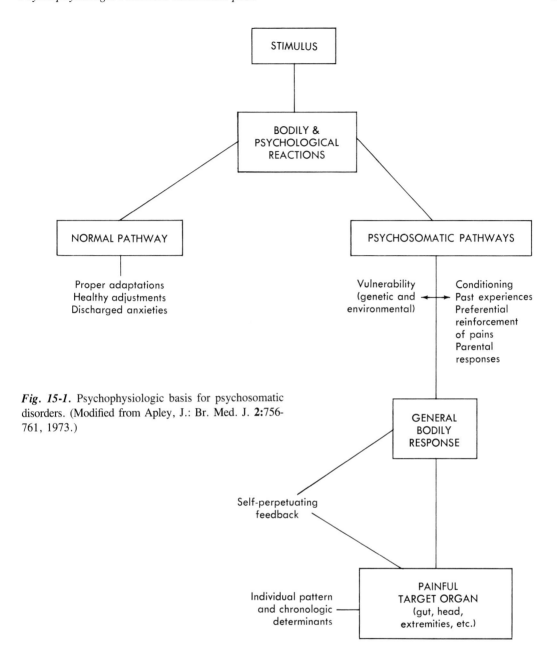

Fig. 15-1. Psychophysiologic basis for psychosomatic disorders. (Modified from Apley, J.: Br. Med. J. **2**:756-761, 1973.)

are not only exceedingly aware of their surroundings, but also have a keen sensitivity to bodily signals, often coupled unfortunately to a low-pain threshold. Many of these features are probably genetically determined. The peak age (Fig. 15-2) for this disorder could be predicted from known age- and sex-related developmental characteristics of children. Specific events or circumstances simply precipitate out the vulnerable subject. That girls develop this condition in greater numbers and at a slightly earlier age than boys most likely relates

to emotional and psychological differences in child development rather than that attributable to physical factors. The 6- to 12-year-old child is very fearful of any encounter that invites loss of newly obtained maturity, or loss of control, and will respond with aggressive behavior. As might be anticipated, such encounters occur frequently when the new school year is started and increases as the school year continues, paralleling the frequency of functional complaints (Fig. 15-3). As a result, school phobias frequently evolve but may also de-

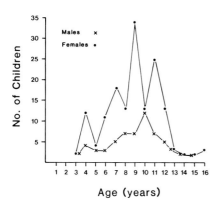

Fig. 15-2. Age and sex distribution of children evaluated for recurrent abdominal pain.

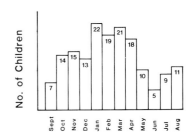

Fig. 15-3. Distribution of children with recurrent abdominal pain seen in the gastroenterology clinic by month of year.

velop without somatic pain. It is during these times of regressive behavior, as the child is trying to regroup and gather new strength to move ahead, that the abnormal degree of dependency between parent (usually mother) and child evolves. Many of these children simply cannot verbally deal with the content of their new conflicts and, in fact, talk through their bodies, thereby placing the focus of attention upon the somatic aspect (abdominal pain), which brings forth a predictable and nonthreatening parental response. Preferential reinforcement of the pain is then dictated by parental responses focusing on the physical symptom. In this learned and conditioned manner, the recurrence of the pain symptom becomes the child's solution to underlying old and new conflicts, using simply what is available to him given his psychologic development and maturity. This relationship between parent and child prevents him or her from moving ahead once again.

Although a high arousal state (dilated pupils) with heightened sympathetic tone (cutaneous vasomotor changes) is observed in most patients with recurrent abdominal pain, neither increased secretion of catecholamines nor decreased peripheral metabolism of these substances has been detected. The same applies to adults with the irritable bowel syndrome, a functional gastrointestinal disorder with features like that seen in children with psychophysiologic recurrent abdominal pain. When studied, plasma levels of dopamine betahydroxylase activity do not change with varying levels of depression, anxiety states, or bowel complaints. Urinary levels of serotonin and homovanillic acid

(HVA) are normal in children with recurrent abdominal pain, suggesting at least an intact metabolic pathway for dopamine to norepinephrine. Unfortunately, very little is presently known about the neurochemistry and neuropharmacology of affective states; however, a relationship between common neurotransmitters of brain and gut is most likely involved in modulating gastrointestinal motility. Such substances now include serotonin, substance P, and enkephalins.

Disordered motility patterns of the distal large bowel have been found in many patients with functional abdominal pain. However, the observed patterns of myoelectric activity have not distinguished the subgroups—those with diarrhea from those with constipation or alternating stool patterns. Repetitive contractions and a high resting pressure zone in the rectosigmoid area are frequently present in these patients. In addition, these patients appear to have an increased sensitivity to visceral discomfort suggesting colonic hyperalgesia. Motility studies done in adults with the irritable bowel syndrome have shown an increased frequency of slow-wave activity (3-per-minute cycling) but with normal motor activity during the unstimulated basal state. Increased slow-wave contractile activity over control patients is noted after stimulation of colonic motor activity with cholecystokinin (CCK) or pentagastrin. However, these contractions are typically nonpropulsive and segmental in nature and impede aboral fecal movement. These are important observations, for they may explain the high incidence of abnormal stooling patterns noted in adults and in many of these children as well. Complaints of obstipation, constipation, or diarrhea are surprisingly common. The distal colonic high pressure zones and disorganized motility patterns presumably result in the delivery of small stool volumes to the rectum and may account for the frequent passage of dry pelletlike stool.

Why a distal colonic abnormality in children should refer pain to the periumbilical area, a pain-sensitive location associated typically with small intestinal dysfunction, is unclear. Rare reports in adults with the irritable bowel syndrome have demonstrated an irregular contractile activity of the small bowel to coincide with attacks of abdominal pain. Perhaps small bowel motor function is also impaired in the child.

A provocative recent report noted a similar predominance of slow-wave activity in 7 of 8 patients serving as controls who, though lacking evidence of abdominal pain or bowel dysfunction, had comparable psychoneurotic traits as the study group with irritable bowel syndrome symptoms. The symptomatic group reflects those individuals with a heightened awareness of bodily signals, rather than the expression of different (quantitative or qualitative) neuromotor activity within the bowel. Just why or how these individuals become more vulnerable to visceral hyperalgesia remains to be elucidated. There are many adults, and probably children as well, who intermittently have identical symptoms but never reveal them to parent or physician. Family experiences with digestive diseases and previously mentioned factors that encourage "illness behavior" are undoubtedly important determinants in the evolution of this condition.

Diagnostic approach

There are no shortcuts to proper diagnosis of the syndrome of recurrent abdominal pain. One must resist mentally screening these patients too quickly into a functional category, though the temptation exists, given the combination of usual age group (5 to 14 years), sex (female predominance 2 to 1), location of the pain (periumbilical), and the general well appearance of the patient, despite the duration and purported severity of the disability. Recall that, by definition, this condition includes not only the exclusion of organic disease but also the elucidation of specific psychological determinants responsible for the perpetuation of the patient's complaint. For without positive and convincing data, most parents will resist the suggestion that repeated psychological factors are the triggering events for the child's somatic pain. One needs to approach this problem by building a strong case to support the contention of psychophysiologic disease, and this requires adequate interviewing time (45 to 60 minutes) that allows the physician to probe the many important facets involved in the problem. It will be most helpful if the caregiver also has an understanding and command of child development and behavioral pediatrics. Armed with the information gleaned from the careful history taking and physical examination, one can confidently summarize for patient and parent a holistic explanation as outlined in Fig. 15-1. The relationship established at the first encounter will have a strong bearing on the prognosis.

The child, and ideally both parents, should be seen in the office for the history taking and the physical examination. Occasionally several interviews may be necessary before this entity can be properly diagnosed and correct treatment recommended.

Observation

During the history taking, the physician will learn much by simply observing the child's behavior and the child-parent interaction. One can quickly sense the child's prevailing mood, be it anger, anxiety, depression, or regression. The facial expressions, changes in mood and affect, tone of voice, nervous tics, or other body movements should be noted as the history taking proceeds. The social maturity of the child can be assessed by these observations. Direct questions to the child provide information to the physician about verbal maturity and ease of expression, as one watches for appropriate affect relative to the content of the questions. Also, one should observe pupil size and vasomotor skin changes during the interview. One can assess parental confidence in the child by noting who answers the questions directed to the child. The parents are often surprised at the child's keen awareness of his environment and also at the intensity of his fears and fantasies when given the opportunity to verbalize in a "safe" setting. Although most children will claim to have pain during the interview session, their behavior, affect, and activity are seldom in keeping with the degree of expressed discomfort.

History taking

History taking is undoubtedly the most important part of the interview, for the physical examination seldom indicates any abnormality.

Pain. The age of onset of the pain is usually between 5 and 10 years with reasonable limits extending from 3 to 16 years. As a rule, one should view a pre–school age child with abdominal pain suspiciously because in this age group organic disease may have confusing or subtle manifestations whereas psychologic factors are less often responsible for the physical complaints. Recently, a slight increase in the number of teen-agers with symptoms more consistent with the adult diagnosis of spastic colon disease (lower abdominal pain and altered bowel function) have been seen in our GI Referral Clinic. A definite female predominance has been noted (2 to 1) as compared to that in previous reports, which found only a slight female predominance with this complaint. Some general aspects of the pain are summarized in Table 15-1. The pain occurs most frequently on a daily basis and is episodic and brief in duration with periods of well-being interspersed. For some children it is severe enough to make them cry or causes sufficient discomfort to alter their activity. A few patients may have continuous mild abdominal discomfort with periodic exacerbations. The pain is usually cramplike, sharp, and colicky, though it may also be described as dull and aching in nature. The pain rarely radiates, but some children feel the discomfort in a symmetric band-like manner across the upper abdomen. The pain lasts from minutes to an hour; rarely does the maximum intensity of discomfort persist for more than 3 hours. The periumbilical area is the primary location of the pain, and the child will usually place his entire hand over the area involved. When instructed to use one finger and point to the site of the pain, the older child typically demonstrates a searching motion with his finger outlining a circle around the umbilicus, whereas the younger child generally places his finger directly into the navel. The pain tends to recur in the same location. So constant are these features that the farther from the umbilicus the pain is, the more likely that an organic cause will be found responsible for the symptom.

The relationship of the attacks of pain to activity, meals, school hours, evening time, bowel habits, and so on is an individual association at best. The child may feel the pain begin immedi-

Table 15-1. Pain features of recurrent abdominal pain in 164 patients (The Children's Hospital, Denver)

	Number	**Percent**
Location		
Periumbilical	100	61
Epigastrium	50	16
Other	14	9
Character		
Sharp, cramplike	82	50
Dull, aching	50	30
Other; mixed	32	20
Frequency		
Daily	83	51
More than once weekly	40	24
1 to 4 weeks	32	20
Less than monthly	9	5
Duration		
Less than 30 minutes	36	22
30 to 60 minutes	32	20
1 to 3 hours	71	43
Over 3 hours	4	2
"Continuous"	21	13

ately upon awakening and even before arising from bed. For others, it starts before breakfast or before the child leaves for school. However, it is equally as common for the pain to occur during school hours or later in the afternoon after returning home. Complaints about pain are frequent before the child falls asleep. However, an important aspect of the pain is that it seldom occurs once the child has fallen asleep, but typically will be reported immediately upon awakening for any reason. It is not unusual for the pain to occur during so-called happy times, serving to make parents consider organic causes more seriously than psychologic ones.

A striking feature of functional abdominal pain of childhood is the failure to obtain any consistent relief from antacids or anticholinergic medications. This leads to increasing frustration on the part of parent and child and serves to magnify the presumed seriousness of the pain episodes, drawing these parties together into a symbiotic relationship. Only rarely will specific dietary eliminations produce a dramatic positive effect, since food allergies or lactose intolerance remain, in our experience, uncommon precipitants for this childhood condition.

Just as inquiry about specific qualities of the

pain is critical in helping to assess whether organic disease may explain the child's symptoms, inquiry about temporally related events going on at the time of onset of the pain is most vital to a diagnosis of functional abdominal pain. It is best to pursue this line of questioning after one begins to gain the confidence of the child and parent after specific questioning about the abdominal symptom. Almost without exception one can find a significant stressful situation that occurred in the child's life about the time the original pain first began. If the precipitating event was an acute illness (25%), one needs to know what diagnosis was considered and how it was treated and the level of concern for the particular illness on the part of the parent, child, and even physician. How did the child deal with the pain? What rituals evolved in coping with the symptom? Many simply "wait it out," lying around the house, watching television, or reading, whereas for others special positions and treatment regimens are described to achieve relief. Heating pads, hot-water bottles, or gentle rubbing of the area or the back by the mother helps some gain relief. The pain-relief measures may become extremely complex as the duration of the illness increases. Even during pain-free periods, the degree of incapacitation seems incredible to most, except the concerned parent. The child withdraws from activities and eventually peers and friends. Unfortunately, school personnel (teachers, nurses) are likewise more concerned with the absolute meaning of the physical complaint than with the underlying triggering factors, furthering the suspicion in the parent's mind that organic disease exists.

It is surprising that the importance of emotional precipitants to the onset of pain episodes may not be considered or appreciated by child or parent. Not infrequently, what the parent perceives as a trivial event, in fact, has developed into a monumental internal emotional conflict for the child, which simply will not go away. Such crises as a serious illness in a parent, a death in the immediate family, older siblings going away to college or into the military, loss of friends or pets, change in environment by a move, or the starting of school should be specifically inquired about, as the content of these potentially psychologic stresses are seldom appreciated or volunteered by the parent for the aforementioned reason.

Associated symptoms. Related symptoms are frequent as the child is carefully scrutinized by

Table 15-2. Major associated symptom or symptoms in recurrent abdominal pain in 164 cases

Symptom	Number	Percent
Bowel dysfunction	48	29
Constipation 31		
Diarrhea 17		
Vomiting	40	24
Tiredness	30	18
Headache	24	15
Pallor	18	11
Dizziness	10	6
Limb pain	3	2
Chest pain	2	1
Weight loss	2	1

the wary parent during pain episodes and between them as well (Table 15-2). The additional complaints tend to be nonspecific and should serve to reinforce for the physician the concept that many of these children feel their whole body is "unwell." They appreciate so many noxious somatic signals. Tiredness and easy fatigue are often reported. Pallor is another common associated symptom reported during the pain episodes. Headache, either during or around the attack of abdominal pain, occurs in 10% to 15% of patients. The child's temperature may be found to be slightly elevated (below 101° F) during attacks. Dizziness, rarely with syncopal episodes, may be reported. Extremity, back, and chest pains may be present at times. Upper gastrointestinal complaints include nausea, vomiting, or belching. Large bowel dysfunction may be present in up to 50% of these patients. Constipation with passage of pelletlike stools is noted most frequently. Diarrhea, either during or after the attacks of pain, is much less a feature in children than in the adult patient with irritable colon syndrome. Generally speaking, it is wise to view suspiciously this last finding, especially if it occurs in the face of documented weight loss or if it is associated with the presence of blood (gross or occult) in the stools.

Despite the duration and severity of the episodes, the child has seldom suffered in terms of weight or growth, a very important bit of information.

Past history. Additional support for the proper diagnosis can be gained when one inquires into other areas. A history of discomforting morning sickness and difficult labor often characterizes the pregnancy. Colic, poor eating habits, and frequent formula changes are often recalled when the neonatal history is obtained. Some combination of undue fears, sleep disturbances, night terrors, enuresis, and difficulties in school is surprisingly common in children with recurrent abdominal pain.

Review of systems. Although a generally unrewarding part of the interview, methodical inquiry about dysfunctional aspects of the remaining organ systems ensures one from overlooking a possible organic cause for the child's pain symptom. Unusual skin rashes or other lesions may suggest an underlying disease condition. Similarly, unexplained pruritus may be associated with an occult abdominal lymphoma or hepatobiliary abnormality. Additional questions about other gastrointestinal complaints may be needed to clarify the important considerations of peptic ulcer disease or inflammatory bowel disease (Crohn's disease). Specifically such matters as pain-food relief, nocturnal pain, jaundice, constipation, diarrhea, and blood in the stool must be considered. Musculoskeletal problems such as recent trauma or known congenital defects of back, spine, or hips should be inquired about. A concurrent history of arthralgia or more importantly arthritis will suggest inflammatory bowel disease, liver disease, or a collagen vascular condition. A pulmonary pathosis can refer pain to the abdomen and may be suspected if shortness of breath, chronic cough, or wheezing is reported.

Detailed questions regarding genitourinary function (frequency, dysuria, enuresis, back or flank pain) are most important, since abnormalities in this system may present in childhood with vague abdominal discomfort. Pain episodes accompanied by a change in consciousness, disorientation or confusion, or excessive drowsiness and sleep may indicate abdominal epilepsy. Unprovoked nighttime vomiting with daytime abdominal pain and headaches suggests increased intracranial pressure or perhaps a brain tumor in the region of the floor of the fourth ventricle.

Family history. This part of the interview should be pursued in detail in that critical information pertaining to the child's genetic vulnerability to develop a psychophysiologic symptom complex will likely be uncovered. Here is the opportunity for the physician to point out that the child is "cut from a similar piece of cloth" as many other family members who likewise are somatic responders

to psychologic stress. A comprehensively recorded diagram of the family tree should be developed as one inquires into the health history of each individual spanning three generations. This technique permits specific questioning about individual family members while also prompting the parent to recall if possible those particular conditions with strong functional associations such as spastic bowel, irritable colon, mucous or spastic colitis, peptic disease (real or supposed), nervous stomachs, anxiety attacks, and mental illness. A positive history for migraines is usually uncovered. More than likely, one will be impressed with the number of family members with chronic medical problems and the frequency of surgical procedures required in these "painful families." The proverb that "the apple doesn't fall far from the tree" can be graphically demonstrated for both parent and child.

Inquiry into the social dynamics of the immediate family unit should be pursued at this time, again with the hope of gaining needed insight into the patient's problem. Discord in the home, be it from a stressed marital relationship because of financial problems, alcoholism, or infidelity, or the result of a recent parental separation, conflicts with siblings, or recent illness in a close family member, are common precipitants for the development of the child's pain symptom. In fact, stresses emanating from the home environment are more than twice as likely to be the source of difficulty than is a deteriorating school situation.

Personality and emotional makeup. Certain personality profiles are commonly found in children with recurrent abdominal pain of functional nature.

The majority of children with recurrent abdominal pain are so-called superachievers and set for themselves very high standards. They tend to tolerate failure very poorly, going about their chores in an obsessive-compulsive manner. The parents frequently describe them as their "best child" in terms of aptitudes, behavior, and maturity. Consequently, they assume many responsibilities more appropriate for an older child. Unfortunately, their emotional development is age appropriate at best, making adaptive responses sometimes very stressful. They may not be particularly demonstrative, but they long for affection. In school they are usually exceptionally good students, and most are the teacher's "pet." They are especially bothered by disruptive classroom behavior of other students, fearful of teachers who frequently yell and make verbal threats to maintain order, and develop overwhelming sympathy to others with physical disabilities. They are extremely frightened by the lack of sensitivity of both adults and other children to moral, ethical, and even religious issues.

Undue fears are especially common, particularly concerning parental health. Fears related to loss of love objects may be compounded by the chronic medical complaints of the immediate family.

Criticism is usually tolerated quite poorly by this group of children because they interpret it as rejection. Seldom do they express anger overtly, preferring to withdraw and pout. They have heightened sensitivity and awareness not only to their external environment but also to physical stimuli arising from within. The anxiety produced by their inability to satisfactorily adapt to these stimuli is vented through their vulnerable target organ, in this instance the gastrointestinal tract. In other children, this anxiety may be expressed through headaches or extremity pain.

A second major category of personality and emotional types is made up of children who are average in intelligence but immature in speech and behavior. They suffer from repeated comparisons to a sibling who has been set as the acceptable standard by the parents. The latter commonly fail to appreciate the individuality of the child and unfortunately set the same high standards for all their children. Such children develop an anxiety reaction when they realize they cannot fulfill the expectations of their parents or environment. Somatization of this anxiety manifests itself as recurrent abdominal pain. In addition, school difficulties, learning disabilities, and school phobias are not unusual.

When given the opportunity to imagine having three wishes come true, the child seldom includes the mention of relief from his physical disability. Instead, the content of the wishes usually contains the important psychodynamic material of the underlying unresolved conflict or conflicts responsible for perpetuating the painful condition. These expressed wishes come as a dreadful shock and surprise to the parent or parents.

Physical findings

Not only is it important for the physician to be thorough, but also a comprehensive examination instills confidence in parent and child that all parts of the body have been examined and are free of disease. The physical examination should be performed both between and during attacks if possible. Despite the chronicity of the complaint, one is struck by the well-being of the patient. Height and weight are not affected by the symptom complex, no matter how protracted. Signs of a heightened anxiety state may be manifested by cold extremities, mottled skin, sweaty palms, evidence of nail and cuticle biting, trichomania, and dilated pupils. Mild systolic hypertension and modest tachycardia may be present initially during the examination.

Abdominal tenderness is verbalized to sudden deep palpation, but guarding is seldom found and usually inconsistent. The discomfort seems vague and diffuse, and hard to localize by the physician. The area of maximum tenderness seldom corresponds with with original location of the subjective pain. The abdominal examination should particularly be viewed by the parent, who is often astounded by the obvious incongruity between the symptom and the freedom of examination.

Generally speaking, more discomfort will be elicited over the course of the colon or in the lower abdomen especially in the area of the descending colon and sigmoid. A ropelike structure, which is sometimes tender and corresponding to the location of sigmoid and descending colon, can be palpated in 20% to 30% of these children.

Laboratory findings and roentgenographic studies

For most patients a few simple laboratory tests can be performed during the initial office visit. Satisfactory results of a complete blood count, sedimentation rate, and urinalysis and studies of stool for occult blood are sufficient to reassure physician and parent that major organic disease does not exist. If pain symptoms are somewhat atypical, especially pertaining to location of the pain, then several urine specimens, including one freshly voided during the pain episode, should be carefully examined for red or white blood cells.

Roentgenographic studies such as abdominal scout films, intravenous pyelogram, voiding cystogram, barium enema, and upper gastrointestinal series are selectively indicated, particularly in those cases where the history and the physical findings suggest organic disease. Likewise, further investigation is indicated when the history is atypical or psychophysiologic determinants are lacking. Recently, a greater use of ultrasonography has been employed when pelvic pathosis, gallstones, dilated biliary structures, or mesenteric cysts are suspected. This noninvasive, radiation-free technique has particular appeal in the evaluation of these sensitive and anxious young children.

For some patients a more complete biochemical survey, including serum electrolytes, calcium, phosphorus, liver-function studies, and amylase and lipid profiles, will be needed. Proctoscopic examination and rectal biopsy are indicated when inflammatory bowel disease is suspected. If Crohn's disease is strongly considered, rectal mucosa tissue should be obtained, even in the face of apparent normal findings. Electron microscopy of biopsy specimens from patients with functional colonic disorders may reveal mucosal edema as the only abnormality.

In difficult and confusing cases, endoscopic examination of the upper gastrointestinal tract can be undertaken in the hope of clarifying the cause of the child's pain. Motility studies have limited clinical usefulness being employed only as a research tool in the study of such patients. A heightened rectosigmoid motility response to prostigmine has been reported in 18 children having recurrent abdominal pain without evidence of organic cause.

Differential diagnosis

The number of possible causes of recurrent abdominal pain is staggering (Table 15-3), but few are likely to escape detection if history taking and physical examination have been thorough. A general approach to the symptom of abdominal pain is discussed in Chapter 1.

The complaint of recurrent abdominal pain in children less than 5 and more than 13 years of age should be carefully regarded, for an organic rather than psychogenic cause is likely to be present.

Genitourinary disease, expecially in the younger pediatric patients, is the most frequent organic cause that may masquerade as recurrent abdominal pain. Results of repeat urine examinations and roentgenographic studies should permit making the diagnosis promptly.

Peptic disease especially in the younger child (less than 5 years) can produce symptoms that mimic this entity. In this age group peptic ulcer pain may be difficult for them to localize. It is often periumbilical rather than epigastric, seldom relieved by eating, and, in fact, may be more severe postprandially. Vomiting is especially common in childhood peptic ulcer disease. If the family history is positive for confirmed peptic ulcer and important psychologic determinants are absent in the history, an upper gastrointestinal series should be performed. Antacids taken 1 and 3 hours postprandially and again at bedtime can be used for 3 to 4 weeks as a therapeutic trial. Either failure to clinically improve, or the persistence of findings on the repeat gastrointestinal series that suggest peptic disease, warrants fiber-optic endoscopic evaluation of the patient.

Chronic constipation can occasionally precipitate crampy, colicky pain, and a therapeutic trial of stool softeners is warranted when such a history is obtained. Mineral oil, bulk laxatives, and a high-fiber diet are especially beneficial. Postprandial pain and tenderness over the left colon are more common in these children. Prolonged transit time has been reported in children with recurrent abdominal pain, but the exact defect in propulsive motility remains uncertain. Early in its course, chronic inflammatory bowel disease (Crohn's disease), may produce colicky abdominal pain, if no other signs are evident. The absence of anemia and of occult blood in the stools, a normal sedimentation rate, and normal results of proctoscopic examination in a well-appearing child most likely exclude this form of chronic inflammatory bowel disease.

In our experience specific food intolerances are a rare cause of recurrent abdominal pain in children. However, one should consider the possibility of lactose intolerance in any nonwhite child presenting with recurrent abdominal pain. Relative deficiencies of intestinal lactase have been demonstrated in up to 40% of black elementary school children and in 75% of black teen-agers. The history of preferential avoidance of milk products may or may not be elicited in these cases. As a rule, diarrhea is seldom documented in the older child with lactose intolerance, but rather cramps, bloating, and increased flatulence are more common complaints. Although children of Jewish descent are eventually at risk to become lactose intolerant, this condition rarely becomes a clinical problem before adulthood when up to 60% to 80% of Jews are reported to be lactase deficient. In two recently published studies using different techniques, lactose intolerance was found in 43% and 29%, respectively, in children with presumed

Table 15-3. Organic causes of recurrent abdominal pain*

Extra-abdominal	Intra-abdominal		
	Gastrointestinal	**Renal**	**Others**
Lead poisoning, porphyria, epilepsy, diabetes, asthma, rheumatic fever, sickle-cell anemia, hyperparathyroidism, familial Mediterranean fever, periodic peritonitis, pulmonary veno-occlusive disease	Malrotation, duplication, congenital or acquired stenosis, peptic disease, hiatal hernia, internal or inguinal hernia, tumors, foreign bodies, volvulus, intussusception, superior mesenteric artery syndrome, celiac-axis compression syndrome, excessive swallowing of air, Crohn's disease, ulcerative colitis, adhesions, chronic constipation, Hirschsprung's disease, celiac disease, nodular lymphoid hyperplasia, lactose intolerance, sorbital malabsorption, Henoch-Schönlein purpura, idiopathic mesenteritis or panniculitis, abdominal wall defects, lymphoma	Pyelonephritis, hydronephrosis, bladder neck obstruction, calculi, ureteropelvic obstruction	Hepatomegaly, splenomegaly, cholecystitis, cholelithiasis, chronic pancreatitis, Fitz-Hugh–Curtis syndrome (perihepatitis)

nonorganic recurrent abdominal pain. A trial period on a lactose-free diet resulted in improvement in 28 of 32 malabsorbers in one series, and in 10 of 11 similar patients in the other study. Unfortunately, in neither report was the diet trial "blinded" or the amount of lactase consumed during the control period quantitated. Because the influence of subjective factors is so great in children with recurrent abdominal pain, critical experimental design is required before the true incidence of lactose intolerance as a cause of recurrent abdominal pain can be ascertained. In our clinical setting a significant percentage of patients (15%) have already found a milk-free diet of no benefit before their referral. The failure to obtain consistent pain relief on a milk-free diet, used in suspicious cases of lactose intolerance, has been disappointing. If improvement does occur by this diet manipulation, the major benefit probably derives from resulting increased bowel motions and passage of softer stools.

That chronic recurrent bouts of abdominal pain are not caused by intussusception may be difficult to determine without use of contrast roentgenographs; in our experience, the pain is more severe in the latter condition, and at the height of an episode there may be abdominal distention and a palpable mass. Henoch-Schönlein purpura and ce-

Table 15-4. Retrospective survey of 21 patients operated on for so-called mesenteric adenitis in terms of recurrent postoperative symptoms

Histologic manifestation	Number	Recurrence
Normal appendix	17	9
Mucosal ulceration	1	0
Fecalith	1	0
Chronic inflammatory changes	2	0

liac disease on rare occasion may have this mode of presentation. Meckel's diverticulum or duplication cysts may rarely be a source of pain. Intermittent volvulus associated with malrotation has also been reported as a cause of recurrent abdominal pain; the pain tends to occur 1 to 2 hours after meals, and the barium enema shows an abnormally located cecum.

Acute left upper quadrant pain may arise from the flexura lienalis, especially if the splenic flexure of the colon lies between the diaphragm, stomach, and spleen. Likewise, interposition of the hepatic flexure of the colon between liver and diaphragm (Chilaiditi's syndrome) may produce the same symptom in the right upper part of the abdomen.

It is important to remember that so-called chronic appendicitis and mesenteric lymphadenitis are highly unlikely causes of recurrent abdominal pain (Table 15-4). Chronic recurrent abdominal pain is, at times, associated with pronounced nodular lymphoid hyperplasia involving the entire colon and rectum (p. 464). These small rounded and oval filling defects of the terminal ileum and large intestine are normally present in children. The relationship between this finding and recurrent abdominal pain is coincidental at best, though some attacks of recurrent abdominal pain start after a febrile illness.

Yersinia enterocolitis usually produces an acute pain episode that mimics appendicitis but on occasion causes a chronic illness that may mimic Crohn's ileitis.

Pinworms are probably never responsible for chronic abdominal pain. Not infrequently they are found in the lumen of an incidentally removed appendix, the latter devoid of any inflammatory reaction. Taeniasis, ascariasis, and giardiasis may give rise to symptoms and can easily be looked for in fresh stool specimens. Abdominal epilepsy is usually part of a syndrome altogether different from the clinical description previously given in children with recurrent abdominal pain. Anemia and the presence of basophilic stippling of the red cells are evidence of chronic lead poisoning; urine studies for coproporphyrins and determinations of blood lead levels may be necessary. Chronic relapsing pancreatitis has presented as recurrent abdominal pain; however, the features of the pain (location and duration) and abnormal results of laboratory tests (white blood cell count and increased serum amylase) should make for easy diagnosis particularly early in its evolution.

Periodic peritonitis (polyserositis, familial Mediterranean fever) is characterized by repeated bouts of abdominal pain, usually accompanied by fever, chest pains, and joint complaints. This condition affects primarily persons of Mediterranean ancestry, with up to 80% having clinical symptoms before 21 years of age. The long duration of the pain (2 to 5 days) combined with elevated temperature and increased leukocyte count and sedimentation rate eliminates any confusion with psychophysiologic cases of recurrent abdominal pain.

Patients with retractile mesenteritis, Weber-Christian disease, collagen-vascular disease (systemic lupus erythematosus, scleroderma, polyarteritis nodosa, and dermatomyositis) may have important abdominal complaints. These patients, however, often have additional extra-abdominal signs and symptoms and tend to look chronically ill. Early in its course diabetes mellitus may masquerade as recurrent abdominal pain perhaps because of episodes of gastric dilatation.

Hyperparathyroidism can present in childhood with episodes of recurrent abdominal pain before evidence for peptic ulcer disease, renal stones, or pancreatitis. Elevated serum calcium levels may be noted on the biochemical survey.

Vague upper abdominal complaints may be the dominant clinical symptoms in older children or teen-agers with gallbladder disease, anatomic aberrations of the extrahepatic biliary structures, Gilbert's disease, or Dubin-Johnson syndrome. Idiopathic or acquired stricture of the common biliary or common hepatic duct, choledochal cysts, and Caroli's disease have been causes of recurrent abdominal symptoms. However, the atypical pain location (right upper quadrant) often with objective pain, or a mass on palpation (and perhaps icterus), should prompt one to use liver-function tests and obtain either or both roentgenographic and ultrasound studies of these structures.

Treatment and prognosis

Treatment of recurrent abdominal pain of psychogenic origin should begin at the initial contact with patient and parents. Their anxiety is often relieved by the thoroughness of the history and of the physical examination and by appropriate exploration of emotional factors leading to somatization. Not infrequently, the initial interview and examination will be sufficiently revealing to convince the parent that children may "talk through their bodies" and that the manifest pain is an expression of an underlying psychologic reaction. The physician can then offer guidance by instructing that harmful stresses that have been elucidated in the child's environment be modified. That these pain episodes are most often anxiety-induced is suggested by the ease with which the patient can be distracted from the pain. The pain episodes should be taken as a "red flag" that something is amiss, and the child can best be helped by a distracting maneuver that permits him time to decompress from the effects of the distressful stimuli. Allowing him to remain nearby while involved with the parent in some simple, helpful task is very therapeutic. Conversation during this time should not be pain oriented but more along the lines of sympathetic encouragement regarding the day's events. Sending the child away to "solo" with his pain is nonproductive, since it deprives him of a unique opportunity to verbalize his many fears, anxieties, stresses, and so on. Drug therapy is, at best, symptom oriented and likewise tends to mask the underlying cause.

Some physicians can provide the proper support and counseling for child and parent (informal psychotherapy). Pointing out to the parent how both of their needs have been excessively captured by this relationship is useful and easily accepted after the initial evaluation has been completed. Others will require the aid of a social worker, psychologist, or psychiatrist, depending on the severity of the psychic disorder and the availability of professional help. Just as the diagnosis should always be made on firm, positive grounds, so too should the approach to and direction of therapy. Our experience indicates that with proper support and treatment, most of the children do quite well, and the frequency of pain episodes diminishes. However, one follow-up study on children with recurrent abdominal pain showed that treatment did not improve the final numbers who eventually became pain free. Those who were treated, however, responded more quickly and had fewer relapses than the untreated group and understood and accepted the association of stress and pain. On the other hand, the untreated group continued to manifest poor adaptability to their vulnerabilities, and they not only had many other nonabdominal disorders (migraine, back pains, "nervous anxiety"), but also their work, marriages, and other activities were negatively affected by their psychophysiologic responses.

A second follow-up study (30 years) found 18 of 34 cases with continued abdominal symptoms. They included such diagnoses as irritable colon syndrome or peptic disease–gastritis syndrome without ulcer (16), and duodenal ulcer (2). A higher incidence of abdominal complaints was likewise found in the offspring of those adults still with symptoms of gastrointestinal dysfunction. Not surprisingly, one third of adults with the irritable bowel syndrome report symptoms starting in childhood.

In a third study, a 5-year follow-up survey of 170 patients at the Mayo Clinic with the diagnosis of nonorganic recurrent abdominal pain found 25% with persistent abdominal discomfort or other psychosomatic complaints. Importantly, 21 of the 69 patients with persisting pain symptoms eventually had a surgical procedure resulting in improvement in six cases. Three patients developed overt Crohn's disease in their study group. Not surprisingly, 92 of 170 patients reported improvement shortly after the initial interview and examination and after having been given the diagnosis of psychophysiologic abdominal pain.

It would appear that prognosis is worse for children whose pain episodes begin before 5 years of age, and worse for males than for females. Treatment is less likely to be helpful if the patient comes from a "painful family" and his symptoms have been going on for over 6 months.

Another less frequently employed technique takes advantage of the hospital setting to break the pain-oriented reward system. The child is required to remain room based, not participate in any recreational programs, and receive a bland diet while "benign neglect" is conveyed by the hospital staff. Visiting by parents, friends, and others is prohibited until the pain is gone and remains absent. One should approach this therapeutic modality with caution because the mother may decompensate with increased longing for the child. Pain generally disappears within 48 hours and seldom recurs in the hospital. Indirectly, much can be learned about the psychodynamics of the home environment by observation of the child's adjustment to the hospital ward and personnel.

REFERENCES

Almy, T.P.: The irritable bowel syndrome. Back to square one? Dig. Dis. Sci. **25**:401-403, June 1980.

Apley, J.: The child with adominal pain, Oxford, England, 1964, Blackwell Scientific Publications.

Apley, J.: Psychosomatic illness in children: a modern synthesis, Br. Med. J. **2**:756-761, 1973.

Apley, J., and Hale, B.: Children with recurrent abdominal pain: How do they grow up? Br. Med. J. **3**:7-9, 1973.

Babb, R.R., and Eckman, P.B.: Abdominal epilepsy, J.A.M.A. **222**:65-66, 1972.

Barr, R.G., Levine, M.D., and Watkins, J.B.: Recurrent abdominal pain of childhood due to lactose intolerance. N. Engl. J. Med. **300**:1449-1452, June 1979.

Berger, H.G.: Somatic pain and school avoidance, Clin. Pediatr. **13**:819-826, Oct. 1974.

Berger, H.G., Honig, P.J., and Liebman, R.: Recurrent abdominal pain: gaining control of the symptom, Am. J. Dis. Child. **131**:1340-1344, Dec. 1977.

Christensen, J.F., and Mortensen, O.: Long-term prognosis in children with recurrent abdominal pain, Arch. Dis. Child. **50**:110-114, 1975.

Deamer, W.C., and Sandberg, D.H.: Recurrent abdominal pain: recurrent controversy, Pediatrics **51**:307-308, 1973.

Dimson, S.B.: Transit time related to clinical findings in children with recurrent abdominal pain, Pediatrics **47**:666-674, 1971.

Fielding, J.F.: The irritable bowel syndrome. I: Clinical spectrum. II: Manometric and cineradiographic studies. III: Hormonal influences, Clin. Gastroenterol. **6**:607-641, Sept. 1977.

Latimer, P., Sarna, S., Campbell, D., and others: Colonic motor and myoelectric activity: a comparative study of normal subjects, psychoneurotic patients, and patients with irritable bowel syndrome, Gastroenterology **80**:893-901, 1981.

Lebenthal, E., Rossi, T.M., Nord, K.S., and Branski, D.: Recurrent abdominal pain and lactose absorption in children, Pediatr. **67**:828-832, June 1981.

Liebman, W.M.: Recurrent abdominal pain in children: a retrospective survery of 119 patients, Clin. Pediatr. **17**:149-153, Feb. 1978.

Oster, J.: Recurrent abdominal pain, headache, and limb pains in children and adolescents, Pediatrics **50**:429-436, 1972.

Ritchie, J.: Pain from distension of the pelvic colon by inflating a balloon in the irritable colon syndrome, Gut **14**:125-132, 1973.

Schmitt, B.D.: School phobia—the great imitator: a pediatrician's viewpoint, Pediatrics **48**:433-441, 1971.

Stone, R.T., and Barbero, G.J.: Recurrent abdominal pain in childhood, Pediatrics **45**:732-738, 1970.

Thompson, D.G., Laidlow, J.M., and Wingate, D.L.: Abnormal small-bowel motility demonstrated by radiotelemetry in a patient with irritable colon, Lancet **2**:1321-1323, 1979.

16 *Parasitic and fungal disease of the gastrointestinal tract*

PARASITIC INFESTATIONS

Geographic and ecologic conditions are important in the prevalence of parasitic infestations. With increased travel and immigration from tropical countries a greater awareness of parasites not usually found in North America is necessary. Sanitary conditions in the community, personal hygiene, food processing, and cooking constitute other factors affecting the epidemiology of infestations.

The host-parasite relationship is variable. In general, the larger the number of parasites in the lumen or in the intestinal wall, the more significant is their pathogenetic effect. The chances of autoinfection vary with the species. It is great in *Enterobius vermicularis* and absent in *Taenia saginata* and in *Ascaris,* since propagation does not take place, with one egg producing one adult.

Intestinal protozoal diseases

Among the dozen intestinal protozoa isolated in American and Canadian children, *Entamoeba histolytica* and *Giardia lamblia* are the only two that are clinically important. Infections with either of these should always be considered in children who have diarrhea, especially when the course is protracted.

Amebiasis

Entamoeba histolytica remains the only proved pathogen among the six species of amebas inhabiting the colon. It has both trophozoite and cyst stages. Ingested cysts from contaminated water, fresh food, or hands rupture in the small intestine and form trophozoites, which mature and inhabit the colon. Ingested trophozoites do not survive in the acid environment of the stomach. It is important to note that water chlorination does not kill cysts; boiling is necessary.

It is more common in subtropic areas, among populations with poor sanitation, and where exposure to fecally transmitted organisms is continual. The recent description of seven cases of amebic liver abscess in children from Arizona suggests that infection with *Entamoeba histolytica* continues to be endemic in the United States. A discussion of amebic liver abscess is found in Chapter 21.

Clinical findings. The large intestine is the site of predilection. Amebas may pass through the bowel walls and invade the liver, lung, and brain. Lesions resemble those of *Shigella* infections or ulcerative colitis (Fig. 16-1, *A*). The diarrheal stools regularly contain blood-streaked mucus, and tenesmus is often noted along with abdominal pain.

A fulminating type of colitis is seen more often in children than in adults, and perforations may occur. The disease is often quite mild or totally asymptomatic even if there is evidence of invasion. A chronic form of the disease gives rise to narrowing of the cecum.

Diagnosis. Because the number of demonstrable amebas in the stools is inconsistent, the diagnosis cannot be ruled out on the basis of a single negative stool report; consequently a minimum of three stool specimens collected during a week should be examined (Fig. 16-1, *B*). Swabbing the rectal mucosa and promptly examining the freshly prepared slide are often useful in detecting the presence of larval or adult stages of the parasite. However, the most reliable examination is done on slides of fresh stool fixed in polyvinyl alcohol and suitably stained. A variety of serologic tests are available: immunofluorescence and countercurrent electrophoresis are the most practical. However, a positive test only indicates amebic invasion at some time during the previous 5 years.

Treatment. Infections with *Entamoeba histolytica* should all be treated, irrespective of symptoms. Although some strains do not appear to be pathogenic and are not tissue invaders, there is no way of differentiating the pathogenic ones from the nonpathogenic. A second reason for treatment is that extraintestinal involvement, particularly the amebic liver abscess, is likely to occur without prior symptomatic involvement of the bowel.

The drug of choice is metronidazole (Flagyl) for symptomatic disease. The dosage in children is 50 mg/day up to a maximum of 2250 mg in 3 divided doses for a period of 10 days. In the absence of symptoms, a contact amebicide such as

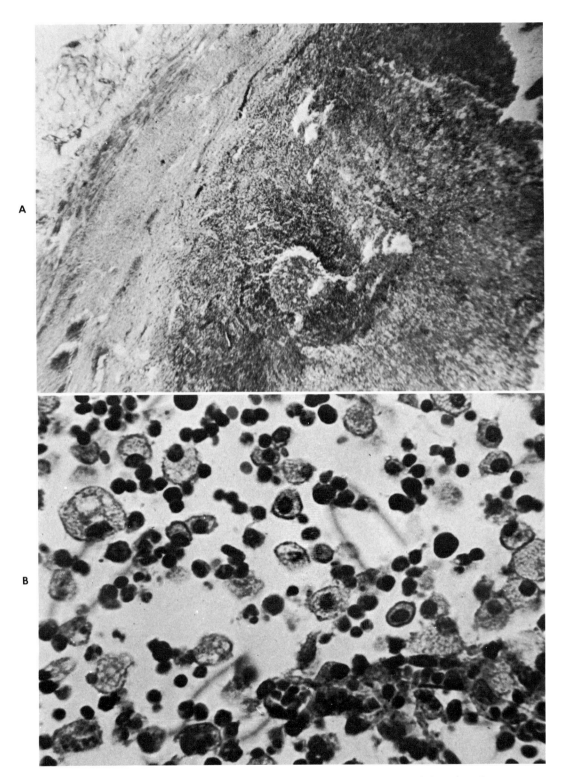

Fig. 16-1. Entamoeba histolytica appendicitis. **A,** Flask-shaped ulcer extends into the submucosa and contains mucopurulent exudate. The architecture of the appendiceal mucosa and submucosa is replaced by necrotic tissue and exudate. **B,** Magnification of the exudate within the ulcer shows a number of spheric hyaline amebic cysts with a refractile wall and a finely granular cytoplasm. (Courtesy I. Kerner, Department of Pathology, Hôpital Sainte-Justine, Montreal.)

diiodohydroxyquin (Diodoquin) 40 mg/kg/day for 3 weeks is indicated.

Giardiasis

Man is the only host and reservoir for the flagellated protozoan *Giardia lamblia,* currently considered as one of the most common causes of infectious diarrhea. Motile trophozoites may be found in duodenal and upper small bowel aspirates. *G. lamblia* is transmitted through ingestion of cysts either from personal contact with an infected individual or from food or water contaminated with infective feces.

A reasonable estimate of worldwide distribution of this disease is 5%. Infestations are especially common in children, and outbreaks of giardiasis are reported in nurseries, day care centers, and institutions. Community epidemics and infestation of groups of tourists (traveler's diarrhea) are described with increasing regularity.

The clinical spectrum is quite broad. The asymptomatic carrier state is common, since a recent study in toddlers suggests a rate of 2%. Susceptibility to infection appears to decrease with age and increase with the size of the infective dose. The administration of 10 to 25 cysts has been shown to infect more than one third of a group of adults, whereas 100 cysts brought on looser stools in all subjects. Cysts begin to be excreted within 9 days after exposure, and they disappear after an average of 18 days. It has been postulated that biliary secretory IgA released into the duodenum could prevent attachment or bring about detachment of the parasite from the microvillus membrane of the duodenum and jejunum.

Clinical findings. The interval between infection and symptoms is commonly about 15 days. The disease may start abruptly and mimic a bout of acute or subacute gastroenteritis. The most consistent pattern is that of anorexia, nausea, a sensation of epigastric fullness, and watery diarrhea. It appears that in most cases the organism, though highly infective, produces an acute self-limited illness that subsides spontaneously within a week to 10 days.

In some cases, diarrhea becomes chronic on an intermittent or continuous basis for a period of a few months. Loss of weight can be impressive; there is abdominal distention with flatulence. The stools become pale, bulky, and malodorous. The failure to thrive and the spruelike picture suggest celiac disease except for the predominance of

polymorphonuclear cells and the presence of acute inflammation involving the epithelial cells and crypts. In other cases, the structural changes can be differentiated from those of celiac disease because the atrophy of the villous architecture is associated with only minimal changes in the epithelial columnar cells. The coexistence of *Giardia* infestation, malabsorption, and immunoglobulin deficiency has been well described. Acquired hypogammaglobulinemia and isolated IgA deficiency are the two immunity deficiencies described with a celiac-like picture, nodular lymphoid hyperplasia, and giardiasis. Diminished host resistance is evident in that the patients most severely affected by giardiasis have underlying immunity deficiencies.

Eradication of the parasite in the majority of patients with giardiasis and acquired hypogammaglobulinemia leads to the disappearance of gastrointestinal symptoms and of malabsorption and to a return of the jejunal architecture toward normal. These dramatic results are particularly important in view of the failure of a gluten-free diet, antibiotics, and repeated gammaglobulin injections observed in such cases.

Diagnosis. Giardiasis should be suspected in immunoglobulin deficiencies, since it is present in close to half the cases. Since it is a frequent cause of chronic diarrhea, it has to be considered in cases of irritable colon syndrome and in the various malabsorption syndromes. The notion of foreign travel or of an epidemic of diarrhea without fever in a day care center is important. Besides person-to-person contact, water is an important mode of transmission. Cysts survive chlorination but are removed if the water-treatment plant uses sedimentation flocculation and filtration.

Cysts should be looked for in two separate stools. The formol-ether technique of concentration greatly increases the chances of a positive examination. Trophozoites can be identified in duodenal aspirates, jejunal biopsy specimens, or impression smears of jejunal mucosa. The last technique is reportedly the most efficient. The smears are air-dried, fixed with methanol, and stained with Giemsa (Fig. 16-2). We have no experience with the "Enterotest," which consists of a recoverable nylon yarn swallowed in a weighted capsule from which the mucus is transferred to a glass slide and properly stained after fixation in methanol.

Treatment and prognosis. All children with giardiasis, whether symptomatic or not, should be

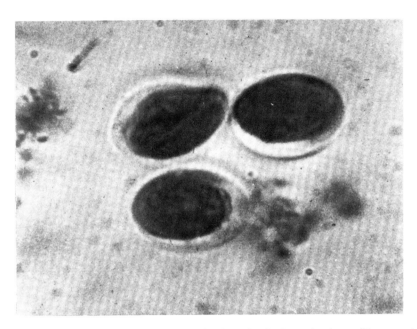

Fig. 16-2. Giardia lamblia cysts. Direct examination of a fresh stool using a Giemsa stain will reveal purplish cysts, whereas epithelial cells are pink. In cases where stools are particularly loose, trophozoites can be identified.

treated for 5 to 10 days. Metronidazole (Flagyl) is the treatment of choice. The adult dosage is 750 mg/day. In the pediatric-age group 35 to 50 mg/kg/day is advocated for 10 days. Quinacrine is a reasonable alternative at a dosage of 6 mg/kg for 5 days (maximum 300 mg/day). On occasion a therapeutic trial of metronidazole in some toddlers with chronic diarrhea and a good epidemiologic history in the absence of laboratory confirmation appear warranted, but they are not generally rewarding.

When the parasite disappears from the stools, symptoms abate completely, and normality of function and structure returns. Treatment failure calls for a second course of metronidazole. Because of the known epidemiology, community outbreaks should prompt screening of the water supply. In endemic or interfamilial cases, fecal-oral spread from person to person calls for the usual hygienic measures, a search for the parasite in household contacts, and treatment when indicated.

Helminthic diseases
Nematodes (roundworms)

Three widespread roundworm infestations are associated with gastrointestinal symptoms or mul-

tisystem involvement—ascariasis, toxocariasis (visceral larva migrans), and oxyuriasis.

Ascariasis. A fourth of the world's population harbors *Ascaris lumbricoides,* but few people are symptomatic because the parasite is well adapted to its human host. Ascariasis is seen throughout North America; however, it is more prevalent in the southern United States. Surveys in the United States suggest that children up to 12 or 14 years of age are as likely to be infected as those of preschool age. Although infestation accounts for 10% to 15% of cases of abdominal emergencies in 4 to 8 year olds in South Africa, the figure in the United States is 0.2%. *Ascaris lumbricoides* has no means of attachment to the intestinal mucosa, but in large numbers they form a bolus of ascarids, which may cause mechanical obstruction, especially since it brings about intestinal spasm. Infective-stage *Ascaris* eggs are ingested when toys or fingers in contact with topsoil contaminated by fecal material are placed in the mouth. The eggs (Fig. 16-3) reach the duodenum and hatch. The larvae enter the intestinal wall, migrate through the liver, are carried to the lungs were they may cause pneumonia with eosinophilia, reach the epiglottis, are swallowed, and become established in the small bowel, where they grow into adult worms and

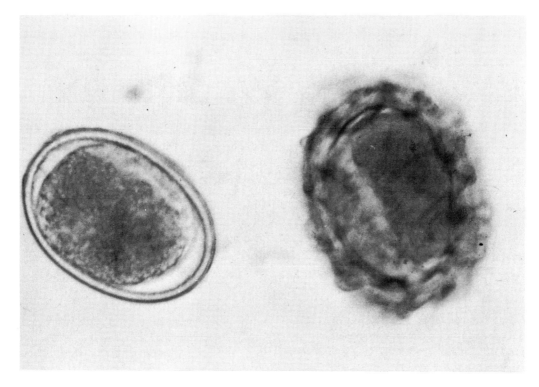

Fig. 16-3. *Ascaris lumbricoides* ova. The ovum on the left has lost its irregular membranous envelope surrounding the chitinous shell. These ova are characterized by a relatively large size and oval shape.

mate. Some may then be evacuated in the feces, be vomited, perforate or obstruct the bowel, or block the extrahepatic biliary tree.

Infestation with *Ascaris* can be symptomless or lead to a range of symptoms including nausea, vomiting, anorexia, loss of weight, a modest degree of malabsorption, insomnia, and irritability. In our experience, the most common complaint is colicky abdominal pain, which can masquerade as recurrent idiopathic abdominal pain of childhood. Pneumonia, hepatomegaly, or jaundice may accompany extraintestinal migration of larvae. The acute symptoms include intestinal obstruction, acute appendicitis, intestinal perforation, or intussusception; however, these complications are rare. In most cases, the mother telephones the physician, saying that her preschool child has vomited or passed a 6-inch pencil-size roundworm.

Ascaris eggs can be detected in feces 2 months after exposure, but only two thirds of clinical cases can be confirmed by a fecal smear. Roentgenograms may demonstrate the parasite. The drug of choice in order of efficacy is pyrantel pamoate, 10 mg/kg in a single dose (Antiminth, 5 ml/25 kg). An alternative treatment is mebendazole (Vermox), 100 mg twice daily for 3 days. The dosage should be adjusted to surface area for children below 2 years of age.

Visceral larva migrans (toxocariasis). Although infestation with *Toxocara* never leads to intestinal symptoms it is discussed in this chapter because the gastrointestinal tract is an essential step in the life cycle of the parasite and because of the public health implications.

Larval toxocariasis is caused by parasitization by the cat nematode, *Toxocara cati,* or by *T. canis,* which is the most common roundworm in the dog. Their life cycle parallels that of the *Ascaris* affecting man. When infective eggs of *Toxocara* are swallowed, they hatch in the upper alimentary tract and may enter the portal system. From the liver, extraintestinal migration may proceed to the lungs, heart, central nervous system, skin, and eyes. Human transmission is through the hand-to-mouth route. Since the percentage of puppies younger than 6 months excreting eggs is very great (90%), the handling of young puppies is epidemiologically important. A recent survey in Montreal public parks has shown that close to 60% of soil samples contained larvae. There is a buildup of the larval population because larvae in the soil are resistant to the winter frost.

Recurrent fever, cough, attacks of asthma, and malnutrition in the presence of hepatomegaly in a child between the ages of 1 and 4 years who has pica are suggestive of visceral larva migrans. In other children, symptoms are completely lacking, and the diagnosis is suspected on the basis of persistent eosinophilia (greater than 25%) and leukocytosis.

Definitive diagnosis rests on the demonstration of larvae lying within hepatic granulomas. The latter consists of giant cells in a chronic inflammatory reaction. Irregular foci of necrosis are common. Convulsions and a picture similar to encephalitis are indicative of central nervous system involvement. The possibility of ocular infestation (retinal granuloma) should always be considered when diagnoses such as retinoblastoma or organizing retinal hemorrhage are entertained. The most consistent laboratory findings include leukocytosis and an eosinophilia of more than 30%. In the invasive stage, a good antibody response ensues with a rise in IgG, IgM, and IgE. Several nonspecific serologic tests have been used, but since they would detect at best only half the cases, they are not recommended. An improved *Toxocara* antigen may soon permit the detection of *Toxocara* antibodies.

Treatment and prognosis. If there is no central nervous system or ocular involvement, visceral larva migrans is considered to be a benign disease. The infestation usually runs a chronic course for about 18 months. Therapy is largely ineffective, though acute signs have been helped with thiabendazole (Mintezol) at a dosage of 25 mg/kg twice a day for 48 hours. Death of the larvae can bring about an aggravation of the inflammatory reaction. Therefore in view of the lack of convincing evidence for the efficacy of thiabendazole it is best not to administer it, and it is frankly contraindicated in cases of retinal granuloma. Corticosteroids should probably be used in severe cases, particularly in patients with extensive pneumonitis, myocarditis, or encephalitis in which their anti-inflammatory effects may prove to be lifesaving.

Oxyuriasis. Oxyuriasis is worldwide in distribution, with children being particularly susceptible.It is said that more than 40% of school-age children harbor pinworms. *Enterobius vermicu-*

laris measures from 2 to 12 mm in length and attaches itself to the mucosa of the cecum and appendix. Gravid female roundworms migrate down the bowel, crawl outside the anal margin, usually at night, and deposit their eggs on the perineal and perianal skin. Reinfection is usually introduced by the finger-mouth mode, since there is a significant degree of pruritus, especially at night. Ingested eggs hatch at the duodenal level, and the larvae migrate to the cecum, where they may invade the appendiceal lumen. Regular deworming of dogs, monitoring of soil and sand, and keeping dogs away from children's play areas are essential measures to reduce the incidence of infestation. However, oxuriasis has never been proved to be a significant cause of appendicitis.

Anal scratching may provoke local perianal infection. Vaginitis is seen in girls, and salpingitis has been reported. Nonspecific symptoms attributed to pinworm infestation include insomnia and irritability. The role of pinworms in the production of recurrent abdominal pain of childhood is no longer accepted. Some cases of enuresis have been attributed to oxyuriasis.

Fecal examination is a poor method of detecting pinworms because eggs are found in only 5% of cases. The most efficient technique entails placing adhesive cellulose tape on the perianal skin for a few seconds and then on a microscopic slide where a drop of toluene has been placed.

Treatment of the entire household and the observance of personal hygiene are usually effective measures of containment. The most effective drug is pyrantel pamoate (Antiminth) in a single dose of 10 mg/kg (5 ml/25 kg). Pyrvinium pamoate (Povan) is also effective in a single dose. The amount recommended is 5 mg/kg (5 ml/10 kg) up to a maximum of 250 mg. It is recommended that all members of the family be treated twice at an interval of 2 weeks.

There is a high rate of reinfection. Hygienic measures such as hand washing, fingernail scrubbing, a daily shower or bath, and a change of underwear are recommended. Ova are resistant to disinfectants; therefore control in schools and institutions is very difficult.

Trichuriasis. *Trichuris trichiura,* a small, slender roundworm commonly known as a whipworm, is exclusively a human parasite. It is widely distributed in the southern United States and is rarely encountered in the nothern parts of North America. In some areas of the world 90% of the

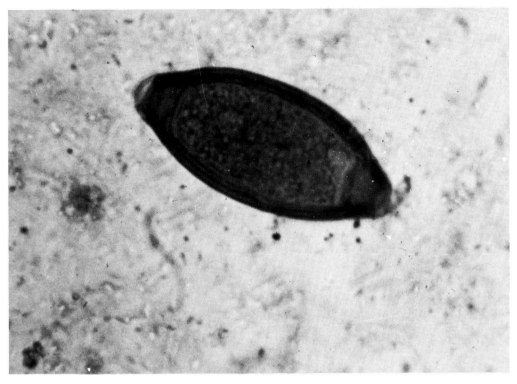

Fig. 16-4. *Trichuris trichiura* ovum. It has dark brown central parts and rather clear terminal knobs. Larvae set free from embryonated eggs penetrate intestinal villi temporarily. They mature into adult worms over a period of 1 to 3 months. Adult worm measures 0.5 cm and has a whiplike anterior extremity (whipworm infection). Worm is small and transparent and measures 3.8 cm in length. It is often coiled like a watchspring.

population may be infected. It is likely the most commonly recognized intestinal helminth in tourists returning from tropical areas, but unless there has been massive infestation, trichuriasis remains asymptomatic.

On being ingested in material on the fingertips or in water, food, or dirt, the eggs hatch in the duodenum and migrate to the cecal area. If large numbers are present, the entire colon may be infested. At the point of attachment of the worms, there may be inflammation, small hemorrhages, and excess mucus.

Massive infestation of the colon produces chronic debilitating diarrhea. Characteristically, it occurs at the age when celiac disease is common (1 to 4 years) and is more likely in malnourished children (Fig. 16-4). There is diarrhea, tenesmus, abdominal pain, and failure to thrive. A hypochromic anemia and slight or moderate eosinophilia are common. Eggs can be demonstrated on a fresh smear of the stools. When invasion of the sigmoidorectal area is massive, proctoscopic examination readily demonstrates the presence of the worms. The bowel mucosa is friable, hyperemic, and edematous and bleeds easily.

Asymptomatic light infections should be left untreated. Moderate and severe infections can be treated with mebendazole (Vermox), 100 mg twice daily for 3 days. A study has shown that in severe trichuriasis a second and a third 3-day course of mebendazole is required.

Cestodes (tapeworms)

Taenia saginata and solium. Taeniasis is produced by either beef *(T. saginata)* or pork *(T. solium)* tapeworms. The beef tapeworm may measure 15 feet or more; its head has four suckers but no rostellar hooklets. Gravid proglottids, or *Taenia* segments, are discharged in human feces. Soil contaminated with eggs (Fig. 16-5) becomes infective for man, cattle, and hogs. The ingested larvae develop into encysted forms mainly in the skeletal muscles (cysticercosis). When humans consume infected meat, the ingested larvae hatch

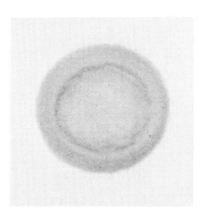

Fig. 16-5. *Taenia* ovum. An unstained egg of *T. saginata* exhibits the sharply distinctive and thick-walled shell with fine striations. The ovum is surrounded by a hyaline membrane.

and then attach and develop in the upper small intestine.

Clinical symptoms caused by *Taenia saginata* infection are minimal. Mild abdominal pain, hunger, and some loss of weight may occur. The usual complaint is the unforgettable experience of evacuating long strips of a flat worm. More serious symptoms may arise if the intestine becomes obstructed by a mass of tangled worms or if detached proglottids obliterate the lumen of the appendix. As is the case for beef tapeworm, man is the only definitive host for the pork tapeworm. The infestation is not usually clinically manifest unless cysticercosis occurs. It is seen with some frequency in immigrants from Asia and Central and South America. Several cases have been seen in Haitians living in Montreal.

T. solium may, in its larval stage, lodge in any tissue (cysticercosis) including the eye and the brain, causing irreparable damage.

The drug of choice for *T. saginata* and *T. solium* is niclosamide (Yomesan), but unfortunately it is no longer available. The alternative is paromomycin (Humatin), 1 gm every 4 hours for 4 doses. The pediatric dosage is 45 mg/kg/day in 4 doses. If the scolex is not passed, it will continue to generate proglottids and the infection will continue. Quinacrine (Atabrine) may be more effective in that the entire worm is excreted. It is less popular because a duodenal tube must be passed to deliver a 1 gm dose in the duodenum. A purgative is usually recommended after drug therapy to ensure rapid expulsion of the worm.

Taeniasis may be prevented by the sanitary dis-

posal of human feces and by freezing or thorough cooking of beef and pork.

Diphyllobothrium latum. The fish tapeworm, *D. latum,* measures 40 to 50 feet in length. The head is spatulate and is provided with a pair of longitudinal sucking grooves. Water contaminated with eggs from infested stools serves as an incubation medium for ciliated embryos eaten by water fleas. The larval stage of the tapeworm is then transmitted to fish, in whose muscular tissues the larval infestation localizes. Raw fish becomes the source of contamination for man, with gefilte fish being a frequent offender.

The symptoms noted with *T. saginata* infection are applicable to infection with *D. latum.* The most important effect of the first tapeworm is its ability to split the vitamin B_{12}–intrinsic factor complex and then to utilize vitamin B_{12}. A megaloblastic anemia with its associated neurologic complications may occur.

Basic control consists in thorough cooking of freshwater fish or freezing it for more than 24 hours. The treatment is the same as for *T. saginata* and *T. solium.*

Hymenolepis nana. *H. nana* measures only 1 to 2 inches in length and is the most common tapeworm in the United States. It occurs most frequently in children living in crowded, unsanitary conditions or in institutions where the chances of direct patient-to-patient infection on ingestion of embryonated eggs are considerable. The worms hatch in the stomach and small intestine and penetrate the lamina propria and develop into cysticercoid larvae. The larvae then migrate into the lumen of the intestine and mature into adult worms.

Large numbers of *H. nana* produce considerable symptoms such as headache, anorexia, intermittent diarrhea, and abdominal pain. The symptoms relate more to the absorption of metabolic waste products of the parasite, particularly in cases of heavy infection. As in other kinds of taeniasis, eosinophilia may be seen. The diagnosis is based on finding characteristic eggs of the *H. nana.*

The treatment is the same as for the other tapeworms. However, in *H. nana* infestations, there are simultaneously not only adult worms in the lumen of the small bowel but also larval forms in various stages of development.

The drug of choice is niclosamide, but since it is no longer available paromomycin (Humatin) is recommended at a dosage of 45 mg/kg/day for 5 to 7 days.

Hydatid disease. The tapeworms *Echinococcus granulosus* and *E. multilocularis* measure only a few millimeters in length and infect dogs. A number of mammals become the intermediate hosts by ingesting dog feces. In turn, the dog will consume meat containing the larvae thereby completing the cycle. Man becomes contaminated by contact with dog feces. The eggs release oncospheres, which will penetrate the mesenteric vessels and implant themselves mainly in the liver and lungs.

The oncospheres trapped in the liver sinusoids develop into bladderlike cysts, which, over a few months, will reach a diameter of 0.5 cm. The fluid of the cyst contains granules that are broad capsules lined with a germinal layer that leads ot the development of a large number of scolices. When a hydatid cyst is ingested by a dog, the embryos are freed from the cyst and grow into adult worms.

Echinococcus granulosus has a worldwide distribution but is more common in the Middle East. The hydatid cysts are usually in the right lobe of the liver and become symptomatic when they reach a size of 10 cm. They may compress adjacent structures or rupture into the biliary tract, or into the peritoneum. The mass may surround itself by a smooth rim of calcification. The most reliable tests are the indirect hemagglutination and the latex agglutination antibody tests. Surgical removal of the intact cyst is the best treatment. When this is not possible, marsupialization and sterilization of its contents with formalin is recommended, though some data show that mebendazole may kill scolices.

Echinococcus multilocularis occurs in Alaska and in northern Canada. Small rodents are intermediate hosts, with the dog being the definitive host. Man acquires the infection by eating contaminated vegetables and berries. In contrast to that of *E. granulosus,* the germinal membrane is not confined within a well-delimited cyst; therefore scolices multiply, invade, infiltrate, and metastasize. The hepatic lesion is widely infiltrative and precludes surgical resection. Mebendazole is the only drug that has been shown to be effective, but up to now there have been only a few reports.

REFERENCES

Ament, M.E.: Diagnosis and treatment of giardiasis, J. Pediatr. **80:**633-637, 1972.

Ament, M.E., and Rubin, S.E.: Relation of giardiasis to abnormal intestinal structure and function in gastrointestinal immunodeficiency syndromes, Gastroenterology **62:**216-226, 1972.

Black, R.E., Dykes, A.C., Sinclair, S.P., and others: Giardiasis in day-care centers: evidence of person-to-person transmission, Pediatrics **60:**486-491, 1977.

Blumenthal, D.S.: Intestinal nematodes in the United States, N. Engl. J. Med. **297:**1437-1439, 1977.

Brandborg, L.L.: Parasitic diseases. In Sleisenger, M.H., and Fordtran, J.S., editors: Gastrointestinal disease, Philadelphia, 1978, W.B. Saunders Co., pp. 1154-1181.

Clinical conference, Brandborg, L.L., moderator.: Giardiasis and traveler's diarrhea, Gastroenterology **78:**1602-1614, 1980.

Hartong, W.A., Gourley, W.K., and Arvanitakis, C.: Giardiasis: clincial spectrum and functional-structural abnormalities of the small intestine mucosa, Gastroenterology **77:**61-69, 1979.

Kamath, K.R., and Murugasu, R.: A comparative study of 4 methods for detecting *Giardia lamblia* in children with diarrheal disease and malabsorption, Gastroenterology **66:**16-21, 1974.

Katz, M.: Parasitic infections, J. Pediatr. **87:**165-178, 1975.

Keystone, J.S., Krajden, S., and Warren, M.R.: Person-to-person transmission of *Giardia lamblia* in day-care nurseries, Can. Med. Assoc. J. **119:**241-248, 1978.

Keystone, J.S., and Murdoch, J.K.: Mebendazole, Ann. Intern. Med. **91:**582-586, 1979.

Krogstad, D.J., Spencer, H.C., and Healy, G.R.: Current concepts in parasitology amebiasis, N. Engl. J. Med. **298:**262-265, 1978.

Marsden, P.D.: Intestinal parasites, Clin. Gastroenterol. **7:**1-239, 1978.

Marsden, P.D.: Ecology of parasites of the human gut. In Circus, W., and Smith, A.N., editors: Scientific foundations of gastroenterology, Toronto, 1978, W.B. Saunders Co.

Osterholm, M.T., Forfang, J.C., Ristinen, T.L., and others.: An outbreak of foodborne giardiasis, N. Engl. J. Med. **304:**24-28, 1981.

Thompson, R.G., Karandikar, D.S., and Leek, J.: Giardiasis: an unusual cause of epidemic diarrhea, Lancet **1:**615-616, 1974.

Wolfe, M.S.: Giardiasis, Pediatr. Clin. North Am. **26:**295-305, 1979.

CANDIDIASIS OF THE GASTROINTESTINAL TRACT

Fungi are normal inhabitants of the human small intestine, and *Candida albicans* is the most prevalent. A recent report suggests that the 20% incidence of rectal colonization by this organism is significantly increased by hospitalization, oral sulfonamides, and systemic antibiotics. *C. albicans* is a budding yeastlike fungus that produces budding blastopores and pseudomycelia in tissue exudates and culture.

The pathogenic role of *C. albicans* in previously healthy individuals is controversial. There is no doubt, however, as to its potential significance in long-term chronic debilitating illness; prolonged treatment with antibiotics, corticosteroids, and immunosuppressives; primary or acquired immune deficiency states; diabetes mellitus; and as a complication of total parenteral nutrition by a central catheter. Under these conditions, colonization of the gastrointestinal tract may give rise to disease locally, but more importantly it may be the reservoir for subsequent disseminated *Candida* sepsis.

Clinical features and pathogenic role

Under conditions in which alterations occur in the host tissue or in the defense mechanisms, *Candida* is commonly found. The esophagus is the segment of the digestive tract that is most heavily infected and more likely to produce symptoms. Candidal esophagitis is a frequent manifestation of chronic mucocutaneous candidiasis and may be associated with laryngeal involvement. The mucosal disease, characterized by erosions and pseudomembranes, may lead to dysphagia, bleeding, and retrosternal pain. Roentgenographic findings may be typical (Fig. 16-6). In the stomach, there may be ulcerations containing *Candida* deep in the ulcer beds; however, few patients have symptoms referable to gastric involvement. In a series of 109 adult patients with malignancies, 22 had evidence of small bowel infection with *Candida;* however, none had symptoms referable to the small bowel. In children dying of leukemia or other malignancies, it is remarkable how few have any symptoms referable to the gastrointestinal tract though, in a large number, there is evidence of fungal infection of the gastrointestinal tract involving mostly the esophagus. Although there is a strong predilection to involvement of the esophagus and stomach, small bowel lesions are occasionally described. Abdominal cramps and watery diarrhea without blood and mucus have been attributed to intestinal candidiasis, but candidiasis as a cause of gastroenteritis remains very unsettled. The coincidence of *C. albicans* and *Salmonella* in a few cases suggested a possible interaction and a pathogenic role for *Candida* when it was shown that diarrhea did not stop until the fungus was eliminated with nystatin. Experimental studies have not shown augmentation of the pathogenicity of Enterobacteriaceae by the presence of *Candida*. Two studies involving cases of protein-calorie malnutrition have shown that with the highly significant increases in bacterial isolations and colony counts from the upper intestinal tract, there were also great increases in *Candida,* particularly in those who had diarrhea. These

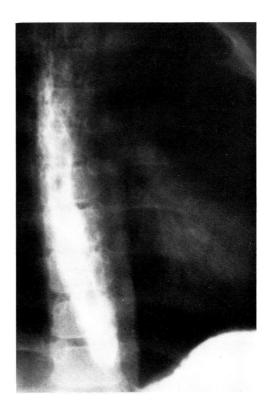

Fig. 16-6. *Candida* esophagitis in a 4-year-old boy with a kidney transplant. The patient experienced severe retrosternal pain and dysphagia. He was treated with amphotericin B, nystatin, and antacids.

findings could very well be of no clinical significance and be totally related to the slow transit time associated with malnutrition. However, a few authors contend that the increased incidence of *Candida* in the gut of these children contributes to the common problem of diarrhea in malnutrition. Since it is known that malnutrition is associated with a depressed cellular immunity, the findings in children with malnutrition are not too surprising. That *Candida* may be primarily involved is unlikely, but it could certainly be opportunistically colonizing the gut already damaged by other microorganisms (bacterial or viral).

It has been previously suggested that *C. albicans* could be primarily involved in causing gastroenteritis in infants. A study of the gastric and small bowel flora in infants with gastroenteritis failed to show a difference in the incidence of isolates but does demonstrate an increased incidence of abundant growth. Of greater significance, perhaps, is the association between abundant growth of *Candida* in the duodenum and depression of

Table 16-1. Extent of gastrointestinal mucormycosis in children

Age	Number	Area of Involvement (%)				Manifestations in the two groups	Underlying condition
		Esophagus	Stomach	Small bowel	Colon		
<1 yr	17	12	59	24	53	Bloody diarrhea Diarrhea Perforation	Malnutrition Prematurity
>1 yr	13	38	85	31	31	Intestinal ob-struction	Malnutrition Malignancy Infection Diabetes

From Michalak, D.M., and others: J. Pediatr. Surg. **15:**320-324, 1980, by permission.

lactase activity at the same level. The authors suggest that the high incidence of decreased disaccharidase activity reported in children with defective cellular immunity may represent another example of the role of *Candida* in either initiating or perpetuating the depression of disaccharidase activity so frequently found in the acute and convalescent phases of gastroenteritis.

Diagnosis

The fungus grows readily on all common laboratory media. A high index of suspicion should be maintained in susceptible patients. The absence of oral thrush does not rule out esophagitis. The presence of symptoms should lead to an esophagogram. Negative roentgenographic findings warrant endoscopy. Mycelia can be demonstrated on biopsy of the esophagus using a silver stain. A stool smear demonstrating the presence of mycelia is suggestive of gastrointestinal fungal infection.

Treatment

At this time, it does not appear warranted to treat with nystatin healthy infants who have diarrhea and stool cultures positive for *Candida*.

Thrush in a patient treated with broad-spectrum antibiotics can be helped with oral nystatin, 250,000 to 500,000 units three times daily. Interruption of the antibiotics is often all that is needed.

In cases of esophageal involvement, Nystatin, 250,000 units suspended in 10 ml of water and administered every 2 hours, may be helpful. Some authors suggest incorporating the drug in a viscous suspension of 0.5% methylcellulose and 0.7% carboxymethylcellulose. Amphotericin B is frequently and successfully used. However the drug

is toxic, intravenous administration is required and relapses occur after the cessation of therapy.

Patients with chronic mucocutaneous candidiasis usually require continuous therapy for their oral, palatal, laryngeal, and esophageal lesions. Topical therapy is unsatisfactory in this disease. Other useful therapeutic approaches include amphotericin B (up to 0.7 mg/kg/day), miconazole nitrate (30 to 60 mg/kg/day), 5-fluorocytosine, transfer factor, and thymosin. Close follow-up study with periodic endoscopy is necessary because symptoms are often minimal until strictures occur.

Mucormycosis

Mucormycosis of the gastrointestinal tract is rare, but one third of cases occur in infants and children. Although 25 years ago it accounted for only 10.5% of fungal infections, its incidence has increased along with that of other mycotic infections.Life-support measures, steroids, chemotherapy, and radiation have undoubtedly contributed to this. Nutritional deficiency, diabetes mellitus, leukemia, solid tumors, burns, renal or hepatic failure, immune defects, and prematurity are some of the underlying conditions that may favor the mycotic invasion. The organisms are ubiquitous saprophytic fungi. The spores gain entry by ingestion of contaminated food (bread and fruit). Gastrointestinal diseases, nasogastric intubation, and procedures leading to ulcerations or trauma facilitate the establishment of the infection.

A recent review of the literature on gastrointestinal mucormycosis in children is summarized in Table 16-1.

The clinical diagnosis is rarely made. The mucormycotic lesion is ulcerating and necrotic with arterial thromboses and a granulomatous inflammatory lesion containing numerous multinucleated giant cells. The organisms can be seen on biopsy material but are more easily identified with a Gomori methenamine silver stain. The disease is rapidly progressive and uniformly fatal unless amphotericin B is started promptly and surgical excision is carried out when indicated. There has been only one survivor in the pediatric age group.

REFERENCES

Barnes, G.L., Bishop, R.F., and Townley, R.R.W.: Microbial flora and disaccharidase depression in infantile gastroenteritis, Acta Paediatr. Scand. **63**:423-426, 1974.

Bishop, R.F., Barnes, G.L., and Townley, R.R.W.: Microbial flora of stomach and small intestine in infantile gastroenteritis, Acta Paediatr. Scand. **63**:418-422, 1974.

Eras, P., Goldstein, M.J., and Sherlock, P.: *Candida* infection of the gastrointestinal tract, Medicine **51**:367-379, 1972.

Gracey, M., Stone, D.E., Suharnojo, M.D., and others: Isolation of *Candida* species from the gastrointestinal tract in malnourished children, Am. J. Clin. Nutr. **27**:345-349, 1974.

Joshi, S.N., Garvin, P.J., and Sunwoo, Y.G.: Candidiasis of the duodenum and jejunum, Gasteroenterology **80**:829-833, 1981.

Kobayashi, R.H., Rosenblatt, H.M., Carney, J.M., and others: *Candida* esophagitis and laryngitis in chronic mucocutaneous candidiasis, Pediatrics **66**:380-384, 1980.

Michalak, D.M., Cooney, D.R., Rhodes, K.H., and others: Gastrointestinal mucormycoses in infants and children: a cause of gangrenous cellulitis and perforation, J. Pediatr. Surg. **15**:320-324, 1980.

Stiehm, E.R.: Chronic mucocutaneous candidiasis: clinical aspects. In Edwards, J.E., Jr, editor: Severe candidal infections, Ann. Intern. Med. **89**:91-106, 1978.

Stone, H.H., Geheber, C.E., Kolb, L.D., and others: Alimentary tract colonization by *Candida albicans,* J. Surg. Res. **14**:273-276, 1973.

Tytgat, G.N., Surachano, S., DeGroot, W.P., and Schelekens, P.T.: A case of chronic oropharyngo-esophageal candidiasis with immunological deficiency: successful treatment with miconazole, Gastroenterology **72**:536-540, 1977.

17 *Selective defects of absorption*

Because of their rarity, most conditions described in this chapter are of minor clinical importance (Table 17-1). Great interest in some of them has arisen because the severe symptoms need to be recognized early if proper treatment is to be given. Taken collectively, transport defects for several specific molecules constitute experiments of nature. They not only illuminate fundamental physiologic processes, but also alert the clinician to the likelihood that some ill-defined pediatric gastrointestinal conditions are possibly caused by selective defects of absorption secondary to inborn errors of intestinal membrane transport.

It is only within the past 15 years that information is available on the mechanism of absorption of amino acids. Transport occurs chiefly through the columnar epithelial cells of the jejunum. Energy dependence and saturation kinetics have been demonstrated. Competition between individual amino acids suggest that there are at least four separate high-capacity systems, each one involving a specific group of amino acids. In addition, there are independent transport systems of lower capacity, probably specific for individual amino acids (Table 17-2).

As discussed in Chapter 10, a significant percentage of dietary amino acids are absorbed as oligopeptides. Therefore the groups of amino acids absorbed less efficiently, because of the low capacity of their own transport system, are proportionately more extensively absorbed as small peptides. In diseases where there is genetic impairment or absence of a specific transport system, the affected individual depends entirely on peptide transport for his supply of those amino acids.

CYSTINURIA

Patients suffering from any of the three recognized forms of cystinuria have in common a propensity to form cystine stones and a renal tubular defect characterized by a renal aminoaciduria involving cystine, lysine, arginine, and ornithine. The gastrointestinal abnormality is related to the selective malabsorption of the amino acids. Clinical nutrition of these patients is normal.

Most patients with cystinuria suffer from type I and cannot actively transport cystine and the dibasic amino acids lysine, arginine, and ornithine across the intestine and kidney. In type II there is detectable transepithelial transport of cystine but none of the dibasics. The defect in type III involves all four amino acids but is milder. Dibasic amino acid malabsorption has no ill effect on the nutritional status of these patients, since they can be transported normally when they are fed as oligopeptides or as proteins.

REFERENCES

Asatoor, A.M., Harrison, R.D.W., Milne, M.D., and Prosser, D.I.: Intestinal absorption of an arginine-containing peptide in cystinuria, Gut **13**:95-98, 1972.

Morin, C.L., Thompson, M.W., Sanford, J.H., and Sass-Kortsak, A.: Biochemical and genetic studies in cystinuria: observations on double heterozygotes of genotype I/II, J. Clin. Invest. **50**:1961-1966, 1971.

LYSINURIC PROTEIN INTOLERANCE

This is a rare autosomal recessive disease characterized by diarrhea and vomiting starting at birth or shortly after weaning in infants who are breast fed. The symptoms are related to the ingestion of large amounts of protein. The low-protein content of human milk prevents the development of symptoms. Later features include aversion to protein, growth retardation, hepatosplenomegaly, muscular weakness, and fragile hair. Large amounts of protein may precipitate coma and convulsions leading to mental retardation.

The defect is unique in that it involves the basolateral membranes of the kidney and of the intestine for the transport of dibasic amino acids. There is hyperdibasic aminoaciduria, low plasma concentrations or arginine, ornithine, and lysine and malabsorption of lysine and arginine. More critical and responsible for the set of symptoms is a functional deficiency of ornithine in the urea cycle leading to hyperammonemia.

Treatment with arginine and lysine supplements has been disappointing. Lysine deficiency is not alleviated whether given as an individual amino acid or as a dipeptide, and arginine tends to exaggerate the diarrhea. A recent report shows that

Table 17-1. Selective defects of absorption

Substrates	Disease entity	Clinical features
Amino acids		
Cystine, lysine, ornithine, argi-nine	Cystinuria	Stone formers; no gastrointestinal symptoms
Lysine, ornithine, arginine	Lysinuric protein intolerance	With familial protein intolerance, diarrhea and vomiting; with lysine malabsorption, failure to thrive
Proline, hydroxyproline, glycine	Iminoglycinuria	No symptoms
Monoamino-monocarboxylic acids	Hartnup's disease	Pellagrous rash, cerebellar ataxia, no symptoms on high-protein diet
Tryptophan	Blue diaper syndrome	Hypercalcemia, blue discoloration of the diaper
Methionine	Methionine malabsorption	Mental retardation, sporadic diarrhea, sweetish smell of urine
Monosaccharides		
Glucose, galactose	Glucose-galactose malabsorption	Diarrhea, dehydration with acidosis
Electrolytes		
Chloride	Congenital chloridorrhea	Diarrhea, alkalosis, hypokalemia
Minerals		
Magnesium	Familial hypomagnesemia	Tetany in neonatal period
Calcium	Vitamin D–dependent rickets	Aminoaciduria, rickets, hypocalcemia
	Familial hypophosphatemic rickets	Rickets, growth failure
Trace elements		
Copper	Menkes' kinky-hair syndrome	Mental retardation, kinky hair, temperature instability
Zinc	Acrodermatitis enteropathica	Diarrhea, dermatitis, alopecia, failure to thrive
Vitamins		
Vitamin B_{12}	Vitamin B_{12} malabsorption	Megaloblastic anemia with pallor, weakness, vomiting, diarrhea, anorexia, failure to thrive
Folic acid	Folic acid malabsorption	Megaloblastic anemia, mental retardation, convulsions

Table 17-2. Transport of amino acids

Group of amino acids	Amino acids transported	Rate of transport
Cystine-dibasic	Cystine, lysine, ornithine, arginine	Rapid
Glycine-imino acids	Glycine, proline, hydroxyproline	Slow
Monoamino-monocarboxylic (neutral amino) acids	Tyrosine, tryptophan, phenylalanine	Very rapid for the three categories
	Alanine, serine, threonine, valine, leucine, isoleucine	
	Methonine, histidine, glutamine, asparagine, cysteine	
Dicarboxylic	Glutamic acid, aspartic acid	Rapid

citrulline (2 to 3 gm/day) along with a diet providing 1 to 2 gm/kg of protein daily prevents hyperammonemia and improves protein nutrition.

REFERENCES

Desjeux, J.F., Rajantie, J., Simell, O., and others: Lysine fluxes across the jejunal epithalium in lysinuric protein intolerance, J. Clin. Invest. **65**:1382-1387, 1980.

Rajantie, J., Simell, O., Rapola, J., and Perheentupa, J.: Lysinuric protein intolerance: a two year trial of dietary supplementation therapy with citrulline and lysine, J. Pediatr. **97**:927-932, 1980.

Rajantie, J., Simell, O., and Perheentupa, J.: Intestinal absorption in lysinuric protein intolerance: impaired for diamino acids, normal for citrulline, Gut **21**:519-524, 1980.

IMINOGLYCINURIA

Impaired renal tubular transport of proline, hydroxyproline, and glycine has been described as a familial disorder. In the few patients who have an associated impairment of intestinal transport, increased concentrations of glycine and of the imino acids have been found in the stools. Proline loading led to a lower serum level of proline in patients than in control subjects. Response to hydroxyproline and glycine was normal.

REFERENCES

Goodman, S.I., McIntyre, C.A., and O'Brien, D.: Impaired intestinal transport of proline in a patient with familial iminoaciduria, J. Pediatr. **71**:246-248, 1967.

Scriver, C.R.: Familial iminoglycinuria. In Stanbury, J.B., Wyngaarden, J.B., and Fredrickson, D.S., editors: The metabolic basis of inherited disease, ed. 4, New York, 1978, McGraw-Hill Book Co.

HARTNUP'S DISEASE

Hartnup's disease is a rare autosomal recessive condition characterized by a pellagrous rash, unusual photosensitivity, and cerebellar ataxia. The clinical features are variable from patient to patient and in the same individual from time to time. The cerebellar ataxia tends to occur when the skin rash is more severe. There is no intellectual deterioration, though emotional instability, delirium, and fainting attacks are described. The clinical manifestations tend to improve with age. These patients are generally of reduced stature.

The disease is characterized by a specific disturbance in the renal tubular reabsorption and in the intestinal absorption of the monoamino-monocarboxylic group of amino acids. Methionine is part of this group but is well absorbed. This perhaps indicates that an independent system for the transport of methionine is functioning.

Nicotinamide deficiency, a consequence of tryptophan malabsorption, accounts for all the clinical features of the disease. As a result of intestinal malabsorption of tryptophan, indoles are formed, absorbed, and excreted in the urine. A recent study has shown a defective absorption of L-histidine that was not present when the same amino acid was fed as a dipeptide; similarly, the absorption of the dipeptide tryptophan and phenylalanine was much greater than when each amino acid was administered in its free form. These results seem consistent with the fact that on a high-protein diet patients with Hartnup's disease remain asymptomatic. Their absorptive disadvantage for certain individual amino acids is counterbalanced by a high-protein diet stimulating their absorption of proteins as oligopeptides. There is a good response to nicotinamide given orally.

REFERENCES

Leonard, J.V., Marrs, T.C., Addison, J.M., and others: Absorption of amino acids and peptides in Hartnup disease, Clin. Sci. Mol. Med. **46**:15P, 1974.

Navab, F., and Asatoor, A.M.: Studies on intestinal absorption of amino acids and a dipeptide in a case of Hartnup disease, Gut **11**:373-379, 1970.

Shih, V.E., Bixby, E.M., Alpers, D.H., and others: Studies of intestinal transport defect in Hartnup disease, Gastroenterology **61**:445-453, 1971.

BLUE DIAPER SYNDROME

A familial form of hypercalcemia with nephrocalcinosis and a defective absorption of tryptophan from the gastrointestinal tract has been reported in two children.

In response to a tryptophan loading test, plasma levels of the amino acid were relatively low. Fecal excretion of tryptophan was excessive. The great increase in the urinary excretion of indolic metabolites such as indican and indole-3-acetic acid showed that a large amount of unabsorbed tryptophan was reaching the colon. Bacterial degradation of tryptophan caused formation of indole, which was absorbed, transformed into indican by the liver, and excreted in the urine. Subsequently, the oxidative conjugation of two molecules of indican formed indigotin (indigo blue), which was responsible for the blue discoloration of the diapers.

REFERENCE

Drummond, K.N., Michael, A.F., Ulstrom, R.A., and Good, R.A.: The blue diaper syndrome: familial hypercalcemia with nephrocalcinosis and indicanuria, Am. J. Med. **37**:928-948, 1964.

METHIONINE MALABSORPTION

A selective absorptive defect of methionine and, secondarily, of branched-chain amino acids and of serine has been described in a few children with mental retardation, sporadic diarrhea, convulsions, and tachypnea. The patients have blue eyes, white hair, and an oasthouse smell, which is characteristic of the urine.

Malabsorption of methionine induces bacterial degradation of methionine in the colon; the reabsorbed alpha-hydroxybutyric acid is then excreted in the urine. A low-methionine diet is effective in coloring the hair and improving the mental status, convulsions, and diarrhea. Methionine precipitates diarrhea and leads to the abnormal excretion of alpha-hydroxybutyric acid in parents and siblings. The disease has all the features of phenylketonuria in addition to those of methionine malabsorption.

REFERENCE

Hooft, C., Timmermans, J., Snoeck, J., and others: Methionine malabsorption syndrome, Ann. Paediatr. **205**:73-104, 1965.

Hooft, C., Carton, D., Snoeck, J., and others: Further investigations in the methionine malabsorption syndrome, Helv. Paediat. Acta **33**:234-349, 1968.

GLUCOSE-GALACTOSE MALABSORPTION

Failure of intestinal hydrolysis of disaccharides or impairment of absorption of monosaccharides results in sugar diarrhea (Chapter 9).

Malabsorption of monosaccharides and disaccharides may be the consequence of intestinal disorders associated with mucosal damage, such as infectious diarrhea or celiac disease. The abnormal intestinal handling of disaccharides may be congenital, as in lactase or sucrase-isomaltase deficiency. The syndrome of glucose-galactose malabsorption is an autosomal recessive defect leading to impaired absorption of the two separate monosaccharides transported by a common mechanism.

The brush border contains a mobile carrier that has binding sites for glucose-galactose and sodium (Fig. 17-1). The presence of sodium (Na^+) increases the affinity of the carrier for glucose and vice versa; therefore both sodium and glucose entry are stimulated by one another. Translocated Na^+ is released by the carrier as Na^+ is pumped out of the cell by an active transport mechanism

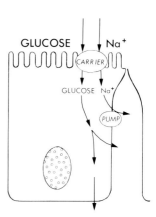

Fig. 17-1. Carrier-mediated glucose-galactose transport.

through the basolateral membrane. This brings about the concomitant freeing of substrate from the carrier, which can be utilized locally or moved out of the cell by passive diffusion. This carrier-mediated transport system is absent in glucose-galactose malabsorption. Some absorption of glucose independent of Na^+ transport has been found in in vitro animal experiments. A disaccharidase-related transport short-circuiting the brush-border glucose-sodium carrier has been evoked to explain this phenomenon (Chapter 10). A jejunal perfusion study in a child with glucose-galactose malabsorption has failed to show that this route could be of physiologic importance.

Clinical findings

The symptoms are essentially the same as in congenital lactase deficiency. Diarrhea starts within a few days after birth, the stools being explosive and watery. Dehydration and metabolic acidosis become severe and can be life threatening. It is a cause of intractable diarrhea. In some cases, the diarrhea becomes less severe after the first few years of life. However, the patient will continue to suffer abdominal discomfort, flatulence, and diarrhea after eating significant amounts of carbohydrates other than fructose.

Diagnosis

Diagnostic methods are essentially the same as in disaccharide malabsorption. The stool pH is acidic, as is commonly found in disaccharidase deficiencies. Reducing substances are invariably present in large amounts (and the breath hydrogen test is positive) after a flat oral glucose or lactose absorption test that precipitates symptoms. Disaccharidase activity is normal, and intestinal structure is intact.

Pathogenesis

Intubation studies demonstrate normal absorption of fructose, contrasting with very poor absorption for glucose and galactose. Autoradiographic studies of mucosal biopsy material show little accumulation of labeled galactose. Complete absence of the active carrier for glucose and galactose or its failure to function is the most likely defect. Intermediate metabolism of glucose and galactose appears to be normal if these monosaccharides are given intravenously. The defective transport of glucose and galactose is not limited to the intestinal cells, since practically all patients with this disorder have glucosuria. A similar defect is present in the renal tubular epithelium, and it is characterized by a low maximal tubular reabsorptive capacity (T_m) for glucose.

Treatment

Drastic exclusion of glucose and galactose from the diet is mandatory. Fructose, the only carbohydrate that can be given safely, can be added at a concentration of 6% to 8% to a carbohydrate-free formula. When the infant is about 7 months old, foods with a low starch and sucrose content can be added according to tolerance. In our one patient with this disorder it was necessary to continue drastic dietary restrictions for the first 2 years. Over a period of 4 years we have seen no amelioration of glucose transport assessed by incubating jejunal mucosa with labeled substrate, but tolerance for glucose-containing carbohydrates has improved.

REFERENCES

Elsas, L.J., Hillman, R.E., Patterson, J.H., and Rosenberg, L.E.: Renal and intestinal hexose transport in familial glucose-galactose malabsorption, J. Clin. Invest. **49**:576-585, 1970.

Fairclough, P.D., Clark, M.L., Dawson, A.M., and others: Absorption of glucose and maltose in congenital glucose-galactose malabsorption, Pediatr. Res. **12**:1112-1114, 1978.

Meeuwisse, G.W., and Melin, K.: Glucose-galactose malabsorption, a clinical study of 6 cases, Acta Paediatr. Scand. **188**(supp.):3-18, 1969.

Stirling, C.E., Schneider, A.J., Wong, M., and Kinter, W.B.: Quantitative radioautography of sugar transport in intestinal biopsies from normal humans and a patient with glucose-galactose malabsorption, J. Clin. Invest. **51**:438-451, 1972.

FAMILIAL CHLORIDE DIARRHEA (CONGENITAL CHLORIDORRHEA, CONGENITAL ALKALOSIS WITH DIARRHEA)

The loss in the stools of alkaline intestinal contents with proportionately less chloride and more bicarbonate than in plasma partly explains the metabolic acidosis associated with most infantile diarrheal states. Chronic diarrhea with striking fecal losses of chloride associated with metabolic alkalosis is a rare familial disorder. More than half of the cases reported so far are from Finland. An acquired and temporary form of the disease has been reported after bowel operations in infants and also in one adult after a bout of intestinal obstruction. It has been suggested that severe potassium depletion may lead to an acquired chloridorrhea that disappears on repletion of potassium. Seven infants with intractable diarrhea associated with metabolic alkalosis, hyponatremia, hypokalemia, hypochloremia, and the excretion of chloride-free urine were recently reported and represent a transient form of the disease.

The intestinal defect is located in the distal ileum and colon. Studies have shown that there is impaired active Cl^- absorption resulting from a defective or absent Cl^-/HCO_3^- exchange mechanism (Fig. 8-2). Chloride is lost in the stools, and osmotic diarrhea develops. Sodium absorption leads to acidification of luminal contents, since H^+ secreted in exchange for Na^+ is not balanced by secreted bicarbonate in exchange for Cl^-. The net result is a reduced rate of fluid absorption and acidification of stools because of a high Cl^- concentration. A defect in the bile acid–concentrating ability of the gallbladder has been described in one patient.

Clinical findings

Polyhydramnios is invariably present. This may be attributable to in utero diarrhea because these babies do not pass meconium after birth.

Diarrhea, abdominal distention (Fig. 17-2), and hyperbilirubinemia are almost invariably present within the first few days. Dehydration is a frequent complication during the early months. A few infants will survive the first months before a diagnosis is made. There is continuing diarrhea or "soft stools," impaired growth, and malnutrition. Diarrhea does not subside with age, but patients

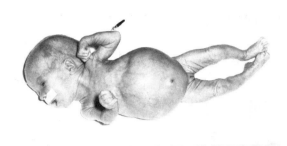

Fig. 17-2. Congenital chloride diarrhea. This newborn shows failure to thrive and severe abdominal distention. (Courtesy Dr. C. Holmberg, Children's Hospital, University of Helsinki, Helsinki, Finland.)

learn to live with their diarrhea and make the necessary social adjustment.

Diagnosis

Diarrhea associated with metabolic alkalosis, hypokalemia, and hypochloremia should make one seriously consider the diagnosis.

Diagnosis is definite if the chloride content of fecal fluid is high. Values are between 50 and 150 mEq/L during the first months and reach 110 to 180 mEq/L subsequently. Normal stools contain 6 to 17 mEq/L of chloride anions. Values in diarrheal stools in other disorders never approach the figures noted in this condition. In fact, in the acidic liquid stools of this familial entity, chloride is more than the sum of sodium and potassium. In contrast, the urine is practically chloride-free.

After a meal, jejunal sodium concentrations are close to those of plasma, whereas chloride concentrations are higher (115 to 120 mEq/L) and bicarbonate are lower (10 mEq/L). In the ileum the sodium concentration is the same as in the jejunum, but because of active chloride absorption and of bicarbonate secretion the chloride concentration drops. As a result, the bicarbonate increases. The sum of the stool Na^+ and K^+ minus the Cl^- concentration provides a more appropriate measure of HCO_3^- (anion gap) because bicarbonate cannot be adequately quantitated since part of it is dissipated as carbon dioxide. The fecal anion gap is very low in chloride diarrhea (Table 17-3).

Management

Insertion of a rectal tube may be necessary to relieve abdominal distention. Antidiarrheal drugs are contraindicated, and dietary changes do not reduce fecal volume. Oral replacement of water and electrolyte losses is done with a 0.7% NaCl and 0.3% KCl solution. Requirements are variable: the average during the first 6 years of life is

Table 17-3. Fecal electrolyte concentrations in familial chloride diarrhea (mEq/L)

Ion	Normal	Chloride diarrhea
Na^+	40	60-75
K^+	80	40
Cl^-	16	125-150
HCO_3^-	30	5

From Holmberg, C., and others: Arch. Dis. Child. **52:**255, 1977.

around 75 mEq/m^2 of NaCl and 45 mEq/m^2 of potassium chloride.

Complications

Despite optimum therapy, which replaces the excessive loss of chloride, sodium, and potassium ions and water, electrolyte balance remains labile, gastrointestinal infections can lead to life-threatening dehydration; extremely rapid losses of potassium may occur. Volvulus has been reported in a few cases. Renal complications characterized by juxtaglomerular hyperplasia, nephrocalcinosis, hyalinized glomeruli, and high level of renin, angiotensin II, and aldosterone do not develop if treatment is initiated early and good control of electrolyte balance is maintained. Growth and development can also be satisfactory.

REFERENCES

Aaronson, I.: Secondary chloride-losing diarrhea, Arch. Dis. Child. **46:**479-482, 1971.

Bakkeren, J., Monnens, L., and Van Os, C.: Defect in bile acid concentrating ability of the gallbladder in congenital chloride diarrhea, Acta Pediatr. Scand. **70:**43-46, 1981.

Bieberdorf, F.A., Gorden, P., and Fordtran, J.S.: Pathogenesis of congenital alkalosis with diarrhea, J. Clin. Invest. **51:**1958-1968, 1972.

Gorden, P., and Levithan, H.: Congenital alkalosis with diarrhea, Ann. Intern. Med. **78:**876-882, 1973.

Holmberg, C., Perheentupa, J., and Launiala, K.: Colonic electrolyte transport in health and in congenital chloride diarrhea, J. Clin. Invest. **56:**302-310, 1975.

Holmberg, C., Perheentupa, J., Launiala, K., and Hallman, N.: Congenital chloride diarrhea, Arch. Dis. Child. **52:**255-267, 1977.

Kaplan, B., and Vitullo, B.: Acquired chloride diarrhea, J. Pediatr. **99:**211-214, 1981.

McReynolds, E.W., Roy, S., and Etteldorf, J.N.: Congenital chloride diarrhea, Am. J. Dis. Child. **127:**566-570, 1974.

FAMILIAL HYPOMAGNESEMIA

The entire role of magnesemia in the body economy is not delineated fully though it is the fourth cation in abundance. Simple ionic diffusion is probably the major mechanism of magnesium absorption though active or facilitated transport has not been ruled out. Hypomagnesemia is difficult to produce in normal man. However, it quite frequently occurs with various gastrointestinal disorders associated with malabsorption and diarrhea, such as celiac disease, short bowel syndrome, and chronic inflammatory bowel disease.

Magnesium depletion is much commoner than has previously been suspected. Because of its close association with potassium in muscle, it should be considered whenever there is potassium depletion. The most important cause of magnesium deficits is diarrhea, particularly in young infants. Muscle weakness and lethargy precede the onset of muscle twitching and frank convulsions.

Clinical findings

There are 8 reported cases of neonatal hypomagnesemia resulting from a selective defect in the intestinal absorption of magnesium.

A recent paper has examined the nature of the precise defect. Perfusion studies in controls suggest that there are two separate systems for magnesium transport in the proximal small bowel—a carrier-mediated system and a simple diffusional process. The data in a 4-year-old child with primary hypomagnesemia suggest that the primary abnormality is a defect in carrier-mediated transport of magnesium from low intraluminal concentrations of magnesium.

The disorder is characterized by repeated tetanic convulsions unrelieved by calcium medication. The onset is usually within the first month of life. Biochemical derangements include, besides hypomagnesemia (less than 0.5 mEq/L), hypocalcemia and hyperphosphatemia. There are no biochemical or histologic signs of generalized malabsorption. Absorption of calcium is normal, but there is a specific defect in the intestinal absorption of magnesium. In a study with ^{28}Mg, the net absorption of magnesium was 8.8% as compared to control values of 55.1%.

Hypocalcemia is a serious complication of hypomagnesemia. Impaired secretion of parathormone, end-organ nonresponsiveness, and a defective calcium-to-magnesium exchange in bone have been postulated as likely mechanisms.

Treatment

Parathormone injections elevate calcium level but fail to raise the magnesium to normal levels. Although vitamin D normally increases the absorption of magnesium, its use has not been effective. Parenteral magnesium chloride or magnesium sulfate can be given intravenously in the acute stage of the disease. Magnesium lactate solution, 10 to 20 mEq/24 hr with meals, has been effective in preventing symptoms and achieving normal serum calcium, though magnesium remains low. In mild to moderate cases of acquired hypomagnesemia, magnesium gluconate may be given orally at a dosage of 1 gm 4 times daily.

REFERENCES

Harris, I., and Wilkinson, A.W.: Magnesium depletion in children, Lancet **2:**735-736, 1971.

Milla, P.J., Aggett, P.J., Wolff, O.H., and Harris, J.T.: Studies in primary hypomagnesaemia: evidence for defective carrier-mediated small intestinal transport of magnesium, Gut **20:**1028-1033, 1979.

Paunier, L., Radde, I.C., Kooh, S.W., and others: Primary hypomagnesemia with secondary hypocalcemia in an infant, Pediatrics **41:**385-402, 1968.

Ponillaude, J.M., Friedrich, A., François, B., and others: Hypomagnésémie congénitale primitive et chronique avec hypocalcémie magnésiodépendante, Arch. Fr. Pediatr. **28:**1021-1040, 1971.

Stromme, J.H., Nesbakken, R., Normann, T., and others: Familial hypomagnesemia, Acta Paediatr. Scand. **58:**433-444, 1969.

Suh, S.M., Tashjian, A.H., Jr., Matsuo, N., and others: Pathogenesis of hypocalcemia in primary hypomagnesemia: normal end-organ responsiveness to parathyroid hormone, impaired parathyroid gland function, J. Clin. Invest. **52:**153-160, 1973.

Woodward, J.C., Webster, P.D., and Carr, A.A.: Primary hypomagnesemia with secondary hypocalcemia, diarrhea and insensitivity to parathyroid hormone, Am. J. Dig. Dis. **17:**612-618, 1972.

VITAMIN D–DEPENDENT RICKETS

Hypophosphatemic, hypocalcemic, and hyperaminoaciduric rickets can result from a dietary deficiency of vitamin D and readily responds to vitamin D given at a dose of 2000 international units (IU) per 24 hours. It may also occur in cases of malabsorption secondary to pancreatic, hepatic, or small bowel disease. Such patients may require larger amounts of vitamin D (5000 to 10,000 units) or, in exceptional cases, may not respond at all. The third form is a genetically inherited defect responsive to treatment when vitamin D is given at a dose of 25,000 to 100,000 IU daily.

A classic study has shown a specific impairment of intestinal calcium absorption in an 18-month-old infant who developed florid rickets on an adequate dietary intake of vitamin D. The malabsorption work-up and a jejunal peroral biopsy were normal in that patient as well as in five others already receiving vitamin D therapy. The calcium balance recorded during a 12-day period demonstrated intestinal malabsorption of calcium, which disappeared when the balance study was redone 9 months after therapy had been initiated.

Once absorbed vitamin D is hydroxylated in the liver to 25-hydroxy-cholecalciferol (25-OH-D_3) and then in the kidney to 1,25-(OH)$_2D_3$. The defect in vitamin D–dependent rickets is a primary deficiency of renal 1-alpha-hydroxylase. It is an autosomal recessive condition that has its onset in the first year of life. Hypophosphatemia, hypocalcemia, elevated alkaline phosphatase, normal serum 25-OH-D_3, aminoaciduria, phosphaturia, and elevated parathormone constitute the typical laboratory findings. Roentgenograms of bones show rickets and signs of hyperparathyroidism. Large amounts of vitamin D or small amounts of 1,25-(OH)$_2D_3$ are effective.

One patient has been described with normal serum 25-OH-D_3 and very high concentrations of 1,25-(OH)$_2D_3$. A reasonable explanation is that there is failure of end-organ response to the dihydroxylated derivative. This condition has been called vitamin D–dependent rickets type II.

REFERENCES

Brooks, M.H., Bell, N.H., Love, L., and others: Vitamin-D dependent rickets type II: resistance of target organs to 1,25-dihydroxyvitamin D, N. Engl. J. Med. **298:**996-999, 1978.

Fraser, D., and Scriver, C.R.: Familial forms of vitamin D–resistant rickets revisited, X-linked hypophosphatemia and autosomal recessive vitamin D dependency, Am. J. Clin. Nutr. **29:**1315-1329, 1976.

Hamilton, R., Harrison, J., Fraser, J., and others: The small intestine in vitamin D dependent rickets, Pediatrics **45:**364-373, 1970.

FAMILIAL HYPOPHOSPHATEMIC RICKETS

Vitamin D–resistant rickets is a sex-linked dominant entity giving rise to rickets or osteomalacia that fails to respond to vitamin D. There is always a severe degree of hypophosphatemia with decreased renal tubular reabsorption of phosphate, as well as a diminished absorption of calcium in all affected children with rickets in the absence of other signs of gastrointestinal malabsorption.

Early studies suggested a reduced absorption of phosphate. This could not be confirmed by others who measured the uptake of phosphate by jejunal mucosal biopsy specimens. However, a recent report shows that five patients treated with 1,25-(OH)$_2D_3$ more than doubled their peak serum concentration of phosphate after a phosphate load. The fact that there was no concomitant change in renal reabsorption of phosphate supports the view that there is an intestinal defect for phosphate.

The disease in its clinical form first becomes manifest, despite a normal intake of vitamin D, when the child starts to walk. Because of the renal tubular defect limited to phosphate, the term "phosphate diabetes" was coined.

1,25-(OH)$_2D_3$ increases the calcemia and improves the absorption of phosphate. When administered with oral phosphate salts, there is great improvement in the mineralization of trabecular bone. However, this treatment regimen does not correct the renal tubular leak of phosphate.

REFERENCES

Brickman, A.S., Coburn, J.W., Kurokawa, K., and others: Actions of 1,25-dihydroxycholecalciferol in patients with hypophosphatemic vitamin D–resistant rickets, N. Engl. J. Med. **289:**495-498, 1973.

Glorieux, F.H., Holick, M.I., Scriver, C.R., and others: X-linked hypophosphatemic rickets: inadequate therapeutic response to 1,25-dihydroxycholecalciferol, Lancet **2:**287-289, 1973.

Glorieux, F.H., Marie, P.J., Pettifor, J.M., and Delvin, E.E.: Bone response to phosphate salts, ergocalciferol and calcitriol in hypophosphatemic vitamin D resistant rickets, N. Engl. J. Med. **303:**1023-1031, 1980.

MENKES' KINKY-HAIR SYNDROME

The kinky-hair syndrome is a rare disorder (1 in 40,000 live births) inherited as a sex-linked trait. The disease becomes manifest within a month or two after birth. Affected babies show temperature instability, coarse facies, long-bone changes, growth retardation, peculiar hair, abnormal tortuosity of arteries, and focal cerebral and cerebellar degeneration. Neurologic impairment rapidly progresses with seizures, spastic quadriparesis, opisthotonos, and decerebration. The hair changes easily alert to the diagnosis. It is scant, whitish, and kinky. Microscopically it shows pili torti, monilethrix, and trichorrhexis nodosa. Death usually occurs by 3 years of age.

These anomalies are the result of a disturbed copper metabolism and, in particular, an impaired copper absorption together with an abnormal copper distribution in various tissues. There is increased copper concentration in the kidneys and intestinal mucosa and a decreased copper concentration in the plasma and liver and in the brain, where it causes irreparable brain damage, which seems to have its onset in utero.

Monoamine oxidases and ascorbic acid oxidase are copper dependent and are necessary for the proper cross-linking of collagen and of keratin. In the patients treated with parenteral cupric acetate, no clinical improvement has been noted. The only worthwhile intervention is tracing the carriers of the disease.

REFERENCES

Buckwall, W.E., Haslam, R.H.A., and Holtz, N.A.: Kinky hair syndrome: response to copper therapy, Pediatrics **52:**653-657, 1973.

Danks, D.M., Campbell, P.E., Stevens, B.J., and others: Menkes' kinky hair syndrome: inherited defect in copper absorption with widespread effects, Pediatrics **50:**188-201, 1972.

Menkes, J.M.: Kinky hair disease, Pediatrics **50:**181-183, 1972.

Nooijen, J.L., De Groot, C.J., Van Den Hamer, C.J.A., and others: Trace element studies in three patients and a fetus with Menkes' disease: effect of copper therapy, Pediatr. Res. **15:**284-289, 1981.

Williams, D.M., Atkin, C.L., Frens, D.B., and Bray, P.F.: Menkes' kinky hair syndrome: studies of copper metabolism and long term copper therapy, Pediat. Res. **11:**823-826, 1977.

ACRODERMATITIS ENTEROPATHICA

It is a rare disorder characterized by symptoms and signs of zinc deficiency. It is caused by a congenital defect of zinc uptake by the intestinal mucosa. A discussion of this disorder and of other causes of zinc deficiency can be found in Chapter 8.

SELECTIVE MALABSORPTION OF VITAMIN B_{12}
Abnormal or absent intrinsic factor

Only one case of abnormal intrinsic factor (IF) has been described. It was shown to bind normally to vitamin B_{12}, but its affinity for ileal re-

ceptors was found to be greatly decreased. There are more than 30 cases of congenital absence of intrinsic factor. Gastric function is normal and remains normal. Hematologic and neurologic signs of vitamin B_{12} deficiency become apparent within the first 3 years of life. The suggestion has been made that some of these patients may have an abnormal intrinsic factor, which remains undetectable by the usual antibody-detecting techniques.

Disorder of intestinal transport of the IF-B_{12} complex

Children suffering from the "Immerslund-Gräsbeck syndrome" have normal amounts of biologically active intrinsic factor but cannot absorb vitamin B_{12} bound to intrinsic factor, though all other parameters of intestinal function are normal. Ileal receptors are present, but there is apparent failure to transport the complex fixed to the microvillus receptor across the intestinal cell. Proteinuria is usually present without other renal abnormality.

With both absorptive defects, pallor, weakness, and anorexia between the ages of 6 and 36 months are the presenting complaints. More than half have vomiting and diarrhea. Growth retardation is noted, along with neurologic signs of vitamin B_{12} deficiency. Megaloblastic anemia is commonly associated with leukopenia and thrombocytopenia. Gastric acidity and histologic state of the small intestine are normal. The Schilling test with and without intrinsic factor is abnormal, and the serum level of vitamin B_{12} is low.

Deficiency of vitamin B_{12}–transport proteins

Congenital deficiency of transcobalamin I has been described but is not associated with clinical disease. This is surprising because it is responsible for the transport of three fourths of the vitamin B_{12} that circulates in human plasma. In contrast, deficiency of transcobalamin II, a vitamin B_{12} binder that functionally appears less important, leads to severe disease very early in life. Within the first few weeks after birth, severe megaloblastic anemia develops, with vomiting, diarrhea, oral ulcerations, and atrophy of the mucosa of the tongue. Leukopenia and thrombocytopenia are common findings. Intestinal mucosal atrophy and agammaglobulinemia were described in one case. Serum vitamin B_{12} is normal, but a disturbed distribution of the vitamin is postulated. In particular, it is believed that vitamin B_{12} is not delivered to the bone marrow. The disease is transmitted according to an autosomal recessive mode of inheritance; intermediate values of transcobalamin II have been found in carriers. There is usually a good response to frequent large doses of vitamin B_{12}.

REFERENCES

Bell, M., Harries, J.T., Wolff, O.H., and others: Familial selective malabsorption of vitamin B_{12}, Arch. Dis. Child. **48:**896-900, 1973.

Corcino, J.J., Waxman, S., and Herbert, V.: Absorption and malabsorption of vitamin B_{12}, Am. J. Med. **48:**562-569, 1970.

Hall, C.A.: Congenital disorders of vitamin B_{12} transport and their contribution to concepts, Gastroenterology **65:**684-686, 1973.

Hitzig, W.H., Dohmann, U., Pluss, H.J., and others: Hereditary transcobalamin II deficiency: clinical findings in a new family, J. Pediatr. **85:**622-628, 1974.

Lanzkowsky, P.: Pediatric hematology-oncology, New York, 1980, McGraw-Hill Book Co.

McKenzie, I.L.: Ileal mucosa in familial selective vitamin B_{12} malabsorption, N. Engl. J. Med. **286:**1021-1025, 1972.

CONGENITAL MALABSORPTION OF FOLIC ACID

Folic acid deficiencies may be secondary to the following well-defined mechanisms: (1) inadequate dietary intake, (2) defective absorption as part of the malabsorption syndrome, (3) increased requirements, and (4) administration of folic acid antagonists such as phenytoin and sulfasalazine.

There are now four reported cases of congenital malabsorption of folic acid with megaloblastic anemia, diarrhea, stomatitis, failure to thrive, weight loss, mental retardation, convulsions, and inability to absorb physiologic doses of folic acid and related compounds. Gastrointestinal function and structure are normal. The disorder became clinically manifest during the first 3 months of life. The absorption of pteroylglutamates and of methyltetrahydrofolic acid is defective. Absorption is not enhanced in the presence of duodenal juice, calf jejunum, or calf pancreas. However, when these children are given large oral doses of folic acid (40 mg/day) or 100 to 250 μg of folic acid intramuscularly daily, they are able to maintain normal serum folate levels. Although the precise defect remains to be identified, the possibility of a genetically determined defect in the folate transport process has been suggested.

REFERENCES

Cooper, B.A.: Megaloblastic anemia in childhood, Clin. Haematol. **5:**640-641, 1978.

Lanzkowsky, P.: Congenital malabsorption of folate, Am. J. Med. **48:**580-583, 1970.

Santiago-Borrero, P.J., Santini, R., Perez-Santiago, E., and others: Congenital isolated defect of folic acid absorption, J. Pediatr. **82:**450-455, 1973.

18 Tumors of the peritoneum, gastrointestinal tract, liver, and pancreas

MESENTERIC AND OMENTAL CYSTS

Mesenteric and omental cysts are rare lesions in infants and children. Mesenteric cysts are said to be five times more common than omental cysts. They arise from the continued growth of congenitally malformed or malpositioned lymphatic tissue. Because fewer than 25% of patients have symptoms within the first 10 years of life, other origins such as trauma or inflammatory obstruction of existing lymph channels have been postulated.

Pathology

The mesentery is made up of two closely juxtaposed layers of peritoneum extending from the posterior abdominal wall to the intestines. Connective tissue, fat, lymphatics, blood vessels, and muscle fibers are sandwiched between these layers. Mesenteric cysts are lined usually with endothelium and often contain muscle and connective tissue. Mesenteric cysts can be quite tense and are commonly multilocular. The fluid they contain may be pale, clear, and of the same composition as plasma, or it may be white and of the

same composition as chyle (Fig. 18-1). It can also be hemorrhagic. Close to 50% of mesenteric cysts occur in the mesentery of the small intestine with most of them being in the ileum. In contrast to duplications, mesenteric cysts have only a contiguity relationship with the bowel.

Clinical features

The extremely variable symptoms associated with mesenteric cysts are related to size, location, and complications. In fact, most cases are asymptomatic, and it is the parents who usually note an increase in the child's abdominal girth. An abdominal mass, usually rounded, smooth, nontender, and mobile, may be palpated. Complications include hemorrhage, rupture, partial or complete intestinal obstruction, and hydronephrosis from ureteral compression. Small cysts can undergo torsion and give rise to a clinical picture resembling acute appendicitis.

Diagnosis

Differential diagnosis is that of an abdominal mass.

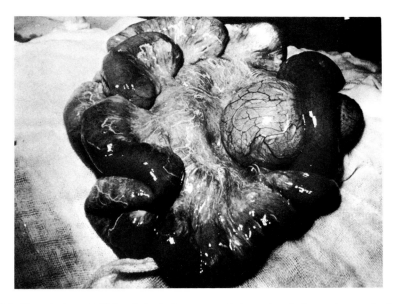

Fig. 18-1. Mesenteric cyst. This relatively large mesenteric cyst projects as a tense spherical mass from the small bowel mesentery. Chylous fluid was removed from the cyst, which had an endothelial lining.

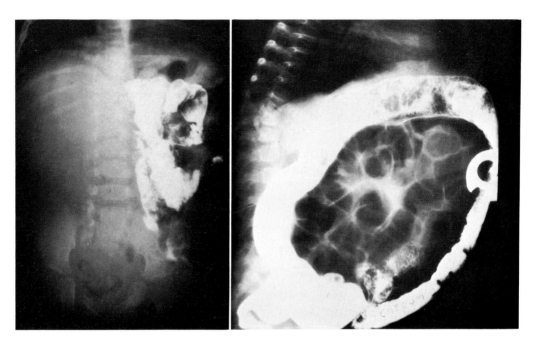

Fig. 18-2. Mesenteric cyst. A large abdominal mass displaces the colon and the distal small bowel. Framing of the mass by the colon and ileum indicates that the mass is intraperitoneal.

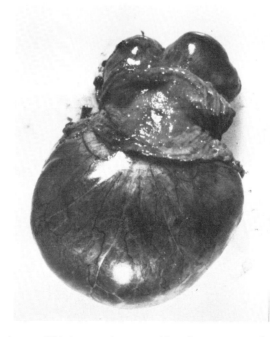

Fig. 18-3. Mesenteric cyst. This large and tense multicystic mass measuring 14.5 × 10.5 × 7.5 cm was removed along with a 10 cm segment of distal jejunum. The mass was restricting the caliber of that loop of small bowel and also of the right ureter. The 4-year-old boy had a history of chronic constipation and abdominal distention interspersed with bouts of severe abdominal pain with vomiting and diarrhea.

X-ray findings

Roentgenograms show displacement of the bowel (Fig. 18-2). The ultrasound examination identifies the cyst as a well-defined sonolucent mass. If the cyst is palpated in the right lower quadrant, it may be diagnosed preoperatively as an appendiceal abscess. Duplication of the bowel with an enteric cyst in the mesentery mimics a mesenteric cyst at exploration. An ovarian cystadenoma may also present as a mesenteric cyst.

Treatment

The cyst should be enucleated when possible. However, when the bowel wall or its vasculature is adherent to the cyst, segmental bowel resection, with wedge resection of the portion of mesentery containing the cyst, is necessary (Fig. 18-3).

REFERENCES

Caropreso, P.R.: Mesenteric cysts, Arch. Surg. **108**:242-246, 1974.

Christensen, J.A., Fuller, J.W., Hallock, J.A., and Sherman, R.T.: Mesenteric cysts, Am. Surg. **41**:352-354, 1975.

Walker, A.R., and Putnam, T.C.: Omental, mesenteric and retroperitoneal cysts, Ann. Surg. **178**:13-19, 1973.

POLYPS OF THE GASTROINTESTINAL TRACT (Table 18-1)

Juvenile polyps

Juvenile polyps are also called retention or inflammatory polyps. They are pedunculated hamartomatous excrescences with a predominance of connective tissue and inflammatory elements over the glandular component. Their stalk is covered by normal colonic mucosa, but their surface is often denuded. The glandular portion shows branching, irregular proliferation, and cystic transformation. The cystic spaces often contain abundant nuclear debris and polymorphonuclear leukocytes besides much mucus (Fig. 18-4). Juvenile polyps are always benign. Most (80%) are within reach of the sigmoidoscope, and two thirds are within the first 10 cm from the anus. Usually, juvenile polyps are solitary. A minority of patients (25%) have two to 12 polyps.

Clinical features

Juvenile polyps are rare before the age of 1 year, but their incidence increases rapidly thereafter and reaches a maximum frequency between 4 and 5 years of age. After this age, polyps become un-

common and are rare after 15 years; autoamputation and self-destruction probably account for this observation. Autoamputation is more common with low-lying polyps because of greater peristaltic force in the rectosigmoid area and contact with harder stools.

Bright red blood in the stools is almost uniformly present. The bleeding is usually intermittent and small in amount, though at times it can be quite profuse and exceptionally exsanguinating. In some cases the bleeding is occult and leads to anemia. Some juvenile polyps have long stalks, predisposing to colocolic intussusception. A more common complication is prolapse of one or more pedunculated polyps through the anus, which may cause prolapse of the rectal mucosa. Some patients complain of diarrhea and tenesmus, but this is more likely with low-lying polyps. Crampy abdominal pain is accounted by traction on the polyp during peristalic activity. Sometimes there is actual passage of identifiable material. Hypoproteinemia and digital clubbing may develop, especially if polyps of large size are present.

The occurrence of juvenile polyps in siblings is not unusual and is of no significance, since adenomatous polyps are the only ones with malignant potential.

Diagnosis

Rectal examination is most important, since more than 30% are located within 10 cm of the anal margin. Most polyps (80%) are within reach of the rectosigmoidoscope. A barium enema should be done (Fig. 18-5) if this examination is negative. Barium air-contrast studies are more helpful than the routine enema (Fig. 18-6). Colonoscopy should be done in selective cases.

Juvenile polyps are usually painless and consequently may be confused with bleeding from a Meckel's diverticulum. This entity usually affects younger children and the blood loss is greater. Since the rectal bleeding is associated with a normal stool pattern, acute or chronic inflammatory bowel diseases are unlikely causes. When pain and tenesmus are present, ulcerative colitis should be ruled out. Blood dyscrasias such as Henoch-Schönlein purpura need to be kept in mind.

Treatment

When faced with a child presenting with hematochezia, the examiner should look for other stigmas of familial adenomatous or hamartoma-

Table 18-1. Polypoid lesions of gastrointestinal tract

Disease	Disease condition	Location	Heredity	Extraintestinal manifestations	Malignancy
Juvenile polyps	Retention or in-flammatory polyp	Colon 70% solitary 80% within 25 cm of anus	None	None	None
Juvenile polypo-sis of colon	Juvenile polyp	Colon, in large numbers	Probably domi-nant	Sometimes other congenital anom-alies	None
Generalized gas-trointestinal juvenile pol-yposis	Juvenile polyp with adenomatous fea-tures	Stomach, small intestine, colon	Dominant	None	Uncommon
Cronkite-Canada syndrome	Juvenile polyp	Stomach, colon, small intestine	None	Alopecia, atrophic nails, brown macular lesions of skin	None
Peutz-Jeghers syndrome	Hamartoma	Stomach, colon, always in small intestine	Dominant	Pigmentation of lips or buccal mucosa	Uncommon (2% to 3%)
Familial ade-nomatous pol-yposis of co-lon	Adenoma	Colon	Dominant	None	Common
Gardner's syn-drome	Adenoma	Colon, sometimes in duodenum and small bowel	Dominant	Soft-tissue and bone tumors (dental abnormalities)	Common
Turcot's syn-drome	Adenoma	Colon	Recessive	Brain tumor	Unknown
Lymphoid polyp-osis (nodular lymphoid hy-perplasia)	Large aggregates of lymphoid tissue	Colon and small intestine	Unknown	None	None

tous polyps. Any polyp within reach of the rec-tosigmoidoscope should be excised for biopsy. If histology confirm that it is a juvenile polyp, noth-ing further should be done. If no lesions are found at rectosigmoidoscopy or if symptoms continue, a barium air-contrast enema should be done.

Colonoscopy under sedation can be used for di-agnosis and polypectomy in those symptomatic cases where rectosigmoidoscopic and roentgeno-graphic examinations show normal results. Al-though it is a safe and efficient procedure, our attitude has been conservative for polyps beyond the reach of the rectosigmoidoscope in cases where a low-lying juvenile polyp has been identified un-less pain or profuse bleeding are present.

Prognosis

Prognosis is excellent because juvenile polyps are never malignant. Occasionally, they may recur.

Juvenile polyposis coli

In rare families, large numbers of juvenile pol-yps may develop in the colon. The pattern of in-heritance appears to be dominant. The rectosigmoid mucosa may be studded with sessile and pe-dunculated polyps, which can be identified roent-genologically or endoscopically throughout the colon. It may cause severe protein loss and ane-mia and, in such cases, requires a proctocolec-tomy. An ileoendorectal pull-through (Soave) is

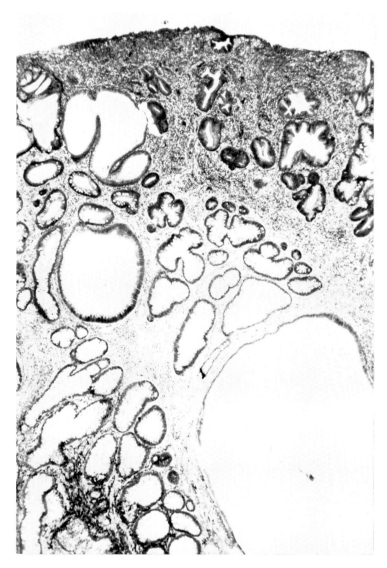

Fig. 18-4. Juvenile polyps are characterized by a surface denuded of epithelial lining and by hyperplastic and cystic glands in a stroma of connective tissue densely infiltrated by an acute and chronic inflammatory reaction.

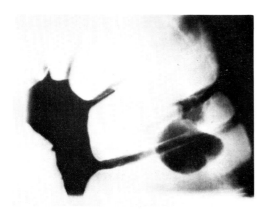

Fig. 18-5. Juvenile polyp of the colon. The stalk is attached to the wall in a pressure film of an ordinary barium enema. Such polyps can be seen only when the colon has been adequately cleansed before the enema is given.

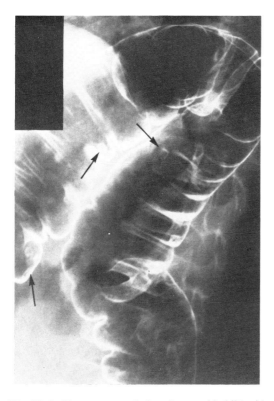

Fig. 18-6. Air-contrast study in a 5-year-old child with unexplained rectal bleeding. Three small polyps, *arrows*, are identified in the transverse and descending colon.

recommended. Some patients have associated congenital anomalies such as hydrocephalus, intestinal malrotation, and mental retardation. The syndrome may be mistaken for familial adenomatous polyposis of the colon, and there may be an increased risk of cancer.

Generalized gastrointestinal juvenile polyposis

This hereditary syndrome involves the stomach, small intestine, and colon. Myriads of typical juvenile polyps can be seen. Some polyps may have adenomatous features. In such cases the closely packed glands are embedded in a sparse stroma and the nuclei show numerous mitoses, hyperchromatic changes, and loss of basal orientation. They may account for the few cases of reported intestinal malignancies. The syndrome appears to be transmitted as a dominant genotype with variable, age-dependent expressivity.

Children affected with this syndrome present with rectal prolapse, bloody diarrhea, anemia, hypoalbuminemia, edema malnutrition, and bouts of abdominal pain secondary to repeated episodes of intussusception. The extensive distribution of lesions makes surgical intervention impossible except for treatment of intussusception and obstruction. In two cases with polyposis limited to the stomach, a subtotal gastric resection was successful in bringing about relief of the anemia and of the protein-losing enteropathy. In contrast to the Peutz-Jeghers syndrome, the polyps do not contain fibromuscular elements, and there is no mucocutaneous melanin pigmentation.

Cronkite-Canada syndrome

A variant of generalized juvenile polyposis has been described by Cronkite and Canada. There are few reports in infants and children of this serious disease giving rise to severe diarrhea, hypokalemia, steatorrhea, and protein-losing enteropathy. The gastric mucosa may resemble that seen in Ménétrier's disease. Extraintestinal manifestations are impressive and characterized by alopecia, nail dystrophy, and brown macular hyperpigmentation of the skin.

Peutz-Jeghers syndrome

The polyps in Peutz-Jeghers syndrome are hamartomas. They are composed of normal epithelium arranged on a branching stroma made up of smooth muscle fibers derived from the tunica muscularis mucosae. The epithelial elements are

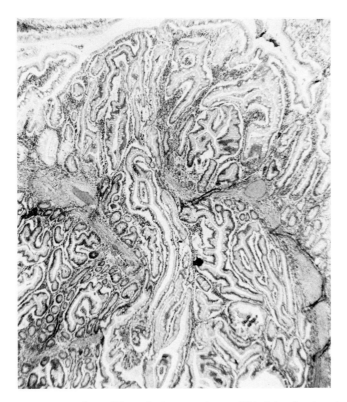

Fig. 18-7. Hamartomatous polyp of Peutz-Jeghers syndrome. This jejunal polyp shows an arborizing fibromuscular stroma and well-differentiated glandular elements.

related to the smooth muscle in the same manner as they are seen in the normal mucosa (Fig. 18-7). The polyps may occur anywhere betweeen the cardiac sphincter and the anus but are regularly present in the small intestine. Although colonic polyps are present in less than 30% of cases, there are indications that they are more frequent in infants and in young children than in adults. The syndrome is inherited through a mendelian dominant gene. Other members of the family are affected in 45% of the cases, either partially (pigmentation or polyps) or completely.

Clinical features

More than 300 cases of Peutz-Jeghers syndrome have been reported. The diagnosis is made before the age of 15 in a third of the cases.

The presence of mucosal pigmentation establishes the diagnosis and usually appears at birth or in infancy. The lips and buccal mucosa are generally involved (Fig. 18-8), as well as the digits. The pigmentation has a tendency to lessen at puberty.

The most common symptom pertaining to the polyposis is recurrent attacks of severe colicky pain, which is attributed to transient intussusception (Fig. 18-9). Vomiting, bleeding, intestinal obstruction, peritonitis are caused by ulceration and infarction of the polyps, which are the leadpoints of intussusception. It is important to note that rectal prolapse and colocolic intussusception may be the mode of presentation in infancy.

Treatment

In unusual instances in which the polyps seem to be fairly well localized to a short segment of intestine, segmental resection should be successful. With the extensive polyposis generally seen, multiple enterotomies will be required throughout the life of most patients. Attempts should be directed to the removal of the larger polyps, which are more likely to be responsible for the symptoms.

Two cases of carcinoma have been reported in pediatric patients, and a few have been reported in adults. In the majority of cases, the malignancies did not appear to be related to the polyps.

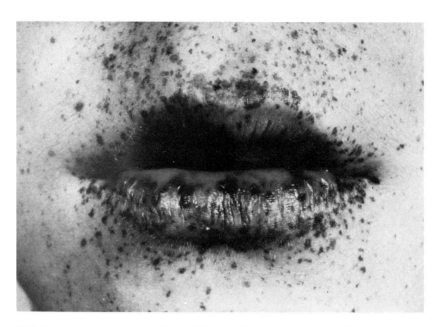

Fig. 18-8. Mucocutaneous pigmentation of Peutz-Jeghers syndrome. A striking increase of melanin deposits is seen on the lips and peribuccal area of this 14½-year-old boy, who suffered repeated bouts of intussusception.

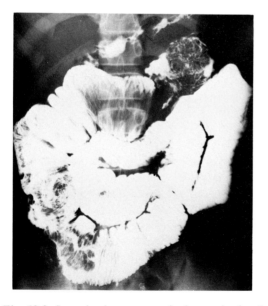

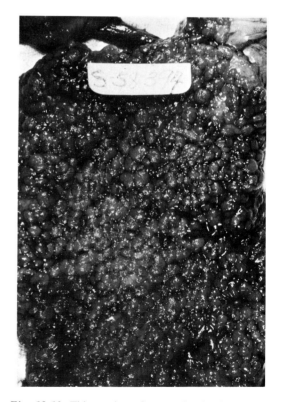

Fig. 18-9. Several polyps are seen in the proximal and distal jejunum of this patient with Peutz-Jeghers syndrome. In these areas, the intestine is dilated and the hamartomas were the lead points for transient intussusception, which developed during the examination. Note the coiled spring appearance in the proximal jejunum.

Fig. 18-10. This portion of resected colon is carpeted with myriads of adenomatous polyps so dense that there is hardly any normal bowel mucosa identifiable between them. The polyps seen here are small mucosal elevations. With time, they can become sessile and then pedunculated.

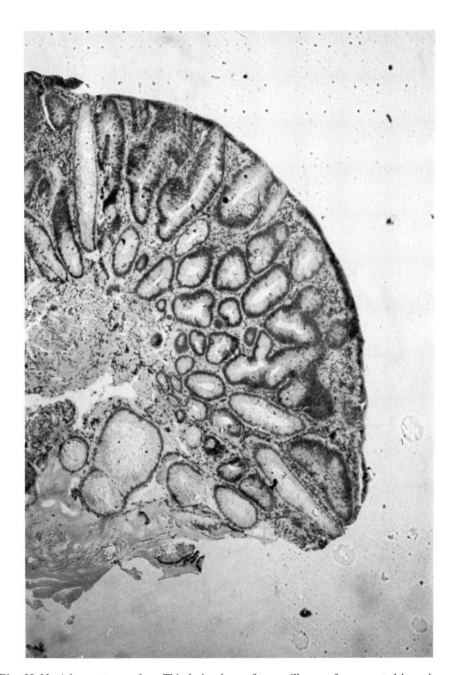

Fig. 18-11. Adenomatous polyp. This lesion has a fine papillary surface carpeted by columnar cells; the crypts are well aligned. The small amount of stroma present is free of inflammation and separates closely packed tubules made up of dense, proliferating epithelium with prominent mitoses. In contrast to the juvenile polyp, cystic changes and inflammation are absent.

Familial adenomatous polyposis of colon

This condition is characterized by the presence in the colon of a large number (300 to 3000) of adenomatous polyps (Fig. 18-10) varying in size from mucosal excrescences to large-stalked polyps (Fig. 18-11). In a few families duodenal adenomas have been reported. A family history of the condition is obtained in roughly two thirds of cases, and the entity is transmitted genetically as a dominant. Each child of a parent with polyposis has a 50:50 chance of developing the disease. About 20% of cases are sporadic. Carcinoma of the colon usually develops before 40 years of age. Information about the time it takes for cancer to develop has been documented (Table 18-2).

Clinical features

The disease has occurred in infants but is more likely to become symptomatic during the late teens. Diarrhea is usually the first symptom; blood loss, anemia, and abdominal pain usually supervene. However, many patients with severe polyposis remain asymptomatic.

Colonoscopic examination will show polyps of various sizes that carpet the colon. Barium enema shows a normal bowel wall with many filling defects (Fig. 18-12).

Treatment

All members of the family should be carefully examined. Because of the natural history of the adenoma-carcinoma sequence, children of an affected parent need not be reexamined by colonoscopy more frequently than every 3 years. A cancer is sometimes present at the time of initial surgery, and in many cases multiple cancers are found. In a series of patients less than 13 years old, cancer was already present in 6%. Subtotal colectomy has been recommended; however, many authors believe that the social advantage of keeping the rectal stump is dangerous, since a carcinoma may develop despite frequent inspection of the stump and fulguration of adenomas. Proctocolectomy with ileostomy, or colectomy with an ileoendorectal pull-through, is the treatment of choice, since any individual who has familial polyposis left untreated will eventually develop carcinoma of the colon. Genetic counseling is essential.

Gardner's syndrome

Gardner's syndrome is a dominantly inherited condition characterized by soft tissue and bone tumors associated with multiple adenomatous intestinal polyps predisposed to malignancy (Fig. 18-

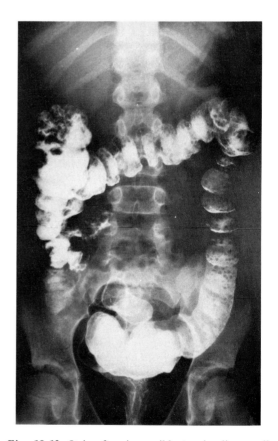

Fig. 18-12. It is often impossible to visualize small polyps when the colon is distended with barium. Postevacuation films and air-contrast films are more informative. Scores of polyps are identifiable in this film by a fine coat of barium adherent to the periphery of the lesions and casting ring shadows of increased density.

Table 18-2. Familial polyposis: length of precancerous phase

Period	Number of cases	Percentage developing cancer
0-5	59	11.9
5-10	29	25.6
10-15	13	31.6
15-20	4	55.6
>20	—	100

Data from Morson, B.C.: Clin. Gastroenterol. **5:**505-525, 1976.

13).Various dental abnormalities have been reported, as well as desmoid tumors and malignancies in sites other than the colon and the duodenum.

The soft-tissue manifestations include epidermoid inclusion cysts, lipomas, fibromas, and epidermoid cysts. The bone tumors (osteomas) usually involve the mandible and sometimes affect other facial bones, the skull, and, occasionally, long bones. The simultaneous occurrence of adenomatous and lymphoid polyposis has been described in a few families. Intestinal symptoms are identical to those described with adenomatous polyposis of the colon. Intestinal polyps, however, are not limited to the colon and may involve the small bowel and the duodenum. Patients with Gardner's syndrome have the same risk of developing colorectal carcinomas as patients with familial adenomatous polyposis of the colon. A review of 83 cases has, in fact, reported malignancy in 50%.

The complete triad of soft-tissue tumors, bone tumors, and intestinal polyps rarely occurs in the first 20 years of life. In fact, soft-tissue tumor is usually the initial manifestation in the first 10 years of life, and bone tumor likely becomes apparent in the second decade. All members of an affected family should be thoroughly examined periodically. A person beyond 40 years of age with no signs of the syndrome is very likely free from the defective gene. Since management is aimed at preventing adenocarcinoma of the bowel, the same aggressive surgical approach as in familial adenomatous polyposis of the colon is indicated.

Detection of adenomas by colonoscopy is recommended before 10 years of age in children of

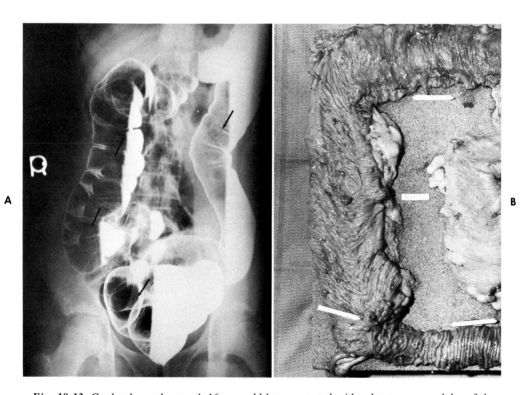

Fig. 18-13. Gardner's syndrome. A 16-year-old boy presented with subcutaneous nodules of the face and scalp but had no gastrointestinal symptoms. An osteoma of the left mandible was found. His father had Gardner's syndrome and died of an adenocarcinoma of the duodenum. **A,** Multiple polyps of various sizes are demonstrated by an air-contrast study of the colon. **B,** On the surgical specimen a number of mucosal polypoid lesions projecting into the lumen of the resected colon are seen. The ones identified in the resected segment of ileum are more discrete and consist of aggregation of lymphoid nodules (nodular lymphoid hyperplasia). Microscopically, the colonic polyps were benign but had the histologic characteristics of adenomatous polyps. (From Duncan, B.R., Dohner, V.A., and Priest, J.H.: J. Pediatr. **72:**497-505, 1968.)

an affected parent or as soon as rectal bleeding or extracolonic manifestations become apparent.

Lymphoid polyposis (nodular lymphoid hyperplasia of colon and rectum)

Microscopic collections of lymphocytes are normal findings in the mucosa and submucosa of the gastrointestinal tract. They may become visible to the naked eye as 1 to 4 mm nodules (follicular hyperplasia). In other situations, their size will be greater than 5 mm and will impart a cobblestone appearance to the intestinal mucosa (nodular lymphoid hyperplasia). Aggregation of lymphoid follicles, known as Peyer's patches, will normally give rise to submucosal nodules in the ileum of children. The roentgenographic findings may be mistaken for Crohn's ileitis or a lymphoma. A pseudolymphoma that presented as a cecal tumor with intussusception was described in a 7-year-old child.

Nodular lymphoid hyperplasia in both the small and the large intestine has been seen in a variety of clinical settings. When it is limited to the small bowel, it may be associated with certain immunoglobulin deficiencies, namely, acquired hypogammaglobulinemia and isolated IgA deficiency. Since, in these two conditions, giardiasis is often present, the relationship between nodular lymphoid hyperplasia and *Giardia lamblia* has been examined. Treatment of the infestation does not bring about a change of the nodular lymphoid hyperplasia. (See also Chapters 12 and 16.)

When limited to the colon, the lesions may be diffuse and involve the entire colon (Fig. 18-14) or may affect only the rectum. Lymphoid polyps have been reported in association with adenomatous polyps in familial adenomatous polyposis and in Gardner's syndrome.

The macroscopic appearance is that of firm, round, submucosal nodules, with smooth or lobulated surfaces. Microscopically these submucosal nodules are made up of lymphoid follicles that distort the normal mucosal architecture. They are composed of mature lymphocytes and a few reticulum cells with or without germinal centers (Fig. 18-15). The lesions may easily be mistaken for those of familial polyposis, ulcerative colitis, lymphosarcoma, or Hodgkin's disease.

Rectal bleeding, nonspecific crampy pain, and diarrhea may occur. Lymphoid polyps can be the lead point for an intussusception. The association between lymphoid polyposis and the presence of

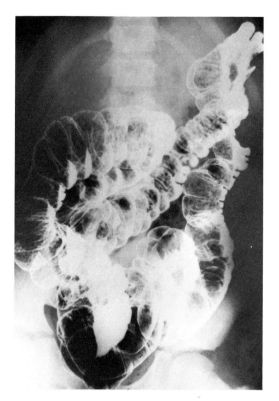

Fig. 18-14. Lymphoid polyposis of the colon. An 11-year-old boy presented with a 5-day history of colicky pain and diarrhea with mucus and blood. Symptoms continued for another week and subsequently disappeared, except for intermittent abdominal pain and loose stools associated with an infection of the upper respiratory tract. Immunoglobulins were normal. There was no family history of polyposis. The barium enema shows a myriad of small polypoid mucosal elevations through the entire colon.

any symptoms has been challenged in both adults and children. Roentgenological and autopsy findings have failed to establish a relationship between the presence of nodular lymphoid hyperplasia and symptoms. It could represent a temporary response to infection (viral) or to an immune aggression. It has been described as occurring after necrotizing enterocolitis, in Hirschsprung's disease complicated by colitis, and in the course of chronic inflammatory bowel disease (Crohn's disease, ulcerative colitis). At endoscopy, the rectal mucosa shows centrally umbilicated protrusions accounted for by the submucosal lymphoid nodules. The rest of the mucosa may be somewhat granular and friable, but there is never any evidence of inflammation or ulceration. Regres-

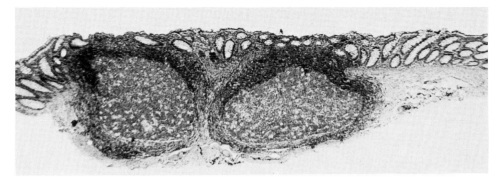

Fig. 18-15. Nodular lymphoid hyperplasia of the colon. Two large lymphoid follicles are seen in the rectal biopsy specimen of a patient with abdominal pain and rectal bleeding. At endoscopy, fine mucosal excrescences were noted. Both follicles occupy a large area in the mucosa and submucosa. The periphery of the follicle on the left is distorting the normal architecture. Crypts and epithelial lining cannot be identified in that area.

sion of symptoms and signs occurs spontaneously. The peak incidence is from 1 to 3 years, with an actual range of 6 months to puberty.

Villous adenoma

In children, the commonest polypoid lesions are juvenile polyps (90%) followed by the lymphoid, Peutz-Jeghers syndrome, and adenomas. The villous adenoma is the rarest. It is a broad-based sessile lesion composed of thickened mucosa disposed in a papillary pattern and lying in a scanty stroma. Nuclear atypia is present, and mucus production is abundant. Mucus diarrhea, fluid and electrolyte depletion, and hypoalbuminemia and rectal bleeding are the usual manifestations. It is a precancerous lesion usually localized in the rectum. Surgical removal should include a margin of normal mucosa.

REFERENCES

Bussey, H.J.R., Veale, A.M.O., and Morson, B.C.: Genetics of gastrointestinal polyposis, Gastroenterology **74:**1325-1330, 1978.

Cameron, G.S., and Lau, G.Y.P.: Juvenile polyposis coli: a case treated with ileoendorectal pullthrough, J. Pediatr. Surg. **14:**536-537, 1979.

Capitanio, M.A., and Kirkpatrick, J.A.: Lymphoid hyperplasia of the colon in children, Radiology **94:**323-327, 1970.

Daum F., Zucker, P., Boley, S.J., and Bernstein, L.H.: Colonoscopic polypectomy in children, Am. J. Dis. Child. **131:**566-567, 1977.

Douglas, J.R., Campbell, C.A., Salisbury, D.M., and others: Colonoscopic polypectomy in children, Br. Med. J. **281:**1386-1387, 1980.

Dozois, R.R., Judd, E.S., Dahlin, D.C., and others: The Peutz-Jeghers syndrome: is there a predisposition to the development of intestinal malignancy? Arch. Surg. **98:**509-517, 1969.

Duncan, B.R., Dohmer, V.A., and Priest, J.H.: The Gardner syndrome: need for early diagnosis, J. Pediatr. **72:**497-505, 1968.

Erbe, R.W.: Current concepts in genetics: inherited gastrointestinal polyposis syndromes, N. Engl. J. Med. **294:**1101-1104, 1976.

Franken, E.A.: Lymphoid hyperplasia of the colon, Radiology **94:**329-334, 1970.

Giltman, L., Cohn, B., and Minkowitz, S.: Pseudolymphoma presenting as a cecal tumor, J. Pediatr. Surg. **11:**565-568, 1976.

Grotsky, H.W., Rickert, R.R., Smith, W.D., and Newsome, J.F.: Familial juvenile polyposis coli, Gastroenterology **82:**494-501, 1982.

Howell, J., Pringle, K., Kirschner, B., and Burrington, J.D.: Peutz-Jeghers polyps causing colocolic intussusception in infancy, J. Pediatr. Surg. **16:**82-84, 1981.

Ippolito, J.R., and Touloukian, R.J.: Colocolic intussusception in an older child, Clin. Pediatr. **17:**720-726, 1978.

Louw, J.H.: Polypoid lesions of the large bowel in children with particular reference to benign lymphoid polyposis, J. Pediatr. Surg. **3:**195-209, 1968.

Mazier, W.P., Bowman, H.E., Sun, K.M., and others: Juvenile polyps of the colon and rectum, Dis. Colon Rectum **17:**523-527, 1974.

McKittrick, J.E., Lewis, W.M., Doane, W.A., and others: The Peutz-Jeghers syndrome, Arch. Surg. **103:**57-62, 1971.

Middleton, P., and Ferguson, W.: Exsanguinating uncontrollable lower GI hemorrhage due to juvenile polyposis coli: report of a case, Dis. Colon Rectum **20:**690-694, 1977.

Morson, B.C.: Genesis of colorectal cancer, Clin. Gastroenterol. **5:**505-525, 1976.

Naylor, E.W., and Lebenthal, E.: Early detection of adenomatous polyposis coli in Gardner's syndrome, Pediatrics **63:**222-227, 1979.

Neitzschman, H.R., Genet, E., and Nice, C.M.: Two cases of familial polyposis simulating lymphoid hyperplasia, Am. J. Roentgenol. Radium Ther. Nucl. Med. **119:**365-368, 1973.

Ranchod, M., Lewin, K.J., and Dorfman, R.F.: Lymphoid hyperplasia of the gastrointestinal tract, Am. J. Surg. Pathol. **2:**383-400, 1978.

Ruymann, F.B.: Juvenile polyps with cachexia: report of an infant and comparison with Cronkite-Canada syndrome in adults, Gastroenterology **57**:431-438, 1969.

Sachatello, C.R., Pickren, J.W., and Grace, J.T., Jr.: Generalized juvenile gastrointestinal polyposis, Gastroenterology **58**:699-708, 1970.

Schaupp, W.C., and Volpe, P.A.: Management of diffuse colonic polyposis, Am. J. Surg. **124**:218-222, 1972.

Shaw, E.B., and Hennigar, G.R.: Intestinal lymphoid polyposis, Am. J. Clin. Pathol. **61**:417-422, 1974.

Sheahan, D.G., Martin, F. Baginsky, S., and others: Multiple lymphomatous polyposis of the gastrointestinal tract, Cancer **28**:408-425, 1971.

Simpson, J.S., Mancer, J.F.K., and Adeyemi, S.D.: Villous adenoma of the rectum: a rare tumor in childhood, J. Pediatr. Surg. **13**:513-516, 1978.

Toccalino, H. Guastavino, E., De Pinni, F., and others: Juvenile polyps of the rectum and colon, Acta Paediatr. Scand. **62**:337-340, 1973.

Utsunomiya, J., Gocho, H., Miyanaga, T., and others: Peutz-Jeghers syndrome: its natural course and management, Johns Hopkins Med. J. **136**:71-82, 1975.

Velcek, F.T., Coopersmith, I.S., Chen, C.K., and others: Familial juvenile adenomatous polyposis, J. Pediatr. Surg. **11**:781-787, 1976.

Watanabe, A., Nagashima, H., Makoto, M., and Ogawa, K.: Familial juvenile polyposis of the stomach, Gastroenterology **77**:148-151, 1979.

Watne, A.L., Johnson, J.G., and Chang, C.H.: The challenge of Gardner's syndrome, CA **19**:275-286, 1969.

Wenzl, J.E., Bartholomew, L.G., Hallenbeck, G.A., and Strickler, G.B.: Gastrointestinal polyposis with mucocutaneous pigmentation in children, Pediatrics **28**:655-661, 1961.

TUMORS OF THE GASTROINTESTIONAL TRACT AND OF APUD CELLS
Gastric tumors

Neoplasms of the stomach are relatively rare in the pediatric age group. A total of 46 cases of gastric teratomas, most of them during the first year of life and all, except one in boys, have been reported. Abdominal distention, bleeding, and a palpable mass are the usual symptoms. Full recovery after surgery can be expected.

Smooth muscle tumors occur during childhood and adolescence. Hematemesis and melena are the usual symptoms. Roentgenographic examination reveals either a polypoid or an ulcer type of lesion. Malignant lesions (leiomyosarcoma) are somewhat more common than the benign 5 to 6 cm sized leiomyomas. Because differential diagnosis of the two lesions is difficult to make, a subtotal gastrectomy is recommended. The place of chemotherapy and of radiotherapy is still de-

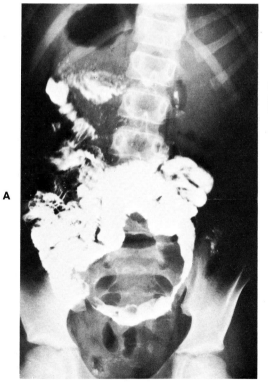

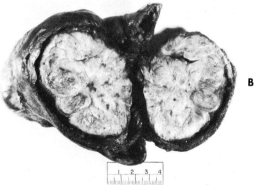

Fig. 18-16. Lymphosarcoma of the small bowel. A 9-year-old girl suffered intermittent abdominal pain for 1 month but had no loss of weight, fever, or anemia. A mobile midline mass was palpable in the lower abdomen. **A,** Roentgenogram shows rigidity and narrowing of a loop of ileum. The differential diagnosis was ileal duplication, but the confusion was settled by surgery. **B,** Surgical specimen shows a large intramural mass of rubbery consistency. The cut surface is relatively pale and assumes a distinct pattern of individual large nodules separated by dense connective tissue.

batable. The prognosis is relatively good. Carcinoma of the stomach is rare.

REFERENCES

Hale, H.W., and Mallo, J.P.: Carcinoma of the stomach in the young, Ann. Surg. **147:**553-557, 1958.

Matias, J.C., and Huang, Y.C.: Gastric teratoma in infancy: report of a case and review of world literature, Ann. Surg. **178:**631, 1973.

Purvis, J.M., Miller, R.C., and Blumenthal, B.I.: Gastric teratoma: first reported case in a female, J. Pediatr. Surg. **14:**86-87, 1979.

Wurlitzer, F.P., Mares, A.J., Isaacs, H., and others: Smooth muscle tumors of the stomach in childhood and adolescence, J. Pediatr. Surg. **8:**421-427, 1973.

Lymphoma of the small intestine

Although there are reports of leiomyoma, leiomyosarcoma, and adenocarcinoma in pediatric patients, most tumors of the small intestine are lymphomas.

There are no reports of gastric lymphomas in children. In children, the ileocecal region is most commonly involved. Abdominal pain, malaise, fatigue, anemia, and diarrhea are the usual symptoms (Fig. 18-16, *A*). A celiac-like picture may be present. Lymphosarcoma is the most frequent lead point for intussusception in children over 6 years of age (p. 109). The tumor arises from the lymphoid tissue of the lamina propria and extends laterally along the submucosal layer (Fig. 18-16, *B*). It may present as a polypoid tumor or may diffusely infiltrate, causing loss of peristalsis and rigidity of the involved segment (Fig. 18-17). In other cases, symptoms of obstruction are produced, since there is a circumferential infiltration of the bowel wall. Prognosis is generally very poor, but patients without lymph node involvement at the time of surgery may do well after combined radiation and chemotherapy. Intraperitoneal lymphosarcoma may compress and invade the bowel wall (Fig. 18-18).

An important association has been established between lymphoma and gluten enteropathy. There is no doubt that the risk of malignant disease in adults with celiac sprue is much greater than in the general population. In close to 60% of those developing a malignancy, the gastrointestinal tract is involved, and lymphomas are diagnosed in almost one third of these tumors. Strict adherence

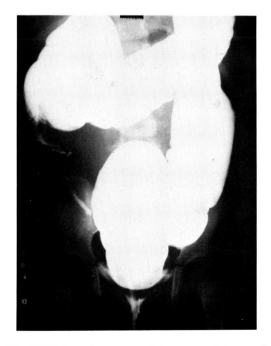

Fig. 18-17. Lymphosarcoma of the cecum. A large soft tissue mass has obliterated most of the cecum, part of the appendix, and the terminal ileum. This is the most common neoplastic lesion of the bowel in pediatric patients.

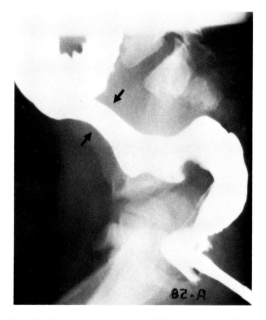

Fig. 18-18. Lymphosarcoma of the rectosigmoid. Extensive circumferential compression of the rectosigmoid causes rigid, pipelike intestinal walls, *arrows*. A tumor mass filled the entire pelvis; the rectosigmoid mesentery was diffusely infiltrated and nodular.

to a gluten-free diet does not seem to reduce the incidence of malignancies (Chapter 10).

REFERENCES

Cooper, B.T., Holmes, G.K.T., and Cooke, W.T.: Intestinal lymphoma associated with malabsorption, Lancet **1**:387-418, 1978.

Freeman, J.: Leiomyoma of small bowel: a case report, J. Pediatr. Surg. **14**:477-478, 1979.

Isaacson, P., and Wright, D.H.: Intestinal lymphoma associated with malabsorption, Lancet **1**:67-70, 1978.

Loehr. W.J., Mujahed, Z., Zahn, F.D., and others: Primary lymphoma of the G.I. tract: a review of 100 cases, Ann. Surg. **170**:232-238, 1969.

Mestel, D.L.: Lymphosarcoma of small intestine in infancy and childhood, Am. Surg. **149**:87-89, 1959.

Wayne, E.R., Campbell, J.B., Koloske, A.M., and Burrington, J.D.: Intussusception in the older child-suspect lymphosarcoma, J. Pediatr. Surg. **11**:789-794, 1976.

Adenocarcinoma and sarcoma of colon and rectum

Although malignant tumor is second only to trauma as a cause of death in the second decade of life, most of the neoplasms encountered are sarcomas, lymphomas, leukemias, and brain tumors. Epithelial neoplasms make up only a small portion of the total. Adenocarcinoma of the colon and rectum is rare during childhood and adolescence. Cases have been reported in the first 3 years of life, but the majority of patients are 10 years of age or older. Boys are more often affected than girls (2 to 1).

Abdominal pain, the usual presenting complaint, is frequently associated with a change of defecation habits and weight loss. Rectal bleeding is somewhat less frequent, but a certain number of patients presenting with this symptom have been erroneously diagnosed as having polyps or hemorrhoidal disease. An abdominal mass may be palpated in more than 50% of cases. The transverse colon and rectosigmoid are the two most frequently affected sites. Few patients having the disease survive for 5 years. The poor prognosis probably relates to the nonspecificity of presenting complaints and more importantly to the large percentage (50%) of these lesions, which are undifferentiated mucin-producing adenocarcinomas.

Certain children have a much greater risk of developing colon cancer, but statistics show that those with familial polyposis, ulcerative colitis, or Crohn's disease very seldom develop a cancer before the age of 20 years. However, we have seen two teenagers who developed malignancies within 5 years of onset of ulcerative colitis. Nevertheless, most cases of colonic and rectal carcinomas develop in a previously normal colon. Since about one third are within reach of the rectosigmoidoscope, endoscopic examinations and barium enemas *must be used more liberally* in examining children with unexplained chronic abdominal pain, abnormal bowel habits, or rectal bleeding.

Smooth muscle tumors of the gastrointestinal tract are rare. Two newborns with intestinal obstruction secondary to a perforation and intussusception have been described. Both had a leiomyosarcoma of the colon that after surgery did not recur.

REFERENCES

Andersson, A., and Bergdahl, L.: Carcinoma of the colon in children: a report of six new cases and a review of the literature, J. Pediatr. Surg. **11**:967-971, 1976.

Caffarena, P.E., Dodero, P., Magillo, P., and Soave, F.: Adenocarcinoma of the rectosigmoid colon in a 10 year old child, J. Pediatr. Surg. **16**:87-89, 1976.

Devroede, G., and Taylor, W.: On calculating cancer risk and survival of ulcerative colitis patients with the life table method, Gastroenterology **71**:505-509, 1976.

Devroede, G.J., Taylor, W.F., Sauer, W.G., and others: Cancer risk and life expectancy of children with ulcerative colitis, N. Engl. J. Med. **285**:17-21, 1971.

Ein, S.H., Beck, A.R., and Allen, J.E.: Colon sarcoma in the newborn, J. Pediatr. Surg. **14**:455-457, 1979.

Golden, G.T., Rosenthal, J.D., and Shaw, A.: Carcinoma of the rectum in adolescence, Am. J. Dis. Child. **129**:742-743, 1975.

Recalde, M., Holyoke, E.D., and Elias, E.G.: Carcinoma of the colon, rectum and anal canal in young patients, Surg. Gynecol. Obstet. **139**:909-913, 1974.

Weedon, D.D., Shorter, R.G., Illstrup, D.M., and others: Crohn's disease and cancer, N. Engl. J. Med. **289**:1100-1103, 1973.

Wennstrom, S., Pierce, E.R., and McKusick, V.A.: Hereditary benign and malignant lesions of the large bowel, Cancer **34**:850-857, 1974.

Tumors of APUD cells
APUD cell system

Unlike that in other endocrine tissues, the APUD (amine content, precursor uptake, and decarboxylation) of the gastrointestinal tract, are not clustered in small discrete organs. Instead, they form a diffuse endocrine system in the mucosa of the stomach, small intestine, and colon, as well as in the pancreas. These cells, derived from the neural crest and responsible for the production of a variety of polypeptide hormones and biogenic amines,

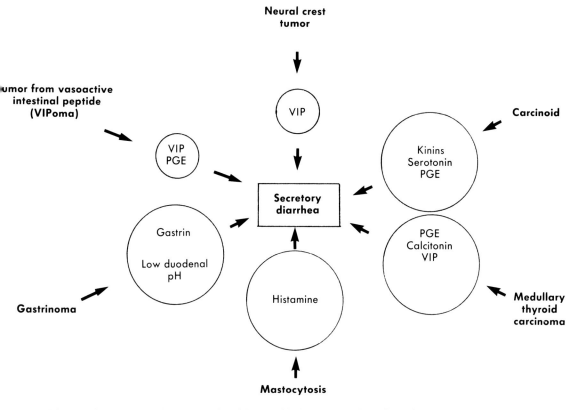

Fig. 18-19. Secretory diarrhea mediated by peptide hormones, biogenic amines, and prostaglandins (PGE). Somatostatinomas have not been included because they have not been described in the pediatric age group.

are also prominent in the brain and in the adrenal medulla, paraganglia, thyroid, skin, and respiratory and urogenital tracts, among other areas. The cells have different functions according to their location and have a spectrum of activity ranging from a neurotransmitter to a true hormonal function. Some products of bioamine- or peptide-producing cells are more closely involved with nerve fibers and myenteric plexuses and are secreted into a synapse (neurocrine) or into the bloodstream (neuroendocrine). Others have a hormonal action and are secreted into the bloodstream (endocrine) or else have a local effect on neighboring cells (paracrine). Disorders of the APUD cell system are frequently responsible for secretory watery diarrhea (Fig. 18-19). Some gut endocrine cells have contact with the lumen of a mucosal gland through microvilli (Fig. 18-20). Their secretory products are stored in granules. Each kind of cell has typical secretory granules producing specific peptides and biogenic amines such as serotonin, histamine, catecholamines, and kinins.

APUD cell tumors of gastrointestinal tract

Carcinoids. Over 90% of carcinoid tumors originate from APUD cells in the gastrointestinal tract. The most frequent sites are the appendix, terminal ileum, and rectum. These tumors display rather consistent morphologic patterns, but the "carcinoid syndrome" is usually associated with the ones involving the ileum.

The spectrum of signs and symptoms of the carcinoid syndrome is quite large and includes diarrhea, crampy abdominal pain, borborygmi, intermittent flushing, telangiectasia, hepatomegaly, asthma-like attacks, and evidence of cardiac valvular lesions. Normally chromaffin cells will convert less than 1% of ingested tryptophan to 5-hydroxytryptamine (serotonin) and subsequently to 5-hydroxyindoleacetic acid (5-HIAA). A large mass

LUMEN

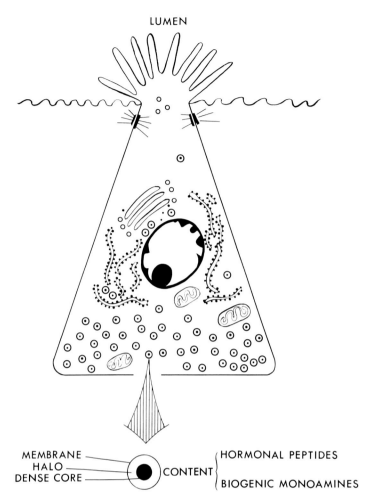

MEMBRANE	CONTENT {	HORMONAL PEPTIDES
HALO		
DENSE CORE		BIOGENIC MONOAMINES

Fig. 18-20. Main features of an APUD (amine precursor uptake and decarboxylation) cell. The apical aspect of the cell is in contrast with the lumen of an intestinal gland through its microvilli. Other cells such as those from oxyntic glands of the stomach are of the closed type and have little contact with the lumen. The secretory granules shown are most numerous around and below the nucleus (Redrawn from Larsson, L.-I.: Scand. J. Gastroenterol. **14**(suppl. 53):1, 1977.)

of tumor cells will convert more than 50% of tryptophan to serotonin, which accounts for most of the symptoms. Nonargentaffin carcinoids are not related to the enterochromaffin cell system, and therefore do not lead to high levels of 5-HIAA. Gastrinomas of the stomach, duodenum, and pancreas fall in this category. Similarly, "hindgut" carcinoids are of the nonargentaffin type and therefore will not produce large amounts of 5-HIAA and will not give rise to the carcinoid syndrome. Histamine may be high, especially in gastric carcinoids. Catecholamines, kinins, prostaglandins, enteroglucagon, and substance P can be found in large amounts in midgut carcinoids, which are generally multihormonal.

The primary tumor is often small (2 to 3 cm), even when metastases are present. In general, both the primary and the secondary tumors tend to progress slowly. An upper gastrointestinal series may reveal a polypoid lesion; sometimes the lesions are multiple and will give rise to a stricture. A liver scan and selective arteriogram may be helpful, but the information obtained by CT scanning is more reliable. The excretion of large amounts (60 to 1000 mg/24 hr) of 5-HIAA ($N <$ 30 mg/24 hr) occurs only in the presence of a metastatic carcinoid. Most carcinoids in the pediatric age group involve the appendix (Fig. 18-21). They are of low-grade malignancy, and they present as acute appendicitis. The prognosis is excel-

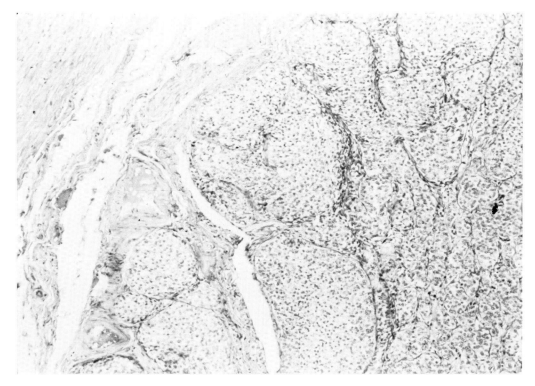

Fig. 18-21. Carcinoid tumor of the appendix in a 6-year-old child. The tumor is lobulated and forms well-identified nests and cords of relatively uniform cells embedded in a rather dense stroma.

lent, despite extension of the tumor through the muscularis mucosae and lymphatics. No recurrences are reported after appendectomy alone.

Three cases of rectal involvement have been reported: all presented with rectal bleeding. They have not been associated with the carcinoid syndrome. Only one case of colonic involvement is known in the pediatric age group. It metastasized to the liver but did not give rise to the carcinoid syndrome; 5-HIAA levels were normal.

Gastrinomas. Although most gastrinomas are found in the head or tail of the pancreas, they can be at times identified in the stomach and duodenum. A short discussion of gastrinomas can also be found in this chapter in the section on functioning pancreatic tumors. A description of the Zollinger-Ellison syndrome is given in Chapter 7.

Extraintestinal APUD cell tumors

Pancreatic endocrine tumors. The endocrine pancreas is an important site for APUD cell tumors, which originate from islet cells. Some are associated with beta cells (insulinoma) or with al-

pha cells (glucagonoma) or from one or several nonbeta and nonalpha cell types now identified by their secretory products. A discussion of pancreatic endocrine tumors is found in the last section of this chapter.

Neural crest tumors. Neural crest tumors account for 8% of pediatric malignant tumors. Ganglioneuromas and ganglioneuroblastomas produce and store large amounts of biogenic amines (catecholamines) and peptides (vasoactive intestinal peptide, VIP) but only 8% to 10% of these patients have diarrhea. Catecholamines and metabolites, such as vanillylmandelic acid (VMA), which are excreted in large amounts in the urine, are not believed to be responsible for the watery diarrhea, hypokalemia, and abdominal distention. These patients may have only hypertension, flushing, and fever.

High plasma and tumor levels of VIP have been described in about 50 patients, 8 of them children. VIP stimulates adenylate cyclase, increases cAMP, and induces electrolyte secretion. It is believed to be the hormonal mediator of pancreatic cholera (WDHA syndrome). Severe unexplained *w*atery *d*iarrhea, *h*ypokalemia, and *a*chlorhydria (hypochlorhydria or normochlorhydria) should prompt a search for a VIP-secreting tumor by a thorough physical examination (Fig. 18-13) and determination of urinary VMA.

Multiple endocrine neoplasia (MEN) syndromes

MEN type 1 (Wermer's syndrome). The MEN type 1 syndrome is inherited as an autosomal dominant. It involves most commonly, the pancreas, parathyroids, pituitary, and adrenals. Thyroid nodules, carcinoids, and neurofibromatosis are also described. The Zollinger-Ellison syndrome is a well-known gastroenterologic presentation of this syndrome. About 30% of adults with Zollinger-Ellison syndrome have in fact MEN type 1. However, this association has not yet been reported in children.

MEN type 2a (Sipple's syndrome). MEN type 2a syndrome is inherited as an autosomal dominant trait and is characterized by the concurrence of medullary thyroid carcinoma, pheochromocytoma, and parathyroid hyperplasia. Although calcitonin and prostaglandins secreted by the medullary thyroid are largely responsible for the "en-docrine diarrhea," high concentrations of VIP have been found in a few cases. In patients with a pheochromocytoma, catecholamines have also been implicated.

MEN type 2b. It is only recently that the combined clinical anomalies of MEN type 2b syndrome and their common neuroectodermal origin have been recognized. A familial pattern is described. These children have the manifestations of type 2a except for parathyroid adenomas. In addition there are skeletal abnormalities, typical facial features, mucosal neuromas on the tongue and diffuse ganglioneuromatosis. Defective peristalsis, perhaps secondary to intestinal ganglioneuromatosis, accounts for the chronic constipation interspersed with bouts of intestinal obstruction, which may lead to surgery. More studies will be needed to determine what role APUD cells could play on the genesis of diffuse hyperplasia of ganglion cells in the gastrointestinal tract and on the mechanism responsible for the constipation. Later in life, as the medullary thyroid carcinoma increases in size and metastasizes," endocrine diarrhea" is the usual intestinal complaint. In contrast to MEN type 2a, medullary thyroid carcinoma is seldom cured by surgical intervention.

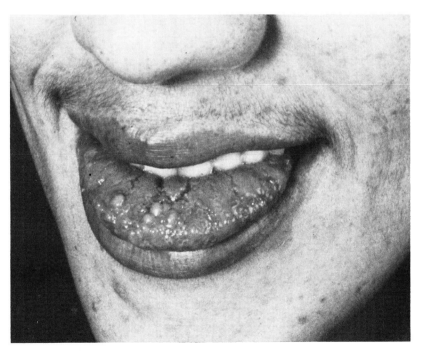

Fig. 18-22. Multiple endocrine neoplasia type 2b. Note the "blubbery" lips and the multiple mucosal neuromas on the tongue.

CLINICAL FINDINGS. The precise number of reported patients with MEN type 2b includes about 100 patients. The disorder is transmitted in an autosomal dominant fashion, but some cases are not familial and represent mutations. The majority of children with this disorder have a characteristic facial appearance that can be recognized as early as the first year of life. The most striking feature is the blubbery lips; the upper lip usually appears to be more prominent. Eversion of upper lids is noted. A marfanoid habitus may be present along with dolichocephaly, micrognathia, pes cavum, and hyperlaxity of joints. Mucosal neuromas are the most constant component of the syndrome. They are found on the lips, tongue (Fig. 18-22), and buccal mucosa. They differ from the neurofibromas of von Recklinghausen's disease by the relative paucity of connective tissue. The medullary thyroid carcinoma involves both lobes and is characterized by the proliferation of C cells, which secrete calcitonin. It usually grows slowly but may be metastatic before giving rise to a palpable nodule.

Diffuse alimentary tract ganglioneuromatosis is a major component of this syndrome because it is present in most cases. There is a striking hypertrophy and proliferation of nerves and nerve plexuses throughout the gastrointestinal tract. The myenteric plexuses are enlarged, and ganglion cells are increased in numbers (Fig. 18-23). Constipation and recurrent bouts of intestinal pseudo-obstruction are important clinical manifestations. They most commonly constitute the initial complaints leading to the first encounter with a physician. It is not known if these symptoms could be secondary to the motor dysfunction associated with ganglioneuromatosis. In other cases, diarrhea alone is present. It is likely that the gastrointestinal tract responds to peptides such as calcitonin and prostaglandins, since diarrhea commonly stops with removal of the medullary thyroid carcinoma. However, we have also noted a disappearance of

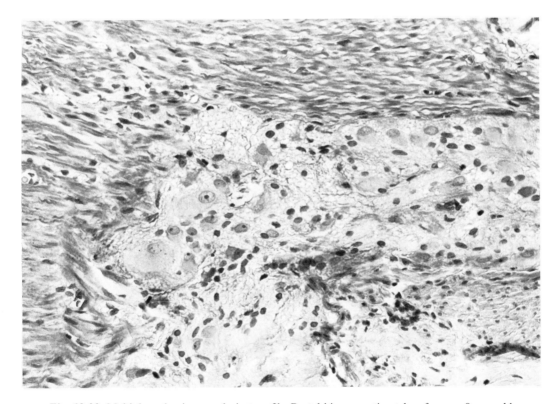

Fig. 18-23. Multiple endocrine neoplasia type 2b. Rectal biopsy section taken from an 8 year old with classic phenotypic features who had a history of chronic constipation that led to three bouts of intestinal obstruction. Auerbach plexuses are prominent and show hyperplastic ganglion cells.

constipation with pseudo-obstruction after surgery.

Megacolon is frequently mentioned in association with MEN type 2b, but its association with Hirschsprung's disease has not been documented. In a pedigree of 106 individuals, we saw 14 cases of medullary thyroid carcinoma and one of pheochromocytoma. Six infants (three girls and three boys) from three related sibships had aganglionic megacolon. In five the extent of the aganglionic bowel did not reach beyond the splenic flexure. Of note is the observation that 10 years after surgery, one of these children started complaining of severe constipation and was found to have a medullary thyroid carcinoma.

DIAGNOSIS. In families with a known history of MEN type 2b, basal and postpentagastrin (0.5 μg/kg) levels of calcitonin should be determined periodically. This test should also be done in infants and children with the typical facial features or in those with constipation associated with recurrent bouts of intestinal pseudo-obstruction. The relationship between Hirschsprung's disease and MEN type 2b syndrome is worthy of note. Our experience suggests that in the event of the recurrence of constipation after surgery for Hirschsprung's disease, the possibility of multiple endocrine neoplasia should be entertained.

TREATMENT AND PROGNOSIS. Medullary thyroid carcinoma is a lethal tumor. A recent survey of 69 patients shows that close to 25% have died of their neoplasm. However, in view of the slow progression of the tumor, 30% of cases with metastatic tumors are alive. There is no effective therapy for medullary thyroid carcinoma, since it is bilateral and multicentric and metastasizes early. Monitoring of calcitonin levels in children and siblings at risk has not yet proved its efficacy. Perhaps prophylactic thyroidectomy should be considered in those with the phenotype. However, they will still be at risk for the development of a pheochromocytoma.

REFERENCES

Buchta, R.M., and Kaplan, J.M.: Zollinger-Ellison syndrome in a nine-year-old child: a case report and review of the entity in childhood, Pediatrics **47**:594-598, 1971.

Carney, J.A., Go, V.L.W., Sizemore, G.W., and Hayles A.B.: Alimentary-tract ganglioneuromatosis: a major component of the syndrome of multiple endocrine neoplasia, type 2b, N. Engl. J. Med. **295**:1287-1291, 1976.

Carney, J.A., Sizemore, G.W., and Hayles, A.B.: Multiple endocrine neoplasia type 2b. In Ioachim, H.L., editor: Pathobiology Annual **8**:105-153, New York, 1978, Raven Press.

Collin, P.P., Schmidt, M., Bensoussan, A., and others: Neurogenic tumors and VIP-induced diarrhea, J. Pediatr. Surg. **14**:525-526, 1979.

Gold, M.S., Winslow, R.R., and Lift, I.I.: Carcinoid tumors of the rectum in children: a review of the literature and reports of a case, Surgery **69**:394-396, 1971.

Jansen-Goemans, A., and Englehardt, J.: Intractable diarrhea in a boy with vasoactive intestinal peptide producing ganglioneuroblastoma, Pediatrics **59**:710-716, 1977.

Kaplan, S.J., Holbrook, C.T., McDaniel, H.G., and others: Vasoactive intestinal peptide secreting tumors of childhood, Am. J. Dis. Child. **134**:21-24, 1980.

Khairi, M.R.A., Dexter, R.N., Burzynski, N.J., and Johnston, C.C.: Mucosal neuroma, pheochromocytoma and medullary carcinoma: multiple endocrine neoplasia type 3, Medicine **54**:89-112, 1975.

Lamers, C.B., Stadil, F., and van Tongeren, J.H.: Prevalence of endocrine abnormalities in patients with the Zollinger-Ellison syndrome and their families, Am. J. Med. **64**:607-612, 1978.

Larsson, L.I.: Gastrointestinal cells producing endocrine, neurocrine, and paracrine messengers, Clin. Gastroenterol. **9**:485-516, 1980.

Lips, C.J.M., Minder, W.H., Leo, J.R., and others: Evidence of multicentric origin of the multiple endocrine neoplasia syndrome type 2a (Sipple's syndrome) in a large family in the Netherlands: diagnostic and therapeutic implications, Am. J. Med. **64**:569-578, 1978.

Mitchell, C.H., Sinatra, F.R., Crast, F.W., and others: Intractable watery diarrhea, ganglioneuroblastoma and vasoactive intestinal peptide, J. Pediatr. **89**:593-595, 1976.

Ryden, S.E., Drake, R.M., and Franciosi, R.A.: Carcinoid tumors of the appendix in children, Cancer **36**:1538-1542, 1975.

Suster, G., Weinberg, A.G., and Graivier, L.: Carcinoid tumor of the colon in a child, J. Pediatr. Surg. **12**:739-742, 1977.

Verdy, M., Choletta, J.P., Cantin, J., and others: Calcium infusion and pentagastrin injection in diagnosis of medullary thyroid carcinoma, Can. Med. Assoc. J. **119**:29-35, 1978.

Verdy, M., Weber, A.M., Bolté, E., and others: Hirschsprung's disease and multiple endocrine type 2b, Gastroenterology **80**:1308, 1981 (abstract).

Systemic mastocytosis

Histamine is a biogenic amine produced by mast cells and also by APUD cells. It has recently been localized to a certain type of enterochromaffin-like cell in the rat gastric mucosa.

Systemic mastocytosis is characterized by diffuse mast cell infiltration of the reticuloendothelial system. A leukemic form has been described. The skin lesions (urticaria pigmentosa) become vesicular and crusty (Fig. 18-24). The lesions tend to be particularly marked on points of pressure. Hepatosplenomegaly is usually present. The pancreas and lymph nodes are also involved. Of 95 pediatric cases, close to 15% have evidence of skeletal involvement (sclerotic or lytic lesions).

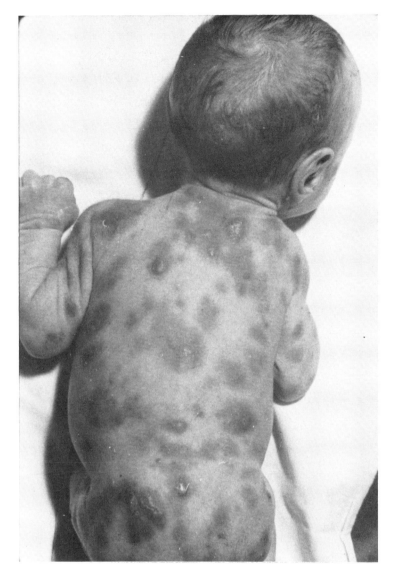

Fig. 18-24. Six-month-old infant with systemic mastocytosis and severe diarrhea. Shortly after birth he developed a generalized pink maculopapular rash that became bullous and crusty. Stroking the skin, even gently, caused a wheal and flare that became vesicular and eventually crusty.

Systemic symptoms include pruritus, flushing, tachycardia, and gastrointestinal symptoms such as nausea, vomiting, diarrhea, peptic disease, fat malabsorption, and weight loss. In adults, the incidence of gastrointestinal manifestations is 15%; it is probably about the same in children. Colonoscopy may permit visualization of lesions. Gastric hypersecretion has been documented along with a rapid gastric emptying time and transit time.

The clinical symptoms and signs of mastocytosis have been attributed to the release of histamine from mast cells. Histamine content of lesions is very high and histaminuria is usually present. Cimetidine decreases gastric acid hypersecretion by blocking the H_2-receptor sites of histamine but does not improve diarrhea. Chlorpheniramine (H_1-receptor blocker) is reportedly effective in decreasing the frequence of bouts of skin lesions. A double-blind study reports effective control of cutaneous gastrointestinal and central nervous system manifestations with oral disodium cromoglycate (100 mg four times daily), which inhibits the calcium-dependent coupled-activation response of mast cells.

REFERENCES

Dantzig, P.I.: Tetany, malabsorption and mastocytosis, Arch. Intern. Med. **135:**1514-1518, 1975.

Gerrard, J.W., and Ko, C.: Urticaria pigmentosa: treatment with cimetidine and chlorpheniramine, J. Pediatr. **94:**843-844, 1979.

Hirschowitz, G.I., and Groarke, J.F.: Effect of cimetidine on gastric hypersecretion and diarrhea in systemic mastocytosis, Ann. Intern. Med. **90:**769-771, 1979.

Lucaya, J., Perez-Candela, V., Aso, C., and Calvo, J.: Mastocytosis with skeletal and gastrointestinal involvement in infancy, Radiology **131:**363-366, 1979.

Parker, C., Jost, G., Bauer, E., and others: Systemic mastocytosis, Am. J. Med. **61:**671-680, 1976.

Soll, A.H., Lewin, K.J., and Beaven, M.A.: Isolation of histamine-containing cells from rat gastric mucosa: biochemical and morphologic differences from mast cells, Gastroenterology **80:**17-27, 1981.

Soter, N.A., Austen, F., and Wasserman, S.I.: Oral disodium cromoglycate in the treatment of systemic mastocytosis, N. Engl. J. Med. **301:**465-469, 1979.

Neurofibromas

The development of digestive tract neurofibromas is well known. However, these multiple tumors are usually small and rarely give rise to symptoms before adulthood. They may be found in the stomach, small bowel, or colon. The most common symptoms are abdominal pain, a palpable mass, gastrointestinal bleeding, or signs of bowel obstruction. Two cases were associated with acquired megacolon. The usually described roentgenographic finding is a sharply demarcated intraluminal filling defect.

Von Recklinghausen's disease

The only consistent features of von Recklinghausen's disease are café-au-lait spots and fibromatous skin tumors. About 25% of adults with multiple neurofibromatosis have gastrointestinal involvement. The most common gastrointestinal symptoms are melena, pain, hematemesis, and constipation. Obstruction rarely occurs. Both neurofibromas and leiomyomas occur. The most frequent site of involvement is the jejunum followed by the stomach.

Leiomyomas and pancreatic rest tumors

Leiomyomas are rare, benign tumors that may arise anywhere in the gastrointestinal tract but are most common in the stomach and jejunum. They may grow primarily in the gut lumen and cause intussusception, or they may grow in the serosa and remain asymptomatic.

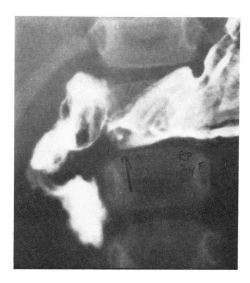

Fig. 18-25. Ectopic pancreas in 6-week-old girl with spitting and single choking episode. Esophagogram and upper gastrointestinal series were obtained to rule out hiatus hernia or gastric outlet obstruction (pyloric stenosis). A filling defect in the antrum was an incidental finding, and the remainder of the study was normal. No treatment at present.

Ectopic pancreatic tissue may be found in various parts of the upper intestinal tract. Most occur in the stomach (Fig. 18-25), duodenum, and jejunum. Symptoms are variable but may mimic pyloric stenosis.

REFERENCES

Buntin, P.T., and Fitzgerald, J.F.: Gastrointestinal neurofibromatosis: a rare cause of chronic anemia, Am. J. Dis. Child. **119:**521-523, 1970.

Hochberg, F.H., Da Silva, A.B., Galdabini, J., and Richardson, E.D., Jr.: Gastrointestinal involvement in von Recklinghausen's neurofibromatosis, Neurology **24:**1144-1151, 1974.

Pous, J.G., and Goalard, C.: Neurofibromatose du mésentère chez l'enfant: étude d'une observation et revue générale, Ann. Chir. Infant. **12:**91-100, 1971.

Strole, W.E.: In Discussion of case 24-1974: weekly clinicopathological exercises, N. Engl. J. Med. **290:**1426-1431, 1974.

VASCULAR MALFORMATIONS OF GASTROINTESTINAL TRACT

There are essentially two types of vascular malformations of the gastrointestinal tract—hemangiomas and telangiectasias. Hemangiomas are true neoplasms in that they represent the outgrowth of ectopic endothelium-lined vascular spaces.

1. The capillary variety is composed of a network of fine, newly formed, closely packed capillaries with

a well-differentiated but somewhat hyperplastic endothelium. They are found throughout the gastrointestinal tract but are more common in the small bowel and perianal skin. More commonly they remain asymptomatic except for those on the perianal skin, which may bleed when traumatized.

2. The cavernous hemangiomas are large thin-walled vessels arising from the submucosal vascular plexus. They may protrude in the lumen as polypoid lesions or may invade the intestine from mucosa to serosa. They usually give rise to bouts of profuse bleeding or to abdominal pain with intussusception being a rare complication.

In a collective review of 61 cases of hemangiomas in the pediatric age group 25% were diagnosed in the first year of life. By 12 years of age, the diagnosis had been made in the majority, but usually after years of bleeding, transfusions, and sometimes unsuccessful surgical explorations. The small bowel was involved in 35% and the colon in 45%, and both colon and small bowel were affected in close to 20%.

Bleeding is the presenting complaint in three fourths of the patients; abdominal pain with intussusception and signs of obstruction may be seen as an initial mode of presentation (Fig. 18-26) in a small minority (10%). Many children may suffer from anemia for several years and have occult blood in their stools before the diagnosis is made. Since nearly 50% of reported patients have cutaneous hemangiomas, intestinal obstruction or bleeding should orient the physician toward the diagnosis. Phleboliths in the pelvis are common in adults. Their presence in children is rare, and they may take years to form. Characteristic findings of multiple, smooth-bordered, intramural, extramucosal filling defects projecting into the bowel lumen confirm the diagnosis.

The "blue-rubber-bleb" nevus disease is characterized by the presence of a bladder-like variety of hemangioma found particularly on the trunk and upper arms. Bleeding hemangiomas of the gastrointestinal tract constitute an important complication. In one family, the disease was transmitted through five generations. Other cases have been sporadic. Cavernous hemangiomas have also been in the gastrointestinal tract in cases of dyschondroplasia (Maffucci's syndrome).

Telangiectasias are not vascular tumors, but ectasias of normal vasculature. The Rendu-Osler-Weber hereditary hemorrhagic telangiectasia syndrome is well known. Its frequency is in the order of 1 to 2 in 100,000. The tip of the tongue, the mucosal surface of the lips, and the face, conjunctivae, ears, fingers, and nail beds are the sites of telangiectases, which will orient the clinician when they are present in patients with painless upper or lower gastrointestinal bleeding (Fig. 18-27). Cirrhosis of the liver occurs in some cases, and there is a high incidence of pulmonary arteriovenous fistula. The CRST syndrome (calcinosis cutis, Raynaud's phenomenon, sclerodactyly, and telangiectasia), a variant of scleroderma likely to be benign, uncommonly gives rise to gastrointestinal bleeding.

Upper and lower endoscopy (colonoscopy) will readily identify local lesions. Biopsies may be followed by profuse bleeding. Fulguration of an isolated polypoid cavernous hemangioma can be done safely. When bleeding is profuse, a selective arteriogram through the superior or inferior mesenteric artery may demonstrate the pathologic vessels. Extensively distributed large hemangiomas may be associated with a consumptive

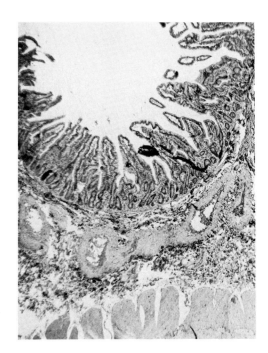

Fig. 18-26. This section of jejunum shows several large, thick-walled blood vessels in the submucosa. The hemangiomatous malformation formed a polypoid mass that was resected from the upper jejunum of an 11-year-old girl who presented with severe bouts of abdominal pain associated with vomiting and anemia.

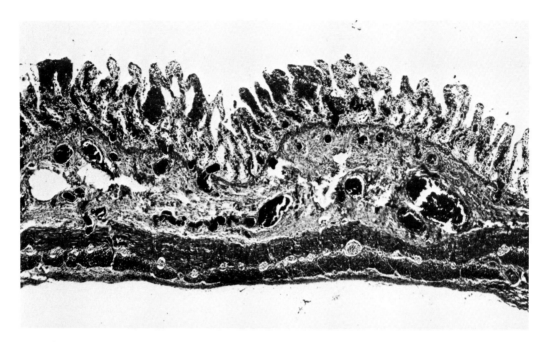

Fig. 18-27. This postmortem section of small bowel was taken from a 1-month-old infant with multiple anomalies and a severe intestinal hemorrhage. Hemorrhagic and autolytic changes are extensive in the lamina propria. The submucosa is fenestrated by a striking number of dilated venules and capillaries.

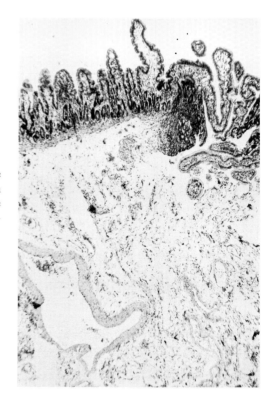

Fig. 18-28. Hemangiomatosis of the small intestine. The vascular malformation of the small intestine was much more extensive and forced multiple enterotomies. The patient was a 17-year-old boy with several hospital admissions for rectal bleeding and anemia.

coagulopathy secondary to the sequestration of platelets and a decrease in fibrinogen.

When lesions are few in number, excision can be undertaken with no problems. With multiple lesions in a limited area, excision of a segment of bowel is warranted. If lesions are widely distributed, it is best to excise the hemangiomas by means of multiple enterotomies (Fig. 18-28). Large, diffuse cavernous lesions in the rectosigmoid can be treated with an abdominoperineal resection followed by a pull-through.

REFERENCES

Abrahamson, J., and Shandling, B.: Intestinal hemangiomata in childhood and a syndrome for diagnosis: a collective review, J. Pediatr. Surg. **8:**487-495, 1973.

Bower, R.J., and Kiesewetter, W.B.: Colo-colic intussusception due to an hemangioma, J. Pediatr. Surg. **12:**777-778, 1977.

Daly, J.J., and Schiller, A.L.: The liver in hereditary hemorrhagic telangiectasia (Osler-Weber-Rendu disease), Am. J. Med. **60:**723-726, 1976.

Holden, K.P.: Diffuse neonatal hemangiomatosis, Pediatrics **46:**411-421, 1970.

Mellish, R.W.: Multiple hemangiomas of the gastrointestinal tract in children, Am. J. Surg. **121:**412-417, 1971.

Morris, S.J., Kaplan, S.R., Ballan, K., and Tedesco, F.J.: Blue-rubber-bleb nevus syndrome, J.A.M.A. **239:**1887, 1978.

Nader, P.R., and Margolin, F.: Hemangioma causing gastrointestinal bleeding, Am. J. Dis. Child. **111:**215-222, 1966.

Shobel, C.T., Smith, L.E., Fonkalsrud, E.W., and Isenberg, J.N.: Ectopic pancreatic tissue in the gastric antrum, J. Pediatr. **92:**586-588, 1978.

HEPATIC TUMORS

Tumors of the liver are relatively rare in pediatric patients, and only large pediatric centers have any significant experience with them. In 1974 a survey of the Surgical Section of the American Academy of Pediatrics collated the information on 375 liver tumors encountered during a 10-year interval. Two hundred fifty-two were malignant, and 123 were benign. In France, a combined pediatric experience from three large centers (Pediatric Liver Unit, Pediatric Surgical Unit, and Pediatric Oncology Service) over a 15-year span produced a cumulative experience of 113 hepatic tumors, of which 48 were primary malignant and 65 were benign. In the Denver area we continue to see two or three new patients each year with a ratio of malignant to nonmalignant lesions of about 3 to 1 (Table 18-3). Five-year survival figures for all stages of malignant hepatic tumors of childhood have been less than 10% in most reported series. On the other hand, for the tumors that can be completely excised by surgery, cure rates of up to

Table 18-3. Experience with primary hepatic tumors in Denver (1970-1981)

Condition	Number
Malignant	
Hepatoblastoma	6
Hepatocellular tumor	7
Lymphoma	1
Rhabdomyosarcoma	1
Benign	
Hamartoma	3
Hemangioendothelioma	2
TOTAL	20

60% can be expected with hepatoblastoma and up to 33% with hepatocellular carcinoma. Radiation and chemotherapy do not improve the chance for survival if the tumor is not amenable to complete removal. Liver replacement by orthotopic transplantation has been extremely disappointing in the treatment of hepatic malignancy. In the two largest experiences (United States and England), recurrence rates of 85% and 70%, respectively, are reported, and presently hepatic transplantation is rarely employed as a treatment option for children with hepatic cancer.

Malignant neoplasms

Incidence figures for malignant liver tumors are difficult to obtain. Of all childhood malignant neoplasms, excluding leukemia, those of the liver account for 0.2% to 5.8%. The incidence is strikingly higher in Japan and China, presumably because of a greater frequency of childhood cirrhosis.

Two major histologic types represent almost all the primary malignant liver tumors in children. Overall, hepatoblastomas are the most common type found in the pediatric age group. These tumors are pathologically similar to the embryonal type of lesion seen in nephroblastoma. Hepatocarcinoma is the second most common histologic type, with other less common lesions being classified as angiosarcoma, mesenchymal tumors, or rhabdomyosarcoma. Some interesting and at times clinically useful information emerges from these two major groups of neoplasms.

Hepatoblastomas

Hepatoblastoma occurs predominantly in the right lobe of the liver (two thirds of the cases in the United States). It has been found in premature infants dying of other causes and may well arise during fetal life. These two observations have led some workers to incriminate the fetal circulation to the liver as being a significant factor in the development of these tumors. The left lobe is supplied with oxygenated blood derived entirely from the umbilical vein, whereas the right lobe is supplied with portal vein blood containing a lower oxygen saturation. The possible relationship between oxygen tensions and their role in "normal" cellular differentiation and division is fruit for intriguing speculation. However, the tumor may arise in the left lobe in over 30% of cases, but being multifocal in others.

Further support for the embryonal origin of these tumors derives from the recovery, in serum of patients with hepatic tumors, of a fetal alpha-l-globulin (fetoprotein). It is present in the serum of 60% to 80% of all patients with hepatomas but not in that of normal persons. This globulin can be detected in the serum of normal fetuses; it disappears shortly after birth but may become detectable in conditions other than hepatomas (neonatal cholestatic syndromes, viral and metabolic hepatitis, and so on).

Other clinical features of hepatoblastoma are a slight predominance in male children (3 to 2) and its likely appearance before 5 years of age. The majority of cases come to diagnosis before 18 months of age though occasional examples have been found in the adolescent.

The absence of clinical symptoms is striking and disturbing. Unfortunately, this particular lesion is usually first appreciated as a hepatic mass during routine examination of the abdomen. At other times only an enlarged liver without a definable tumor is palpated at routine examination of the abdomen. More often, it is not recognized until it has grown to such size as to produce significant abdominal enlargement. Most lesions are greater than 10 cm in size at the time of diagnosis. If the tumor is detected late, a history of anorexia, listlessness, fever, weight loss, and so forth may be obtained. Sometimes the history indicates that the tumor undergoes a rapid growth spurt just before diagnosis. At the time of diagnosis, this lesion is usually large and focal, without evidence of metastases (Fig. 18-29).

Results of routine liver function tests are generally normal, and the few abnormalities occasionally present are inconsistent and seldom of any diagnostic value. The presence of alpha-fetoprotein in the patient's serum may be most helpful.

Hepatocarcinoma

Hepatocarcinoma has interesting clinical associations that are poorly understood. It occurs much more frequently in boys than in girls (3 to 1). Most cases occur before school age and again during adolescence. Children with underlying liver disease, particularly cirrhosis, seem to be predisposed to this neoplasm but not to the same extent as adults with cirrhosis. Hepatocarcinoma has been seen in postnecrotic cirrhosis, biliary cirrhosis, and so-called cryptogenic cirrhosis. An increased incidence of this tumor is also reported in patients with alpha-l-antitrypsin–deficient cirrhosis. One needs to be aware of the occasional development of hepatocarcinoma in children requiring long-term anabolic androgen therapy (particularly C17-alkylated androgens) for aplastic anemia. A recently reported case of Fanconi's anemia treated with oxymetholone developed a rapidly fatal hepatocellular carcinoma within 2 months of treatment.

Although yet to be reported in the pediatric age patient, oral contraceptive–associated liver tumors (benign adenoma) are at added risk to malignant transformation. A worldwide review of this association found 10 (8%) malignant tumors in 117 women taking birth control pills from 6 months to over 5 years.

Abdominal enlargement with vague discomfort or sharp pain are the predominant clinical symptoms, perhaps more because of patient age and awareness than anything specific in the patterns of tumor growth. This neoplasm carries a poorer prognosis than hepatoblastoma does because it can be multifocal and tends to metastasize early (Fig. 18-30).

These lesions are associated with anomalies and endocrinopathies in some children. Virilization in males has been reported and appears to result from gonadotropin activity within the tumor. Leydig-cell hyperplasia, without spermatogenesis is found on testicular biopsy. A recent experience with a young teen-age male presenting with bilateral gynecomastia and elevated serum estrogen level revealed a hormone-secreting hepatocarcinoma in the right lobe of the liver as causative. Other curious abnormalities include hemihypertrophy, congenital absence of the kidney, and macroglossia. We have seen a child with hepatocarcinoma and associated hepatic glycogenosis (with normal glycolytic enzymes), renomegaly caused by severe cystic glomerular disease, and a de Toni-Fanconi syndrome. The original diagnosis of von Gierke's

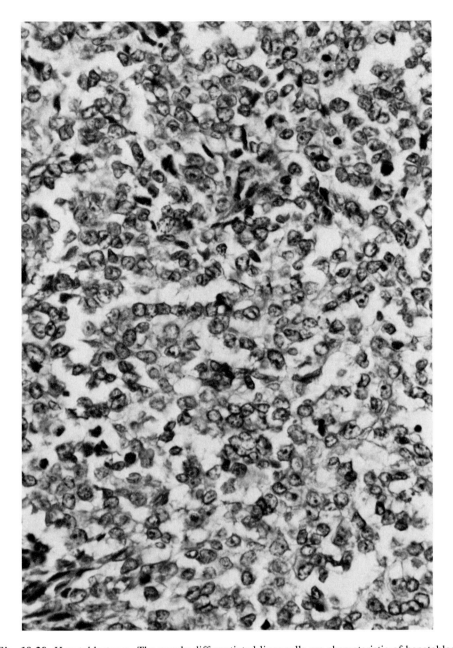

Fig. 18-29. Hepatoblastoma. The poorly differentiated liver cells are characteristic of hepatoblastoma. A 5-month-old male infant had an abdominal mass at routine well-baby examination. The mass seemed continguous with the liver and extremely firm to palpation. A determination of the fetal alpha-1-globulin was elevated; a liver scan was interpreted as abnormal; the intravenous pyelogram was normal. At exploration, an 8 cm mass occupying most of the right lobe of the liver was identified and removed en bloc by right lobectomy.

disease was obviously incorrect, though the clinical and laboratory features were similar.

Abdominal distention and pain usually in the right upper quadrant or the presence of a mass most often leads to diagnosis. Depending on the delay in diagnosis, anorexia, fatigue, weight loss, or pallor may or may not be present.

As with hepatoblastoma, results of liver function tests are normal or mildly abnormal. A times, hypoglycemia may be striking. Increase of blood cholesterol was believed to be suggestive of this type of hepatic neoplasm; however, as with results of many other liver function tests in this condition, it too, has lacked consistency to be of di-

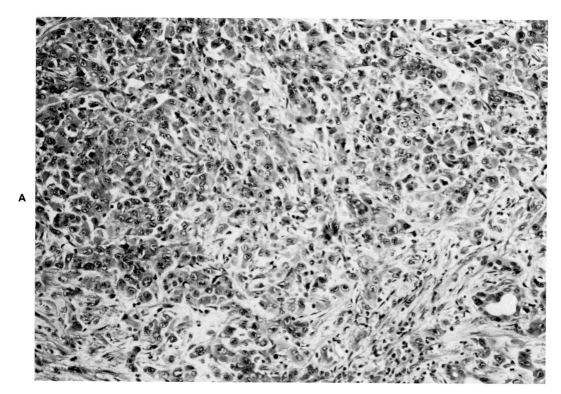

Fig. 18-30. Hepatocarcinoma. **A,** In an autopsy specimen from a 10-year-old girl, a portion of the tumor (lower right) is adjacent to compressed portal zone. **B,** High-power magnification shows the tumor cellularity of **A.** This child suffered abdominal pain for a month before admission to hospital, and progressive abdominal enlargement ensued. A large, firm mass filling the entire upper abdomen was palpated. The child died shortly after surgery from a massive intratumor hemorrhage.

agnostic value. Hyperuricemia may be present in some patients. It appears that increase of serum fetoprotein will apply to hepatocarcinoma as well as to hepatoblastoma.

Investigative studies

Once an abdominal tumor is discovered at physical examination, certain laboratory and roentgenographic procedures are indicated while the patient is being prepared for surgery. In particular, differentiation from other, more common abdominal tumors is obviously needed. Neuroblastoma or Wilms' tumor can often be differentiated from hepatic tumor by proper roentgenographic techniques and interpretation. Intravenous pyelogram remains the single most useful tool in determining the existence of these lesions.

Interpretation of three-way plain films of the abdomen with particular attention to the displacement of intra-abdominal structures from their normal anatomic locations can be used to ascertain the source of the tumor. Eighty percent of the lesions can be suspected by this technique alone. The additional findings of intrahepatic calcifications and upward displacement of the hemidiaphragm are helpful clues. Chest and metastatic bone surveys are indicated when tumor is suspected. Ten percent of cases will have pulmonary metastases at a time of diagnosis. A much greater experience has improved the usefulness of nuclear-medicine liver scans in the pediatric age group, especially in the prediction of abnormalities caused by "cold" space-occupying lesions, typical of most hepatic tumors.

Abdominal CT scanning is extremely sensitive in the detection of intrahepatic tumors unless the lesion is very well differentiated and has a density comparable to that of the neighboring normal liver tissue (Fig. 18-31). Postoperatively, this diagnostic aid is most useful in assessment of the rate of liver regeneration in patients subjected to lobectomy.

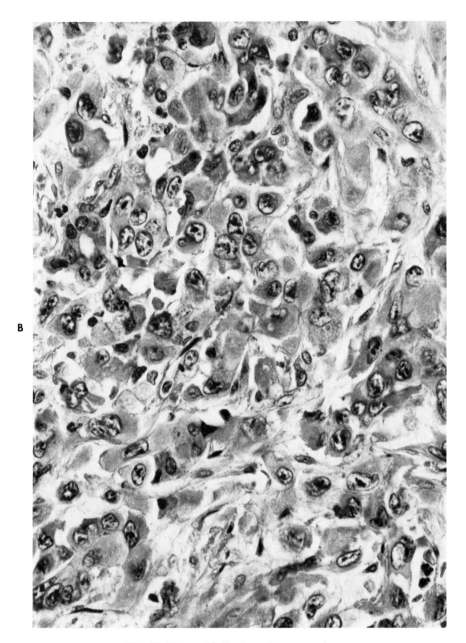

Fig. 18-30, cont'd. For legend see opposite page.

Perhaps a more useful adjunct in evaluating patients with suspected intrahepatic space-occupying lesions is arteriography. In the younger child (less than 1 year) the aortic flush method is employed, whereas selective hepatic arteriograms can usually be obtained in the older patient and will provide information regarding vascular anatomy and resectability. We view the specific abnormal vascularization pattern as the single most informative evidence signifying an intrahepatic tumor (Fig. 18-

32). A venacavogram is indicated when previous investigations suggest a posteriorly located lesion.

Percutaneous liver biopsy may be extremely dangerous in patients with hepatic neoplasms because rupture of the distended capsule of the liver or tumor may cause massive intratumor or extratumor hemorrhage. The child should have a roentgenographic metastatic survey before surgery. Laparotomy is undertaken for final diagnosis.

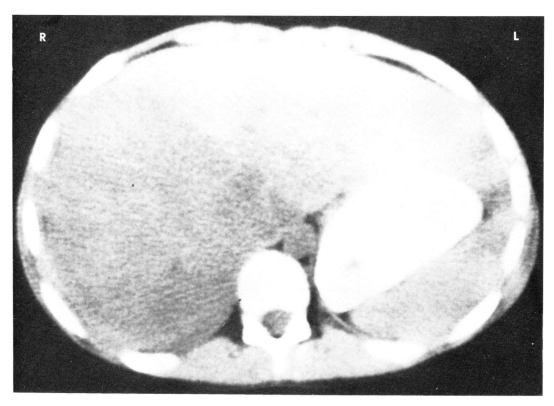

Fig. 18-31. Abdominal CT scan revealing a large, mixed-density contrast-enhancing mass lesion occupying the greater portion of the right lobe of the liver. Barium-filled structure is stomach. This study was obtained in a 15-year-old boy with a 1-year history of bilateral gynecomastia, intermittent right upper quadrant pain, and moderate hepatomegaly. Elevated serum estrogen level was found.

Differential diagnosis

Other abdominal lesions are capable of producing hepatomegaly or a mass or both. If an abdominal mass is palpable. Wilms' tumor, neuroblastoma, neuroblastoma with hepatic metastases, pancreatic pseudocysts, choledochus cysts, and mesenteric cysts deserve consideration. Usually the lesion is distressingly firm, so that malignancy seems likely. If hemorrhage into the lesion has occurred (peliosis), the tumor may feel cystic. The relationship of the tumor to the liver can be appreciated by its fixed position at rest and movement during inspiration as the liver descends. The margins of these tumors can sometimes be easily defined, or they may be contiguous with the liver edge, making clinical demarcation difficult.

About 70% of hepatic neoplasms are confined to, or arise from, the right lobe. If a distinct lesion cannot be defined by palpation, asymmetric hepatomegaly may provide a useful clinical clue. When liver enlargement is diffuse, cardiac, hematologic, nutritional, metabolic, and infectious causes may be considered.

Treatment and results

Long-term survival is possible only if the tumor can be entirely resected at surgery. Not uncommonly, the wide resection may involve removal of 40% to 60% of liver tissue. The remaining hepatic mass must have a normal arterial and portal blood supply to survive. When complete resection is possible, survival figures for hepatoblastoma now approach 60% and 33% for hepatocarcinoma.

It is important that the pathologist be aware of the variant pattern of hepatocellular carcinoma, fibrolamellar carcinoma (fibrolamellar oncocytic hepatoma), a tumor associated with a more favorable prognosis. The distinctive histologic features

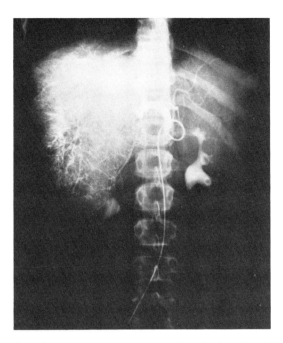

Fig. 18-32. Selective hepatic artery angiogram in case described in Fig. 18-31 revealing dilated, somewhat tortuous intrahepatic vessels in the right lobe of the liver. Early and intense "staining" but without vascular puddling favors the diagnosis of hepatoma over hemangioma.

of this lesion include deeply eosinophilic neoplastic hepatocytes, presumably because of their mitochondrion-rich cytoplasm, surrounded by mature collagen fibers arranged in a lamellar fashion. Recurrence of disease is usually found in the lungs or locally in the abdomen in neighboring nodes or viscera.

Significant complications also occur in patients requiring hepatectomy. Substantial intraoperative blood loss is the most worrisome and may be responsible for cardiac arrest. Postoperatively, subphrenic abscess formation, bowel obstruction, biliary fistula, and air embolization are all reported with variable frequency. Hypoglycemia needs to be guarded against, as does hypoalbuminemia.

Ancillary treatment of patients with hepatic carcinoma include radiation (1000 to 3000 rads) with or without chemotherapy. This approach may be of value in selected cases of hepatoblastoma where it is necessary to first reduce the tumor size and permit subsequent surgical resection. Otherwise, neither of these adjunctive therapies offer much to the long-term survival figures for lesions that are not completely resectable. Chemotherapeutic agents include vincristine, 5-fluorouracil, cyclophosphamide (Cytoxan), and actinomycin D.

The most common cause of death in children who are not amenable to complete resection is almost always secondary to the consequences of local tumor extension into intra-abdominal organs and viscera. For some, death is caused by liver failure. Distant metastases to the lungs with progressive respiratory failure is also a common cause of death. For others intratumor or intra-abdominal hemorrhage, or sepsis, or both, may be the terminal event. In nonoperative cases 90% of children with hepatoblastoma will die within 12 months of diagnosis, whereas 80% of those with hepatocellular carcinoma will be dead within 1 year.

Provided that the vascular supply to the remaining liver is adequate, complete hepatic regeneration can be expected within 6 postoperative months despite massive resection. This can be followed by serial liver scans, which also serve to detect recurrences within the regenerating liver. Extrahepatic intra-abdominal recurrence is best detected by CT scan.

The disheartening results of surgery for these tumors are not easy to explain, for often the tumors are well localized, resected margins are free of tumor, and no distant metastases can be found during the initial survey. Results of surgery for other embryonal tumors (nephroblastomas) noted for their tendency to spread late have been better than for the hepatic group. A number of recent improvements in surgical technique have reduced the postoperative morbidity in patients subjected to hepatic lobectomy. These include early ligation of the troublesome hepatic veins, inflow and outflow hemostasis, finger fracture of the liver, and Plasmanate infusions. The delay in ligation of all hepatic veins draining the tumor before manipulation probably contributes to venous seeding with tumor cells and perhaps accounts for the subsequent appearance of metastases.

The late recurrence of disease after liver transplantation or even simple lobectomy strongly indicates that surgery alone will not improve survival rate of these patients. Techniques permitting better visualization or identification of metastases need to be developed, as do more effective chemotherapeutic agents. These techniques combined with early diagnosis may yield a greater number of survivors.

Benign tumors

Most benign tumors in pediatric patients are congenital in origin (Table 18-4), with some manifesting symptoms within the first 3 to 6 months of life. Benign tumors during childhood seldom arise from either liver or duct cells. Although benign tumors may be discovered during abdominal surgery for other causes, most pediatric cases are recognized as a result of their large size, producing abdominal enlargement and hepatomegaly. Since these large tumors may also produce compression symptoms in neighboring abdominal structures, discovery of the primary cause is not infrequently serendipitous. Some benign tumors (hemangioendothelioma, adenoma) may cause pain secondary to thrombosis, infarction or intratumor hemorrhage (peliosis), or rupture into the peritoneal cavity. Others (mesenchymal cystic hamartomas) may cause abdominal pain attributable to rapid accumulation of intratumor fluid. Hemangioendothelioma may be the unsuspected cause in the infant with congestive heart failure, or thrombocytopenia with excessive bleeding and bruising. Although rare in children, multiple nodular hyperplasia of the liver can produce portal hypertension.

General laboratory studies of liver function are normal as is the alpha-fetoprotein test. Diagnosis

Table 18-4. Types of benign liver tumors reported by the Surgical Section of the American Academy of Pediatrics, 1974

Hemangioma	38
Hamartoma	37
Hemangioendothelioma	16
Adenoma	7
Focal nodular hyperplasia	4
Cholangiohepatoma	1
Epithelioid epithelioma	1
Benign cyst	10
Hydatid cyst	6
Eosinophilic granuloma	1
Lymphangioma	2
TOTAL	123

is strongly suspected by the results of the radionuclide liver scan, CT scan, or ultrasound, or by the characteristic vascular pattern unique to many of these lesions seen during selective arteriography.

Confirmatory diagnosis requires surgery and intraoperative biopsy. Percutaneous liver biopsy may be hazardous, especially in extensive vascularized tumors, and is not recommended. As with malignant neoplasms, surgical excision is the treatment of choice. Unfortunately, some benign tumors are not resectable, being either too extensive in size of multicentric in origin. Other therapeutic modalities (radiation, prednisone) can be used in cases of large hemangioma or diffuse hemangioendothelioma.

Although a number of varieties of benign hepatic tumors occur, based upon frequency of occurrence, only four warrant inclusion and discussion at this time.

Hamartomas

Hamartoma, one of the most common of the benign lesions, must be differentiated from the malignant group because expected survival is substantially different. This lesion accounts for 10% of all hepatic tumors and about one third of the benign varieties. Actually, some pathologists argue against including hamartoma in the discussion of tumors, since, strictly speaking, it is an anomaly of development, a malformation, rather than a true neoplasm. Within this lesion, a variety of normal hepatic elements are abnormally represented in terms of architecture and anatomic relationships. However, most of these lesions tend to be solid and therefore present as a mass similar to the neoplastic lesions. Some hamartomas can be cystic, or contain cystic elements, which can mislead the pathologist and the surgeon. The presence of normal elements of embryonic nature in disorderly array and of benign histologic appearance is typical of this lesion. These tumors may be enormous, leading to abdominal enlargement, and yet the only symptoms produced are related to the pressure effects and resulting disturbance in function of neighboring structures. Therefore early diagnosis is usually first entertained after abdominal palpation, which results in recognition of the symptomless mass. This lesion may occur at any age, but the majority come to diagnosis before school age.

The presence of a negative alpha-fetoprotein test only suggests that the intrahepatic mass is benign. Preoperatively, arteriography remains the procedure of choice for identifying hepatic hamartomas that clinically may be confused with malignant lesions. In contrast to the findings seen in hepatoblastoma and hepatocarcinoma, the portal venous phase of the arteriogram shows tumor exclusion, indicating a primary arterial vascularization characteristic of hepatic hamartomas. Cystic hamartomas may be suspected by the results of ultrasonography and arteriography.

Treatment of hamartoma is surgical: simple excision is possible if the lesion proves to be cystic or pedunculated. The benign nature of the lesion can sometimes be identified early in the course of surgery, in which the tumor mass may be removed by finger separation of the capsule from the neighboring normal liver parenchyma. Since many hamartomas are nonencapsulated, hepatic lobectomy is required for complete removal. In those rare instances where the risks of complete surgical removal appear too great, it is prudent to leave these benign lesions in place. Barring unforeseen complications, cure should be achieved in these fortunate patients after surgical removal. Neither recurrences nor malignant transformation is reported.

Hemangioendotheliomas and cavernous hemangiomas

Hemangioendotheliomas and cavernous hemangiomas are benign lesions frequently diagnosed before 3 to 4 months of age because of the presence of significant hepatomegaly with or without cutaneous hemangiomas. They are a rare cause of hepatic tumors and vary from single lesions of huge size (giant cavernous hemangioma or solitary angioma) to multinodular and infiltrative lesions varying from microscopic size to large nodules. This latter variety is the type frequently associated with cutaneous lesions (Fig. 18-33). Some pathologists include this group of lesions with hamartomas.

These lesions can produce systemic and hematologic symptoms as well as local abdominal pressure and discomfort. Commonly (45%), the patient has cutaneous evidence of hemangiomas and may occasionally present with congestive heart failure or cholestatic jaundice in infancy. Splenomegaly may be noted. Gastrointestinal bleeding from bowel lesions may occur, and cyanosis develops from significant arteriovenous shunting within the lesions. Bruits may be heard over the head, lungs, liver, or abdomen in such patients and are a useful clinical finding. Intrahepatic calcification may be seen on routine abdominal films or by CT scan. Sequestration of platelets and resulting thrombocytopenia occurs, so that petechiae and ecchymoses may be the initial features in some patients. A microangiopathic hemolytic anemia may be present in some cases. Fatal hemorrhage accounts for some deaths and congestive heart failure for others.

Distressingly, the multinodular lesions are usually not well defined and tend to be infiltrative, a feature that frequently renders them nonresectable.

When the aforementioned physical and laboratory findings are present in an infant with or without hepatomegaly, an organized radiologic evaluation is critical before surgery. The total body opacification phase of the intravenous pyelogram should be observed, since it may show single or multiple mottled collections of the contrast medium within the liver suggesting an abnormal vascular lesion. Provided that the lesions are greater than 1 cm, a radionuclide liver scan using technetium-99m sulfur colloid will reveal the hemangioma as "cold" spots. This can be followed by either an indium-113m or a stannous pyrophosphate technetium-tagged red blood cell study to further define the vascular nature of these lesions. Either of these techniques is useful in following the subsequent course and evolution of these particular tumors. Finally, angiography can be carried out as the definitive study, since it will demonstrate pathonomonic features indicating the existence of benign vascular tumors. The arterio-

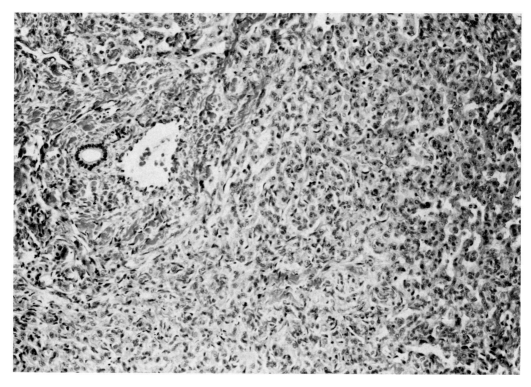

Fig. 18-33. Hemangioendothelioma (infiltrative). Liver biopsy specimen was taken from a 5-month-old child with cutaneous hemangiomas, hepatosplenomegaly, and gastrointestinal bleeding. A hemangioma-like process surrounds the portal region. Most of the liver was infiltrated by this lesion.

graphic findings of significance include enlarged feeding hepatic artery, hypervascularity of the lesion or lesions, vascular lakes, and large early-draining hepatic veins.

Most isolated hemangiomas are amenable to surgical excision provided that the patient's cardiac status is not a contraindication to anesthesia. In these latter examples and in those with extensive solitary infiltrating lesions, or when the disease is multicentric, digitalis, prednisone, and radiation therapy (500 to 1000 rads) are commonly employed before surgical considerations. Since the hepatic artery is not an end artery, ligation of this vessel is of questionable value; however, in cases of intractable heart failure, the more aggressive approach may be necessary. Whenever possible, however, caution and conservatism should prevail in the management of such patients when simple surgical excision cannot be accomplished.

In unfortunate cases the healing or regression of these infiltrative hemangiomas can leave the liver disorganized and fibrotic (Fig. 18-34). Portal hy-

pertension and its vagaries may eventually develop. Large solitary angiomas may not show spontaneous regression.

Nodular hyperplasia

This tumor is an uncommon cause of hepatic neoplasm in the pediatric age group. To some authors it is believed to represent another hamartomatous condition. In most instances it is discovered as an incidental finding at surgery performed for other reasons, or even at autopsy. Less than 20% of cases have symptoms attributable to this tumor, with abdominal pain being the most common complaint. Typically, focal nodular hyperplasia of the liver is comprised of solitary circumscribed nodules of normal-appearing hepatic cells separated by collagenous septa. Bile ductules may be prominent within the fibrous septa and inflammatory cells consisting of lymphocytes and occasionally neutrophils may be present. These features serve to distinguish this lesion from hepatic adenoma. At times the nodules may be multiple (multiple nodular hyperplasia) and up to 5 to 6

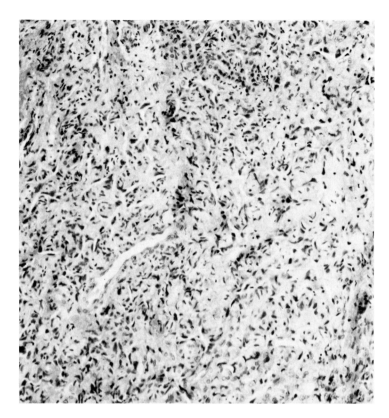

Fig. 18-34. Hemangioendothelioma (after radiation). Repeat liver biopsy specimen taken a year after radiation therapy to the liver shows cleftlike spaces associated with hemosiderin-laden cells and dense, collagenous connective tissue.

cm in size. In the latter instance, the lesions tend to be in the perihilar area, and compression of portal structures is belived responsible for the rare complication of portal hypertension.

The cause of this condition is unknown. Some relate its evolution to an embryologic defect, others to an abnormal reparative process in areas of liver injury, whereas some implicate an abnormal vascularization or blood-flow phenomenon in response to an unknown stimulant. It is curious that a similar lesion has been noted in women taking oral contraceptives. The association of nodular hyperplasia and other hamartomatous lesions is provocative, since this tumor is found with other congenital defects, including cavernous hemangioma of the liver, genitourinary abnormalities, and hemihypertrophy, and in Felty's syndrome. An unusual case of focal nodular hyperplasia has been reported in type-1 glycogen-storage disease associated with vasoconstrictive pulmonary hypertension. Besides focal nodular hyperplasia of the liver, benign adenomas and even hepatocellular carci-

noma have been reported in this form of glycogen-storage disease.

In almost all instances, this is a benign condition and needs no specific therapy. The lesion is not premalignant. Surgical resection should be avoided, except in the most unusual cases where obstruction to neighboring structures occurs.

Nonparasitic, solitary cysts

Nonparasitic, solitary cysts are nonneoplastic, cystic lesions of the liver; they are an infrequent cause of an abdominal mass. As with malignant tumors of the liver, these lesions tend to arise more frequently from the right lobe, where they may be found in a subcapsular position or attached by a pedicle.

Solitary liver cysts occur at any age, are usually asymptomatic, and are slightly predominant in females. Abdominal pain provoked by pressure on neighboring viscera may be the presenting complaint in some patients; in others, spontaneous rupture, hemorrhage, suppuration, and leakage of contents into the peritoneal cavity may be a spectacular mode of presentation. The cysts vary in size, and calcifications have been reported. Fluid may be present in large quantities and has the appearance of bile-stained serous secretion. Indeed, the lining cells usually have features of a glandular epithelium (mucous or ciliated), though nonglandular epithelium and absence of epithelium have been reported.

The interior of the cyst may be divided into communicating chambers by trabeculations and septa, but the capsule is well defined, thick, and amenable to surgical removal.

Preoperative diagnosis can be suspected after radiologic studies have been done, including radioactive liver scans and ultrasound.

Surgical diagnosis and removal is required to ensure complete cure.

REFERENCES

Atkinson, G.O., Kodroff, M., Sones, P.J., and Gay, B.B.: Focal nodular hyperplasia of the liver in children: a report of three new cases, Radiology **137:**171-174, 1980.

Clatworthy, H.W., Jr., Schiller, M., and Grosfeld, J.L.: Primary liver tumors in infancy and childhood: 41 cases variously treated, Arch. Surg. **109:**143-147, 1974.

Craig, J.R., Peters, R.L., Edmundson, H.A., and Omata, H.: Fibrolamellar carcinoma of the liver: a tumor of adolescents and young adults with distinctive clinico-pathologic features, Cancer **46:**372-379, 1980.

Everson, R.B., Museles, M., Henson, D.E., and Grundy, G.W.: Focal nodular hyperplasia of the liver in a child with hemihypertrophy, J. Pediatr. **88:**985-987, June 1976.

Exelby, P.R., Filler, R.M., and Grosfeld, J.L.: Liver tumors in children in the particular reference to hepatoblastoma and hepatocellular carcinoma: American Academy of Pediatrics Surgical Section Survey—1974, J. Pediatr. Surg. **10:**329-337, June 1975.

Geist, D.C.: Solitary non-parasitic cyst of the liver: a review of the literature and report of two patients, Arch. Surg. **7:**867-880, 1955.

Ishak, K.G., and Glunz, P.R.: Hepatoblastoma and hepatocarcinoma in infancy and childhood: report of 47 cases, Cancer **20:**396-422, 1967.

Ishak, K.G., and Rabin, L.: Benign tumors of the liver, Med. Clin. North Am. **59:**995-1013, July 1975.

Ito, J., and Johnson, W.W.: Hepatoblastoma and hepatoma in infancy and childhood, Arch. Pathol. **87:**259-266, 1969.

Kew, M.C., Kirschner, M.A., Abrahams, G.E., and Katz, M.: Mechanism of feminization in preliminary liver cancer, N. Engl. J. Med. **296:**1084-1088, 1977.

Klatskin, G.: Hepatic tumors: possible relationship to use of oral contraceptives, Gastroenterology **73:**386-394, Aug. 1977.

McLean, R.H., Moller, J.H., Warwick, W.J., and others: Multinodular hemangiomatosis of the liver in infancy, Pediatrics **49:**563-573, 1972.

Meadows, A.T., Naiman, J.L., and Valdes-Dapena, M.: Hepatoma associated with androgen therapy for aplastic anemia, J. Pediatr. **84:**109-110, 1974.

Nebesar, B.A., Tefft, M., and Filler, R.M.: Correlation of angiography and isotope scanning in abdominal diseases of children, Am. J. Roentgenol. Radium Ther. Nucl. Med. **109:**323-340, 1970.

Nuernberger, S.P., and Ramos, C.V.: Peliosis hepatis in an infant, J. Pediatr. **87:**424-426, Sept. 1975.

Pizzo, C.J.: Type I glycogen storage disease with focal nodular hyperplasia of the liver and vasoconstrictive pulmonary hypertension, Pediatrics **65:**341-343, Feb. 1980.

Rosenfield, N., and Treves, S.: Liver-spleen scanning in pediatrics, Pediatrics **53:**692-697, 1974.

Rotman, M., John, M., Stowe, S., and Inamdar, S.: Radiation treatment of pediatric hepatic hemangiomatosis and coexisting cardiac failure, N. Engl. J. Med. **302:**852, April 1980.

Slovis, T.L., Berdon, W.E., Haller, J.O., and others: Hemangiomas of the liver in infants, Am. J. Roentgenol. Radium Ther. Nucl. Med. **123:**791-801, April 1975.

Stromeyer, F.W., and Ishak, K.G.: Nodular transformation (nodular "regenerative" hyperplasia) of the liver: a clinicopathologic study of 30 cases, Hum. Pathol. **12:**60-71, 1981.

Weinberg, A.G., Mize, C.E., and Worthen, H.G.: The occurrence of hepatoma in the chronic form of hereditary tyrosinemia, J. Pediatr. **88:**434-438, March 1976.

PANCREATIC TUMORS

Infrequent, congenital developmental cysts (cystadenomas) usually affect the body and tail of the pancreas. They may grow to large size and cause symptoms by extrinsic pressure, but the function of the pancreas is not compromised. Pseudocysts are dealt with in Chapter 28.

Table 18-5. Clinical findings in 28 patients with nonfunctioning malignant pancreatic tumors

Condition	Number
Abdominal pain	14
Abdominal mass	12
Icterus	9
Steatorrhea	8
Anorexia	8
Vomiting	6
Anemia	6
Weight loss	6
Fever	4
Melena	2
Hematemesis	2

With permission from Welch, K.J.: The pancreas. In Ravitch, M.M., and others, editors: Pediatric surgery, ed. 3, Chicago, 1979, Year Book Medical Publishers, Inc.

Neoplasms involving the pancreas are exceptional in the pediatric age group and can be divided into nonfunctioning and functioning (islet cell) tumors.

Nonfunctioning tumors

A review of the literature on malignant tumors of the pancreas in children reveals a total of 28 cases up to 1978. All cases were carcinomas except for a 2-year-old child with cystadenosarcoma. Nonfunctioning islet cell carcinomas and adenocarcinomas accounted for the majority of the cases. Four patients were below 1 year of age and 14 were 6 years and younger. The variety and the nonspecificity of early symptoms and signs make an early diagnosis very difficult (Table 18-5). The one case seen at Hôpital Sainte-Justine presented with anemia, weight loss, and unexplained fever (Fig. 18-35).

Ultrasonography, computed tomography, endoscopic retrograde cholangiopancreatography, and selective angiography facilitate an earlier diagnosis and may in the future ameliorate the 5-year survival figure. In the series described, there were only seven survivors. However, five survivors had a nonfunctioning islet carcinoma, a survival rate of 55%, whereas all nine cases with adenocarcinomas died rapidly. A total pancreatoduodenectomy is the only chance for a cure. Radiation and chemotherapy are not believed to be particularly effective but are advocated.

Functioning tumors

Endocrine pancreatic tumors usually but not always give rise to clinical syndromes through their production of hormonal or neuronal peptides (Table 18-6). These tumors arising from pancreatic islets may contain an admixture of different endocrine cell types. Immunocytochemistry and radioimmunochemistry reveal that these tumors contain a variety of peptides, but they generally give rise to one particular clinical syndrome.

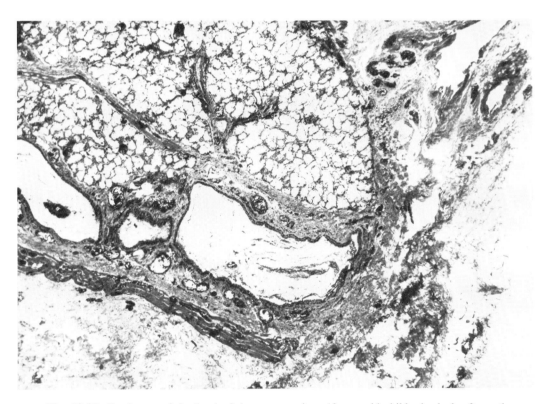

Fig. 18-35. Carcinoma of the head of the pancreas in a 12-year-old child who had a 3-month history of abdominal pain, weight loss, anemia, and icterus. Postmortem examination showed widespread metastases of an anaplastic adenocarcinoma.

Table 18-6. Syndromes, clinical findings, and peptide hormones in endocrine pancreatic tumors

Syndromes	Clinical findings	Hormonal diagnosis
Gastrinoma	Zollinger-Ellison syndrome	Pronounced hypergastrinemia, gastrin determination after calcium infusion
Carcinoid tumor	(See section on carcinoid tumors)	Increased urinary excretion of serotonin and of 5-HIAA
Insulinoma	Hypoglycemia, lethargy, seizures with CNS damage	Hyperinsulinism in face of hypoglycemia
Glucagonoma	Diabetes, necrotizing migratory dermatosis, part of multiple endocrine neoplasia syndrome	Hyperglucagonemia
VIPoma (pancreatic cholera)	Watery diarrhea, hypokalemia, hypochlorhydria or achlorhydria (WDHA)	High plasma levels of VIP, pancreatic polypeptide in tumor, prostaglandins in tumor
Somatostatinoma	Abnormal glucose tolerance test, steatorrhea, hypochlorhydria	Large quantities of somatostatin in tumor

Insulinomas and nesidioblastosis

There are numerous causes of hypoglycemia in the pediatric age group. Hyperinsulinism, responsible for only 1% of the cases, may be attributable to beta-cell hyperplasia, beta-cell secretory defects, nesidioblastosis, and insulinomas. A high incidence of brain damage is reported if the diagnosis of hyperinsulinism is not made promptly. A number of patients are misdiagnosed and treated for protracted seizures.

Nesidioblastosis is characterized by diffuse scattering of disorganized islet cells most likely derived from the pancreatic ductal epithelium. A familial occurrence has been reported: it appears to be an autosomal recessive condition. It accounts for a fourth of the cases of hyperinsulinism for which surgery has to be carried out. Hypoglycemia fails to respond to medical therapy (glucose, glucagon, diazoxide). It is reported in neonates with Beckwith's syndrome and in a few cases of sudden infant death syndrome. Upon operation, an 85% to 90% distal pancreatectomy should be carried out. Somatostatin infusions have been recently reported to be effective in reducing insulin release in the preoperative phase.

Insulinomas are reported with increased frequency. There are probably close to 100 published cases. The tumor is round, firm, and encapsulated. In three fourths of the cases it is located in the body or tail of the pancreas. Multiple adenomas are also well known. Ectopic adenomas occur rarely (2%) but have been found in the liver, duodenum, stomach, and spleen as well as in a Meckel's diverticulum. Most are benign adenomas, but there are two reports of malignant islet cell tumors.

A subtotal (85%) pancreatectomy is a safer procedure even in cases where an adenoma is identified in view of the possibility that there could be more than one insulinoma.

Gastrinomas and islet cell hyperplasia

Although gastrinomas have been reported in the stomach and duodenum, most originate from a single or multiple (75%) pancreatic non–beta-cell islet tumor. In rare cases, the Zollinger-Ellison syndrome is caused by diffuse pancreatic islet cell hyperplasia or to benign G-cell hyperplasia of the pyloric antrum. Most gastrinomas are malignant.

Peptic ulceration (see Chapter 7) is the predominant feature, with diarrhea occurring in 30% to 80%. The peptic ulcers may be multiple, usually recur rapidly, and occupy atypical locations such as the jejunum. Gastrinomas are usually small, but a CT scan may at times be helpful. Angiography is seldom helpful. At surgery, identification of a tumor is possible in only half the cases; furthermore, the gastrinomas are multifocal in 70%, and more than 60% are metastatic at the time of operation. Gastrinomas are slow growing, and control of the peptic ulcer diathesis and of the diarrhea when present is satisfactory with cimetidine. Total gastrectomy is indicated if "medical" gastrectomy fails. Excision of identifiable gastrinomas is indicated though chances are that tumor is already present elsewhere at the time of operation. Fewer than 25 cases have been described in the pediatric literature, with the most (75%) in boys. The youngest patient was a 5-year-old child who also had the Marden-Walker syndrome (mental retardation, micrognathia, blepharophimosis, low-set ears, kyphoscoliosis, and mild joint contractures).

VIPomas (tumors secreting vasoactive intestinal peptide) and islet cell hyperplasia

Recent reviews of the pancreatic cholera syndrome (WDHA) in adults reveal that less than 25% of the cases are attributable to a well-localized pancreatic non–beta islet cell tumor (malignant in 40% of reported cases) or to diffuse hyperplasia. All pediatric cases have been caused by neural crest tumors except for one infant who was symptomatic from birth with refractory watery diarrhea and who underwent a 95% pancreatectomy. In this case plasma and pancreatic tissue concentrations were very high and there was hyperplasia of the islands of Langerhans. Histochemical studies revealed that the proliferating cells were of the nonbeta type.

REFERENCES

Case records of the Massachusetts General Hospital (Case 30-1978), N. Engl. J. Med. **299:**241-248, 1978.

Cubilla, A.L., and Fitzgerald, P.J.: Classification of pancreatic cancer (non endocrine), Mayo Clin. Proc. **54:**459-467, 1979.

Garcia, J.C., Carney, J.A., Stickler, G.B., and others: Zollinger-Ellison syndrome with neurofibromatosis in a 13 year old boy, J. Pediatr. **98:**982-984, 1978.

Ghishan, F.K., Soper, R.T., Nassif, E.G., and Younoszai, M.K.: Chronic diarrhea of infancy: non beta islet cell hyperplasia, Pediatrics **64:**46-49, 1979.

Ginsberg-Fellner, F., and Rayfield, E.J.: Metabolic studies in a child with a pancreatic insulinoma, Am. J. Dis. Child. **134:**64-67, 1980.

Grosfeld, J.L., Clatworthy, H.W., and Hamondi, A.B.: Pancreatic malignancy in children, Arch. Surg. **101:**370-375, 1970.

Gundersen, A.E., and Janis, J.F.: Pancreatic cystadenoma in childhood: report of a case, J. Pediatr. Surg. **4:**478-481, 1969.

Hirsch, H.J., Loo, S., Evans, N., and others: Somatostatin inhibition of insulin and gastrin hypersecretion in pancreatic islet-cell carcinoma, N. Engl. J. Med. **296:**1323-1326, 1977.

Knight, J., Garvin, P.J., Danis, R.K., and others: Nesidioblastosis in children, Arch. Surg. **115:**880-882, 1980.

Krejs, G.J., Orci, L., Conlon, J.M., and others: Somatostatinoma syndrome: biochemical, morphologic and clinical features, N. Engl. J. Med. **301:**285-293, 1979.

Modlin, I.M.: Endocrine tumors of the pancreas, Surg. Gynecol. Obstet. **149:**751-769, 1978.

Moynan, R.W., Neerhout, R.C., and Johnson, T.S.: Pancreatic carcinoma in childhood, J. Pediatr. **65:**711-720, 1964.

Schwartz, S.S., Rich, B.H., Lucky, A.W., and others: Familial nesidioblastosis: severe neonatal hypoglycemia in two families, J. Pediatr. **95:**44-53, 1979.

Taxy, J.B.: Adenocarcinoma of the pancreas in childhood: report of a case and a review of the English language literature, Cancer **37:**1508-1518, 1976.

Welch, K.J.: The pancreas. In Ravitch, M.M., Welch, K.J., Benson, C.D., Aberdeen, E., and Randolph, J.G., editors: Pediatric surgery, ed. 3, Chicago, 1979, Year Book Medical Publishers, Inc.

19 *Prolonged obstructive jaundice*

The infant with prolonged obstructive jaundice (neonatal cholestatic syndrome) frequently poses a diagnostic dilemma for the physician, who must decide whether the jaundice is attributable to medical or surgical causes. Unfortunately, in up to 15% of cases this diagnostic dilemma may be insoluble by routine clinical, laboratory, and radiologic studies, and at times even after histologic examination of the tissue. Several reasons exist for this observed difficulty. The most important one seems to emanate from the limited number of responses, either physiologic or anatomic, that the closely interdependent structures (hepatocytes, small intrahepatic bile ductules, and large extrahepatic bile ducts) are capable of expressing in the face of a great variety of insults. The physiologic events that predictably follow either hepatocyte or bile duct injury of any cause almost always include a diminution in bile flow, decreased hepatocyte clearance of bilirubin and bile acids, and morphologic evidence of cholestasis. Adding to the difficulty in resolving this diagnostic dilemma is the observation that the pathologic lesion may be very similar in 10% to 15% of cases, whether the cause of the cholestasis is either intrahepatic or extrahepatic disease. Rather than attributing this observation only to the limitation of responses by the injured liver, one could also argue that certain causes may in fact produce a continuous morphologic expression of disease, and factors other than cause (genetic, gestational age at the time of insult, secondary toxic metabolites, maternal health, and so on) may influence the appearance of the final pathologic lesion that occurs in the neonatal cholestatic syndrome. Despite the existence of these diagnostic handicaps in assessment of the infant with neonatal cholestasis, the underlying site of obstruction can be assigned with confidence to either an intrahepatic or extrahepatic location by careful interpretation of clinical, laboratory, radiologic, and histologic evaluation in 85% to 90% of cases, thereby clarifying the need for immediate diagnostic surgical exploration (minilaparotomy) or continued medical management.

The reasons for promptly resolving this diagnostic dilemma are equally as compelling for certain medical causes of cholestasis as for promptly correcting any surgical cause that may exist. Specifically, there are several medical entities (galactosemia, congenital fructose intolerance) that manifest neonatal cholestasis and are amenable to precise therapeutic measures. Such therapy when instituted early in the course of illness leads to immediate improvement and also offer a favorable long-term prognosis. On the other hand, not all cases of extrahepatic cholestasis will be permanently helped by surgery, but the chances are greatest if surgery is performed early in life. It would appear that restoration of bile flow needs to be accomplished before the first 2 to 3 months of life, lest reversal of the progressive biliary cirrhosis not occur. This observation seems particularly important for patients with "noncorrectable" biliary atresia who are subjected to hepatic portoenterostomy (Kasai procedure).

In the face of such potential confusion and the concurrent pressures to quickly resolve the diagnostic dilemma, one could ask why not simply explore all cases of the neonatal cholestatic syndrome? Arguments to the contrary are numerous. First, a sizable number of these infants would be subjected to an unnecessary operation, since intrahepatic causes occur as frequently as extrahepatic ones in producing the neonatal cholestasis. Furthermore, exploratory laparotomy is probably detrimental to patients with intrahepatic cholestasis, particularly when the causes are genetic or metabolic in nature. Also, surgery, which should resolve the cause of the prolonged jaundice, may fail to do so, depending on the expertise of the surgeon, pathologist, and radiologist in dealing with these conditions. In one study a combination of surgical exploration, liver biopsy, and operative cholangiogram failed to identify the underlying lesion in 5% of cases. It is from an awareness of these various factors that the goals of the "ideal" work-up in a child with neonatal cholestasis were derived. Such a work-up should (1) seek to identify, wherever possible, the specific or associated

Table 19-1. Neonatal cholestatic syndromes–causes and associations

Congenital infectious causes	Genetic and metabolic associations	Miscellaneous associations
Cytomegalovirus*	Galactosemia	Hemolytic disease
Rubella virus*	Tyrosinemia	Bacterial sepsis
Herpesvirus	Congenital fructose intolerance	Pyelonephritis
Hepatitis B virus*	Alpha-1-antitrypsin deficiency*	Hyperalimentation
Echoviruses 14 and 19	Cystic fibrosis	Congestive heart failure
Coxsackievirus B	Niemann-Pick disease	Hypoplastic left heart syndrome
Toxoplasmosis	Trisomy 17, 18, and 21	Postnecrotizing enterocolitis, gastroschisis, omphalocele
Syphilis	Turner's XO 45 syndrome	Neonatal hypopituitarism
	Menke's syndrome	"Inspissated bile syndrome"(without
	Byler's disease	hemolysis)—perinatal shock, respiratory
	Aagenaes's syndrome	distress syndrome, acidosis
	Cholestasis in North American Indians	Generalized hemangiomatosis
	Trihydroxycoprostanic acid (THCA)–associated cholestasis	
	Zellweger's syndrome	
	Polysplenia syndrome†	

*Rarely reported with biliary atresia.
†Frequently associated with biliary atresia.

cause, (2) abolish unnecessary surgical exploration, and (3) avoid excessive delay in identifying and surgically correcting any obstructing anatomic lesion.

The hospital setting is best suited for the rapid evaluation of these children. A thorough work-up including liver biopsy can most often be accomplished in 3 to 5 days and a decision then made to either continue medical treatment or undertake surgical exploration. Given the degree of urgency in diagnosing either a medical or surgical cause of jaundice, it behooves the physician to seek out those clinical clues that might suggest a cholestatic cause whenever jaundice is noted during routine well-child examinations. For some children, unfortunately, a recognition that cholestasis exists may have been delayed over 2 to 3 months before they reach the hospital for complete evaluation. The reasons for this delay can be numerous. Lack of awareness by parents that dark-colored urine or light-colored stools are abnormal and have significance is not surprising, especially if the patient is the firstborn. The initial well-baby visit may be scheduled at 2 weeks, a time when clinical jaun-

dice may be attributed to benign causes (physiologic jaundice, breast-milk jaundice) without complete clinical assessment. The infant may not be seen again until 8 weeks of age, since few show overt signs of the underlying illness. Naturally, should the caregiver employ a casual approach to the jaundice during these first months of life with incomplete consideration to the entire range of diagnostic possibilities, inadequate laboratory assessment will follow, invariably causing further delay. On the other extreme, this incomplete but hurried approach may result in unnecessary surgical exploration.

If a complete preoperative evaluation is to be carried out, the physician faced with the neonate presenting with prolonged jaundice must become familiar with those clinical clues, available laboratory and roentgenologic tests, and therapeutic maneuvers that can increase his accuracy of diagnosis in identifying one of the large number of specific causes or associated conditions, that may cause the neonatal cholestatic syndrome. Although identification of a specific cause is made in only 25% of cases, the search is most impor-

Table 19-2. Laboratory and roentgenologic studies useful in evaluating neonates with cholestasis

Blood	Urine	Bacteriologic, virologic, and serologic studies	Liver function	Stool	Special studies	Radiology and other
Complete blood count, red blood cell smear	Routine analysis	Bacterial cultures from nose, blood, urine, and spinal fluid as clinically indicated	Total and fractionated bilirubin, serially	Bile	^{131}I–rose bengal (in 3-day stool collection)	Skull
Coombs' test, blood type	Bile		SGOT, SGPT, gamma glutamyl transpeptidase (GGT)	Trypsin	Bile acids (qualitative or quantitative)	Long bones
Reticulocyte count	Urobilinogen	Viral cultures (throat, urine, stool)	Alkaline phosphatase		Sweat chlorides	Upper gastrointestinal series
Platelet count	Amino acid screen	TORCH complex	Cholesterol		Peroxide hemolysis	Ultrasonography of gallbladder and portal structures
Prothrombin time	Organic acid screen	VDRL test	Serum protein electrophoresis		Abnormal, low-density lipoprotein (LP-X); lecithin-cholesterol acyltransferase (LCAT)	Hepatobiliary scintigraphy (^{99m}Tc-diethyl-IDA, or DIDA; PIPIDA)
Partial thromboplastin time		HBsAg in mother and child	Serum alpha-1-antitrypsin activity		Alpha-1-fetoprotein (AFP)	
Fibrinogen levels		Immunoglobulins	Serum 5′-nucleotidase		Galactosemia screen	
					24-hour duodenal fluid collection	

tant, since a positive result generally implies a nonsurgical cause for the cholestasis. Even in the absence of a specific one, the thorough preoperative evaluation when coupled with the results of a nonsurgical liver biopsy should be sufficiently discriminating to allow one to correctly assign such an infant to either an intrahepatic or an extrahepatic category in up to 95% of cases. A list of the viral, bacterial, and protozoal causes, as well as genetic and metabolic causes, and a large group of miscellaneous conditions that seem to predispose the neonate to cholestasis is shown in Table 19-1. Of these, only the polysplenia syndromes (situs inversus, levocardia, absence of the inferior vena cava) are consistently associated with extrahepatic biliary atresia. The routine laboratory and roentgenographic studies presently used in identifying some of these predisposing conditions are listed in Table 19-2 and subsequently discussed in greater detail. Provided that no contraindications to percutaneous liver biopsy exist, the procedure should be carried out as soon as possible. Specific indications for diagnostic "closed" liver biopsy and indications for "open" biopsy appear in the next column.

Indications for percutaneous liver biopsy

Age less than 3 months
Chance of establishing an etiologic diagnosis
Stools not completely acholic
Radionuclide scan or ^{131}I–rose bengal excretion not suggesting biliary atresia
No contraindications (bleeding, diathesis, ascites, liver too firm)

Indications for open liver biopsy

Age greater than 3 months
Contraindications to closed biopsy exist (any age)
Histologic lesion seen at closed biopsy clearly atresia-like
Histologic lesion seen at closed biopsy "equivocal" and patient nearly 3 months of age
Medical failure; persistent cholestatic jaundice after 4 weeks of therapy and stools acholic
Evidence for metabolic disease strong; enzyme assays needed
Mass lesion on upper gastrointestinal series or water density mass found by ultrasonography

The interpretation of the histologic lesion observed in liver tissue can then be coupled with the clinical, laboratory, and roentgenologic studies to improve the predictive diagnostic accuracy and to

Table 19-3. Discriminating clinical and pathologic features of intrahepatic and extrahepatic neonatal cholestasis

	Intrahepatic	Extrahepatic
Clinical features	Preterm, small for gestational age	Full term, average (weight) for gestational age
	Ill-appearing	Relatively well
	Hepatosplenomegaly	Hepatomegaly (firm to hard)
	Other organ involvement	
	Incomplete cholestasis (stools with some bile color)	Complete cholestasis (acholic stools beyond 10 days)
	Associated causes identified (infections, metabolic, familial, and so on)	Polysplenia syndrome
Liver lesion (features arranged in decreasing order of occurrence)	Cholestasis	Cholestasis
	Lobular disarray	Neoductular proliferation (angulated, distorted, elongated)
	Hepatocellular necrosis	Portal and perilobular fibrosis
	Giant-cell transformation	Bile lakes
	Portal inflammation	Normal lobular architecture
	Minimal fibrosis	Rare giant cells
	Rare neoductular formation	Rare inflammatory cell response
	Pseudogland formation	
	Steatosis	
	Extramedullary hematopoiesis	

allow for proper disposition. The more important discriminating clinical and pathologic features of intrahepatic and extrahepatic cholestasis are listed in Table 19-3. If the infant is under 8 to 10 weeks of age and the body of evidence suggests an intrahepatic cause for the cholestasis, a trial of medical therapy is indicated for the next 2 to 4 weeks. If the infant is under 8 weeks of age and the accumulated evidence does not allow separation between intrahepatic and extrahepatic causes and provided that the original liver biopsy tissue showed lack of significant fibrosis, we elect to treat medically, using cholretics for the next 2 to 4 weeks, and then reevaluate the patient with liver function studies, serum bile acids, and the use of a biliary technetium-tagged radionuclide (DIDA being our preference) or the ^{131}I–rose bengal excretion test and liver biopsy. All results are then compared to the original findings. Failure to obtain objective evidence that now resolves the diagnostic dilemma at 10 to 12 weeks of age generally calls for exploratory laparotomy, operative cholangiogram, and repeat open liver biopsy. We feel strongly that this overall approach to the neonate with cholestasis will hasten the correct diagnosis and reduce the frequency of unnecessary surgical explorations. With little regard for age, however, exploratory surgery is undertaken in those infants with obstructive jaundice when one of the following situations exists: (1) if, after thorough investigation, no specific cause has been identified, but, most importantly, the interpretation of the "closed" liver biopsy and accompanying laboratory and radiographic studies strongly suggest extrahepatic obstruction; (2) if a mass lesion is noted on upper gastrointestinal series or an echo-free density suggesting choledochal cyst is seen by ultrasound examination; (3) when contraindications to percutaneous needle liver biopsy exist; (4) in any case yielding equivocal information when the infant is 10 to 12 weeks of age or older; or (5) when a large surgical specimen of liver tissue is needed as in those rare diagnoses requiring enzyme determinations to confirm suspected metabolic etiology. It cannot be overemphasized that whenever diagnostic minilaparotomy is undertaken to resolve the cause of neonatal cholestasis, it should be performed by a surgeon with sufficient experience and competence that will allow for extending the surgery to accomplish a definitive surgical drainage procedure should extrahepatic disease be discovered.

Laboratory and roentgenographic investigations

No single laboratory test can consistently be relied on to unequivocally resolve the diagnostic dilemma for the physician faced with the problem of prolonged obstructive jaundice in the neonate. However, one develops confidence in the significance and trend of certain laboratory results, especially when they correlate with the clinical and histologic data.

Over the years, many new tests have received temporary enthusiasm only to be discarded at a later time. On the other hand, certain specific tests have been developed to aid in the diagnosis of some of the more recently described causes of prolonged neonatal jaundice.

The following list includes those tests and procedures that are usually necessary unless specific diagnosis can be made by other information.

Hematologic tests

Complete blood count, red blood cell smear
Coombs' test, blood type
Reticulocyte count
Platelet count
Prothrombin time
Partial thromboplastin time
Fibrinogen levels

The results of these tests should enable one to rule out hemolytic causes contributing to the mixed hyperbilirubinemia. Coagulation studies are especially useful because they often reflect the earliest recognizable abnormalities in those cases of severe neonatal hepatitis. This group of tests may also reveal an underlying hemolytic anemia, with recognizable "burr" cells and fragmented red blood cells seen on the peripheral smear. This may occasionally be observed in the "idiopathic" variety of giant-cell hepatitis.

Bacteriologic, virologic, and serologic tests

Bacteriologic cultures from nose, throat, blood, urine, and spinal fluid, as clinically indicated
Viral cultures (throat, urine, stool)
TORCH complex test
VDRL test
HBsAg in mother and child
Immunoglobulin levels

Viral cultures should be obtained for cytomegalovirus and, when indicated, herpes simplex virus and enteroviruses (coxsackievirus B, echovirus) as well. One can obtain serologic screening for toxoplasmosis, rubella, cytomegalovirus, and herpes simplex by sending the neonate's serum to the Center for Disease Control (CDC) in Atlanta, Georgia, and requesting the TORCH complex test. Syphilis must always be considered and ruled out with the VDRL and *Treponema pallidum* immobilization (TPI) tests.

We routinely test infants' serum for HBsAg by radioimmunoassay. If maternal testing previously identified her as either a chronic carrier of HBsAg or having acquired HBsAg during pregnancy, cord blood is also evaluated for this hepatitis marker.

An elevated IgM value of greater than 60 mg/dl has been taken as presumptive evidence of an in utero infection and statistically implies that the underlying cause for the jaundice requires medical rather than surgical treatment. However, in utero acquired cytomegalovirus, rubella, and HBsAg infection have been found in rare cases of extrahepatic biliary atresia, thereby weakening the significance of an elevated IgM level in patients with prolonged obstructive jaundice.

Liver function tests

Total and fractional bilirubin, serially
SGOT, SGPT, gamma glutamyl transpeptidase (GGT)
  or alkaline phosphatase, cholesterol level
Serum protein electrophoresis
Serum alpha-1-antitrypsin activity
Serum 5'-nucleotidase

No single liver function test can consistently differentiate surgical from medical obstructive jaundice. Serum bilirubin determinations may be helpful, but one cannot rely on the absolute value or the ratio of direct- to indirect-reacting bilirubin to help in determining the cause of jaundice. A fluctuating bilirubin level is likewise nondiagnostic, but clearing of the jaundice over a 3-month period is incompatible with the diagnosis of extrahepatic biliary atresia. Likewise, neither the degree of elevation of serum transaminase values has correlated with the underlying disease process, nor the alkaline phosphatase and cholesterol values, especially early. An elevated value for the enzyme 5'-nucleotidase or gamma glutamyl transpeptidase (GGT) is consistent with hepatobiliary injury and more specific than the elevated routine alkaline phosphatase value. Both enzymes seem to parallel the degree of bile duct injury and proliferation and are not influenced by rapid bone growth as alkaline phosphatase is. Since proliferation of bile ducts is a constant feature of biliary

atresia, values for 5'-nucleotidase (values greater than a range of 25 to 30 IU/L) have been reported to be consistent with atresia, whereas lower values are indicative of neonatal hepatitis. At present there is less information available regarding the discriminatory value of GGT in this regard.

Serum protein electrophoresis may yield certain clues toward the identification of the underlying process. A low serum albumin level may indicate significant underlying liver cell injury, or on occasion it may be found in young jaundiced infants with cystic fibrosis. The absence or a very low level of the alpha-1-globulin fraction should suggest alpha-1-antitrypsin deficiency disease.

A number of neonates with prolonged obstructive jaundice have alpha-1-antitrypsin deficiency, making a quantitative determination of this protease inhibitor a mandatory part of the laboratory work-up. Not only will there be immediate genetic implications, but also medical management can be promptly instituted once such a neonate is identified. Up to now only an exceptional case of alpha-1-antitrypsin deficiency has been associated with biliary atresia, whereas a few others have been reported in association with small or hypoplastic extrahepatic biliary ducts.

Urinalysis

Routine
Bile
Urobilinogen
Amino acid screen
Organic acid screen

Of great importance is promptly recognizing the presence of proteinuria and reducing sugars. Routine screen for urine glucose in a pediatric patient should always be done with Clinitest tablets (and, if possible, followed with glucose oxidase tape) so as not to miss the diagnosis of a treatable disease, galactosemia. Some but not all cases of congenital fructose intolerance will be detected by Clinitest of the urine, since fructosuria may be present along with proteinuria.

Generally speaking, the persistent absence of urobilinogen in the urine is suggestive of jaundice requiring surgical rather than medical treatment but, unfortunately, not in the neonate. In 10% to 15% of cases of intrahepatic cholestasis bile flow may be completely obstructed for 2 to 3 months or longer, thereby giving the same urine results as those expected with atresia.

Serum amino acid and organic acid screening

will aid in detecting those cases of tyrosinemia and congenital fructose intolerance with significant liver disease.

Stool analysis

Bile level
Fecal chymotrypsin

A truly acholic stool is significant and easy to recognize. However, the significance of the stool with some degree of color is difficult to assess, since the source of origin of the bile pigment products remains uncertain. in fact, further testing may fail to confirm the presence of bile in the light yellow or pale green stools. The presence of a strongly positive test for bile in the stool is significant and except in extremely unusual situations unlikely to be found in cases of jaundice requiring surgical treatment. On the other hand, the absence of urobilinogen from the stool may be normal in neonates.

Stool chymotrypsin determinations are relatively easy to perform. Persistent absence of fecal chymotrypsin is suggestive of pancreatic insufficiency, particularly cystic fibrosis, a condition that on occasion is associated with the neonatal cholestatic syndrome.

Special tests

^{131}I–rose bengal
Bile acids (qualitative or quantitative) in serum and urine
Sweat chlorides
Peroxide hemolysis
Abnormal, low-density lipoprotein (LP-X); lecithin-cholesterol acyltransferase (LCAT)
Alpha-1-fetoprotein (AFP)
Galactosemia screen
24-hour duodenal fluid collection

Despite a variety of modifications applied to the ^{131}I–rose bengal test, by itself it continues to have limited usefulness in consistent differentiation between obstructive jaundice of severe nature in the neonate, but still requiring medical management, and that requiring surgery. It is of maximal value only when the excretion results, be they measured by scanning of the liver and abdomen or by counting of the stool radioactivity in a 3-day collection period, give normal results. Decreased or absent excretion of the radioactivity is consistent only with an obstructive process to bile flow but does not provide information that permits the phy-

sician to localize the level of the defect (intrahepatic versus extrahepatic). Unfortunately, errors in diagnosis are not uncommon, and the procedure may yield false high excretion values that delay necessary surgery. A useful technical modification of the ^{131}I–rose bengal test does away with the stool and urine collections, which are somewhat difficult in small infants. Information is obtained by scanning of the liver an hour after administration and then 4 to 6 hours later. In nonobstructive jaundice, radioactivity in the intestinal tract should be greater than that in the liver and thus is appreciated when the entire abdomen is scanned, but the amount of radioactivity required is 50 times (50 μCi) greater than the 1 μCi used for the method requiring stool collections.

Other modifications include pretreatment of the jaundiced neonate with phenobarbital and cholestyramine, drugs that can increase bile flow and thereby increase the sensitivity of the test. The results of serial ^{131}I–rose bengal determinations performed in the jaundiced patient maintained on such therapy may aid in differentiation of the nature of the underlying process.

Determination of the serum bile acid level is now available in kit form, but it has limited usefulness in helping to resolve the diagnostic dilemma posed by cholestatic syndromes. Total blood bile acids are elevated in all cases regardless of underlying cause. The early impression that intrahepatic and extrahepatic disease could be differentiated by a ratio of primary bile acids (cholate/chenodeoxycholate) was not substantiated by subsequent testing of the large number of such infants.

Pilocarpine iontophoresis for measuring sweat chlorides is the method of choice, though adequate collection of sweat (more than 50 mg) may not be possible until the child is 4 to 6 weeks old. Values greater than 60 mEq/L of chloride on successive tests are diagnostic of cystic fibrosis.

Like so many other tests, the peroxide hemolysis test has failed to consistently differentiate "obstructive" neonatal hepatitis from biliary atresia and therefore has limited usefulness in our opinion. Later in the course, it may be used as an indirect measurement of serum vitamin E levels.

The presence of an abnormal, low-density lipoprotein (LP-X) in the jaundiced neonate is another indicator of cholestasis but is also of limited usefulness. The LP-X is present in 15% to 20%

of infants with severe intrahepatic cholestasis, as well as in all those with extrahepatic atresia, and therefore this test suffers from the same shortcomings as so many other laboratory tests. It remains to be confirmed that the simultaneous estimation of lecithin-cholesterol acyltransferase (LCAT) activity in plasma in the presence of LP-X will consistently differentiate from intrahepatic and extrahepatic cholestasis.

Likewise the measurement of alpha-1-fetoprotein (AFP) has lacked the specificity to distinguish between all examples of intrahepatic or extrahepatic neonatal cholestasis. More importantly, this protein is consistently found in very high concentration in the serum of children with hereditary tyrosinemia, and we have noted its presence in a case of congenital fructose intolerance.

Galactosemia should be ruled out by a red blood cell assay of galactose-1-phosphate uridyltransferase activity in any jaundiced infant with a history of vomiting, irritability, and failure to thrive. It should also be strongly entertained whenever the liver biopsy shows evidence of steatosis. It is particularly important to remember that one cannot rely only on a negative result of urine-reducing sugars, especially early in this disease.

Some believe that the 24-hour duodenal fluid collection with attention to the color of the returned fluid discriminates between intrahepatic and extrahepatic causes of neonatal cholestasis. This procedure requires the fluoroscopic placement of a small (size 8 French) feeding tube just distal to the second portion of the duodenum. Fluid is collected by gravity over the next 12-hour period while the child is fasting. If no bile pigment is noted in the return during this initial time, the infant is then fed a glucose electrolyte solution (Pedialyte) every 2 hours for the subsequent 12 hours. Failure to obtain duodenal fluid with obvious bile pigment coloration after 24 hours has been taken as an indication that a surgical cause of jaundice exists. A trial of intravenous cholecystokinin (1 mg/kg) or magnesium sulfate given through a tube can be tried as a bile-flow stimulant before one decides on surgery. If duodenal fluid return does reveal bile pigment, a percutaneous needle biopsy is still recommended to obtain histologic verification, since both false-positive and false-negative results have been noted. Fluctuating bile-pigment color in the duodenal fluid is commonly observed in intrahepatic cholestasis.

Radiology

Skull roentgenograms
Roentgenograms of long bones
Upper gastrointestinal series
Ultrasonography of the gallbladder and portal structures
Hepatobiliary scintigraphy

Intracranial calcifications may be present in 50% of patients with congenital toxoplasmosis and in a lesser number of infants with cytomegalovirus infection.

Characteristic changes in the metaphyses of the long bones are present in some patients with congenital rubella.

The presence of a congenital choledochal cyst (less than 5% of the time) or other rare anomaly of the extrahepatic bile ducts might be suspected if the first and second portions of the duodenum show an extrinsic pressure deformity. For this reason an upper gastrointestinal series has traditionally been part of the investigation of neonates with prolonged obstructive jaundice, but an ultrasound study has definite advantages and has replaced contrast radiography in the routine evaluation of such patients. This noninvasive technique will reliably permit identification of a choledochal cyst, thereby immediately resolving any diagnostic dilemma so that surgery can be promptly undertaken. It remains to be determined whether this technique can clearly differentiate all cases of intrahepatic from extrahepatic causes. The presence of a gallbladder and common bile duct can only be taken as presumptive evidence that patency of the entire extrahepatic biliary system exists. For example, since proximal dilatation of the patent ducts is seldom noted in biliary atresia, this technique may have difficulty in identifying some variations in biliary atresia, particularly distal duct atresia. It also remains to be seen whether ultrasound is sufficiently sensitive to identify hypoplastic but patent extrahepatic ducts.

An evaluation of the hepatobiliary system by radiopharmaceuticals (hepatobiliary scintigraphy) has become extremely popular over the last several years. This technique has the potential to differentiate hepatocellular disease and intrahepatic small-duct cholestasis, as well as to permit evaluation of medium and large-sized extrahepatic bile ducts. In the recent past, the ^{131}I–rose bengal test remained the standard hepatobiliary radiopharmaceutical means for evaluation of patency of the extrahepatic biliary system. More recently, the technetium 99m–labeled agents have essentially replaced the ^{131}I–rose bengal excretion test. The ^{99m}Tc–diethyl iminodiacetic acid (DIDA) is said to be superior to many other similar products and has the highest hepatocyte-extraction efficiency (48% to 56%). Experimental data suggest that this product is handled by the bilirubin transport system rather than by the pathway for clearing bile acids. The sensitivity of this test permits recognition of partial biliary obstruction because of structural abnormalities such as choledochal cyst or stenosis of the extrahepatic duct system. When complete obstruction exists, no activity is detected in the intestines. It remains to be seen whether the DIDA scan will differentiate all examples of severe intrahepatic cholestasis, especially those where bile flow into the intestines is absent yet patent extrahepatic ducts exist. Early in the course of neonatal cholestasis the degree of hepatocyte clearance of the radioisotope may reflect the underlying integrity of liver cell function and thereby suggest the underlying disease process. For example, hepatocyte function is believed to be well preserved early in the course of biliary atresia, and therefore prompt uptake by the liver coupled with failure to excrete the radioisotope into the intestines can be taken as presumptive evidence for an extrahepatic obstructing lesion (Fig. 19-1). Poor hepatocyte clearance indicates liver cell damage, which suggests intrahepatic disease, and patency of the extrahepatic ducts is confirmed by the detection of the isotope in the intestinal tract (Fig. 19-2).

Pathology

Many efforts have been made to divide neonatal cholestasis into subgroups based on certain specific features of the histologic picture with the hope of assigning a specific cause. The results have at times been confusing and have not solved the problem.

Attempts to consistently differentiate the two major categories (intrahepatic versus extrahepatic) of obstructive neonatal jaundice solely on the basis of histologic findings obtained by liver biopsy, either open or closed, improves with experience and can approach 95% accuracy. A summary of the typical histologic findings in intrahepatic versus extrahepatic causes is presented in Table 19-3. The findings are arranged in order of frequency and therefore significance. Some overlapping between these two major groups may occur. A common diagnostic error is often the result of misinterpretation of varying degrees of portal bile duct neoproliferative changes that occur in ''hepatitis'' and alpha-1-antitrypsin deficiency.

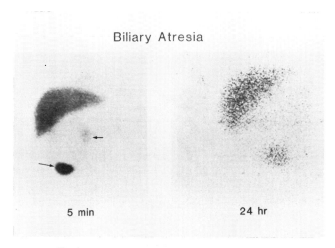

Biliary Atresia

5 min   24 hr

Fig. 19-1. ^{99m}Tc-DIDA (^{99m}Tc–diethyl iminodiacetic acid) images obtained after 5 minutes and again at 24 hours from a 2-month-old infant with complete cholestasis. The early image (at 5 minutes) shows excellent hepatic clearance of the isotope from the vascular pool suggesting intact hepatocyte function. Radioactivity is also seen in the kidney and bladder, *arrows*. The delayed image (24 hours) again shows radioactivity remaining in the liver and bladder, but none in the gastrointestinal tract. The diagnosis of biliary atresia was confirmed at surgery.

Open versus closed biopsy. Percutaneous liver biopsy has been employed with less hesitancy in the very young infant, thereby permitting accumulation of a sizable experience for review in this area.

In the absence of abnormal coagulation studies, percutaneous biopsy may safely be performed without significant (less than 1%) morbidity and without mortality. With experience, adequate tissue (more than three portal zones and central veins) can usually be obtained (Chapter 32). We generally are able to use some tissue for appropriate cultures (bacterial and viral), electron microscopy, and special qualitative chemical studies when needed. The concern regarding obtainment of representative tissue for evaluation by this technique remains, but the problem also exists after open biopsy, especially if the liver is cirrhotic and only a wedge of tissue is taken. Despite some of these shortcomings, a conservative approach using clinical, laboratory, and percutaneous liver biopsy remains the one of choice for the majority of infants during the first 2 to 3 months of life.

Unfortunately, not all patients with prolonged obstructive jaundice are candidates for percutaneous liver biopsy. The presence of a significant degree of ascites or of a coagulation defect resistant to correction with vitamin K and to fresh frozen plasma (10 ml/kg) calls for an open biopsy. The risk of postbiopsy bleeding is definitely increased in the face of advanced cirrhosis and a "stiff" capsule when a closed biopsy is done. The problem of obtaining representative tissue from a cirrhotic liver by the percutaneous route is significant, for penetration into the liver is made more difficult by subcapsular fibrosis and bile duct proliferation. Even when the operator appears to accomplish adequate depth of penetration, inadequate tissue may be obtained because of packing of the distal end of the biopsy needle with subcapsular fibrous tissue. Finally, in the face of suspected cirrhosis one could argue for resolving the diagnostic dilemma with minimal delay. In these cases, rapid clarification of the underlying lesion can best be accomplished by diagnostic laparotomy.

REFERENCES

Alagille, D.: Differentiation of extra- and intrahepatic neonatal cholestasis. In Javitt, N.B., editor: Neonatal hepatitis and biliary atresia, Department of Health, Education, and Welfare publ. no. 79-1296, pp. 187-190, 1979.

Andres, A.M., Lilly, J.R., Altman, R.P., and others: Alpha$_1$-fetoprotein in neonatal hepatobiliary disease, J. Pediatr. **91**:217-221, 1977.

Neonatal Hepatitis

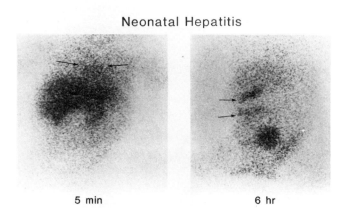

5 min   6 hr

Fig. 19-2. ^{99m}Tc-DIDA images obtained from a young infant with neonatal cholestatic syndrome. Substantial radioactivity remains in the vascular compartment *(arrows around the heart)* after 5 minutes—a possible indication of impaired hepatocyte function. Although biliary excretion is delayed, radioactivity does appear in the gastrointestinal tract by 6 hours, *arrows.* (From Ohi, R., Klingensmith, W.C., and Lilly, J.R.: Clin. Nucl. Med. **6**:297, 1981.)

Andres, J.M., Mathis, R.K., and Walker, W.A.: Liver diseases in infants. I. Developmental hepatology and mechanisms of liver dysfunction, J. Pediatr. **90:**686-697, 1977.

Balistreri, W.F., Suchy, F.J., Farrell, M.K., and Heubi, J.E.: Pathologic versus physiologic cholestasis: elevated serum concentration of a secondary bile acid in the presence of hepatobiliary disease, J. Pediatr. **98:**399-402, 1981.

Brough, A.J., and Bernstein, J.: Conjugated hyperbilirubinemia in early infancy, Human Pathol. **5:**507-516, 1974.

Danks, D.M., Campbell, P.E., Jack, I., and others: Studies of the aetiology of neonatal hepatitis and biliary atresia, Arch. Dis. Child. **52:**360-367, 1977.

Greene, H.L., Helinek, G., Moran, R., and O'Neill, J.: A diagnostic approach to prolonged obstructive jaundice by 24-hour collection of duodenal fluid, J. Pediatr. **95:**412-414, 1979.

Hays, D.M., Woolley, M.M., Synder, W.H., Jr., and others: Diagnosis of biliary atresia: relative accuracy of percutaneous liver biopsy, open liver biopsy and operative cholangiography, J. Pediatr. **71:**598-607, 1967.

Javitt, N.B.: Cholestasis in infancy: status report and conceptual approach, Gastroenterology **70:**1172-1181, 1976.

Javitt, N.B., Keating, J.P., Grand, R.J., and Harris, R.C.: Serum bile acid patterns in neonatal hepatitis and extrahepatic biliary atresia, J. Pediatr. **90:**736-739, 1977.

Johnston, D.I., Mowat, A.P., Orr, H., and Kohn, J.P.: Serum alpha-fetoprotein levels in extrahepatic biliary atresia, idiopathic neonatal hepatitis and alpha-1-antitrypsin deficiency (PiZ), Acta Paediatr. Scand. **65:**623-629, 1976.

Klingensmith, W.C., Fritzberg, A.R., Spitzer, V.M., and Koep, L.J.: Clinical comparison of ^{99m}Tc-diethyl-IDA and ^{99m}Tc-PIPIDA for evaluation of the hepatobiliary system, Radiology **134:**195-199, Jan. 1980.

Lawson, E.E., and Boggs, J.D.: Long-term follow-up of neonatal hepatitis: safety and value of surgical exploration, Pediatrics **53:**650-655, 1974.

Majd, M., Reba, R.C., and Altman, R.P.: Hepatobiliary scintigraphy with ^{99m}Tc-PIPIDA in the evaluation of neonatal jaundice, Pediatrics **67:**140-145, 1981.

Melhorn, D.K., Gross, S., and Izant, R.J., Jr.: The red cell hydrogen peroxide hemolysis test and vitamin E absorption in the differential diagnosis of jaundice in infancy, J. Pediatr. **81:**1082-1087, 1972.

Nahmias, A.J.: The TORCH complex, Hosp. Pract., pp. 65-72, May 1974.

O'Brien, M.L., Buist, N.R.M., and Murphey, W.H.: Neonatal screening for alpha₁-antitrypsin deficiency, J. Pediatr. **92:**1006-1010, 1978.

Poley, J.R., Smith, E.J., Boon, D.J., and others: Lipoprotein-X and the double ^{131}I-Rose Bengal test in the diagnosis of prolonged obstructive jaundice, J. Pediatr. Surg. **7:**660-669, 1972.

Shiraki, K.: Hepatic cell necrosis in the newborn, Am. J. Dis. Child. **119:**395-400, 1970.

Simon, J.B., and Poon, R.W.M.: Lipoprotein-X levels in extrahepatic versus intrahepatic cholestasis, Gastroenterology **75:**177-180, 1978.

Sveger, T.: Liver disease in alpha₁-antitrypsin deficiency detected by screening of 200,000 infants, N. Engl. J. Med. **294**(24):1316-1321, 1976.

Taylor, K.J.W., and Rosenfield, A.T.: Grey-scale ultrasonography in the differential diagnosis of jaundice, Arch. Surg. **112:**820-825, 1977.

Young, C.Y.: Serum 5'-nucleotidase in neonatal hepatitis and biliary atresia: preliminary observations, Pediatrics **50:**812-815, 1972.

TEXTBOOKS

Alagille, D., and Odièvre, M.: Liver and biliary tract disease in children, New York, 1979, John Wiley & Sons, Inc.

Chandra, R.S.: The liver and biliary system in infants and children, New York, 1979, Churchill-Livingston.

Javitt, N.B., editor: Neonatal hepatitis and biliary atresia: an international workshop, Department of Health, Education, and Welfare publication no. 79-1296, 1978.

Mowat, A.P.: Liver disorders in childhood, London, 1979, Butterworth & Co. (Pubs.) Ltd.

NEONATAL INTRAHEPATIC CHOLESTASIS
General considerations and pathophysiologic mechanisms

Neonatal cholestasis is recognized clinically by the presence of jaundice, hepatomegaly, dark-colored urine that stains the diaper, and stools that vary in color from normal to partially or completely acholic. The serum bilirubin reveals an elevation of the direct-reacting bilirubin fraction (greater than a range of 1.5 to 2 mg/dl). An elevated serum bile acid value of greater than 10.0 μM/L is confirmatory of this diagnosis. Assignment of the infant's illness to the broad category of intrahepatic cholestasis (versus that of extrahepatic cholestasis) implies that patency of the extrahepatic biliary system exists, though bile flow may be minimal or absent. In the neonate, numerous causes have been identified that lead either to an impairment of biliary secretion from the hepatocyte into the canaliculus or to a flow of bile from within the canaliculus to interlobular, and eventually the extrahepatic ducts. An identifiable etiology (infectious, metabolic, genetic, toxic, and so on) is found in up to 25% of cases (Table 19-1). However, within this large group of recognized causes, great nonspecificity exists between the results of laboratory and radiologic studies, as well as the appearance of the pathologic lesion seen on liver biopsy.

The mechanism by which intrahepatic cholestasis occurs is better understood for those examples in which known causes have been identified. Direct hepatocyte injury with nuclear or cytoplasmic organelle disruption, as seen with infections from herpesvirus and enterovirus, results in diminished hepatocyte adenosine triphosphate (ATP) production and often cell death. In other situations the combination of neonatal hypoxia and shock results in frank liver cell necrosis. In less severe insults, the primary injury is to the endoplasmic reticulum so that bile formation or its flow within the canaliculus is hindered. The accumulation of toxic intermediates, as occurs in inborn errors of metabolism (galactosemia, congenital fructose intolerance, tyrosinemia) impairs hepatocyte mitochondrial function, reduces available cellular energy, and leads to cholestasis. Once cholestasis develops, the accumulated bile acid metabolites within hepatocytes may in turn interfere with the canalicular bile flow. The deleterious impact upon the hepatocyte's energy-dependent system not only impairs bile formation but more than likely also reduces the transport of intrahepatocyte constituents of bile, resulting in the accumulation of bilirubin and bile acids within the hepatocytes (morphologic cholestasis). Any injury to the sinusoidal and intercellular surface of the liver plasma membrane (basolateral membrane) will damage the energy-dependent sodium-potassium ATPase pump and diminish bile flow. Bile acid uptake by the hepatocyte requires a functional carrier-mediated, sodium-dependent pump (symport). Bacterial endotoxins are believed to act primarily at the canalicular surface, affecting the bile salt–independent portion of bile flow. Again, accumulated bile salts, especially sulfated monohydroxy derivatives (lithocholic acid), may directly injure the canalicular membrane and are thought capable of impairing the contractile function of actin-containing myofibrils that surround the canaliculus.

The mechanism by which so-called idiopathic cases of neonatal intrahepatic cholestasis produce their biochemical and pathologic impact remains unknown, but the final common pathway of bile secretion or flow is likewise affected. It remains to be seen whether as-yet unrecognized maternal virus infections acquired in utero and passed to the fetus are responsible for this large group of unknown causes of cholestasis. Up to now the fetal acquisition of maternal hepatitis B virus disease is an unusual cause of neonatal cholestasis at least in this country, and hepatitis A virus disease likewise seems to be a most unusual cause.

Other pathophysiologic mechanisms have previously received consideration and certainly warrant continued study. One theory speculates that the primary event leading to cholestasis in the majority of cases may be a temporary (or permanent) defect in bile acid metabolism or bile acid transport, either genetically or environmentally acquired, that develops in utero. Such a defect could result in accumulation of monohydroxy bile acids within the liver, products known to cause cholestasis and, together with the reduction of bile flow, could in turn incite the noted hepatocyte response (lobular disarray, giant-cell transformation, and so on), as well as produce gross and ultrastructural aberrations of the intrahepatic and extrahepatic bile ducts. Serum sulfated lithocholate values are elevated in neonates with cholestasis from both intrahepatic and extrahepatic causes. Although sulfation is believed to be an effective detoxifying mechanism for cholestatic bile acids, recent animal studies have shown that they do not lose their cholestatic potential when conjugated with glycine as opposed to taurine.

The eventual pathologic lesion might reflect the temporal vulnerability of these developing hepatobiliary structures, a hypothesis consistent with the previously proposed concept that the entities "idiopathic" intrahepatic cholestasis, paucity of the interlobular bile ducts, and extrahepatic biliary atresia may in fact be part of a continuum, perhaps having a common cause. As previously mentioned, pathologic features of these entities may coexist in the same patient, either at the time of the initial diagnostic studies, later as the disease process evolves, or occasionally at autopsy. The observation that serum bile acid patterns (chenodeoxycholic/cholate) are similar in intrahepatic and extrahepatic causes of neonatal cholestasis is consistent with this hypothesis.

Another unproved hypothesis, which remains somewhat attractive, proposes that neonatal intrahepatic cholestasis may reflect liver damage caused by soluble antigen-antibody complexes that have been sequestered by the fetal reticuloendothelial system, particularly in the liver. A form of isoimmunization to fetal hepatocyte or bile duct epithelium proteins may occur in the mother, with formation of maternal antibodies or soluble antigen-antibody complexes then reaching the fetus through the placenta.

Perinatal or neonatal hepatitis from known infectious causes

General considerations. Neonatal infection may occur by transplacental spread, by the ascending route from vaginal or cervical structures into the amniotic fluid, or by swallowed contaminated products during delivery such as maternal blood or urine and later from breast milk or contaminated hands. Infectious agents particularly associated with neonatal intrahepatic cholestasis include cytomegalovirus (CMV), herpesvirus, rubella, echovirus 11, 14, or 19, coxsackievirus A or B, adenovirus, hepatitis B virus (HBV), syphilis spirochete, and toxoplasmosis sporozoon. The hepatocyte injury caused by these infecting agents ranges from massive hepatic necrosis (herpesvirus) to focal necrosis and mild inflammation as seen in cytomegalovirus disease or hepatitis B virus disease. Direct injury to hepatocyte organelles and the resulting compromise to energy-dependent functions is believed to be responsible for accumulation of intrahepatocyte bilirubin and bile acids and for canalicular bile stasis. In general, cholestasis from infective agents is suggested by the infant who feeds poorly, appears ill, and is failing to thrive.

Clinical findings. Clinical symptoms from these infectious causes usually appear in the first 2 weeks of life but may be delayed for as long as 2 to 3 months of age. Jaundice has been noted in the first 24 hours of postnatal life or may become obvious later after a temporary anicteric period. Loss of appetite, poor suck, lethargy, and vomiting are frequent clinical observations in the affected infant. Stool color may be normal to pale, but seldom acholic. Dark-colored urine that stains the diaper is usually reported. The liver is enlarged with a uniform, somewhat firm consistency. Splenomegaly is variable. For certain infectious agents, a maculopapular or petechial rash may be present. In less severe cases, failure to thrive may be the major complaint, jaundice subclinical, and the clue to underlying liver disease taken from the finding of hepatomegaly. Other unusual presentations also include hypoproteinemia with anasarca (nonhemolytic hydrops), or hemorrhagic disease of the neonate.

Laboratory findings. The blood count may show normal results, or neutropenia. Thrombocytopenia is common especially in very ill infants, and signs of mild hemolysis may be present suggesting disseminated intravascular coagulation. Mixed hyperbilirubinemia, elevated transaminases, abnormal clotting studies, mild to severe acidosis, and elevated cord blood or serum IgM levels (greater than 60 mg/dl) are consistent with congenital in-

fection. Viral cultures should be obtained of throat, urine, stool, and cerebrospinal fluid. Specific serologic tests comparing infant and maternal levels are usful (TORCH titers), as are skull and long-bone roentgenograms, in which one looks for intracranial calcifications or "celery stalking" in the metaphysis of the humerus, fibula, or tibia respectively.

Pathology. The histologic features on liver biopsy tissue obtained by the percutaneous route are likely to be consistent with those of intrahepatic causes of cholestasis, but only occasionally will the findings suggest a specific infectious cause. Exceptions include the presence of intracytoplasmic inclusions of cytomegalovirus (Cowdry type I bodies) in hepatocytes or bile duct epithelial cells, whereas intranuclear acidophilic inclusions strongly implicate herpesvirus infection of the liver. A variable degree of lobular disarray is typical. The normal cordlike arrangement of liver cells is lost because of ballooned pale hepatocytes, giant-cell transformation, focal necrosis, and collapse of the reticulin-supporting network. Portal changes are not striking, but modest neoductular proliferation and mild fibrosis can be seen in some cases.

Differential diagnosis. Infectious causes of intrahepatic cholestasis need to be especially differentiated from genetic-metabolic causes (inborn errors), since the clinical presentations within these groups of conditions may be very similar. Particularly galactosemia, congenital fructose intolerance, and tyrosinemia should be immediately considered and ruled out by selective tests (see elsewhere). Alpha-1-antitrypsin deficiency and cystic fibrosis may be alternative possiblilities. Specific physical features should be sought when one is considering certain familial causes of intrahepatic cholestasis (Alagille's syndrome), or if consideration is being given to the diagnosis of Menke's syndrome or Zellweger's syndrome. In contrast to the aforementioned differential diagnostic considerations, infants with extrahepatic causes for cholestasis are usually born after a term gestation, are seldom ill, and have stools that are persistently acholic in appearance, but the enlarged liver is firm to hard. In up to 95% of cases, when these clinical aspects are combined with the histologic appearance of the liver, intrahepatic cholestasis from proved or presumed infectious agents will be correctly considered without the need for exploratory surgery.

Treatment. Most forms of viral neonatal hepatitis are treated symptomatically by the correction of existing fluid and electrolyte disturbances, coagulation abnormalities (vitamin K, partial exchange transfusion, fresh frozen plasma) and provision of adequate calories by the oral or peripheral route. If cholestasis remains persistent, additional medical treatment is needed (see "idiopathic" neonatal cholestasis, p. 526). Steroids are probably contraindicated, and specific antiviral agents have not produced consistent benefit. Obviously, penicillin should be employed if syphilis is suspected. Specific antibiotic treatment is needed for those rare cases of bacterial hepatitis, or if an associated urinary tract infection is etiologic. Hyperimmune hepatitis B serum (0.05 ml) is strongly recommended to neonates born of an HBV-infected mother.

Prognosis. Multiorgan involvement is commonly associated with neonatal hepatitis caused by viral agents and, unfortunately, portends a poor outcome. Death is from hepatic failure, intractable acidosis, or intracranial hemorrhage, especially in herpesvirus and echovirus disease, but exceptional in congenital cytomegalovirus or rubella infections. Hepatitis B virus disease may be a rare cause of fulminant neonatal viral hepatitis. On the other hand, recovery from such transplacental acquired diseases may be complete, or with sequelae, especially neurologic. Persisting liver disease varies from mild chronic hepatitis to portal fibrosis or even cirrhosis. Chronic cholestasis may lead to dental enamel hypoplasia, biliary rickets, severe pruritus, and xanthoma.

Herpesvirus

In utero infection is recognized at birth by the cutaneous presence of grouped vesicles, early onset seizures, and hypothermia with mild to absent icterus. Occasional survivors of this form of herpesvirus infection are reported but with high incidence of neurologic sequelae (50% to 80%).

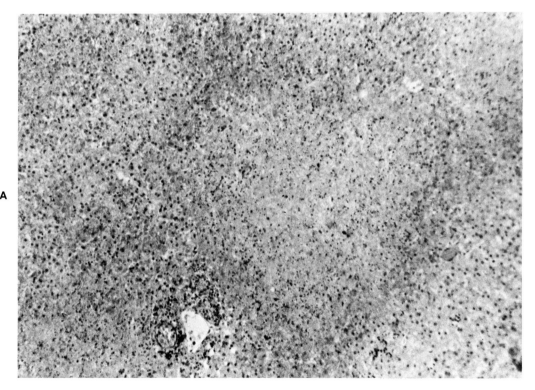

Fig. 19-3. Neonatal herpesvirus hepatitis in a 1-month-old infant dying of disseminated neonatal herpesvirus disease. **A,** Liver tissue shows focal coagulative necrosis with minimal inflammatory response. The infant's clinical features were primarily those of gastrointestinal bleeding with sepsis, and jaundice was minimal. Subsequent inspection of the perineum of the infant's mother showed herpetic lesions, from which herpesvirus was grown in tissue culture. (Courtesy G. Mierau, research technologist, The Children's Hospital, Denver.)   *Continued.*

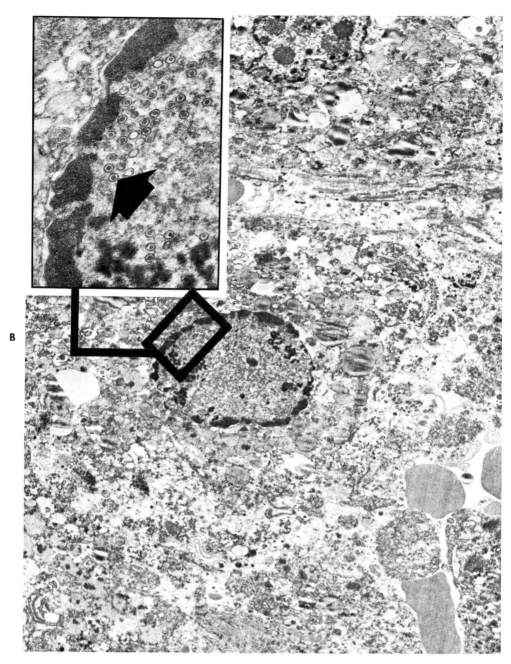

Fig. 19-3, cont'd. **B,** Electron microscopy demonstrates the characteristic intranuclear inclusions, *arrow,* compatible with particles of the herpes group of virus obtained from the liver tissue.

Perinatally acquired disease from maternal genital herpes often presents at 1 to 3 weeks of age with a shocklike picture, pallor, lethargy, spontaneous hemorrhage, and seizures. Jaundice becomes apparent almost simultaneously with the cutaneous manifestations. Death is rapid because of a combination of disseminated intravascular coagula- tion, hemorrhage, and hepatic coma. The patho- logic appearance of the liver shows coagulative necrosis with intracellular inclusions (Fig. 19-3). Treatment with vidarabine (ara-A) has not been of proved benefit. Delivery of an at-risk infant by cesarean section is indicated when maternal geni- tal herpes exists.

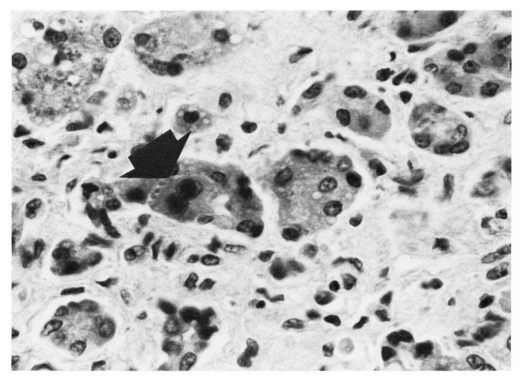

Fig. 19-4. Congenital cytomegalovirus hepatitis. Liver tissue of an autopsy specimen from a 1-month-old child presenting with petechiae, hepatosplenomegaly, and jaundice shows the viral inclusion within a bile duct epithelial cell, *arrow*.

Cytomegalovirus hepatitis

The liver injury caused by this agent may reflect isolated organ involvement or be part of the more typical global presentation that includes petechial rash, jaundice, hepatosplenomegaly, microcephaly, retinopathy, hemolytic anemia, thrombocytopenia, and intracerebral calcifications. Cytomegalovirus may be acquired in utero, or at birth from swallowed contaminated fluids, or during the neonatal period from exposure to infected maternal breast milk, saliva, or urine.

When neonatal hepatitis is an isolated manifestation, hepatomegaly and jaundice are the prominent clinical findings. A liver biopsy specimen shows variable inflammation, deranged lobular architecture with ballooned liver cells, and rarely giant-cell transformation. When present, intracytoplasmic inclusions (Cowdry type I bodies) in hepatocytes or bile duct epithelial cells are probably diagnostic (Fig. 19-4). The diagnosis may also be made in the absence of histologic proof when either in utero cytomegalovirus is grown from neonatal secretions (saliva, urine) or a rise in indirect hemagglutination titers is demonstrated. A pronounced elevation in the alkaline phosphatase has been noted in neonatal cytomegalovirus disease.

The prognosis is poor in those infants manifesting cytomegalovirus septicemia with multiorgan involvement. Portal fibrosis, with or without neoductular proliferation and at times biliary cirrhosis, evolves in those examples of isolated hepatic involvement. Unfortunately, no specific treatment is available.

Congenital rubella hepatitis

Hepatomegaly and jaundice, when noted in association with other congenital anomalies (cataracts, microcephaly, cardiac lesions), are very suggestive of congenital rubella. Liver involvement is not always found despite the presence of other organ anomalies. The hepatic lesion shows minimal focal hepatocyte damage, cholestasis, portal inflammation, and, in unusual cases, significant portal fibrosis. The diagnosis is made by

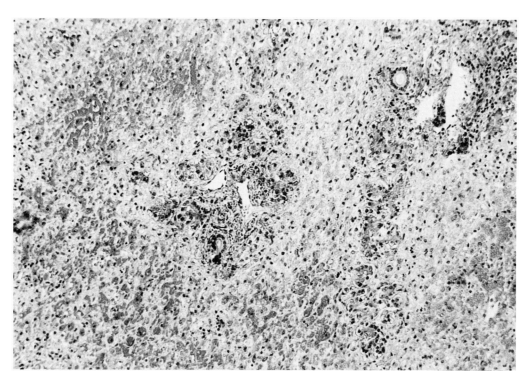

Fig. 19-5. Liver tissue from an infant dying of severe hepatic necrosis and failure caused by acquired (post–exchange transfusion) HB-Ag disease. Massive hepatocyte necrosis with minimal inflammation is seen in the pathologic specimen.

serologic studies and in some cases by virus isolation.

Neonatal hepatitis B virus disease

Infection with this agent may occur at any time during perinatal life, but the greatest risk to the neonate occurs when acute maternal disease with hepatitis B virus occurs either during the last trimester of pregnancy, or at the time of delivery. Most often neonatal acquisition occurs when contaminated maternal body fluids (blood) is swallowed during delivery or later from saliva or from serosanguineous secretions coming out of an injured nipple in breast-fed babies.

The neonatal liver disease caused by hepatitis-B virus is extremely variable. Fulminant hepatic necrosis has been reported, particularly with the use of intrapartum or postpartum transfusions of infected blood or blood products. In such cases rapidly progressive jaundice, stupor, shrinking liver size, and coagulation abnormalities dominate the clinical picture. Respiratory and circulatory failure follows soon thereafter. Histologically, the liver shows massive hepatocyte necrosis, collapse of the

reticulum framework, minimal inflammation, and occasionally pseudoacinar structures of the remaining hepatocytes (Fig. 19-5). Rare survivors are reported with restitution of the liver architecture toward a near-normal appearance.

More commonly, less severe examples of neonatal hepatitis B virus disease produce focal hepatocyte necrosis and mild portal inflammatory changes. Cholestasis is both intracellular and canalicular. Chronic persistent hepatitis may follow for many (5 to 7) years with serologic evidence of persistent antigenemia (HBsAg) and mildly elevated transaminases and then spontaneously resolve. Progression to liver cirrhosis is most unusual with this form of neonatal liver disease. Since infants born of mothers with markers of infectivity (HBsAg, HBeAg, HBcAb, DNA polymerase) are at high risk to become chronic carriers, they should receive hyperimmune hepatitis B serum (0.05 ml) immediately after delivery and repeated at least at 1 month of age. Three doses of hepatitis B vaccine (0.5 ml) can then be given by intramuscular injection starting at 2 to 3 months of age. The second dose is given 1 month and the third dose 6 months after the initial dose. The present recommendation of the American Academy of Pediatrics Committee on Infectious Diseases is that mothers with hepatitis B virus markers of infectivity not breast-feed their newborns, provided that artificial formulas and adequate refrigeration are available. If hepatitis B virus is locally endemic, as in underdeveloped nations, such mothers should be permitted to breast-feed their infants. With the availability of the new hepatitis B vaccine these recommendations will probably be altered in the near future.

Other neonatal viral hepatitis agents

Fulminant hepatic necrosis has been associated with enteroviruses, particularly echoviruses 11, 14, and 19 as well as coxsackievirus B. In addition, adenovirus and varicella have produced a similar clinicopathologic picture. An underlying defect in the infant's immunologic system deserves consideration in these exceptional cases. The diagnosis is best made by proper virologic and serologic studies of both mother and infant.

Syphilis

In utero acquired syphilis is easily recognized by the findings of skin rash, bony changes, and hepatomegaly. Jaundice is present and the liver tissue reveals significant perilobular and interlobular fibrosis with scattered round-cell infiltration. In less classic examples, the diagnosis can be confirmed by positive serologic testing when liver biopsy material shows only nonspecific features of viral hepatitis (focal necrosis, portal inflammation, and minimal or focal fibrosis). Severe in utero hepatic involvement from syphilis should be suspected in a neonate presenting with nonhemolytic hydrops.

Toxoplasmosis

Although many infants with congenital toxoplasmosis are jaundiced, specific hepatic findings are not common. Features of cholestasis may be the result of the septicemia (toxins?), rather than direct hepatic injury by the organism. Rarely does the liver show fibrosis or cirrhosis, with a portal mononuclear infiltrate being most common. The presence of microcephaly, choreoretinitis, and intracranial calcifications strongly point to toxoplasmosis as etiologic, and a positive dye test (Sabin-Feldman) confirms the diagnosis. Hemagglutinating antibodies and fluorescent antibodies rise early and persist thereafter. Specific toxoplasmosis IgM antibodies in the infant are also diagnostic. Direct treatment for this infection employs sulfadiazine (100 to 150 mg/kg/day) and pyrimethamine (1 mg/kg/day) for 30 days.

Neonatal bacterial hepatitis

Most bacterial infections are transplacental from intercurrent amnionitis, arising from ascending spread from intercurrent vaginal or cervical infection. The onset is abrupt, usually within 48 to 72 hours of life, and signs of sepsis manifested by noticeable lethargy or shock. Jaundice, which appears early, is seen in 25% of cases and is of a "mixed" variety. The liver rapidly enlarges and histologic features show a diffuse hepatitis, with or without microabscess or macroabscess formation. The most common organisms are *Escherichia coli, Listeria monocytogenes,* and group B streptococci. Isolated neonatal liver abscesses from *E. coli* or *Staphylococcus aureus* are often associated with a history of umbilical vein catheterization. Bacterial hepatitis and neonatal liver abscesses require large-dose specific antibiotic treatment and rarely surgical drainage. Deaths are very common, but those fortunate survivors show no long-term consequences of the liver disease.

Neonatal jaundice with urinary tract infection

The typical appearance of jaundice in these infants is between the second and fourth weeks of life. Most cases are males, and a history of decreased appetite and lethargy is reported. Fever may be present. Stools are normal to partially acholic in appearance. Jaundice generally follows an anicteric period and hepatomegaly is invariably present on the physical examination. Except for the pronounced hyperbilirubinemia (mixed variety), other liver function tests may be normal or minimally deranged. Leukocytosis, however, is present and pyuria confirmed by culture techniques. The liver histologic appearance shows cholestasis with variable neoductular proliferation, minimal fibrosis, and a slight inflammatory response. The mechanism for the liver impairment is unknown, though the toxic action of bacterial products (endotoxins) on canalicular bile flow has been incriminated. Treatment of the urinary tract infection leads to a prompt resolution of the cholestasis without hepatic sequelae. Radiographic and urologic studies to rule out structural anomalies within the genitourinary tract are mandatory.

REFERENCES

Balagtas, R.C., Bell, C.E., Edwards, L.D., and Levin, S.: Risk of local and systemic infections associated with umbilical vein catheterization: a prospective study in 86 newborn patients, Pediatrics **48:**359-367, 1971.

Balistreri, W.F., Tabor, E., and Gerety, R.J.: Negative serology for hepatitis A and B viruses in 18 cases of neonatal cholestasis, Pediatrics **66:**269-271, 1980.

Bernstein, J., and Brown, A.K.: Sepsis and jaundice in early infancy, Pediatrics **29:**873-882, 1962.

Boyer, J.L.: Newer concepts of mechanisms of hepatocytic bile formation, Physiol. Rev. **60:**303-326, 1980.

Bulova, S.I., Schwartz, E., and Harrer, W.V.: Hydrops fetalis and congenital syphilis, Pediatrics **49:**285-287, 1972.

Dresler, S., and Linder, D.: Noncirrhotic portal fibrosis following neonatal cytomegalic inclusion disease, J. Pediatr. **93:**887-888, 1978.

Dupuy, J.M.: Hepatitis B in children. II. Study of children born to chronic HBs-Ag carrier mothers, J. Pediatr. **92:**200-204, 1978.

Escobedo, M.B., Barton, L.L., Marshall, R.E., and Zarkowsky, H.: The frequency of jaundice in neonatal bacterial infections, Clin. Pediatr. **13:**656-657, 1974.

Esterly, J.R., Slusser, R.J., and Ruebner, B.H.: Hepatic lesions in the congenital rubella syndrome, J. Pediatr. **71:**676-685, 1967.

Gerety, R.J., and Schweitzer, I.L.: Viral hepatitis type B during pregnancy, the neonatal period and infancy, J. Pediatr. **90:**368-374, 1977.

Hamilton, J.R., and Sass-Kortsak, A.: Jaundice associated with severe bacterial infection in young infants, J. Pediatr. **63:**121-132, 1963.

Hughes, J.R., Wilfert, C.M., Moore, M., and others: Echovirus 14 infection associated with fatal neonatal hepatic necrosis, Am. J. Dis. Child. **123:**61-67, 1972.

Lake, A.M., Lauer, B.A., Clark, J.C., and others: Enterovirus infections in neonates, J. Pediatr. **89:**787-791 1976.

Nahmias, A.J., and Visintine, A.M.: Herpes simplex. In Remington, J.S., and Klein, J.O., editors: Infectious diseases of the fetus and newborn infant, Philadelphia, 1976, W.B. Saunders Co.

Ng, S.H., and Rawstron, J.R.: Urinary tract infections presenting with jaundice, Arch. Dis. Child. **46:**173-176, 1971.

Numazaki, Y., Oshima, T., Tanaka, A., and others: Demonstration of IgG EA (early antigen and IgM MA (membrane antigen) antibodies in CMV infection of healthy infants and in those with liver disease, J. Pediatr. **97:**545-549, 1980.

Oppenheimer, E.H., and Hardy, J.B.: Congenital syphilis in the newborn infant: clinical and pathologic observations in recent cases, Johns Hopkins Med. J. **129:**63-82, 1971.

Philip, A.G.S., and Larson, E.J.: Overwhelming neonatal infection with ECHO 19 virus, J. Pediatr. **82:**391-397, 1973.

Phillips, M.J., Oda, M., Mak, E., and others: Microfilament dysfunction as a possible cause of intrahepatic cholestasis, Gastroenterology **69:**48-58, 1975.

Prince, A.M.: Use of hepatitis B immune globulin: reassessment needed, N. Engl. J. Med. **299:**198-199, 1978.

Saxoni, F., Lapatsanis, P., and Pantelakis, S.N.: Congenital syphilis: a description of 18 cases and re-examination of an old but ever-present disease, Clin. Pediatr. **6:**687-691, 1967.

Shiraki, K., Yoshihara, N., Sakurai, M., and others: Acute hepatitis B in infants born to carrier mothers with the antibody to hepatitis B e antigen, J. Pediatr. **97:**768-770 1980.

Strauss, L., and Bernstein, J.: Neonatal hepatitis in congenital rubella, Arch. Pathol. **86:**317-327, 1968.

White, J.G.: Fulminating infection with herpes-simplex virus in premature and newborn infants, N. Engl. J. Med. **269:**455-460, 1963.

Wyllie, R., and Fitzgerald, J.: Bacterial cholangitis in a 10-week-old infant with fever of undetermined origin, Pediatrics **65:**164-167, 1980.

Zimmerman, H.J., moderator: Clinical Conference: Jaundice due to bacterial infection, Gastroenterology **77:**362-374, 1979.

Zimmerman, H.J.: Intrahepatic cholestasis, Arch. Intern. Med. **139:**1038-1045, 1979.

Inborn errors of metabolism and familial, "toxic," and miscellaneous causes of intrahepatic cholestasis

Within this heterogenous grouping of causes of intrahepatic cholestasis reside critical conditions that demand both early diagnosis and institution of specific dietary treatment if reversal of the liver injury and clinical symptoms is to occur. Also of importance within this broad group of conditions are entities that will require genetic counseling to parents once the diagnosis is established.

Galactosemia, hereditary fructose intolerance, and tyrosinemia

Intrahepatic cholestasis attributable to these inborn errors of metabolism presents as part of a distinct clinical syndrome. Typically vomiting, lethargy, poor feeding, and irritability often precede the appearance of jaundice. Seizures caused by hypoglycemia may occur. Firm hepatomegaly is constant, and not surprisingly the infant is considered to be septic. Indeed, gram-negative organisms can be cultured from the blood in perhaps over 25% of cases, especially in infants with galactosemia. Liver tissue obtained percutaneously will suggest "metabolic liver disease" by the presence of steatosis, canalicular bile plugging, prominent pseudoacinar arrangement of hepatocytes, and periportal fibrosis in the absence of an acute inflammatory process (Fig. 19-6). These three entities are discussed in detail in the section on metabolic liver disease as causes of cirrhosis (see Chapter 24). If hypoglycemia is refractory, hypopituitarism with jaundice should be considered in the differential diagnosis.

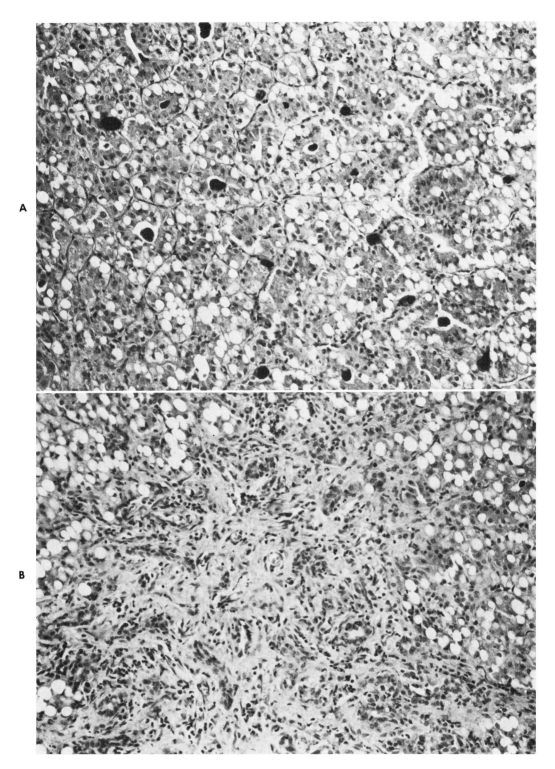

Fig. 19-6. Neonatal ''metabolic'' liver disease. This liver biopsy section was obtained from a 2-month-old infant with jaundice, failure to thrive, hypoglycemia, hypophosphatemia, and increased amounts of urinary metabolites of tyrosine. **A,** Lobular disarray with pseudoglandular formation, steatosis, bile plugging in intralobular ducts, and minimal inflammation characterize this type of hepatocyte injury. Absence of hepatic fructose-1-aldolase was biochemically confirmed. **B,** Unfortunately, significant portal fibrosis is already present at this young age.

Alpha-1-antitrypsin deficiency

In two large prospective newborn screening programs, neonatal cholestasis was found associated with homozygous alpha-1-antitrypsin deficiency (PiZZ) in 11% and 5% of cases respectively. Retrospective investigation of a heterogenous group of pediatric liver patients revealed an incidence from 5% to 35% to be associated with alpha-1-antitrypsin deficiency.

The infant with neonatal cholestasis and alpha-1-antitrypsin deficiency lacks specific clinical features. Rather, the neonate homozygous for this condition appears at added risk to other "triggering" causes of liver injury. In many instances the events that expose the infant's vulnerability take place in utero, in that up to 45% of these affected newborns are reported to be small for gestational age. After delivery, a history of poor feeding with mild failure to thrive and intermittent irritability are common symptoms that accompany the discovery of icterus at 3 to 12 weeks of age. Jaundice has been noted both earlier and later in other cases. Since alpha-1-antitrypsin deficiency has now been reported in association with extrahepatic causes of neonatal cholestasis (biliary atresia, severe hypoplasia of common bile duct), serum quantitative levels of this glycoprotein is mandatory in all cases of neonatal cholestasis.

Liver biopsy material obtained from symptomatic patients during the neonatal period shows a continuum of disease from that suggesting intrahepatic disease to that of extrahepatic causes of cholestasis. The long-term prognosis may correlate with the early histologic lesion, portal fibrosis, and neoductular proliferation imparting a poorer prognosis. In some cases reduced numbers of interlobular bile ducts may also be noted. One should remember that alpha-1-antitrypsin globules may not be observed in hepatocytes before 8 to 10 weeks of life (Fig. 19-7). A more complete discussion of alpha-1-antitrypsin deficiency disease is given in Chapter 24.

Cystic fibrosis

This autosomal recessive disease only on rare occasion presents as cholestasis in the neonatal period and then most often in association with meconium ileus. In such cases the diagnosis should not be difficult. On the other hand, a positive family history of cystic fibrosis, or persistent absence of stool trypsin and chymotrypsin, favors the diagnosis when meconium ileus is not part of the early clinical presentation. Otherwise, the lack of adequate sweat production in the neonate often causes delay in the diagnosis. Laboratory studies show nonspecific liver-function abnormalities, but the finding of a mild anemia or hypoproteinemia should be taken as clues to the underlying diagnosis of cystic fibrosis. These latter abnormalities are particularly common in infants fed a soybean-based formula or fed exclusively on the breast.

Liver biopsy material obtained from the jaundiced neonate with cystic fibrosis most often reveals both intrahepatocyte and canalicular cholestasis, nonspecific periportal alterations, neoductular proliferation, widening of the portal zones by fibrous tissue, and chronic inflammatory cells. In general, the lobular architecture is preserved. Giant cells are rarely noted. Within this nonspecific histologic picture, only the additional finding (in less than 50% of cases) of excess biliary mucus appearing as inspissated granular eosinophilic material within the interlobular bile ducts is strongly suggestive of cystic fibrosis (Fig. 19-8). Although a nonspecific finding, the presence of steatosis should always suggest a metabolic-genetic cause such as cystic fibrosis. Excessive amounts of hemosiderin within hepatocytes have also been taken as evidence of cystic fibrosis (see Fig. 27-5). At other times features seen in the liver biopsy may be indistinguishable from extrahepatic biliary obstruction, and in fact upon surgical exploration, plugging of the common bile duct by sludged inspissated viscid bile may be found. Lastly, the best known lesion in cystic fibrosis, focal biliary cirrhosis, may be present early in life (10%) but rarely manifests liver function abnormalities and therefore seldom is a cause of neonatal cholestasis. Unless the infant succumbs to other gastrointestinal complications (meconium ileus), the neonatal cholestasis of cystic fibrosis invariably resolves and generally does so without liver damage. It seems reasonable that some of these infants in fact develop focal biliary cirrhosis that progresses to the more serious entity of multinodular biliary cirrhosis. The latter eventually causes symptoms in 5% to 10% of cases, usually in the teen-ager or young adult. Occasionally signs of portal hypertension and hepatic decompensation present before 10 years of age. A more complete discussion of cystic fibrosis and the hepatobiliary disease appears in Chapter 28.

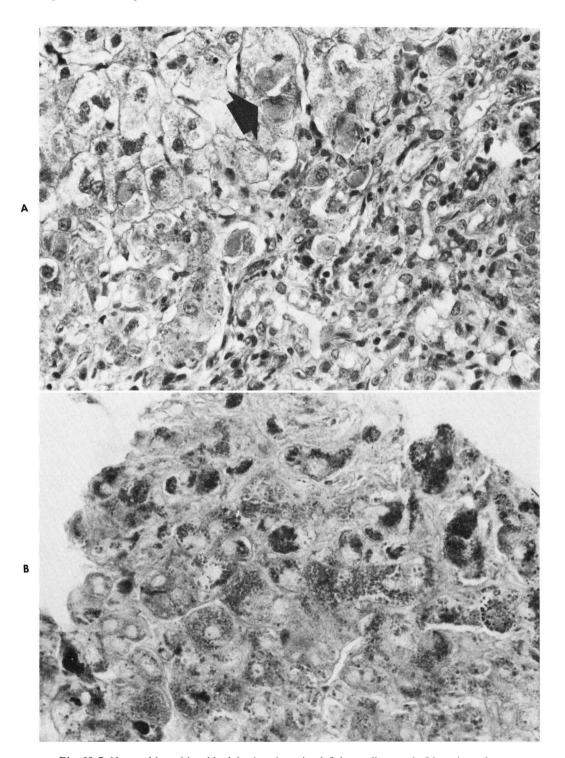

Fig. 19-7. Neonatal hepatitis with alpha-1-antitrypsin–deficiency disease. **A,** Liver tissue from an infant with cholestatic jaundice revealed lobular injury and hepatocyte disorganization, giant cell formation, cholestasis, and eosinophilic deposits, *arrow,* suggesting the diagnosis. **B,** Periodic acid–Schiff (PAS) stain clearly demonstrates the hepatocyte accumulation of alpha-1-antitrypsin. Gradual resolution of the jaundice occurred, but clinical signs of cirrhosis became evident by the time the child was 2 years of age.

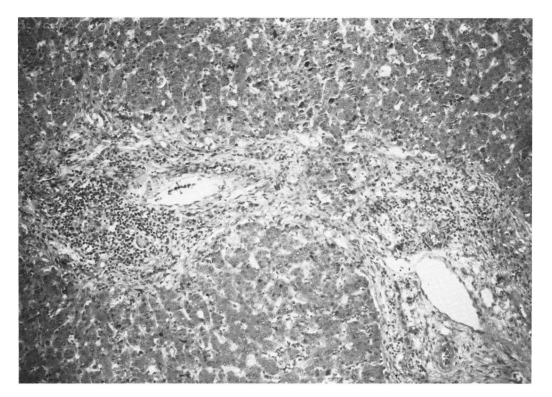

Fig. 19-8. Liver disease in a jaundiced infant with cystic fibrosis. The liver biopsy section shows pronounced canalicular bile plugging. The portal zones are widened by a combination of excess collagen, neoductular proliferation, and a round cell infiltrate. The lobular architecture is preserved and giant cells are absent. These findings mimic those noted in extrahepatic causes of neonatal cholestasis.

Niemann-Pick disease

Prolonged cholestatic jaundice in the neonatal period may be the earliest manifestation of this disorder of sphingomyelin metabolism. It is not surprising that the typical foamy-appearing Niemann-Pick cells seen in liver biopsy material are occasionally mistaken for hepatocyte giant-cell transformation and the cholestasis attributed to other causes of neonatal liver disease (Fig. 19-9). Mild lobular disarray and cholestasis may be the only abnormalities seen in various portions of the liver tissue. Laboratory tests reveal modest elevation of serum bilirubin (mixed variety) and aminotransferases (SGOT and SGPT). Cholestasis is clinically incomplete, and stools are pale to normally colored; thus confusion is eliminated with extrahepatic causes. The jaundice generally disappears within 3 to 6 months. The neurologic sequelae rather than the liver involvement inevitably determine the eventual prognosis (see also Chapter 24).

Byler's disease

This familial and often fatal form of severe cholestasis can present in the neonatal period. A history of previously affected children is the most important clinical information. Consanguinity is common, and many cases have been reported in the Amish kindred in this country and from small communities in southern France. An intrahepatic process is suggested early, since the cholestasis is usually incomplete, with partially colored stools being noted. Clinically, hepatomegaly and early (3 to 4 months) pruritus are present in these jaundiced infants. Elevated serum bilirubin levels, bile acids, alkaline phosphatase, and prolonged retention of Bromsulphalein in the face of a normal serum cholesterol level is the typical biochemical pattern noted in laboratory screening of these patients. Recently, an unusual bile acid, hyocholic acid, has been found in these patients but not in nonfamilial cases of cholestatic liver disease. The

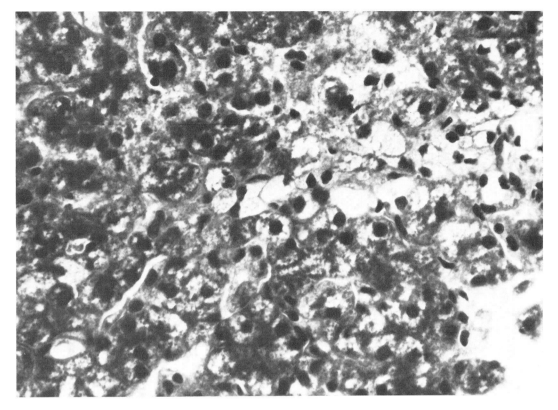

Fig. 19-9. Niemann-Pick disease. Foamy Kupffer cells are clustered among near-normal hepatocytes. Biopsy specimen was obtained from a 2-month-old infant with mild cholestasis. Diagnosis was confirmed by white blood cell enzyme analysis. (Trichrome stain, ×450.)

significance of this observation remains to be determined, since we have found hyocholic acid to be more related to the severity of the liver damage than to the type of cholestatic liver disease. Histologic examination of liver tissue shows pronounced cholestasis, widened portal zones with fibrous tissue, and chronic inflammatory cells. Giant cells are infrequently reported. Bile ducts are normal, decreased, or proliferative. Features of cirrhosis may be found in many after one year of age. The disease is refractory to the standard therapeutic measures employed in the treatment of intrahepatic cholestasis, the course being punctuated by persistent or recurrent bouts of jaundice associated with severe pruritus typically triggered by intercurrent infections. Failure to thrive becomes evident, and progression to cirrhosis with death caused by liver failure is usual before 3 to 6 years of age. Some children survive to adolescence. Somewhat similar clinical and biochemical manifestations have been reported in children from

a strongly consanguineous group of North American Indians living in Canada.

Other, rare familial-genetic disorders associated with neonatal cholestasis syndrome and normal or increased numbers of intrahepatic bile ducts

> Zellweger's (hepatocerebrorenal) syndrome (Fig. 19-10)
> Turner's syndrome (XO) (Fig. 19-11) or mosaic with isocentric X chromosome
> Hereditary lymphedema with recurrent cholestasis (Aagenaes's syndrome)
> Generalized hemangiomatosis
> Benign recurrent familial cholestasis

Each of these conditions should be recognized by the characteristic physical features, family history, or chromosomal studies. Cholestasis is usually mild; stools are normal or partially acholic. Pathologic features on liver biopsy are not spe-

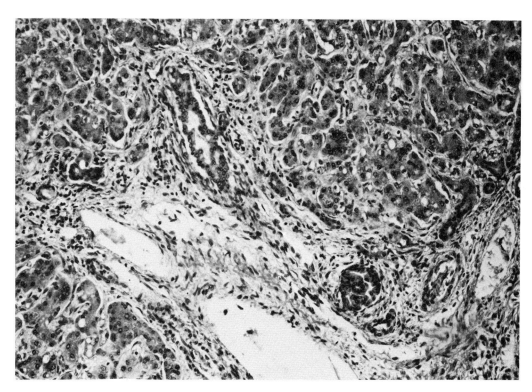

Fig. 19-10. Liver tissue obtained at autopsy from a neonate with the clinical features of cerebro-hepatorenal syndrome of Zellweger. Cholestatic jaundice was present till death, with only mild alterations of other liver function tests. The biopsy section shows lobular disarray, pseudoglandular orientation of some hepatocytes, mild portal fibrosis, and normal proliferating bile ducts.

cific. Infants with Zellweger's syndrome have a poor overall prognosis and usually die very young. The prognosis for the remaining conditions will depend on the severity of injury to the other organs involved.

"Toxic" causes for neonatal cholestasis

Neonatal "gut shock" conditions. Perinatal events that result in hypoperfusion of the gastrointestinal tract (hypoxia, anoxia, shock) not infrequently are followed in 1 to 2 weeks by evolving cholestasis in addition to laboratory evidence that indicates mild hepatocyte injury (elevated aminotransferases). This sequence of events is particularly observed in premature infants with severe congenital heart disease or the respiratory distress syndrome complicated by severe hypoxia, hypoglycemia, shock, and acidosis. Other perinatal conditions that also predispose to subsequent cholestasis (in from 25% to 50% of cases) are the gastrointestinal lesions of ruptured omphalocele, gastroschisis, and necrotizing enterocolitis. The mechanism for the cholestasis is unclear, but he-

patocyte and canalicular injury secondary to intestinal "toxic" products gaining access to the portal or systemic circulation is suggested. This is not surprising, since these gastrointestinal conditions are often associated with injury to the intestinal microcirculation—events that lead to increased permeability of the damaged mucosa to bacterial antigens, toxic degradation products, or dietary antigens.

The role of anesthetic agents, a variety of medications, intercurrent septic episodes, and hyperalimentation solutions are frequently complicating aspects in the histories of such neonates, all having direct or potentiating properties to produce cholestasis.

Liver-function studies reveal mixed hyperbilirubinemia, surprisingly high gamma glutamyl transpeptidase or alkaline phosphatase values, but only mild elevation of aminotransferase levels. Stools are normal to pale but seldom persistently acholic. Liver biopsy reveals cholestasis in hepatocytes and in canalicular structures. Mild portal and stellate fibrosis is commonly seen in the ab-

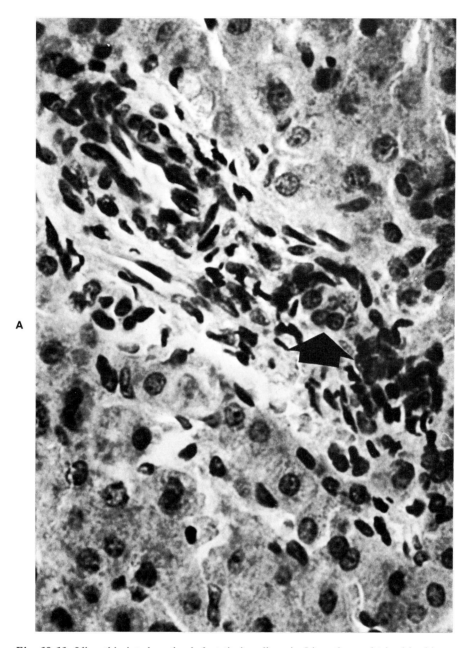

Fig. 19-11. Idiopathic intrahepatic cholestatic jaundice. **A,** Liver tissue obtained by biopsy was deeply bile stained. The portal region shows minimal inflammation with either absent or abnormal bile ducts, *arrow*. This percutaneous liver biopsy section was taken from a 3-week-old child with clinical features of Turner's syndrome (XO) who had persistent obstructive jaundice since birth. The infant's stools were continuously acholic, and the urine was devoid of urobilinogen. Serum bilirubin levels were as great as 17 mg/dl, with a predominance of the direct-reacting fraction. Hepatosplenomegaly was present on physical examination, though evidence of isoimmunization or anemia was absent. An attempt to increase bile flow with cholecystokinin was unsuccessful. Tentative diagnosis was that of early development of hypoplasia of the intrahepatic bile ducts.

Continued

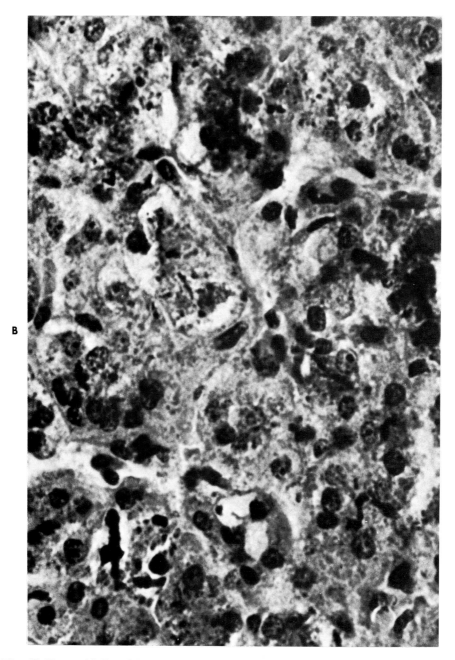

Fig. 19-11, cont'd. **B,** High-power view of a liver lobule in **A** shows the severe cholestatic jaundice within hepatocytes and canaliculi.

sence of significant inflammatory response. At times eosinophils may dominate the inflammatory lesion (Fig. 19-12, *A*). The lobular architecture is usually preserved and hepatocyte necrosis uncommon in milder cases. Neoductular proliferation is likewise absent or minimal.

Differential diagnosis. A history of premature birth associated with respiratory, metabolic, or anatomic intestinal complications immediately fa-

vor an intrahepatic cause for the cholestasis. In addition, the presence of normal or fluctuating-colored stool is reassuring in this regard. As is often the case, attributing the cholestasis to any one cause is most difficult in these sick neonates. The role of parenteral hyperalimentation usually poses the greatest clinical conflict especially in the infant unable to accept oral feedings.

Treatment. Judicious use of choleretics (choles-

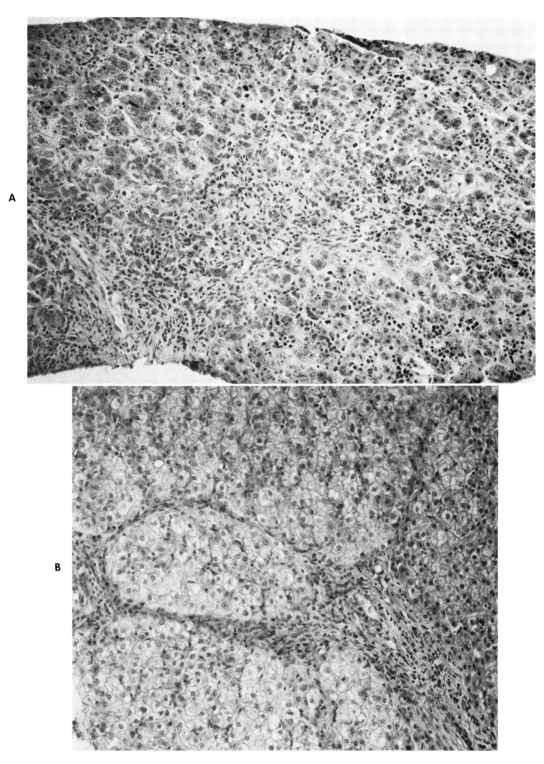

Fig. 19-12. Cholestatic syndrome developing in a neonate after a severe episode of necrotizing enterocolitis. **A,** Needle liver biopsy section reveals pronounced cholestasis within hepatocytes and canaliculi, lobular disarray, extramedullary hematopoiesis, and mild perilobular necrosis. **B,** Repeat liver biopsy section taken at time of second operation done to restore bowel continuity (6 months later). Grossly, the liver had a micronodular appearance, and histologic examination reveals intralobular septa and perilobular fibrosis, suggesting early cirrhosis. No signs of cholestasis were found.

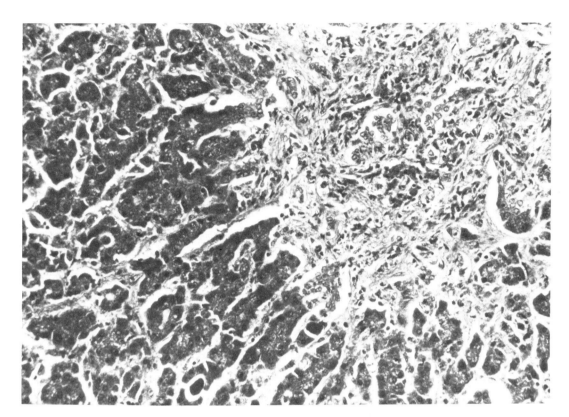

Fig. 19-13. Hyperalimentation liver disease. Liver biopsy section taken from a 3-month-old infant with short-bowel syndrome after surgery requiring central hyperalimentation almost continuously from birth. Rising bilirubin levels and progressive firm hepatomegaly were the cause for this biopsy. Fibrous tissue widening of the portal region and fingerlet fibrous extensions into the lobule are seen associated with pronounced cholestasis both in hepatocytes and canaliculi. (× 100.)

tyramine, phenobarbital) coupled with nutritional support is the mainstay of treatment until the cholestasis resolves. In some cases this may take 3 to 6 months. When total parenteral nutrition is required, the amino acid concentration of the solution should probably be less than 2 gm/dl. The present data suggests that Intralipid 10% can be continued as a caloric supplement in these cholestatic infants.

Prognosis. Complete resolution of the hepatic abnormalities is the rule, but portal fibrosis with perilobular or interlobular stellate can be seen on follow-up biopsies (Fig. 19-12, *B*). Cirrhosis is exceptionally reported.

Prolonged parenteral nutrition. Most often cholestasis becomes manifest after 2 or more weeks of intravenous total parenteral nutrition (TPN). The incidence is about 25% to 40% of cases treated by TPN. The premature infant is especially vulnerable to this complication of TPN even when the history of other predisposing conditions mentioned with neonatal "gut-shock" categories is lacking. The duration of exposure to the protein components of hyperalimentation solution is the most important factor predisposing to cholestasis. The histologic findings in TPN-induced cholestasis includes isolated hepatocyte necrosis, ballooning degeneration, widening of the portal zones by fibrous tissue, but little inflammation (Fig. 19-13). A predominance of eosinophils may be noted in areas of extramedullary hematopoiesis. Kupffer cells may be loaded with PAS-positive material (Fig. 19-14). If Intralipid 10% has been used, foamy lipidlike pigment material may be seen in Kupffer cells, wandering macrophages, or macrophages forming pseudoxanthomas. Laboratory abnormalities include an early rise in serum bile acids, followed by rising direct-reacting bilirubin fraction and finally elevation of aminotransferases.

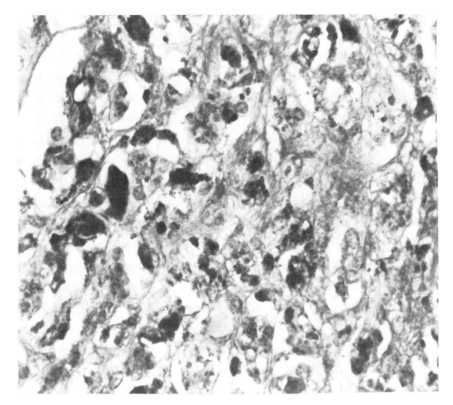

Fig. 19-14. Hyperalimentation liver disease. Liver tissue from an infant on 5 months of continuous central hyperalimentation. Biopsy section shows ballooning degeneration of hepatocytes, intrahepatic cholestasis, and irregular-shaped, PAS-positive granular material in Kupffer cells. (PAS stain, after diastase, ×400.)

The mechanism for TPN-induced cholestasis is unsettled. Diminished stimulation to bile flow from prolonged absence of oral feeds, direct toxic effect of additives in the hyperalimentation solution, an improper ratio of neutral to aromatic amino acids, and taurine-deficient solutions have all been considered potential cholestatic "toxic" factors. Intralipid 10% is not believed to be either causative or additive. Fortunately, the prognosis is very good since resolution of the liver abnormalities occurs with 1 to 4 months once TPN is discontinued. Residual portal fibrosis and occasionally cirrhosis have been found on follow-up liver biopsy specimens, especially in neonates requiring prolonged (more than 3 to 4 months) of TPN.

"Inspissated bile syndrome." The accumulation of bile in canaliculi and small- to medium-sized intrahepatic bile ducts occurs in the face of significant hemolytic diseases of the newborn (Rh, ABO). Some workers believe that unconjugated bilirubin may also be a "cholestatic" agent under these special circumstances. Others believe that an underlying hepatic injury must be present to allow for this clinical syndrome to evolve. The presence of mixed hyperbilirubinemia is typical, and hepatocyte cholestasis with or without additional evidence of cellular injury is seen by routine microscopy. Variable degrees of hepatocyte necrosis, occasional to extensive giant-cell transformation, balloon liver cells, and pronounced extramedullary hematopoiesis are surprising findings in some cases (Fig. 19-15). When hemolysis has been severe, the cholestasis may seem complete, with acholic stools passed by the infant. Serum levels of bilirubin can reach 30 to 40 mg/dl, with the majority being direct reacting. When the inspissation of biliary material occurs in the extrahepatic ducts, the differentiation between intrahepatic disease and biliary atresia may be extremely difficult. A trial with a choleretic (cho-

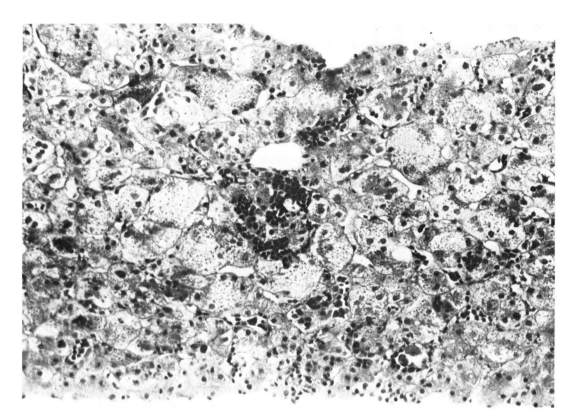

Fig. 19-15. Liver tissue from a 7-week-old infant with nonisoimmune hemolytic disease and cholestatic jaundice clinically believed to have "inspissated bile syndrome." Noticeable giant-cell transformation, hepatic lobule disarray, and cholestasis suggest that the hepatic and hematologic disorder may have had a common cause. Note the cluster of extramedullary hematopoietic tissue. (×100.)

lestyramine or phenobarbital) is indicated when hemolytic disease is confirmed and variable degrees of success are reported. Once the stools return to normal color, patency of the extrahepatic biliary tree is assured. Sometimes small bile-colored "plugs" are identified in the infant's stools at the time the stool color becomes normal. Although most cases slowly improve over 2 to 6 months, persistence of complete cholestasis for over 6 to 8 weeks requires further studies to determine if laparotomy and exploration of the extrahepatic biliary tree is necessary. Irrigation of the common duct is rapidly curative when obstructing inspissated biliary material can be dislodged by this method.

Idiopathic and nonfamilial intrahepatic cholestasis (giant-cell hepatitis)

By far the largest number of cases of neonatal intrahepatic cholestasis fall into this category. They are characterized primarily by the lack of identification of predisposing conditions or any specific cause despite an exhaustive search, and the somewhat common histologic picture. Probably up to 75% of cases of neonatal intrahepatic cholestasis fall within this category. The cholestasis may be mild to extremely severe such that in 10% of cases it may be clinically and biochemically indistinguishable from extrahepatic causes. The features seen on liver biopsy, however, may be especially helpful in resolving this diagnostic dilemma when lobular disarray and extensive giant-cell transformation are seen accompanied by a prominent portal inflammatory response (Fig. 19-16). Generally speaking, it is unusual in the first 2 months of life to see either significant neoductular proliferation or important portal fibrosis in biopsy material from such cases, findings that typically and especially dominate the histologic lesion of extrahepatic causes of biliary atresia. In less obvious cases a

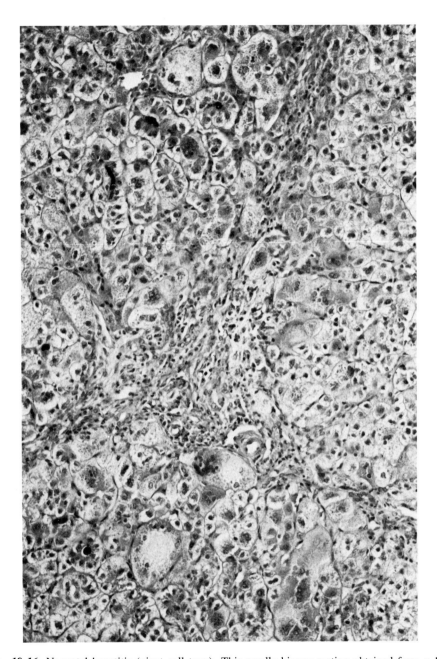

Fig. 19-16. Neonatal hepatitis (giant cell type). This needle biopsy section obtained from a 10-week-old jaundiced infant shows virtually all the pathologic criteria to support the continued use of medical management. Lobular disorganization, pseudoductules, cholestasis (canalicular and hepatocytic), numerous giant cells, yet minimal portal changes are noted.

clinical history that includes a small-for-gestational age or premature infant, poor feeding, emesis, or failure to thrive is most consistent with intrahepatic causes of cholestasis. Obviously the presence of normal or intermittently normal color to the stools is probably the most helpful information that can rule out a surgical condition for the cholestasis.

Those cases suspected of "idiopathic" intrahepatic cholestasis should have a trial of choleretics (cholestyramine, phenobarbital), in addition to vitamin (A, D, K, and E) and nutritional support. Should evidence of persisting complete cholestasis be documented after 4 to 6 weeks of treatment by either passage of acholic stools or failure to excrete a biliary technetium-tagged radionuclide (DIDA), a repeat liver biopsy is warranted. The decision can then be made regarding need for minilaparotomy and intraoperative cholangiogram. In such examples a small but patent extrahepatic biliary tree (hypoplastic bile ducts) is frequently demonstrated at surgery and is probably the result of diminished bile flow rather than the cause. Cholecystostomy has been employed with improvement in cholestasis, but recurrences do occur when this form of drainage is discontinued. In such cases it is prudent for the surgeon not to undertake extensive exploration of these portobiliary structures.

Treatment. Once a patent extrahepatic tree is confirmed, therapy should include choleretics (cholestyramine, 250-500 mg 4 times daily), phenobarbital (3-5 mg/kg/day in 2 divided doses), a special formula containing medium-chain triglycerides (Portagen or Pregestimil), supplemental fat-soluble vitamins (A, D, E, and K) in water-miscible form. This therapeutic program is continued as long as biochemical testing reveals significant cholestasis. Therapy with cholestyramine demands monitoring of serum electrolytes for evidence of metabolic acidosis (elevated chloride and diminished bicarbonate levels). Other complications of this product include intestinal obstruction, hypernatremia, and prolonged prothrombin times. Serum barbiturate levels should also be checked periodically, especially in the younger infants to confirm that one is in the therapeutic range.

Prognosis. The long-term consequences of these idiopathic varieties seem to correlate best with the duration of the cholestasis. In general, a failure to resolve the cholestatic picture within the first year of life is associated with progressive liver disease and evolving cirrhosis. Sometimes this progression occurs in association with a reduction in the number of interlobular bile ducts (paucity of interlobular bile ducts) overlapping with those cases assigned to the category of "anatomic" but nonsyndromic forms of intrahepatic cholestasis (see below). With time, perilobular and intralobular fibrosis continue and portal hypertension ensues. Splenomegaly and esophageal varices confirm this eventuality. Finally ascites, usually associated with a rise in the serum bilirubin level, heralds the onset of hepatic failure. Death can be expected within 6 to 12 months.

Rarely, the "idiopathic" variety of persistent neonatal cholestasis may not lead to progressive liver disease, yet severe pruritus and growth retardation are common, at least during childhood. In addition, long-standing vitamin E deficiency may usher in a neurologic syndrome characterized by ataxia, areflexia, loss of vibratory and position sensation, and ophthalmoplegia.

Anatomic type of intrahepatic cholestasis (paucity of interlobular bile ducts)

This specific category of intrahepatic cholestasis is characterized by diminished numbers of interlobular bile ducts and additionally in some by a diminished number of portal zones. The early and sometimes even late liver biopsy specimens also show the expected features of hepatocyte and canalicular cholestasis. The extrahepatic biliary system is patent, though not infrequently the ducts may be of diminished caliber (hypoplastic) as a result of decreased bile flow. In addition, this particular category of intrahepatic cholestasis may be associated with physical and visceral abnormalities that allow the separation into two distinct subgroups, syndromic and nonsyndromic types, each with an apparently different prognosis. The mechanism for development of paucity of the intrahepatic bile ducts is unclear. Some cases clearly follow the pathologic lesion of giant-cell hepatitis, others occur in association with alpha-1-antitrypsin deficiency disease, whereas others follow idiopathic giant-cell hepatitis. One could argue whether the initial inflammatory process that surrounds the small interlobular bile ducts in these patients is a primary process, or it is secondary to the hepatocyte's inability to excrete normal or abnormal bile acid derivatives or bile pigment. In most cases serial biopsy specimens have shown that after resolution of the inflammatory process, there is a concomitant disappearance of the intra-hepatic portal bile ducts.

Syndromic variety—hepatic, cardiac, and vertebral dysplasia (Alagille's syndrome, arteriohepatic dysplasia). The children who constitute this group are easily recognized by their characteristic facies, a subtle finding in the neonatal period but becoming more obvious with age (Fig. 19-17). The forehead is prominent just as the nasal bridge is. The eyes are deepset, and hypertelorism is commonly found. The chin is small and slightly pointed at least early in life and may project forward. The children tend to range in the lower percentiles of height and weight. In the neonatal period the cholestasis is usually incomplete and stools retain a normal coloration. Pruritus may be evidenced by irritability with itching after 4 months of age. Physical examination also reveals an enlarged, firm, and somewhat smooth-edged liver. Splenomegaly is absent in most; if present, it is proportionate to the degree of portal hypertension and indicates an underlying cirrhosis. Cardiac murmurs are frequent and consistent with either central or peripheral pulmonic stenosis. Xanthomas are rarely seen early in the disease. In time they appear in the creases of the palms and can eventually be found on the extensor surfaces of the arms and legs (Fig. 19-18) and on the nape of the neck. The skin appears thickened and somewhat loose, especially on the dorsum of the hands. The fingers may be short, and the thumbs seem broad. Digital clubbing and some cyanosis also develop in some children. For others the cholestasis is subclinical and goes undiscovered until later in childhood,

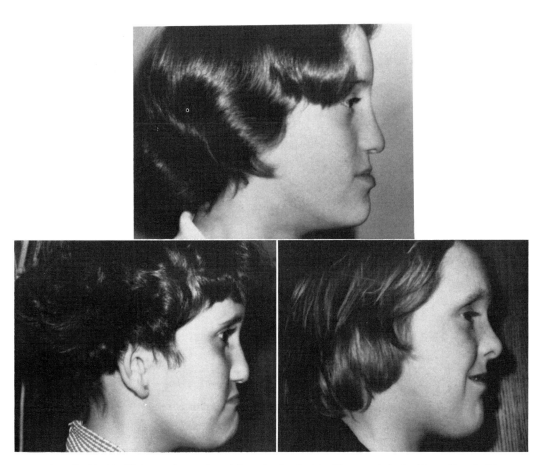

Fig. 19-17. Alagille's syndrome (arteriohepatic dysplasia). Characteristic facial profile of older children with syndromic form of paucity of the interlobular bile ducts. Prominent forehead, high insertion of nasal bridge, deep-set eyes, relatively small maxilla.

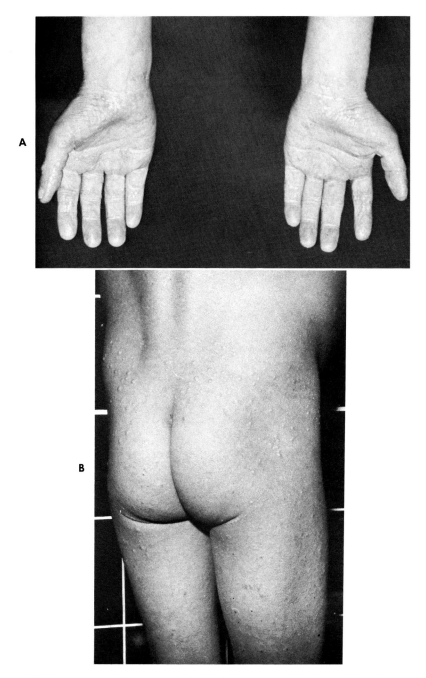

Fig. 19-18. Intrahepatic biliary hypoplasia. **A,** Palmar view of a 5-year-old boy's hands shows xanthomas in the creases and on the thenar eminence. **B,** Cutaneous xanthomas. Also note the small scabbed excoriations on the thighs.

when they come to diagnosis while being investigated for unexplained pruritus or xanthomas but without clinical icterus. If mild jaundice was present initially, it cleared early in life or was attributed to some other cause. In this subgroup of children, the liver is seldom enlarged and splenomegaly is rare. Isolated reports of familial examples of other syndromic forms of neonatal cholestasis may well be variants of this condition.

Laboratory features. Mild elevations of serum bilirubin are present (2 to 8 mg/dl) with more than half being direct reacting. The alkaline phosphatase and gamma glutamyl transferase (GGT) is greatly elevated as is the cholesterol level, especially early in life. Serum bile acids are always elevated. Transaminases are slightly increased; coagulation studies are normal as are the serum proteins.

Pathologic lesion. Pathologic findings in this condition are extremely variable in all age groups. The primary early lesion (neonatal) is characterized by bile stasis, which usually predominates the clinical and histologic picture. Portal zones are fewer in number than normal. Bile may be found in hepatocytes, small canaliculi, and some small interlobular bile ducts. Disruption of the lobular architecture is unusual though some cases do show ballooned hepatocytes, mild giant-cell transformation, and pseudoglandular arrangement of hepatocytes (Fig. 19-19). The portal inflammatory response may be sent or striking, whereas fibrosis is rarely present. Bile ducts in the portal zone may be absent or proliferated initially. When present, they appear abnormal, and frequently polymorphonuclear cells can be found surrounding them or even within the bile duct epithelial cells suggesting pericholangitis (Fig. 19-20). When pres-

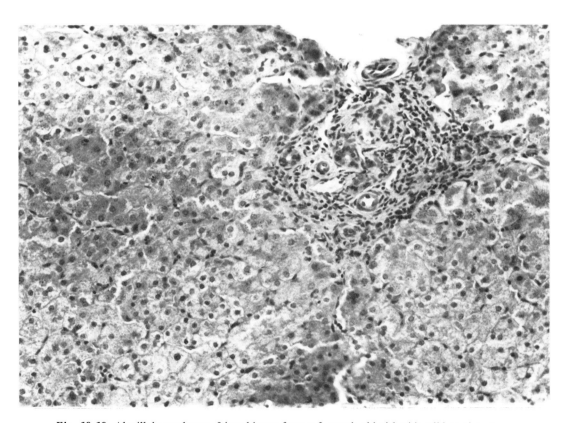

Fig. 19-19. Alagille's syndrome. Liver biopsy from a 3-month-old girl with mild persistent neonatal cholestatic syndrome. The lobular architecture is somewhat disorganized. Ballooned hepatocytes are present as is intrahepatic cholestasis, especially apparent in the periportal giant cells. The portal area contains several bile ductules and a mixed cellular reaction. Some inflammatory cells seem to be directly associated with the bile duct epithelium. (×100.) Subsequent liver biopsies showed the evolution of the hepatic disorder in this case (see Figs. 19-20 and 19-21).

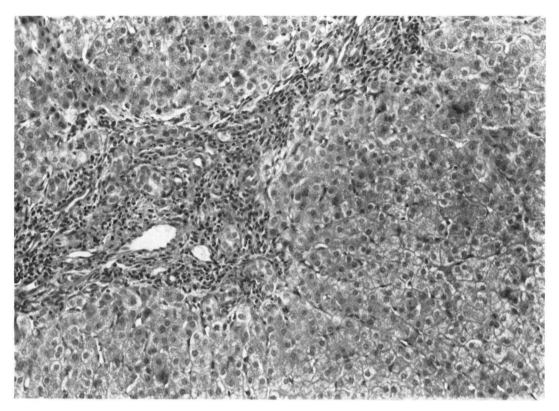

Fig. 19-20. Evolving histopathologic appearance in Alagille's syndrome. Liver biopsy section obtained at 13 months from patient described in Fig. 19-19 because of mild persistent cholestasis and early skeletal rickets. Giant-cell change is no longer evident, and the lobular architecture is near normal. The expanded portal region still demonstrates increased, but normal-appearing bile ducts, a lymphocytic infiltrate, and a slight extension of portal connective tissue. (× 100.)

ent, portal bile ducts are usually devoid of bile, collapsed, or difficult to recognize, and the ductular epithelial cells are often distorted and swollen.

Serial liver biopsy specimens are most informative, and in some patients one can witness gradual disappearance of the portal and interlobular bile ducts, perhaps as a consequence of the intercurrent inflammatory process (Fig. 19-21). At times the original features seen on liver biopsy are solely those of "idiopathic" intrahepatic cholestasis, with moderate or severe cholestatic jaundice present. This same progressive disappearance of the intrahepatic portal bile ducts may be found in the presence of cholestasis but in the absence of periductular inflammation, emphasizing the toxic role of abnormal bile acids or their derivatives. It is curious that a similar lesion has been noted in the transplanted liver, perhaps as a consequence of the rejection reaction.

The histologic lesion is also variable in the older patient who comes to the same diagnosis (Fig. 19-22). Fibrosis may be totally absent in some, whereas in others it is severe enough to produce portal hypertension (biliary cirrhosis). Likewise, cholestasis may or may not be present; in fact, the fewer bile ducts present, the less likely that cholestasis will be found. In some patients the results of liver histology appear so normal that diagnosis can be missed by a casual observer (Fig. 19-23).

Other abnormalities. The *cardiovascular* abnormalities are variable, with pulmonary artery stenosis, either proximal or peripheral, being the most common. Other cardiac lesions found include atrial septal defect, coarctation of the aorta, tetralogy of Fallot, and so on. *Vertebral arch defects* seen on spine films are characterized by incomplete fusion of the vertebral body or anterior arch (butterfly deformity) and diminished interpedical distance in the thoracicolumber region.

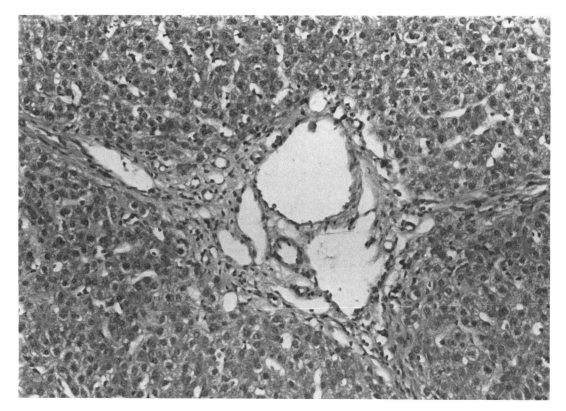

Fig. 19-21. Alagille's syndrome. Liver biopsy section obtained at age 6 years from patient described in Figs. 19-19 and 19-20. Portal zone is without bile ducts. The inflammatory lesion is absent, and the hepatic lobules appear normal ($\times$ 100). Clinically the child is anicteric but remains troubled by pruritus. Bile acids are elevated.

Other abnormalities described in this syndrome are manifest later in life. These include *growth retardation* in the face of normal growth hormone levels. A *weak, high-pitched voice* can be appreciated in some children. *Eye* findings (posterior embryotoxon), *renal* abnormalities (dysplastic kidneys or tubular ectasia), and *neurologic* features (areflexia, ataxia, ophthalmoplegia) eventually develop in some children.

Differential diagnosis. Once liver tissue has revealed paucity of the interlobular bile ducts, the main consideration is the correct assignment of the child to either the syndromic or nonsyndromic subgroup. Most examples of the latter tend to evolve as a consequence of neonatal "idiopathic" hepatitis, or less commonly in association with alpha-1-antitrypsin deficiency disease complicating neonatal cholestasis. When the typical facies is lacking, as in the neonatal period, a search for other organ involvement (spine, heart, eye, and so on) may allow for assigning the infant to the proper category. A familial but nonsyndromic form (the THCA syndrome) has been found to produce a precursor of cholic acid, trihydroxycoprostanic acid (THCA), suggesting that qualitative determination of serum and urine bile acids may be worthwhile in this sorting process. The importance of proper categorization of these infants stems from the observation that long-term prognosis is quite different between the syndromic and nonsyndromic groups.

Treatment. High-dose cholestyramine (4 to 12 gm/day) is beneficial in controlling the pruritus and aiding in the resolution of xanthomas, but its value has been contested. Phenobarbital is useful as adjunctive therapy to lower both the serum bilirubin and bile acid levels. The serum cholesterol level diminishes to normal or near-normal levels by 5 years of age. Good nutrition started early in life, together with supplemental water-miscible forms

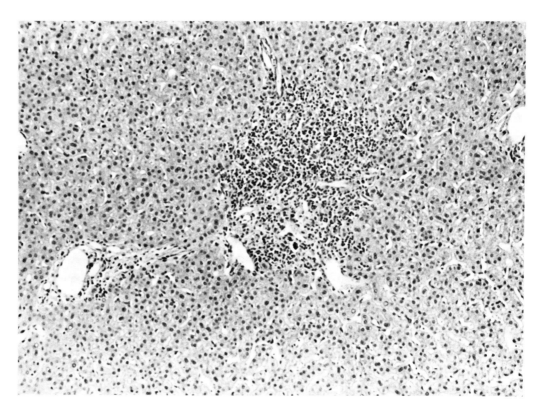

Fig. 19-22. Intrahepatic biliary hypoplasia. Two portal regions here best demonstrate the focal nature of the persisting inflammatory reaction. Neither portal region has an identifiable bile duct. The lobular architecture is preserved and fibrosis absent. This liver biopsy section is from a 3-year-old boy with persistent jaundice and pruritus. His neonatal course was complicated by persistent obstructive jaundice, which operative cholangiography and liver biopsy subsequently proved to be caused by neonatal hepatitis. Slow but incomplete resolution of his initial symptoms and biochemical features suggesting obstructive jaundice (increased serum bilirubin, 5.3 mg/dl, and alkaline phosphatase and cholesterol) were indications for this liver biopsy.

of fat-soluble vitamins, is especially important to prevent rickets and subsequent neurologic sequelae. Periodic serum vitamin E levels should be checked because some children may have extraordinarily poor absorption of this supplemental vitamin product.

Prognosis. Patients with the syndromic form of intrahepatic cholestasis have a relatively favorable prognosis. In most, clinical and biochemical evidence of jaundice disappears by 4 to 5 years of age or sooner and pruritus usually by adolescence. The liver becomes free of cholestasis in most cases and reveals absent or minimal fibrosis despite persistent biochemical abnormalities (elevated bile acids and GGT) even after many years. Possibly the most bewildering aspect of this entity is demonstrated by those patients with normal serum bilirubin but elevated serum bile acids, in

the face of complete absence of bile duct structures in the biopsy material. The excretory pathway for the normal conjugated bilirubin load is unknown in these patients. It is usual to find some bile in the gallbladder at laparotomy while fecal bilirubin derivatives are present in normal amounts. This may imply that other areas of the liver not represented in the biopsy specimen indeed have functioning bile ducts that handle the entire bilirubin load for these patients.

Survival into adulthood is common in these cases. Eventually the liver becomes more firm and slowly recedes in size. Although hypogonadism has been noted, fertility is not obviously affected. The cardiac, vertebral, renal, or eye abnormalities seldom affect longevity, but the slow progression of the liver disease toward cirrhosis occurs in some unfortunate examples (Fig. 19-24). The long-term

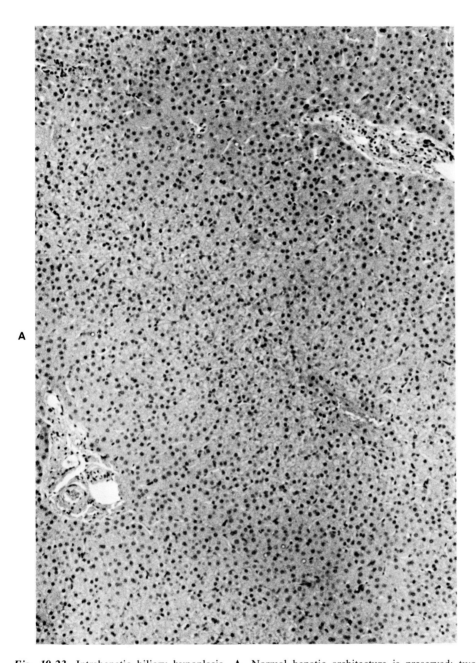

Fig. 19-23. Intrahepatic biliary hypoplasia. **A,** Normal hepatic architecture is preserved; two portal regions and one central vein are identifiable. This liver biopsy section was obtained from a 2-year-old child who complained of intermittent pruritus and on physical examination was noted to have three isolated xanthomas. Jaundice was absent, and the liver was of normal size. A history of prolonged neonatal jaundice was obtained, but a specific diagnosis was not made at that time.

Continued.

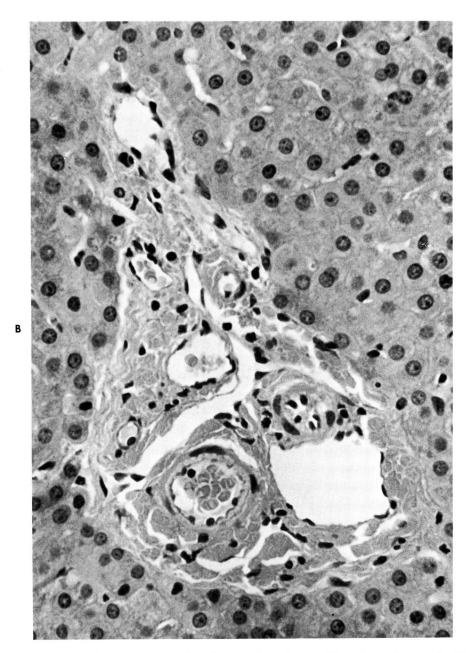

Fig. 19-23, cont'd. **B,** High-power view of a typical portal zone of liver shows absence of a bile duct.

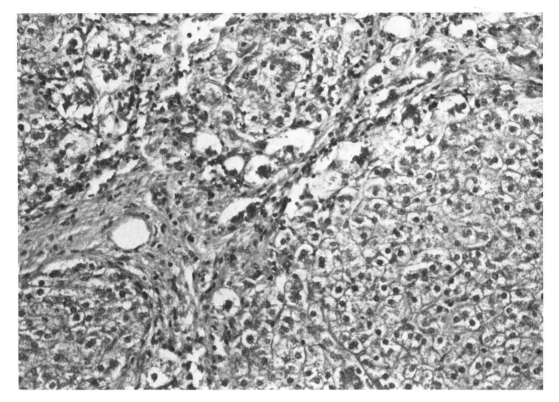

Fig. 19-24. Alagille's syndrome. Liver biopsy section obtained from 16-year-old patient shown in Fig. 19-17, *C,* while undergoing splenorenal shunt surgery for complications of portal hypertension. This area of the biopsy section shows a portal zone devoid of bile ducts associated with adjacent hepatocytes reflecting variable injury. Other areas showed perilobular fibrosis and cirrhosis. (×100.)

outcome for those children developing a vitamin E–deficient neurologic syndrome remains to be determined.

Nonsyndromic form with paucity of interlobular bile ducts. These infants demonstrate the usual features of cholestasis, the latter may be sufficiently severe as to cause confusion with possible extrahepatic causes when results of clinical and biochemical studies are considered. However, needle liver biopsy is generally discriminating and shows those features consistent with intrahepatic cholestasis. These include some combination of lobular disarray, giant-cell transformation, portal inflammation, and minimal fibrosis, all in conjunction with significant hepatocyte and canalicular cholestasis. Portal interlobular bile ducts may be sparse, collapsed, or difficult to identify because of surrounding edema and the inflammation reaction. Follow-up liver biopsy specimens may show resolution of the inflammatory components,

dense portal fibrous tissue, and absence of interlobular bile ducts (Fig. 19-25). Familial examples do occur, but, except in cases associated with alpha-1-antitrypsin deficiency, the search for an etiologic agent is predictably unrewarding. Follow-up liver biopsies at 1 to 3 years will reveal resolution of the portal inflammatory process, rare interlobular bile ducts, persistent cholestasis, and progressive fibrosis in most. No other organ systems are involved, and pruritus, xanthomas, thickened skin on hands and feet, short stature, and developmental delays are typical consequences of the entity. Qualitative serum bile acids may be abnormal in some cases, with trihydroxycoprostanic acid (a precursor of cholic acid) being found in a family with two such affected infants.

The long-term prognosis is not favorable, even with the use of choleretics, vitamin, and nutritional support. Biliary cirrhosis and liver failure usually occur before adolescence.

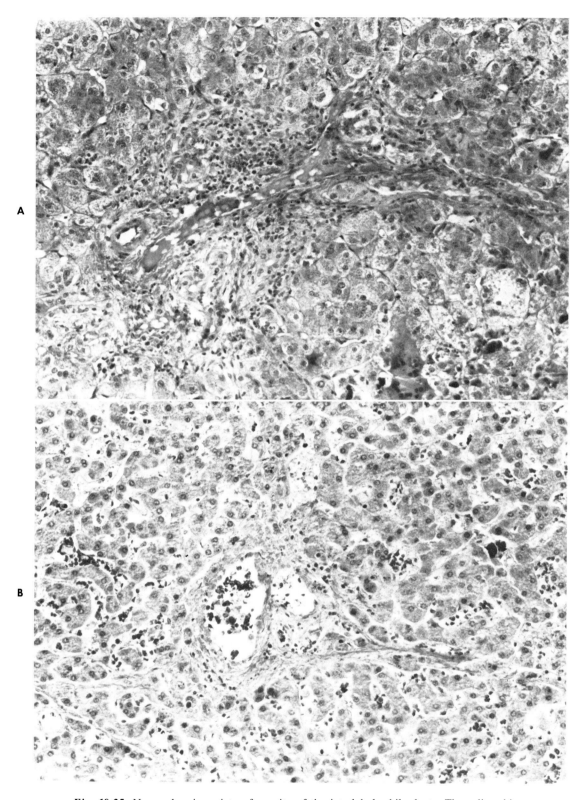

Fig. 19-25. Nonsyndromic variety of paucity of the interlobular bile ducts. These liver biopsy specimens were obtained at 2 months and 6 years, respectively. Cholestatic jaundice persisted until death. **A,** Lobular disarray associated with giant cells and cholestasis. Inflammatory changes are minimal, whereas bile ducts are difficult to recognize. **B,** Follow-up biopsy specimen obtained at autopsy (6 years of age). Portal region without bile ducts or inflammation. Only a single duct was found in 100 portal zones counted. From many portal zones delicate fibrous strands could be seen coursing between the hepatic plates. (**A** and **B,** ×100.)

REFERENCES

Aagenaes, O., Van Der Hagen, C.B., and Refsum, S.: Hereditary recurrent intrahepatic cholestasis from birth, Arch. Dis. Child. **43:**646-657, 1968.

Aagenaes, O.: Hereditary recurrent cholestasis with lymphedema: two new families, Acta Paediatr. Scand. **63:**465-471, 1974.

Alagille, D., Odièvre, M., Gautier, M., and Dommergues, J.P.: Hepatic ductular hypoplasia associated with characteristic facies, vertebral malformations, retarded physical, mental, and sexual development, and cardiac murmur, J. Pediatr. **86:**63-71, 1975.

Andres, J.M., and Walker, W.A.: Effect of *Escherichia coli* endotoxin on the developing rat liver. I. Giant cell induction and disruption in protein metabolism, Pediat. Res. **13:**1290-1293, 1979.

Applebaum, M.N., and Thaler, M.M.: Reversibility of extensive liver damage in galactosemia, Gastroenterology **69:**496-502, 1975.

Beale, E.F., Nelson, R.M., Bucciarelli, R.L., and others: Intrahepatic cholestasis associated with parenteral nutrition in premature infants, Pediatrics **64:**342-347, 1979.

Berjanover, Y., Sharp, B., Whitney, J.O.W., and others: Transplacentally induced liver injury due to lithocholate: canalicular Na, K-activated ATPase and membrane microviscosity in newborns, Pediat. Res. **12:**430, 1978 (Abstract).

Bernstein, J., Chang, C.-H., Brough, A.J., and Heidelberger, K.P.: Conjugated hyperbilirubinemia in infancy associated with parenteral alimentation, J. Pediatr. **90:**361-367, 1977.

Bloomer, J.R., and Boyer, J.L.: Phenobarbital effects in cholestatic liver disease, Ann. Intern. Med. **82:**310-317, 1975.

Brown, M.R., and Putnam, T.C.: Cholestasis associated with central intravenous nutrition in infants, N.Y. State J. Med. **78:**27-30, Jan. 1978.

Case Records of the Massachusetts General Hospital, N. Engl. J. Med. **302:**1405-1413, 1980.

Clayton, R.J., Iber, F.L., Ruebner, B.H., and McKusick, V.A.: Byler disease, Am. J. Dis. Child. **117:**112-124, 1969.

Coen, R., and McAdams, A.J.: Visceral manifestation of shock in congenital heart disease, Am. J. Dis. Child. **119:**383-389, 1970.

Crocker, A.C., and Farber, S.: Niemann-Pick disease: a review of 18 patients, Medicine **37:**1-95, 1958.

Danks, D.M., Tippett, P., Adams, C., and Campbell, P.: Cerebro-hepato-renal syndrome of Zellweger, J. Pediatr. **86:**382-387, 1975.

Danks, D.M., Campbell, P.E., Smith, A.L., and Rogers, J.: Prognosis of babies with neonatal hepatitis, Arch. Dis. Child. **52:**368-372, 1977.

Dunn, P.M., and Chir, B.: Obstructive jaundice, liver damage and Rh haemolytic disease of the newborn, Jewish Mem. Hosp. Bull. N.Y. **10:**94-124, 1965.

Hadchouel, M., and Gautier, M.: Histopathologic study of the liver in the early cholestatic phase of alpha-1-antitrypsin deficiency, J. Pediatr. **89:**211-215, 1976.

Hardwick, D.F., and Dimmick, J.E.: Metabolic cirrhoses of infancy and early childhood, Perspect. Pediatr. Pathol. **3:**103-144, 1976.

Heathcote, J., Deodhar, K.P., Scheuer, P.J., and Sherlock, S.: Intrahepatic cholestasis in childhood, N. Engl. J. Med. **295:**801-805, 1976.

Herman, S.P., Baggenstoss, A.H., and Cloutier, M.D.: Liver dysfunction and histologic abnormalities in neonatal hypopituitarism, J. Pediatr. **87:**892-895, 1975.

Isenberg, J.N., Hanson, R.F., Williams, G., and others: A clinical experience with familial paucity of intrahepatic bile ducts associated with defective metabolism of trihydroxycoprostanic acid to cholic acid: Liver Diseases in Children (Hépatologie infantile), INSERM **49:**43-56, 1975.

Jacob, A.I., Goldberg, P.K., Bloom, N., and others: Endotoxin and bacteria in portal blood, Gastroenterology **72:**1268-1270, 1977.

Larochelle, J., Mortezai, A., Belanger, M., and others: Experience with 37 infants with tyrosinemia, Can. Med. Assoc. J. **97:**1051-1055, 1967.

Levin, S.E., Zarvos, P., Milner, S., and Schmaman, A.: Arteriohepatic dysplasia: association of liver disease with pulmonary arterial stenosis as well as facial and skeletal abnormalities, Pediatrics **66:**876-883, 1980.

Levy, H.L., Sepe, S.J., Shih, V.E., and others: Sepsis due to *Escherichia coli* in neonates with galactosemia, N. Engl. J. Med. **297:**823-825, 1977.

Linarelli, L.G., Williams, C.N., and Phillips, M.J.: Byler's disease: fatal intrahepatic cholestasis, J. Pediatr. **81:**484-492, 1972.

Manginello, F.P., and Javitt, N.B.: Parenteral nutrition and neonatal cholestasis, J. Pediatr. **94:**296-298, 1979.

Mathis, R.K., Andres, J.M., and Walker, W.A.: Liver disease in infants. II. Hepatic disease states, J. Pediatr. **90:**864-880, 1977.

Molland, E.A., and Purcell, M.: Biliary atresia and the Dandy-Walker anomaly in a neonate with 45,X Turner's syndrome, J. Pathol. **115:**227-231, 1975.

Mowat, A.P., Psacharopoulos, H., Williams, R., and others: Prognosis in childhood of liver disease associated with alpha-1-antitrypsin deficiency, type PiZZ, Gut **18:**978, 1977 (Abstract).

O'Brien, M.L., Buist, N.R.M., and Murphey, W.H.: Neonatal screening for alpha$_1$-antitrypsin deficiency, J. Pediatr. **92:**1006-1010, 1978.

Odièvre, M., Gautier, M., Hadchouel, M., and Alagille, D.: Severe familial intrahepatic cholestasis, Arch. Dis. Child. **48:**806-812, 1973.

Odièvre, M., Martin, J.P., Hadchouel, M., and Alagille, D.: Alpha$_1$-antitrypsin deficiency and liver disease in children: phenotypes, manifestations, and prognosis, Pediatrics **57:**226-231, 1976.

Odièvre, M., Gentil, C., Gautier, M., and Alagille, D.: Hereditary fructose intolerance in childhood, Am. J. Dis. Child. **132:**605-608, 1978.

Odièvre, M., Hadchouel, M., Landrieu, P., and others: Long-term prognosis for infants with intrahepatic cholestasis and patent extrahepatic biliary tract, Arch. Dis. Child. **56:**373-376, 1981.

Oppenheimer, E.H., and Esterly, J.R.: Hepatic changes in young infants with cystic fibrosis: possible relation to focal biliary cirrhosis, J. Pediatr. **86:**683-689, 1975.

Postuma, R., and Trevenen, C.L.: Liver disease in infants receiving total parenteral nutrition, Pediatrics **63:**110-115,1979.

Riely, C.A., Cotlier, E., Jensen, P.S., and Klatskin, G.: Arteriohepatic dysplasia: a benign syndrome of intrahepatic cholestasis with multiple organ involvement, Ann. Intern. Med. **91:**520-527, 1979.

Riely, C.A.: Familial intrahepatic cholestasis: an update, Yale J. Biol. Med. **52**:89-98, 1979.

Rosenstein, B.J., and Oppenheimer, E.H.: Prolonged obstructive jaundice and giant-cell hepatitis in an infant with cystic fibrosis, J. Pediatr. **91**:1022-1023, 1977.

Ruebner, B.H., Bhagavan, B.S., Greenfield, A.J., and others: Neonatal hepatic necrosis, Pediatrics **43**:963-970, 1969.

Sardemann, H., and Tygstrup, I.: Prolonged obstructive jaundice and haemangiomatosis, Arch. Dis. Child. **49**:665-667, 1974.

Scriver, C.R., Silverberg, M., and Clow, C.L.: Hereditary tyrosinemia and tyrosyluria: clinical report of four patients, Can. Med. Assoc. J. **97**:1047-1050, 1967.

Sharp, H.L., Carey, J.B., White, J.G., and Krivit, W.: Cholestyramine therapy in patients with a paucity of intrahepatic bile ducts, J. Pediatr. **71**:723-736, 1967.

Sharp, H.L., and Mirkin, B.L.: Effect of phenobarbital on hyperbilirubinemia, bile acid metabolism, and microsomal enzyme activity in chronic intrahepatic cholestasis of childhood, J. Pediatr. **81**:116-126, 1972.

Sondheimer, J.M., Bryan, H., Andrews, W., and Forstner, G.G.: Cholestatic tendencies in premature infants on and off parenteral nutrition, Pediatrics **62**:984-989, 1978.

Stellard, F., Watkins, J.B., Szczepanik-Van Leeuwen, P., and Alagille, D.: Hyocholic acid: an unusual bile acid in Byler's disease, Gastroenterology **77**:A42, 1979 (Abstract).

Stiehl, A., Thaler, M.M., and Admirand, W.H.: The effects of phenobarbital on bile salts and bilirubin in patients with intrahepatic and extrahepatic cholestasis, N. Engl. J. Med. **286**:858-861, 1972.

Sveger, T.: Alpha$_1$-antitrypsin deficiency in early childhood, Pediatrics **62**:22-25, 1978.

Valman, H.B., France, N.E., and Wallis, P.G.: Prolonged neonatal jaundice in cystic fibrosis, Arch. Dis. Child. **46**:805-809, 1971.

Vileisis, R.A., Inwood, R.J., and Hunt, C.E.: Prospective controlled study of parenteral nutrition-associated cholestatic jaundice: effect of protein intake, J. Pediatr. **96**:893-897, 1980.

Watson, B.H., and Miller, V.: Arteriohepatic dysplasia, Arch. Dis. Child. **48**:459-466, 1973.

Weber, A.M., Tuchweber, B., Yousef, I., and others: Severe familial cholestasis in North American Indian children: a clinical model of microfilament dysfunction? Gastroenterology **81**:653-662, 1981.

Weinberg, A.G., and Bolande, R.P.: The liver in congenital heart disease, Am. J. Dis. Child. **119**:390-394, 1970.

Wenger, D.A., Barth, G., and Githens, J.H.: Nine cases of sphingomyelin lipidosis: a new variant in Spanish-American children, Am. J. Dis. Child. **131**:955-961, 1977.

Williams, C.N., Kaye, R., Baker, L., and others: Progressive familial cholestatic cirrhosis and bile acid metabolism, J. Pediatr. **81**:493-500, 1972.

EXTRAHEPATIC CHOLESTASIS
Biliary atresia

Extrahepatic biliary atresia accounts for at least 50% of all cases of prolonged obstructive jaundice in the neonate, but the absolute incidence is said to be about 1 in 8000 to 1 in 14,000 live births. There appears to be an increased incidence in Orientals (fourfold to fivefold), with a female/male ratio of 2 in 1, which is not seen in Caucasians. In the latter, males are affected as frequently as females. Several epidemiologic prospective studies have suggested a time-space clustering of cases of extrahepatic biliary atresia, though specific environmental or infectious correlates are lacking. Although not quite statistically significant, one study evaluating etiologic factors in biliary atresia found the maternal history to involve previous miscarriages and the use of birth-control pills at the time conception.

Up to now, only speculation exists about the cause and the mechanism by which this entity develops in the child. Whereas in intrahepatic cholestasis proved in utero or perinatally acquired infectious causes may approach 15% to 20% of cases, identification of an in utero infecting agent is extremely rare in extrahepatic biliary atresia. Attempts to produce extrahepatic biliary atresia in experimental animals have been unsuccessful, and uncertainty exists about which experimental animals, if any, exhibit the same embryonic development of the bile ducts as man does. Extrapolation of the experimental data will remain doubtful until this dilemma is resolved.

At first glance one might suspect that biliary atresia is a congenital malformation of the bile duct system of the liver. A number of observations, however, suggest that such a simplistic explanation may be unrealistic. Probably the most potent counterargument comes from the rarity of biliary atresia in fetuses, in stillborns, or in neonates coming to autopsy for other reasons. Although up to 25% of infants with biliary atresia are said to have minor or major malformations, especially of the vascular system (absence of the inferior vena cava, preduodenal portal vein, anomalous hepatic arterial supply), the rarity of this entity in association with pancreatic duct atresia is taken as evidence against an underlying congenital aberration of the developing primitive bile duct system as causative. Furthermore, the delayed onset of clinical features (jaundice) and evolving signs of complete cholestasis (normal to eventually acholic stool color) suggests that the process occurs after the immediate neonatal period and argues against the simplistic, maldevelopment theory.

There is a definite attractiveness in a hypothesis incriminating an in utero insult to the hepatobiliary system—be it infectious, vascular, or chemical, either singly or in combination—in which the resultant obliterative sclerosing process of the larger bile ducts is a progressive postpartum event. The first passed stools are usually normal in color, a sign again suggesting early patency of the ducts. In exceptional cases the stools may remain of normal color for up to 2 months or longer before becoming acholic in appearance. Furthermore, the presence of patent intrahepatic bile ducts found in the region of the porta hepatis again suggests the obliterative process to be a postpartum event, rather than attributable to a congenital absence of the primitive bile duct. It is also interesting that with a trend to earlier surgical intervention, a greater percentage of "correctable" forms of biliary atresia are being observed. The completeness of the obliterative process will determine the time of appearance of clinical features as well as the severity of the intrahepatic lesion. Indeed, this concept is compatible with the theory that the entities neonatal hepatitis, biliary atresia, and even choledochal cyst are on a continuum and represent variable expressions of a neonatal obstructive cholangiopathy, but probably from different specific causes. The final lesion is undoubtedly influenced by genetic, environmental, and temporal factors.

Certainly, histologic features of idiopathic neonatal cholestasis with significant giant cell transformation may be seen occasionally in neonates whose subsequent diagnosis is that of biliary atresia. This histologic lesion has been reported in perhaps 10% of patients, especially when liver biopsy was obtained early (less than 2 to 3 months). Examples of either idiopathic neonatal hepatitis or biliary atresia have been found in patients with a choledochal cyst, again suggesting that the insult may affect all levels of the hepatobiliary system.

For some time, the hypothesis of failure of recanalization had many supporters who believed that the embryologic process generating patency of ducts failed to occur. Today, most workers believe that the pathologic lesion develops after canalization has occurred, for a central collapsed ductal structure, or glandlike structures containing small but patent lumens, can often be found in the so-called atretic remnants, visually or microscopically. A variety of combinations have been reported in extrahepatic biliary atresia, from complete obliteration of the entire extrahepatic system (most common) to partial and segmental obliterations. Whether these examples are manifestations of basic structural differences or the varied successes in the

resolution process cannot be answered at present. At times, a combination of extrahepatic atresia and paucity of the intrahepatic ducts is found. Awareness of the lesions that may be encountered and their accurate recognition at the time of surgery considerably influence operative morbidity and mortality.

Clinical features

The development of obstructive jaundice in the neonate poses one of the most difficult problems in pediatrics and sets into motion a diagnostic search of considerable magnitude, much of which has been covered in the previous discussion dealing with neonatal intrahepatic cholestasis. Biliary atresia can be immediately suspected if a work-up reveals the presence of cardiovascular anomalies with malrotation of the bowel or abdominal heterotaxia, levocardia, and so on. These findings suggest the polysplenia syndrome, the only abnormality most consistently associated with biliary atresia.

In the classic case of neonatal biliary atresia, the infants are products of term gestation and the appearance of jaundice is delayed for 2 to 3 weeks. It may first be recognized by the physician rather than the parent during the first or second well-baby visit. On the other hand, infants with well-documented cases of biliary atresia have been noted to become jaundiced during the first few days of life when it is mistakenly believed to represent physiologic jaundice. Dark urine staining the diaper is often seen and reported by the mother. However, she may not appreciate that the acholic stools are abnormal, especially if the child is her first. Not infrequently, the stools are somewhat pale yellow, tan, or buff colored, presumably because the shed bilirubin-laden intestinal mucosa cells are incorporated into the stool. However, once they become acholic, little variation in color is subsequently observed.

Unless the diagnosis is greatly delayed, the infant with extrahepatic biliary atresia seldom looks very ill, though some degree of failure to thrive will be apparent on graphic representation of the infant's height and weight. The jaundice may be more green than yellow. Again, depending on the delay in diagnosis, early evidence of digital clubbing (subungual edema) may be seen with or without cyanosis. Xanthomas have been reported early in the disease, but this has not been a common finding in our experience. The liver is typically enlarged and generally quite firm to hard. The spleen, however, is seldom palpable early (less than 3 weeks), presumably since portal hypertension takes time to develop in this disease. Instead, the presence of an enlarged spleen within the first few weeks can be taken as presumptive evidence that an intrahepatic cause is responsible for the prolonged obstructive jaundice.

Pruritus may be directly observed if the infant scratches or digs at his skin. More often, the mother or the nurses relate that the infant is quite irritable and difficult to comfort. The irritability is believed to be the result of increased serum bile acids, which uniformly occur in these children.

Later in the disease a rachitic rosary and widened epiphyses may occur as a consequence of vitamin D deficiency. A high-output cardiac murmur can be heard over the entire precordium and lung fields. Decreased peripheral vascular resistance and arteriovenous shunting partially accounts for the altered hemodynamic state (p. 751). Auscultatory findings consistent with peripheral pulmonary stenosis may also be appreciated in some.

Laboratory tests

It is obvious from the previous discussion of laboratory investigation of prolonged obstructive jaundice that no single laboratory test exists that will consistently permit the exclusive diagnosis of extrahepatic biliary atresia from other causes of this clinical picture. This particularly applies to those confusing cases of idiopathic intrahepatic cholestasis in which the obstructive component dominates the clinical and laboratory picture.

Tests most consistently found to be abnormal in cases of biliary atresia include increased serum levels of total cholesterol, alkaline phosphatase, and gamma glutamyl transpeptidase, with modest elevation of serum aminotransferases. The ^{99m}Tc-DIDA excretion study done early in the course shows excellent hepatic clearance of the isotope but no activity in the gastrointestinal tract even after 24 hours (Fig. 19-1). Values of serum 5'-nucleotidase are usually greater than 25 IU/L. Generally speaking, the peroxide hemolysis is abnormal and alpha-1-fetoprotein is normal or slightly elevated. Other routine liver function tests are extremely unreliable indicators of the underlying lesion. Despite complete cholestasis, the prothrombin time is seldom prolonged at the time of diagnosis.

The consistent passage of stools devoid of measurable bile or urobilinogen is highly suggestive of biliary atresia. A slow but steady rise in the serum bilirubin level with equal increase of direct and indirect fractions was believed to be compatible with extrahepatic biliary atresia. However, like so many observations in this disease, it has not survived the test of time and experience.

In the absence of a choledochal cyst discovered by ultrasound examination, the results of presently available laboratory and radiographic tests are unable to identify other existing anomalies of the bile duct system and therefore do not permit sorting out those patients with extrahepatic causes who possibly might be helped by surgery.

Histologic lesion

Biopsy material from the liver may be obtained either by the percutaneous route or at the time of surgical exploration. The arguments concerning open and closed biopsy have been discussed earlier in this chapter (p. 497).

The percutaneous biopsy will permit the proper diagnosis to be made in more than 90% of patients with extrahepatic biliary atresia. Material obtained by this method is strongly suggestive of biliary atresia if the following histologic features are present in addition to the cholestasis: neoductular proliferation, portal and perilobular fibrosis, bile lakes, and preservation of the basic hepatic architecture. Other histologic features found in extrahepatic biliary atresia that are variable and less specific are listed in Table 19-3.

The speed with which the characteristic histologic lesion develops seems to vary from patient to patient, but almost all patients certainly show significant morphologic changes by 2 months of age (Fig. 19-26).

The basic pathologic lesion found in the remnants of the extrahepatic biliary system suggests an inflammatory process. Luminal obliteration, various degrees of degeneration of bile duct epithelium, intraductal and periductal inflammation, and sclerosis are typical findings (Fig. 19-27). At times the lesion in the extrahepatic biliary tree is segmental, suggesting different levels of injury or varied successes at resolution. Proliferating glandlike small bile duct radicals lined by cuboid epithelium may be found in the fibrous strands removed at the time of surgery. It is unclear whether they represent an effort at recanalization (Fig. 19-28).

Some workers believe that after portoenteros-

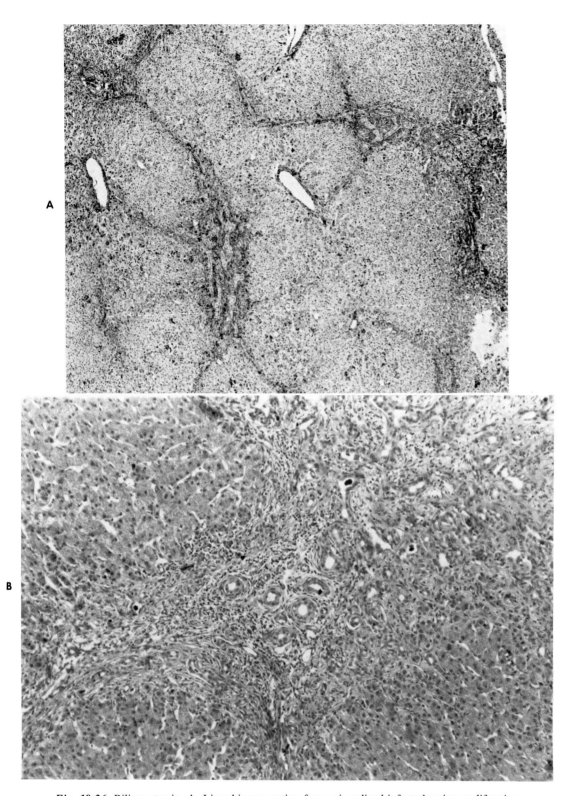

Fig. 19-26. Biliary atresia. **A,** Liver biopsy section from a jaundiced infant showing proliferating bile ducts and early portal and perilobular fibrosis while the overall hepatic architecture is preserved. **B,** High-power view of portal zone with normal-appearing adjacent lobules.

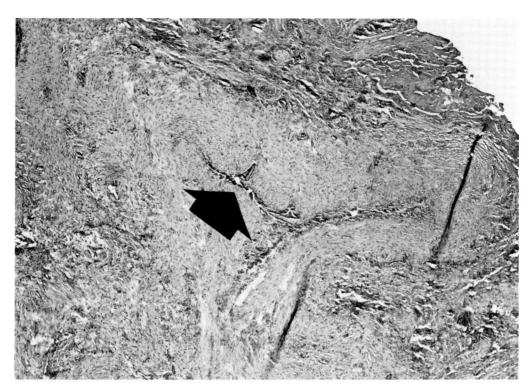

Fig. 19-27. Biliary atresia. Histologic section through the fibrous biliary tree remnant found at surgical exploration in a 2-month-old jaundiced infant. A small, collapsed bile duct is present, *arrow,* surrounded by intraductal and periductal fibrosis. Chronic inflammatory cells are present in small numbers.

tomy, the likelihood of bile drainage indeed correlates with the histologic lesion observed in the proximal portion of the resected remnants. The greatest likelihood of success (sustained bile drainage) is found when a columnar epithelium–lined central bile duct structure is present within the pathologic lesion that shows periductal fibrosis with or without an accompanying chronic inflammatory reaction. Others have noted that the quantity and quality of bile flow will correlate with the presence or absence of a "reasonable" bile duct structure (over 150 μm) in tissue taken from the porta hepatis. The severity of intrahepatic fibrosis and the degree of neoductular proliferation may also correlate with the histologic appearance of the extrahepatic bile duct remnants, but the degree of intrahepatic fibrosis does not correlate with the age at diagnosis.

Diagnosis

Once biliary atresia is strongly suspected from the clinical, laboratory, roentgenologic, and histologic assessment, surgical exploration is under-

taken as soon as possible. When the diagnosis has been greatly delayed, a brief preoperative period of nutritional rehabilitation and correction of existing coagulation abnormalities may be necessary. The minilaparotomy should be performed by a pediatric surgeon both experienced and skilled in treating this condition.

The laparotomy must include at least an adequate liver biopsy specimen and an operative cholangiogram (if the gallbladder is present) as a minimal reward for undertaking the procedure. Most pediatric surgeons agree on the early surgical maneuvers after entering the abdomen. Once the gallbladder is identified, fluid is aspirated to determine whether it contains normal bile. The presence of bile in the gallbladder implies patency of the proximal duct system, and the operative cholangiogram performed in this situation attempts to determine whether the distal biliary duct system is patent. Visualization of radiopaque medium in the duodenum is acceptable evidence that the distal extrahepatic ducts are not obstructed (Fig. 19-29). If complete patency of the extrahepatic

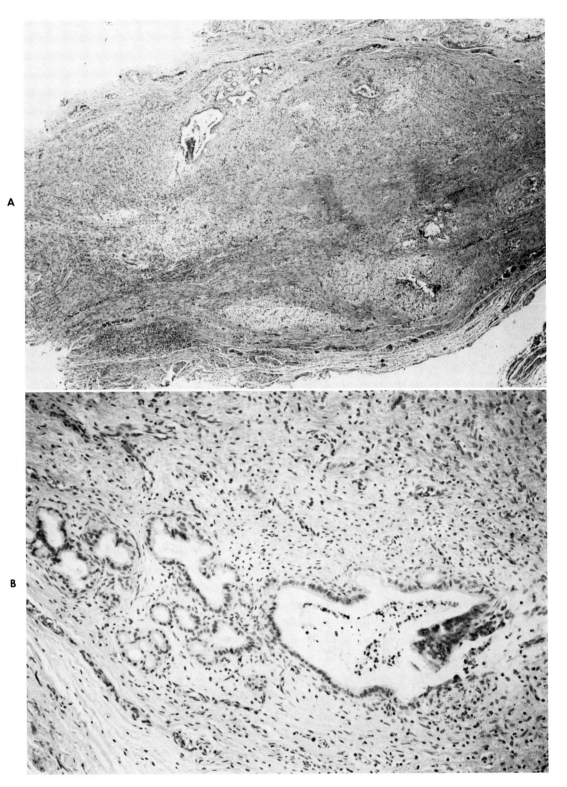

Fig. 19-28. Biliary atresia. **A,** Histologic section through the fibrous biliary tree remnant removed in preparation for the Kasai procedure. Note the small glandular bile ducts surrounded by fibrous scar tissue. Chronic inflammatory cells are present. **B,** High-power view shows relatively normal bile duct epithelium within the proliferating ductules.

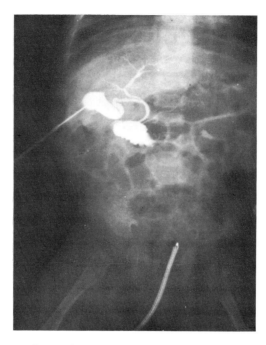

Fig. 19-29. Normal operative cholangiogram in an infant with prolonged obstructive jaundice. Complete opacification of the extrahepatic biliary system is seen. Dye is also noted within the liver radicles, duodenum, and pancreatic duct.

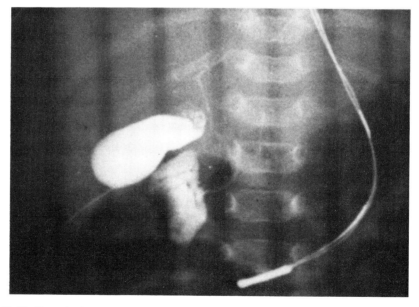

Fig. 19-30. Hypoplastic extrahepatic bile ducts. Operative cholangiogram in an infant suspected of having biliary atresia. At surgery a normal-sized gallbladder containing white mucus was found. The bile ducts are threadlike but patent from the liver hilum to the duodenum. Except for obtainment of a liver biopsy (wedge and needle) specimen, no additional surgical procedure is indicated in these cases.

biliary system is confirmed, the surgeon should obtain both a wedge liver biopsy and a needle biopsy specimen taken from the apex of the wedge. Because possibilities do exist for patchy representation of the underlying hepatic disease, a biopsy specimen from both hepatic lobes is recommended whenever possible. The operative procedure is then terminated.

If the surgeon encounters a small, collapsed, atretic-appearing gallbladder devoid of normal bile but containing white bile, he should still try to obtain a cholangiogram. Such a gallbladder of disuse has been seen in cases of severe intrahepatic cholestasis associated with neonatal hepatitis or paucity of the intrahepatic bile ducts. A patent extrahepatic biliary system will be visualized by the cholangiogram, though the extrahepatic ducts may appear small and hypoplastic (Fig. 19-30). In such cases, the procedure is terminated after the liver biopsy material is obtained.

When the gallbladder is absent or atretic and a cholangiogram cannot be made, the incision is then extended and the surgeon carefully continues a dissection of the structures within the porta hepatis up to the liver hilum with the hope of identifying a usable bile duct for anastomosis to the bowel. Should no suitable structure be found for the anastomosis, the definitive drainage procedure will require a hepatoportoenterostomy (Kasai's operation). If the gallbladder is absent or atretic, the likelihood of finding a usable proximal duct appears to be less than 10%.

Surgical treatment

The most common anatomic variety of extrahepatic biliary atresia is that in which the entire system, from porta hepatis to duodenum, is atretic. This represents almost two thirds of the entire group. The dismal earlier results in these patients subjected to either hepatoenterostomy (approximation of cut liver surface to opening in bowel) or creation of internal biliary fistulas using Vitallium tubes have been responsible for the abandonment of these procedures.

Some patients secrete bile postoperatively through the rubber drain left in the region of the porta hepatis, and when the abdomen is reentered, the exact site of origin of the bile cannot be found. In such cases, a hepatoenterostomy had also been used with variable success.

Since 1959, when Kasai and co-workers first began to publish their success in obtaining bile flow after hepatic portoenterostomy in patients with biliary atresia, renewed enthusiasm for employing aggressive corrective surgery in these so-called noncorrectable cases has occurred in many countries around the world. Kasai's procedure involves ligating the distal common duct remnant and using this as a guide. Dissection and resection of the remaining extrahepatic bile ducts follows and includes that of the hepatic radicals as well as of the fibrous mass at the porta hepatis. Resection of this most proximal segment includes a ''button'' of tissue about 2 to 3 mm deep and 10 mm across. The gross and microscopic findings in the resected fibrous ''button'' just within the liver capsule may correlate with both the quantitative and qualitative aspects of subsequent bile excretion, and probably with prognosis. The bile-drainage tract is a hepatic portojejunostomy in Roux-en-Y fashion, preferably with a section of jejunum 40 to 50 cm in length used for the latter. Although the bowel–to–porta hepatis anastomosis flouts the important surgical principle of having a mucosa-to-mucosa anastomosis, bile begins to drain in 1 to 4 weeks in well over half the patients. Over the years a host of variations of the original bilidigestive anastomosis have been published, some directly related to the finding of patent extrahepatic remnants, but the majority are surgical maneuvers to diminish the high incidence 40% to 50%) of subsequent cholangitis.

The Denver group has used an intestinal Roux-en-Y anastomosis in which a cutaneous double-barreled enterostomy is constructed by Mikulicz's technique. The externally draining portojejunostomy is believed to have reduced the incidence of episodes of cholangitis, while also permitting observation and study (quantitative and qualitative) of the bile effluent. Bile from the proximal segment may be re-fed by tube into the distal stoma until such time as reestablishment of bile flow to the main gastrointestinal tract is accomplished. The latter is done by crushing of the intestinal spur with a Gross-Mikulicz clamp, and the procedure thereby spares the infant a second major operation (Fig. 19-31).

The importance of early surgical intervention has now been reinforced by the results of short-term data from Kasai and co-workers, who report biliary drainage success rates of 80% to 90% in patients operated on before 60 days of age, but falling to 20% if the operation is delayed beyond 90 days. Other pediatric surgeons likewise experi-

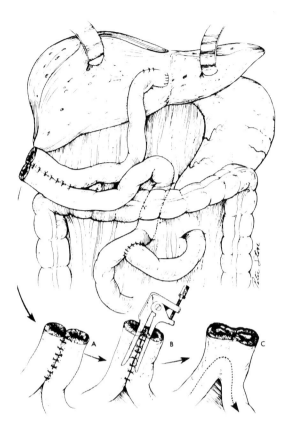

Fig. 19-31. The biliary-enteric anastomosis currently being performed in Denver for patients with biliary atresia. After excision of the extrahepatic bile ducts, the terminal side of a long (30 cm) Roux-en-Y intestinal segment is anastomosed to the stump of the transected duct in the liver hilum. A Mikulicz anastomosis is placed in the middle of the Roux-en-Y segment and exteriorized as a double-barreled enterostomy. *Insets,* Creation and subsequent management of the Mikulicz enterostomy. (From Lilly, J.R., and Altman, P.R.: Surgery **78:**76, 1975.)

enced in performing this operation continue to report 40% to 50% successful bile drainage even in children operated on between 2 and 3 months of age. Most agree, however, that obtainment of successful bile flow after 120 days is unlikely. It is interesting that these improved figures for continuous bile drainage by hepatoportoenterostomy are now higher than previously noted after the anastomosing of a patent segment of the extrahepatic bile duct to bowel in so-called correctable cases of biliary atresia. It has become apparent that, unless the patent distal remnant contains normal-appearing bile, hepatoportoenterostomy, even in these patients, may well be the procedure of

choice. In the past some surgeons believed that by allowing any useful biliary radical a chance to enlarge and dilate before the definitive procedure was carried out, they might offer a greater chance for subsequent success. In light of the present experience, early surgical intervention that permits establishment of bile drainage appears to offer the best chance for long-term survival, and the previous approach involving "second-look" surgery in infants with biliary atresia is no longer warranted.

If, at the time of the original surgery, the surgeon finds a portion of the extrahepatic biliary system patent and suitable for anastomosis (less than 10% to 20% of cases), either a portocholedochojejunostomy or cholecystojejunostomy can be attempted, depending on the existing anatomy.

Complications of biliary atresia surgery. Complications attending hepatic portoenterostomy are substantial and often life threatening. The most feared complication is that of postoperative cholangitis, which occurs in probably 50% of cases and as high as 100% (in one reported series) when normal-appearing bile ducts were found at the level of the porta hepatis. It would appear that cholangitis occurs especially in the face of sustained patency of the biliary digestive anastomosis (Fig. 19-32). The mechanism of cholangitis is poorly understood though ascending infection through the intestinal conduit to the porta hepatis by gastrointestinal organisms seems to be most plausible. Interestingly, septicemia is extremely rare and organisms have rarely been cultured from liver tissue obtained during bouts of cholangitis. Some workers believe that as a result of portoenterostomy an obstruction to hepatic-lymphatic drainage (lymphangitis) may predispose to episodes of intrahepatic cholangitis. Unfortunately, these attacks not only produce an acute febrile illness characterized by high fever, chills, leukocytosis, and rising bilirubin, but also hasten any ensuing liver damage and thereby accelerate the process of biliary cirrhosis. Episodes of cholangitis more commonly occur during the first postoperative year and thereafter diminish in frequency (four or five episodes versus two or three episodes per year). During attacks, the volume of bile flow invariably decreases, an event that can easily be appreciated if a cutaneous enteric conduit is present. Aminoglycoside antibiotic therapy generally leads to prompt resolution of the process with defervescence of fever and return of bile flow. Treatment

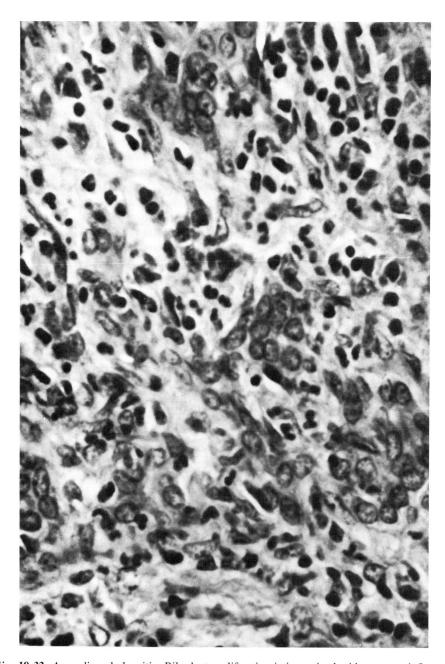

Fig. 19-32. Ascending cholangitis. Bile duct proliferation is intermixed with an acute inflammatory reaction. This child had prolonged obstructive jaundice during the newborn period and was found to have complete extrahepatic biliary atresia. Dissection was carried out to the liver hilum. Hepatojejunostomy was performed to the hilum of the liver when spontaneous flow of bile was noted coming from the original drain site. The child had done reasonably well until 1 year before hospital admission, when he experienced recurrent episodes of fever and intermittent pruritus leading to present admission and liver biopsy.

is continued for 10 to 14 days. Prophylaxis against cholangitis is now routine in most centers during the first year of life, with a combination of an antibiotic (trimethoprim-sulfamethoxazole, ampicillin, cephalosporin) and a choleretic (phenobarbital) being employed.

Another important complication that follows hepatic portoenterostomy is redeposition of fibrous tissue at the anastomotic site resulting in cessation of bile flow. Reoperation is feasible but requires a tedious, time-consuming dissection, with removal of the scar and resection of a new button of tissue from the liver hilum. Resumption of bile flow may be expected in 25% of reoperated cases. Although while peritonitis resulting from leakage of the biliary digestive anastomotic site may occur, it is more commonly reported in cholecystojejunostomy than with hepatic portoenterostomy.

Other complications of hepatic portoenterostomy more than likely reflect the natural history of this evolving pathologic process. Most disturbing is the continued progression of intrahepatic fibrosis that results in biliary cirrhosis, events that may occur despite adequate bile flow and clearing of the infant's jaundice. It is unclear at what stage this relentless progression to biliary cirrhosis may be consistently halted or reversed by the surgical drainage procedure. Some authors believe that progression of the liver disease represents a reaction to a "fibrogenetic" factor specific to congenital biliary atresia. Although the degree of fibrosis appears to increase with the age of the patient, the degree of increase is not consistent for all patients. One has to be impressed with the severity of the hepatic lesion seen in some unfortunate infants even before 8 weeks of age, implying other genetic or environmental determinants. A trend toward earlier surgical intervention (before 2 months) and long-term follow-up study of this particular age group should, we hope, answer the question of whether the evolving cirrhosis is attributable to progression of the underlying disease process, regardless of successful restoration of bile flow. It is likewise disappointing to find abnormal intrahepatic duct structures on transhepatic cholangiography even after resolution of jaundice. The ducts are often ectatic, dilated, and tortuous and reveal an abnormal drainage pattern.

Postoperatively, notwithstanding "adequate" bile flow, growth and nutrition may be compromised in these patients. In some children normal volume of bile (200 to 300 ml/day) may not occur until 6 to 12 months postoperatively, and even with refeeding of the bile through the distal stoma, fat malabsorption and steatorrhea are primarily responsible for the poor growth and gain, especially during the first year of life. Early on, fat-soluble vitamin D deficiency is first suspected by roentgenographic evidence of rickets. Later, the older child often shows bony changes of osteoporosis. Intestinal malabsorption of vitamin D rather than impaired hepatic conversion of the vitamin to 1,25-dihydroxy-vitamin D_3 is believed to be the mechanism by which rickets develops in biliary atresia, but a pathophysiologic explanation for the delayed appearance of osteoporosis remains to be clarified.

Other complications of the disease process include persistence of portal hypertension and the subsequent development of splenomegaly with hypersplenism and esophageal varices. Hemorrhage from these varices is surprisingly rare early in the postoperative course. In some centers spontaneous regression of esophageal varices has been observed in children surviving to school age years.

Although 100% of infants with biliary atresia not corrected by surgery will die (only 1% survive to 4 years of age), undertaking surgery of the Kasai type is no small decision. The operation has far-reaching effects on both the infant and family. The need for repeated hospitalizations especially during the first year of life, with or without subsequent surgery, substantially contributes to the early developmental delays especially in gross motor skills. The majority of families can be expected to have difficulty in coping with the ongoing medical and surgical crisis, and the almost continuous stress parallels the high incidence of marital discord and subsequent divorce. Significant financial hardships posed by relocation close to a regional medical center undoubtedly contributes to the marital discord.

Prognosis after hepatoportoenterostomy. Without doubt this operation has substantially extended the survival of many infants with biliary atresia, with some authors reporting 3-year survival rates of 35% to 65%. The Japanese experience reports 48 infants who have survived free from jaundice for more than 5 years after surgery, five in this small group being older than 10 years, the eldest a young adult. In the French experience of 33 survivors, 22 were reported to be completely jaun-

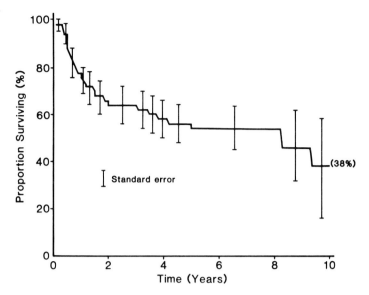

Fig. 19-33. The proportion of surviving patients with biliary atresia after ''corrective'' surgery over varying time periods as reported by the Biliary Atresia Registry to the Committee of the Section on Surgery of the American Academy of Pediatrics in 1981.

dice free and their long-term prognosis was believed to be good. Seventeen of these children were 3 or more years of age, and five were over 5 years. The surgical results in 47 consecutive cases of extrahepatic biliary atresia reported from England showed effective bile drainage and return of serum bilirubin concentrations to normal in 38% of patients. However, 16 jaundice-free survivors continued to show abnormal liver function tests with almost all having persistence of a firm-to-hard enlarged liver and palpable spleen. Complications of portal hypertension manifested by esophageal hemorrhage was reported in one child, but the mean age of follow-up study in the group was only 20 months, with a range from 3 to 65 months.

The current Denver experience shows an overall 3-year survival of 38%, rising to 66% in those children operated on before 2 months of age and when the external enteric conduit for biliary drainage was utilized. In the group followed for at least 3 years, five were noted to have esophageal varices, with one resolving spontaneously at 45 months of age, and one patient who bled from varices subsequently had sclerotherapy as prophylaxis. Recent actuarial figures from the entire United States experience reporting biliary atresia data to the Surgical Section of the American Academy of Pediatrics projects a 38% 10-year survival postoperatively (Fig. 19-33). The best predictors for long-term survival after portoenter-

ostomy are (1) surgery before 10 to 12 weeks, (2) presence of a large bile duct (more than 150 μm) in the porta hepatis, and (3) bile bilirubin concentration greater than 8.8 mg/dl 3 months after surgery.

Another long-term concern in patients surviving with ''stable'' biliary cirrhosis is the small but apparent increased risk to develop hepatic carcinoma. Hepatocellular carcinoma and carcinoma in situ has been found in the livers removed in preparation for orthotopic liver transplantation. In addition, cholangiocarcinoma has also been reported in infants surviving surgery for biliary atresia.

In those unfortunate children who fail to obtain sustained bile flow, biliary cirrhosis ensues quite rapidly and death from hepatic failure usually occurs before 18 months of age. Not infrequently, progressive and intractable ascites, with derangement of fluid and electrolyte balance, contribute to the patient's final demise. Terminally, an intercurrent infection and sepsis usher in disseminated intravascular coagulation, severe acidosis, and hemorrhage.

For a number of years it was believed that the Kasai hepatic portoenterostomy procedure might be considered a useful first-stage procedure for treatment of biliary atresia. It was hoped that infants subjected to that operation would grow to sufficient size before requiring orthotopic liver transplantation for a "permanent" cure. Unfortunately, orthotopic liver transplantation has not afforded the long-term benefits, except in a very limited number of patients. In the largest series dealing with pediatric patients subjected to liver replacement for biliary atresia, only eight of the 48 were alive 1 year after transplantation. The early difficulties with obtainment of better survival figures in this patient group were attributable to technical problems, requiring the anastomosis of small structures, improper donor organ size, the finding of coexisting vascular and intestinal anomalies (absent inferior vena cava, preduodenal portal vein, anomalous hepatic artery, intestinal malrotation, and situs inversus). However, prevention of rejection reaction by immunosuppression still poses considerable problems for these patients. Septic episodes and hepatic abscess formation occur with distressing frequency in these immunosuppressed children. Even with immunosuppressive therapy and organ survival, a distressing finding from follow-up biopsies (or at autopsy) in some of the donor organs has been the disappearance of interlobular bile ducts, hepatocyte and canalicular cholestasis, and septal fibrosis. As with Kasai's procedure, the need for repeat hospitalizations contributes to severe growth and developmental delays adding to the psychologic burden for both child and family. Hope continues, however, that the difficulties will be overcome with time, and therein another chance for survival for infants subsequently failing a hepatic portoenterostomy operation will be maintained.

Medical aspects of treatment

Continued attention to nutritional needs of these children is particularly important during the first year of life. Certainly, until bile flow is adequate, the children should be fed a formula containing medium-chain triglycerides (Portagen or Pregestimil) to minimize fat malabsorption and maximize caloric utilization. The infants also need supplementation with water-miscible forms of vitamins A, E, and K. For those infants showing a progressive decrease in density of bone by roentgenographic examination, 1,24-dihydroxy-vitamin D_3 can be given on a daily basis at a dosage of 0.20 μg/kg.

Although of unproved value, prophylactic antibiotics during the first year of life are routinely employed. Trimethoprim-sulfamethoxazole, ampicillin, or a cephalosporin are the most common antibiotics utilized. Aminoglycosides (gentamicin, amikacin, 25 mg/kg/day) and recently metronidazole (Flagyl) have been employed to treat episodes of cholangitis. Checking blood levels of these agents ensures obtainment of maximum effect.

Choleretic agents may have a role in the postoperative period to facilitate bile flow and theoretically reduce the incidence of ascending cholangitis. Phenobarbital, 3 to 5 mg/kg/24 hr, or cholestyramine, 2 to 4 gm/24 hr, is a useful drug in this regard.

The consequences of portal hypertension generally require no special treatment during the first several years of life. Likewise, hypersplenism seldom poses any difficulties for the patient. Since the esophageal varices may spontaneously regress by 4 to 5 years of age, prophylactic portocaval shunting is not recommended. In the unusual infant who bleeds from varices, endosclerosis of the varices (see Chapter 25) may be undertaken as a reasonable delaying tactic while one awaits their spontaneous regression. Antacids or cimetidine is of no proved value in the prevention of esophageal hemorrhage. However, the parents of these children should be provided with a list of products known to contain salicylates so that they may be assiduously avoided during intercurrent febrile illnesses and respiratory infections.

The appearance of ascites portends a poor prognosis. Initially, the ascites may be intermittent or persistent but is generally responsive to medical measures that include limiting the dietary sodium intake or the use of diuretics. Spironolactone (Aldactone) and furosemide (Lasix) are generally effective agents in treating this complication. A complete discussion of ascites as a complication of chronic liver disease is found in Chapter 24.

Enrollment of the child in a physical therapy program will serve to prevent significant gross motor delays, a finding common in these children especially during the first 1 to 2 years. Actively involving the parents in a home stimulation program is extremely worthwhile because it serves to reestablish maternal-child bonding through non–illness dependent relationships. Regional centers engaged in biliary atresia surgery are capable of providing such support systems for family members, either individually or in groups, with discussions led by clinical social workers and psychiatric personnel where appropriate.

Utilizing this overall medical and surgical treat-

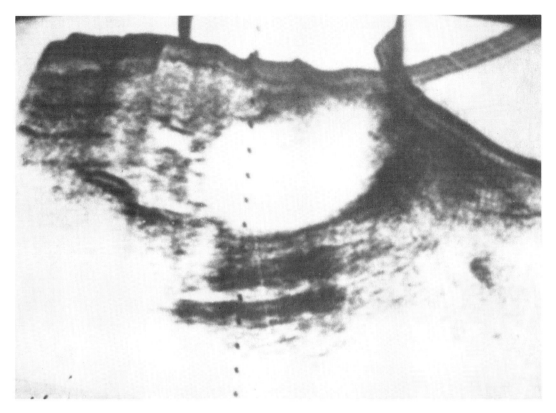

Fig. 19-34. Choledochal cyst. This large echo-free mass demonstrated by ultrasound examination in a 6-week-old infant with persistent cholestasis. A dilated biliary duct is also apparent.

ment program, the majority of the surviving older children can lead reasonably normal lives, attending preschool and participating in age-appropriate activities along with their peers.

Certainly not all children operated on for biliary atresia will demonstrate prolonged survival, but the survival rates continue to improve as does the overall quality of life. Without surgery, the disease is invariably fatal in most children before they reach 18 months of age.

Choledochal cyst

This lesion is a rare cause of extrahepatic biliary obstruction in the neonatal period and is found in 1% to 3% of cases presenting with obstructive jaundice. The cystic dilatation of the common duct may conform anatomically to that typically observed in the older child (type 1-Alonzo-Lej classification) and may be detected by abdominal palpation as a subhepatic mass. These lesions can be easily identified by ultrasound examination (Fig. 19-34) or suspected by the mass effect it creates upon the duodenum during upper gastrointestinal

roentgenology (Fig. 19-35). These large cysts are associated with dilatation of the proximal bile ducts and complete distal obstruction, findings best appreciated by the operative cholangiogram. The hepatic pathologic appearance shows those features consistent with extrahepatic obstruction (neoductular proliferation and portal fibrosis), but, interestingly, coexistent lobular disarray and giant-cell transformation may also be present. Whenever possible, these lesions are best treated by a cyst resection and hepatojejunostomy or choledochojejunostomy (see Chapter 26). Provided that recurrent episodes of cholangitis are few, the prognosis is very good, with resolution of the jaundice and restoration of the normal liver architecture expected.

When associated with neonatal cholestasis, smaller cyst formation (less than 2 cm) involving the extrahepatic biliary tree is more than likely to be a variant of biliary atresia. Indeed, the cholangiogram performed through the cyst lumen often shows abnormal-appearing proximal biliary ducts of small caliber having an irregular and beaded

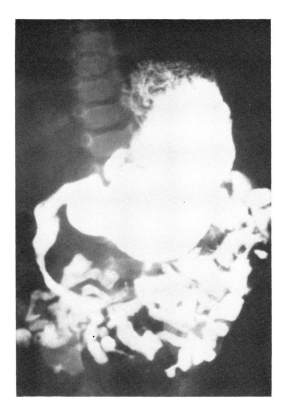

Fig. 19-35. Barium-contract upper gastrointestinal series in an infant with cholestatic syndrome. A large extrinsic mass is noted that widens the duodenal C-loop while also pulling the duodenal bulb downward. A choledochal cyst was found at surgery.

configuration. In these cases the failure to visualize the duodenum by intraoperative cholangiography is consistent with accompanying atresia of the distal duct system (Fig. 19-36). Unless these small cysts contain normal-appearing bile, most surgeons experienced in this field will perform a hepatic portoenterostomy rather than use either the cyst or a proximal duct structure for the biliary digestive anastomosis. Again, the hepatic histologic appearance is typically that expected in extrahepatic obstruction, but 10% of cases do show features also encountered in intrahepatic cholestasis. The long-term prognosis for this group of infants is similar to that discussed previously for all infants with biliary atresia subjected to hepatic portoenterostomy.

Spontaneous perforation of extrahepatic bile ducts

Spontaneous perforation of the extrahepatic bile duct is the one extrahepatic condition that can mimic certain causes of intrahepatic cholestasis. The confusion with possible intrahepatic causes

derives from the infant's clinical presentation that frequently includes irritability, vomiting, failure to thrive, low-grade fever, and abdominal distention. These signs and symptoms evolving over the first month of life in a jaundiced neonate are consistent with infectious causes of intrahepatic cholestasis, certain metabolic causes, or cholestasis associated with a urinary tract infection. However, the finding of a normal liver size in the face of acholic stools may help separate this particular entity from the aforementioned causes of neonatal cholestasis. If, in addition, ascites is detected either by physical examination or ultrasound, the physician should suspect spontaneous perforation of the extrahepatic bile ducts. Aspiration of the ascitic fluid will promptly confirm the diagnosis by revealing bile-colored material. Additional clinical features sometimes include the presence of bile-stained hydroceles and, if present, the umbilical hernia as well. Liver-function studies are generally normal with the exception of the elevated serum bilirubin level. Abdominal scanning after the ^{131}I–rose bengal test or the recently em-

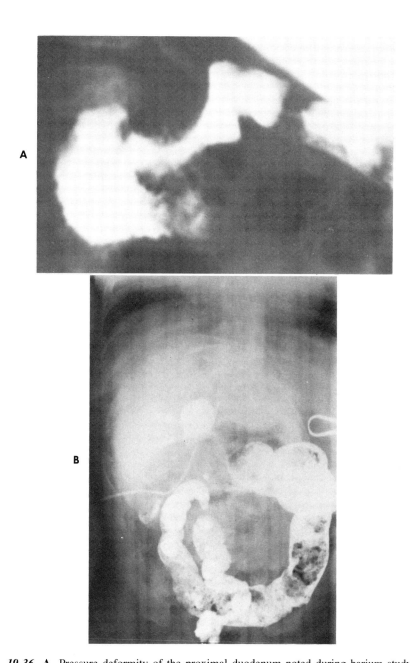

Fig. 19-36. **A,** Pressure deformity of the proximal duodenum noted during barium study of the upper gastrointestinal tract, which was performed as part of the "routine" work-up of a patient with a neonatal cholestatic syndrome. **B,** Operative cholangiogram performed on the same infant reveals the dilated biliary structure, which failed to communicate with the duodenum, requiring a choledochojejunostomy.   *Continued*

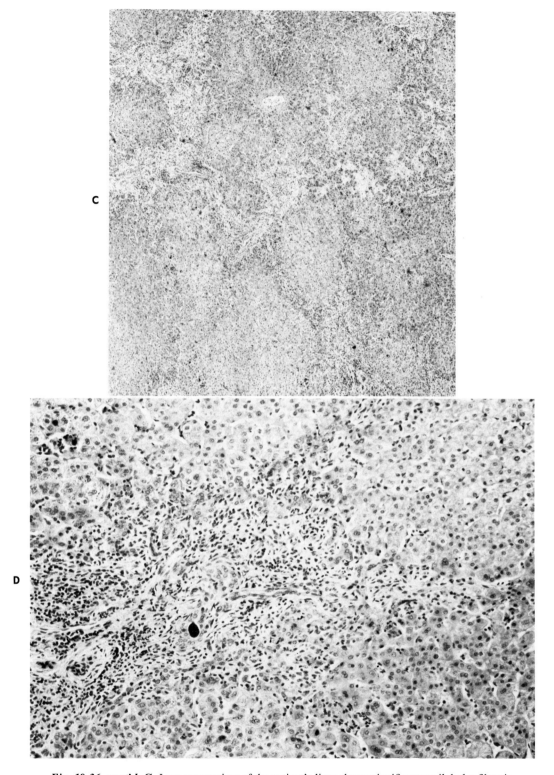

Fig. 19-36, cont'd. **C,** Low-power view of the patient's liver shows significant perilobular fibrosis (6 weeks of age) with a moderate portal inflammatory response. **D,** High-power view shows normal hepatocytes, portal reaction, and plugged bile duct.

ployed DIDA scan likewise should be diagnostic. Occasionally the bile accumulates in the subhepatic region as a "false" sac, whereby it may mimic that of a neonatal choledochal cyst.

Surgery is immediately undertaken both to ascertain the site of the perforation and to uncover any predisposing conditions that may be associated with this lesion. The site of perforation in almost all cases is reported to be at the junction of the cystic and common ducts. An embryologic defect and resulting malformation in the duct wall is believed to predispose to local weakness and subsequent rupture. The events that lead up to rupture of this mural defect are unknown, but abnormal dynamics of bile flow within the extrahepatic system during the first few months of life is suggested, since most cases occur during this time period. Occasional examples have also been associated with stenosis of the distal portion of the common duct, obstructing stones or sludged bile.

When the abdomen is entered, a cholecystogram is usually performed to identify the pathologic condition and site of perforation. The inflammed porta hepatis is not explored, but rather soft-rubber drains are left in the area of the perforation and the abdomen is closed. Most surgeons prefer to leave a catheter in the gallbladder for follow-up studies to determine healing of the perforation. Thereafter the drains and cystostomy catheter may be removed. Postoperatively the infants are kept on antibiotics, yet rarely is the bile found free in the abdomen infected. Some employ parenteral hyperalimentation to minimize bile flow until such time that follow-up studies reveal healing of the perforation. Otherwise, those products devoid of fat (Vivonex, nonfat skim milk) may be offered orally. A recent report recommends cholecystojejunostomy as the surgical drainage procedure of choice when accompanying obstruction of the distal common bile duct is encountered.

Intrinsic bile duct obstruction

This condition is probably the least common cause of extrahepatic biliary obstruction in the neonate. Most cases occur after severe hemolytic disease (Rh, ABO, and so on) resulting in inspissation of viscid bile and formation of granular concretions and occasionally gallstones, all capable of occluding the distal portion of the common duct. The clinical picture is that of complete cholestasis (acholic stools). Ultrasound study may reveal dilated proximal bile duct structures as the

DIDA scan also may. The preoperative suspicion is enhanced by a history of hemolytic disease, in which case a brief trial of choleretics, such as cholestyramine and phenobarbital, can be employed provided that the liver biopsy specimen does not show advancing portal fibrosis. A trial of repeated intravenous cholecystokinin given every 8 hours for 1 or 2 days may be useful.

Although the diagnosis may be suspected clinically, almost all will require surgery and an intraoperative cholangiogram for confirmation. Underlying stricture or stenosis of the distal common duct will also be revealed by this study. After opening of the common duct the inspissated material is irrigated and removed, and contrast medium then instilled into the T-tube drain confirms patency of the extrahepatic system into the duodenum. The T tube is removed after 3 weeks.

REFERENCES

Andrews, W.S., Pau, C.M., Chase, P., Foley, C., and others: Fat soluble vitamin deficiency in biliary atresia, J. Pediatr. Surg. **16**(3):284-290, 1981.

Barkin, R.M., and Lilly, J.R.: Biliary atresia and the Kasai operation: continuing care, J. Pediatr. **96**:1015-1019, 1980.

Barlow, B., Tabor, E., Blanc, W.A., and others: Choledochal cyst: a review of 19 cases, J. Pediatr. **89**:634-940, 1976.

Berenson, M.M., Garde, A.R., and Moody, F.G.: Twenty-five year survival after surgery for complete extrahepatic biliary atresia, Gastroenterology **66**:260-263, 1974.

Bernstein, J., Braylan, R., and Brough, A.J.: Bile-plug syndrome: a correctable cause of obstructive jaundice in infants, Pediatrics **43**(2):273-276, 1969.

Chandra, R.S.: Biliary atresia and other structural anomalies in the congenital polysplenia syndrome, J. Pediatr. **85**:649-655, 1974.

Chandra, R.S., and Altman, R.P.: Ductal remnants in extrahepatic biliary atresia: a histopathologic study with clinical correlation, Pediatrics **93**:196-200, 1978.

Draz, S., Barajas, L., and Fonkalsrud, E.W.: Reversibility of biliary cirrhosis due to bile duct obstruction, J. Pediatr. Surg. **6**:256-263, 1971.

Dunn, P.M.: Obstructive jaundice and haemolytic disease of the newborn, Arch. Dis. Child. **38**:54-61, Feb. 1963.

Gautier, M., Jehan, P., and Odièvre, M.: Histologic study of biliary fibrous remnants in 48 cases of extrahepatic biliary atresia: correlation with postoperative bile flow restoration, J. Pediatr. **89**:704-709, 1976.

Ghishan, F.K., LaBrecque, D.R., Mitros, F.A., and others: The evolving nature of "infantile obstructive cholangiopathy," J. Pediatr. **97**:27-32 1980.

Harris, V.J., and Kahler, J.: Choledochal cyst: delayed diagnosis in a jaundiced infant, Pediatrics **62**(2):235-237, 1978.

Hays, D., and Snyder, W., Jr.: Untreated biliary atresia, Surgery **54**:373-375, 1963.

Hays, D.M., Woolley, M.M., Snyder, W.J., Jr., and others: Diagnosis of biliary atresia: relative accuracy of percutaneous liver biopsy, open liver biopsy and operative cholangiography, J. Pediatr. **71**:698-607, 1967.

Hitch, D.C., Shikes, R.H., and Lilly, J.R.: Determinants of survival after Kasai's operation for biliary atresia using actuarial analysis, J. Pediatr. Surg. **14**(3):310-314, 1979.

Howard, E.R., Johnston, D.I., and Mowat, A.P.: Spontaneous perforation of common bile duct in infants, Arch. Dis. Child. **51**:883-886, 1976.

Howard, E.R., and Mowat, A.P.: Extrahepatic biliary atresia, Arch. Dis. Child. **52**:825-827, 1977.

Hughes, R., and Mayell, M.: Cholelithiasis in a neonate, Arch. Dis. Child. **50**:815-816, 1975.

Kasai, M.: Treatment of biliary atresia with special reference to hepatic porto-enterostomy and its modifications, Progr. Pediatr. Surg. **6**:5-52, 1974.

Kasai, M., Kimura, S., Asakura Y., and others: Surgical treatment of biliary atresia, J. Pediatr. Surg. **3**:665-675, 1968.

Kobayashi, A., and Ohbe, Y.: Choledochal cyst in infancy and childhood, Arch. Dis. Child. **52**:121-128, 1977.

Kobayashi, A., Utsunomiya, T., Ohbe, Y., and others: Ascending cholangitis after successful surgical repair of biliary atresia, Arch. Dis. Child. **48**:697-703, 1973.

Kooh, S.W., Jones, G., Reilly, B.J., and Fraser, D.: Pathogenesis of rickets in chronic hepatobiliary disease in children, J. Pediatr. **94**:870-874, 1979.

Krovetz, L.J.: Congenital biliary atresia: I. Analysis of 30 cases with particular reference to diagnosis. II. Analysis of the therapeutic problem, Surgery **47**:453-489, 1960.

Kulkarni, P.B., and Beatty, E.C., Jr.: Cholangiocarcinoma associated with biliary cirrhosis due to congenital biliary atresia, Am. J. Dis. Child. **131**(4):442-444, April 1977.

Landing, B.H.: Considerations of the pathogenesis of neonatal hepatitis, biliary atresia and choledochal cyst: the concept of infantile obstructive cholangiopathy, Progr. Pediatr. Surg. **6**:113-139, 1974.

Lilly, J.R.: Surgical jaundice in infancy, Ann. Surg. **186**(5):549-558, Nov. 1977.

Lilly, J.R., and Altman, R.P.: Hepatic portoenterostomy (the Kasai operation) for biliary atresia, Surgery **78**:76-86, 1975.

Lilly, J.R., Altman, R.P., Schröter, G., and others: Surgery of biliary atresia, Am. J. Dis. Child. **129**(12):1429-1432, Dec. 1975.

Lilly, J.R., and Starzl, T.E.: Liver transplantation in children with biliary atresia and vascular anomalies, J. Paediatr. Surg. **9**(5):707-714, Oct. 1974.

Lilly, J.R., Weintraub, W.H., and Altman, R.P.: Spontaneous perforation of the extrahepatic bile ducts and bile peritonitis in infancy, Surgery **75**:664-673, 1974.

Miyata, M., Satani, M., Ueda, T., and Okamoto, E.: Long-term results of hepatic portoenterostomy for biliary atresia: special reference to postoperative portal hypertension, Surgery **76**:234-237, 1974.

Nakai, H., and Landing, B.H.: Factors in the genesis of bile stasis in infancy, Pediatrics **27**:300-307, Feb. 1961.

Odièvre, M.: Long-term results of surgical treatment of biliary atresia, World J. Surg. **2**:589-594, 1978.

Odièvre, M., Valayer, J., Razemon-Pinta, M., and others: Hepatic portoenterostomy or cholecystostomy in the treatment of extrahepatic biliary atresia, J. Pediatr. **88**:774-779, 1976.

Ohi, R., Shikes, R.H., and Lilly, J.R.: Bile flow and ductular histology in biliary atresia, Gastroenterology **77**:A30, 1979.

Psacharopoulos, H.T., Howard, E.R., Portmann, B., and Mowat, A.P.: Extrahepatic biliary atresia: preoperative assessment and surgical results in 47 consecutive cases, Arch. Dis. Child. **55**:851-856, 1980.

Sharp, H.L., Krivit, W., and Lowman, J.T.: The diagnosis of complete extrahepatic obstruction by rose bengal ^{131}I, J. Pediatr. **70**:46-53, 1967.

Silverberg, M., and Davidson, M.: Nutritional requirements of infants and children with liver disease, Am. J. Clin. Nutr. **23**:604-613, 1970.

Starzl, T.E., Koep, L.R., Halgrimson, C.G., and others: Fifteen years of clinical liver transplantation, Gastroenterology **77**:375-388, 1979.

Starzl, T.E., Koep, L.J., Schröter, G.P., and others: Liver replacement for pediatric patients, Pediatrics **63**(6):825-829, June 1979.

Weber, A., and Roy, C.C.: The malabsorption associated with chronic liver disease in children, Pediatrics **50**:73-83, 1972.

Whitington, P.F., and Black, D.D.: Cholelithiasis in premature infants treated with parenteral nutrition and furosemide, J. Pediatr. **97**(4):647-649, 1980.

20 *Nonhemolytic noncholestatic hyperbilirubinemia syndromes*

PHYSIOLOGIC JAUNDICE OF THE NEWBORN
Mechanisms in physiologic jaundice

The fetus normally maintains low levels of serum bilirubin, and several factors are now believed responsible for this physiologic state in utero (Fig. 20-1). Inhibition of maturational events prevents activation of the fetal hepatic enzymes, glucuronyl transferase and uridine diphosphate glucuronide dehydrogenase (UDPG dehydrogenase), thereby preventing the formation of significant amounts of bilirubin glucuronide in utero. These observations have been repeatedly confirmed in a variety of mammals, including man.

The mechanism for this inhibition is not completely understood, but many workers believe that a progestational steroid, pregnanediol, plays a significant role in suppressing glucuronyl transferase in utero. Recently, it has been suggested that activation of hepatic conjugation enzymes is substrate dependent. Under normal conditions the rapid placental transfer of unconjugated bilirubin (substrate) from fetus to mother is capable of maintaining the physiologic state. The ability of fat soluble, nonpolar bilirubin to diffuse easily across cell membranes is facilitated at this maternal-fetal interface, perhaps because of the greater concentration of circulating albumin in the maternal blood. The ability of the placenta to clear unconjugated bilirubin, but not the glucuronide of bilirubin, is undoubtedly extremely important in preventing the fetus from developing significant levels of hyperbilirubinemia. Hepatocyte uptake is to a large degree dependent on the concentration of the intracellular ligandin (Y protein) whose concentration is extremely low during fetal life and rises rapidly just before or shortly after delivery. This protein may be substrate inducible (by bilirubin), but under normal conditions, effective placental clearing of fetal bilirubin keeps the hepatic contribution for clearing this substance in reserve.

The physiologic inter-relationships between placental function, fetal unconjugated serum bilirubin level, and hepatic bilirubin uptake and conjugating activity are nicely emphasized by the observations that in instances of severe Rh isoimmunization, the placental capacity to handle bilirubin production can be overcome; as fetal serum levels rise, direct-reacting bilirubin (glucuronide) is produced by the fetal liver and can be detected in cord blood. The highest levels have been reported in babies born after intrauterine blood transfusions. It is also curious that some elevation of direct-reacting bilirubin can be occasionally detected in the cord blood of postmature babies, a condition not infrequently associated with a dysplacental state (falling maternal estriols).

The clamping of the umbilical cord immediately after delivery separates the new-born infant from mother and placenta, leaving the development of physiologic jaundice in the newborn to be determined primarily by the balance achieved between bilirubin production from breakdown of red blood cells and other heme sources, and rapid maturation and effectiveness of the hepatic glucuronide conjugation mechanism. Undoubtedly, in a manner as yet unexplained, genetic and environmental factors play a role in governing the appearance and the magnitude of the bilirubin rise. The newborn wastes little time in adjusting to his new environment.

Bilirubin production parallels the rapid increase in reticuloendothelial tissue activity of heme oxygenase, the rate-limiting enzyme, in breaking down the heme molecule into biliverdin. Apparently, the concentration of biliverdin reductase is sufficiently high in newborn tissues to accomplish the rapid conversion of biliverdin to bilirubin. Not only is the neonate suddenly faced with handling large amounts of bilirubin from the degradation of hematopoietic heme, but he must also cope with a large percentage of nonerythropoietic heme (myoglobin, cytochromes, catalase) that temporarily accompanies the adjustment to extrauterine life.

Meanwhile, hepatic glucuronyl transferase activity, virtually absent during intrauterine life, begins to increase rapidly within the first 2 weeks of life. In addition, the concentration of specific intracytoplasmic binding ligandins increases, thereby facilitating the rapid transfer of albumin-bound

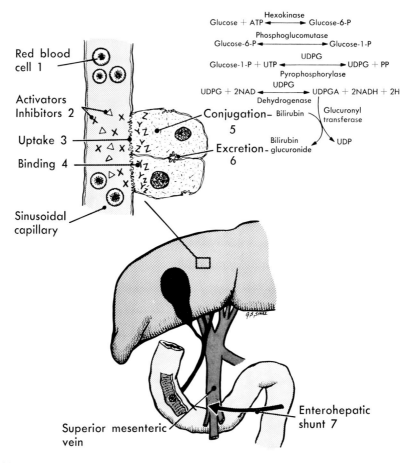

Fig. 20-1. Factors known or believed to be involved in the nonhemolytic hyperbilirubinemia syndromes: physiologic jaundice of the newborn (**1, 2, 3, 4, 5, ?6, 7**); breast-milk hyperbilirubinemia (**2,5**); Crigler-Najjar syndrome (**5**); Gilbert's syndrome (**?1, ?2, 3, ?4, 5, ?6, ?7**); Dubin-Johnson syndrome (**?2, ?3, 6**); Rotor's syndrome (**3, 6**).

Key: **1,** Red blood cell breakdown—production of bilirubin.
       2, Serum factors (inhibitors, activators, glucose concentration, others).
       3, Uptake (across hepatic sinusoid membrane).
       4, Binding (intracellular Y and Z proteins).
       5, Conjugation (glucuronyl transferase deficiency, partial or complete).
       6, Excretion (intracellular transport to bile canaliculus).
       7, Enterohepatic shunt.

bilirubin across the hepatic cell membrane, which in turn prevents the efflux of bilirubin back into the plasma. Ligandin and Z protein may be necessary for the intracellular transport of bilirubin to the endoplasmic reticulum, the site of action of the enzyme uridine diphosphoglucuronyl transferase. Bilirubin monoglucuronide is formed at this location, but recent evidence suggests that bilirubin diglucuronide is formed at another intracellular site, perhaps the hepatic membrane in the region of the bile canaliculus. The products of bili-

rubin conjugation reach the biliary system after transfer across this specialized portion of the hepatocyte, the bile canaliculi. The secretory process is energy dependent and probably carrier mediated. The rapidly increasing concentration in the neonate of another enzyme, beta-glucuronidase, may also be important in the elimination of bilirubin diglucuronide from the hepatocytes.

Obviously, the development of physiologic jaundice is multifactorial and needs to be considered within the framework of those concepts dealing with the increased production of bilirubin products, the release from "inhibitors," the activation and maturation of the bilirubin uptake, binding, conjugating, and secreting systems within the liver, and the efficiency of the excretory system outside the liver. The rapidity with which the normal full-term infant activates his hepatic conjugating system of bilirubin is emphasized by the fact that the average serum bilirubin level at 3 days of age is only about 7 mg/dl. Calculations with figures for red blood cell breakdown per day (derived from estimated fetal red blood cell life-span of 90 days), total hemoglobin mass, and bilirubin space would predict over three times this amount (26 mg/dl) if no conjugation of bilirubin took place.

In the normal full-term infant, bilirubin levels reach a maximum (6 to 12 mg/dl) between the fourth and the sixth day of life. Although premature infants have the same bilirubin level at birth as full-term infants, their bilirubin values tend to reach higher levels (11 to 15 mg/dl) by the fifth or sixth day. Of particular interest is the fact that conjugated bilirubin in both premature and full-term infants begins to appear at the same time after birth, with levels being maintained below 1.5 mg/dl in normal conditions. Although some believe this fact emphasizes the in utero role played by inhibitors on a supposedly dormant hepatic conjugating system, the same observation could also support the theory of substrate activation of the hepatic conjugating system. As previously mentioned, this proposed method of activation fails to occur in utero except in special situations (severe Rh sensitization), because of rapid and effective placental transfer of unconjugated bilirubin. However, substrate activation could also be delayed postnatally should a temporary abnormality of the specific hepatic plasmamembrane receptor sites for unconjugated bilirubin prevent the transfer of this organic anion into the hepatic cell. Obviously, a large bilirubin load (hemolysis) may overwhelm the maturational events necessary to maintain the neonate's bilirubin levels within the "physiologic" range. The hepatic cell membrane allows bilirubin to pass in either direction; the fraction not bound to intracellular ligandin is free to return to the bloodstream. Slow maturation of Y protein or its competitive inhibition by other organic anions (such as steroids, fatty acids, glutathione, thyroid hormones, and sulfonomides) obviously can affect serum bilirubin levels. Although Z protein is said to be present in adult lev-

els at birth, its functional capacity may not be mature at this time. This could be an important determinant of the hepatocyte's ability to clear bilirubin, especially after saturation of Y protein is accomplished during times of large bilirubin loads.

A variety of factors can influence the effectiveness by which conjugation of bilirubin to a diphosphoglucuronide form takes place within the hepatocyte. The formation of uridine diphosphoglucuronic acid is in itself a complex enzymatic reaction and requires glucose, amino acids, and energy, any of which may be in short supply in some neonates. Insufficient glucuronide formation may in part explain the hyperbilirubinemia noted in conditions associated with abnormal glucose homeostasis (postmaturity, infants of diabetic mothers, upper bowel obstruction, and so on).

The plasma clearance of unconjugated bilirubin by the liver also depends on the rate of hepatic conjugation and hepatic excretion. Reflux of unconjugated bilirubin from the liver cell into the plasma can occur in the face of defective conjugation and excretion of bilirubin. The rate of rise of serum bilirubin levels is greater in patients with inability to clear bilirubin from the hepatocytes than in those whose hepatic excretion of bilirubin is normal. An enzyme important in facilitating excretion of conjugated bilirubin from the body is beta-glucuronidase, found in low concentrations in serum of neonate infants but developing rapidly after birth. Some believe that even this enzyme is possibly induced by the substrate bilirubin diglucuronide formed within the liver cells. Beta-glucuronidase is capable of hydrolyzing bilirubin diglucuronide that reaches the gut into its fat-soluble form, unconjugated bilirubin, which in turn can be readily absorbed through the intestinal mucosa. The availability of substrate (conjugated bilirubin) for beta-glucuronidase activity may be related to the absence of seemingly significant numbers of intestinal bacteria in the lumen of the bowel during the first few days of life. Once bacterial colonization has occurred in the intestinal tract, bacterial enzyme reduction of bilirubin to urobilinogen occurs rapidly, so that little conjugated bilirubin is available for beta-glucuronidase action.

In some neonates the enterohepatic shunt of unconjugated bilirubin may contribute in a significant way to development of physiologic jaundice. Since meconium contains a large absorbable bilirubin load (80 to 100 mg) at birth, any unusual delay (greater than 24 hours) in passage of this material has the potential to significantly add to the enterohepatic contribution that requires hepatic clearance. The enterohepatic circulation of bilirubin (and bile salts) has been modified by use of agents such as agar, cholestyramine, or charcoal in different experimental studies. When agar, known to be capable of sequestering bilirubin, was fed to one group of neonates, it prevented development of physiologic jaundice; a control group reached expected levels for serum bilirubin. Whether agar affects serum bilirubin levels solely by blocking the enterohepatic shunt or by also promoting an exudative enteropathy of serum unconjugated bilirubin cannot be differentiated at this time.

The relationship between infant feeding and the development of physiologic jaundice is poorly understood, yet curious. Early feeding can prevent significant neonatal hyperbilirubinemia from developing in infants of diabetic mothers, normal premature infants, and full-term infants as well. Although glucose serves as the source of glucuronic acid formation (Fig. 20-1), lowering of bilirubin levels in similar infants has been achieved with 0.45% saline solution and distilled water as well. Perhaps the early oral alimentation hastens intestinal bacterial colonization, which then reduces the contribution of enterohepatic shunting in the development of physiologic jaundice. A relationship between fasting and serum bilirubin levels has been found in patients with Gilbert's disease, an entity with certain similarities to physiologic neonatal jaundice. Whether bilirubin production, carrier-mediated transport, or conjugation of bilirubin is influenced by "breaking the fast" in Gilbert's disease is not known, but an effect on the enterohepatic shunt seems unlikely.

Finally, shunting of blood away from the liver by way of the ductus venosus may influence hepatic clearance of bilirubin under certain circumstances peculiar to the newborn and thereby influence the serum levels of unconjugated hyperbilirubinemia. Examples include delayed closure of the ductus in premature infants, in newborn infants with respiratory distress, or when umbilical venous catheters are used.

It is obvious that many factors are probably involved in physiologic neonatal jaundice. Although delayed maturation or activation of glucuronyl transferase has been singled out as the primary defect, a complex interrelationship and dependency exist even under ideal physiologic conditions between bilirubin production, binding, uptake, conjugation, and excretion of this anion. It is worth remembering that physiologic jaundice does not occur in animals lacking glucuronyl transferase (Gunn rat), an observation emphasizing the complexity of the problem.

Significance

General considerations. In the infant born after a full-term, uncomplicated pregnancy there is little need for concern, since bilirubin levels in physiologic jaundice seldom reach 15 mg/dl. Occasionally, bilirubin values higher than 20 mg/dl can be found in these otherwise asymptomatic full-term infants, and controversy exists about what, if anything, should be done in this situation. The problem is obviously more difficult when it develops in small infants, in whom the serum level of unconjugated bilirubin carries greater potential significance. The lowered albumin-binding capacity or bilirubin binding to secondary sites on the albumin molecule, hypoxia, acidosis, and increased permeability of the blood-brain barrier are abnormalities frequently associated with prematurity and capable of influencing the susceptibility to neurologic complications of high bilirubin levels from whatever cause. No firm rule can cover all possible situations, but 25 mg/dl in full-term infants and 15 to 20 mg/dl in premature infants of uncomplicated pregnancies are maximal levels believed to be tolerated without subsequent neurologic residua. Bilirubin levels exceeding these values should be treated by exchange transfusions.

Certain guidelines are necessary to reassure the clinician that one is dealing with physiologic rather than pathologic jaundice. First, the evolution of hyperbilirubinemia should not be obvious before 24 to 36 hours of age. Jaundice that is clinically evident before this time should be considered pathologic, and a search for its cause should be immediately undertaken. In particular, hemolysis caused by isoimmunization attributable to Rh or other red cell antigens (ABO incompatability), glucose-6-phosphate dehydrogenase deficiency, defects in the glycolytic pathway of the red cells, hemoglobinopathies, unstable hemoglobins, and spherocytic hemolytic anemia need to be ruled out. Drug-induced hemolytic anemias also need to be considered and ruled out when hemolysis and jaundice are noted in the newborn. Vitamin K analogs (Synkavite), primaquine, and sulfamethoxypyridazine have been offenders when used in susceptible individuals. Second, bilirubin levels exceeding 12 mg/dl in full-term infants and greater than 15 mg/dl in premature infants must be viewed suspiciously. Again, hemolytic causes, infection, excessive red blood cell load and destruction from maternal-fetal transfusions or late clamping of the cord, excessive bruising, cephalohematomas, dehydration, hypoglycemia, and so on need to be considered and ruled out by appropriate studies. Third, persistent unconjugated hyperbilirubinemia beyond the eighth day of life in full-term infants and beyond the twelfth to fourteenth day in prematures may be attributable to an easily identifiable, benign cause, such as breast-milk jaundice. On occasion, however, it may be caused by more serious but treatable conditions, such as galactosemia or hypothyroidism, where early diagnosis and treatment are related to good outcome. At the same time, one must also consider the more concerning diagnosis of the Crigler-Najjar syndrome. Last, alarm is justified for other reasons if the conjugated bilirubin fraction is greater than a range of 1.5 to 2 mg/dl. This finding usually implies either hepatocyte injury that prevents bile secretion into the canaliculus, or its excretion from the biliary system into the intestine (see Chapter 19). However, it may occasionally arise in the absence of demonstrable hepatocyte injury, whereby the excessive bilirubin load is believed to overwhelm the functional capacity of secretory and excretory pathways of hepatocytes. This phenomenon is most often seen in association with hemolytic disease and has been termed the ''inspissated bile syndrome.''

Bilirubin toxicity. Although bilirubin toxicity may be demonstrable to only few biologic tissues, the impact on the newborn's nervous system is the most important. For reasons that are yet unclear, bilirubin deposition has a predilection to the neuronal elements of the basal ganglia, but it can also be found in other areas of the brain. Bilirubin's toxic effect is believed to be a result of interference with cellular respiration and disruption of those important energy-dependent organelle functions. The severest expression of bilirubin encephalopathy is kernicterus, with clinical signs becoming apparent in affected neonates by the third to seventh day of life. The Moro reflex is difficult to elicit or is absent. Yawning, opisthotonos, and a weak, high-pitched cry are also noted, especially in full-term babies. Premature babies have a more subtle clinical presentation with apnea and bradycardic episodes, hypotonicity, sluggishness, poor feeding, and emesis—signs and symptoms that suggest sepsis. The subclinical impact of neonatal bilirubin encephalopathy may be appreciated later in childhood when delayed motor development, spastic cerebral palsy, cognitive learning disorders, and nerve deafness become manifest.

Because an imprecise relationship exists between the evolution of the signs and symptoms of bilirubin encephalopathy and the maximum serum bilirubin levels, some controversy remains as to under what circumstances or conditions should the clinician intervene. Although no firm rule can cover all possible situations, attempts to keep bilirubin levels in otherwise well full-term infants below 20 mg/dl are recommended, and keeping levels below 15 mg/dl in otherwise well preterm infants is likewise a safe assumption. Because the risk to kernicterus is especially related to the immaturity of the blood-brain barrier, the very early preterm baby carries the greatest vulnerability at lower bilirubin levels. Furthermore, the premature infant is frequently delivered with the perinatal handicaps of hypoxia, acidosis, or hypotension, events associated with increased risk of kernicterus, therefore necessitating early and more energetic attempts to keep the bilirubin levels at even lower levels. Disagreement exists as to which laboratory measurement, if any, best predicts the infant's risk to kernicterus. Total bilirubin levels, residual binding capacity, free bilirubin, or ''easily'' dissociated bilirubin that is bound to secondary sites on the albumin molecule have all been assessed as possible predictors to the risk of kernicterus. Obviously, many of these laboratory tests are not available to the practitioner, and therefore the assessment of clinical findings coupled with the total bilirubin level remains for most the basis for intervention.

Treatment

Physiologic jaundice is considered a benign condition and requires no specific treatment; however, cases are plentiful in which physiologic jaundice reaches bilirubin levels that are above the acceptable limits that define this entity, posing a threat of kernicterus and therefore requiring intervention. Treatment considerations should be based upon the specific cause and the urgency of the situation.

Exchange transfusion. The most rapid and efficacious method for treating hyperbilirubinemia is by standard exchange transfusion. It is the treatment of choice when hemolytic causes are responsible for the jaundice, and exceedingly high concentrations of serum bilirubin may evolve very quickly. Some clinicians incorporate a preexchange albumin infusion (1 gm/kg), with the hope of further binding free bilirubin, to facilitate the transfer of tissue bilirubin into the blood where it will be removed by the ensuing exchange transfusion. To be most effective, the exchange transfusion should be carried out within the following hour.

When performed by trained personnel in the newborn nursery, exchange transfusions in a carefully monitored infant should carry minimal morbidity. Attention to details of umbilical vein catheter placement, the volume of removed and replaced blood, and maintenance of temperature control are factors that contribute to good outcome results.

Phototherapy. Phototherapy continues to be the most frequently employed modality to lower serum bilirubin. It is also used prophylactically, when the likelihood of higher bilirubin levels is anticipated, or as adjuvant treatment where the clinical situation portends an increased risk to kernicterus at all bilirubin levels. Controlled studies have shown a pronounced effect by this therapy, especially in smaller, nonerythroblastotic infants.

The effect of light in the degradation of bilirubin has been known for some time. In the presence of oxygen, the exposure of bilirubin to radiant energy produces pigmented, nontoxic, water-soluble degradation products (biliverdin, dipyroles, and others), which are easily eliminated by hepatic and renal pathways in either free of conjugated forms. These products of photooxidation do not seem to affect bilirubin-binding sites on albumin. Increased amounts of unconjugated bilirubin and other conjugated and unconjugated water-soluble products of bilirubin have been found in duodenal bile in infants subjected to phototherapy for unconjugated hyperbilirubinemia.

To accomplish this result one should place the naked infant, with shielded eyes, under a group of fluorescent blue lights with the predominant wavelength of 460 nm, at a distance of 40 cm from the skin surface. Serial bilirubin determinations every 8 to 12 hours are required because the assessment of jaundice by visual observation of skin color becomes extremely unreliable during phototherapy. A rebound in the bilirubin levels may be noted if phototherapy is discontinued prematurely. Most infants with exaggerated physiologic jaundice require 3 to 5 days of phototherapy depending on the underlying cause.

No deleterious effects have been reported in human beings with short-term exposure to the therapy, but ophthalmic lesions have been found in experimental newborn animals so treated. The so-called bronze-baby syndrome after phototherapy has been described and may be caused by retention of these pigments in the face of impaired hepatic excretory function. Passage of loose, dark green stools is frequently noted in babies treated with phototherapy, and it likewise reflects the passage of large amounts of bilirubin breakdown products. It is possible that these products of bilirubin degradation increase secretory activity as well as motility and have a cathartic effect as unabsorbed bile acids do in other disease states (Crohn's disease, ileal resection). There is no solid evidence to suggest that these degradation products interfere with intestinal lactase activity. The use of a lactose-free formula is not helpful. Transient and less troublesome complications also reported with phototherapy include a generalized macular rash and lethargy. Since insensible water loss may increase during phototherapy, the infant is best kept in a humidified atmosphere during the treatment period.

Phenobarbital. The use of phenobarbital in the treatment of unconjugated hyperbilirubinemic states has enjoyed modest success. This drug will enhance microsomal protein synthesis and stimulate those enzyme activities associated with smooth endoplasmic reticulum, including glucuronyl transferase. It would appear that ligandins are also increased by phenobarbital. Both events therefore serve to promote the uptake and conjugation of bilirubin, and bile flow is further stimulated by the effect of this agent upon the nonbile salt-dependent portion of bile flow. Consequently, a reduction in serum bilirubin levels can be expected with the use of this drug. Interestingly, recent studies have shown that phenobarbital is singularly more effective in reducing bilirubin levels and shortening the duration of hyperbilirubinemia in neonates when it is given to the mother before delivery, but losing its effectiveness in this regard when given to the newborn after delivery. The unpredictable nature of drug metabolism in neonates demands careful monitoring of blood levels and appropriate adjustment of dosage to achieve ideal pharmacokinetic benefits. Since phenobarbital indeed carries some definite risks (lethargy, apnea, clotting abnormalities, and hypersensitivity reactions), its use in a traditionally benign condition (physiologic jaundice) is difficult to justify except in unusual circumstances. A more proper application of phenobarbital usage in hyperbilirubinemic states might involve infants with Crigler-Najjar syndrome type II and exceptional cases with severe breast-milk jaundice. The bile flow–promoting property of the drug is useful in those examples of neonatal hyperbilirubinemia complicated by elevated direct-reacting fraction (cholestatic jaundice) (see Chapter 19).

Other agents and measures. The prophylactic use of products capable of binding bilirubin conjugates in the intestine and thereby reducing the enterohepatic bilirubin load has likewise enjoyed brief popularity. Activated charcoal (which binds bilirubin), given orally within 4 hours but not later than 12 hours after birth, reduced serum bilirubin levels under those of controls. Cholestyramine resin, a chelating agent that binds bilirubin, did not lower serum bilirubin levels when given with formula to premature infants. Agar powder (USP) given with feedings (250 mg every 4 hours), commencing at 20 hours of age, has prevented significant physiologic jaundice from developing. Wherever possible, early introduction of fluids, proper hydration, and correction of underlying hypoglycemia will aid in reducing maximum levels of serum bilirubin. Wherever applicable drugs that depress glucuronyl transferase activity should be eliminated. Novobiocin, for example, is a potent inhibitor of this enzyme, and its use results in considerable amounts of unconjugated bilirubin. Other drugs increase the breakdown of red blood cells in certain inherited conditions (glucose-6-PD deficiency) and thereby raise bilirubin levels. Some drugs increase the risk of kernicterus by competing for bilirubin-albumin–binding sites (see following list).

*Drugs capable of in vitro displacement of bilirubin from albumin on polidexide (Sephadex) G-25 columns**

> Caffeine and sodium benzoate[†]
> Sodium salicylate
> Diazepam (Valium)[‡]
> Tolbutamide (Orinase)
> Sulfisoxazole (Gantrisin)
> Furosemide (Lasix)
> Sodium oxacillin (Prostaphlin)
> Hydrocortisone
> Gentamicin (Garamycin)
> Digoxin
> Sodium meralluride (Mercuhydrin)
> Sulfadiazine

In addition, drugs administered to the mother at the time of delivery may reach the newborn through the transplacental passage; later these same agents, which are usually psychotropic, sedative, and tranquilizing, reach the neonate via breast milk and unfavorably influence the availability of albumin-bilirubin–binding sites. Such drugs as morphine and vitamin K analogs can influence bilirubin levels by competing for organic anion transport and protein binding at the hepatic cell level.

*Data from Stern, L.: Pediatrics 49:916-918, 1972.
†Generic and trade names are listed in order of quantitative displacement exhibited; concentrations of drugs used were those of in vivo levels resulting from manufacturers' recommended dosages.
‡Injectable preparation only.

REFERENCES

Bakken, A.F.: Bilirubin excretion in newborn human infants. I. Unconjugated bilirubin as a possible trigger for bilirubin conjugation, Acta Paediatr. Scand. **59:**148-152, 1970.

Behrman, R.E., and others: Preliminary report of the committee on phototherapy in the newborn infant, J. Pediatr. **84:**135-147, Jan. 1974.

Bratlid, D.: Reserve albumin binding capacity, salicylate saturation index, and red cell binding of bilirubin in neonatal jaundice, Arch. Dis. Child. **48:**393-397, 1973.

Gartner, L.G., Lee, K., Vaisman, S., and others: Development of bilirubin transport and metabolism in the newborn rhesus monkey, J. Pediatr. **90:**513-531, 1977.

Harper, R.B., Sia, C.G., and Kierney, C.M.P.: Kernicterus 1980: problems and practices viewed from the perspective of the practicing clinician, Clin. Perinatol. **7:**75-92, 1980.

Hsia, D.Y., and Porto, S.: Neonatal jaundice. In Popper, H., and Schaffner, F., editors: Neonatal jaundice: progress in liver diseases, vol. 3, New York, 1970, Grune & Stratton, Inc.

Karp, W.B.: Biochemical alterations in neonatal hyperbilirubinemia and bilirubin encephalopathy: a review, Pediatrics **64:**361-368, 1979.

Kopelman, A.E., Brown, R.S., and Odell, G.B.: The "bronze" baby syndrome: a complication of phototherapy, J. Pediatr. **81:**466-472, 1972.

Levi, A.J., Gatmaitan, Z., and Arias, I.M.: Deficiency of hepatic organic anion-binding protein: impaired organic anion uptake by liver and "physiologic" jaundice in newborn monkeys, N. Engl. J. Med. **283:**1136-1139, 1970.

Levine, R.: Bilirubin: worked out years ago? Pediatrics **64:**380-385, 1979.

Lucey, J.F.: Neonatal jaundice and phototherapy, Pediatr. Clin. North Am. **19:**827-839, 1972.

Lucey, J.F.: Comment: Another view of phototherapy, J. Pediatr. **84:**145-147, 1974.

Maisels, M.J.: Neonatal jaundice. In Avery, G.: Neonatology, Philadelphia, 1981, J.B. Lippincott Co.

Maurer, H.M., Wolff, J.A., Finster, M., and others: Reduction in concentration of total serum-bilirubin in offspring of women treated with phenobarbitone during pregnancy, Lancet **2:**122-124, July 20, 1968.

Oh, W., and Karecki, H.: Phototherapy and insensible water loss in the newborn infant, Am. J. Dis. Child. **124:**230-232, 1972.

Poland, R.L., and Odell, G.B.: Physiologic jaundice: the enterohepatic circulation of bilirubin, N. Engl. J. Med. **284:**1-6, 1971.

Reyes, H., Levi, A.J., Gatmaitan, Z., and Arias, I.M.: Studies of Y and Z, two hepatic cytoplasmic organic anion–binding proteins: effect of drugs, chemicals, hormones, and cholestasis, J. Clin. Invest. **50:**2242-2252, 1971.

Schmid, R.: Bilirubin metabolism: state of the art, Gastroenterology **74:**1307-1312, 1978.

Stern, L., Khanna, N.N., Levy, G., and Yaffe, S.J.: Effect of phenobarbital on hyperbilirubinemia and glucuronide formation in newborns, Am. J. Dis. Child. **120:**26-31, 1970.

Wallin, A., Jalling, B., and Boreus, L.O.: Plasma concentrations of phenobarbital in the neonate during prophylaxis for neonatal hyperbilirubinemia, J. Pediatr. **85:**392-397, 1974.

Wennberg, R.P., Schwartz, R., and Sweet, A.Y.: Early versus delayed feeding of low birth weight infants: effects on physiologic jaundice, J. Pediatr. **68:**860-866, 1966.

Whitington, P.F.: Effect of jaundice phototherapy on intestinal mucosal bilirubin concentration and lactase activity in the congenitally jaundiced Gunn rat, Pediatr. Res. **15:**345-348, 1981.

BREAST-MILK HYPERBILIRUBINEMIA

Prolonged unconjugated hyperbilirubinemia in nursing neonates was recognized in the early 1960s. Since then several studies have appeared to confirm this observation, but there is yet no agreement on the nature of the responsible factor present in breast milk.

From 5% to 15% of women secrete milk capable of inhibiting glucuronyl transferase activity in vitro, whereas only 1% or 2% of nursing infants actually demonstrate prolonged unconjugated hyperbilirubinemia. With rare exception, the inhibitory factor in the maternal milk does not result from ingestion of drugs. In some instances, oxytocic agents, perhaps through an effect on prostaglandin E_2 concentration, may produce an additive effect on the inhibitor factor in maternal milk. The observation that two thirds of breast-fed siblings of jaundiced infants likewise developed prolonged jaundice during breast feeding, whereas formula-fed siblings were unaffected, suggests a genetically determined vulnerability. The mode of inheritance remains unclear, as do the factors dictating penetrance, since an abnormal family history in neonates of first-degree relatives is usually lacking for breast-milk hyperbilirubinemia.

In most infants affected by breast milk, the jaundice develops slowly; it is quite apparent by the end of the first or early part of the second week. No sex predilection has been noted. Maximum total bilirubin values have been as high as 27 mg/dl, with most being between 10 and 20 mg/dl. Maximum direct-reacting bilirubin is seldom above 2 mg/dl. The infants are unaffected by the elevated bilirubin levels, which may persist for as long as 3 months and then spontaneously regress to normal values despite continued breast feeding. Appetite remains good, weight gain and growth are maintained, and neurologic signs are absent. No infant has shown any sequelae to this form of jaundice at subsequent follow-up examination.

One should not assume that all breast-fed infants who develop unconjugated hyperbilirubinemia fit into this category. Some infants may have more severe physiologic jaundice; others may be noted to have hypothyroidism, upper small bowel obstruction (pyloric stenosis), Crigler-Najjar syndrome, or sepsis. A missed hemolytic state may at times also be the responsible cause in a nursing infant. Should serum bilirubin levels reach worrisome levels (greater than 20 mg/dl), temporary discontinuation of breast feeding for only 2 to 4 days is generally required to obtain a fall in the bilirubin level to a more "acceptable" value. A 50% reduction is not uncommonly found. Resumption of breast feeding is followed by a small rebound effect of 2 to 5 mg/dl. There is little reason for completely discontinuing breast feeding in these jaundiced infants.

The major controversy about breast-milk hyperbilirubinemia concerns the nature of the inhibitory substance in the mother's milk. Early studies showed that milk from mothers whose nursing infants were hyperbilirubinemic was capable of inhibiting glucuronyl transferase activity in vitro, but, occasionally, inhibitory action was also observed using milk from mothers of nonjaundiced infants. Much confusion from published reports can be attributed to the use of both differing in vitro systems (guinea pig, rat, and human liver slices) for testing inhibitor activity and differently handled (fresh versus stored) breast-milk samples. The latter often leads to the improper assignment of "control" milk simply upon the basis of the absence of prolonged jaundice in the nursing infant. It is now known that storage of presumed "control" milk may convert to "inhibitory" milk. In addition, the early studies employed *o*-aminophenol rather than bilirubin as the substrate for measuring glucuronyl transferase activity in most in vitro systems that showed the inhibitory effect of breast milk. Subsequent studies using bilirubin as the substrate in a system employing human liver slices provided contrary results. Furthermore, fresh milk samples may or may not demonstrate inhibitory activity in vitro despite the presence of prolonged unconjugated hyperbilirubinemia in the nursing infant.

At present two factors in breast milk have received the most attention as likely candidates responsible for the inhibitory effect upon bilirubin conjugation in the nursing neonate. First, an unusual isomer of the natural steroid in breast milk, pregnane-3α,20β-diol, has been isolated from the milk of mothers whose nursing infants develop this clinical syndrome. This isomer has been identified in the urine of these same mothers during the period of nursing but not later. It has not been identified in the mothers' serum, and indeed their serum does not inhibit *o*-aminophenol conjugation in vitro but may affect bilirubin conjugation in rat liver slice preparations.

Controversy exists concerning both the existence of this isomer and the results obtained in normal infants fed the material. Administration of this inhibitory steroid to two normal infants produced unconjugated hyperbilirubinemia in one study, whereas administration to 20 infants in a different study failed to produce any significant rise in bilirubin levels over those of the controls. Urinary excretion, indicating absorption, of the steroid isomer was found in the latter study. Breast milk, shown to have a high degreee of inhibitory activity in vitro, has not always revealed the presence of the steroid isomer by standard chromato-graphic techniques. Once again, an unsuccessful in vitro attempt to demonstrate the inhibitory effect of various concentrations of either pregnane-3α,20β-diol or pregnane-3α,20α-diol when added to human liver slice preparations has recently been published.

Present evidence suggests that the inhibitory activity noted in stored breast milk obtained from nursing mothers of jaundiced infants may possibly be attributable to elevated levels of nonesterified fatty acids liberated by lipoprotein lipase, an enzyme whose activity is not entirely suppressed by storage at temperatures of 4° C or lower and normally requires cofactor activation by bile salts. Indeed, free fatty acid concentrations are higher in stored milk obtained from the sixth postpartum day on, and they parallel the observed increase in activity of lipoprotein lipase activity. However, these inhibitory levels of free fatty acids (greater than 4 mEq/L) were no different from stored milk from mothers either nursing jaundiced infants or nursing nonjaundiced infants. Although fresh milk samples from mothers of jaundiced infants have been reported to demonstrate increased lipoprotein lipase activity, the concentration of free fatty acids was surprisingly normal. Once again, fresh breast milk failed to demonstrate consistently any inhibitory activity in several in vitro systems tested. The mechanism by which free fatty acids interfere with bilirubin conjugation has not been precisely defined. Free fatty acids have been shown to affect Z-protein binding of sulfobromophthalein sodium while not influencing the binding of other organic anions to Y-protein ligandins. Both an inhibitory effect of free fatty acids on glucuronyl transferase activity and an enhancing effect on the enterohepatic circulation has been suggested. Heating breast milk to 56° C for 15 minutes or longer inactivates lipoprotein lipase action and prevents the subsequent appearance of higher levels of free fatty acids in stored breast milk. In unusual situations when bilirubin levels reach unusually high values in the nursing infant (greater than 17 mg/dl), some recommend that the breast milk be heated as soon as it is collected and then fed to the infant by conventional bottle means.

Laboratory studies have shown that the inhibitor in the milk appears to be absent from colostrum, particularly in whites, and fluctuates in quantity from day to day. Clinical observations of affected babies tend to support this experimental data. The effect of the milk inhibitory substance on the severity and duration of the hyperbilirubinemia probably depends on many factors besides the quantity ingested from mothers's milk. Some of these variables have been discussed in the section on physiologic jaundice of the newborn, earlier in this chapter. Genetic or environmental factors also may play a significant role in breast milk jaundice. Early-onset breast-milk jaundice has been noted in some native American tribes (Navajo). The quantity of mature hepatic glucuronyl transferase available for bilirubin conjugation is another variable.

Breast-milk hyperbilirubinemia should not be confused with the rare syndrome called transient familial neonatal hyperbilirubinemia (Lucy-Driscoll syndrome), which is believed to result from a gestational substance present in the mother's serum and the infant's as well. In the latter entity hyperbilirubinemia is not related to breast feeding, for the serum bilirubin rapidly reaches worrisome levels within the first few days of life. Neurologic signs and sequelae have been reported. The serum of mother and affected infant is capable of greatly inhibiting glucuronyl transferase activity in vitro; this effect is present in the mother's serum for about 2 weeks after delivery.

REFERENCES

Adlard, B.P.F., and Lathe, G.H.: Breast milk jaundice: effect of 3α-20β-pregnanediol on bilirubin conjugation by human liver, Arch. Dis. Child. **45:**186-189, 1970.

Arias, I.M., Wolfson, S., Lucey, J.F., and McKay, R. Jr.: Transient familial neonatal hyperbilirubinemia, J. Clin. Invest. **44:**1442-1450, 1965.

Cole, A.P., and Hargreaves, T.: Conjugation inhibitors and neonatal hyperbilirubinemia, Arch. Dis. Child. **47:**415-419, 1972.

Foliot, A., Ploussard, J.P., Housset, E., and others: Breast milk jaundice: in-vitro inhibition of rat liver bilirubin–uridine diphosphate glucuronyltransferase activity and Z protein–bromosulfophthalein binding by human breast milk, Pediat. Res. **10:**594-598, 1976.

Gartner, L.M., and Arias, I.M.: Studies of prolonged neonatal jaundice in breast-fed infants, J. Pediatr. **68:**54-66, 1966.

Gartner, L.M., and Lee, K.S.: Effect of starvation and milk feeding on intestinal bilirubin absorption, Gastroenterology **76:**A-13, Nov. 1979.

Newman, A.J., and Gross, S.: Hyperbilirubinemia in breast-fed infants, Pediatrics **32:**995-1001, 1963.

Odièvre, M., and Luzeau, R.: Lipolytic activity in milk from mothers of unjaundiced infants, Acta Paediatr. Scand. **67:**49-52, 1978.

Poland, R.L.: Breast-milk jaundice, J. Pediatr. **99:**86-88, 1981.

Ramos, A., Silverberg, M., and Stern, L.: Pregnanediols and neonatal hyperbilirubinemia, Am. J. Dis. Child. **111:**353-356, 1966.

Saland, J., McNamara, H., and Cohen, M.I.: Navajo jaundice: a variant of neonatal hyperbilirubinemia associated with breast feeding, J. Pediatr. **85:**271-275, 1974.

Severi, F., Rondini, G., Zaverio, S., and Bruschelli, M.: Prolonged neonatal hyperbilirubinemia and pregnane-3(alpha),-20(beta)-diol in maternal milk, Helv. Paediatr. Acta **25:**517-521, 1970.

Stiehm, R.E., and Ryan, J.: Breast-fed jaundice, Am. J. Dis. Child. **109:**212-216, 1965.

NEONATAL UNCONJUGATED HYPERBILIRUBINEMIA CAUSED BY UPPER GASTROINTESTINAL OBSTRUCTION

Although unconjugated hyperbilirubinemia occurs in association with upper bowel obstruction in the neonate, it is most commonly seen in hypertrophic pyloric stenosis, where the incidence is reported to be from 3% to 10%. In over half the cases the jaundice is noted to begin within the first week of life and to persist until the time of diagnosis. In some, discernible icterus is reported after the first week or so, whereas in others it may reappear after an initial clearing. The levels of bilirubin are usually 5 to 10 mg/dl, with unusual cases achieving higher values. Jaundice clears quickly after surgical alleviation of the obstruction.

For now, the diminished enzyme activity of uridine diphosphoglucuronyl transferase found in liver biopsy specimens obtained during corrective surgery is believed to explain the hyperbilirubinemia in most patients. Other factors certainly may contribute to the elevated bilirubin levels. A net decrease in the infant's intake and the accompanying malnutrition may in turn deplete glycogen stores and glucose availability for glucuronide formation. The relative starvation also leads to increased lipolysis, and the resulting elevation of free fatty acids has the potential to inhibit bilirubin uptake and subsequent conjugation by glucuronyl transferase.

It is interesting to speculate that at least some of these patients may in fact eventually prove to have Gilbert's disease. Their vulnerability (decreased glucuronyl transferase activity) is simply precipitated out during the neonatal period by the relative fasting imposed by the upper bowel obstruction. The incidence of jaundice in pyloric stenosis is not too dissimilar from that reported in the general population for Gilbert's disease.

The unconjugated hyperbilirubinemia that occurs in association with more complete upper bowel obstructive lesions (duodenal atresia, annular pancreas, jejunal atresia) is difficult to assign to a cause-and-effect relationship because of its early appearance. The onset of jaundice in these examples of complete small bowel obstruction has been noted at 3 to 5 days of age rather than at a later time as mentioned when it occurs in most examples of pyloric stenosis. Some cases are simply examples of an exaggerated expression of physiologic jaundice that accompanies dehydration, malnutrition, and hypoglycemia as part of the early neonatal course in such patients.

REFERENCES

Chaves-Carballo, E., Harris, L.E., and Lynn, H.B.: Jaundice associated with pyloric stenosis and neonatal small-bowel obstruction, Clin. Pediatr. **7**:198-202, 1968.

Dodge, J.A.: Infantile hypertrophic pyloric stenosis in Belfast, 1957-1969, Arch. Dis. Child. **50**:171-178, 1975.

Woolley, M.M., Felsher, B.F., Asch, M.J., and others: Jaundice, hypertrophic pyloric stenosis and glucuronyl transferase, J. Pediatr. Surg. **9**:359-363, 1974.

UNCONJUGATED HYPERBILIRUBINEMIA AND CONGENITAL HYPOTHYROIDISM

On occasion, persistent unconjugated hyperbilirubinemia may be a dominant clinical feature of congenital hypothyroidism. In these cases prolonged jaundice persists to the third to sixth week of life when a gradual evolution of more obvious features of the hypothyroid state appear. The jaundice clears relatively quickly once treatment of the deficiency has begun.

Because the early diagnosis of this treatable condition is essential to improved outcome results, the clinician must be on guard in all cases of prolonged jaundice irrespective of the type of infant feeding employed. Proper thyroid function studies are mandatory in such cases. It is reassuring that in most states the routine neonatal screening test presently employed includes an assessment of thyroid function. However, occasional delays, or errors in final diagnosis can still be anticipated, and therefore repeat thyroid-function studies are indicated in unexplained cases of prolonged unconjugated hyperbilirubinemia.

The exact mechanism for the observed elevation of unconjugated bilirubin is unknown. Although hepatic ligandin levels increase in animals rendered hypothyroid, presumably because of impaired degradation of this protein, an underlying structural or functional defect that interferes with

the hepatic clearance of bilirubin in hypothyroid states cannot be ruled out.

REFERENCES

Smith, D.W., Klein, A.M., Henderson, J.R., and Myrianthopoulos, N.C.: Congenital hypothyroidism: signs and symptoms in the newborn period, J. Pediatr. **87**:985-962, Dec. 1975.

Weldon, A.P., and Danks, D.M.: Congenital hypothyroidism and neonatal jaundice, Arch. Dis. Child. **47**:469-471, June 1972.

FAMILIAL UNCONJUGATED HYPERBILIRUBINEMIAS

Crigler-Najjar syndrome (type I and type II, chronic nonhemolytic unconjugated hyperbilirubinemia)

Crigler-Najjar syndrome is fortunately not often encountered, for the diagnosis is likely to be missed in the neonatal period until signs and symptoms of kernicterus are already apparent in these jaundiced children. The severe form (type I) of the disease produces a rapidly rising serum level of unconjugated bilirubin within the first few days of life. The diagnosis can be suspected when evidence for hemolysis is lacking, liver function studies are normal, and continuous therapeutic efforts including exchange transfusion and phototherapy are necessary to maintain serum bilirubin levels below a range of 20 to 25 mg/dl. A history of consanguinity may be obtained suggesting an inborn error of metabolism; likewise, a history of previously encountered significant neonatal jaundice may be present in the family pedigree. The rate of rise and the magnitude of unconjugated bilirubin (13 to 48 mg/dl) are probably responsible for the high incidence of neurologic sequelae and kernicterus seen in these neonates.

The high serum levels of unconjugated bilirubin result from an absence of uridine diphosphoglucuronyl transferase (and possibly other transferases) needed to conjugate bilirubin to the monoglucuronide form. The selectiveness of this particular genetic defect has been supported by recent studies showing that intravenously administered bilirubin monoglucuronide can be readily excreted into the bile of patients with Crigler-Najjar syndrome (also demonstrated in the Gunn rat) implying intact secretory pathways. Liver tissue from these patients indeed lacks uridine diphosphoglucuronyl transferase activity, but the enzyme bilirubin glucuronoside-glucuronosyl transferase required for the formation of bilirubin diglucuronide is present in normal amounts. As might be expected, in vivo experiments have shown that bilirubin diglucuronide appears in the bile of patients with Crigler-Najjar syndrome after bilirubin monoglucuronide infusion.

Two forms of Crigler-Najjar exist, called type I and type II. Type I disease is inherited as an autosomal recessive similar to that seen in the animal counterpart (Gunn rat), and homozygotes for this disease have a complete absence of monoglucuronide-conjugating activity for bilirubin and an absence of glucuronide-conjugating activity for other anions such as menthols, corticosteroids, and salicylates. Heterozygotes have normal serum bilirubin levels, but an impairment of glucuronide formation can be demonstrated when one uses other anionic substrates besides bilirubin (such as menthol) for loading experiments.

The few type I patients who survive the initial insult of hyperbilirubinemia and kernicterus remain jaundiced throughout life and have colorless bile devoid of bilirubin glucuronide. Their feces have normal color with fecal-urobilinogen values only slightly diminished. The ability of unconjugated bilirubin to weep across the intestinal mucosa probably explains the presence of the stool urobilinogen. This same mechanism may be largely responsible for maintaining the constant level of serum bilirubin noted in surviving patients. Furthermore, this observation has led to the successful use of cholestyramine as a treatment adjuvant to phototherapy in surviving patients. A few patients with type I disease have survived without kernicterus even to late teen-age years or early adult life, whereas other long-term survivors have manifested significant neurologic deficits. At autopsy the brains of late surviving patients reveal neuronal damage and gliosis. Bilirubin staining is absent, contrary to the findings seen in the brains of neonates dying with kernicterus.

The treatment of surviving patients with Crigler-Najjar type I disease remains extremely difficult, and at best the prognosis is guarded. It would appear that neurologic sequelae of bilirubin encephalopathy may inexplicably develop at any age. On occasion a deterioration in the patient has been attributed to an intercurrent viral infection.

Early in life, exchange transfusion coupled with phototherapy is the most predictable means of maintaining the serum bilirubin level below 20 mg/dl, the level believed likely to result in brain damage. With advancing age, phototherapy becomes an increasingly difficult modality to employ, especially in the older infant and young child, where cooperation and compliance is less than optimum and efforts to enforce prolonged periods of phototherapy may well result in a psychologic disturbance in the affected child. Consequently, bilirubin levels invariably rise and again reach plateau at a higher level. Even with supplemental cholestyramine therapy, a daily minimum of 12 hours of phototherapy is required for optimum results. Cholestyramine binds bilirubin (and bile acids) in the lumen of the intestine in an irreversible manner, thereby reducing the contribution of this substance to the circulation by way of the enterohepatic shunt. Doses between 4 and 8 gm/day of cholestyramine have had variable but positive effects in maintaining a lower serum bilirubin concentration and therefore reducing the time the child must spend under phototherapy. Agar, likewise, has the potential to bind bilirubin in the gut lumen, but it has only had limited clinical application in patients with Crigler-Najjar type I disease. As expected phenobarbital has no effect in lowering serum bilirubin levels in patients with Crigler-Najjar type I disease. The effectiveness of ongoing therapy should also be gauged by periodic neurologic and developmental testing, in addition to obtainment of objective indicators from measurement of albumin-bilirubin saturation levels.

Experimentally, enzyme induction in homozygote jaundiced Gunn rats has been achieved by use of grafts of rat hepatoma cells or normal rat kidney tissue. The human kidney likewise contains glucuronyl transferase activity but in concentrations believed to be too low to expect enzyme induction from grafting techniques. Direct liver implants from normal animals into the enzyme-deficient Gunn rats have produced contradictory results. Attempts at seeding the liver by use of portal vein injections with enzyme-replete liver cells has produced some promising early data, resulting in lowering of serum bilirubin levels in immunologically suppressed Gunn rats.

The early reports of this syndrome were derived from observations of seven children of two families. Consanguinity between parents existed, and six of the seven children developed kernicterus. Since then, over 50 cases that fit the clinical pattern of type I Crigler-Najjar syndrome have been described. Our experience with type I Crigler-Najjar syndrome is limited to two children in one family. The first child developed neurologic manifestations at 18 months of age (ataxia, slurred speech) and finally succumbed to the complications attending a severe rejection reaction of the auxiliary (heterotopic) liver transplant at 22 months of age. This child was the third infant of a non-consanguineous marriage with a normal family history. Over the first 18 months of life, serum-unconjugated bilirubin eventually reached a plateau at 30 to 34 mg/dl despite therapeutic efforts including phenobarbital and phototherapy. Lower levels (15 to 20 mg/dl) chould be maintained by plasmapheresis, but technical difficulties prevented chronic employment of this modality. Attempts at creating a permanent arteriovenous fistula were hampered by small vessel size and thrombosis of the shunt. In the hope of accomplishing either enzyme induction or enzyme transfer, the decision to utilize auxiliary liver transplantation was made. During the time the auxiliary liver functioned (48 hours), bilirubin levels rapidly fell to normal, but after rejection the serum bilirubin levels unfortunately rose to higher than pretransplantation values.

The second infant of this family was initially treated with exchange transfusion and then continuous phototherapy and cholestyramine until approximately 8 months of age. Initially bilirubin levels ranged from 15 to 20 mg/dl but gradually increased to levels approaching 40 to 50 mg/dl by 8 months of age. Neurologic evaluation revealed evidence of kernicterus by 6 months of age, with opisthotonos, decreased reflexes, and a seizure disorder. At 11 months of age the child had acute respiratory disease and expired soon thereafter. Postmortem examination revealed microcephaly, cholelithiasis, and chronic cholecystitis. As expected, the liver was grossly normal. Sections of the brain revealed absence of pigment staining in the various nuclear groups, and microscopically degenerative changes were noted throughout the central nervous system, characterized by neuronal loss, duplication, and gliosis.

It would appear that survival of these infants without neurologic sequelae will have to await perfection of techniques that allow for either enzyme transfer or induction. Auxiliary or orthotopic transplantation still must await improvements in overcoming rejection reactions. Meanwhile, extracorporeal phototherapy, or a newly described hemoperfusion over albumin-conjugated agarose columns may hold promise for the future.

Another group of patients manifesting chronic nonhemolytic hyperbilirubinemia have been identified as a homogenous group based on clinical, biochemical, genetic, and pharmacologic observations. These patients, with a milder form of Crigler-Najjar syndrome (type II), have lesser elevations of serum bilirubin (8 to 22 mg/dl) and survive to adult life without neurologic sequelae. They are handicapped only by the cosmetic impact of jaundice. Bile from these patients is pigmented and contains conjugated bilirubin monoglucuronide. It would appear that bilirubin diglucuronide is not formed and therefore cannot be detected in the bile of patients with type II Crigler-Najjar syndrome. Analysis of enzyme activity of glucuronyl transferase in liver biopsy specimens from several families suggest that this conjugation defect is inherited as an autosomal dominant trait with variable penetrance.

A very important point that differentiates type I and type II patients is the latter group's dramatic lowering of serum bilirubin in response to orally administered phenobarbital (6 to 10 mg/kg/24 hr). Type I patients show no response either in vivo or in vitro after prolonged ingestion of the drug. Serum bilirubin levels in type II patients usually level off at about 2 or 3 mg/dl after 10 to 20 days of treatment with phenobarbital. Discontinuance of the drug results in a return of the serum bilirubin to pretreatment levels after 1 to 2 weeks.

The exact mechanism by which phenobarbital enhances bilirubin conjugation is not completely known. It is assumed that an increase of glucuronyl transferase occurs as a result of stimulation of protein synthesis within the hepatic cell. Phenobarbital, and other substances as well, is capable of causing proliferation of smooth endoplasmic reticulum, which in turn leads to an increase of enzyme activity. The genetic information for making glucuronyl transferase is believed to be absent in type I patients and in the animal counterpart (Gunn rat). Neither lowering of serum bilirubin nor conjugation of bilirubin occurs in vivo and in vitro respectively, evidence that induction of conjugation mechanisms by hepatic tissue has not occurred. To explain their ability to respond to phenobarbital, a qualitatively different, or partial, defect is suggested for patients with type II disease. Why bilirubin in these patients is incapable of enhancing its own biotransformation within the hepatocyte is unclear. Certainly, in the experimental animal unconjugated bilirubin is capable of inducing UDP-glucuronyl transferase and facilitates conjugation and excretion. Therefore, it is unlikely that the beneficial therapeutic effect of phenobarbital in type II patients is simply caused by induction of UDP-glucuronyl transferase. Some authors have shown that phenobarbital increases the quantity of the hepatic organic anion-binding protein Y, which facilitates removal of unconjugated bilirubin from the serum. However, failure of type I patients to demonstrate even a lowering of serum bilirubin after drug therapy raises some doubt as to the importance of the Y protein in Crigler-Najjar syndrome. Remember, however, that the effect of phenobarbital on the liver extends beyond its effect on the smooth endoplasmic reticulum and the associated microsomal enzymes. Increased rate of transport of other organic anions from plasma to bile can be seen, as well as increased excretion of endogenous bile acids. Even such exogenous drugs as rose bengal have accelerated excretion in phenobarbital-treated subjects. Whether a combination of these known effects of phenobarbital is responsible for lowering the serum bilirubin in patients with type II Crigler-Najjar syndrome, or another, as yet unidentified, function of this drug is responsible, remains to be determined. This may include alteration of the enzyme's primary or secondary structure, cellular environment, or an effect on the regulatory function of other organelles.

Besides the deficiency of glucuronyl transferase, no other abnormality can be found in these patients to explain the unconjugated hyperbilirubinemia. Studies of red blood cell survival have yielded normal values. The liver is histologically normal, and other conjugated derivatives are excreted normally into the bile.

The milder forms may be difficult to differentiate from other examples of chronic unconjugated hyperbilirubinemia not caused by hemolysis. Such entities as Gilbert's disease, post–viral hepatitis syndrome, shunt hyperbilirubinemia, and bilirubin-uptake impairment caused by drugs (flavaspidic acid) may all mimic the clinical condition of milder forms of type II Crigler-Najjar syndrome. In fact, present evidence suggests that Crigler-

Najjar type II and Gilbert's disease represent varied expressions of a common genetic defect.

REFERENCES

Arias, I.M., Gartner, L.M., Cohen, M., and others: Chronic nonhemolytic unconjugated hyperbilirubinemia with glucuronyl transferase deficiency, Am. J. Med. **47:**395-409, 1969.

Arrowsmith, W.A., Payne, R.B., and Littlewood, J.M.: Comparison of treatments for congenital nonobstructive nonhaemolytic hyperbilirubinaemia, Arch. Dis. Child. **50:**197-201, 1975.

Berk, P.D., Wolkoff, A.W., and Berlin, N.I.: Inborn errors of bilirubin metabolism, Med. Clin. North Am. **59:**803-816, July 1975.

Blaschke, T.F., Berk, P.D., Scharschmidt, B.F., and others, Crigler-Najjar syndrome: an unusual course with development of neurologic damage at age eighteen, Pediatr. Res. **8:**573-590, 1974.

Gollan, J.L., Huang, S.N., Billing, B., and Sherlock, S.: Prolonged survival in three brothers with severe type 2 Crigler-Najjar syndrome; ultrastructural and metabolic studies, Gastroenterology **68:**1543-1555, 1975.

Gordon, E.R., Shaffer, E.A. and Sass-Kortsak, A.: Bilirubin secretion and conjugation in the Crigler-Najjar syndrome type II, Gastroenterology **70:**761-765, 1976.

Mukherjee, A.B., and Krasner, J.: Induction of an enzyme in genetically deficient rats after grafting of normal liver, Science **182:**68-70, Oct. 1973.

Odièvre, M., Trivin, F., Eliot, N. and Alagille, D.: Cases of congenital nonobstructive, nonhaemolytic jaundice: successful long-term phototherapy at home, Arch. Dis. Child. **53:**81-82, 1978.

Thaler, M.M., and Schmid, R.: Drugs and bilirubin, Pediatrics **47:**807-810, 1971.

Wolkoff, A.W., Chowdhury, J.R., Gartner, L.A., and others: Crigler-Najjar syndrome (type I) in an adult male, Gastroenterology, **76:**840-848, 1979.

Wranne, L.: Congenital non-hemolytic jaundice, Acta Paediatr. Scand. **56:**552-556, 1967.

Gilbert's disease (idiopathic unconjugated hyperbilirubinemia, constitutional hepatic dysfunction)

Gilbert's disease is probably the most common cause for mild, chronic or intermittent unconjugated hyperbilirubinemia that occurs in the absence of overt hemolysis and intrinsic liver disease in up to 5% of whites. However, the low levels of serum bilirubin (mean values about 3 mg/dl) and the benign and intermittent course can make diagnosis difficult. Although clinical jaundice may be recognized in the pediatric age group, the low level of awareness for the disease invariably results in delayed diagnosis. The diagnosis may be suspected in the neonatal period by analysis of UDP-glucuronyl transferase activity in liver biopsy samples taken from infants with moderate and prolonged hyperbilirubinemia. Enzyme activity in some of these infants have been reported to be comparable to that found in an older family member with a proved diagnosis of Gilbert's disease. In one large series the reported mean age for recognition of icterus was 18 years (range, 10 to 38 years), with diagnosis delayed for an average of 6 years. It is equally common for the icterus to be detected serendipitously by routine laboratory screening for associated nonspecific complaints such as abdominal pain, fatigue, anorexia, or malaise. It is not surprising that many of these patients have been misdiagnosed as having hepatitis.

The contrary is also true, in that some patients first suspected of having Gilbert's disease were subsequently shown to have post–viral hepatitis syndrome when percutaneous liver biopsy was performed. Indeed, without careful studies it may be difficult to separate other entities characterized by mild, chronic unconjugated hyperbilirubinemia from Gilbert's disease.

Gilbert's disease is believed to be familial and most likely inherited as an autosomal dominant with variable penetrance and expressivity. Males are more often affected than females (4:1).

Etiology

The defect in Gilbert's disease may be multifactorial, but the most consistent biochemical abnormality is the persistent partial reduction of hepatic bilirubin uridine diphosphate glucuronyl transferase (UDPG-T) activity to a range of 10% to 30% of normal. Other evidence also suggests that an abnormality of hepatic plasma membrane–binding sites for unconjugated bilirubin exists. The role of hepatic organic anion-binding proteins as possible contributors to defective bilirubin uptake and transport across the hepatic cell membrane still needs further study. Data derived from experiments concerned with the hepatic transport of organic ions other than bilirubin show that sulfobromophthalein (Bromsulphalein, BSP) concentration at 45 minutes is abnormal in some of these patients. BSP disappearance curves suggest a defective hepatic uptake in a certain number; in others, the defect seems to involve a later step in the transport process. The early (K_1) BSP clearance is normal, but the delayed (K_2) component is slow, with retention in the order of 15% or less. Bili-

rubin-clearance studies suggest a relative decrease in the efficiency of adding the second glucuronide to the bilirubin molecule in patients with Gilbert's disease. Some workers believe that patients with unconjugated hyperbilirubinemia who also show a hepatic uptake defect to a variety of organic anions (sulfobromophthalein and indocyanine green) either represent a disease different from Gilbert's or perhaps show an unusual expression of the latter condition.

Increased production of bilirubin from reduced red blood cell survival has been suggested as a possible significant factor in maintaining mild unconjugated hyperbilirubinemia. Almost 50% of patients with Gilbert's disease have been noted to have a slightly reduced red blood cell survival, but in the face of normal hepatic function another mechanism must exist to explain the hyperbilirubinemia. Again, hepatic uptake and membrane-transfer abnormalities seem likely in this disease, in which case even the slightest increase in bilirubin formation may be significant.

The late onset of this disease has suggested to some that it may even reflect an acquired condition, developing in susceptible subjects as a consequence of an infection such as viral hepatitis.

The accentuation of jaundice with intercurrent illness and with fasting is an intriguing phenomenon in Gilbert's disease. A curious observation about the relationship between the degree of hyperbilirubinemia and caloric intake has been repeatedly observed. Caloric deprivation produces a reciprocal rise in serum unconjugated bilirubin, but the mechanism is unclear. The withdrawal of fat from the diet seems to be critical in the hyperbilirubinemia observed with fasting. Intravenous administration of lipid (Intralipid) during the fasting period also inhibits the expected rise in unconjugated bilirubin in Gilbert's disease. Fasting may cause increased bilirubin production (enhanced heme oxygenase activity) or impairment of membrane binding or carrier-mediated transport of bilirubin. Although UDPG-T levels remain unchanged, hepatic uridine diphosphate glucuronic acid formation may be compromised as a result of depletion of glycogen stores; however, intravenous glucose perfusion does not alter the effect of fasting. Caloric deprivation is likely to occur during illness, prolonged physical exertion, or emotional upset, conditions previously noted to be associated with recurrence of jaundice.

Clinical features

Mild, fluctuating levels of jaundice are seldom recognized clinically in these patients. Almost 70% of patients report other symptoms such as malaise, fatigue, and abdominal pain as the reason for seeking medical attention. Since the bilirubin is primarily unconjugated, the urine is of normal color; on the other hand, sufficient conjugation and excretion of bilirubin does occur to produce stools of normal color. Except for scleral icterus, the remainder of the physical examination is normal.

Diagnosis

With the realization that acquired diseases could also cause unconjugated hyperbilirubinemia, more stringent requirements must be met before the diagnosis of Gilbert's disease can be made. For the diagnosis of Gilbert's disease the following criteria should be fulfilled. A mildly elevated unconjugated bilirubin level documented by several tests, especially after a 48-hour low-calorie (400 kcal) and low-fat diet. A rise in serum total bilirubin concentration of 1.4 mg/dl or greater can be expected. A nicotinic acid provocation test (50 mg, intravenous) has been used in adults to assist in making the diagnosis of Gilbert's disease. The characteristic threefold increase, and prolongation of unconjugated hyperbilirubinemia for 120 to 180 minutes typically follows the administration of this substance in Gilbert's patients. Normal individuals show a twofold increase of bilirubin up to 90 minutes before declining. The mechanism involved in response to nicotinic acid appears to be an increased endogenous conversion of heme to bilirubin, especially in the spleen. This phenomenon contributes an additional load to the already compromised underlying defect of uptake and conjugation. Pretreatment with phenobarbital can temporarily diminish or eliminate the nicotinic acid effect upon unconjugated hyperbilirubinemia.

The patient should have normal liver function tests (transaminase, alkaline phosphatase, BSP), normal hematologic studies (hemoglobin, hematocrit, red blood cell smear, reticulocyte count, and red blood cell osmotic fragility), normal physical examination (except minimal icterus), and normal hepatic histologic appearance. If necessary, one can analyze for UDPG-T activity, which is reduced in this condition to 10% to 30% of normal. This should eliminate other possible conditions that can imitate Gilbert's disease, such as shunt hyperbilirubinemia, post–viral hepatitis syndrome, compensated hemolytic state, and type II Crigler-Najjar syndrome. Complete differentiation from mild forms of the latter entity may be extremely difficult at times and require enzyme analysis of liver biopsy material.

Treatment

Most patients are minimally disturbed by the vague abdominal pain or by the cosmetic effect of the scleral icterus and therefore require no treatment. The disease is benign; the liver histologic appearance remains normal throughout the duration of the illness. Should scleral icterus or skin pigmentation become bothersome, phenobarbital, 6 to 10 mg/kg/24 hr, has been employed with success. The main side effect of the drug, drowsiness, is overcome when it is used in graded increments. Bilirubin levels often return to normal, constitutional complaints may or may not vanish, and the response to fasting can be overcome when the larger dose is used.

REFERENCES

Arias, I.M.: Chronic unconjugated hyperbilirubinemia without overt signs of hemolysis in adolescents and adults, J. Clin. Invest. **41**:2233-2245, 1962.

Black, M., and Sherlock, S.: Treatment of Gilbert's syndrome with phenobarbitone, Lancet **1**:1359-1362, 1970.

Felsher, B.F., Rickard, D., and Redeker, A.G.: The reciprocal relation between caloric intake and the degree of hyperbilirubinemia in Gilbert's syndrome, N. Engl. J. Med. **283**:170-172, 1970.

Fromke, V.L., and Miller, D.: Constitutional hepatic dysfunction (CHD; Gilbert's disease): a review with special reference to a characteristic increase and prolongation of the hyperbilirubinemic response to nicotinic acid, Medicine **51**:451-464, 1972.

Gollan, J.L., Bateman, C., and Billing, B.H.: Effect of dietary composition on the unconjugated hyperbilirubinaemia of Gilbert's syndrome, Gut **17**:335-340, 1976.

Goresky, C.A., Gordon, E.R., Shaffer, E.A., and others: Gilbert's syndrome: no longer an uptake defect? Gastroenterology **76**:1497-1498, 1979.

Israels, L.G., Sunderman, H.J., and Ritzman, S.E.: Hyperbilirubinemia due to alternate path of bilirubin production, Am. J. Med. **27**:693-702, 1959.

Lake, A.M., Truman, J.T., Bode, H.H., and others: Marked hyperbilirubinemia with Gilbert's syndrome and immunohemolytic anemia, J. Pediatr. **93**:812-814, 1978.

Levi, A.J., Gatmaitan, Z., and Arias, I.M.: Deficiency of hepatic organic anion-binding protein, impaired organic anion uptake by liver and ''physiologic'' jaundice in newborn monkeys, N. Engl. J. Med. **283**:1136-1139, 1970.

Powell, L.W., Hemingway, E., Billing, B.H., and Sherlock, S.: Idiopathic unconjugated hyperbilirubinemia (Gilbert's syndrome): a study of 42 families, N. Engl. J. Med. **277**:1108-1112, 1967.

FAMILIAL NONCHOLESTATIC CONJUGATED HYPERBILIRUBINEMIA
Dubin-Johnson syndrome

An inherited disorder of bilirubin secretion, Dubin-Johnson syndrome is seldom recognized in the pediatric age group unless it is known to exist in one of the parents. The disease is now believed to be transmitted as an autosomal recessive trait with variable penetrance and expressivity.

The primary lesion in this disorder remains unknown. Hepatic lysomal enzymes are reportedly intact. Although suspected, a structural defect in the bile canalicular membrane has not been appreciated by electron microscopic examination of liver tissue. The possibility exists that other yet undiscovered enzymes involved in organic anion secretion may be lacking in patients with Dubin-Johnson syndrome.

This condition is recognized by certain distinctive features, and an occasional overlap with other syndromes of chronic nonhemolytic hyperbilirubinemia has been reported. The serum bilirubin levels in Dubin-Johnson syndrome are usually below 6 mg/dl of plasma, but they may range from normal to 19 mg/dl. A slight predominance of the direct-reacting fraction (60% of total bilirubin) is usually present, since the conjugated bilirubin regurgitates out of the hepatic cell into the capillary sinusoids. The gross and histologic appearance of the liver is unique in that a dark yellow-brown or black pigment is quickly recognized in a centrilobular location. This material has the physical and chemical properties of catechol-derived melanin and is believed to be derived from the metabolic breakdown products of epinephrine, which cannot be secreted into the bile.

Indeed, it is the defective capacity of the hepatic cells to transport and secrete certain organic anions that is considered to be the primary abnormality in the Dubin-Johnson syndrome. Patients have a reduced hepatic capacity to secrete conjugated bilirubin and glutathione-conjugated bilirubin, BSP, methylene blue, rose bengal, and iodocyanine green. Failure to visualize the gallbladder with radiopaque dyes, such as iopanoic acid, in these patients is also attributable to the hepatic secretory defect. However, this abnormality of hepatic cells does not involve secretion of all other organic anions. Bile acids, the major organic anion in human bile, are secreted and excreted normally and account for the absence of hepatocyte cholestasis in these patients.

Some pediatric patients have come to diagnosis after developing clinical jaundice subsequent to an intercurrent illness, or when certain drugs known to impair or compete for hepatic anion secretory sites have been employed. In particular, the anabolic steroid norethandrolone and certain oral contraceptives such as norethynodrel (Enovid) can result in elevated conjugated serum bilirubin levels suggesting the diagnosis. Pregnancy may also precipitate the diagnosis.

Clinical and laboratory features

The paucity of abnormal clinical features contributes to difficulty in recognition and diagnosis. Its fluctuating and intermittent low levels of serum bilirubin may not be clinically recognized. The vague abdominal complaints that characterize the condition are nonspecific and intermittent and rarely suggest the possibility of Dubin-Johnson syndrome to the physician. During exacerbations, the liver becomes palpable and tender and the urine darkens in most patients. Signs of chronic liver damage does not occur in this entity. Pruritus is absent.

Mild elevation of serum bilirubin is present (2 to 8 mg/dl of plasma), with direct-reacting fraction predominating. Prolonged retention of sulfobromophthalein is the only other standard liver function test that is abnormal. Conjugation with glutathione is commonly found. Transaminase, serum proteins, bile acids, alkaline phosphatase, and flocculation tests are normal. By standard methods, failure to visualize the gallbladder with oral cholecystographic agents is common.

Urinary chemistry may be helpful in diagnosis. Patients with Dubin-Johnson syndrome have an abnormal urinary coproporphyrin excretion pattern, eliminating increased amounts of isomer I and decreased amounts of isomer III, thereby reversing the usual urinary ratio of these substances that is found in normal individuals. Studies in the phenotypically normal family members revealed identical urinary excretion patterns only at quantitatively intermediate levels, suggesting heterozygocity. This obervation has been taken as evidence that in this condition an autosomal recessive inheritance pattern is operating.

Liver histology

The striking appearance of liver tissue obtained from patients with Dubin-Johnson syndrome deserves special comment in that this feature is often diagnostic. The gross specimen is strikingly speckled with alternating areas of dark yellow-green to black because of the accumulation of a pigment, believed to be melanin, and normal light-colored areas. This material is located in the centrilobular areas and, according to electron microscopic studies, appears to be concentrated within the lysosomes. Cholestasis is absent in uncomplicated cases because bile acid excretion is normal. Otherwise, the liver histologic appearance is normal by routine and electron microscopy.

Diagnosis

The diagnosis of this entity requires the findings of the previously mentioned clinical, laboratory, and histologic features. The two-phase BSP clearance and urinary coproporphyrin ratio are most helpful. The normal results of alkaline phosphatase, gamma glutamyl transpeptidase (GGT), and bile acids rules out cholestatic conditions. Some confusion can exist at times when the unconjugated serum bilirubin fraction is primarily elevated and yet the patient's liver biopsy reveals the typical pigment deposits of Dubin-Johnson syndrome. A few patients with Dubin-Johnson syndrome have been shown to have decreased hepatic uptake of injected bilirubin, whereas 20% of family members of two probands were found to have slight serum elevation of unconjugated but not of conjugated bilirubin.

Treatment

No treatment is needed for this disease; the prognosis is excellent. Phenobarbital has recently been shown to significantly lower the total and direct-reacting serum bilirubin in some patients with Dubin-Johnson syndrome. This drug simultaneously elevates the maximum transport of BSP. It remains unclear why other patients with this entity have not responded similarly to phenobarbital administration. Absence of hepatic damage is the rule in long-standing examples of the disease. Because the jaundice may be exaggerated by severe physical exertion, alcoholism, drugs, infections, and surgery, these should be avoided if possible. For unknown reasons increased fetal loss has been reported in Dubin-Johnson syndrome.

REFERENCES

Billing, B.H., Williams, R., and Richards, T.G.: Defects in hepatic transport of bilirubin in congenital hyperbilirubinemia: an analysis of plasma bilirubin disappearance curves, Clin. Sci. **27**:245-257, 1964.

Cornelius, C.E., Arias, I.M., and Osburn, B.I.: Hepatic pigmentation with photosensitivity: a syndrome in Corriedale sheep resembling Dubin-Johnson syndrome in man, J. Am. Vet. Assoc. **146**:709-713, 1965.

DiZoglio, J.D., and Cardillo, E.: The Dubin-Johnson syndrome and pregnancy, Obstet. Gynecol. **42**:560-563, 1973.

Dubin, I.N., and Johnson, F.B.: Chronic idiopathic jaundice with unidentified pigment in liver cells: new clinico-pathologic entity with report of 12 cases, Medicine **33**:155-197, 1954.

Gartner, L.M., and Arias, I.M.: Pharmacologic and genetic determinants of disordered bilirubin transport and metabolism in the liver, Ann. N.Y. Acad. Sci. **151**:833-841, 1968.

Scully, R.E., Galdabini, J.J., and McNeely, B.U.: Case records of the Massachusetts General Hospital, N. Engl. J. Med. **299**:592-598, 1978.

Shani, M., Seligsohn, V., and Ben-Ezzer, J.: Effect of phenobarbital on liver function in patients with Dubin-Johnson syndrome, Gastroenterology **67**:303-308, 1974.

Wolkoff, A.W., Cohen, L.E., and Arias, I.M.: Inheritance of the Dubin-Johnson syndrome N. Engl. J. Med. **288**:113-117, 1973.

Rotor's syndrome

This rare inherited disease, which, like Dubin-Johnson syndrome, leads to elevated serum levels of conjugated bilirubin, is rarely diagnosed in the pediatric age group. It appears to be transmitted as a recessive trait, with males and females being equally affected. Although Rotor's syndrome has certain features in common with Dubin-Johnson syndrome, recent data indicates that it may be best to consider them separate entities rather than variants of the same disease.

The major features of Rotor's syndrome distinguishing it from Dubin-Johnson syndrome are that (1) pigment is absent from the hepatocytes and (2) different hepatic organic anion excretory pathways may be affected. For example, the oral cholecystogram is normal in Rotor's syndrome, in contrast to that in Dubin-Johnson syndrome. Evidence that hepatic uptake may also be involved to a greater degree in Rotor's syndrome is suggested by qualitative differences in BSP clearances. Although serum clearance is greatly abnormal in both conditions, in Rotor's syndrome the dye retention remains predominantly unconjugated but it is conjugated in Dubin-Johnson syndrome. Furthermore, studies of plasma clearance of indocyanine green and unconjugated bilirubin revealed considerable retention of these anions as well. A reduced hepatic storage capacity with compromised secretory function of certain organic anions appears basic to this condition, in contrast to that in patients with Dubin-Johnson syndrome. Lastly, urinary coproporphyrin excretion patterns are nonspecific and similar to that seen in cholestatic liver disease. The mild increase in total urinary coproporphyrins also show an increased level of isomer I, but not to the levels reported in Dubin-Johnson syndrome.

Jaundice is mild (less than 10 mg/dl of plasma) and fluctuates, with the conjugated and the free bilirubin fractions being present in equal proportions. Fatigue, emotional upsets, infections, and exercise all may increase the serum bilirubin level. The nonspecific complaints of abdominal pain noted in Dubin-Johnson syndrome are absent in patients with Rotor's syndrome. Surprisingly, jaundice may decrease during pregnancy.

Except for the serum bilirubin and BSP abnormalities, other tests of liver function are generally normal. Hematologic evidence of hemolysis is lacking. Liver biopsy specimens appear normal by light microscopy, with an increase in numbers of pericanalicular lysosomes noted by electron microscopy.

Rotor's syndrome, like Dubin-Johnson syndrome, has a good prognosis for life and requires no specific treatment.

REFERENCES

Arias, I.M.: Studies of chronic familial non-hemolytic jaundice with conjugated bilirubin in serum with and without an unidentified pigment in the liver cells, Am. J. Med. **31:**510-518, 1961.

Haverback, B.J., and Wirtschafter, S.K.: Familial non-hemolytic jaundice with normal liver histology and conjugated bilirubin, N. Engl. J. Med. **262:**113-117, 1960.

Kawasaki, H., Kimura, N., Irisa, T., and Hirayama, C.: Dye clearance studies in Rotor's syndrome, Am. J. Gastroenterol. **71:**380-388, 1979.

Rotor, A.B., Manahan, L., and Flurentin, A.: Familial non-hemolytic jaundice with direct van den Bergh reaction, Acta Med. Philipp. **5:**37-49, 1948.

Wolkoff, A.W., Wolpert, E., Pascasio, F.N., and Arias, I.M.: Rotor's syndrome, Am. J. Med. **60:**173-179, 1976.

Wolpert, E., Pascasio, F.M., Wolkoff, A.W., and Arias, I.M.: Abnormal sulfobromophthalein metabolism in Rotor's syndrome and obligate heterozygotes, N. Engl. J. Med. **296:**1099-1100, 1977.

21 *Acute liver disease*

ACUTE VIRAL HEPATITIS
General discussion

The number of reported cases of viral hepatitis in the United States in 1980 was 59,996, with 29,087 attributable to type A, 19,015 to type B, and 11,894 unspecified. There were 8413 cases of hepatitis A, 2671 of hepatitis B, and 3271 unspecified that occurred in patients under 18 years of age. It is estimated that these figures may represent only 25% of the absolute numbers because most cases are anicteric and therefore unrecognized, whereas others are simply not reported by physicians to public health agencies. Newer serologic tests can aid in the diagnosis of symptomatic patients who are either mildly jaundiced or even anicteric and can increase the number of hepatitis patients identified during endemic and epidemic outbreaks when subjected to thorough epidemiologic surveillance. The anticipated increase in hepatitis B virus cases in the past few years has been partly realized because of newer serologic testing methodology. An increase in the "hepatitis reservoir" has also occurred as a result of promiscuous sexual practices and the widespread use of illicit drugs administered parenterally, particularly in the teen-age and young-adult population and in the homosexual community. Reported hepatitis B cases now approach a range of 19,000 to 20,000 per year, with a fatality placed at 1% to 2%. Underreporting is less of a problem than previously noted. Contamination of water and food by virus B hepatitis is now potentially significant because transmission of this hepatitis virus, once believed to occur only by the parenteral route (serum hepatitis), can now be accomplished by nonparenteral routes (oral, venereal). Person-to-person spread can occur from objects such as shared razors and toothbrushes.

Traditionally, viral hepatitis has been divided into two distinct types of illnesses, infectious hepatitis (type A) and serum hepatitis (type B). The separation was primarily made on clinical grounds, with a diagnosis of infectious hepatitis being made in the absence of a positive history of inoculations, need for blood or blood products, ingestion of certain drugs, or recent immunizations. The acute onset of jaundice in a patient with a known exposure to other similarly affected persons usually meant that the patient had infectious hepatitis. Jaundice developing in a person with a history of recently eating so-called high-risk foods such as clams and oysters or drinking contaminated water has also been taken as resulting from infectious rather than serum hepatitis. It is now apparent that previous distinctions used to separate infectious and serum hepatitis are no longer tenable in light of new information. With the discovery of human hepatitis virus B in patients' serums as the specific agent responsible for some cases of this disease, classical differentiation between serum and infectious hepatitis had to be abandoned.

Within the space of 5 years, current research activity has added immeasurably to our understanding of the pathobiology of hepatitis A and hepatitis B virus–induced liver disease. These two agents, together with cytomegalovirus, infectious mononucleosis virus, Ebstein-Barr virus, and herpesvirus, are currently the major known etiologic agents of acute viral hepatitis in man that can be precisely evaluated. Undoubtedly, other hepatitis viruses (non-A, non-B) exist, but they cannot at present be distinguished by current epidemiologic or clinical features. As was learned with hepatitis A and B viruses, any rapid progress will depend on the identification of immunologic markers of these new and yet-to-be-discovered infectious agents. Meanwhile, presumed "infectious hepatitis," which cannot be specifically proved to be caused by hepatitis A virus (or other known agents) might best be relegated to the broad category of viral hepatitis type A.

Hepatitis A virus

Based upon the recommendation of the World Health Organization Expert Committee on Viral Hepatitis, hepatitis A virus (HAV) and its specific antibody, anti-HAV, is the presently accepted terminology and replaces the previously used terms: infectious hepatitis, short-incubation hepatitis, MS-1 strain (Willowbrook), HA-Ag, anti-HA.

Etiologic agent. Hepatitis A virus is a 27 nm particle present in feces and blood during the late incubation period and during the acute phase of the illness. It can be aggregated and identified from these sources by immune electron microscopy using antibody obtained from patients recovering from HAV disease. The hepatitis A virus is clearly immunologically distinct from hepatitis B virus (HBV).

Hepatitis A virus is a nonenveloped particle and apparently without a distinct virus core. Excess virus coat material has not been found in any body fluids. The virus is relatively heat stable, remaining infectious after 1 hour at 60° C, and is completely resistant to alternate freezing and thawing procedures. Based upon the physicochemical properties that have been examined, the virus has been classified with the RNA-containing enterovirus subgroup, picornavirus.

Hepatitis A virus has worldwide distribution, but up to now immunologic comparisons of different strains, obtained from widely separated geographic borders or from various body fluids, have shown antigenic homogeneity. No strain differences have been elicited up to now.

Marmoset monkeys remain the most widely used experimental animal to study the HAV. Chimpanzees raised in captivity or known to be anti-HAV negative are the only other nonhuman primate susceptible to this virus. Both animals can be infected by inoculation of fecal filtrates containing the virus particles. It is interesting that the serial passage of HAV in marmosets seems to alter the virus and enhance virulence. A shortened incubation period, increased susceptibility, and higher levels of virus titers are found in the livers of subsequently infected animals. Over the years the virus has proved difficult to grow in tissue culture, and only recently has the success of propagation of the virus been reported using explanted marmoset liver cell culture, as well as in fetal rhesus monkey kidney cells. Surprisingly, propagation of the virus by this technique is not cytopathogenic to the cell lines.

Epidemiology. Hepatitis A virus appears to have worldwide distribution, but the natural perpetuation of the virus is believed to reside outside the human host. Chronic carriage of the virus in humans, if it exists at all, seems to be extremely rare. The extrahuman reservoir, however, is unknown, though the fauna residing in contaminated water supplies is suspect. Prevalence of exposure to HAV increases with age and decreasing socioeconomic levels. Although close to 50% of persons can be shown to have antibody to HAV by 30 to 40 years of age, only 3% to 5% of these individuals can recall an illness consistent with acute viral hepatitis. That most HAV infections are inapparent had been suspected from many clinical observations, but most clearly demonstrated in the beautifully conducted long-term studies by Dr. Krugman and his co-workers at the Willowbrook State Home for the Retarded. As might be suspected, antibodies to HAV commonly appear before early adult age in underdeveloped countries where sanitary conditions are primitive and poverty widespread. This contrasts with the relative lack of serologic evidence of immunity to HAV in pediatric patients growing up in modernized communities including the larger urban cities (Fig. 21-1). In the United States children from lower socioeconomic levels and living in urban communities are reported to have a prevalence rate of anti-HAV in from 8% to 30% depending on age, whereas a 2% prevalence rate of this antibody has been found in upper-class children under 15 years of age (Table 21-1).

A decreasing incidence of acute viral hepatitis A disease has been noted over the past 5 to 10 years, and the previously observed fall-winter prevalence for school children no longer is evident. Because of the general susceptibility of children to HAV, common-source outbreaks are more frequently reported in this age group and are especially likely to occur in day care centers, schools, and residential facilities for the mentally retarded. Generally speaking, anicteric disease and milder illness is the rule in the younger patient.

The fecal-oral route of transmission is the most common and especially explains the high level of infectivity noted in institutions and crowded facilities, such as those for the mentally retarded. Indirect exposure to the virus also occurs in common-source outbreaks and is usually traced to the ingestion of contaminated seafood such as shellfish, that is, clams and oysters. Food handlers incubating HAV are notorious in their potential for simultaneously exposing a large vulnerable population. The importance of the enteric infectivity of this virus is also emphasized by recent observations that, overall, sexual promiscuity does predispose to enhanced transmission of HAV, such as that found in homosexual men who engage in oral-anal sexual contact. Reports that anti-HAV titers are not higher in homosexual males than in a control group matched for age and socioeco-

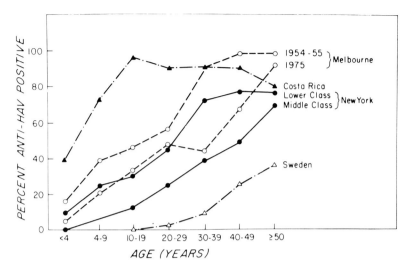

Fig. 21-1. Prevalence of exposure to hepatitis A virus (HAV) expressed as the percentage positive for antibody to HAV (anti-HAV) as a function of age. Note the contrasts between, **A,** lower- and middle-class populations in New York City; **B,** a developing country, Costa Rica, and an advanced, modern urban society, Sweden; and, **C,** populations in Melbourne sampled 20 years apart. (From Dienstag, J.L.: In Popper, H., and Schaffner, F., editors: Progress in liver diseases, New York, 1979, by permission of Grune & Stratton, Inc.)

Table 21-1. Antibody to hepatitis A antigen (anti-HAV) in children

Characteristic	Number tested	Number anti-HA positive	Percentage that are positive
Age (years)			
<5	34	3	8.8
5-9	33	8	24.2
≥10	39	12	30.8
Race			
White	54	9	16.7
Black	52	14	26.9
HBsAg or anti-HBs			
Negative	97	17	17.5
Positive	9	6	66.7

From Stevens, C.E., and others: J. Pediatr. **91:**436-438, 1977.

nomic class, may not hold from one urban city to the next. Neither does multiple exposure to blood products seem to increase the risk for HAV disease. The accidental transmission by percutaneous injection has been shown experimentally, but rarely is this a significant problem in clinical practice. These latter observations probably correlate well with a very brief viremia that occurs in HAV disease. Urine obtained from patients during the early appearance of jaundice and tested for infectivity has given positive results in studies done at Willowbrook. Controversy exists as to whether respiratory secretions from infected patients may represent another possible route for transmitting HAV disease.

Of all the body excretory products, the feces remain the most important reservoir source for transmitting HAV. Unfortunately, the fecal viral shedding commences during the incubation period when the individual is symptom free. Increasing amounts of virus continue to be present when nonspecific prodromal symptoms become apparent, and the amount peaks before the diagnosis of hepatitis is usually suspected vis-à-vis the appearance of jaundice. By this time the exposure of susceptible contacts to the virus has unknowingly been accomplished. One can assume that all household contacts have in fact been exposed. The feces remain an infectious source material for the virus, albeit at lower concentrations of virus for up to 16 days after the appearance of jaundice and dark urine. Based on recent evidence, chronic fecal carriage fortunately does not seem to occur.

Pathogenesis and postinfection immune responses to HAV. Because most individuals gain exposure to HAV disease by way of oral ingestion

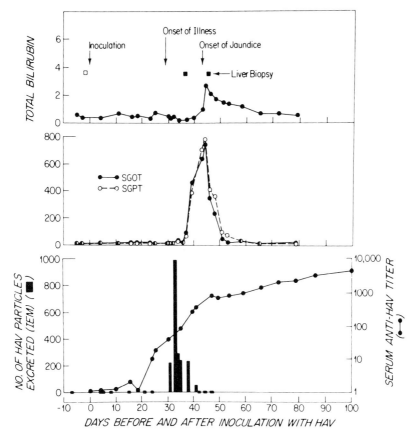

Fig. 21-2. Pattern of fecal excretion of hepatitis A virus (HAV) and development of antibody to HAV (anti-HAV) in relation to other indicators of acute viral hepatitis in a patient with experimental HAV infection. □, No hepatic lesions; ■, hepatic features compatible with acute viral hepatitis. (From Dienstag, J.L.: In Popper, H., and Schaffner, F., editors: Progress in liver diseases, New York, 1979, by permission of Grune & Stratton, Inc.)

of contaminated substances, replication of the virus in the intestinal tract has long been postulated. However, intraenterocyte localization of virus has not been observed in animal studies. Localization and incubation of the virus in gut-associated lymphoid tissue in orally infected hosts remains a distinct possibility, but this premise has not been sufficiently studied.

Whether by the oral or by the parenteral route of exposure, the virus undergoes a 2 to 4-week incubation period. It can first be found in the host's liver after 1 to 2 weeks of exposure and reaches peak concentrations in this organ by 3 to 4 weeks. Intrahepatocyte virus can be demonstrated by immunofluorescence before fecal shedding and also before the brief viremia that occurs later during the incubation period. Replication of HAV takes place primarily in the hepatocyte cytoplasm from

whence it is released into the blood via sinusoids or into the bile via the bile canaliculi. The majority of virus reaching the intestinal lumen and appearing in the feces is probably derived by the latter route. Peak shedding of virus in the feces occurs during the clinical prodrome and before biochemical evidence of hepatitis can usually be detected. Morphologic evidence of hepatocyte injury lags behind both the finding of fecal shedding of virus, as well as the elevated aminotransferase serum levels. These events are summarized in Fig. 21-2. Deposition of virus by viremic spread most likely explains its extrahepatic presence in other organs such as the spleen, salivary glands, pancreas, and kidney.

The host humoral immune response is apparent by laboratory testing at the time clinical symptoms commence, with anti-HAV titers reaching peak levels some 2 to 3 months after the illness. Antibody levels decline somewhat thereafter but continue to confer lifelong immunity to the host. Reexposure to HAV in such an individual with low to barely detectable levels of anti-HAV may result in an amnestic antibody response, but without evidence for viral replication or hepatitis.

The early-appearing antibody, which can be detected by radioimmunoassay (RIA) or enzyme-linked immunosorbent assay (ELISA) techniques, is associated with the IgM class of antibodies. This antibody poses some problems in interpretation, since the known prevalence rate of anti-HAV in the pediatric population is between 3% and 30%. In addition, the acute-phase titer may be very high, and convalescent serum from such a patient may not reveal a discernible titer rise. A late-appearing antibody of the IgG class does develop within 1 to 4 weeks after the acute illness and is readily detectable by the sensitive immune adherence hemagglutination assay (IAHA). Determination of this antibody is most helpful in arriving at a serologic diagnosis of acute HAV disease. A positive test for IgM-specific anti-HAV by either RIA or ELISA, and a simultaneously negative IAHA assay during the acute illness can be considered adequate presumptive evidence for HAV disease when only a single specimen is available. Paired serums, taken 3 weeks apart and showing a rise in titer of anti-HAV by IAHA, are likewise confirmatory of acute HAV disease. At present the routine application of immune electron microscopy to detect early-appearing anti-HAV coproantibody of the IgA class is not practical for most hospital laboratories. In hepatitis A viral disease, the host's immune response to HAV infections is rarely associated with antigen-antibody complex phenomena, though depressed serum complement levels have occasionally been reported in individuals manifesting arthralgias and skin rashes. Also, in contrast to HBV infections, the host's cellular immune response does not appear to be important in the evolution of the pathologic lesions found in HAV disease. Current data suggests that HAV appears to be cytopathic without involvement of host immunocytes, but instead the severity of illness and the ensuing cellular destruction seem to depend on the intensity of virus replication.

Except in rare cases (less than 1 in 1000), the host's circulating (humoral) immune response is sufficient to eradicate the virus before significant hepatic injury. Exceptionally is the HAV the cause of fulminant hepatic necrosis with resulting hepatic encephalopathy and death. Hepatitis A virus is not responsible for perpetuation of chronic active hepatitis, since the virus is not present in liver biopsy material, feces, or blood of these individuals. Neither can the virus be found in the host manifesting biochemical and histologic features of chronic persistent hepatitis as a consequence of proved HAV disease.

Hepatitis B virus

The presently approved nomenclature for hepatitis B virus and its respective components and specific antibodies, as recommended by the World Health Organization Expert Committee on Hepatitis, is as follows:

Hepatitis B virus (Dane particle)	HBV
Hepatitis B surgace antigen	HBsAg
Hepatitis B surface antibody	anti-HBs
Hepatitis B core antigen	HBcAg
Hepatitis B core antibody	anti-HBc
Hepatitis B e arttigen	HBeAg
Hepatitis B e antibody	anti-HBe
Hepatitis B surface antigen subtypes	HBsAg/abw
	HBsA/ayw
	HBsA/adr
	HBsA/ayr

Etiologic agent. Hepatitis B virus (HBV) consists of an antigenic outer lipoprotein envelope or shell (HBsAg) and an inner core, also with antigenic specificity (HBcAg). The nuclear material within the core is double-stranded DNA, containing DNA polymerase activity. The complete HBV is 42 nm in size and is the so-called Dane particle. Immune electron microscopy has shown that the hepatitis virus surface antigen material (HBsAg) is manufactured in the hepatocyte cytoplasm in association with the endoplasmic reticulum, and in excess quantity. Immunofluorescent studies have shown this excess surface antigen material to be closely associated with the hepatocyte plasma membrane. The HBcAg is synthesized primarily in the hepatocyte nucleus, but some of this material may also be seen in the endoplasmic reticulum of the cytoplasm. HBcAg has not been identified outside of hepatocytes. Unused excess surface antigen leaves the hepatocytes and gains access to the circulation, where it appears as spheric particles 20 nm in diameter, or as filamentous forms also 20 nm in diameter and of varying lengths (100 to 200 nm). These circulating antigenic particles are believed to be empty shells and probably non-infectious material

The complete virus (Dane particle) is probably assembled in the cytoplasm of infected hepatocytes and subsequently released into the circulation, where together with excess HBsAg material, they can be identified in almost every body fluid. For unknown reasons, HBV has not been demonstrated in the feces of infected hosts. It is most curious that both the replication of these components and the assembly of the complete virus can be accomplished without apparent hepatocyte injury. Another identifiable HBV antigen is the e antigen, which is present in the serum of infected patients shortly after the appearance of HBsAg, and often before any rise in transaminases can be detected by laboratory testing. The HBeAg usually disappears during the prodromal illness but may persist in some individuals who are chronic carriers of HBsAg. The e antigen is a distinctly separate antigenic material from the HBsAg, but its exact location on or in the Dane particle remains uncertain. Some workers believe that the e antigen might in fact be host derived, developing as a result of HBV infection. The finding of HBeAg in the serum of chronic carriers serves as an important marker of infectivity because of its concurrent association with Dane particles in the host. Once antibodies (anti-HBe) to this particular antigen appear in the serum, the e antigen disappears, and simultaneously one cannot find Dane particles in the circulation.

The morphologic complexity of the HBV is compounded somewhat by antigenic subtypes now recognized with the surface antigen material. These antigenic structures (spheric particles, filamentous forms, the surface of the Dane particle) share a common group-specific antigen, *a,* along with two other sub-determinants, either *b* or *y, w* or *r*. Each subtype reveals differing antigenic reactivities, but they do not produce any unique clinical expression of hepatitis. These genotypes, which are mutually exclusive, have value in epidemiologic assessment of HBV disease, since distinct geographic distribution patterns have been observed for these subtypes.

Epidemiology. Hepatitis B virus has worldwide distribution with a carrier rate in the United States general population between 0.1% to 0.3%. This figure varies with age, environmental factors, socioeconomic status, customs and mores of a given society, and an individual's occupation. The prevalence of anti-HBs in middle-class suburban children is said to be about 5%, whereas a 15% prevalence rate was found in adults screened from a similar socioeconomic background. Man appears to be the primary reservoir for this virus, and person-to-person spread the most common means of acquisition. The role and magnitude of virus-harboring arthropods as vectors in the spread of this disease remains under study. Acquisition of this viral agent was once believed possible only by the parenteral route (serum hepatitis). It is interesting that probably less than 25% of cases of posttransfusion hepatitis can be proved to be caused by HBV disease. It is now known that transmission of infection to susceptible individuals can be accomplished by a variety of ways, since almost all body fluids and secretions (except possibly the feces) may contain the virus. The presence of hepatitis B surface antigen in saliva, tears, sweat, nasopharyngeal secretions, urine, genital secretions, and possibly mother's milk obviously provides ample opportunity for nonparenteral spread. At particular risk are close family contacts, neonates born of carrier mothers, and clients and staff of custodial institutions for retarded children. Other groups at particularly high risk for acquisition of HBV infection include hospitalized patients and their health care providers, laboratory personnel, both the patients and staff of hemodialysis units, military populations, sexual partners of chronic HBsAg carriers, and individuals requiring frequent transfusions of blood products, such as hemophiliacs or those with hereditary hemoglobinopathies. Immune-suppressed patients or cancer patients on chemotherapy likewise have an increased risk to acquire HBV infections. Evidence for HBV disease in all of these aforementioned groups approaches three- to fivefold the incidence found in the general population.

As expected, most pediatric cases of HBV infection are acquired by the nonparenteral route. This is certainly true in developed countries where parenteral exposure to the HBV from blood and blood products is most unusual because of careful screening of donors. Since the reported frequency of HBsAg-carrier mothers with markers of infectivity is well below 1% in most of these nations, transplacental acquisition of the virus is also unusual. In underdeveloped parts of the world and

Table 21-2. Immunopathogenic mechanisms

System	Immunologic localization	Mediation
I. Antibody-dependent complement-mediated cytolysis	Ab	Complement
II. Antibody-directed cellular cytotoxicity	Ab	K cells
III. T lymphocyte–mediated cytotoxicity	T cell	T cell
IV. Macrophage-mediated cytolysis	a. Nonspecific	Macrophage
	b. T recognitive factor	Macrophage
V. Immune complex injury	Nonspecific at local site	Complement
		K cells
		B cells

From Edgington, T.S., and Chisari, F.V.: Am. J. Med. Sci. **270:**213-227, 1975.

especially in the islands of the South Pacific, markers of previous HBV exposure, or a carrier state, develop within the first 5 years of life at a frequency not expected until adulthood in developed countries of the world.

Evidence of acute active or prior HBV infection is found in close to 8% of asymptomatic, urban adolescents. Higher figures (50% to 80%) are reported where the parenteral use of illicit drugs is common and in those engaged in homosexual activity (25% to 30%).

The magnitude of HBV infection versus that of hepatitis A virus disease is most likely a reflection of the higher carrier rate in asymptomatic individuals. This may vary from 40% to 90% in neonatally acquired disease and from 5% to 10% in those infected as adults. In institutional settings, HBsAg carriage is from 5% to 15%. It has been noted that children with trisomy 21 in custodial care facilities are especially vulnerable to become carriers of HBsAg.

Pathogenesis and postinfection host immune responses. The natural history of HBV infection has been more precisely defined, since the development and application of highly sensitive immunologic techniques provided a means to identify the HBV and its components in the infected host. These techniques also permitted the elucidation of the sequence of immunologic events that occur after exposure to the virus.

After parenteral acquisition of the HBV, there is an incubation period, which may be as short as 6 days, but typically is from 3 to 10 weeks. In unusual cases the incubation period may be as long as 6 months before evidence of disease becomes apparent. Infection by the oral route is believed to require a greater infective dose of virus and a slightly longer incubation period before the illness becomes manifest. When the virus reaches the hepatocytes, virus replication begins with synthesis of core material (HBcAg) taking place in the nuclei, with surface coat antigen (HBsAg) material being manufactured in the endoplasmic reticulum of the infected hepatocytes. Synthesis of the complete virion (Dane particle) takes place in the cytoplasm and by a mechanism still undiscovered, and the virus, along with excess surface antigen material, gains access to the sinusoid circulation. This replication and synthetic activity of HBV takes place either with no, or very minimal, cytopathogenic impact upon the hepatocytes. Hepatocellular injury, which is histologically similar to that seen in HAV disease, is dependent on the nature and intensity of the host's immune response to the HBV infection. As will be seen, both a humoral and a cellular immune response develops, and it is directed against intrahepatic specific viral antigens (HBsAg, HBeAg, HBcAg) and perhaps against membrane-bound viral and host neoantigens (liver-specific lipoprotein, altered hepatocyte plasma membrane, and so on). These events are most likely the cause of the ensuing hepatic injury. A variety of immunopathogenetic mechanisms have been implicated (Table 21-2). Laboratory evidence of acute HBV disease may include the presence of HBsAg, of Dane particles by immune electronmicroscopy, of hepatitis B–specific DNA polymerase activity, HBeAg, and at times HBsAg immune complexes in the blood of such a patient.

Humoral immune response. The sequence of events related to the appearance of humoral immunity in a typical case of HBV infection has been well defined. It varies somewhat depending on whether the host makes a full recovery or develops chronic infection with this virus. Coincident with the rise in aminotransferases and a decline in DNA polymerase activity is the appearance of anti-HBc as the earliest immunologic marker of host response to the infection. This antibody may be identified by complement fixation and radioimmunoassay as well as by immune electron microscopy. Anti-HBe appears in the serum soon thereafter, either before or after the appearance of anti-HBs, the latter at times demonstrable early during biochemical evidence of liver disease and at other times not until several months later. For diagnostic reasons it is important to recall that at times anti-HBs may not be detectable by routine laboratory testing for some months after HBsAg disappears from the blood. HBsAg is most readily identified by radioimmunoassay, and passive-hemagglutination techniques provide extreme sensitivity when testing for the presence of anti-HBc or HBeAg in the serum, all serving as evidence for HBV exposure.

The seroconversion from HBsAg to anti-HBs is usually synonymous with clearing and resolution of the disease. In unusual circumstances serologic negativity for HBs antigen (also anti-HBs negative) may be noted in some patients with chronic persistent hepatitis or chronic active hepatitis. These individuals usually have persisting high titers of anti-HBc indicating ongoing viral replication. Once anti-HBs appears, it then confers lifelong specific immunity against reinfection by HBV.

The early-appearing anti-HBe follows the disappearance of HBeAg in the blood and circulating Dane particles. There is some evidence to support the concept that anti-HBe also suppresses hepatitis B core replication in the hepatocyte, which in turn accounts for the simultaneous disappearance of Dane particles. On the other hand, anti-HBe has no effect on the production and release of the excess antigenic coat material (HBsAg). It would appear that anti-HBe is important in both the elimination of virus and the simultaneous production of cytopathogenic changes. Anti-HBc, on the other hand, does not seem to have a role in either eliminating the virus or in causing hepatocyte injury. Anti-HBc is usually short lived but remains present in chronic HBV infection and is indicative of ongoing viral replication in liver cells. As mentioned previously, in rare instances anti-HBc may be present in infected but HBsAg-negative individuals.

Cell-mediated immune response. In contrast to HAV infection, HBV disease also invokes a cell-mediated immune response from the host. This can be demonstrated by several different techniques including leukocyte migration–inhibition assays, lymphocyte stimulation, and cytotoxicity against HBsAg-coated target cells. The exact contribution of cell-mediated immunity versus that of humoral antibody in elimination of both the virus and the circulating antigens remains under study. Cell-mediated immunity is present at the time HBsAg is cleared from the serum and liver tissue, and then it gradually disappears. When chronic HBV infection evolves, evidence for persistent cellular immune reaction against HBsAg remains in the host. That severe hepatic necrosis does occur in agammaglobulinemic patients strongly suggests an important role for cell-mediated cytolysis.

The pathologic impact of humoral and cell-mediated immunity varies from submicroscopic injury, manifest only by biochemical evidence of hepatitis (elevated aminotransferase levels), to a liver lesion showing either focal, massive, or bridging necrosis, with or without changes consistent with chronic aggressive hepatitis. Depending on unknown factors, infection may be insufficiently eliminated and persists (HBsAg-positive) without hepatocyte damage, or with histologic evidence of chronic persistent or chronic aggressive hepatitis. Fortunately, HBV infection is most often completely eradicated by the stimulated immune response and usually does so without producing clinical symptoms in the host.

In summary, the appearance in the serum of HBsAg is soon followed by anti-HBc, anti-HBe, and finally anti-HBs, the last indicating termination of the HBV infection and providing lifelong immunity.

Immune-complex phenomenon. Generally speaking, the clinical and biochemical expression of liver injury that occurs in a typical pediatric case of HBV infection is indistinguishable from that seen in HAV disease. A prodrome of constitutional complaints, followed by icterus and then by recovery, is the expected course with either of these hepatotrophic viruses. However, in 5% to 15% of adult cases of HBV infection, an atypical prodromal illness with predominant extrahepatic manifestations is reported (Table 21-3). The clinical picture may be indistinguishable from serum sickness. A similar clinical spectrum may occur in children, but incidence figures are not well es-

Table 21-3. Extrahepatic manifestations of hepatitis B viral disease

Condition	Frequency of HBsAg positive	Clinical and pathologic findings	Immune response
Serum sickness	10% to 20%	Rash, fever, polyarthralgia, arthritis	Circulating immune complexes (HBsAg-IgM, HBsAg-IgG) Reduced $C'H_{50}$, C'_3, C'_4 in serum and joints
Glomerulonephritis	Up to 30% or more in children	Hematuria, proteinuria, membranoproliferative or membranous type of lesion	Nodular deposits of HBsAg, IgG, and C' on glomerular basement membrane
Polyarteritis nodosa	30% to 40%	Serum sickness–like onset, progress to peripheral neuropathy, hypertension; eosinophilia found; fibrinoid necrosis and perivascular inflammation of small arteries and arterioles	HBsAg persists; reduced $C'H_{50}$; circulating complexes of HBsAg–anti-HBs; deposits of HBsAg, IgM, IgG, and C'_3 in vessels

Modified from Gocke, D.J.: Am. J. Med. Sci. **270:**49-52, 1975.

tablished. Arthralgia or arthritis is less commonly seen than a skin rash, which is described as a papular acrodermatitis usually on the face, buttocks, and the extensor surfaces of the arms and legs. This may be associated with mild lymphadenitis and fever and has been called the Gianotti-Crosti syndrome. At times the skin rash may also be urticarial and have features of angioedema. Both manifestations (joints and skin) are generally transient in nature and resolve when jaundice appears. This is coincident with a documented rise in anti-HBs and increasing serum complement levels. In chronic HBsAg disease, an overload of immune complexes deposited in renal glomeruli can produce a histologic lesion consistent with membranous glomerulonephritis, though other renal lesions have also been described. In fact, one report states that hepatitis B virus infection may account for up to 30% of unexplained cases of chronic glomerulonephritis in children. In adults the deposition of these immune complexes in blood vessel walls gives rise to an illness indistinguishable from that of idiopathic periarteritis nodosa. These cryoprecipitable complexes, which are capable of activating both the classic and the alternate complement pathways, have been isolated in the serum of patients undergoing these serum sickness–like reactions. Such complexes are complement fixing and often contain IgG, IgM, and IgA, along with C_3, C_4, C_5, HBsAg, and anti-HBs.

Differences in the nature and extent of the host's immune response also plays an important part in the evolution of the various manifestations seen in HBV disease. For example, excess anti-HBs is seen in fulminant hepatic necrosis and the polymyalgia rheumatica syndrome. On the other hand, excess HBsAg is seen in the Gianotti-Crosti syndrome and polyarteritis. The early appearance of the humoral immune response during the incubation period is associated with the formation of immune complexes in such individuals and probably accounts for the extrahepatic manifestations. To what extent these complexes are also responsible for hepatocyte injury remains to be determined.

The long-term effects of the carrier state vary from a benign entity called chronic persistent hepatitis to the more worrisome conditions of chronic active hepatitis or the gradual progression to cirrhosis. Of no small concern is the observation that the risk of hepatic carcinoma evolving later in life is substantially increased in individuals with HBsAg chronic liver disease.

Clinical findings

Although the basic manifestations are quite consistent, the severity of the disease varies considerably and is probably related to the quantity of virus involved in the original exposure and to the host's immune response and capacity to localize, neutralize, or prevent substantial replication and subsequent spread. Most childhood cases of hepatitis produce minimal symptoms and are usually anicteric. A mild clinical prodrome can easily be confused with a gastrointestinal "flulike" illness, and no doubt proper diagnosis is seldom made in these cases because many are handled over the telephone.

When the classic form of presentation is available, the diagnosis is seldom missed. The first 5 to 7 days of the illness are characterized by slight to moderate fever, extreme anorexia, nausea and vomiting, asthenia, malaise, and easy fatigability. In the pediatric age group, neither diarrhea is common, nor pruritus. A similar symptom complex may or may not be present in the family. Abdominal pain, especially in the epigastric area and right upper quadrant, occurs in some patients.

Physical examination at this time may reveal only one important finding—tender hepatomegaly. It may be detected if the physician carefully observes the facial expression of the child while gently percussing over this structure with a finger or gently with the fist. At times, tenderness is elicited on deep inspiration that permits the liver edge to flip over the examining fingers. The child may verbally deny pain, but it seldom will be hidden from his facial expression. During the early part of the prodrome, jaundice is not present and splenomegaly may or may not be noted. Occasionally a serum sickness–like syndrome including a macular rash, urticarial lesions, arthralgias, or arthritis may antedate the appearance of clinical jaundice, these symptoms most often being noted in hepatitis B virus disease.

Suddenly the patient or the parent recognizes jaundice, usually as scleral icterus. A history of passage of dark urine and light stools preceding the jaundice can be obtained, and a proper diagnosis is usually made. At this time, physical examination finds the liver to be enlarged and uniformly tender. Splenomegaly is found in 10% to 15% of the cases during the icteric phase. Less obvious sites that may reveal the presence of underlying jaundice include the underside of the tongue and the tympanic membranes.

Over the next several days the jaundice may increase in severity, but the patient begins to feel better, an observation that has valuable prognostic significance. Most often the appetite returns, nausea and fever disappear, and the patient becomes cheerful. A diuresis may be reported. All this may occur during the time when laboratory evidence suggests worsening of the liver disease (rising serum bilirubin and transaminase). This divergent course between the patient's complaints and the laboratory findings is the hallmark of benign viral hepatitis and generally carries a good prognosis. The physician should become suspicious about the course of the illness should jaundice deepen while symptoms of anorexia, nausea, vomiting, or fever persist or worsen.

As indicated, the second phase of hepatitis (icteric phase) follows a dome-shaped pattern with gradual increase in the intensity of the jaundice before its slow resolution, with the entire time of jaundice typically being less than 4 weeks. A predominantly "cholestatic" form of hepatitis may evolve in some patients and is characterized by laboratory findings that suggest an extrahepatic biliary obstructive process (high direct-reacting bilirubin fraction, greatly elevated alkaline phosphatase or gamma glutamyl transpeptidase, and total cholesterol). Severe pruritus often accompanies this form of hepatitis.

Persistence of jaundice beyond 4 weeks is cause for concern unless only low-grade unconjugated hyperbilirubinemia exists (posthepatitis syndrome). It is not unusual for a mild, short-lived relapse of both clinical symptoms and slight jaundice to occur after 10 to 12 weeks of the illness. This complication is said to occur in about 15% of patients and is not considered worrisome. The laboratory abnormalities may again resolve quickly, or slowly over the next 6 to 12 months. This form of hepatitis has been called "two-phase" or "relapsing" hepatitis. On the other hand, either persistence or recurrence of anorexia, fever, or vomiting with deepening of jaundice should always be viewed with alarm; this mode of presentation is seen in 50% of children who go on to develop subacute or fulminating hepatitis, or some 60% of children who develop chronic active hepatitis.

The recovery phase of acute hepatitis varies. It generally takes from 1 to 3 months before clinical and routine laboratory abnormalities become normal and the patient enjoys complete well-being without malaise and fatigue. Children generally recover quite promptly, so that any delay in the resolution of this clinical syndrome should also be viewed suspiciously.

For years, the acuteness of the onset of symptoms was believed useful in differentiating "infectious" from "serum" hepatitis. An acute onset of clinical symptoms was more consistent with the former diagnosis, whereas a less spectacular, insidious onset was believed to be characteristic of the latter entity. This clinical differentiation has not held up now that the specific diagnosis of both type A and type B hepatitis is possible by specific testing.

It is most important to appreciate the fact that acute hepatitis has a predictable sequence that the physician can anticipate. Deviations from the usual course should be viewed as evidence that the illness may not be benign-acute, or perhaps that the diagnosis is erroneous. Liver disease in children and young adults should not be viewed with the equanimity implied by the term "catarrhal jaundice" (meaning 'cold in the liver'). Fulminating hepatitis with coma and death, chronic hepatitis, chronic active hepatitis, and eventually cirrhosis and hepatic decompensation follow this "benign" disease with sufficient frequency to warrant complete respect for this entity.

Diagnosis

The diagnosis of hepatitis is usually made in the typical case simply by the clinical features of a flulike prodrome, jaundice, and an enlarged, tender liver. Laboratory tests are indicated not only to identify hepatitis virus A or B disease but also to rule out other possible viral causes. In addition, laboratory tests can establish the presence of other conditions that produce a hepatitis-like illness (Wilson's disease or alpha-antitrypsin deficiency), useful information for prognosis and treatment.

If jaundice is absent but the patient has clinical symptoms (anorexia, malaise, fatigue), the first clue to proper diagnosis may come from additional historical information. Obviously, the knowledge of a recent outbreak of hepatitis in the patient's environment is most helpful. Fecal-oral spread from person-to-person contact or exposure to a common source of the disease is the usual mode of transmission. Children in crowded environments such as day care centers or residential facilities of mentally retarded are at particular risk to acquire both type A and type B hepatitis virus. A history of exposure to a similarly affected person is present in 20% to 30% of cases of hepatitis. Further inquiry must often be made about other specific exposures that potentially carry a high risk of hepatitis virus A disease. Besides contact with persons known to have hepatitis, drinking water of questionable purity, eating of certain shellfish

(clams, oysters), a recent history of inoculations, parenteral use of illicit drugs, transfusions, and ingestion of drugs are events that may provide epidemiologic diagnostic information. With the young child, the history of exposure is obtained less often than that reported with adults, for many cases seem to be subclinical or extremely mild in this age group. This is not true for the teen-ager, from whom a history of known exposure can usually be obtained.

Additional clues to proper diagnosis can come from knowledge of the time factor between possible exposure and the new symptoms. Symptoms that begin within 15 to 40 days after definite exposure to cases of hepatitis suggest hepatitis virus A disease, and presumably the serum should be HBsAg negative. However, rare examples of HBsAg seroconversion have now been reported to occur within 10 days of exposure. On the other hand, symptoms that begin 50 to 160 days after a suspected exposure are probably caused by hepatitis B virus disease, and the serum is likely to reveal the presence of HBsAg or anti-HBc, or both, and demonstrate DNA polymerase activity. Unfortunately, a large number of cases fall between these two incubation periods, and therefore serologic testing is needed.

The laboratory can aid in specific diagnosis, especially when the clinical syndrome is mild and jaundice is faint or absent. In addition, laboratory tests of liver function may provide information as to the severity of the underlying disease, while at times suggesting other possible causes. Finally, liver biopsy is likely to provide the most useful information but is seldom needed or indicated in suspected viral hepatitis that follows the traditional course.

Laboratory findings

Most laboratories now do a battery of liver-function tests, or a so-called liver profile, even when only a few test results are usually necessary. Proper interpretation and utilization of the screening panel results will require both knowledge and understanding of the sensitivity, specificity, and selectivity of each individual test. This should allow the clinician to accurately extrapolate the potential severity of the underlying hepatic disease.

At best, only rough correlation exists between the structural alterations and corresponding biochemical abnormalities that reflect liver cell injury. For example, changes in the bile secretory apparatus (dilated bile canaliculi, changes in the Golgi apparatus, bile pigment in cell) are associated with cholestasis and therefore can be related to the elevated serum bilirubin and alkaline phosphatase levels. Alterations in the synthesis of hepatic proteins (albumin) parallel the degree of injury to the endoplasmic reticulum. Disruption of hepatocyte membrane has been believed responsible for the elevations in serum transaminase activity, but actually this may be secondary to defective organelle binding of these enzymes, which then permits their free passage out of the cell. It is not surprising that the other vague but constant clinical findings of hepatitis, such as fatigue, malaise, and anorexia, are not accounted for by any of the present studies, and much of this disease remains unexplained.

Complete blood count, platelet count, and Coombs' test. Hemoglobin, hematocrit, and white blood cell count are most often normal in the usual case of viral hepatitis. A decrease in granulocytes and increased numbers of "atypical"lymphocytes is not infrequent. Rarely, pancytopenia or aplastic anemia can develop in viral hepatitis. High white blood cell counts (more than 25,000 mm^3) and thrombocytopenia may be seen in fulminating hepatitis. A sudden fall in hematocrit caused by hemolysis may be seen in some patients with hepatitis who also have glucose-6-phosphatase dehydrogenase (G-6-PD) deficiency in their red blood cells. Hemolysis in the absence of G-6-PD deficiency but in the presence of liver disease should again make the physician suspect Wilson's disease.

A positive Coombs' test is more likely to signify chronic hepatitis, particularly chronic active hepatitis. In addition, burred red blood cells (acanthocytes) when seen in the peripheral blood smear signify chronic or severe liver disease.

Sedimentation rate. Although many physicians use the sedimentation rate as a guide to ongoing inflammation, it certainly is less specific than some of the other tests available to assess hepatocyte injury. The sedimentation rate is usually normal in acute HBV disease but tends to be elevated in HAV disease. Serial measurements may be used to follow patients under treatment for chronic active liver disease.

Urinalysis. Screening the urine for bilirubin is particularly worthwhile in those patients with a nonspecific "flulike" illness, but who also demonstrate tenderness in the epigastrium or right upper quadrant. Bilirubinuria is often present before clinical jaundice is noted, and urobilinogen is likewise present unless obstruction is severe, at which times stools are acholic.

Serum bilirubin. The rising serum bilirubin in hepatitis lags slightly behind the rise in serum transaminase. It generally reaches a peak after 5 to 10 days of clinical jaundice, with maximum levels between 5 and 15 mg/dl. In most patients, peak bilirubin levels are found at the time the patient begins to show symptomatic improvement. The elevated serum bilirubin level tends to decline slowly over the next 3 to 6 weeks, with an occasional transient exacerbation (15%) at the 8 to 10 week period. Prolongation of the elevated serum bilirubin, especially if over half is direct reacting, is cause for concern and deserves additional evaluation of the patient. This is particularly true if one also notes a simultaneous elevation of the serum alkaline phosphatase or gamma glutamyl transpeptidase. Particularly, extrahepatic biliary causes for these biochemical abnormalities should be considered, including the presence of a choledochal cyst, cholelithiasis, or an unsuspected stricture of the common duct. At times drug-induced cholestatic liver disease may give an identical biochemical pattern. Similarly, levels that initially rise above 15 mg/dl in a patient who is not improving indicate severe hepatic damage as seen in submassive necrosis or fulminating hepatitis. Posthepatitis hyperbilirubinemia of the indirect-reacting type is rare in children but may persist for months. Bilirubin clearance, rather than increased production, seems to be the underlying problem. This may possibly cause diagnostic confusion with the congenital type of unconjugated hyperbilirubinemia, Gilbert's disease.

Serum transaminases (SGOT, SGPT). Results of serum aminotransferase activity remain the most sensitive indicators of active, ongoing hepatocellular injury. Either the aspartate aminotransferase (AST, formerly serum glutamic oxaloacetic transaminase, SGOT) or the alanine aminotransferase (ALT, formerly serum glutamic pyruvic transaminase, SGPT) can be measured by most laboratories. The AST (SGOT) is usually part of the automated serum-screening method employed in most hospital and commercial laboratories. This particular transaminase has less specificity and selectivity than that of the ALT (SGPT) but is technically more reliable, and therefore it is extremely useful in the pediatric age population for the detection of mild liver injury and in subsequent monitoring of the disease course. In mild and anicteric cases of hepatitis A virus disease the AST may be the earliest and only abnormality detectable, becoming positive 7 to 10 days before symptoms appear. In hepatitis B virus disease, abnormalities in serum transaminase are noted after the appearance of (and sometimes after the disappearance of) HBsAg. DNA polymerase activity, HBeAg, and anti-HBc are usually present when the serum transaminases begin to rise.

The correlation between the severity of the liver injury and the AST value is not very good if the figure is below 3000 IU. Values above this are more often seen in submassive hepatic necrosis and fulminating hepatitis and therefore warrants concern and further studies. Isoenzyme determination of AST that reveals an increased ratio of the mitochondrial fraction to cytosol fraction is said to correlate with the severity of the hepatocellular injury. This laboratory determination is seldom necessary, however, because other markers of severe injury indicating widespread necrosis are available by simpler tests, such as results obtained from measurement of the prothrombin time and fibrinogen levels.

The rise in transaminase is usually abrupt, remains stable for several days, and then begins to fall quite promptly. In hepatitis A the elevation of transaminase lasts about 10 to 21 days, whereas in hepatitis B it is more likely to last from 20 to 30 days.

A secondary rise in the serum transaminase may occur as a supposedly normal event in 15% to 20% of patients after 8 to 10 weeks of disease and should not be viewed with alarm. A persistent, low-grade elevation of the serum transaminase, when seen in the absence of persistent antigenemia and of other biochemical abnormalities, is consistent with a benign course and warrants no further studies or intervention for the first 3 months of the disease. Mild biochemical abnormalities of AST may be found in as many as 30% of children after the resolution of other clinical findings of disease. Persistence of elevated transaminase in the face of persistent antigenemia has potentially greater significance for chronicity and should be further investigated by laboratory and perhaps liver biopsy.

Serum alkaline phosphatase. The alkaline phosphatase value is seldom helpful in the usual types of viral hepatitis because it is frequently normal or slightly elevated. In the pediatric population, particularly in the young infant and adolescent, it loses both sensitivity and specificity because of the contribution of bone alkaline phosphatase from osseous activity. Falsely high values for children may also be noted when the determination is obtained from the biochemical screen (SMA-12). However, a greater than 50% rise in alkaline phosphatase should make the clinician suspect biliary tract abnormalities, especially if the elevated bilirubin level is primarily direct-reacting. High levels of serum alkaline phosphatase may also be found in the unusual cases of "cholestatic hepatitis" or in those cases of liver disease from infectious mononucleosis. We have also seen persistently high liver alkaline phosphatase values in cases of portal fibrosis (with or without cirrhosis), presumably because of an in utero cytomegaloviral infection.

Gamma glutamyl transpeptidase (GGT). The availability of this laboratory test has been especially welcomed in aiding the evaluation of pediatric liver disease. Gamma glutamyl transpeptidase (GGT) is associated with the microsomal portion of the cytoplasm, bile duct epithelial cells, and renal, small bowel, and choroid plexus epithelial cells, and it appears to be involved in amino acid transport across the cell membrane. Other than in the neonatal period, when a transient elevation is reported, the GGT is not influenced thereafter by age or by osseous activity. The serum level of GGT is believed to parallel the liver fraction of the serum alkaline phosphatase and conveys a great deal of sensitivity in the assessment of hepatobiliary disease. It may be elevated five- to tenfold early in the course of mild biliary tract disease when alkaline phosphatase serum values may be normal. It is also extremely useful in screening anicteric hepatitis, especially when obtained with serum transaminase studies. Normal values for GGT militate against hepatobiliary disease. Caution is suggested when one is interpreting slightly elevated values for GGT in patients taking anticonvulsant medication, in insulin-dependent diabetics, or during the nephrotic syndrome. In these cases spurious elevation of the GGT may occur, but underlying liver disease may also coexist. Assessment with GGT has greater usefulness in hepatobiliary disease than measurement of 5'-nucleotidase does.

Tests for acute hepatitis A viral disease

Anti-HAV. Whenever possible this test should be obtained during the acute icteric phase of the illness, with simultaneous determination of the IgM-specific antibody by radioimmunoassay (RIA) or enzyme-linked immunosorbent assay (ELISA), and of IgG-specific antibody by immune adherence hemagglutination assay (IAHA). The presence of high-titer IgM-specific antibody to HAV, and a low or absent IgG antibody titer to the same virus can be taken as presumptive evidence for acute HA-induced disease. Serially, a fall in IgM antibody and a rise in IgG antibody remains the most conclusive evidence for diagnosis. These tests are now widely available and can be performed by certain commercial and centralized public health laboratories.

Tests for acute hepatitis B virus disease

HBsAg. Serologic evidence for HBsAg activity should be sought because clinical separation of acute HBV disease from that of HAV is not reliable. The identification of HBV disease may have epidemiologic significance and allows the physician to passively immunize contacts with specific immune globulin. It is important to remember that antigenemia (HBsAg) may appear early in the illness and be very transitory in some patients; therefore its presence needs to be sought as early as possible in cases of suspected hepatitis. Where the disease is common, family members may be screened for HBsAg if administration of hyperimmune globulin is being considered. In addition, maternal HBsAg should always be determined if hepatitis is diagnosed in a child under 1 year of life. Most laboratories use the highly sensitive radioimmunoassay for this determination.

HBeAg. Screening for the presence of this HBV antigen is seldom required in the index case with acute viral hepatitis. Rather, the major usefulness of this test derives from the positive relationship that exists between the presence of HBeAg and the potential infectivity of an individual who has become a chronic carrier of HBsAg. Indeed, persistence of HBeAg appears to be associated with chemical and morphologic evidence of chronic hepatitis. It is especially important to screen for the presence of maternal e antigen when one is assessing the risk of vertical acquisition of HBV disease by the neonate from the carrier mother.

Screening for the presence or absence of HBeAg in chronic carriers of HBsAg is also important from a public health point of view. At particular risk of becoming chronic carriers of HBsAg besides neonates born of carrier mothers are patients with Down's syndrome, leukemia, and lymphoma.

Anti-HBc. This serologic marker may occasionally be necessary when an illness suspected as possibly caused by HBV is recognized late into its course, at a time when HBsAg has already disappeared, yet before anti-HBs is measurable by routine laboratory testing. Persistent high titers of anti-HBc usually indicate ongoing intrahepatic viral replication.

Anti-HBs. This antibody is seldom detectable before 3 to 4 months after the appearance of the acute disease. Anti-HBs may not appear in some cases for up to 1 year after disappearance of HBsAg. In those who become chronic carriers of HBsAg, anti-HBs does not develop.

Anti-HBe. This test is seldom indicated in acute liver disease and is apparently a difficult assay to perform. Occasional usefulness of this information again has to do with assessment of the potential activity of an HBsAg-carrier present. The presence of anti-HBe in carrier mothers correlates with a decreased risk of fetal acquisition of HBV but is not 100% protective.

Mononucleosis spot test. This simple test has a high degree of accuracy (95%) and at times may provide an unsuspected diagnosis that can explain the hepatosplenomegaly and lymphadenopathy.

Prothrombin time. The prothrombin time remains very useful in assessing the severity of initial liver injury and also in following the success of regeneration of the severely damaged liver. Therefore, one should strongly consider obtaining this laboratory test when either clinical suspicion or biochemical results suggest severe liver injury. In acute hepatitis the prothrombin time is normal in probably 95% of cases. It may, however, be slightly prolonged in those patients presenting with a history of pronounced anorexia or vomiting for over 5 days, or having been on a broad-spectrum antibiotic. In these examples, the prothrombin time can be expected to return to normal 12 to 24 hours after the intramuscular administration of 5 to 10 mg of vitamin K. Prolongation of the prothrombin time (less than 50% of normal) signifies widespread hepatic damage, especially if the prolongation is vitamin K resistant.

Serum protein electrophoresis. This laboratory determination is useful both in the acute illness and in following the course of the disease. The serum albumin value is seldom depressed (less than 3.5 gm/dl) in acute viral hepatitis because of its relatively long half-life of 15 to 25 days. Values greater than 3.5 gm/dl can be expected in over 80% of the cases of acute hepatitis. After 8 days of disease, values of serum albumin may be reduced by 25% of normal, probably because of both decreased protein intake and ongoing hepatic injury. Likewise, the gamma globulin fraction is normal to slightly elevated (less than 2 gm/dl). Later into the illness, a depressed serum albumin level may well indicate a massive hepatic injury or an expanded vascular volume because of an oliguric state, or it may be the first clue to an underlying chronic liver disease. A coincident rise and persistence of the hyperbilirubinemic state, in the face of a falling serum albumin, almost always suggests massive hepatic injury. An elevated gamma globulin (greater than 2.5 gm/dl) is suggestive of chronic active hepatitis and may be present within the first 3 to 4 weeks of obvious disease.

Attention to the alpha-1 fraction of the electrophoretic strip is also suggested, since in acute infectious hepatitis there is an increase with values greater than 0.2 gm/dl. Lower levels, however, should suggest alpha-1-antitrypsin–deficiency liver disease.

Alpha-1-antitrypsin. Serum alpha-1-antitrypsin levels should be determined in cases of neonatal cholestasis, when a family history of nonalcoholic liver disease is obtained, when the acute disease process fails to resolve as expected, and when the alpha-1-globulin fraction of the serum electrophoretic pattern is noted to be less than 0.2 gm/dl. It should also be obtained when signs of underlying chronic liver disease are present on physical examination. Serum levels of alpha-1-antitrypsin that are in the homozygote or heterozygote range call for an alpha-1-antitrypsin protease inhibitor phenotyping. Almost all cases of alpha-1-antitrypsin deficiency liver disease are associated with protease inhibitor phenotype PiZZ.

Serum ceruloplasmin. We urge the use of the ceruloplasmin test in all cases of suspected acute liver disease in pediatric patients greater than 5 years of age and especially when a known exposure is lacking in the history. In the absence of a low serum protein level, a low ceruloplasmin level is strongly suggestive of Wilson's disease. Al-

though rare, Wilson's disease can be present despite a normal serum ceruloplasmin value, in which case urine and hepatic copper studies may be indicated (see Chapter 24).

Antinuclear antibodies (ANA). A positive result from this test usually signifies severe or chronic liver disease, but it is also warranted when the acute disease deviates from the expected normal course (p. 596). A positive ANA factor in the serum is suggestive that the underlying liver disease may be rapidly evolving into the chronic aggressive form of hepatitis. This pathologic lesion is characterized by an inflammatory response rich in plasma cells and lymphocytes believed to be responsible for the immunologic reactions. Of patients with chronic active hepatitis, more than 25% will have positive ANA or other immunochemical markers present in their serum at some time during their disease.

Lactic dehydrogenases (LDH). LDH determination is useful only if the respective LDH isoenzymes are also reported. An elevation in the hepatic isoenzyme fraction provides confirmatory rather than any specific diagnostic information in the face of known liver injury.

Serum electrolytes, pH, and blood gases. These tests are occasionally indicated, especially if vomiting and anorexia are dominant features of the prodrome. The values are usually normal, but the presence of a respiratory alkalosis should make one suspicious of severe liver injury or chronic disease (cirrhosis).

Blood glucose. Pronounced hypoglycemia is seen in severe hepatic necrosis, whereas normal to slightly diminished values are found in typical viral hepatitis measured when the patient is fasting. Impairment of glycogen synthesis and faulty gluconeogenesis provide the most likely explanation for these observations in acute viral hepatitis.

Thymol turbidity. A disturbance in the stability of serum proteins is reflected in the turbidity or flocculation tests. They have generally fallen into disfavor, primarily because of their poor reproducibility and their inability to provide additional helpful information. In the studies reported from the Willowbrook State Institution, a rise in the thymol turbidity was consistent with short-incubation hepatitis A virus disease (MS-1, infectious), whereas in patients with long-incubation hepatitis B virus disease (MS-2) the thymol turbidity did not rise.

Pathologic lesion

There are indications for performing a liver biopsy in acute hepatitis, but they are not numerous. Because the clinical and laboratory features of acute hepatitis are sufficiently distinct to make a correct diagnosis, a tissue diagnosis is seldom needed. However, patients who follow an atypical course or in whom diagnosis is uncertain deserve a tissue diagnosis (Fig. 21-3).

In the typical histologic lesion consistent with acute viral hepatitis, single-cell or focal, spotty necrosis of liver cells can be found scattered throughout the lobules in a random manner. A mild, predominantly mononuclear inflammatory reaction is seen around these areas of focal necrosis in the hepatic lobules. Lesser numbers of polymorphonuclear cells and eosinophils are also present. A central vein phlebitis is a useful diagnostic finding when present. The portal areas are widened by inflammatory response of variable degree. Mild ductular proliferation can also be seen, whereas fibrosis is lacking. The limiting plate of the lobule remains intact, and the overall hepatic architecture is preserved. Other typical findings in acute viral hepatitis include balloon cells, acidophilic bodies (Councilman bodies), multinucleated hepatocytes, and increased numbers of mitoses within liver cells. Kupffer cells are usually prominent, being distended with cellular debris and at times viruslike particles. Kupffer cells may in fact seem to occlude the sinusoids in extreme cases. A ground-glass appearance of the hepatocyte cytoplasm suggests hepatitis B virus disease. Cytoplasmic HBsAg material will stain positively with orcein or aldehyde fuchsin. Variable degrees of bile stasis are always present either in the liver cells or in bile canaliculi.

In contrast to the immense contribution of immune electron microscopy in localizing particles of hepatitis virus B within serum and hepatocytes of infected individuals, routine electron microscopy of liver tissue has not been as helpful as anticipated in clarifying structural-clinical relationships of hepatitis. The changes seen by light microscopy are perhaps more impressive. Ultrastructural abnormalities include dilatation of the profiles of the rough endoplasmic reticulum, depletion of glycogen bodies, decreased hepatocyte sinusoid microvilli, collagen fibrils in the space of Disse, and abnormal basement membrane formation. Nuclei, lysosomes, and mitochondria show fewer constant abnormalities. One cannot differentiate hepatitis A virus disease from hepatitis B virus disease on the basis of the ultrastructural changes within the hepatocyte found during the acute disease. It would appear that more subtle functional abnormalities of the surviving hepatocytes better explain the degree of clinical abnormalities seen in acute hepatitis.

In more severe forms of viral hepatitis, the histologic lesion usually parallels the clinical course of the patient. Fulminant hepatic necrosis with collapse is easily recognized when one notes the abnormal proximity of either portal zones or central veins to each other. In these severe examples recognizable liver cells are few and scattered and often orient themselves into a pseudoacinar or pseudoductular arrangement. The mononuclear inflammatory reaction is usually scattered through the area of necrosis (Fig. 21-4). A severely affected lobule may border on a lobule that reveals a few areas of focal necrosis. Another variation seen in the severe form of acute viral hepatitis is the histologic lesion characterized by bands of necrosis that bridge portal zones or connect portal zones to central veins. This intralobular and interlobular bridging represents a severe form of the disease and has been called subacute hepatic necrosis, or bridging necrosis (Fig. 21-5). Similar lesions may be found in less severe cases of acute viral hepatitis and in fulminating hepatitis as well. This pathologic finding carries a worse prognosis both for initial mortality and later morbidity (cirrhosis). Massive hepatic necrosis as seen in fulminating hepatitis is discussed in Chapter 23.

The histologic lesion of chronic aggressive hepatitis may be found early (3 to 4 weeks) in a clinical syndrome believed to be caused by acute viral hepatitis. Disruption of the limiting plate and the presence of piecemeal necrosis immediately separate this lesion from those found in acute benign hepatitis or even chronic persistent hepatitis. Details of the distinguishing features of chronic aggressive hepatitis are discussed in Chapter 24. In fortunate individuals serial biopsies have been consistent with good outcome upon resolution to the normal histologic appearance. For others, this lesion may evolve to that noted observed in patients with chronic active hepatitis.

Pathologic lesions have also been found in organs other than the liver, a fact suggesting that both hepatitis A and B (and perhaps other agents) produce a generalized systemic disease. Mild but definite abnormalities have been reported in the

Text continued on p. 596.

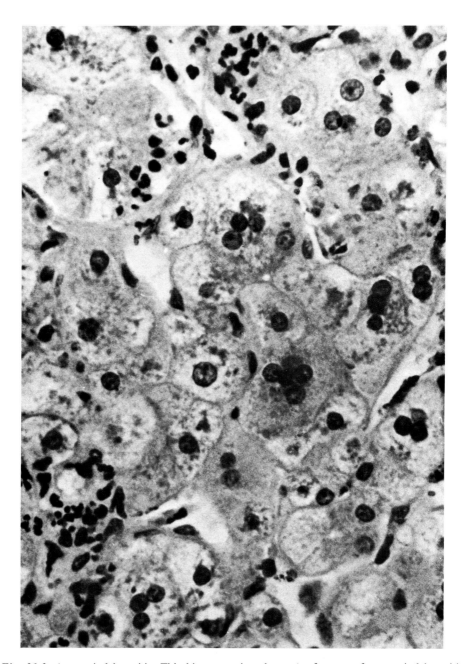

Fig. 21-3. Acute viral hepatitis. This biopsy section shows the features of acute viral hepatitis characterized by multinucleated giant cells, bile stasis, and the acute inflammatory reaction that can be seen within the hepatic lobule. This 5-year-old child suddenly developed anorexia and low-grade fever and was noted to be jaundiced. Physical examination revealed an enlarged, tender liver and moderate icterus. Biochemical abnormalities included a serum bilirubin of 8.9 mg/dl and SGOT of 1500 IU with a normal prothrombin time and serum protein electrophoresis. Percutaneous liver biopsy was done after 4 weeks of illness. Gradual resolution followed over the next several weeks.

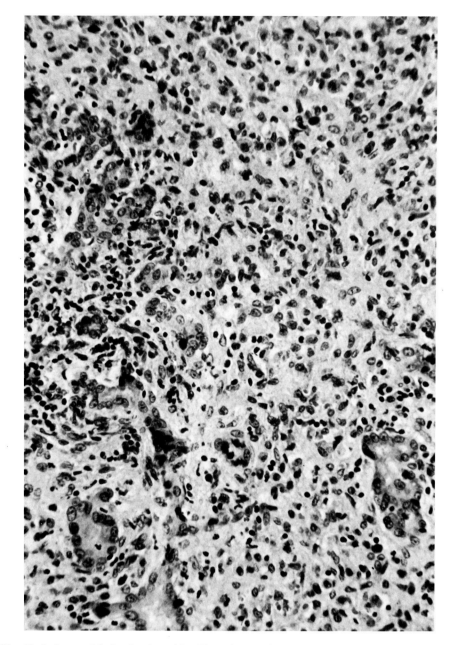

Fig. 21-4. Severe fulminating hepatitis. The microscopic appearance of the liver demonstrates severe hepatocellular disarray, balloon hepatocytes, and necrosis with acute inflammatory reaction. This 11-month-old infant was well until 7 days before admission, when he became anorexic and vomited on several occasions. The following day the child was noted to be distinctly icteric; in addition, an enlarged liver was palpable at the time of examination. The child was subsequently hospitalized and over the next 6 days became progressively more jaundiced, lethargic, and semicomatose. Death occurred within 2 weeks of disease onset.

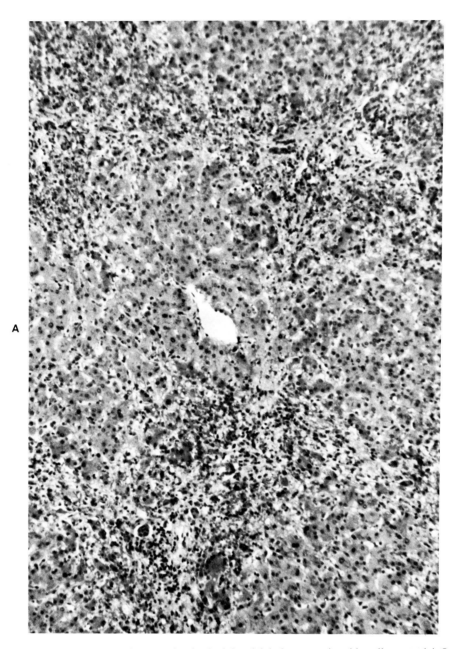

Fig. 21-5. Subacute hepatic necrosis. **A,** Peripheral lobular necrosis with collapse and inflammation is seen producting the lesion of portoportal "bridging." An 8-year-old girl was admitted with what was believed to be viral hepatitis. A severe bleeding disorder unresponsive to medical management occurred, and the child died.

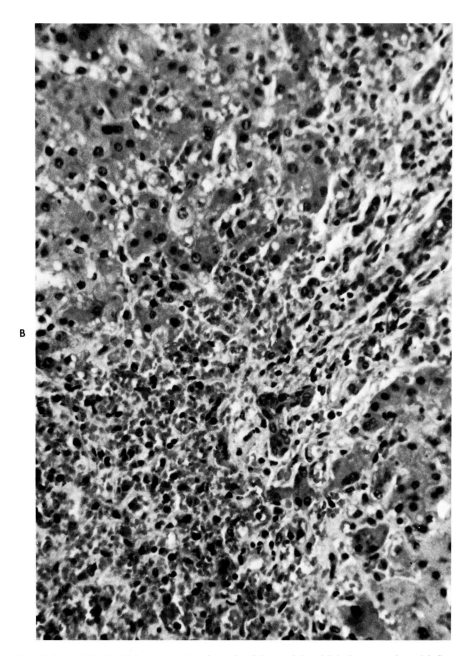

Fig. 21-5, cont'd. B, High-power view from **A** of the peripheral lobular necrosis and inflammatory process.

kidney (tubules and glomeruli), gastrointestinal tract (blunting of villi, increased numbers of goblet cells), and bone marrow (delayed maturation of red blood cell precursors).

Management

Rest. There is no solid evidence that demonstrates conclusively that bed rest, absolute or partial, influences the rate of recovery or the final outcome of acute viral hepatitis. Indeed, data obtained from two similar groups with acute hepatitis showed no difference in duration of the disease when one group was subjected to strenuous activity and the other to light activity. It makes more sense to allow the child or teen-ager an option regarding bed rest. The sick child who feels ill will usually go to bed voluntarily, and the older teen-ager may quickly yield to the suggestion. Once clinical improvement appears, it may be difficult to keep the patient at bed rest if he chooses to be up. Gradual ambulation and graded increments of activity seem a reasonable approach to regaining physical strength and stamina, but again this approach has little bearing on the rate of healing of the liver disease.

Diet. As with bed rest, compulsive, if not ritualistic, dietary programs have evolved over the years, again without solid data to prove that adherence to one diet or the other influences the severity, clinical course, or final outcome of acute viral hepatitis. The traditional low-fat, high-carbohydrate diet has been most popular, simply because it is palatable rather than for any special intrinsic value. Because anorexia and nausea are such striking features of early hepatitis, patients given foods high in fat content usually have intensification of these symptoms because of gastric retention rather than worsening of liver disease. Once the patient's anorexia vanishes, he may select and tolerate eggs, buttered toast, and meats without difficulty. Patients who receive and can tolerate a higher fat diet actually seem to improve more quickly than a control group given the restricted fat diet. Here again, the data would dictate that the patient be permitted to choose his own diet within reasonable limits, so as to provide adequate daily carbohydrate (4 gm/kg) and protein (1 gm/kg).

Other than for vitamin K, there is little evidence to suggest that vitamin supplementation truly offers much to the patient with acute hepatitis. If the disease occurs in previously malnourished patients or in some teen-agers with poor dietary habits, vitamin supplementation with a water-soluble product (Poly-Vi-Sol) is advisable.

Drugs. The patient with acute viral hepatitis occasionally requires an antiemetic drug when vomiting is severe. Intravenous fluids usually suffice, but at times antihistamines such as diphenhydramine (Benadryl) may be helpful. There is no indication for use of corticosteroids early in the disease, and indeed a number of studies have shown that this drug does not favorably influence the course of acute viral hepatitis. Increased hepatocellular necrosis with increased morbidity and mortality accompanies the enhanced viral replication in liver and lymphoid tissues in corticosteroid-treated mice. Impairment of reticuloendothelial function and inhibition of interferon production are other known effects of cortisone. There is concern that treatment with corticosteroids may also favor persistence of HBV in the host. Furthermore, corticosteroids have been shown to be potentially detrimental in acute liver injury by their inhibitory effect on lysosomal release of hydrolytic enzymes whose function is to prevent the deposition of collagen. In the event that the clinical disease is prolonged (over 4 weeks) or laboratory tests suggest chronic active hepatitis not caused by HBV, the use of steroids may then be indicated.

Gamma globulin. Administration of conventional or hyperimmune hepatitis B virus gamma globulin to the ill patient, even in large doses, has no apparent influence on the course of the disease, whether because of hepatitis virus A or B. However, all close contacts are at risk and should receive intramuscular gamma globulin as soon as possible. (See the discussion of prevention on p. 598.)

Follow-up study

Biochemical and clinical assessment must be part of the follow-up study of patients recovering from acute viral hepatitis and is outlined in Fig. 21-6. One cannot rely solely on the patient's history or the physical examination. Biochemical proof of healing of the liver injury demands transaminase and bilirubin determinations every other week until normal results are obtained. Persistent elevations of transaminase or bilirubin for greater than 2 months must be viewed suspiciously and additional studies obtained, even when clinical symptoms are not remarkable. At this time one should also obtain a serum protein electrophoresis and an

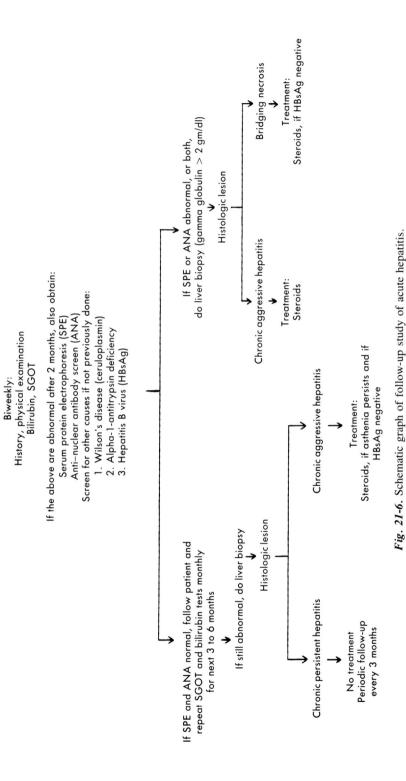

Fig. 21-6. Schematic graph of follow-up study of acute hepatitis.

antinuclear antibody test. If other possible causes for acute hepatitis have not previously been considered in the laboratory evaluation, then a serum ceruloplasmin, alpha-1-antitrypsin determination, and HBsAg screen are indicated. A liver biopsy should be performed at this time if the gamma globulin fraction is found elevated to greater than 2.0 gm/dl or the antinuclear antibody test (ANA) is positive. The histologic lesion of chronic aggressive hepatitis in such a setting requires commencement of specific therapy (see Chapter 24). A normal gamma globulin value and a negative ANA, in the face of persistent abnormalities of the transaminase and bilirubin, are usually found commensurate with a histologic lesion similar to that of acute viral hepatitis, and has been called "chronic persistent hepatitis" (Fig. 24-1). This clinicopathologic entity may take 6 to 12 months to resolve and occasionally even longer. Between the 3- and 6-month follow-up period we recommend monthly biochemical evaluation of the patient. At the end of 6 months (after the acute stage of the disease) prognostic and therapeutic decisions can best be made after examination of liver tissue, and a biopsy is therefore recommended. The disease, consistent with the histologic diagnosis of chronic persistent hepatitis, requires no specific treatment and only clinical and biochemical follow-up study perhaps every third month. Lesions showing features of chronic aggressive hepatitis again demand repeat of the serum protein electrophoresis and ANA. Once again, if either of these studies is abnormal, steroid therapy is indicated. What to do when the combination of biochemical and immunologic markers of chronic-active liver disease is negative but the hepatic lesion is consistent with this diagnosis, remains controversial. A trial of steroids is probably justified in non-HBsAg cases especially if the patient reports persistent asthenia.

Complications

As previously described, departure from the clinical course so characteristic of benign viral hepatitis suggests an impending complication of this disease. The complications may be separated into two major groupings. In one group the disease runs a long course, in which prolongation of the clinical symptoms and laboratory abnormalities do eventually subside in a benign manner. In the other group the disease leads quickly to death or is severe and prolonged, with recovery most often attended by cirrhosis.

Those patients with prolonged disease, as evidenced by biochemical and pathologic criteria, is discussed in the section on chronic hepatitis (Chapter 24); those with fulminant hepatic necrosis leading to hepatic coma and death are discussed in the section of fulminating hepatitis (Chapter 23).

The incidence of complications arising from hepatitis A virus disease is only about 0.1% to 0.2% of cases. Persistent hepatitis as a complication of hepatitis B virus disease has been reported to occur in a frequency of 0% to 50%, with 5% to 10% being most common. Mild hepatitis running a chronic persistent course and chronic aggressive hepatitis with and without cirrhosis have now been documented as consequences of persistent antigenemia. Rarely, chronic glomerulonephritis, either membranoproliferative or of the membranous type, evolves and is associated with the deposition of immune complexes or may be a consequence of chronic antigenemia. The development of polyarteritis nodosa as a consequence to chronic HBsAg carriage is fortunately extremely rare in childhood. Survivors of fulminant hepatic necrosis may go on to postnecrotic cirrhosis, an unfortunate complication of hepatitis discussed at length in Chapter 24.

A rare but often fatal complication of acute viral hepatitis is the development of aplastic anemia. Males are more likely to be affected than females (9 to 1), and most are young children. Pancytopenia can follow the hepatitis by 1 to several weeks even when there is clinical improvement. The mechanism is unknown, but an autoimmune response by the host to the initial viral injury has been proposed. Death in most cases is from massive hemorrhage. At present, bone marrow transplantation offers the best chance for long-term survival.

Prevention

With the identification of hepatitis B virus as the agent responsible for "serum" hepatitis, prevention of this form of liver disease has been bolstered immeasurably. Its immediate application has been in blood banking, whereby all donor blood is screened for HBsAg. This applies to the whole blood and blood products (plasma, fibrinogen, albumin), since the latter have long been implicated as agents capable of causing hepatitis. Since hepatitis B virus disease can be transmitted by the oral route as well as parenterally, individuals employed in occupations in which the potential for mass contamination exists are usually screened for this antigen. This might include, for example, food handlers, dentists, surgeons, and medical staff working in dialysis and oncology units.

Meanwhile, strict attention to likely sources of contamination will prevent most new cases of hepatitis. Careful attention to personal hygiene with thorough hand washing, especially when one is around known cases of hepatitis, will reduce the fecal-oral route of transmission substantially. Hospitalized patients are best isolated, and personnel administering to the patient's needs should wear gowns. Linens, dishes, silverware, and bedpans should be handled with care, cleansed in detergent soaps, and autoclaved when possible. Again, hand washing is critical. Disposable needles and syringes should be used once and discarded. Preferably, disposable eating utensils and bedpans should be employed. A reduction in water-borne and food-borne outbreaks depends on strong community and public health department measures in each locale. The rising number of cases of hepatitis in drug addicts and male homosexuals is cause for great concern, and continued education as to the dangers of hepatitis seems to be another way to constructively reach this group.

Passive immunity to hepatitis A virus disease is quite effective; conventional immunoglobulin is given in a dose of 0.02 to 0.06 ml/kg for close exposure contacts, or 0.01 to 0.02 ml/kg for casual contacts. The disease may be prevented or modified significantly in about 80% to 90% of cases when the immune serum globulin (ISG) is given soon after the exposure.

Even when both the clinical and the biochemical expression of hepatitis is significantly attenuated by the use of immune serum globulin, an IgG-specific antibody often develops and serves to be protective against subsequent exposures (passive-active immunity). At present, immune serum globulin is not recommended for casual school contacts (other pupils or teachers) or an occasional household visitor, unless historical facts implicate a specific exposure event that might result in infection. Immune serum globulin may be administered to those exposed in common-source

outbreaks such as food and water but has not been recommended to subjects exposed in food-borne outbreaks from restaurants after the index case has been identified. Likewise, it can be recommended for those exposed in closed institutional settings, but not for hospital personnel caring for hepatitis A patients. Rather attention to sound hygienic practices is usually sufficient to protect one against acquiring hepatitis A disease. Gamma globulin given before exposure to hepatitis A virus is probably protective for a long as 6 months.

Passive immunity to HBV can be achieved when HBV hyperimmune gamma globulin (hepatitis B immune serum globulin, HBIG) is used in special settings. Hyperimmune gamma globulin, 0.5 ml, should be given intramuscularly within 48 hours to neonates born of mothers with acute HBV disease during the last trimester of pregnancy through the time of delivery. It should also be given to neonates born of mothers who are chronic carriers of HBsAg with markers of infectivity (HBsAg positive, anti-HBc positive, DNA polymerase activity, anti-HBe negative). Repeat doses should be planned for these infants at 1 month and perhaps again at 3 and 6 months of age unless the infant can be given the new hepatitis B vaccine (Heptavax·B). HBIG in a dose of 0.5 ml/kg should be given to individuals who received "low-dose" exposure by needle stick inoculation or through an open wound. A second dose is then given 30 days later and is usually preventive in such cases. A similar dose of hepatitis B immune globulin can be given to sexual contacts when one partner is HBsAg positive and the other has neither detectable surface antigen nor anti-HBs. Preexposure prophylaxis against hepatitis B with HBIG is not recommended at present. Repeated failure of this product to provide passive-active immunization militates against long-term usefulness for those individuals at increased risk for acquisition of the virus. Although HBIG has been given to patients and staff of renal dialysis units and to blood-bank personnel, and indeed does reduce the incidence of acquired HBV infection, its chronic and repeated use is not without danger of host sensitization to foreign proteins.

Active immunization against HBV

A recently completed double-blinded hepatitis B vaccine efficacy trial in homosexual males has yielded extremely successful results. The vaccine

Table 21-4. Transmission of HBV from HBsAg carrier to newborn

Country of study*	Number	Positive infants	Vertical transmission (%)
Stevens (Taiwan)†	158	63	40
Okada (Japan)†	11	8	73
Kohler (U.S.A.)	7	6	86
Schweitzer (U.S.A.)	21	1	5
Skinhøj (Denmark)	52	0	0
Gerety (U.S.A.)	36	3	8
Dupuy (France)‡	17	8	67

*Stevens, C., et al.: N. Engl. J. Med. **252:**771, 1975; Okada, K., et al.: N. Engl. J. Med. **294:**746, 1976; Kohler, P.F., et al.: N. Engl. J. Med. **291:**1378, 1974; Schweitzer, I.L., et al.: Gastroenterology **65:**277, 1973; Dupuy, J.M., et al.: J. Pediatr. **92:**200, 1978; Gerety, R.S., et al.: J. Pediatr. **90:**368, 1977.
†Higher transmission rates in endemic areas.
‡Only 1 in 8, or 16%, became persistent carrier.

currently employed was derived from formalin-inactivated, highly purified HBsAg particles obtained from serum of asymptomatic chronic carriers and after pilot testing was completed in chimpanzees and human volunteers. In the field trial, vaccine was administered initially, with booster dose given at 1 month and again at 6 months. The antibody response (anti-HBs) was of high titer in 96% of the recipients, declining somewhat over the next several months, but levels remained protective for up to 18 months. The vaccine (Heptavax·B) has proved to be extremely safe, with complaints about soreness at the injection site being the major side effect. It is now available and has a tremendous potential in prophylaxis of individuals in high-risk occupations and those who reside in geographic locations around the world where the virus is so prevalent. The immunization schedule consists of three doses of vaccine given intramuscularly: the first when elected, the second 1 month later, and the third 6 months after the first dose. The neonate and children less than 10 years of age receive 0.5 ml each time and older children and adults 1 ml per dose. The role of the vaccine in post-exposure prophylaxis needs additional study. The potential benefits to accrue from this obviously include a substantial reduction in the pool of HBsAg carriers, lessening the numbers of cases of chronic liver disease and, we hope, thereby reducing as well the subsequent high incidence of carcinoma of the liver in such patients.

Neonatal HBV disease

In the United States, where the carrier rate of HBsAg is less than 1%, neonatal acquisition of HBV disease from carrier mothers is said to be as low as 5% to 10%. This is in contrast to the islands of the South Pacific where 40% to 50% of mothers are carriers and neonatal acquisition is closer to 95% (Table 21-4). A variety of factors (racial origin, geographic location, and environmental factors), acting in poorly understood ways, are involved in producing incidence figures of this magnitude for both carriage and acquisition of HBsAg. Since the neonate tolerates HBV infection quite well (exceptions are recognized), the major concern for the acquisition of HBV disease is an epidemiologic one, since a high percentage of these infants become chronic carriers of HBsAg. This phenomenon is presumably a result of their ineffective immune response to clear the virus and the subsequent development of tolerance. Recent data from Japan indicates that clearing of the HBsAg acquired during the neonatal period may eventually occur between 5 and 8 years of age when the appearance of anti-HBs can finally be demonstrated.

It is generally agreed upon that most cases of neonatally acquired HBV disease result from the ingestion of contaminated amniotic fluid, vaginal secretions, or placental and uterine maternal blood during the time of delivery rather than by transplacental spread. It is interesting that babies delivered by cesarean section from carrier mothers have the same acquisition rate of HBsAg as those born vaginally. Postnatal acquisition is most likely from routine maternal-child rearing practices. Breast feeding is also a potential mode of transmission of the virus, though breast milk collected in the absence of a nipple tear is an unlikely source of the virus. It is surprising that the vertical transmission rate from mother to child is not higher than what has been observed.

HBsAg is seldom found in cord blood, or in the serum of the neonate born of chronic-carrier mothers. When transplacental spread does occur, it is associated with acute maternal infection during the third trimester or at the time of delivery. Furthermore, the incidence of transplacental spread is greater when the mother, in addition to being a carrier of HBsAg, also has markers of infectivity such as HBeAg and anti-HBc. The presence of anti-HBe does not necessarily militate against neonatal acquisition of the carrier state. In less-developed countries the fetus is also at particular risk to acquire transplacental HBsAg after in utero transfusion or transfusions for severe hemolytic disease. It would appear that most neonatal cases of HBV disease leading to fulminant disease have occurred in these settings.

It is reported that infants born of HBsAg-carrier mothers have no increased risk to teratogenicity because of maternal infection, though there is an increased risk for premature delivery, especially if acute maternal hepatitis occurs during the last trimester. Not infrequently, premature labor and delivery occurs at the height of the illness when maternal levels of HBsAg are noted to be extremely high.

As previously mentioned, HBsAg acquisition by the neonate is seldom associated with serious consequences. Antigenemia usually appears after 6 to 8 weeks of postnatal life when biochemical evidence of hepatitis can be documented. Clinical symptoms of hepatitis are seldom reported. However, liver injury can be seen in some biopsy material, characterized by minimal focal necrosis with a mild portal inflammatory response of mononuclear cells. Only on rare occasions has neonatal infection resulted in fulminant hepatic necrosis or been responsible for chronic ongoing liver disease (chronic active hepatitis, chronic persistent hepatitis) or cirrhosis.

Public health and preventive measures

At present the American Academy of Pediatrics recommends that carrier mothers should not breast feed their neonates if other acceptable milk substitutes are available. Although the milk itself may contain HBsAg, it is of low titer, and greater virus acquisition during breast feeding may actually come from serum or blood released from cracks in the areolar tissue. Whenever possible, the neonate should receive intramuscular HBIG, 0.5 ml, immediately after delivery, and certainly within the first 48 hours post partum. This may be repeated at 1, 3, and perhaps again at 6 months of age unless the infant can be given the newly developed hepatitis B vaccine. The first dose of this product (0.5 ml intramuscularly) is recommended at 3 months of age.

It is also recommended that newborn units develop a written policy for handling potentially infective neonates. The following are suggested items to be addressed:

1. One should wear gloves at all times when handling the infant.
2. One should thoroughly cleanse the skin, especially before any inoculations, such as vitamin K, are given to the infant.
3. Needle and blood precautions should be undertaken.
4. Laboratory workers should be alerted to the possible infectiousness of specimens from such an infant by specially labeling tubes containing the infant's blood or body fluids.
5. Mandatory use of gloves and gowns and diligent attention to hygienic measures by nonnursery personnel need to be enforced.

Other virus-producing hepatitis-like illnesses

Generally these following viral agents produce a predominantly systemic illness with multiorgan involvement. When the liver is involved in the systemic process, the injury tends to be focal rather than diffuse, and laboratory abnormalities usually reveal minimally elevated bilirubin, consistent with seldom-observed clinical jaundice. Transaminase activity, however, tends to be increased 2 to 3 times above normal. Agents capable of producing a hepatitis-like illness are numerous and include infectious mononucleosis virus, cytomegalovirus, herpesvirus, adenovirus, coxsackieviruses, rheovirus, certain echoviruses, and the rubella virus. Arbovirus infection (yellow fever) produces an important hepatitis illness in certain endemic portions of the world. Unusual agents that may also produce a viral hepatitis–like illness include protozoa, toxoplasmosis, and *Rickettsia psittaci*.

Infectious mononucleosis. This illness is caused by a human herpesvirus IV, also called the "Epstein-Barr virus." Acquisition is usually by person-to-person spread via contaminated respiratory secretions, and after a relatively long incubation period of 30 to 40 days, clinical illness begins and usually includes moderately high fever, sore throat, significant symmetric adenopathy, and malaise. Splenomegaly is found in over 25% of the patients, and the liver is slightly enlarged but seldom tender. Manifestations of other organ-system involvement are frequent and appear in the bone marrow, central nervous system, lungs, and skin. On rare occasion this illness may produce a clinical spectrum suggesting Reye's syndrome.

Although jaundice is most uncommon, biochemical abnormalities of hepatic involvement can be demonstrated in 25% to 50% of patients. The serum transaminase activity tends to be elevated out of proportion to the marginal alteration in serum bilirubin levels. In addition, the serum alkaline phosphatase may be substantially increased. On liver biopsy, as many as 80% to 90% of the patients are said to show histologic abnormalities. The pathologic lesion usually includes a mononuclear cell inflammatory response around the portal tracts, rare intralobular cytolysis, and Kupffer cell hyperplasia. Cholestasis is rare, and if the biopsy is taken during the recovery stage, an increase in mitotic activity is typically present. Except in very rare cases of massive hepatic necrosis associated with the infectious mononucleosis virus, the liver damage heals without residual effects, but this may take from 3 to 8 months.

The diagnosis can be suspected in the teen-ager and young adult from clinical and physical findings. It is confirmed by examination of the peripheral blood, coupled with a demonstration of a positive-heterophil antibody test (MonoSpot test). The peripheral smear shows the presence of many atypical lymphocytes (Downey cells) in the face of a pronounced leukocytosis. In addition, a specific antibody for the Epstein-Barr virus can be demonstrated by complement fixation test (CF). The rise in CF titer in paired serums can be considered as confirmatory evidence for the disease.

Differential diagnosis may at times include cytomegalovirus disease or hepatitis A or B virus disease.

There is no specific treatment for infectious mononucleosis infections. Antibiotic treatment is warranted when group A hemolytic streptococcal pharyngitis is found complicating the underlying disease. The use of steroids in the adolescent and young adult who manifest persistent lassitude and malaise remains controversial.

Cytomegalovirus. Human cytomegalovirus has worldwide distribution, and inapparent exposure to this agent occurs with increasing frequency paralleling one's age. From 1% to 2% of neonates are infected presumably by contamination from maternal sources. By 2 years of age 5% to 10% of children in urban settings have antibodies, 20% by 15 years of age, and 50% to 60% of adults likewise show serologic evidence of previous exposure to cytomegalovirus infection.

Gestationally acquired cytomegalovirus disease is usually in the disseminated form, with effects obvious in the skin, central nervous system, lymphoid tissue, and liver. Isolated examples of subclinical hepatic disease probably occur as well, though it is more frequent in postnatally acquired infection. Moderately severe and symptomatic cytomegalovirus infection in postnatal life and later childhood includes a febrile illness with a rubella-like rash, adenopathy, and hepatosplenomegaly as typical accompanying features. Laboratory studies are most likely to show a lymphocytosis and thrombocytopenia, which may suggest childhood leukemia, lymphohistiocytosis, or infectious mononucleosis. However, the heterophil (MonoSpot) is normal and the bone marrow is nondiagnostic. Liver-function tests tend to be mildly disturbed, especially the transaminases, with less effect seen in serum bilirubin values. Diagnosis may be made on liver biopsy when cytomegalovirus inclusions are found in hepatocytes or more commonly in bile ductular epithelial cells (Fig. 19-4). The hepatic pathologic condition is variable with minimal focal necrosis, intrahepatocyte cholestasis, and occasional giant-cell transformation being shown. The portal infiltrate is usually mononuclear in nature. A neoductular proliferative response with or without accompanying portal and perilobular fibrosis are seen at other times. A less severe form of cytomegalovirus infection manifesting as an acute febrile illness without rash has also been reported.

The most dramatic expression of this disease is usually seen in the immune-compromised host including transplant patients or in cancer patients on chemotherapy. In these individuals, the virus may remain dormant and periodically produce symptomatic disease.

Whenever possible, proof of infection should include isolation of the virus from freshly obtained secretions (urine, throat, gastric) and serologic testing for IgG-EA (early antigen), which is considered a marker for active cytomegalovirus replication. Another early marker of infection that may likewise be sought by serologic testing is IgM-MA (membrane antibody). The likelihood of recovering cytomegalovirus from culture techniques and demonstrating the presence of antibodies seems to be higher when the infected infant has a hepatitis-like clinical illness or when hepatosplenomegaly is found. However, the relationship between liver disease, the recovery of the virus, and the presence of antibody did not apply to neonates who had biliary atresia. It is surprising that the histologic lesion in some infants may be unremarkable and often without demonstrable viral inclusions, despite other clinical evidence for active cytomegalovirus infection. Generally speaking, a greater degree of liver involvement tends to follow acquired postnatal infection.

Treatment is symptomatic because antiviral agents have not proved efficacious in eradicating this particular agent.

Yellow Fever. This illness is caused by an arbovirus *(Flavivirus),* group IV disease, and occurs in endemic outbreaks in enzootic areas in South America and Africa. The mosquito is the vector for this virus and the incubation period is usually 4 to 6 days. The clinical illness begins with a febrile course, headache, myalgia, and lethargy. In more severe cases, where the mortality may be 5% to 10%, injury to the myocardium and complications of renal failure are at fault. In these patients hepatic involvement is revealed by the presence of jaundice and tender hepatomegaly. The liver histopathologic condition in the severe form usually includes a midzonal lobular necrosis, minimal inflammatory response, and variable steatosis. Upon recovery, the liver injury tends to heal without scarring.

The diagnosis can be confirmed by a specific complement fixation and hemagglutination antibody test. There is no specific treatment for this disease, but prevention can be achieved by vaccination. The major differential diagnosis to be considered when hepatic and renal involvement are dominant is leptospirosis.

REFERENCES

Andiman, W.A.: The Epstein-Barr virus and EB virus infection in childhood, J. Pediatr. **95:**171-182, 1979.

Beasley, R.P., Stevens, C.E., Shiao, I.S., and Meng, H.C.: Evidence against breast-feeding as a mechanism for vertical transmission of hepatitis B, Lancet **2:**740-741, 1975.

Bianchi, L., and Gudat, F.: Immunopathology of hepatitis B. In Popper, H., and Schaffner, F., editors: Progress in liver diseases, vol. 6, New York, 1979, Grune & Stratton, Inc.

Blumberg, B.S., and London, W.T.: Hepatitis B virus and the prevention of primary hepatocellular carcinoma, N. Engl. J. Med. **304:**782-784, 1981.

Bodenbender, R.H.: Hepatitis and aplastic anemia, Am. J. Dis. Child. **122:**440-441, 1971.

Boyer, J.L., and Klatskin, G.: Pattern of necrosis in acute viral hepatitis: prognostic value of bridging (subacute hepatic necrosis), N. Engl. J. Med. **283:**1063-1071, 1970.

Carter, A.R.: Cytomegalovirus disease presenting as hepatitis, Br. Med. J. **3:**786, 1968.

Conrad, M.E., Schwartz, F.D., and Young, A.A.: Infectious hepatitis—a generalized disease: a study of renal, gastrointestinal and hematologic abnormalities, Am. J. Med. **37:**789-801, 1964.

Corey, L., and Holmes, K.K.: Sexual transmission of hepatitis A in homosexual man, N. Engl. J. Med. **302:**435-438, 1980.

Derso, A., Boxall, E.H., Tarlow, M.J., and Flewett, T.H.: Transmission of HBsAg from mother to infant in four ethnic groups, Br. Med. J. **1:**949-952, 1978.

Dienstag, J.L.: Hepatitis B virus infection: more than meets the eye, Gastroenterology **75:**1172-1174, 1978.

Dienstag, J.L.: Hepatitis A virus: identification, characterization and epidemiologic investigations. In Popper, H., and Schaffner, F., editors: Progress in liver disease, vol. 6, New York, 1979, Grune & Stratton, Inc.

Dienstag, J.L.: Toward the control of hepatitis B, N. Engl. J. Med. **303:**874-876, 1980.

Dupuy, J.M., Giraud, P., Dupuy, C., and others: Hepatitis B in children. II. Study of children born to chronic HBsAg carrier mothers, J. Pediatr. **92:**200-204, 1978.

Edgington, T.S., and Chisari, F.V.: Immunologic aspects of hepatitis B virus infection, Am. J. Med. Sci. **270:**213-227, 1975.

Fauerholdt, L., Asnaes, S., Ranek, L., and others: Significance of suspected ''chronic aggressive hepatitis'' in acute hepatitis, Gastroenterology **73:**543-548, 1977.

Feinstone, S.M., and Purcell, R.H.: New methods for the serodiagnosis of hepatitis A, Gastroenterology **78:**1092-1094, 1980.

Fennell, R.S., III, Andres, J.M., Pfaff, W.W., and Richard, G.A.: Liver dysfunction in children and adolescents during hemodialysis and after renal transplantation, Pediatrics **67:**855-861, 1981.

Francis, T.I., Moore, E.L., Eddington, G.M., and Smith, J.A.: Clinicopathologic study of human yellow fever, Bull. W. H.O. **46:**659-667, 1972.

Gerety, R.J., and Schweitzer, I.L.: Viral hepatitis type B during pregnancy, the neonatal period, and infancy, J. Pediatr. **90:**368-374, 1977.

Gocke, D.J.: Extrahepatic manifestations of viral hepatitis, Am. J. Med. Sci. **270:**49-52, 1975.

Jhaveri, R., Rosenfeld, W., Salazar, J.D., and others: High titer multiple dose therapy with HBIG in newborn infants of HBsAg positive mothers, J. Pediatr. **97:**305-308, 1980.

Kleinknecht, C., Levy, M., Peix, A., and others: Membranous glomerulonephritis and hepatitis B surface antigen in children, J. Pediatr. **95:**946-952, 1979.

Kilpatrick, Z.M.: Structural and functional abnormalities of the liver in infectious mononucleosis, Arch. Intern. Med. **117:**47-53, 1966.

Krugman, S., Overby, L.R., Mushahwar, I.K.: Viral hepatitis, type B: studies on natural history and prevention reexamined, N. Engl. J. Med. **300**:101-106, 1979.

Krugman, S., Hollinger, F.B., Mosley, J.W., and Maynard, J.E.: Immunoprophylaxis for viral hepatitis: other views, Gastroenterology **77**:186-191, 1979.

Krugman, S.: The newly licensed hepatitis B vaccine, J.A.M.A. **247**:2012-2015, 1982.

Levy, R.N., Sawitsky, A., Florman, A.L., and Rubin, E.: Fatal aplastic anemia after hepatitis: report of five cases, N. Engl. J. Med. **273**:1118-1123, 1965.

Litt, I.F., Cohen, M.I., Schonberg, S.D., and Spigland, I.: Liver disease in the drug-using adolescent, J. Pediatr. **81**:238-242, 1972.

Madigan, N.P., Newcomer, A.D., Campbell, D.C., and Taswell, H.F.: Intense jaundice in infectious mononucleosis, Mayo Clin. Proc. **48**:857-862, 1973.

Numazaki, Y., Oshima, T., Tanaka, A., and others: Demonstration of IgG EA (early antigen) and IgM MA (membrane antigen) antibodies in CMV infection of healthy infants and in those with liver disease, J. Pediatr. **97**:545-549, 1980.

Oleske, J., Minnefor, A., Cooper, R., and others: Transmission of hepatitis B in a classroom setting, J. Pediatr. **97**:770-772, 1980.

Papaevangelou, G., and Hoofnagle, J.H.: Transmission of hepatitis B virus infection by asymptomatic chronic HBsAg carrier mothers, Pediatrics **63**:602-605, 1979.

Reesink, H.W., Reerink-Brongers, E.E., Lafeber-Schut, B.J.T., and others: Prevention of chronic HBsAg carrier state in infants of HBsAg-positive mothers by hepatitis B immunoglobulin, Lancet **2**:436-437, Sept. 1, 1979.

Repsher, L.H., and Freebern, R.K.: Effects of early and vigorous exercise on recovery from infectious hepatitis, N. Engl. J. Med. **281**:1393-1396, 1969.

Robinson, W.S., and Lutwick, L.I.: The virus of hepatitis, type B: Parts I, II, N. Engl. J. Med. **295**:1168-1236, 1976.

Rubenstein, D., Esterly, M.B., and Fretzin, D.: The Gianotti-Crosti syndrome, Pediatrics **61**:433-437, 1978.

Segool, R.A., Lejtenyi, C., and Taussig, L.M.: Articular and cutaneous prodromal manifestations of viral hepatitis, J. Pediatr. **87**:709-712, 1975.

Schaffner, F.: The structural basis of altered hepatic function in viral hepatitis, Am. J. Med. **49**:658-668, 1970.

Simon, J.B., and Patel, S.K.: Liver disease in asymptomatic carriers of hepatitis B antigen, Gastroenterology **66**:1020-1028, 1974.

Spero, J.A., Lewis, J.H., Fisher, S.E., and others: The high risk of chronic liver disease in multitransfused juvenile hemophiliac patients, J. Pediatr. **94**:875-878, 1979.

Szmuness, W., Stevens, C.E., Oleszko, W.R., and Goodman, A.: Passive-active immunization against hepatitis B: immunogenicity studies in adult Americans, Lancet **1**:575-577, 1981.

Tabor, E., Jones, R., Gerety, R.J., and others: Asymptomatic viral hepatitis types A and B in an adolescent population, Pediatrics **62**:1026-1030, 1978.

Tabor, E., April, M., Seeff, L.B., and Gerety, R.J.: Acute non-A, non-B hepatitis: prolonged presence of the infectious agent in blood, Gastroenterology **76**:680-684, 1979.

Tisdale, W.A.: When to hospitalize the hepatitis patient, Hosp. Pract., pp. 35-41, Oct. 1967.

Trepo, C.G., Magnius, L.O., Schaefer, R.A., and others: Detection of e antigen and antibody: correlations with hepatitis B surface and hepatitis B core antigens, liver disease, and outcome in hepatitis B infections, Gastroenterology **71**:804-808, 1976.

Zuckerman, A.: Hepatitis B: nature of the virus and prospects for vaccine development. In Popper, H., and Schaffner, F., editors: Progress in liver diseases, vol. 5, New York, 1976, Grune & Stratton, Inc.

BACTERIAL HEPATITIS

Primary bacterial hepatitis not associated with ascending cholangitis or underlying liver disease is an extremely rare pediatric condition. An occasional case may occur in the perinatal period. Here, direct bacterial seeding of the liver usually results in a hepatitis-like lesion associated with microabscess or macroabscess formation and, unfortunately, grave consequences. These infants are extremely ill, easy to go into shock, pale, ashen in color, lethargic, hypothermic, and possibly icteric. In most, the infection is acquired in utero, especially associated with premature rupture of the membranes or during delivery from swallowing infected amniotic fluid and vaginal secretions. Transplacental spread may also occur. Ascending spread by omphalitis or insertion of a contaminated umbilical vein catheter is causative in other cases. Bacterial culture of liver tissue grows the same organism obtained from the blood of these septic neonates, the most common being *Escherichia coli, Listeria monocytogenes,* and *Streptococcus* group B, for the prenatally acquired disease, and *Staphylococcus aureus* in postnatal cases. If recognized early, the rapid progression of this condition may be abated by prompt antibiotic treatment. If not, septic shock and consumptive coagulopathy frequently precede cardiorespiratory failure as the terminal event in most cases (75%).

In the older child and adolescent, rare causes of bacterial hepatitis have been infection with *Brucella* and *Mycobacterium* (tuberculosis), organisms that lead to a granulomatous hepatic lesion. On occasion, septicemic *Clostridia perfringens* may seed the liver with subsequent gas production possible in the abscess cavities.

The most important bacterial liver infection in the teen-age girl is *Neisseria gonorrhoeae* perihepatitis (Fitz-Hugh-Curtis syndrome). This occurs most often as an extension of pelvic inflammatory disease and is heralded by fever and right upper quadrant pain, but shoulder-tip and pleuritic pain may also be reported. As many as one third of cases with acute salpingitis may have liver involvement. Careful auscultation over the subcostal portion of the liver may reveal the presence of a friction rub. The liver is slightly tender and variably enlarged. Pelvic findings of acute salpingitis are present in most cases. About the liver, the greatest concentration of organisms is on and within the liver capsule, though occasionally they may penetrate into the subcapsular zone, and there produce a local inflammatory lesion. Liver biopsy is contraindicated in suspected cases for fear of introducing organisms into the deeper hepatic tissue.

Diagnosis can be suspected from the clinical presentation and history of dysmenorrhea, menorrhagia, or vaginal discharge. The pelvic examination reveals a painful inflammatory process, and results of vaginal and cervical cultures are positive. The response to antibiotic treatment also serves to confirm the diagnosis when culture proof is lacking (15% to 20%). The differential diagnosis may include acute pyelonephritis, cholecystitis, cholelithiasis, hepatitis, and at times pneumonia and pleurisy. Recent reports suggest that *Chlamydia trachomatis* may also be causative of this syndrome. Laboratory findings include leukocytosis, elevated sedimentation rate, transaminases, and sometimes bilirubin. An oral cholecystogram often fails to visualize the gallbladder during acute perihepatitis infections, but it should appear normal by ultrasound examination.

Persons with disseminated forms of gonococcal disease are best treated as inpatients using penicillin, given intravenously 10 million units daily until symptoms subside, followed by ampicillin, 0.5 gm orally four times daily. The duration of treatment should be no less than 7 days. Outpatient management is also possible when one uses 4.8 million units of aqueous penicillin divided in two injection sites, followed by an oral loading dose of ampicillin, 3.5 gm, and 1 gm of probenecid. Thereafter, ampicillin at 0.5 gm four times daily for 7 additional days is employed.

Failure to improve on treatment, confusion about the diagnosis and persistence of right upper quadrant pain are all indications for diagnostic and possibly therapeutic laparoscopy. Direct visualization and fulguration of the perihepatic adhesions can be accomplished by this procedure. The coagulated adhesions can then be separated by use of laparoscope scissors or blunt dissection. Prompt relief of symptoms can be expected.

REFERENCES

Kimball, M.W., and Knee, S.: Gonococcal perihepatitis in a male, N. Engl. J. Med. **282:**1082-1083, 1970.

Litt, I.F., and Cohen, M.I.: Perihepatitis associated with salpingitis in adolescents, J.A.M.A. **240:**1253-1254, 1978.

Reichert, J.A., and Valle, R.F.: Fitz-Hugh-Curtis syndrome: a laparoscopic approach, J.A.M.A. **236:**266-268, 1976.

Wang, S.P., Eschenbach, D., Holmes, K.K., Wager, G., and Grayston, J.T.: *Chlamydia trachomatis* infection in Fitz-Hugh-Curtis syndrome, Am. J. Obstet. Gynecol. **138:**1034-1038, 1980.

Weinstein, L.: Bacterial hepatitis: a case report on an unrecognized cause of fever of unknown origin, N. Engl. J. Med. **299:**1052, 1978.

LEPTOSPIRAL LIVER DISEASE

This spirochete is an unusual cause of acute liver disease in North America, and even in endemic areas less than 10% of leptospiral disease involves the liver. Infection is most often acquired by exposure to contaminated water and occasionally by direct contact to the animal vector. The organism enters the human host through the skin or respiratory tract. Wild rodents and domestic animals harbor this organism and are primarily responsible for transmission of the spirochete to man.

The diagnosis should be considered when a history of biphasic illness is elicited, and the child has findings of a maculopapular or petechial rash, conjunctivitis, meningeal signs, hepatomegaly, and slight icterus. Since the primary pathologic lesion in this disease is a vasculitis, other organ systems may also be involved.

Routine laboratory abnormalities include leukocytosis and elevated sedimentation rate. Liver function tests are variably disturbed with elevation of transaminases and bilirubin. With muscle involvement creatinine phosphokinase (CPK) may likewise be elevated. If meningeal signs are present, a cerebrospinal fluid pleocytosis can be found. Urine examination will reveal white and red blood cells with proteinuria in more severely affected cases. The liver biopsy specimen can show features of nonspecific hepatitis that is usually mild and diffuse, with rare cytolysis.

Specific diagnosis can be made when the organism is found in the blood early in the disease, or in the urine at a later time (14 to 30 days) by either dark-field or phase-contrast microscopy. Leptospiral agglutinins can be identified by serologic testing and appear after the first week or two of illness. Early treatment with penicillin (50,000 units/kg/day) in divided doses can be given for 7 to 10 days, but its role in ameliorating the course of this condition is questionable.

Anicteric cases can be expected to have a benign course. The presence of obvious liver involvement correlates with a poor prognosis with increased mortality. These latter patients generally have renal and cardiac involvement, which adds significantly to the final morbidity and mortality.

REFERENCES

Wong, M.L., Kaplan, S., Dunkie, L.M., and others: Leptospirosis: a childhood disease, J. Pediatr. **90:**532-537, 1977.

PYOGENIC LIVER ABSCESS

Fortunately, pyogenic liver abscess is not common in pediatric patients. In a large pediatric hospital this diagnosis accounted for only 3 of 100,000 admissions. A compilation of cases of pyogenic hepatic abscesses from a number of large general hospitals found 7% occurred in patients under 20 years of age. The incidence of this condition obtained from autopsy of pediatric patients from all causes is said to be about 0.35%. If one excludes those cases associated with defective neutrophil function (chronic granulomatous disease), the male predominance previously noted in this condition is no longer apparent. Most pediatric cases are likely to develop in the pre–school age child (Table 21-5).

Lack of awareness for this rare entity is suggested by a report stating only 2 of 27 patients with hepatic pyemia had been suspected before the patient's death. Under normal circumstances the hepatic reticuloendothelial system is remarkably effective in clearing portal venous or hepatic arterial blood of bacteria that transiently may find their way into the circulation. Undoubtedly, widespread use of effective antibiotic therapy has substantially reduced bacterial seeding from such conditions as pyoderma, burns, and osteomyelitis. In addition, only a few cases now seem to result from either penetrating liver injury or perforation of the bowel. Although the diagnosis of acute appendicitis in the child under 2 years of age is seldom made before perforation, pylephlebitis, and hepatic pyemia remain rare complications. Again, prompt specific antibiotic therapy combined with proper surgical drainage of the abdomen has protected the child from hepatic pyemia in all these conditions. Umbilical vein catheterization, a procedure now limited almost exclusively to neonatal

Table 21-5. Clinical and pathologic findings in 40 children without chronic granulomatous disease who developed hepatic abscess

Condition	Number of children
Sex	
Male	22
Female	18
Age (years)	
0-1	18
1-5	9
5-10	8
10-20	5
Cause of infection	
Sepsis	16
Contiguous infection	10
Cryptogenic	8
Trauma	4
Biliary	2
Portal	0
Underlying process	
Leukemia	7
Recurrent infections	2
Sickle-cell anemia	1
Immunosuppressive drugs	1
Aplastic anemia	1
Type of lesion	
Solitary	20
Multiple, small or microscopic	20
Survival	
Survived	14
Died	10

From Chusid, M.J.: Pediatrics **62:**554, 1978.

exchange transfusion, has the potential for bacterial seeding of the liver with subsequent development of multiple hepatic abscesses, especially in the left lobe. Detailed attention to aseptic technique remains imperative when one is employing this procedure in the neonate.

In contrast to adults in whom biliary obstruction or cryptogenic cases dominate, hepatic abscess formation in pediatric patients most often evolves from generalized sepsis occurring in children with congenital or acquired immunodeficiency states or other expressions of compromised host resistance. The latter examples include those children on chemotherapy and immunosuppressive agents. One third to one half the cases in pediatrics occur in the slightly older child with defective leukocyte function (chronic granulomatous disease).

Direct seeding through the portal vein may also occur in inflammatory bowel disease, especially regional enteritis, but fortunately this is a rare event. Although more common in adults, spread through the biliary duct system can also be responsible for hepatic pyemia even in the pediatric patient. Children subjected to biliary tract–drainage procedures for congenital biliary atresia or choledochal cyst that employs an intestinal conduit (Roux-en-Y) are potentially at risk for development of hepatic pyemia. Although ascending cholangitis is a frequent postoperative complication of portoenterostomy (Kasai's procedure), vigorous antibiotic therapy seems to prevent hepatic abscess formation. However, hepatic pyemia is not infrequently found as a complication of orthotopic liver transplantation despite the use of similar antibiotic prophylaxis. In this immunosuppressed host, the transplanted organ may also be temporarily impaired (Kuppfer cell function) in regard to bacterium-clearing properties. Children with a known underlying hemolytic condition who developed unexplained fevers should be suspected of having possible hepatic pyemia, for ascending cholangitis from obstructing cholelithiasis may be at fault.

Abdominal trauma with penetrating injuries may cause direct bacterial contamination of the liver surface or substance. Nonpenetrating abdominal injury can also be responsible for pyogenic abscess formation presumably because of subsequent bacterial seeding in unsuspected areas of hemorrhage or in devitalized hepatic tissue. As in adults, cryptogenic cases, those not caused by generalized sepsis or direct spread from contiguous structures, do occur in pediatric patients and are typical of those in patients with chronic granulomatous disease. In many cases, identifying the factor or factors responsible for decreasing the liver's focal resistance to bacterial infection has not been possible. However, intrinsic disease conditions such as amebic abscess, hydatid cysts, tumor, and ischemia should always be considered because they predispose this organ to bacterial seeding within the areas of focal hepatic injury.

The probability of developing either a single abscess or multiple abscesses seems to be influenced by the site of the antecedent infection. Contamination of an umbilical vein catheter or ascending spread from omphalitis more likely will result in multiple abscess formation. If portal vein invasion is suspected as the mode of infection, a solitary liver abscess in the right lobe is likely. A patient with biliary tract disease or with bacterial sepsis is likely to have multiple liver abscesses in both lobes. Injury to the stomach or pancreas often results in a solitary abscess of the left lobe, whereas children with chronic granulomatous disease typically have a solitary lesion in the right lobe.

Clinical features, laboratory tests, and diagnosis

The difficulty in diagnosis of hepatic pyemia stems from lack of awareness of this condition rather than from subtleties in clinical or laboratory findings. Some persons believe that the pathobiologic manifestation of this condition is changing and that less than 25% to 50% of patients now fit the classical description of the signs and symptoms attending this entity. Delay in diagnosis from 1 to 4 months is not unusual in reported cases. Whether the disease evolves as a consequence of a known antecedent infectious process or insidiously in a supposedly well person, spiking fevers (with or without chills), abdominal pain, and variable hepatomegaly eventually appear. Great systemic toxicity may not be present. The diagnosis is easier if these complaints develop in association with or after an abdominal condition (bowel perforation, gastric or biliary surgery, penetrating abdominal injuries, inflammatory bowel disease), especially if jaundice appears and the liver rapidly enlarges. However, the diagnosis may not be so obvious if a period of well-being intervenes. Before the development of newer evaluation methods, the diagnosis of pyogenic liver abscess in such cases was not made until autopsy in up to 60%, despite the presence of fever and hepatomegaly.

Indeed, when the onset is insidious, the early symptoms may be nonspecific with recurrent fevers, malaise, nausea, anorexia, and abdominal pain (usually right upper quadrant) being frequent complaints. As delay in diagnosis continues, weight loss becomes a common finding and makes one consider an underlying tumor. Physical examination usually reveals an ill-appearing patient with pallor or, in 10% to 25% of patients, jaundice. The most striking physical finding in the older child is tenderness over the subcostal portion of the liver or, at times, in the intercostal spaces. The liver may be slightly enlarged but not easily appreciated because of guarding over this area. At times a mass may be palpated in the right upper quadrant. Loss of diaphragmatic excursion associated with normal or deep respiration may be detected by percussion.

Initial laboratory studies reveal a variable degree of anemia and leukocytosis. However, a normal leukocyte count does not exclude the diagnosis of pyogenic liver abscess. The sedimentation rate is always elevated. Nonspecific alterations in liver function occur in half the cases including mild elevation of transaminases, bilirubin, serum alkaline phosphatase, or gamma glutamyl transpeptidase. More significant elevations of bilirubin and alkaline phosphatase are likely to ·be seen when biliary tract disease is responsible for the development of the liver abscess. Hypoalbuminemia is frequently noted in patients with symptoms of long duration. Although not part of routine laboratory investigations of these patients, an elevated serum vitamin B_{12} level is believed to be a useful aid in diagnosis. Blood cultures obtained as part of the septic workup may be positive in up to half the cases.

Hepatic pyemia carries a 100% mortality if unrecognized and untreated. Once the diagnosis is entertained, it must be ruled out by more sophisticated laboratory and radiologic studies. Other conditions that may mimic this clinical presentation include hepatic amebic abscess, infected hydatid cyst, rapidly expanding hepatic carcinoma with central hemorrhage or necrosis, and subphrenic or subhepatic pyogenic abscesses from other causes.

Roentgenograms. Routine roentgenograms of the chest should be taken during both inspiration and expiration. The right hemidiaphragm is elevated and limited in excursion. Atelectatic changes at the right base may be visible with or without a pleural effusion. The liver may appear enlarged. Occasionally the diagnosis can be entertained when upright abdominal plain films are viewed and intrahepatic gas bubbles or air-fluid levels in the right upper quadrant are seen.

Radioisotope liver scan. A radioisotope scan is the most useful tool in the diagnosis of hepatic abscess, with an overall accuracy of 80% to 85% (Fig. 21-7). False-negative results are more common than false-positive ones. Multiple small (less than 2 cm) lesions are most likely to be missed by these techniques. Either a technetium-99m sulfur colloid or a gallium-67 citrate scintiscan is the most frequently used isotope. The abscess cavity shows up as either a focal "cold" spot with the former isotope, or a "hot" filling defect with the latter. Scanning in both anterior, posterior, and lateral views is recommended.

Ultrasonic liver scan. The presence of either a "cold" or "hot" focal defect on liver scan cannot be used to differentiate liver abscess from other conditions that replace normal liver tissue, such as primary or metastatic neoplasm, benign solid space-occupying lesions, or cystic disease. Ultrasonography can distinguish between solid- and fluid-filled cavities, thereby differentiating between solid tumors and fluid-containing cysts or abscesses. This technique has additional value in following the course of the disease after treatment because it is noninvasive and involves no radiation exposure to the patient.

Hepatic angiography. Selective catheterization of the hepatic artery in children can be accomplished in most pediatric centers by the femoral artery–aorta–celiac access route. This procedure can often allow visualization of lesions less than 2 cm in size, which may be missed by radioisotope liver scan. An avascular pyogenic abscess causes stretching and displacement of intrahepatic vessels. At times the lesion may be better visualized during the sinusoid phase of the angiogram when the avascular lesion is outlined by a zone of hyperemia forming a rim of contrast material ("halo" effect). It is recommended that this procedure be done before exploratory surgery in patients with positive scans, not only to further increase accuracy of diagnosis, but also to provide the surgeon with specific information about the vascular anatomy to the liver. This will become particularly important if hepatic lobectomy is required for abscess removal.

Needle aspiration. Although not widely used, needle aspiration of a hepatic abscess under careful fluoroscopic control may be attempted. The material should be promptly examined for parasites and cytologic types and submitted for aerobic and anaerobic bacteriologic culture and sensitivity studies.

Treatment

If not treated, pyogenic hepatic abscess is fatal in all cases. A combination of surgical drainage and antibiotics can result in cures in 50% to 75% of patients, particularly if the lesion is solitary and the diagnosis is not made too late. Fortunately, over 50% of the cases will have a solitary abscess amenable to specific therapy. Delaying diagnosis

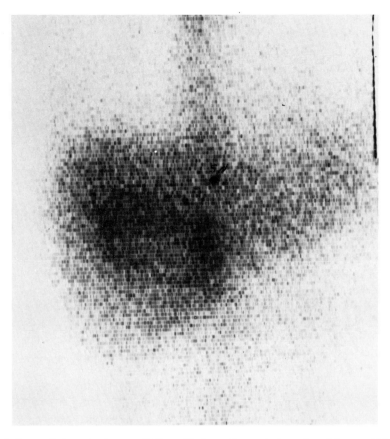

Fig. 21-7. Pyogenic hepatic abscess. Gallum-67 citrate liver scintiscan in a 14-year-old boy with previously unexplained fevers, weight loss, and tender hepatomegaly. The scan shows a large intrahepatic abscess (zone of increased density) occupying much of the right lobe. Surgical drainage and antibiotics led to eventual cure.

is often found in the reports with high mortality figures.

Whenever indicated, the patient should be given whole blood, plasma, or albumin to improve his clinical condition before surgery. Although somewhat controversial, the surgical approach to the liver abscess usually involves transperitoneal drainage. This decision is best made after consideration of the possible underlying cause for the hepatic abscess and the intrahepatic location of the process by radiographic evaluation. At laparotomy the external surface of the liver may look normal, but fluctuance may be palpable. Fluid obtained by needle aspiration should be sent for necessary bacteriologic cultures (aerobic and anaerobic) and antibiotic sensitivities. In addition, the material should be examined for the presence of amebas or other organisms. Fluid that contains a distinct odor of infection usually indicates the presence of anaerobic organisms. At times, partial

or complete lobectomy may be required, especially for solitary deep intrahepatic abscesses or multiple lobar abscesses.

Adhering to the basic principle of ensuring adequate drainage, one should leave the tube in the abscess cavity, which may thereafter be used to irrigate the cavity (with or without antibiotic solution). The technique of following resolution of the lesion by injection of radiopaque material through the tube has fallen into disfavor with the availability of ultrasonography. The drainage tube is removed when only a sinus tract remains.

The most common organism recovered in the pediatric population is *Staphyloccus aureus*. Other aerobic organisms occasionally noted include *Enterobacter, Streptococcus viridans,* enterococcus, and *Klebsiella*. Indigenous bowel anaerobes such as *Bacteroides, Clostridium,* and streptococci may also occur. Accordingly, a combination of oxacillin or methicillin, given intravenously 100 mg/kg/

24 hr in 4 divided doses, and chloramphenicol, 100 mg/kg/24 hr in 3 divided doses, can be employed. Peak chloramphenicol blood levels should be checked during the course of therapy. The results of bacteriologic sensitivity testing will dictate necessary changes in the selection of antibiotics. The drugs are continued 4 to 6 weeks for those patients treated by surgical drainage. A lesser period of treatment is suggested if the abscess or abscesses have been totally excised.

Complete surgical drainage of multiple hepatic abscesses is usually impossible. These patients have an extremely high mortality even with aggressive specific antibiotic therapy.

Complications and prognosis

Early recognition, possible only by increased awareness and selection of high-yield diagnostic studies, should give the patient with solitary liver abscess a reasonably good prognosis. Although proper surgical drainage and antibiotics in treatment of solitary lesions yield survival rates of over 75%, the figures for all types of hepatic abscess conditions vary from 30% to 50%. Metastatic spread of the abscess to other organs (lungs, brain, peritoneum, pericardium) severely diminishes chances for survival, as multiple lesions scattered throughout the liver do.

Liver failure, septic shock with hypotension, or peritonitis, is a terminal event in those patients who have intraperitoneal rupture of the abscess and subsequently die.

REFERENCES

Barbour, G.L., and Juniper, K., Jr.: A clinical comparison of amebic and pyogenic abscess of the liver in sixty-six patients, Am. J. Med. **53:**323-334, 1972.

Bingaman, R., Riley, H.D., Jr., and Bhatia, M.: Hepatic abscess 12 years after corrective surgery for congenital bile duct atresia, Clin. Pediatr. **15:**482-485, 1976.

Chusid, M.J.: Pyogenic hepatic abscess in infancy and childhood, Pediatrics **62:**554-559, 1978.

Kaplan, S.L., and Feigin, R.D.: Pyogenic liver abscess in normal children with fever of unknown origin, Pediatrics **58:**614-616, 1976.

Madayag, M.A., Lefleur, R.S., Braunstein, P., and others: Radiology of hepatic abscess, N.Y. State J. Med. **75:**1417-1423, 1975.

Nolan, J.P.: Bacteria and the liver, N. Engl. J. Med. **299:**1069-1071, 1978.

Palmer, E.D.: The changing manifestations of pyogenic liver abscess, J.A.M.A. **231:**192, 1975.

Ranson, J.H.C., Madayag, M.A., Localio, S.A., and Spencer, M.D.: New diagnostic and therapeutic techniques in the management of pyogenic liver abscesses, Ann. Surg. **181:**508-517, 1975.

Ribaudo, J.M., and Ochsner, A.: Intrahepatic abscesses: amebic and pyogenic, Am. J. Surg. **125:**570-574, 1973.

Rubin, R.H., Swartz, M.N., and Malt, R.: Hepatic abscess: changes in clinical, bacteriologic and therapeutic aspects, Am. J. Med. **57:**601-610, 1974.

Satiani, B., and Davidson, E.D.: Hepatic abscesses: improvement in mortality with early diagnosis and treatment, Am. J. Surg. **135:**647-650, 1978.

Shulman, S.T., and Beem, M.O.: An unique presentation of sickle cell disease: pyogenic hepatic abscess, Pediatrics **47:**1019-1022, 1971.

AMEBIC LIVER ABSCESS

A continued but gradual increase in the frequency of amebic liver abscess has been noted in the United States over the past several years. Throughout the country endemic foci of the disease have been found since the Southeast Asian conflict and also in the southern border states, where a high concentration of Mexican nationals and farm workers are concentrated. Poor sanitation and crowded living conditions predispose to amebiasis, with person-to-person transmission considered most important. Not infrequently, other close relatives of the index case will be found to be carriers of this organism. In addition to a noted male predominance, other undefined variables may be at play to explain the higher likelihood of recurrence in some individuals. Pediatric examples of this disease have been found in children as young as 6 weeks of age. With the continued increase in worldwide tourism, which includes travel to areas where a high incidence of disease-producing strains of *Entamoeba histolytica* are endemic, a greater index of suspicion needs to be maintained if prompt diagnosis and improved treatment results are to be expected. Since mortality is very much related to delayed institution of specific therapy, urgency in diagnosis is apparent.

Amebic liver abscess occurs as a complication of invasive colonic disease in 1% to 8% of all patients. Shortly after amebas reach the liver, presumably by the portal route, a focal destruction of liver tissue begins, with subsequent coalescence leading to formation of an abscess cavity. It is surprising that the surrounding liver tissue neighboring upon the abscess is remarkably free of signs of inflammation.

Clinical features, laboratory tests, and diagnosis

In the usual case, signs and symptoms of acute illness are characterized by a moderate to high

Table 21-6. Main clinical features in 400 consecutive admissions with amebic liver abscess

Features	Percentage
Length of history	
0-2 weeks	59
2-4 weeks	20
4-12 weeks	16
12 weeks	5
Symptoms	
Pain	99
Right hypochondrium	73
Right side of chest	28
Epigastrium	21
Right shoulder	9
Previous dysentery	19
Present diarrhea or dysentery	14
Cough	11
Dyspnea	4
Signs	
Tenderness in right hypochondrium	85
Liver palpable and tender	80
Fever	75
Signs at right lung base	47
Localized intercostal tenderness	38
Epigastric tenderness	22
Localized swelling over liver	10

From Adams, E.B., and MacLeod, I.N.: Medicine **56:**315, 1977.

temperature, chills, nausea, mild weight loss, and an intense aching abdominal pain in the right upper quadrant in three fourths of the cases (Table 21-6). Prodromal respiratory symptoms with cough, pleuritic chest pain or shoulder-tip pain, and malaise may be the subtle complaints of a patients who harbors an amebic liver abscess that has extended into the right hemidiaphragm. Less often, the amebic abscess may be present for a long time (months) with few symptoms, but as the disease progresses, the aforementioned clinical symptoms eventually develop. Diarrhea is occasionally reported in these patients, but seldom is the stool specimen positive for *Entamoeba histolytica* trophozoites. For most patients they cannot recall a gastrointestinal prodrome though *E. histolytica* invasion of the gut produces a colitis-like picture in many.

Physical examination usually reveals an ill- and toxic-looking patient. Decreased diaphragmatic excursion and diminished breath sounds in the posterior lower right hemithorax may be noted,

especially if the lesion has eroded through the diaphragm. Deep respiratory efforts may be guarded because of pleuritic pain. Hepatomegaly, either into the abdomen or up into the chest is typical, and tenderness to both palpation and percussion can be demonstrated, especially in the right hypochondrium. Subcutaneous edema and intercostal tenderness may be found over an abscess cavity of large size (greater than 20 cm). The right lobe is the site of the amebic abscess in over 90% of cases. Abscesses located along the inferior aspect of the liver or in the left lobe may present as a tender mass in the epigastrium and suggest pancreatic pseudocyst or intragastric tumor. Lesions located in the superior aspect of the left lobe of the liver may involve the pericardium and produce a "friction rub" heard in the left side of chest. Clinical jaundice is seldom detected. On occasion rectal examination will reveal Hematest-positive stool.

Routine laboratory tests show a polymorphonuclear leukocytosis with mild, normochromic, or hypochromic anemia, absence of peripheral eosinophilia, and an elevated sedimentation rate. Liver function studies are generally normal or mildly disturbed, with modest elevation of the serum transaminases, bilirubin, and alkaline phosphatase. That a greater disturbance in liver function studies does not occur is probably attributable to the absence of hepatic inflammation in the area surrounding the amebic abscess. Upright abdomen and chest roentgenograms are abnormal in up to 75% of cases and reveal an elevated hemidiaphragm, with or without an underlying pulmonary infiltrate or pleural effusion. Diagnostic confusion is usually between pyogenic liver abscess, hepatic tumors, *Echinococcus* cyst, lobar pneumonia, and at times tuberculous pleural effusion (Fig. 21-8).

Localization of the abscess is best accomplished by liver scintiscan technique using technetium-99m sulfur colloid or ultrasonography, both of which provide almost immediate diagnostic information (Fig. 21-9). In unusual circumstances gallium-67 citrate may be used, particularly if superimposed bacterial infection is suspected. Selective angiography occasionally is required to detect multiple, small (less than 2 cm) lesions.

Confirmation of the diagnosis is most often obtained from results of serologic testing, needle aspiration of the abscess, and the patient's response to the simultaneous use of tissue amebicidal drugs. The indirect hemagglutination assay (IHA) has been

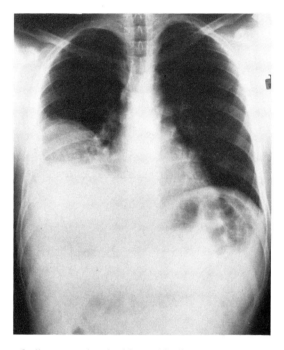

Fig. 21-8. Pulmonary findings associated with amebic liver abscess. Chest radiograph obtained in a 16-year-old boy complaining of fevers, weight loss, cough, and right-sided abdominal and chest pain. He was initially treated with antibiotics for suspected pneumonia but failed to improve.

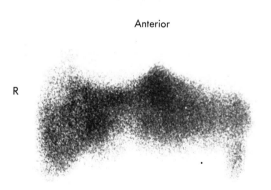

Fig. 21-9. ^{99m}Technetium–sulfur colloid scan performed in the patient discussed in Fig. 21-21. A large filling defect is seen in the superior aspect of the right lobe of the liver.

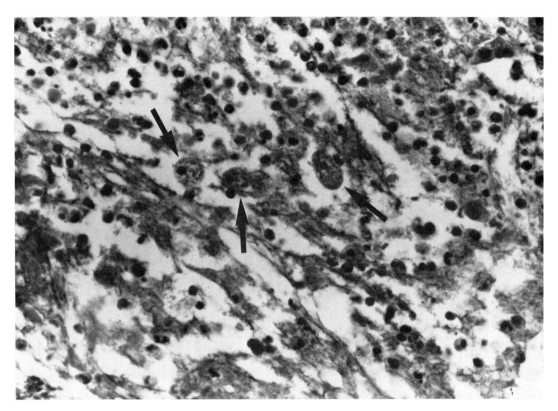

Fig. 21-10. Amebiasis. Phagocytic amebas containing red blood cells, *arrows,* are shown in a cellular coagulum obtained from scrapings of the abscess wall located in the infrahepatic area. The patient was a young Mexican national presenting with fever and an acute abdomen. Abdominal ultrasound exam localized the lesion before surgery. ($\times 250$.)

the mainstay of serologic diagnosis for many years and is available from the Parasitology Division of the National Center for Disease Control in Atlanta, Georgia. This test has a high degree of sensitivity (positive titers being greater than 1:128) in about 95% of patients with invasive amebiasis. However, the test does have some shortcomings. Results may not be available for 2 to 3 weeks, since most specimens require handling and shipping, with increased risk to loss or breakage of the specimen. High antibody titers may remain for many years after previous exposure to the parasite; therefore the specificity of the test (false positive) may be reduced for any person. The commercially available agar-gel immunodiffusion precipitant (GDP) test can be performed by most laboratories and has the advantage of having a low cost and requiring relatively simple techniques. The GDP test apparently detects a different antibody that is of shorter duration (in most cases not detectible after 6 months) than that detected by the IHA. In addition, this procedure yields rapid results, often within 24 hours, and maintains a high degree of sensitivity (90% to 95%) as does the IHA. Furthermore, the use of the GDP test means a higher positive predictive value; that is, an elevated GDP titer indicates that the patient indeed has the disease. It is recommended that both tests be performed whenever possible, because they are complementary.

In countries with a large experience with invasive amebiasis, needle aspiration of the abscess is undertaken for diagnosis and frequently gives some immediate relief of clinical symptoms. Clinically defining the area of maximal tenderness (by palpation and percussion), aided further by localization of the abscess by radioisotope scans, will permit successful entry into the abscess cavity with minimal risk. The finding of amebas (25% to 80%) in the aspirated fluid is immediately diagnostic. The material is classically described as similar to "anchovy sauce" but unfortunately is often variable in color and consistency. If a strong odor to the fluid is noted, bacterial contamination is suggested. Aerobic and anaerobic cultures should routinely be carried out.

Once the diagnosis of amebic abscess is suspected, whether or not needle aspiration is performed, medical therapy should be instituted at once. The clinical response is seen in most cases within 48 to 72 hours, aspiration or surgery is obviated, and diagnosis then rests upon results of serologic testing. If a surgical approach to the abscess is needed, a biopsy, or scrapings taken from the inner surface of the abscess wall, provides the highest likelihood of yielding trophozoites of *E. histolytica* (Fig. 21-10).

Treatment

A variety of successful treatment protocols is now available. In uncomplicated amebic abscesses, oral metronidazole (Flagyl), 30 to 50 mg/kg/24 hours in 3 divided doses for 7 to 10 days, is presently the most frequently employed regimen. It is suggested that informed consent be obtained when this drug is used in pediatric patients even though the mutagenicity observed in bacteria and the carcinogenic potential documented in rodents have not been found in human studies. Intravenous metronidazole is now available (15 mg/kg infused over 1 hour, to be followed by 7.5 mg/kg every 6 hours also infused in 1 hour) and can be used when the drug cannot be given orally and contraindications to the use of other available agents exist. Some workers follow the week of metronidazole treatment with a 2-week course of chloroquine (10 to 20 mg/kg/day in 1 or 2 divided doses). In severe cases, with impending extension of the disease, or cases complicated by pulmonary or pericardial spread, a combination of intramuscular dehydroemetine (which is less toxic than emetine) at 1 to 1.5 mg/kg/24 hours for 5 to 10 days and chloroquine for a total of 21 days is recommended. Patients must be carefully observed for neurologic and cardiac toxicity. Disappearance of the abscess, which may take from 4 to 6 months, can be followed by liver scintiscan or ultrasonography. Provided that the patient is asymptomatic, the slow resolution of the abscess cavity is not a cause for concern.

Surgical drainage of the amebic abscess is rarely indicated once medical treatment is instituted. If concern about rupture of a large abscess exists or the patient's pain is unusually severe, needle aspiration under fluoroscopy is the procedure of choice, resulting in rapid clinical improvement. Repeat aspirations are rarely necessary. Occasionally the amebic abscess becomes secondarily infected (10% to 20%), in which case surgical drainage will be necessary. However, since the signs and symptoms of a noninfected abscess are similar to those containing bacteria, it is best for one to wait 3 days while observing the effect of antiamebic drug therapy before considering other invasive procedures. One must keep in mind that a clinical response to metronidazole does not necessarily confirm the diagnosis of an amebic abscess since the drug has very potent antibacterial properties against anaerobic gram-negative organisms.

Complications

Erosion through the diaphragm with rupture of the abscess into the right side of the chest is the most common complication of this disease. Here it may undergo loculation as an amebic empyema, or spread into lung tissue. A hepatobronchofistula may develop, leading suddenly to the production of voluminous sputum or hemoptysis, with surprising improvement in the patient's clinical condition. Accumulation of fluid in the pleural space can be needle aspirated. Chest-tube drainage is not required unless secondary bacterial infection is present in the empyema fluid. Rupture of the abscess into the peritoneal cavity presents as an ''acute abdomen'' and surgical exploration and drainage is indicated. Supradiaphragmatic extension and rupture of an abscess from the left lobe of the liver can result in suppurative amebic pericarditis and tamponade, requiring emergency measures. Needle aspiration of the pericardial sac is usually sufficient to alleviate the acute symptoms, though surgical drainage may be required in refractory cases. The sudden appearance of abdominal pain followed by melena may suggest rupture of the abscess into a loop of intestine or into the biliary duct system (hemobilia), both rare complications of amebic abscess. Hematogenous spread through the veins of Batson may be responsible for the development of amebic brain abscess, a very rare complication of the hepatic involvement.

Prognosis

The prognosis is excellent in the absence of complications, for complete functional and anatomic restoration of the liver can be expected with medical treatment. The pulmonary involvement likewise heals without pleural thickening or fibrosis of the lung parenchyma. Prognosis in peritoneal rupture of an amebic abscess is better than what follows bowel perforation from invasive amebic disease, presumably because of the absence of bacterial contamination in the former. Although the case-fatality ratio increases with the associated complications, mortality and morbidity can still be reduced once adequate therapy is instituted. The lowest mortality (1%) for uncomplicated cases is reported from centers with the greatest clinical experience, and where the index of suspicion for this entity is acutely high. Otherwise, overall mortality figures are from 10% to 20%. Extension into the chest, peritoneal cavity, or pericardium has yielded case-fatality figures of 6.7%, 18.4%, and 29.6%, respectively, from a large South African experience.

Finally, recurrences of invasive amebic disease are distinctly possible, for antibody in itself seems not to be protective.

REFERENCES

Adams, E.B., and MacLeod, I.N.: Invasive amebiasis. I. Amebic dysentery and its complication; II. amebic liver abscess and its complications, Medicine **56:**315-334, 1977.

Barbour, G.L., and Juniper, K.: A clinical comparison of amebic and pyogenic abscess of the liver in sixty-six patients, Am. J. Med. **53:**323-334, 1972.

Brandt, H., and Tamayo, R.P.: Pathology of human amebiasis, Hum. Pathol. **1:**351-385, 1970.

Cohen, H.G., and Reynolds, T.B.: Comparison of metronidazole and chloroquine for the treatment of amoebic liver abscess: a controlled trial, Gastroenterology **69:**35-41, 1975.

Crane, P.S., Lee, Y.T., and Seel, D.J.: Experience in the treatment of two hundred patients with amebic abscess of the liver in Korea, Am. J. Surg. **123:**332-337, 1972.

Dykes, A.C., Ruebush, T.K., II, Gorelkin, L., and others: Extraintestinal amebiasis in infancy: report of three patients and epidemiologic investigations of their families, Pediatrics **65:**799-803, 1980.

Harrison, H.R., Crowe, C.P., and Fulginiti, V.A.: Amebic liver abscess in children: clinical and epidemiologic features, Pediatrics **64:**923-928, 1979.

Jenkinson, S.G., and Hargrove, M.D., Jr.: Recurrent amebic abscess of the liver, J.A.M.A. **232:**277-278, 1975.

Jessee, W.F., Ryan, J.M., Fitzgerald, J.F., and Grosfeld, J.L.: Amebic liver abscess in childhood, Clin. Pediatr. **14:**134-146, 1975.

McCarty, E., Pathmanand, C., Sunakorn, P., and Scherz, R.G.: Amebic liver abscess in childhood, Am. J. Dis. Child. **126:**67-70, 1973.

Patterson, M., Healy, G.R., and Shabot, J.M.: Serologic testing for amoebiasis, Gastroenterology **78:**136-141, 1980.

Strauss, R.G., and Bove, K.E.: Fever, shock and hepatomegaly in a 13-month-old boy, J. Pediatr. **87:**819-823, 1975.

Wadlington, W.B., Faber, R., and O'Neill, J.A., Jr.: Recent experience with hepatic amebiasis, Clin. Pediatr. **14:**163-170, 1975.

OTHER PARASITIC CAUSES OF ACUTE LIVER DISEASE

A variety of parasitic infections may involve the liver and biliary tract but are seldom causative in children living in the Western Hemisphere. With increasing world travel and the recent immigration of large numbers of Southeast Asians into this country, a heightened awareness of these conditions becomes necessary.

Liver flukes, particularly *Clonorchis sinensis* and *Fasciola hepatica,* have a predilection for the bile ducts where the adult organism matures. Here they may produce an acute illness indistinguishable from cholecystitis, complicated cholelithiasis, hydrops of the gallbladder, ascending cholangitis, or toxic hepatitis. Fever, right upper quadrant pain, and hepatomegaly are typical findings common to these conditions as are the abnormal results of liver function studies. These findings and a pronounced leukocytosis, with impressive eosinophilia (35% to 50%) in a patient with a history of recent travel to or from an endemic area, should suggest nonamebic, parasitic disease of the biliary tree. The diagnositc procedure of choice is transhepatic cholangiography, but results can be confusing, suggesting obstructive calculus disease of the common bile ducts (in fact, mature flukes) and surgery undertaken. The parasites are then discovered after common duct exploration. If liver biopsy is obtained, the flukes can be seen on microscopic examination in liver granuloma. The ova may be found in the duodenal fluid and in stool examined during the acute stages of the disease. Intermittent and progressive biliary obstructive disease often leads to cirrhosis, especially with *Clonorchis sinensis* involvement.

Currently, drug treatment with dehydroemetine (1 mg/kg/day) for 10 days is recommended, but the efficacy remains questionable. An increased risk to cholangiosarcoma is reported in adults with long-standing involvement with either of these organisms.

Hydatid disease of the liver is caused by the dog tapeworm, *Echinoccus granulosus,* when the adult worm produces an asymptomatic mass in the right lobe of the liver. Signs of acute liver disease become manifest from compression and obstruction of the neighboring biliary tree, which in turn results in right upper quadrant pain, jaundice, and a hepatic mass discovered by physical examination. These clinical signs and symptoms may also suggest hepatic abscess, hydrops of the gallbladder, cholecystitis, or ascending cholangitis. Rupture of the cyst into the abdominal cavity produces the clinical picture of an "acute abdomen" of any other cause.

Hepatic scintiscans and ultrasound studies will help to identify the hepatic lesion as a fluid-filled cyst. Calcifications may be seen at the periphery of the cavity. As in amebiasis, eosinophilia is infrequent in this condition. Diagnosis is best confirmed by serologic testing (immunoelectrophoresis and hemagglutination). Complete removal of the cyst by surgery remains the treatment of choice.

Hepatic involvement (granulomas, portal fibrosis) with systemic parasitic disease is commonly seen in *malaria, visceral larva migrans* (see Chapter 16), and *visceral leishmaniasis,* but involvement of the liver seldom affects the final outcome of these patients. However, liver disease from *Schistosoma* infection does eventually produce significant portal and periportal fibrosis, resulting in portal hypertension of the presinusoid, noncirrhotic type. Since these lesions develop slowly, they are rarely diagnosed in the pediatric age group.

REFERENCES

Barros, J.L.: Hydatid disease of the liver, Am. J. Surg. **135:**597-600, 1978.

Hou, P.C., and Pang, L.S.C.: *Clonorchis sinensis* infestation in man in Hong-Kong, J. Pathol. Bacteriol. **87:**245-250, 1964.

Mahmoud, A.A.: Schistosomiasis, N. Engl. J. Med. **297:**1329-1331, 1977.

DRUG- OR TOXIN-INDUCED LIVER DAMAGE

Although the numbers of pediatric cases presenting with serious toxic liver disease and requiring hospital admission remain small, one is surprised how often the history of acute liver disease is complicated by the ingestion of or exposure to potential hepatotoxins. The list of such agents seems to expand exponentially. It has been stated that in a United States household, an average of 17 over-the-counter drugs can be found in addition to five prescription medications, many having potential hepatotoxic activity. For the pediatric

population an additional risk is posed by the likelihood of accidental ingestion of toxic quantities of a drug or by acquisition of abnormal amounts because of medication errors of overdosage or by self-poisonings. Multiple drug usage can result in hepatotoxicity by unsuspected drug interactions.

This situation has been further complicated for physicians caring for teen-age children because their risk of exposure to hepatotoxins has become significant by virtue of the expanded drug scene. This now includes agents that may be sniffed, ingested, or taken parenterally. The number of such drugs or toxins capable of producing liver damage is substantial.

Physicians are not without fault if they prescribe medications without complete awareness of the potential adverse side effects of the agent or agents either by itself or in conjunction with other drugs that may already be in the household. In response to this growing problem, a number of drug consultation centers have been established across the United States to serve as a readily available repository of valuable drug information for consumers and health care providers. From this source, information about both prescription and over-the-counter drugs can be obtained and, when appropriate, the pharmacologic and toxicologic aspects of environmental toxins and poisons including treatment recommendations. In the Rocky Mountain region, one can reach the Rocky Mountain Drug Consultation Center of Denver, Colorado, by calling the following toll-free number: 1-800-332-6475.

That the liver is not more frequently included in toxic aggressions by orally ingested agents is surprising, since portal blood carries the highest concentration of such products after their absorption from the gastrointestinal tract. The intimate relationship between structure and function is certainly exemplified by this particular organ and best explains this phenomenon. The liver is endowed with certain unique capabilities that involve the alteration of lipid-soluble, nonpolar agents, to more water-soluble polar derivatives, which facilitate their eventual renal elimination. An oxidative reaction is catalyzed by hepatocyte drug-metabolizing enzymes, the mixed-function oxidases (Fig. 21-11). These are enzymes located in the smooth endoplasmic reticulum and the most important group referred to as the cytochrome P-450 system. The resulting hydroxylation products can then be easily conjugated to their sulfated or glucuro-

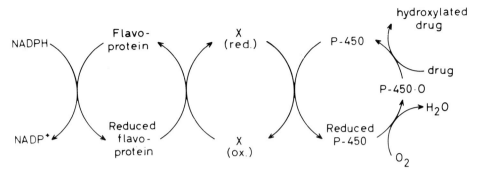

Fig. 21-11. The liver microsomal electron transport system. The flavoprotein is usually termed "NADPH–cytochrome c reductase" and is reduced by NADPH. Fe^{++}-protein is a nonheme iron-protein, and cytochrome P_{450} is the final oxidase of the system. (From Rane, S., and Sjöqvist, F.: Pediatr. Clin. North Am. **19**:37, 1972.)

nide form; the more polar compounds can then be excreted by the kidneys. Other intrahepatocyte-conjugating pathways also exist; an important one in drug metabolism utilizes glutathione, either directly or after other intermediary reactions. The liver also is capable of self-inducing alternate pathways for biotransformation of certain toxins ("metabolic adaptation"), particularly with continued exposure to some agents. This may explain the transient hepatic injury pattern reported early in the course, but one that disappears with continued exposure to the agent (oral contraceptives). Keep in mind that the reverse effect is also possible by similar biotransformation pathways, these producing heightened drug toxicity. This may be expressed as an acute injury pattern during continuous drug ingestion or may remain latent until reexposure occurs as in halothane-induced hepatic damage.

Maintaining the functional integrity of this important hepatic enzyme system is not a simple matter. A variety of factors influence both the qualitative and quantitative aspects of the mixed-function oxidases, a fundamental one being genetic in nature. Pharmacogenetic studies have recently shown that a genetic defect in the function of the cytochrome P-450 system exists in certain individuals and in turn explains the varying drug metabolic reactions noted in these patients when taking phenytoin (Dilantin) or isoniazid. In addition, the functional integrity of the mixed-function oxidase system is affected by such variables as the patient's age, general nutritional status, presence or absence of underlying liver disease, hepatic blood flow (portal hypertension), or the simultaneous ingestion of substances known to serve as "activators" of the drug-metabolizing enzymes. These and undoubtedly other, yet-to-be-discovered variables play an important role in toxic liver injury. It has been long recognized that the type and extent of the hepatic damage produced by a toxin is affected by the dose and duration of exposure, and now even these considerations must be interpreted within the framework of the "functional state" of the mixed-function oxidases.

Mechanisms of damage

Some previous distinctions (Table 21-7) used to differentiate liver damage caused by either presumed drug-induced sensitivity reactions or toxin-induced causes are no longer applicable. Further studies into the mechanism of action of both classes of "hepatotoxins" have revealed evidence that similarities exist in their production of hepatic cell injury. Although the physicochemical properties of the agent in question may dictate some specificity to their initial metabolic pathway, many in fact seem to share a common final event before producing hepatic damage. After the enzymatic interaction with the mixed-function oxidases, certain drugs and toxins are transformed into products having heightened bioactivity (arylated, alkylated, or acylated intermediates), which allows for the binding of these by-products to vital cellular macromolecules. The cellular damage that results is believed to be primarily caused by this latter process but by yet-undefined mechanisms. For example, even carbon tetrachloride (CCl_4), a well-known protein poison and chemical hepatotoxin, undergoes biotransformation before it can exert a toxic effect on the liver cell. It is first cleaved into free radicals, CCl_3 and Cl, by the

Table 21-7. Some previously considered distinctions between drug-induced and toxin-induced liver damage

	Drugs	Toxins
General method of action	Hypersensitivity route	Protoplasmic poisons
Individual susceptibility	Not common	Constant
Dose-injury relationship	Unpredictable	Proportionate and predictable
Interval from exposure to effect	Variable, but usually long	Short and predictable
Histologic lesion	Variable	Characteristic
Reproducible in animals	No	Yes
Systemic manifestations	Yes	Rare

cell's drug-metabolizing enzyme system associated with the smooth endoplasmic reticulum. The liberated CCl_3 then binds covalently to the hepatocyte lipid and protein macromolecules interfering with organelle function and finally producing the characteristic lesion recognized as that consistent with CCl_4 poisoning. In a somewhat similar fashion, the previously considered idiosyncratic drug-induced hepatic injury observed in some patients taking isoniazid (INH) can now be attributed to the hepatic bioactivation of a toxic metabolite, acetylhydrazine, produced in excess quantity by the cytochrome P-450 system in these individuals. The acetylation activity of the mixed-function oxidases also appears to be under genetic control, and individuals that are either fast or slow "acetylators" have now been identified. Fast acetylators of INH are at risk to develop hepatic damage by this drug. Variations in the hepatocyte-hydroxylation enzyme system also appear to be under genetic control. A primary fault of hydroxylating capacity leads to toxic blood levels of phenytoin (Dilantin), resulting in hepatic and extrahepatic reactions that develop while patients are taking therapeutic doses of the drug.

The incompatibility of certain drug combinations manifested by hepatotoxicity can often be explained by the influence of one of the agents upon the mixed-function oxidases. Certain drugs such as phenobarbital, phenytoin, meprobamate, and rifampin are known to induce a proliferation of the smooth endoplasmic reticulum and lead to heightened activity of the drug-metabolizing enzyme system. A patient taking one of these drugs is predisposed to manifest hepatic damage when exposed to another drug with hepatotoxic potential, even when administered in therapeutic doses.

Dose-related toxicity is well exemplified by acetaminophen (and probably phenacetin) metabo-

lism (Fig. 21-12). Therapeutic amounts of acetaminophen are easily handled by the usual conjugation routes in the liver. Up to a point, even excesses of hydroxylated acetaminophen can be conjugated without ill consequences using glutathione and then excreted as mercapturic acid. After depletion of glutathione to levels 60% to 80% of normal, covalent binding of the arylated metabolites of acetaminophen to other hepatic macromolecules takes place and hepatocyte injury ensues. Here again, pretreatment of the host with phenobarbital enhances the likelihood of hepatic injury, as the increased formation of toxic metabolites (acetaminophen-mercapturate) has been measured in the urine of such individuals.

Other mechanisms besides biotransformation to alkylating or arylating agents are also important in certain cases of toxic hepatic injury. Competitive binding by certain drugs to either carrier or transport enzyme systems can displace normally produced biologic products which in turn produce cellular damage, either directly or indirectly. The interference with organic anion transport by drugs such as rifampin, novobiocin, sulfobromophthalein, and cholecystographic agents may produce hyperbilirubinemic states, sometimes in association with cholestasis. Competitive interference with the excretion of bilirubin and bile acids plays a role in the hepatic cholestasis that occurs after phenothiazine ingestion. This is reminiscent of the mechanism by which hepatic injury occurs in galactosemia and in congenital fructose intolerance. When challenged with the sugar in question, patients with these inborn errors of metabolism accumulate endogenously produced toxic substrates, which in turn inhibit or interfere with normal hepatocyte function and lead to hepatic injury.

The steatosis noted in association with certain toxic agents is probably caused by lipoperoxida-

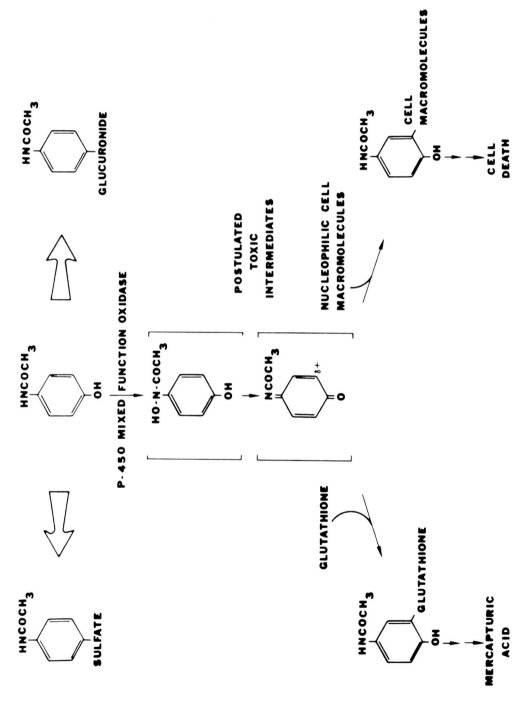

Fig. 21-12. Pathways of acetaminophen metabolism to normal and postulated toxic intermediates. (From Mitchell, J.R., et al.: In Popper, H., and Schaffner, F., editors: Progress in liver diseases, New York, 1976, Grune & Stratton, Inc.)

tion reactions that produce intermediate products and that subsequently interfere with the hepatocyte role in fatty acid metabolism. Bioactivation products by the liver cells may interfere with synthesis of the lipid-carrier protein (apoprotein), or the formation of the phospholipid moiety, thereby allowing for accumulation of intrahepatic triglyceride. Toxins, such as carbon tetrachloride, that are capable of lipoperoxidation also interfere with the oxidation of fatty acids in the mitochondria and further add to the accumulation of intrahepatocyte fat.

Some agents produce their initial toxic effect by simply interfering with the organelles involved in protein synthesis. Puromycin acts by disrupting transfer-RNA activity, whereas actinomycin D, aflatoxins, D-galactosimine, and amanthine seem to affect primarily messenger-RNA activity. Some agents can inhibit the translation of proteins from messenger RNA and produce hepatic damage. Cycloheximide, emetine, and diphtheria toxins are examples of this type of protein synthesis inhibition. Interference with the initial step in protein synthesis by sequestration of ATP, thereby preventing the amino acid activation to aminocyl-AMP, is believed to be the primary mechanism by which ethionine acts in producing hepatic injury.

In light of these newly discovered mechanisms of action, allergic hypersensitivity-induced hepatic injury by drugs now appears to be a less frequent cause than originally believed. It is quite likely that the drug-tissue reaction produces chemically reactive by-products that subsequently bind to macromolecules and subsequently induce an immunologic response in the host. Either humoral or tissue-bound hypersensitization may then become manifest during continuous use of the drug in question or upon reexposure to it. Although now considered rare, hypersensitivity reactions should still be suspected if (1) systemic signs such as fever, exanthem, and arthralgias exist; (2) peripheral eosinophilia is noted; (3) hepatic and extrahepatic symptoms develop after a latency period with continued drug use, or even after its discontinuation; (4) reintroduction of the suspected offender reproduces the symptom complex; or (5) historically the agent is known to produce untoward side effects of a hypersensitivity nature in only a small percentage of individuals (less than 1%). Sulfonamides, penicillin and its derivatives, and perhaps halothane-induced

liver injury remain examples of this mechanism in action.

By unclear mechanisms, the physical effects of therapeutic x irradiation to the liver can produce a reproducible pattern of hepatic injury. This organ is especially vulnerable to irradiation during periods of rapid growth, as occurs in infancy and early childhood, or after partial hepatectomy, when increased numbers of mitotic figures are known to be present. It is believed that the amount of liver mass irradiated, rather than the dose, is important in dictating the intensity of the injury. During the postirradiation period, rapid hypertrophy of the nonirradiated portion of the liver may have heightened vulnerability to chemotherapeutic agents with hepatotoxic potential. This is especially true of actinomycin D, a drug frequently used in combination with radiation of Wilms' tumor. It is suggested that this chemotherapeutic agent be withheld for the first 1 to 2 months after irradiation and surgery for right-sided Wilms' tumor in childhood.

Clinical features

So nonspecific are the clinical features of toxic liver disease that often only a high degree of awareness of this possibility, or through disciplined history taking, will the clinician arrive at the correct explanation for the patient's symptoms. Fever, anorexia, nausea with or without vomiting, and lassitude may be reported in mild forms. Pruritus, with or without overt jaundice or dark urine, may dominate the patient's symptom complex especially in phenothiazine-induced cases. Abdominal discomfort with vague or sharp pains in the epigastrium or right upper quadrant may occur in those persons developing drug-induced neoplastic lesions, or during the postirradiation period after the liver area was included. At other times extrahepatic manifestations dominate the clinical picture, especially in the face of massive toxic liver damage. Various combinations of symptoms, including circulatory collapse with shock, renal failure, gastrointestinal hemorrhage, neuropsychiatric disturbances, and coma with obtundation, may be seen accompanying the severe hepatic necrosis in cases of acetaminophen and iron overdosage, or after repeated exposures to halothane anesthesia, the ingestion of the mushroom *Amanita phalloides,* carbon tetrachloride, white phosphorus, and certain other environmental hepatotoxins. Ongoing hepatic injury may be discovered during the investigation of a patient complaining of fevers, rash, and arthralgias, from extrahepatic manifestations of the drug-hypersensitivity reaction.

In most cases of toxic liver injury, hepatomegaly is not a constant finding on physical examination. Tenderness of the liver edge is even less often elicited. Both of these physical findings, however, can usually be demonstrated in examples of hepatic injury occurring primarily at the level of the postsinusoid hepatic venous drainage system. Examples of this phenomenon include veno-occlusive disease produced by the accidental ingestion of *Senecio* alkaloids, especially after the drinking of certain herbal decoctions. Veno-occlusive disease may evolve in the postirradiation state. In such cases, ascites may also be present. Splenomegaly may develop in veno-occlusive injury but is otherwise seldom noted in toxic liver injury.

Laboratory studies

Variable but nonspecific elevations of serum aminotransferase activity, with or without a modest elevation of serum bilirubin, is most frequent. These mild laboratory indicators of hepatic injury are often present in the absence of overt clinical symptoms. An elevation of the serum alkaline phosphatase or gamma glutamyl transpeptidase and bilirubin may be even noted, especially from those agents capable of producing a cholestatic lesion. A peripheral eosinophilia can be seen in examples of drug-induced hypersensitivity reactions. Serum antimitochondrial antibodies are occasionally reported in cholestasis-associated hepatic injury. Positive lupus erythematosus cell preparations have been found in cases of methyldopa and oxyphenisatin-induced chronic active liver disease. In cases of severe hepatic injury with massive necrosis, abnormalities in coagulation are demonstrable by prolongation of the prothrombin and partial thromboplastin time, often accompanied by a decrease in the fibrinogen concentration. Quantitative serum levels of some hepatotoxins can be determined by specific toxicologic screening tests and are useful in cases believed to be caused by aspirin, acetaminophen, anticonvulsants, and chemotherapeutic agents.

Pathology

By light microscopy, the spectrum of liver injury from hepatotoxins is certainly more limited than the numbers of agents with this capability. Some toxics with considerably different chemical and pharmacologic activity produce similar-appearing lesions, whereas certain related groups of drugs or toxins effect a similar and reproducible injury pattern. At times the localization of the injury, seen microscopically, corresponds to the presumed subcellular site of action of the toxin. Despite the fact that, at best, only a few hepatotoxins produce a "diagnostic" histopathologic lesion, the constellation of nonspecific findings on biopsy will often point to the possibility that a hepatotoxic agent might be involved. These findings include hydropic swelling of hepatocytes, a ground-glass appearance, or more irregular clumping of the cytoplasm that is believed caused by the proliferation of the smooth endoplasmic reticulum. In addition, contrasts in the intensity of nuclear staining, variable steatosis, minimal necrosis, and a slight increase in numbers of mitotic figures are frequently observed in this nonspecific reaction. The inflammatory response is absent or minimal, with macrophages being the dominant cell type even when hepatic cytolysis is present. The aforementioned lesion can especially be found in individuals taking phenobarbital.

A more comprehensive list of agents frequently used in pediatric patients and the corresponding histologic injury pattern noted is shown in Table 21-8. Some examples of toxin-induced hepatic injury are shown in Table 21-9.

A *focal hepatitis*-like lesion can be seen with such drugs as aspirin, isoniazid, penicillin, methotrexate, oxacillin, carbenicillin, and recently cimetidine. More extensive hepatic *zonal necrosis* is found in carbon tetrachloride and white or yellow phosphorus poisoning, being centrilobular in the former and perilobular in the latter. Injury to the vascular endothelial lining results in *centrilobular hemorrhage with cellular necrosis* as occurs after the ingestion of herbal remedies containing *Senecio* alkaloids or of foods contaminated with high concentrations of aflatoxins. A similar histologic lesion is seen after high doses of radiation therapy to the liver.

So-called *bridging necrosis,* accompanied by a substantial inflammatory response of mononuclear cells, has been reported in adults taking methyldopa or using laxatives containing oxyphenisatin. A similar lesion has been found after repeated exposures to halothane anesthesia, propylthiouracil, methimazole, and isoniazid. Along this same con-

Table 21-8. Some frequently encountered drugs capable of producing liver injury

Drug	Parenchymal necrosis			Cholestasis	Inflammation		Steatosis
	Focal	Extensive	Zonal		Portal	Diffuse	
Acetaminophen (poisoning)	+		+++	+			+
Amethopterin (methotrexate)			+				+
Ampicillin	+			+	++		
Azathioprine (Imuran)	++	+		+	+	+	
Chlordiazepoxide (Librium)	+			++	+		
Chlorpromazine (Thorazine)	+			+++	++		
Chlorpropamide (Diabinese)	+			+++	++		
Cimetidine	+			+			
Dantrolene sodium	++	+		++	++		
Diazepam (Valium)				++	+		
Erythromycin estolate (Ilosone)			+++	+			
Furosemide (Lasix)	++			+	+		
Gold therapy	+			++	+		+
Griseofulvin	+			+++	+		
Halothane		+++	++	++	++	+++	
Imipramine (Tofranil)	+				++	++	
Indomethacin			+++	++	++	++	++
Iron (poisoning)		+++	+++		+		
Isoniazid	+			+	+		
6-Mercaptopurine	+	+	++	+	+	++	++
Methimazole (Tapazole)	+			++	++		+
Methotrexate	++				+		
Methyldopa (Aldomet)	+		+++	+++	+++	+	+
Methyltestosterone				+++	+	+	
Nicotinamide			+	+	+		
Nitrofurantoin (Furadantin)	+			+++	+		
Norethandrolone (Nilevar)				+++	+		
Oxacillin	+			++			
Oxyphenisatin	++			+	+	++	
Para-aminosalicylic acid (PAS)	++			+	+++		
Penicillin	+			+	+		

	Parenchymal necrosis			Cholestasis	Inflammation		Steatosis
	Focal	Extensive	Zonal		Portal	Diffuse	
Phenobarbital			++		+		+
Phenylbutazone (Butazolidin)	+				+		
Phenytoin (Dilantin)	++			+ to +++	+	+	
Propoxyphene (Darvon)	++			+++	++	+	++
Rifampin		++	+				++
Salicylates	++	+			++		++
Sulfonamides	+++	+		++	+		+
Tetracyclines							
Oral (with coexistent renal disease)			+		++		++ to +++
Intravenous				+	+		+++
Triacetyloleandomycin (Cyclamycin)	+			++	+		
Tromethamine			+++		+++		
Valproic acid (Depakene)	+	++	++	+	+	+	+
Vitamin A	+			+	+		++
Vitamin B$_3$			+	+	+		+

Table 21-9. Some frequently encountered toxins capable of producing liver injury

Toxins	Parenchymal necrosis			Cholestasis	Inflammation		Steatosis
	Focal	Extensive	Zonal		Portal	Diffuse	
Arsenic	+		+++	+	++		+
Beryllium	+		+++		++		
Carbon tetrachloride			+++			+	++
Iron		++	+++		+++		+
Phosphorus			+++		++	+	
Senecio alkaloids			+++		++		
Tetrachlorethanes			+++				+++

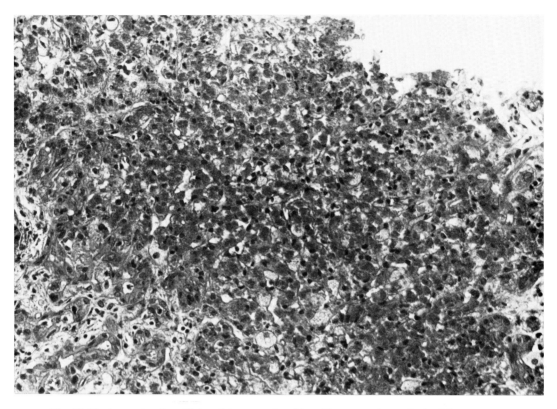

Fig. 21-13. Acetaminophen (Tylenol) hepatopathy. Liver biopsy specimen obtained from a young teen-ager 96 hours after self-poisoning with unknown quantity of the drug. Plasma acetaminophen level was greater than 300 μg/ml on admission, 72 hours after ingestion. Serum bilirubin was 15 mg/dl, and aminotransferase values were over 5000 IU. The prothrombin was prolonged and failed to correct with vitamin K. Liver biopsy specimen obtained after administration of fresh frozen plasma (10 ml/kg). Histologic appearance reveals some ballooned liver cells, large zones of shrunken necrotic hepatocytes with nuclear pyknosis, and the absence of inflammatory cells. (×100.)

tinuum of hepatic injury, a more aggressive histologic lesion, characterized by piecemeal necrosis, has also been seen with methyldopa and oxyphenisatin use, as well as with the antispasticity agent dantrolene sodium. *Centrilobular to generalized lobular hepatic necrosis* may be seen in severe acetaminophen (Fig. 21-13) and iron poisoning, in halothane reexposure, and after ingestion of *Amanita phalloides,* a poisonous mushroom. Less often, such injury patterns may be seen after extensive exposure to environmental toxins such as trichloroethylene, tetrachloroethylene, and trinitrotoluene.

A predominantly *cholestatic* liver-injury picture with or without features of acute hepatitis is typical of hepatic damage seen with phenothiazine-containing agents, and 17-alpha-substituted tes-

tosterone derivatives. Estrogenic oral contraceptives are notorious for producing a mixed hepatic injury pattern, predominantly cholestatic but with focal necrosis of hepatocytes. Reports of significant cholestatic liver injury have been found in children taking erythromycin estolate, nitrofurones, gold therapy for juvenile rheumatoid arthritis, and phenytoin (Fig. 21-14).

Certain hepatotoxins result in a predominant *steatosis* of the liver. This may be the small-droplet variety (microvesicular steatosis) as occurs after exposure to hypoglycins from ingestion of the akee fruit (Jamaican vomiting sickness) and at times with the anticonvulsant valproic acid (Depakene). The lesions mimic the histopathologic condition seen in Reye's syndrome. Mixed small- and large-droplet steatosis occurs after high-dose intrave-

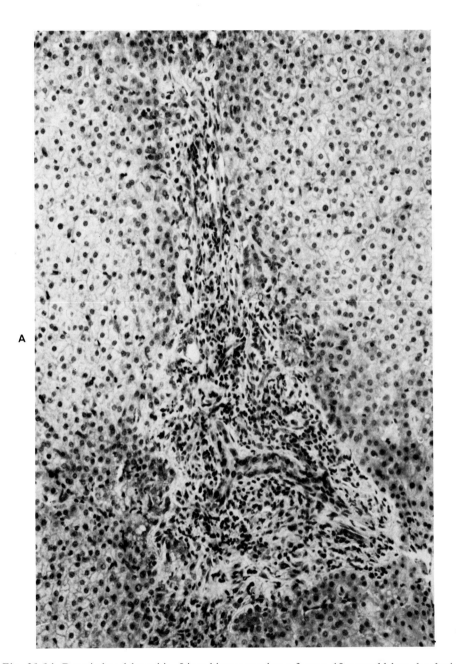

Fig. 21-14. Drug-induced hepatitis. Liver biopsy specimen from a 10-year-old boy developing jaundice 6 weeks after starting phenytoin (Dilantin) therapy for a seizure disorder. **A,** Inflammatory response is predominantly portal and pericholangiolar. *Continued.*

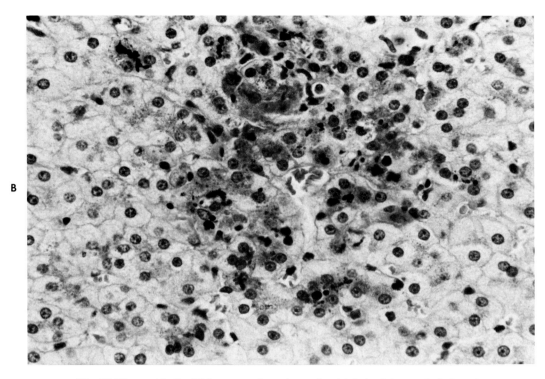

***Fig. 21-14, cont'd.* B,** High-power view shows focal lobular injury and cholestasis.

nous tetracycline therapy and also after chronic intake of excessive doses of vitamin A. For unclear reasons ethanol-induced hepatic steatosis is extremely rare in the pediatric population despite the reality of alcoholism existing in some junior and senior high school age students. A variable amount of fat accumulation predictably accompanies the hepatic injury from carbon tetrachloride and other environmental agents capable of acting as cellular protein poisons.

Changes of *neoplasia* can occur from a variety of substances with hepatotoxic potential. Chronic vinyl chloride exposure is associated with a high incidence of hepatic angiosarcoma. Benign nodular hyperplasia and adenomas can occur with chronic oral contraceptive use. Hepatomas may develop after the long (and short) term employment of androgen therapy in Fanconi's anemia.

Hepatic *granulomatous* changes may be induced by toxic substances, particularly beryllium, sulfonamides, hydralazine, and phenylbutazone. They may also be part of a foreign-body reaction in response to physical contaminants (talc) employed in the solubilization of parenterally administered illicit drugs (Fig. 21-15).

Last, *cirrhosis* changes caused by long-term use of hepatotoxic agents are more difficult to assign to a cause-and-effect relationship, but such progression is suspected with hepatic damage induced from methyldopa, oxyphenisatin, vitamin A, and continuous use of methotrexate (Fig. 21-16).

Diagnosis

As previously alluded to, a history of exposure to a potential hepatotoxin must be sought in all cases of clinically suspected acute liver disease, when otherwise unexplained biochemical tests suggest hepatic injury, and where suspicion is aroused by certain features noted on liver biopsy obtained for other reasons. Confirmation of involvement of hepatotoxic agents can at times be obtained by toxicologic screening tests of blood and occasionally urine. Indirect evidence can also be obtained when one observes clinical and biochemical improvement of the withdrawal from exposure. Confirmation is possible by the careful reintroduction of the suspected offender, though doing so is not without risk. This may be considered in special circumstances, particularly when no other choice of drug essential to the patient's treatment is available.

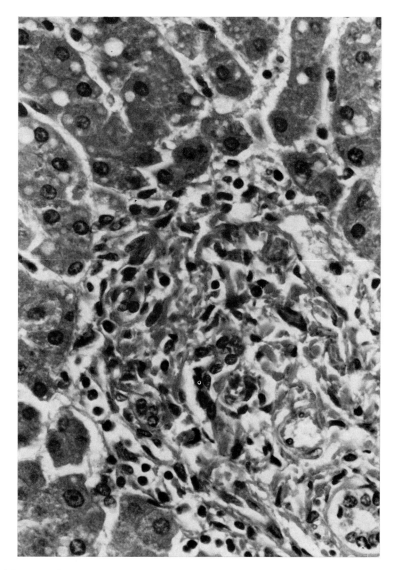

Fig. 21-15. Hepatic granuloma caused by physical contaminants (talc) incorporated into illicit drugs administered parenterally. Liver biopsy specimen obtained from a teen-age drug addict with abnormal liver function studies but HBsAg negative. The portal macrophage reaction is associated with evidence of phagocytosis of foreign material, best seen by polarized light. Steatosis of hepatocytes is also apparent. (×450.)

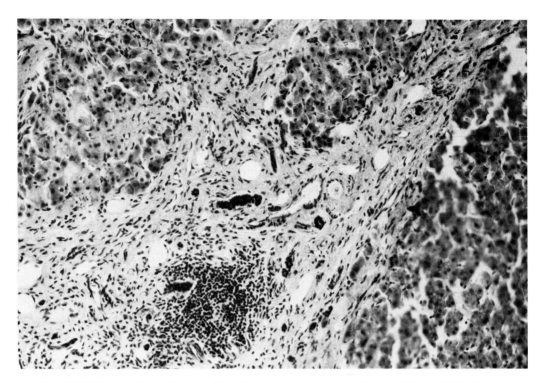

Fig. 21-16. Drug-induced cirrhosis. Liver biopsy specimen from a 9-year-old boy with leukemia previously treated for several years with methotrexate (amethopterin). The development of splenomegaly and hypersplenism (in the absence of other hematologic evidence of exacerbating leukemia), low serum albumin, and prolonged sulfobromophthalein retention prompted this biopsy. Evidence of cirrhosis is present, with portal fibrosis, intralobular septa, and nests of chronic inflammatory cells.

Treatment

Withdrawal of the offending agent is usually indicated as the primary thrust of treatment. This position may be tempered if it is known that the hepatic liver injury is mild and nonprogressive or that the drug is a necessary modality for the patient's overall well-being. Simply lowering the dosage of the drug may lead to resolution of both clinical symptoms and biochemical abnormalities and is especially applicable for those individuals who are "fast" acetylators and "slow" hydroxylators. Continued use of the drug in anticipation of the induction of new hepatic metabolic pathways for drug biotransformation is not recommended. Steroid therapy continues to have no proved value in drug-induced hypersensitivity reactions.

In cases of severe liver damage, employment of the supportive therapies described for the treatment of fulminant hepatic failure are often necessary (Chapter 23). Reducing the blood concentration of the circulating toxin is sometimes needed and can be accomplished by exchange transfusion, hemoperfusion over charcoal, dialysis, or forced diuresis with or without the use of chelating agents.

Glutathione administration is of no value, since it is not taken up by the liver cell. Currently, a large multicentered study in the United States is determining the effectiveness of N-acetylcysteine (Mucomyst) as an adjunct to therapy in the prevention of acetaminophen-induced liver injury. As previously noted with cysteamine, N-acetylcysteine is taken up by liver cells, where it is believed capable of binding with the toxic (arylated) metabolites of acetaminophen, thereby preventing hepatic injury. An oral loading dose of N-acetylcysteine, 140 mg/kg, followed by a maintenance amount of 70 mg/kg every 4 hours for 12 consecutive doses is employed. Early data suggest optimal results when the drug is administered within 10 to 12 hours of ingestion and in those persons with blood levels of acetaminophen greater than 200 mg/dl at 4 hours after ingestion.

Prognosis

Generally, the prognosis is good once the exposure to the offending hepatotoxin is eliminated. One can be less certain about this for environmental agents whose hepatotoxicity may have a long latency, as noted in vinyl chloride exposure and subsequent development of angiosarcoma. Progression to cirrhosis during continuous drug usage is possible with isoniazid by itself, or in combination with rifampin, continuous methotrexate usage, methyldopa, oxyphenisatin-containing laxatives, and occasionally acetaminophen and salicylates. Biliary cirrhosis is extremely rare but may occur after the continued use of phenytoin in toxic doses, phenothiazines, tolbutamide, and methyltestosterone. Resolution of the hepatic injury usually follows examples that result in veno-occlusive–like changes, as seen after the ingestion of *Senecio* alkaloids and from x radiation therapy. Where massive hepatic necrosis occurs, the prognosis is more likely to be dictated by the severity of the extrahepatic complications affecting the cardiovascular system, central nervous sytem, gastrointestinal tract, and kidneys. Full restoration of hepatic structure and function can, however, follow liver injuries of this magnitude.

REFERENCES

Aiges, H.W., Daum, F., Olson, M., and others: The effects of phenobarbital and diphenylhydantoin on liver function and morphology, J. Pediatr. **97**:22-26, 1980.

Black, M.: Acetaminophen hepatotoxicity, Gastroenterology **78**:382-392, 1980.

Chiprut, R.O., Viteri, A., Jamroz, C., and Dyck, W.P.: Intrahepatic cholestasis after griseofulvin administration, Gastroenterology **70**:1141-1143, 1976.

Coe, R.W., and Bull, F.E.: Cirrhosis associated with methotrexate treatment of psoriasis, J.A.M.A. **206**:1515-1520, 1968.

Dienstag, J.L.: Halothane hepatitis, allergy or idiosyncrasy? N. Engl. J. Med. **303**:102-104, 1980.

Gerber, N., Dickinson, R.G., Harland, R.C., and others: Reye-like syndrome associated with valproic acid therapy, J. Pediatr. **95**:142-144, 1979.

Gleason, W.A., deMello, D.E., deCastro, F.J., and Connors, J.J.: Acute hepatic failure in severe iron poisoning, J. Pediatr. **95**:138-140, 1979.

Goldstein, L.I., and Ishak, K.G.: Hepatic injury associated with penicillin therapy, Arch. Pathol. **98**:114-117, 1974.

Grishan, F.K., LaBrecque, D.R., and Younoszai, K.: Intrahepatic cholestasis after gold therapy in juvenile rheumatoid arthritis, J. Pediatr. **93**:1042-1043, 1978.

Hamlyn, A.N., Douglas, A.P., James, O.F.W., and others: Liver function and structure in survivors of acetaminophen poisoning, Dig. Dis. **22**:605-610, 1977.

Jacques, E.A., Buschmann, R.J., and Layden, T.J.: The histopathologic progression of vitamin A–induced hepatic injury, Gastroenterology **76**:599-602, 1979.

Kalow, W., and Inaba, T.: Genetic factors in hepatic drug oxidations. In Popper, H., and Schaffner, F., editors: Progress in liver diseases, vol. 5, New York, 1976, Grune & Stratton, Inc.

Krowchuk, D., and Seashore, J.H.: Complete biliary obstruction due to erythromycin estolate administration in an infant, Pediatrics **64**:956-958, 1979.

Lilly, J.R., Hitch, D.C., and Javitt, N.B.: Cimetidine cholestatic jaundice in children, J. Surg. Res. **24**:384-387, 1978.

Maddrey, W.C., and Boitnott, J.K.: Drug-induced chronic hepatitis and cirrhosis. In Popper, H., and Schaffner, F., editors: Progress in liver diseases, vol. 6, New York, 1979, Grune & Stratton, Inc.

McIntosh, S., Davidson, D.L., O'Brien, R.T., and Pearson, H.A.: Methotrexate hepatotoxicity in children with leukemia, J. Pediatr. **90**:1019-1021, 1977.

McVeagh, P., and Ekert, H.: Hepatotoxicity of chemotherapy following nephrectomy and radiation therapy for right-sided Wilms' tumor, J. Pediatr. **87**:627-628, 1975.

Menard, D.B., Gisselbrecht, C., Marty, M., and others: Antineoplastic agents and the liver, Gastroenterology **78**:142-164, 1980.

Mihas, A.A., Holley, P., Koff, R.S., and Hirschowitz, B.I.: Fulminant hepatitis and lymphocyte sensitization due to propylthiouracil, Gastroenterology **70**:770-774, 1976.

Mitchell, J.R., and Jollow, D.J.: Metabolic activation of drugs to toxic substances, Gastroenterology **69**:392-410, 1975.

Nogen, A.G., and Bremner, J.E.: Fatal acetaminophen overdosage in a young child, J. Pediatr. **92**:832-833, 1978.

O'Gorman, T., and Koff, R.S.: Salicylate hepatitis, Gastroenterology **72**:726-728, 1977.

Olans, R.N., and Weiner, L.B.: Reversible oxacillin hepatotoxicity, J. Pediatr. **89**:835-838, 1976.

Pessayre, D., Bentata, M., Degott, C., and others: Isoniazid-rifampin fulminant hepatitis, Gastroenterology **72**:284-289, 1977.

Perez, V., Schaffner, F., and Popper, H.: Hepatic drug reactions. In Popper, H., and Schaffner, F., editors: Progress in liver diseases, vol. 4, New York, 1972, Grune & Stratton, Inc.

Peterson, R.G., and Rumack, B.H.: Treatment of acute acetaminophen poisoning with *N*-acetylcysteine, J.A.M.A. **237**:2406, 1977.

Rumack, B.H., and Peterson, R.G.: Acetaminophen overdose: incidence, diagnosis and management in 416 patients, Pediatr. **62**(supp.):898-903, 1978.

Rumack, B.H., and Matthew, H.: Acetaminophen poisoning and toxicity, Pediatrics **55**:871-876, 1975.

Stein, M.T., and Liang, D.: Clinical hepatotoxicity of isoniazid in children, Pediatrics **64**:499-505, 1979.

Suchy, F.J., Balistreri, W.F., Buchino, J.J., and others: Acute hepatic failure associated with the use of sodium valproate, N. Engl. J. Med. **300**:962-966, 1979.

Tysell, J.E., Jr., and Knauer, C.M.: Hepatitis induced by methyldopa (Aldomet), Am. J. Dig. Dis. **16**:849-855, 1971.

Villeneuve, J.P., and Warner, H.A.: Cimetidine hepatitis, Gastroenterology **77**:143-144, 1979.

Wilkinson, S.P., Portmann, B., and Williams, R.: Hepatitis from dantrolene sodium, Gut **20**:33-36, 1979.

22 *Reye's syndrome*

In 1963, an Australian pathologist, R.D.K. Reye, brough into focus a clinicopathologic entity in children, characterized by an encephalopathy associated with noninflammatory fatty infiltration of several organs, particularly the liver and kidneys. With tremendous rapidity Reye's syndrome (RS), as it subsequently became known, suddenly emerged as the most common noninfectious cause of encephalopathy in the pediatric-age group and carried with it a distressingly high mortality. The number of documented cases now is well over 1000, which represents a doubling of cases reported in the past 5 to 6 years. It remains to be seen if this exponential increase of Reye's syndrome cases will continue, or if there will be a leveling off or even a decrease in the incidence over the next several years. As with any new condition, a variety of factors can usually be implicated to explain the early rise in numbers of reported cases. First, an increased awareness by pediatric care-givers and subsequently by the general medical community has led to early recognition and accurate identification of a cluster of clinical symptoms that suggest this condition, many of which are "mild" Reye's syndrome cases. In earlier years these latter examples perhaps would not have reached medical care or, if seen by a physician, would have been misdiagnosed as a "toxic" encephalopathy of unknown cause. Currently, a significant thrust in public education is taking place emanating from local lay organizations consisting of parents of Reye's syndrome victims and from larger foundations (National Reye's Syndrome Foundation), both types utilizing additional help from various news media sources. Because of heightened parental awareness of the symptoms suggesting Reye's syndrome, especially during epidemics, parents are indeed seeking early medical attention for their ill children. The dissemination of epidemiologic and demographic data from local and state health department agencies occurred after outbreaks of Reye's syndrome within their respective catchment areas, especially during the 1970s. This collation of statewide reporting on a national scale (Bureau of Epidemiology, National Center for Disease Control, Atlanta, Geor-

gia) began in 1973, and by 1977 the reporting of important epidemiologic observations once again furthered public and physician awareness of Reye's syndrome.

Based upon the results of retrospective review of autopsy materials (such as the liver, brain, and kidney) from children dying before the 1960s with a final diagnosis such as acute toxic encephalopathy, acute nonsuppurative encephalitis, acute serous encephalitis, infantile diarrhea with encephalitis, and acute brain swelling, Reye's syndrome indeed seems to be a new disease condition. Although many features in the clinical history of these cases were noted to be consistent with those reported in Reye's syndrome (vomiting, altered consciousness), microvesicular steatosis of the liver and kidney, the pathologic hallmark of this syndrome, was seldom found. Epidemiologists, geneticists, and other workers have been intrigued and puzzled by the recent emergence of this disease condition. In the continued absence of identification of a specific infectious cause, environmental factors, often implicated in other diseases over the past 30 years, again beg for active incrimination in this entity as well.

Epidemiology

Reye's syndrome has now been reported in most parts of the world but seems most prevalent in the United States, Canada, United Kingdom, Australia, Southeast Asia (Thailand), and the Union of South Africa. The greatest reported experience from the European continent has come from Czechoslovakia, with only infrequent reports emanating from France.

Almost from the time of the original description of Reye's syndrome, the disease was noted to occur more frequently in white, school-age children living in suburban or rural areas, rather than from inner-city children living in urban centers. Outbreaks of Reye's syndrome predictably surface in the older school-age child during seasonal (winter) epidemics of influenza virus or in the slightly younger school-age child when varicella-zoster viral outbreaks are common during the spring and summer months. Both influenza virus

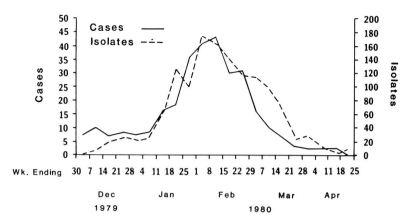

Fig. 22-1. Reported Reye's syndrome cases by week of onset of prodrome, and influenza B isolates by week of report, United States, November 30, 1979, to April 25, 1980. (From Morbid. Mortal. Weekly Rep. **29**:321, 1980.)

and varicella-zoster infection have age-specific affinities, and this best explains the difference in age ranges noted above. Sporadic cases of Reye's syndrome occur throughout the year, affect all age children, and seem to be temporally associated with a variety of viral agents. These instances reveal a less distinct geographic distribution of cases between urban and rural areas. In the preschool- and school-age child, the predominance of white (up to 90%) over Hispanics (10%) and blacks (2%) is quite striking. However, two recent reports have noted no racial predominance in the young infant (less than 12 months of age) with Reye's syndrome, and interestingly, most of these cases emanate from the inner-city population rather than the rural community.

In the past 10 years, nationwide outbreaks of Reye's syndrome have been epidemiologically associated with influenza B epidemics in 1973-1974, 1976-1977, and 1979-1980 and with the influenza A (N_1) epidemic in 1978-79. From December 1, 1979, to April 30, 1980, the most recent influenza B epidemic in this country, the U.S. Center for Disease Control reported 304 patients with confirmed Reye's syndrome (Fig. 22-1) in which 75% had associated respiratory symptoms, 15% diarrhea, 15% varicella. The overall case mortality for Reye's syndrome was put at 25% during this epidemic.

Although this concentration of Reye's syndrome patients seems impressive, it appears in fact to be an unusual complication of influenza B infection, with the estimated incidence being somewhere between 1 in 2000 and 1 in 100,000. In an epidemiologic study from Michigan, the maximum reported incidence of Reye's syndrome cases was stated to be between 30.8 to 57.8 per 100,000 cases of influenza B. In contrast, minimum and maximum rates of Reye's syndrome associated with influenza A (H_1N_1) infections were calculated at 2.5 to 4.3 cases per 100,000 influenza A infections. Present data suggest that not all influenza A viruses are similarly predisposed to produce outbreaks of Reye's syndrome. Despite reports of sizable community outbreaks of influenza A (H_3N_2) during the winters of 1975-1978, a significant clustering of Reye's syndrome cases was not seen. It remains unlikely that the influenza virus, especially B, has unique properties that lead to Reye's syndrome. Rather, the high attack rate of influenza viruses to produce clinical illness in susceptible children (greater than 25%) may fortuitously include those somehow predisposed to manifest Reye's syndrome. How the "unmasking" of susceptibles takes place remains unknown. Although not common, multiple cases of Reye's syndrome can occur in the same household, but recurrence of the disease has been reported in an occasional child after presumably different viral infections.

That a higher incidence of Reye's syndrome cases comes from the rural area or noncentral part of a city, rather than the urban inner-core settings, during influenza epidemics of similar proportion in all locations has led to speculation that factors outside a large city environment might somehow predispose to the evolution of this entity (Table 22-1). A simultaneous exposure to exogenous toxic substances, on either an acute or a chronic basis,

Table 22-1. Incidence of Reye's syndrome in 1974 in population younger than 18 years in Michigan.

Area	Total population	Total white population	Number of cases of Reye's syndrome	Number of cases of Reye's syndrome	
				Per 100,000 population	Per 100,000 white population
Rural	907,632	891,873	28	3.08	3.13
Other urban	310,541	291,972	1	0.32	0.34
Urbanized	2,031,525	1,638,976	16	0.79	0.98

Corey, L., and others: J. Infect. Dis. **135:**398, 1977.

which may include naturally occurring toxins (aflatoxins), herbicides, insecticides, chemical fertilizers, or spray-dispersal emulsifiers, can possibly result in an enhancing effect of the antecedent or concurrent viral illness that accompanies the history of Reye's syndrome. Additional support for this position comes from several previous epidemiologic observations. The clustering of Reye's syndrome cases reported in 1969 and 1971 from rural areas in northeastern Thailand were distinctly correlated with the latter part of the rainy seasons, a time when heightened contamination of food (rice) by aflatoxin B_1 is found. This toxin is produced by certain strains of the fungus *Aspergillus flavus,* which has worldwide distribution (see the discussion of etiology, p. 635). An outbreak of Reye's syndrome in Nova Scotia in 1972 was believed to be temporally associated with a recently completed insecticide spraying program against the spruce budworm. It is curious that the toxin-induced clinical pathologic picture seen in Jamaican vomiting sickness, clearly the result of ingested hypoglycin, mimics that of Reye's syndrome.

Though physicians and public health officers are aware that environmental factors may play an important role in the pathogenesis of Reye's syndrome, thorough epidemiologic investigation during several outbreaks has failed to reveal a common environmental toxin or exposure.

Proposed etiology and pathophysiologic mechanisms

Genetic and metabolic vulnerability. The concept of an underlying metabolic vulnerability continues to be popular for a number of reasons. First, the condition remains relatively rare in the face of widespread "unmasking" of potentially vulnerable subjects during specific viral epidemics, particularly influenza B. Second, an incidence of the disease higher than expected and higher than what can be explained by chance alone has been noted in siblings. Third, the similarity of the clinicopathologic expression of acute Reye's syndrome to other known inheritable defects in enzyme metabolism is striking and provocative. However, if a genetic and metabolic defect exists, the nature of which remains unknown, it will also have to explain the apparent age-related temporary vulnerability of this pediatric condition. Although the occurrence of Reye's syndrome in infancy (less than 6 months) is unusual, it does happen, but the magnitude of the vulnerability definitely increases with age, since the majority of cases occur during early school-age years between 5 and 12. One theory suggests that the at-risk individual undergoes an enhancement or conditioning process during these critical years. Some workers in this field believe that this is brought about by chronic exposure to subtoxic levels of environmental agents and, independently or in conjunction with specific viral infections, these conditioning events produce a temporary abnormality in the maturation process required for normal cellular responses to subsequent stresses. A reduced capacity to produce and respond to interferon inducers may be a mechanism by which certain toxics alter the host's response to viral infections. It is known that the young animal (rat) is more vulnerable to the effects of virus infection if "primed" by exposure to insecticides. In fact, the disease that evolves is not what one expected, but rather a Reye's syndrome–like picture is produced instead. It remains to be clarified, however, what underlying genetic predisposition is required to produce this temporary vulnerability. If genetic factors are not necessary, the vulnerability could be an acquired phenomenon by a chance sequence of interrelated events that eventually produce Reye's syndrome. At present neither chromosomal studies, nor HLA typing, nor dermatoglyphic examination of Reye's syndrome patients has uncovered evidence to support an underlying genetically linked vulnerability.

As suggested above, the observation that the clinical, biochemical, and pathologic picure of Reye's syndrome is also found in other pediatric inborn errors of metabolism has continued to provide the impetus that would, we hope, uncover in patients with Reye's syndrome a similar underlying explanation. Particularly, a great deal of effort has been directed toward establishment of a link between Reye's syndrome and enzymatic defects in the urea cycle (Fig. 22-2). As in Reye's syndrome, symptomatic patients with carbamoyl phosphate synthetase I (CPS) deficiency and those with either form of ornithine transcarbamoylase (OTC) deficiency manifest central vomiting and altered consciousness, and blood studies invariably reveal hyperammonemia, elevated transaminases, and hypocitrullinemia. Analysis of liver biopsy tissue during acute Reye's syndrome has indeed revealed a quantitative reduction, but not an absence, of both of these mitochondrial enzymes. However, the suspected lack of specificity of these observations in patients with Reye's syndrome and the differences in pathologic condition have been substantiated by recent data. Neither the microvesicular steatosis nor the ultrastructural changes in the mitochondria, believed to be relatively specific for Reye's syndrome, are present in the liver tissue of symptomatic patients with either the hemizygous lethal form (X-linked) of OTC deficiency or the heterozygote female with recurrent clinical symptoms. Similarly, liver tissue taken from patients with CPS deficiency lacks the histologic picture of Reye's syndrome. Therefore the hyperammonemia, common to all these entities (Reye's included), is a necessary prerequisite neither for the hepatocyte mitochondrial injury, nor for the low-enzyme levels of OTC or CPS. Rather, other factors must be responsible for the mitochondrial damage in Reye's syndrome, and the reduced activities of OTC and CPS noted are apparently secondary to these unknown events. The infrequent documentation of significant levels of orotic acid in the urine of patients symptomatic with Reye's syndrome makes doubtful the evolution of important OTC deficiency. Orotic acid is predictably present in the urine of symptomatic OTC-deficient patients and is believed to represent the metabolic end product of accumulating excess carbamoyl phosphate. Under conditions of increased protein load or intercurrent infection, OTC-deficient individuals produce excess carbamoyl phosphate, which leaks out of the mitochondria, to be further metabolized by cytoplasmic enzymes to orotic acid (Fig. 22-2). Experimentally, orotic acid does interfere with lipoprotein synthesis and theoretically could contribute to the fatty acid accumulation at least in patients with Reye's syndrome, but again microvesicular steatosis is not present in significant amounts in liver tissue of patients who have OTC. It is possible, however, that the reduced activity of these urea-cycle enzymes plays an important but not primary role in the hyperammonemia of patients with Reye's syndrome.

Several other known inborn errors of metabolism produce a somewhat similar cluster of clinical-biochemical-pathologic abnormalities as that seen in Reye's syndrome. These conditions usually present in infancy and are similarly triggered by either an intercurrent illness or a dietary indiscretion that stresses the infant's underlying biochemical defect. Clinical symptoms usually include vomiting, followed by seizures or altered consciousness, and the serum ammonia and transaminases are elevated. Hepatic steatosis may in fact be seen on liver biopsy in these entities. This group includes those with defects in the metabolism of the branched-chain amino acids, isovaleric acid and valine, and disordered metabolism of methylmalonate and propionate. The resulting organic acidemia, consisting primarily of short- and medium-chain fatty acids or dicarboxylic organic acids, is believed responsible for the clinical pathologic condition. In contrast to Reye's syndrome, these disease conditions usually occur in infancy and are manifested by recurrent episodes of crises, seizure disorders, and mental and developmental retardation. Although levels of total fatty acids are elevated in Reye's syndrome, the values for short- and medium-length fatty acids do not approach the levels reported in the above entities. In Reye's syndrome the free fatty acidemia is believed to be a phenomenon secondary to failing glyconeogenesis and increased lipolysis. An additional contribution to the fatty acidemia in Reye's syndrome comes from a decrease in lipoprotein formation and interference with beta oxi-

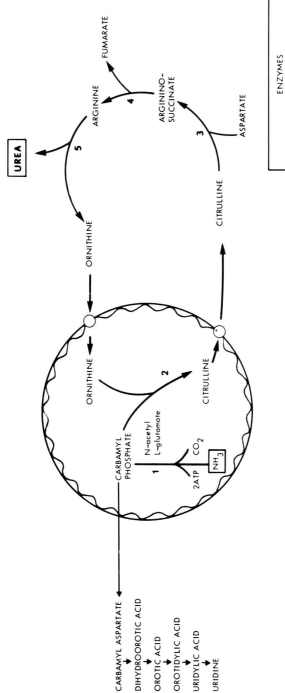

Fig. 22-2. The urea-cycle and alternate pathways for the elimination of ammonia. Intramitochondrial enzymes believed to be low in Reye's syndrome are carbamylphosphate synthetase I and ornithine transcarbamylase, resulting in hypocitrullinemia and elevated blood ammonia. *1,* Carbamyl phosphate synthetase I; *2,* ornithine transcarbamylase; *3,* argininosuccinate synthetase; *4,* argininosuccinate lyase; *5,* arginase. (Modified from Gelehrter, T.D., and Snodgrass, D.J.: N. Engl. J. Med. **290:**430-433, 1974, by permission.)

dation of fatty acids at the mitochondrial level.

Another inborn error of metabolism that may mimic Reye's syndrome is systemic carnitine deficiency. A microvesicular steatosis is reported during the acute episodes, which are manifested by vomiting and encephalopathy. The biochemical abnormalities include elevated transaminases, hyperammonemia, and hypoglycemia. The consequences of carnitine deficiency produce an impairment in the intracellular transport of fatty acids into the mitochondria, negating sufficient beta oxidation of fatty acids. A failure in ATP production occurs, and since ATP is needed in the initial step of the urea cycle (Fig. 22-2), increasing levels of ammonia accumulate. However, carnitine deficiency has not been found in liver tissue obtained from patients with Reye's syndrome. On the contrary, both free carnitine and total carnitine levels are elevated three to 10 times in the liver cells of patients with Reye's syndrome.

Although an underlying inborn error of metabolism is an attractive explanation for the unique vulnerability of patients who develop Reye's syndrome, it seems difficult to accept this concept, given the temporary nature of this disease and the infrequency of recurrences, despite an apparent constancy of exposure to both viral infections and environmental conditions.

Exogenous factors. That either single, or multiple, exogenous factors exert a synergistic effect during the illness associated with Reye's syndrome has been emphasized repeatedly from epidemiologic studies showing the geographic clustering and rural distribution of cases, especially during epidemics associated with influenza B infections.

Viral infection. Almost all cases of Reye's syndrome are associated with a presumed or proved viral illness. Symptoms of Reye's syndrome almost always begin shortly after apparent recovery from an antecedent illness and less frequently are superimposed upon those of the viral infection. Although most cases of Reye's syndrome are associated with the myxovirus group (influenza B and A) and varicella-zoster virus (chickenpox), a host of other viruses have been incriminated in sporadic cases. These include enteroviruses, the Epstein-Barr virus, polio virus, rheoviruses 1 and 2, coxsackieviruses A and B, adenovirus, herpesvirus, and mumps virus. If, however, the viral infection indeed alters the host, it must do so very early during the infection and in a very subtle manner, since neither histologic evidence of inflammation is present, nor has virus isolation from the critically involved organs (liver, brain, kidney) been successful. The temporary ''dysfunctional'' state perhaps remains dormant and awaits another yet unknown triggering event before the entire disease process evolves.

Up to now, nothing special has been identified about the influenza or varicella-zoster groups that could account for the high prevalence of Reye's syndrome during epidemics of these infections. The substantial attack rate (virulence) of both these agents in susceptible children has been known for a long time (25% to 75%) and probably explains the association of Reye's syndrome during large outbreaks of tbse infections; by sheer numbers they simply serve to ''unmask'' those at risk to develop Reye's syndrome.

Environmental toxins. The potential importance of this component in the evolution of Reye's syndrome continues to deserve maximum attention. The abrupt onset of the clinical picture suggests a toxic cause, especially in the face of a noninflammatory histologic appearance. The demographic data suggest that environmental factors could explain the greater number of cases seen in rural communities than that in urban ones during epidemics of influenza B infection. A chronic, subtoxic exposure of the host may be more important than a sudden acute environmental alteration in this disease condition. In fact, an acute exposure phenomenon has been associated with but one outbreak of Reye's cases (Nova Scotia) and was believed related to a previous insecticide-spraying campaign. Chronic subtoxic exposure to ingested or inhalant environmental toxics, such as insecticides, herbicides, chemical fertilizers, and dispersing agents might be more frequent in rural children and somehow predispose them to Reye's syndrome.

Two naturally occurring toxins clearly produce a Reye's syndrome–like illness. *Aflatoxin B_1* produced by the fungus *Aspergillus flavus* has been implicated in the endemic outbreaks of Reye's syndrome in young children living in rural areas of Thailand. This toxin is found in high concentration in the food and water supply of rural communities after the rainy seasons. Indeed, high concentrations of aflatoxin were present in the tissues of 22 of 23 children dying of Reye's syndrome after such an epidemic. Although *aflatoxin B_1* had been found in the blood and urine of children during acute Reye's syndrome, the amounts are not significantly different from those in controls. In the United States, aflatoxin-contaminated food sources, especially in the southeastern part of the country, include grain products such as cornmeal and cornbread, some cereals, occasionally nuts, peanut butter, and hypoallergenic milk substitutes. Chronic ingestion in endemic areas might allow for a slow accumulation of aflatoxin in the liver of the at-risk group. Although aflatoxin exposure of this small magnitude is itself unlikely to be responsible for Reye's syndrome, the toxin is suspected to be one of the interrelated factors considered necessary to bring about the full expression of the disease.

The other naturally occurring exogenous toxin that upon ingestion produces a Reye's syndrome–like illness is the compound *hypoglycin,* a substance found in the unripe fruit of the akee, *Blighia sapida.* The active metabolite methylenecyclopropylacetic acid acts by inhibiting the transport of fatty acids into the mitochondria and also inhibits the dehydrogenation of 6- to 10-carbon dicarboxylic CoA esters. Failure of complete oxidation of these products allows for their accumulation, and a large, but specific urinary excretion of both dicarboxylic acids and short-chain fatty acids can be used to identify this hypoglycin-induced illness. However, neither methylenecyclopropylacetic acid nor increased amounts of these dicarboxylic urinary metabolites are found during the acute phase of Reye's syndrome.

Although a definite cause and effect concerning the direct role of environmental toxins in producing Reye's syndrome is still lacking, a synergistic effect between toxins and viruses remains a distinct possibility. Examples of enhanced and altered expression of viral disease, with increased fatality, can be produced by pretreatment of especially young animals with such agents as DDT, organophosphates, polychlorinated biphenyls, solvents, and emulsifiers. Many of these agents are common to rural areas, but again the demographic data fail to show an unusually high level of exposure to any of the substances during outbreaks of Reye's syndrome.

Drugs. That certain medications may be playing a role in the evolution of Reye's syndrome has been suspected since the early recognition of this entity. Two classes of drugs have received the most attention—antiemetic and antipyretic agents.

Because vomiting is an almost constant clinical feature of Reye's syndrome, it is not surprising that antiemetic products have frequently been employed in an effort to abate this symptom. That these products administered orally, or as a rectal suppository, can increase the morbidity or mortality in Reye's syndrome has never been proved by any controlled study, but the possibility cannot be eliminated at present. Many of these antiemetic agents also contain phenathiazines, barbiturates, and antihistamines, all capable of altering the level of consciousness or producing extrapyramidal signs, either of which may be confused with the central nervous system manifestations of acute Reye's syndrome. Furthermore, many of these agents contain ingredients that have a hepatotoxic potential, and in this altered host an "activated" metabolic state might exist in the hepatocytes, which then favors the evolution of Reye's syndrome.

Of the two most widely used antipyretics, aspirin (ASA) rather than acetaminophen may be playing an unknown role in the development of Reye's syndrome. A recently conducted case control study of Reye's syndrome by the Ohio State Department of Health found increased use of salicylates during the antecedent illness in Reye's syndrome cases in comparison to that in controls (97% versus 71%), whereas acetaminophen was used less frequently in Reye's syndrome than that in controls (16% versus 32%). Similar studies with smaller numbers of patients in Arizona and Michigan also yielded essentially the same results. Although ASA has hepatotoxic potential for some individuals even in therapeutic doses, significant elevations of serum salicylate levels are seldom found during the acute phases of Reye's syndrome. This is not surprising since most often the aspirin is taken during the antecedent illness, which has resolved 3 to 7 days earlier, and the drug usage discontinued. But even when the acute Reye's syndrome begins superimposed upon the intercurrent illness, elevated salicylate levels are most unusual. The concept of drug hepatotoxicity developing with therapeutic dosage is plausible if a metabolically activated or even dysfunctional state exists in the hepatocyte at the time the drug is ingested. Although a causal relationship cannot be inferred, the similarity of known derangements reported in patients with Reye's syndrome and those produced by ASA toxicity is striking. Aspirin is capable of uncoupling oxidative phosphorylation, especially the oxidation of cytochrome *c,*

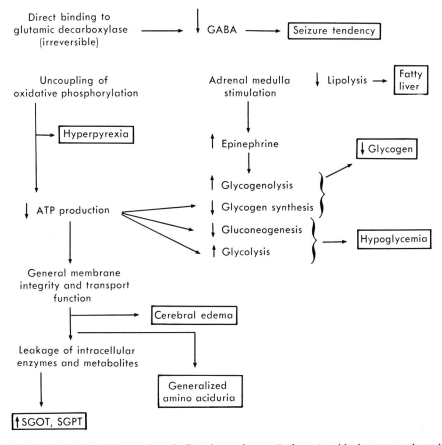

Fig. 22-3. Similarity of observations in Reye's syndrome *(in boxes)*, with the proposed mechanisms for the toxic effects of aspirin.

the terminal phosphorylation step, and may result in decreased ATP production. Salicylate also inhibits succinic acid dehydrogenase whose activity is depressed in patients with Reye's syndrome. In addition, ASA is believed capable of interfering with the transport of cytoplasmic ornithine into the mitochondria. Many findings of Reye's syndrome could fit into this mechanism (Fig. 22-3). Certainly, decreased glycogen synthesis, decreased gluconeogenesis and increased glycolysis result in hypoglycemia and hypoglycorrhachia. Again, loss of cell-membrane integrity results in defects in cell transport mechanisms and can in turn cause cerebral edema, elevated transaminase levels, and generalized aminoaciduria, all frequently noted in patients with Reye's syndrome. The American Academy of Pediatrics has taken the position that aspirin-containing products be avoided in children suspected of having an influenza-like illness or chickenpox.

Endogenous factors. Ever since the constancy of biochemical abnormalities was recognized in the acute phase of Reye's syndrome, there have been attempts to identify the exact role of these endogenously produced substances in Reye's syndrome. The large number of metabolic derangements identified in these patients reflects the magnitude of the disturbance in homeostasis that evolves during the illness. Determining the exact sequence of metabolic events responsible for these findings is handicapped by the known interaction of many identified accumulating substrates. Some have similar modes of action; others act synergistically to produce secondary and tertiary disturbances in cellular function. Up to now, the two endogenously produced toxins that have received the greatest attention include ammonia and free fatty acids.

Ammonia. Hyperammonemia is a biochemical requirement in the definition of Reye's syndrome. This protein derivative accumulates very early in the evolution of the disease, probably as a result of widespread tissue breakdown, especially muscle, but also from the host's generalized efforts at gluconeogenesis. The substantial nitrogen load in turn overwhelms the metabolic pathway for urea formation, perhaps already handicapped from concomitant mitochondrial injury in hepatocytes, as reflected in decreased activity of the enzymes carbamoyl phosphate synthetase and ornithine transcarbamoylase. A large urinary excretion of nitrogen results, but not in the form of urea. As mentioned previously, the increase in ammonia is not by itself believed responsible for the mitochondrial damage in hepatocytes. Other cellular events, perhaps those related to the impaired metabolism of fatty acids, affects mitochondrial function.

A major toxic role for the increased ammonia levels in Reye's syndrome has been assigned to the evolving encephalopathy because a reliable correlation exists between the serum ammonia level upon admission, the depth of coma, and the subsequent outcome of the patient. A heightened sensitivity of neuronal function to increased circulating ammonia levels has been postulated in patients with Reye's syndrome and has been likened to that observed in the portal encephalopathy of chronic liver disease. Whether these reactions are directly or indirectly mediated by ammonia is unknown, but potentiation is likely from other circulating toxins. However, the capacity of deaminated serum from patients with Reye's syndrome to adversely affect mitochondrial function has been noted in recent in vitro studies, which, if confirmed, would weaken the argument that elevated blood ammonia levels are playing a primary role in the ongoing events of patients with Reye's syndrome.

Fatty acids. It is still not known whether the free fatty acidemia consistently found in Reye's syndrome reflects the primary and crucial triggering event in the evolution of this condition. The data reported from experimental animal studies show that the administration of short- and medium-chain fatty acids convincingly induces an encephalopathy and pathologic lesion similar to Reye's syndrome. However, it remains difficult to transpose those observations to humans with Reye's syndrome where the host has been altered by a variety of additional factors (virus, drugs, exogenous toxins). The free fatty acidemia of patients with Reye's syndrome is believed primarily to be the result of excessive lipolysis in adipose tissue stores in response to gluconeogenic demands by

the ill host. Indeed, elevations in blood cortisol, growth hormone, glucagon and epinephrine, and insulin levels are commonly found during the acute phase of this disease. As happens with the increased nitrogen load, the excessive production of free fatty acids likewise finds relative impairment of hepatocyte function, and steatosis ensues. The mitochondrial injury, which is believed to include impairment of beta oxidation of fatty acids, may be self-perpetuating by substrate accumulation, though this has not been proved. It is surprising that a decrease in available ATP, which should result from presumed uncoupling of mitochondrial oxidative phosphorylation by free fatty acids, has not been confirmed in liver tissue obtained from patients with Reye's syndrome during the acute illness. Furthermore, in vitro studies fail to demonstrate a reversal of mitochondrial respiratory function alterations produced by Reye's syndrome serum after binding of free fatty acids by addition of albumin. Another alternative to impaired beta oxidation is that intrahepatic lipid accumulates as a consequence of elevated orotic acid concentrations. This metabolic by-product of the urea cycle, in turn, can interfere with prebetalipoprotein and betalipoprotein formation, for without the availability of these apoprotein moieties, lipid cannot be exported out of the hepatocyte. The accumulation of free fatty acids, either directly or synergistically with other metabolic intermediates also having detergent-like properties, further damages the mitochondrial membrane, impairs the urea cycle, and in turn leads to the accumulation of ammonia.

The present evidence favors the likelihood that these two major endogenous "toxins," ammonia and fatty acids, synergistically produce the encephalopathy of Reye's syndrome. Together they are capable of inhibiting oxidative metabolism and the energy-producing needs of neurons and brain capillary endothelium cells, which in turn favors the development of cerebral edema and coma.

Reye's "serum factor." That the mitochondrial injury may yet be caused by circulating factors other than ammonia or free fatty acids has come from recent in vitro studies. Serum from patients with Reye's syndrome obtained during the acute phase of the illness was still capable of impairing the respiratory function of rat liver mitochondria after deamination, and after incubation with bovine serum albumin to bind free fatty acids. The "serum factor" was also present after ultrafiltration that eliminated substances of greater than 2000 molecular weight and seemed to act in a concentration-dependent manner, either as an uncoupling agent at the latter steps of the electron-transport chain (stage IV respiration), or by alteration of the sodium flux in mitochondria. A substance with these properties, accumulating in the serum of patients with Reye's syndrome, would be capable of disrupting the energy-linked function in mitochondria, and neuronal tissue may be the most sensitive, since central vomiting and encephalopathy are the first clinical symptoms to appear. Cerebral edema may be a consequence of this "serum factor" affecting cellular energy functions, or sodium fluxes, and thereby altering capillary endothelium lining permeability of the blood-brain barrier. Cases of predominantly central nervous system involvement of Reye's syndrome with minimal liver enzyme elevation are not uncommon, especially since increased awareness and sensitivity to this diagnosis has been forthcoming. However, as previously noted, the resulting energy deficiency (of ATP) at the mitochondrial level has been entertained, but not proved, by analysis of liver tissue taken from patients with Reye's syndrome during the height of their illness.

Again, one cannot ignore the possibility that other already identified endogenous "toxins" (ammonia and short-chain free fatty acids), accumulating from mitochondrial injury, play a synergistic role in the presence of the "serum factor."

AMP-hypoxanthine-salvage defect. The data from another experimental model using platelet-rich plasma obtained from patients with Reye's syndrome suggest that the abnormality in energy formation comes about from a disturbance in purine metabolism that results in lack of salvage of AMP to ATP. This impaired synthesis (or wastage) of ATP is accompanied by high losses of hypoxanthine (in urine?) and an elevation in serum pyrophosphate. In this particular model, low ATP and ADP levels were consistently found in patients with Reye's syndrome during the height of their encephalopathy while AMP, hypoxanthine, and xanthine values were within the normal range. There is some evidence suggesting that accumulation of pyrophosphate can also affect the anabolic activities of ATP by substrate inhibition.

Abnormal serum amino acid pattern. The hyperaminoacidemia in Reye's syndrome consists especially of elevated levels of glutamine, alanine, α-amino-*N*-butyrate, and lysine. Although other amino acids such as tyrosine and valine may also be elevated, this finding tends to occur in more severe cases. The role of elevated aromatic amino acids, especially tyrosine and its metabolite tyramine (a reflection of the disturbance in hepatic function), has also been considered as possibly an important substrate in the encephalopathy of this disease. The use of this secondary pathway of tyrosine metabolism could singly be attributable to overloading of the usual metabolic pathway with 4-hydroxyphenylpyruvic acid, or in combination with a deficiency of the necessary enzyme tyrosine transaminase (Fig. 22-4). In addition, reduced levels of brain dopamine and norepinephrine, with increased octopamine concentration, have been found in patients with Reye's syndrome suggesting increased use of the alternate pathway of tyrosine to tyramine and thence to octopamine. This last metabolite (octopamine) has been assigned a role in the encephalopathy of classic chronic liver disease by a "false" neurotransmitter mechanism. The accumulating "false" neurotransmitters, octopamine and tyramine, may then act to displace dopamine from brain tissue, which in turn accumulates in ventricular fluid of patients with Reye's syndrome. The finding of increased prolactin levels in both the serum and ventricular fluid of patients with Reye's syndrome may also reflect the reduction in brain (hypothalamic) dopamine concentration, since dopamine and catecholamines are believed to exert an inhibitory effect upon prolactin release by the anterior pituitary gland. The correlation between blood tyramine levels and the severity and duration of encephalopathy seen in Reye's syndrome is similar to that ascribed to the elevated blood-ammonia levels.

An unrelated but important observation derived from studies of the hyperaminoacidemia in Reye's syndrome was that the pattern found could differentiate those cases that might otherwise be confused with acute salicylism. The amino acid pattern in the latter condition tends to be normal, even when biochemical evidence of hepatic damage (elevated transaminase and hyperammonemia) is present.

Endotoxins. Using the *Limulus* assay, endotoxin-like activity has been found in the plasma and cerebrospinal fluid of children with Reye's syndrome. Presumably, increased circulating endotoxin is the result of heightened production from the gut flora, especially during times of stress, but, more importantly, it occurs in the face of im-

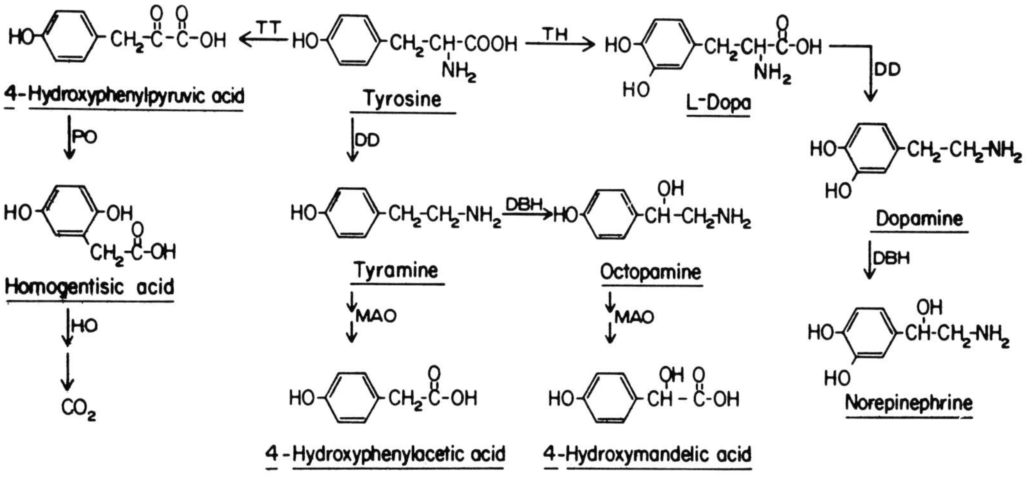

Fig. 22-4. Biosynthesis and metabolism of tyramine. In the enzyme system: *TT,* tyrosine transaminase; *TH,* tyrosine hydroxylase; *DD,* dopa decarboxylase; *PO,* 4-hydroxyphenylpyruvic acid oxidase; *HO,* homogentisic acid oxidase; *MAO,* monoamine oxidase; *DBH,* dopamine β-hydroxylase. (From Faraj, B.A., et al.: Pediatrics **64:**76-80, copyright, 1979, American Academy of Pediatrics.)

paired hepatic clearing function. Central hyperventilation is a known response to small doses of endotoxin reaching the brain. The degree of serum endotoxin-like activity is believed to bear a relationship to the severity of the encephalopathy, based upon observations of clinical features and electroencephalogram indices. Far-reaching effects of endotoxins are mediated by release of vasoactive substances, which in turn interfere with mitochondrial respiratory function, events implicated in the physiopathologic disturbances previously discussed in Reye's syndrome.

Clinical and laboratory features

There is typically a recognizable progression of the clinical syndrome. The child is usually young (most patients are between 3 months and 16 years). Antecedent or accompanying illness has been either a mild respiratory infection (influenza-like) or chickenpox. The child seems to be recovering or is actually well again, when vomiting of a pernicious nature ensues, and in the absence of a significant elevation of fever the patient becomes confused, agitated, and stuporous, within 2 to 8 hours. Occasionally, the vomiting is intermittent over a 24-hour period or longer. In the very young infant, the disease may be ushered in by seizures or an apneic episode. Physical examination reveals an agitated, confused, semicomatose patient with peculiar, rapid, and somewhat deep respira-

tions, which alternate with pauses of 5- to 10-second duration of very quiet breathing (Biot's respiration). Signs of dehydration are present, and the pupils are often slightly dilated and react slowly to light. Chest examination is normal, there is no jaundice, and the liver may be of normal size to mildly enlarged. Hyperreflexia and up-going toes are common neurologic findings. Although the child seems comatose, a reaction (withdrawal) to deep pain can usually be obtained. Sudden changes in posture are common. As the level of consciousness continues to decrease, spontaneous or stimulated posture responses may assume a decorticate, or the more worrisome decerebrate position. At times a seizure, particularly in the young child, may supervene and be followed by flaccidity. Constancy of occurrence of the clinical data from our earliest cases is shown in Table 22-2. The relative percentages of these findings have remained essentially the same over the years. The staging of the patient with regard to the level of coma is derived from the neurologic assessment at the time of admission and serially thereafter. Several classification systems exist, with most centers now using a modified Lovejoy scheme (Table 22-3). Accuracy in assigning the proper grade of coma to the patient has both therapeutic and prognostic implications.

The following results of certain laboratory studies are also required for the diagnosis of Reye's

Table 22-2. Clinical data in Reye's syndrome*

Clinical aspects	Number of patients
Historical features	
Age (years)	
Less than 2	6
2-5	10
6-10	9
11-16	9
Sex	
Males	15
Females	19
Prodromal illness	
Upper respiratory infection, "flulike"	27
Chickenpox	6
Mumps	1
Mode of onset	
Vomiting	31
CNS symptoms (lethargy, delirium, combative seizures, syncope, coma)	34
Physical findings	
Stage of coma on admission	
I	0
II	2
III	24
IV	8
Abnormal respirations (Kussmaul-like)	21
Jaundice	0
Hepatomegaly	8
Dilated pupils	31
Reactive-brisk	7
Reactive-sluggish	18
Nonreactive	6
Deep tendon reflexes	
Hyperactive (3 +, 4 +)	23
Babinski's sign	
Positive	26

*Based on 34 consecutive cases seen at The Children's Hospital and St. Anthony's Hospital, Denver.

Table 22-3. Criteria for clinical staging of coma in patients with Reye's syndrome at time of admission

Stage		Signs and symptoms
	0	Alert, oriented, normal response to painful, tactile, verbal, and visual stimuli
Precoma state	I	Drowsy, responds to commands but indifferent, usually remains awake
	II	Very lethargic, lapses into sleep when not disturbed, agitated responses to stimulation, disoriented, confused vocal responses, abnormal respiratory pattern, hyperventilates with agitation, hyperreflexic, pupils respond briskly
Coma	III	Predominantly comatose, does not verbalize or respond to command; inappropriate motor responses to local painful stimuli and generalized in nature, assumes decorticate or decerebrate posturing; pupils dilated, with sluggish responses to light; central hyperventilation, hyperreflexia, Babinski's sign often present; oculovestibular reflex (ice water caloric test) and oculocephalic reflex (doll's eye) preserved; infant and younger child may show Cheyne-Stokes or Biot's breathing pattern
	IV	Deep coma; decerebrate posturing and ridigity predominates; loss of oculovestibular (doll's eye) reflex, negative isocaloric test, absent pupillary response, absent pain response, corneal reflexes gone
	V	Flaccid, respirations irregular and gasping at times, pupils fixed and dilated, cardiovascular instability (hypotension, arrhythmia), signs of herniation (anisocoria, Cushing's sign)

Modified from Lovejoy, F.H., and others: Am. J. Dis. Child. **128**:36-41, 1974.

syndrome: (1) sterile spinal fluid, with less than 10 white blood cells per milliliter, and normal spinal fluid protein and sugar levels—if hypoglycemia exists, the latter may be commensurably lower; (2) elevated serum transaminase activity (SGOT) of at least twofold; (3) elevated blood-ammonia level over 1½ times normal (simultaneously checked against control); (4) prolongation of the prothrombin time (greater than 2 standard deviations from the mean). Many workers believe that at least three of these specific laboratory studies should be abnormal before one can make the diagnosis of Reye's syndrome. It is important to keep in mind, however, that on occasion manifestations affecting predominantly the central nervous system may evolve so rapidly that transaminase values may not be significantly elevated.

Other commonly found laboratory results in Reye's syndrome include the following:

1. Negative toxicology screen of blood and urine (If salicylates, phenothiazine, or acetaminophen is detected, these studies should be repeated serially.)
2. Bilirubin normal or less than 3 mg/dl
3. Mixed metabolic acidosis and respiratory alkalosis
4. Variable hypoglycemia (especially in younger patients)
5. Elevated creatine phosphokinase (CPK) and lactic dehydrogenase LDH values
6. Normal or elevated blood urea nitrogen
7. Mild leukocytosis
8. Hypophosphatemia
9. Serum and urine ketones present
10. Hyperaminoacidemia, especially of alanine, glutamine, α-amino-N-butyrate, and lysine

Other rare laboratory abnormalities include elevation of the serum amylase, evidence of a consumption coagulopathy (thrombocytopenia, decrease in factor VIII levels, and presence of fibrin split products). Serum complement activity may be depressed, especially C_1; rarely the BUN may be elevated above 30 mg/dl.

The EEG is diffusely abnormal with high-voltage slow-wave activity predominating. The type or grade of EEG pattern correlates with the various levels of precoma state or coma. Representative laboratory data from 34 patients presenting with Reye's syndrome is shown in Table 22-4.

Pathologic lesion. Stricter attention to the pathologic definition of Reye's syndrome has become necessary because of the increased numbers of so-called "mild" Reye's cases, coupled with the observation that other entities may in fact mimic at least the clinical features of this disease. Pathologic confirmation is also essential in those examples with recurrences of this clinical syndrome.

Brain. The severity of the global metabolic encephalopathy is believed to underlie the development of cerebral edema. Variable degrees of intracranial hypertension are present in almost all patients with clinical signs and symptoms of encephalopathy. The extreme examples of cerebral edema parallel the magnitude of the initial functional disturbance in these patients, which in turn probably determines the outcome for most patients. Grossly the brain is swollen, with fullness

Table 22-4. Laboratory data in Reye's syndrome*

Investigative tests	Number of patients
Blood	
SGOT elevated	33/33
Ammonia elevated	20/26
Prothrombin time prolonged	25/29
Bilirubin (less than 3 mg/dl)	26/27
Glucose (less than 60 mg/dl)	10/31
Salicylate present	10/27
Electroencephalogram	
Diffuse, slow, high-voltage	16
Other patterns	9
Virus isolations	
Myxovirus	1
Influenza A_2 England	1

*Based on 34 consecutive cases seen at The Children's Hospital and St. Anthony's Hospital, Denver.

and flattening of the gyri. Evidence of brainstem herniation, most frequently temporal (uncal), cerebellar, or tonsillar, may be present in autopsy cases and can explain certain clinical events. The histopathologic finding of diffuse cerebral edema is certainly consistent with many of the clinical features noted in these patients, that is, breathing abnormality, alternating decorticate and decerebrate posturing, pupillary abnormality, and hyperreflexia, though a circulating "toxin" may likewise be causative.

Microscopically, a mixed picture of diffuse neuronal edema and bland ischemic necrosis of neurons is most common, particularly in the periventricular area, cerebrum, and brainstem. Anoxic changes also include karyorrhexis, perineuronal and perivascular clearing, and nerve-fiber separation. Wallerian degeneration of white matter and transsynaptic degeneration can be found. Occasionally, focal microinfarctions are noted, and fatty vacuolation around small blood vessels are present in some patients. The endothelial cells of the brain microcirculation are usually hypertrophied and edematous. Electron microscopy of brain tissue shows altered mitochondria, with expansion of the matrix base and a striking reduction in the intramitochondrial dense bodies. At times the pathologic lesion of the brain cannot be distinguished from that commonly seen in "respirator brains." Many of these features are characteristic of a nonperfused organ. However, even in the severe examples, much of the neuronal injury is believed to be reversible, since most survivors will recover without neurologic deficits.

The opportunity for study of premortem routine and electron microscopic changes in the brain of patients with Reye's syndrome has only recently been available from therapeutic craniectomy procedures. Once again, mitochondrial alterations, astrocyte swelling, and myelin blebs have been noted, but no other unusual features have been found.

Liver. The striking changes in the liver are essential to accurate diagnosis (Fig. 22-5), but the entity can be strongly suspected without liver biopsy, especially during community outbreaks of the disease, if the previously described clinical history, physical findings, and results of critical laboratory tests are confirmatory. Some individuals recommend liver biopsy in all cases of suspected Reye's syndrome, whereas others make it mandatory only in special instances. When the presenting history is confusing or suggests other possible diagnoses such as ingestion of toxics and when recurrent episodes of a similar nature have been reported, in our opinion a liver biopsy is mandatory for specific diagnosis. In addition, we would recommend it in very young children or infants less than 6 months of age or the older adolescent and young adult where the disease is uncommon.

Percutaneous liver biopsy can be employed with minimal risk in these patients after particular attention to existing abnormal parameters of coagulation and their correction as indicated. We have not had difficulty with this procedure if the prothrombin time is greater than 40% and the partial thromboplastin time is not longer than 60 to 70 seconds (normal less than 45 seconds). On those occasions when bleeding studies are more severely affected, percutaneous liver biopsy can be done without anticipated complications immediately after the administration of fresh frozen plasma (10 ml/kg). In unusual circumstances a two-volume exchange transfusion may also precede the biopsy.

The liver tissue obtained by percutaneous biopsy can be recognized as abnormal by simple gross inspection in most cases. The tissue is pale and almost white in appearance, making one wonder at times whether it is indeed liver. Microscopically, diffuse microvesicular steatosis of the swollen hepatic cells is most apparent. The nuclei are not displaced, and the cytoplasm is pale, fatty,

and lacelike. Necrosis and inflammation are strikingly absent or minimal and when present are found in a portal to periportal distribution. Glycogen is virtually absent from the liver cells.

A much greater experience is available in assessment of the hepatic ultrastructural changes occurring during the course of the disease. The smooth endoplasmic reticulum is proliferated. Golgi saccules are empty, and peroxisomes are increased. The mitochondrial changes seen in liver biopsy specimens obtained early in Reye's syndrome include swelling and expansion of the matrix space, pleomorphism, alterations in the matrix substance itself, and loss of intramitochondrial dense bodies. These observations have been attributed to a chemically mediated process, though specificity has been questioned. The rapid reversibility of the ultrastructural changes has been noted, but unfortunately these events may not correlate positively with the final outcome. The liver biopsy taken after institution of medical therapies (hypertonic glucose, insulin, and so on) may show features suggesting improvement of metabolic function (Fig. 22-6).

Kidneys. The proximal tubule cells of the kidney are microscopically swollen and contain fat vacuoles. Recently, examples of acute tubular necrosis have been reported on biopsy from patients experiencing acute renal failure during the evolution of their disease. Whether this represents a different entity, or possibly the result of hypovolemia and osmotherapy, has not been determined.

Other organs and tissues. Other parts that may be involved in Reye's syndrome include *cardiac* and *skeletal muscle* and the *pancreas*. The pancreas has also been noted to show evidence of hemorrhagic necrosis with foci of ductal ectasia, inspissation of eosinophilic secretions, and edema suggesting acute pancreatitis.

Differential diagnosis

Although not always mutually exclusive, a pediatric patient presenting with evidence of an acute encephalopathy, who by history has been ill or is just recovering from an illness, conjures up somewhat different diagnostic possibilities than the same child said to be well and afebrile at the time symptoms of central nervous system dysfunction commenced (Table 22-5).

In the latter instance (well child) one should strongly consider the possibility of an *ingestion or exposure to some toxic substance or drug*. Human

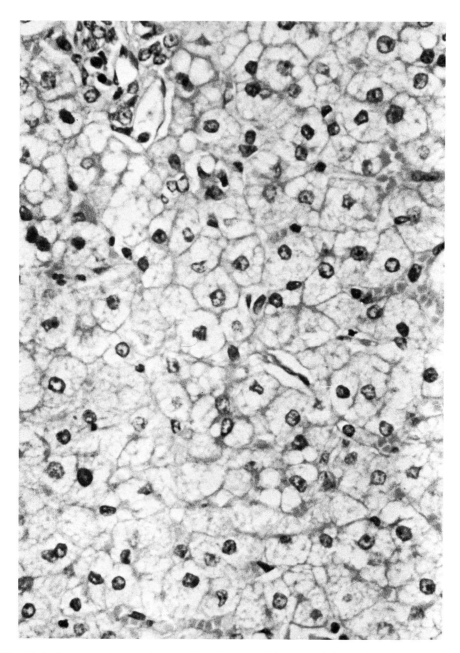

Fig. 22-5. Reye's syndrome. Autopsy liver from a child dying of this entity. The entire liver showed diffuse hepatic steatosis with random pyknosis. Overt degerative change or acute inflammatory reaction is absent. The lipid is generally diffuse with some vacuole formation, and the nuclei are centrally located within the cell. Five days before admission the child developed a mild upper respiratory infection with minimal fever and seemed to be improving. Six hours before admission, vomiting commenced and the child rapidly became stuporous. Physical examination revealed a semicomatose child with Kussmaul respirations who responded only to deep pain. There was no obvious icterus, acetone-like odor was present on the breath, and the liver was palpable 3 cm below the right costal margin. The deep tendon reflexes were hyperactive, and a bilateral positive Babinski's sign was present. The spinal fluid was acellular with a glucose content of 18 mg/dl. The blood glucose was 21 mg/dl. SGOT was 898 IU, bilirubin was 0.5 mg/dl, and prothrombin time was 15 seconds with a control of 12 seconds. Despite a variety of supportive measures including dexamethasone (Decadron), intravenous mannitol, cooling, and a 2-volume exchange transfusion, the patient died within 24 hours of admission. In addition to the typical hepatic lesion, pronounced cerebral edema and fatty vacuolization in the renal tubules were also noted in the autopsy material.

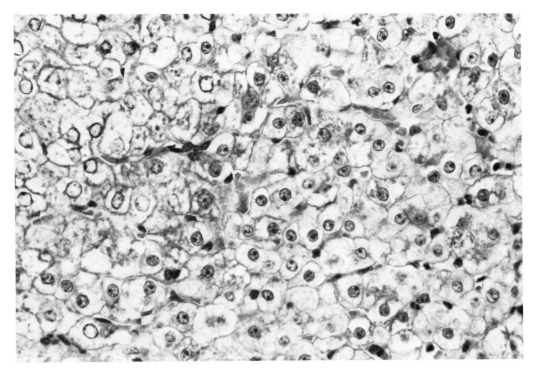

Fig. 22-6. Reye's syndrome. Percutaneous liver biopsy section from a child with clinical and biochemical features of Reye's syndrome only 24 hours after initiation of therapy (hypertonic glucose, insulin, and so on). Pale hepatocytes with minimal steatosis predominate, but glycogen nuclei and mitotic figures suggest improving liver function. Indeed, this child was awake and oriented 18 hours after the biopsy.

Table 22-5. Diagnostic considerations in encephalopathy of children

Previously well	Previously unwell
Toxic or drug ingestion or exposure	Meningitis (bacterial, viral, and so on)
Head trauma (known or "missed") (subdural or epidural hematoma)	Encephalitis
	Reye's syndrome
	Endotoxins or viral antigens (systemic febrile illness) (focal infection)
Hypoglycemia	Metabolic derangement (electrolytes, Ca^{++}, Mg^{++}, glucose)
Cardiac arrhythmias with hypoxia	
Postictal state	Toxic or drug exposure
Confusional migraine	Hypertension (renal disease)
Hypertensive crisis	Fulminant hepatic failure (hepatic encephalopathy
Reye's syndrome	Portal encephalopathy
	Congenital heart disease
	Status epilepticus or postictal state
	Latent inborn error of metabolism

exposure to naturally occurring endemic toxins (hypoglycins, aflatoxins) or the more globally used herbicides, insecticides, solvents, and hydrocarbons can produce a Reye's syndrome–like picture. Likewise, central nervous system symptoms may be the predominant toxic expression of drugs taken in therapeutic dosage or from overdose, be it accidental or self-induced. One should consider possible *head trauma,* either recent or old, as cause of the acute encephalopathy. So-called "missed" head trauma, where parents or other family members are unaware of the previous injury, is not uncommon in the pediatric population. A disturbance in carbohydrate metabolism with resulting *hypoglycemia* certainly may produce central nervous system manifestations. Although infrequently a cause of encephalopathy in a well child, *inborn errors of metabolism* may need to be considered and ruled out. These include the inheritable enzyme deficiencies in the urea cycle previously alluded to, certain organic acidemias (isovaleric, propionic, glutaric, methylmalonic) and carnitine deficiency. All have the ability to mimic the clinical features of Reye's syndrome.

On the other hand, *bacterial or viral infections of the central nervous system* need to be primarily considered in the unwell child developing an encephalopathy. Bacterial meningitis, viral encephalitis, brain abscess, or subdural empyema are possible explanations for the encephalopathy. In addition, a consideration should be given to such entities as *systemic febrile illnesses,* including meningococcemia, toxic-shock syndrome, relapsing fever, and even malaria. *Focal infections with a systemic component,* as from bacterial endotoxins or viral antigens, may produce an encephalopathic-like picture. In the face of an intercurrent illness, *metabolic derangements* in fluid and electrolytes or an imbalance in carbohydrate homeostasis may evolve and present with central nervous system symptoms. Renal hypertension from *acute or chronic renal disease* may present with an encephalopathy but again more often in a child who has been previously unwell. Rarely, *acute fulminant liver disease* with hepatic encephalopathy may occur before the appearance of clinical jaundice. An intercurrent illness may sufficiently stress the child with an underlying *congenital heart defect* and usher in a hypoxic encephalopathy. It is not uncommon for an intercurrent illness to unmask an *inborn error of metabolism* such as those mentioned above, and, once again, *toxin* and drug causes for the encephalopathy should be considered even in the unwell child with central nervous system symptoms.

The number of possibilities in the differential diagnosis of Reye's syndrome can often be reduced expediently by careful history taking, with special attention to the specifics of the present illness, and often by garnering of information about the child's past history and family history. Physical examination will also help to further sort toward the most likely diagnosis. Attention to the patient's vital signs on admission, presence of any unusual odors, respiratory pattern, evidence of trauma about the head or remainder of the body, the presence of meningeal signs, scleral icterus, liver size, and neurologic examination are most prudent and informative in this regard.

The results of laboratory studies and, when appropriate, an examination of liver biopsy material should permit clarification of the correct diagnosis. Bacteriologic culture of blood, cerebrospinal fluid, and urine will almost always be necessary. Toxicologic screening studies of blood and urine

are likewise most often required and should check particularly for the presence of salicylates, acetaminophen, phenothiazines, tricyclic antidepressants, anticonvulsants (phenytoin, phenobarbital, valproic acid, glutethimide (Doriden), and propoxyphene (Darvon). Other important blood tests to help in differentiating the specific causes of the Reye's syndrome–like illnesses should include examination of blood pH, electrolytes, calculation of the anion gap, blood glucose, BUN, liver function, blood ammonia, and coagulation. Evidence for hemolysis can be checked by examination of the peripheral blood smear. The urine should be surveyed for the presence of ketones and protein and screened for organic acids including orotic acid. In difficult or confusing cases, a liver biopsy may be extremely useful for one to arrive at the correct diagnosis. Most often, examination by light microscopy is sufficient, whereas at times electron microscopy of liver tissue is needed. Specific biochemical studies on frozen hepatic tissue may be required before the diagnostic dilemma can be resolved.

Treatment

Except for the mildest of cases, the requirements for treating Reye's syndrome have the potential to become extraordinarily complex. Since patients with Reye's syndrome may progress to deeper levels of coma over the first 24 to 72 hours of the illness, once initial stabilization of the patient has been achieved, referral to a pediatric center with intensive (critical) care capabilities is strongly recommended. Stabilization for most patients might involve blood-volume expansion with crystalloid to correct hypotension or dehydration, restoration of blood glucose levels, oxygen, antiseizure medications (phenytoin), or sedation with short-acting barbiturates, but osmotherapy (mannitol) and endotracheal intubation with assisted ventilation may be needed in more severe cases showing rapid progression to deeper levels of coma.

For the past few years a change in direction and emphasis of treatment has certainly contributed to the improved survival figures now reported for patients with Reye's syndrome. Undoubtedly, increased awareness of this entity and increased reporting of milder cases coming to treatment early in the course of the illness have also been responsible for the reduced, overall mortality figures. However, for those patients reaching the advanced stages of coma (stages III to V), the increased survival figures are a testimonial to improvements in critical care medicine, especially the objective management of cerebral edema vis-à-vis continuous direct measurement of intracranial pressure. The application of intracranial monitoring devices for use in pediatric-age patients has sustained the impetus and has shifted the primary focus of therapy in Reye's syndrome away from reduction of circulating toxins (ammonia and free fatty acids) by exchange transfusion, peritoneal dialysis, plasmapheresis, to maintenance of a normal intracranial pressure (ICP), cerebral perfusion pressure (CPP), and adequate oxygenation of the brain. At present, the lack of a specific etiologic agent and incomplete understanding of the sequence of pathologic events in this condition necessitate the use of therapeutic regimens that remain primarily supportive, but overall care should also be anticipatory in nature wherever possible. The added incentive to employ more invasive management in the severely affected patient comes from the observation that the mitochondrial injury and resulting generalized disturbance of cellular function is a reversible process, and survival of such carefully monitored and treated patients is attended by the high likelihood of full or near complete recovery.

Standard procedures and initial therapy

1. Base-line values of vital signs (blood pressure, pulse, respiration, temperature), patient's weight, a composite neurologic score based upon respiratory pattern, coma level and type of response to stimuli, pupil size and response to light, and urine output and ECG pattern should be promptly recorded. One should plan to repeat neurologic watch scores on an hourly basis, and the overall schedule for collecting this data can be adjusted depending on the patient's subsequent course.

2. Placement of intravenous, intra-arterial, central venous pressure lines, a nasogastric tube, and a bladder catheter should be accomplished as soon as possible.

3. Patients should be positioned with the head elevated to at least 30 degrees. Coordinating patient care activities will reduce the frequency of sudden changes in intracranial pressure.

4. Initially the patient should take nothing by mouth (NPO) and careful records of intake and output maintained.

5. The choice of intravenous fluids and rate of administration will depend upon clinical assessment of the degree of dehydration, existing hypovolemia, the results of serum electrolytes, BUN, and blood glucose values. The presence of a contracted vascular volume is confirmed when a low central venous pressure (CVP) and a decreased mean arterial blood pressure are found.

Initial expansion of the vascular volume can be accomplished by use of a solution of normal saline and 10% dextrose given 10 to 20 ml/kg over 1 hour. This "flush" may be repeated once again to accomplish the desired expansion of vascular volume (CVP 5 to 8 cm H_2O, mean blood pressure above 65 mm Hg). Thereafter, a 0.25 to 0.5 normal solution in 10% to 15% dextrose solution can be given at a rate to keep the sugar-free urine output at 1 to 2 ml/kg/hr and at a specific gravity of less than 1.020. Slightly lower than maintenance fluid volumes can be calculated from the patient's timed urine output plus 200 ml/m^2/day (for insensible fluid losses) and replace it in a 4-hour time period. Keep in mind that urinary losses of fluid and electrolytes may be substantial if osmotherapy is simultaneously employed, and more frequent replacement of these losses (every 2 hours) may be necessary to prevent a fall in the central venous pressure. The glucose concentration in the administered fluid should be adjusted to keep blood glucose values at 150 to 200 mg/dl or just below the level that produces glucosuria. If possible, one should avoid rapid fluctuations in blood glucose.

Sodium concentration in the replacement fluid should be adjusted to achieve serum levels of 140 to 145 mEq/L. The measurement of urine sodium losses can serve as a very useful guide in this regard. Potassium replacement is best given as a phosphate salt unless the serum phosphorus level is greater than 5.5 mg/dl or the serum calcium is found to be less than 8 mg/dl.

6. Vitamin K (3 to 5 mg) can be given intramuscularly and repeated in 12 hours if indicated. Should invasive procedures be contemplated or significant clinical bleeding is apparent, the abnormalities in coagulation are best corrected with an infusion of 10 ml/kg of fresh frozen plasma over 1 to 2 hours.

7. When the patient is in lighter stages of coma, the serum osmolality can be maintained at 315 to 320 mOsm/L. Adjusting the blood glucose concentration is sometimes sufficient to achieve this range of osmolality without additional anti-cerebral edema agents being resorted to.

8. Core temperature should be kept at 36.5° to 37° C by use of a heating or cooling blanket. Ideally, temperatures should be recorded from an esophageal probe, which is especially useful in those patients in deeper levels of coma.

9. Seizures are best treated with phenytoin (Dilantin) given slowly by intravenous infusion at 10 mg/kg. Repeat doses of 5 mg/kg every 12 hours can be further adjusted to achieve therapeutic blood levels by the results of direct assay.

10. Antibiotics (ampicillin, 200 mg/kg) is given intravenously if aspiration or pneumonia has occurred.

11. Sedation can be achieved by use of morphine sulfate 0.1 mg/kg and repeated as necessary.

12. Antacids can be administered through the nasogastric tube to achieve a gastric pH of greater than 3.5 units.

13. An electroencephalogram should be obtained initially. Brainstem-evoked potentials are particularly useful in those patients with progressive disease. The initial-pattern EEG has some correlation with outcome and is also valuable in evaluation of the effectiveness of presumed coma-producing blood levels of barbiturates.

Invasive procedures and therapies for patients in stage III to V coma

1. Endotracheal intubation should be carried out in those patients entering into or already noted to be in coma levels III to V. This procedure is best carried out by anesthesiology personnel using intravenous pancuronium bromide (Pavulon), 0.1 mg/kg, for muscle relaxation, often in combination with a short-acting barbiturate such as thiopental. Thereafter the patient's breathing is maintained by artificial ventilation to yield PaO_2 values of 100 to 150 mm Hg and a $PaCO_2$ of 23 to 25 mm Hg.

2. An intracranial direct-pressure recording device should be inserted by the neurosurgeon. One may choose either the subdural screw bolt, the Holter ventricular catheter, or the epidural placement of the Ladd fiberoptic intracranial pressure–monitoring device, depending on the experience of those involved in caring for these patients. As most patients are in the semiupright position, the zero pressure point is obtained by calibration of the device at the level of the ear. Prophylaxis with oxacillin or methicillin, 100 mg/kg/24 hr given every 4 hours, is recommended with the use of these devices.

3. Anti–cerebral edema efforts should be utilized to keep intracranial pressure (ICP) below 15 to 20 mm Hg and the cerebral perfusion pressure (CPP = Mean arterial blood pressure − Intracranial pressure) at not less than 40 to 50 mm Hg. Somewhat higher levels of intracranial pressure may be tolerated for brief periods of time provided that cerebral perfusion pressure remains adequate.

a. *Manual hyperventilation* for 2 to 3 minutes per spike episode is most efficacious in promptly lowering intracranial pressure. Manual hyperventilation should also be used in a prophylactic manner just before one carries out any noxious stimulus that is known to cause a rise in intracranial pressure, such as suctioning of the patient's endotracheal tube.

b. *Intravenous mannitol,* at 0.25 to 1 gm/kg, can be given over 20 to 30 minutes as the agent of choice for reducing sustained (or rebound) elevations of intracranial pressure. Large doses (2 gm/kg) of mannitol may be necessary in selected patients and be given every 2 to 4 hours provided that the serum osmolarity does not remain over 340 mOsm/L and urine output remains adequate. However, the dose of mannitol should be the lowest required to obtain the desired results. Abrupt cessation of this treatment after 3 or 4 days of its continued use increases the risk to hyperosmolar encephalopathy. Brain cells adapt rapidly to a hyperosmolar external environment by formation of "idiogenic" osmoles from presumably amino acids. Isotonic fluid can then shift into these "hyperosmolar" brain cells causing a rebound elevation of the intracranial pressure.

When the patient is in stage III to V coma and intracranial pressure is stubbornly above 15 to 20 mm Hg, serum osmolarity should be kept at 325 to 340 mOsm/L.

c. *Glycerol* (1.5 gm/kg) has been used as another adjuvant for treating cerebral edema and can be given through the nasogastric tube every 4 hours. Although less rebound effect is said to occur with glycerol than with mannitol, it seems to be less effective in producing as prompt a decrease in intracranial pressure. Larger doses may be tried.

d. Neurosurgical doses of *dexamethasone* (Decadron), 0.5 mg/kg every 6 to 8 hours, are still used by many workers. Although the value of this agent appears marginal in reducing cytotoxic cerebral edema, its use is recommended when an intraventricular monitoring device is employed.

e. A brisk *diuresis* may help lower the intracranial pressure, especially if hyperexpansion of the vascular volume is evident from rising central venous pressures, or excessive weight gain is noted with or without edema. Furosemide (Lasix), 1 to 2 mg/kg, can be given intravenously for this purpose.

f. The value of the *barbiturate coma* in treating both the encephalopathy and the raised intracranial pressure in severely affected patients awaits the results of a multicentered collaborative control study presently underway. A short-acting barbiturate, pentobarbital, can be successfully employed as an adjuvant in treating those patients who fail to respond to previously mentioned therapeutic efforts and intracranial pressure remains dangerously high. A loading dose of the drug can be given by slow intravenous infusion at 5 mg/kg over 30 minutes and repeated four times if neither significant hypotension nor alteration in cardiac function has occurred. The blood barbiturate level of 25 to 30 μg/ml is desirable though levels as high as 40 μg/ml may at times be necessary to achieve the desired result. Maintenance doses of 2 mg/kg/hr of the barbiturate given over a 15-minute interval is usually necessary thereafter and can be adjusted pending results of blood levels. Confirmation of barbiturate coma can also be obtained from the results of an electroencephalogram.

g. *Removal of cerebrospinal fluid* can be accomplished by use of the intraventricular catheter and is especially helpful in the management of sudden spikes of intracranial pressure not sufficiently lowered by manual hyperventilation.

h. *Bifrontal decompression craniectomy* has been used in some pediatric centers when all other measures have failed to control sustained elevations of intracranial pressure. Bone flaps are removed and stored and subsequently replaced 3 months after recovery.

4. In the slightly older child, placement of a pulmonary artery catheter (Swan-Ganz) is suggested and can provide valuable information regarding cardiac function, especially during barbiturate coma.

5. Efforts to lower the hyperammonemia have included both conservative and invasive therapies. The nonabsorbable antibiotic neomycin, at a dose of 500 mg every 6 hours, is given through the nasogastric tube. This drug may reduce the contribution of ammonia produced by bacterial action on intraluminal proteins and blood. The use of lactulose as another means of lowering the blood ammonia levels has not been regularly employed. The rationale for using the amino acid citrulline to reduce blood ammonia levels (by combining with aspartate) came from the observation that hypocitrullinemia exists in patients with Reye's syndrome, perhaps as a result of reduced levels of the enzyme transcarbamoylase. Since this enzyme is needed for normal citrulline production, with citrulline then being involved in the removal of a cytoplasmic ammonia group (that is, ammonia [NH_3] $\rightarrow$ glutamate $\rightarrow$ aspartate + citrulline $\rightarrow$ ornithine + urea), it seemed advantageous to provide this amino acid exogenously (Fig. 22-2). Citrulline given in doses of 100 mg/kg over several courses had been attributed to the survival of a few such treated patients. Unfortunately, the studies were poorly controlled in that peritoneal dialysis and exchange transfusions were simultaneously employed. An important objection to the use of this agent has been raised, in that the possibility also exists that citrulline may raise blood ammonia levels if the presumed carbamoyl phosphate synthetase deficiency also exists in Reye's syndrome. In this situation citrulline may then become an ammonia donor. The use of the amino acid precursor ornithine has also been suggested from experimental studies, which show that higher than physiologic levels of this amino acid may be necessary in patients with Reye's syndrome to saturate the enzyme ornithine transcarbamoylase to form citrulline. No control studies using either of these amino acids have been published at present.

More invasive therapies to reduce blood ammonia levels have included peritoneal dialysis, exchange blood transfusion, plasmapheresis, and a combination of hypothermia with total-body washout. Again, the small number of patients and lack of controls matched for severity of disease has rendered interpretation of the results claiming improved survival figures most difficult.

6. Reduced body temperature (hypothermia) to 32° to 33° C has not achieved much popularity in the treatment of the encephalopathy of Reye's syndrome. The potential risks with this modality again outweigh any proved advantage. Deleterious side effects from hypothermia include significant hypotension, excessive oxygen consumption from shivering, and the potential for rebound encephalopathy during warming. The decrease in core temperature seen during barbiturate coma may be acceptable provided that the shivering response is prevented by muscle relaxants pancuronium bromide (Pavulon), and cerebral perfusion pressure is maintained at all times. Hypothermia is contraindicated in the young infant where the homeostatic balance seems to be more delicate, and the margin of safety is much less than that in the older child.

Clinical course and complications

From the time of admission some progression of the encephalopathy to a deeper level of coma is likely to occur in up to 75% of these patients. Since those passing rapidly through the deeper stages of coma carry a higher mortality, prompt treatment intervention should be undertaken. Fortunately, the majority of patients who stabilize in the precoma stages (0 to 2) will show signs of clinical improvement once rehydration efforts are instituted, glucose homeostasis is restored, and a modest use of osmotherapy is offered. Within 24 to 48 hours after admission this patient group is usually ready for oral feedings, and full recovery rapidly follows over the subsequent 48 hours. Complications are extremely rare in these milder cases.

About 25% of patients presenting at admission in deeper levels of coma (stages III to V) remain stable or worsen rapidly or slowly over the ensuing days as the disease runs its full course. In this latter group the finding of *refractory elevation of intracranial pressure* is the most dreaded early complication of Reye's syndrome. Clinical signs of herniation of brain tissue may be noted, and anoxic brain damage will rapidly follow the serious compromise to cerebral perfusion pressure. *Impaired cardiac function* from hypovolemia, cardiac muscle injury, or arrhythmias may suddenly develop and require specific medications to maintain the desired mean arterial blood pressure. Weighing the patient twice a day can provide an early indication about the development of *sudden inappropriate vasopressin* secretion, a not uncommon consequence of brain injury. A rapid weight gain, rising central venous pressure, and decrease in serum sodium and serum osmolarity favor this diagnosis and demand adjustment in fluid management. On the other extreme, *diabetes insipidus* may develop but is more often a late complication, especially in patients in deep coma with suspected hypoxic brain damage. The known effects of the drug vasopressin upon the cardiovascular system needs to be appreciated when one is treating this complication, particularly in patients with Reye's syndrome. *Renal failure* either of a functional nature or from acute tubular necrosis may be seen in some patients and, if severe, will require peritoneal dialysis as an additional treatment modality. *Acute pancreatitis* may complicate Reye's syndrome and result in the sequestration of significant amounts of fluid in the abdomen and retroperitoneal space. It should be suspected when unexplained discrepancies exist in the fluid management of these patients. Serum amylase determination and pancreatic ultrasound can confirm the diagnosis. Evolving *neurogenic pulmonary edema* should be suspected when a falling PaO_2 is reported. The appearance of blood-tinged material during suctioning of the endotracheal tube, auscultatory findings of rales, and bilateral alveolar infiltrates on chest roentgenogram can confirm the diagnosis. A prompt diuresis with use of furosemide (Lasix) (1 to 2 mg/kg intravenously) or mannitol (1 gm/kg over 15 to 20 minutes) along with a simultaneous increase in the inspiratory-flow oxygen concentration (F_iO_2) is usually therapeutic. Cautiously raising the level of positive-end expiratory pressures (PEEP) to 3 to 5 cm of water may also be tried, provided that the intracranial pressure does not rise to concerning levels. It is believed that phenobarbital treatment of the encephalopathy may lessen the likelihood of neurogenic pulmonary edema. *Hypophosphatemia* should be corrected promptly. Not only can it impair the oxygenation of tissues by raising the affinity of oxyhemoglobin, but it may also be responsible for acute respiratory failure in some patients. Lesser, but confusing neurologic consequences of hypophosphatemia include muscle weakness, hyporeflexia, and even paresis.

Complications of invasive procedures and ag-

Table 22-6. Relationship between survival, ammonia levels, and therapy in Reye's syndrome.

	Patients with ammonia level < 300 µg/dl			Patients with ammonia level > 300 µg/dl		
		Those who died			Those who died	
	Total	Number	Percent	Total	Number	Percent
Supportive care only	79	17	22	24	14	58
Exchange transfusion	31	10	32	25	16	64
Dialysis	14	7	50	25	16	64
Exchange transfusion and dialysis	4	2	50	1	1	100
TOTAL	128	36	28	75	47	63

From Corey, L., and others: Pediatrics **60**:708, 1977.

gressive treatment modalities can significantly affect the clinical course of patients with Reye's syndrome. These risks often parallel the increased complexity of care but can be kept to a minimum when treatment is supervised by experienced individuals trained in critical care medicine.

The numbers of in-dwelling lines and monitoring devices employed in the management of these patients pose the distinct possibility of *superimposed infections*. A *consumptive coagulopathy* may evolve as an early sign of sepsis. Sudden *changes in fluid balance or excessive manipulation* of the patient must be guarded against, lest the results produce undesirable spike increases in the intracranial pressure. Too rapid withdrawal of treatment modalities may likewise produce damaging results. In this regard an organized plan for weaning the patient from invasive monitoring and treatment is necessary. Weaning can be begun if the patient has stabilized with normal or near-normal values for 24 hours (intracranial pressure less than 20 mm Hg, cerebral perfusion pressure greater than 50 mm Hg). If barbiturates have been utilized, these should be reduced by one half the dose every 8 hours and discontinued after 24 hours. Ventilator adjustments should be made to gradually raise the $Paco_2$ to 30 mm Hg, and if tolerated, muscle-relaxation drugs can be discontinued and the patient allow to breathe on his own with ventilation assistance as needed. Small doses of mannitol may still be required to counteract intracranial pressure spikes noted during these manipulations. Thereafter the Swan-Ganz catheter, intracranial pressure–monitoring device, and arterial lines may be removed. Endotracheal extubation can follow, though some patients may require reintubation and assisted ventilation for an addi-

tional 3 to 7 days because of significant muscle weakness and easy fatigability that follows prolonged coma. Thereafter the remainder of the support systems can be discontinued and the patient orally alimented. Continued use of oxacillin or methicillin for 7 to 10 days is suggested after intracranial catheter removal. A followup CT scan is suggested at 3 to 6 months for those individuals having an intraventricular cannula to rule out an evolving porencephalic cyst.

Prognosis

The prognosis correlates best with the final depth of coma and the admission or peak concentration of blood ammonia levels (Table 22-6). Prognosis is said to be worse for those patients rapidly passing through three or more stages to deeper levels of coma.

Patients not progressing beyond stage II and who have blood ammonia concentrations less than 300 mg/dl have up to a 95% chance for full recovery, barring any unusual complicating events. Patients reaching stage III and IV coma with blood ammonia concentrations greater than 300 mg/dl have from 25% to 85% survival rates depending on the series reported. Improved survival figures in this particular group continue to parallel the commitment to invasive monitoring and treatment within intensive care units; therefore it seems to justify the added risk attending such therapies. Few survivors are reported from patients reaching stage V coma. The overall case fatality figures reported by the National Center for Disease Control have gone from 41% in 1974 to 23% in 1977-1978. Not all of this decrease in mortality is explained simply by an increased awareness of the diagnosis, or admission to the hospital in earlier stages of the dis-

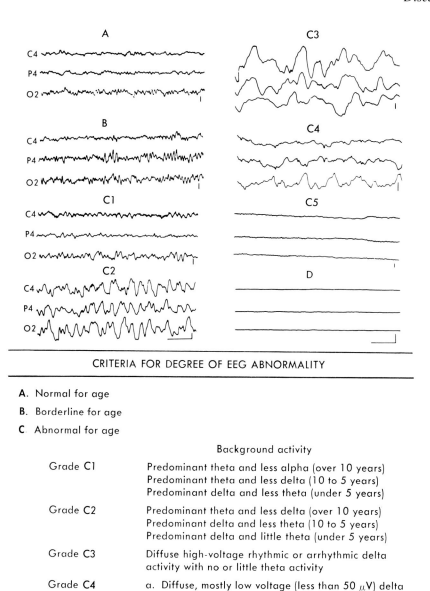

CRITERIA FOR DEGREE OF EEG ABNORMALITY

A. Normal for age

B. Borderline for age

C. Abnormal for age

		Background activity
Grade C1		Predominant theta and less alpha (over 10 years) Predominant theta and less delta (10 to 5 years) Predominant delta and less theta (under 5 years)
Grade C2		Predominant theta and less delta (over 10 years) Predominant delta and less theta (10 to 5 years) Predominant delta and little theta (under 5 years)
Grade C3		Diffuse high-voltage rhythmic or arrhythmic delta activity with no or little theta activity
Grade C4		a. Diffuse, mostly low voltage (less than 50 μV) delta activity with no or little theta activity b. Suppression-burst activity
Grade C5		Nearly isoelectric activity

D. Electrocerebral silence

Fig. 22-7. Examples of EEG patterns frequently encountered in patients with Reye's syndrome. (Modified from Aoki, Y., and Lombroso, C.T.: Neurology **2**:333-343, 1973.)

ease, because case-fatality ratios also decreased within individual stages of coma.

It has also been noted that when biochemical evidence for both liver and skeletal muscles is present (high SGOT and CPK, elevated LDH of muscle origin) this likewise indicates a poor prognosis. However, most of these patients will also have blood ammonia levels greater than 300 mg/dl.

The appearance of the EEG on admission and serially thereafter likewise has some prognostic value in Reye's syndrome patients (Fig. 22-7).

The overall morbidity figures in the survivors are from 10% to 30%, with the sequelae being of greater magnitude and permanence for those remaining in the deeper levels of coma for long times (5 to 7 days). The younger the child, the greater the likelihood of neuropsychological sequelae. Fifty percent of surviving infants are reported with handicaps that include mental retardation, seizure disorder, spastic hemiparesis, blindness, and developmental delays. The older child may have a temporary language and perceptual motor deficit that can compromise their learning capabilities in a classroom setting. Permanent deficits in cognitive learning skills have also been reported after recovery from Reye's syndrome.

Recurrences of this disease are rare but have been reported. Some persons have had up to five repeat episodes of acute Reye's syndrome, confirmed on each occasion by biochemical and histologic data. However, we urge that all patients with recurrences be screened for an underlying inborn error of metabolism as previously mentioned (see the discussion of etiology, p. 632).

REFERENCES

Aprille, J.R., Austin, J., Costello, C.E., and Royal, N.: Identification of the Reye's syndrome 'serum factor,' Biochem. Biophys. Res. Commun. **94:**381-389, 1980.

Barker, G.A.: The role of decompressive craniectomy in Reye's syndrome, J. Natl. Reye's Syndrome Found. **1:**73-79, 1980.

Bobo, R.C., Schubert, W.K., Partin, J.C., and Partin, J.S.: Reye's syndrome: treatment by exchange transfusion with special reference to the 1974 epidemic in Cincinnati, Ohio, J. Pediatr. **87:**881-886, 1975.

Bove, K.E., McAdams, A.J., Partin, J.C., and others: The hepatic lesion in Reye's syndrome, Gastroenterology **69:**685-697, 1975.

Brunner, R.L., O'Grady, D.J., Partin, J.C., and others: Neuropsychologic consequences of Reye syndrome, J. Pediatr. **95:**706-711, 1979.

Caillie, M., Morin, C.L., Roy, C.C., and others: Reye's syndrome: relapses and neurological sequelae, Pediatrics **59:**244-301, 1977.

Chapoy, P.R., Angelini, C., Brown, W.J., and others: Systemic carnitine deficiency: a treatable inherited lipid-storage disease presenting as Reye's syndrome, N. Engl. J. Med. **303:**1389-1394, 1980.

Cooperstock, M.S., Tucker, R.P., and Baublis, J.V.: Possible pathogenic role of endotoxin in Reye's syndrome, Lancet, **1:**1272-1274, June 7, 1975.

Corey, L., Rubin, R.J., and Hattwick, M.A.W.: Reye's syndrome: clinical progression and evaluation of therapy, Pediatrics **60:**708-714, 1977.

Corey, L., Rubin, R.J., Thompson, T.R., and others: Influenza B–associated Reye's syndrome: incidence in Michigan and potential for prevention, J. Infect. Dis. **135:**398-407, 1977.

Corey, L., Rubin, R.J., Hattwick, M.A.W., and others: A nationwide outbreak of Reye's syndrome, Am. J. Med. **61:**615-625, 1976.

Corey, L., Rubin, R.J., Bregman, D., and Gregg, M.B.: Diagnostic criteria for influenza B–associated Reye's syndrome: clinical vs. pathologic criteria, Pediatrics **60:**702-707, 1977.

Crocker, J.F.S., Lee, S.H.S., Rozee, K.R., and Digout, S.C.: Pesticide emulsifiers as a contributing factor in Reye's syndrome: their effect on the interferon response in-vivo, J. Natl. Reye's Syndrome Found. **1:**120-125, 1980.

Crocker, J.F.S., Rozee, K.R., Ozere, R.L., and others: Insecticide and viral interaction as a cause of fatty visceral changes and encephalopathy in the mouse, Lancet **2:**22-24, July 6, 1974.

Crocker, J.F.S., Ozere, R.L., Safe, S.H., and others: Lethal interaction of ubiquitous insecticide carriers with virus, Science **192:**1351-1353, 1976.

DeLong, G.R., and Glick, T.H.: Encephalopathy of Reye's syndrome: a review of pathogenetic hypotheses, Pediatrics **69:**53-63, 1982.

DeVivo, D.C., Keating, J.P., and Haymond, M.W.: Reye syndrome: results of intensive supportive care, J. Pediatr. **87:**875-880, 1975.

Ellis, G.H., Mirkin, L.D., and Mills, M.C.: Pancreatitis and Reye's syndrome, Am. J. Dis. Child. **133:**1014-1016, 1979.

Faraj, B.A., Neuman, S.L., Caplan, D.B., and others: Evidence for hypertyraminemia in Reye's syndrome, Pediatrics **64:**76-80, 1979.

Fishman, R.A.: Brain edema, N. Engl. J. Med. **293:**706-711, 1975.

Fleisher, G., Schwartz, J. and Lennette, E.: Primary Epstein-Barr virus infection in association with Reye syndrome, J. Pediatr. **96:**935-937, 1980.

Friend, M., and Trainer, D.O.: Polychlorinated biphenyl: interaction with duck hepatitis virus, Science **170:**1314-1316, 1970.

Gall, D.G., Cutz, E., McClung, H.J., and Greenberg, M.L.: Acute liver disease and encephalopathy mimicking Reye syndrome, J. Pediatr. **87:**869-874, 1975.

Glasgow, A.M., Eng, G., and Engel, A.G.: Systemic carnitine deficiency stimulating recurrent Reye syndrome, J. Pediatr. **96:**889-891, 1980.

Greene, H.L., Wilson, F.A., Glick, A.D., and others: Hepatic ATP concentrations and glycolytic enzyme activities in Reye syndrome, J. Pediatr. **89:**777-780, 1976.

Gregersen, N.: Studies on the effects of saturated and unsaturated short-chain monocarboxylic acids on the energy metabolism of rat liver mitochondria, Pediat. Res. **13:**1227-1230, 1979.

Halsey, N.A., Hurwitz, E.S., Meiklejohn, G., and others: An epidemic of Reye syndrome associated with influenza A (H_1N_1) in Colorado, J. Pediatr. **97:**535-539, 1980.

Heick, H.M.C., Shipman, R.T., Norman, M.G., and James W.: Reye-like syndrome associated with use of insect repellent in a presumed heterozygote for ornithine carbamoyl transferase deficiency, J. Pediatr. **97:**471-473, 1980.

Hilty, M.D., Romshe, C.A., and Delamater, P.V.: Reye's syndrome and hyperaminoacidemia, J. Pediatr. **84:**362-365, 1974.

Hilty, M.D., McClung, H.J., Haynes, R.E., and others: Reye syndrome in siblings, J. Pediatr. **94:**576-579, 1979.

Huttenlocher, P.R., and Trauner, D.A.: Reye's syndrome in infancy, Pediatrics **62:**84-90, 1978.

Iancu, T.C., Mason, W.H., and Neustein, H.B.: Ultrastructural abnormalities of liver cells in Reye's syndrome, Hum. Pathol. **8:**421-431, 1977.

Johnson, G.M., Scurletis, T.D., and Carroll, N.B.: A study of sixteen fatal cases of encephalitis-like disease in North Carolina children, N.C. Med. J. **24:**464-473, 1963.

Kaul, A., Cohen, M.E., Broffman, G., and others: Reye-like syndrome associated with Coxsackie B₂ virus infection, J. Pediatr. **94:**67-69, 1979.

LaBrecque, D.R., Latham, P.S., Riely, C.A., and others: Heritable urea cycle enzyme deficiency: liver disease in 16 patients, J. Pediatr. **94:**580-587, 1979.

Ladisch, S., Lovejoy, F.H., Hierholzer, J.C., and others: Extrapulmonary manifestations of adenovirus type 7 pneumonia simulating Reye syndrome and the possible role of an adenovirus toxin, J. Pediatr. **95:**348-355, 1979.

Lansky, L.L., Kalavsky, S.M., Brackett, C.E., and others: Hypothermic total body washout and intracranial pressure monitoring in stage IV Reye syndrome, J. Pediatr. **90:**639-640, 1977.

Lloyd, K.G., Davidson, L., Price, K., and others: Catecholamine and octopamine concentrations in brains of patients with Reye syndrome, Neurology **27:**985-988, 1977.

Lovejoy, F.H., Smith, A.L., Bresnan, M.J., and others: Clinical staging in Reye syndrome, Am. J. Dis. Child. **128:**36-41, 1974.

Lumeng, L., Green, H., and Fitzgerald, J.: The serum factor in Reye's syndrome and its effects on mitochondrial metabolism and function in vitro, Gastroenterology **76:**1291, 1979 (Abstract).

Margolis, L.H., and Shaywitz, B.A.: The outcome of prolonged coma in childhood, Pediatrics **65:**477-483, 1980.

Milley, J.R., Nugent, S.K., and Rogers, M.C.: Neurogenic pulmonary edema in childhood, J. Pediatr. **94:**706-709, 1979.

Nelson, D.B., Kimbrough, R., and Landrigan, P.S.: Aflatoxin and Reye's syndrome: a case control study, Pediatrics **66:**865-869, 1980.

Newman, J.H., Neff, T.A., and Ziporin, P.: Acute respiratory failure associated with hypophosphatemia, N. Engl. J. Med. **296:**1101-1103, 1977.

Newman, S.L., Faraj, B.A., Caplan, D.B., and others: Prolactin and the encephalopathy of Reye's syndrome, Lancet **2:**1097-1100, 1979.

Orlowski, J.P., Johannsson, J.H., and Ellis, N.G.: Encephalopathy and fatty metamorphosis of the liver associated with cold-agglutinin autoimmune hemolytic anemia, J. Pediatr. **94:**569-575, 1979.

Pegelow, C., Goldberg, R., Turkel, S., and Powars, D.: Severe coagulation abnormalities in Reye syndrome, J. Pediatr. **91:**413-416, 1977.

Reye, R.D.K.: Encephalopathy and fatty degeneration of the viscera: a disease entity in childhood, Lancet **2:**749-752, 1963.

Roe, C.R., Schonberger, L.B., Gelbach, S.H., and others: Enzymatic alterations in Reye's syndrome: prognostic implications, Pediatrics **55:**119-126, 1975.

Ryan, N.J., Hogan, G.R., Hayes, A.W., and others: Aflatoxin B₁: its role in the etiology of Reye's syndrome, Pediatrics **64:**71-75, 1979.

Schubert, W.K., Partin, J.C., and Partin, J.S.: Encephalopathy and fatty liver (Reye's syndrome). In Popper, H., and Schaffner, F., editors, Progress in liver diseases, vol. 4, New York, 1972, Grune & Stratton, Inc.

Shaywitz, B.A., Venes, J., Cohen, D.J., and Bowers, M.B.: Reye syndrome: monoamine metabolites in ventricular fluid, Neurology **29:**467-472, 1979.

Shaywitz, B.A., Rothstein, P., and Venes, J.L.: Monitoring and management of increased intracranial pressure in Reye syndrome: results in 29 children, Pediatrics **66:**198-204, 1980.

Sinatra, F., Yoshida, T., Applebaum, M., and others: Abnormalities of carbamyl phosphate synthetase and ornithine transcarbamylase in liver of patients with Reye's syndrome, Pediatr. Res. **9:**829-833, 1975.

Snodgrass, P.J., and DeLong, G.R.: Urea-cycle enzyme deficiencies and an increased nitrogen load producing hyperammonemia in Reye's syndrome, N. Engl. J. Med. **294:**855-860, 1976.

Starko, K.M., Ray, C.G., Dominguez, L.B., and others: Reye's syndrome and salicylate use, Pediatrics **66:**859-864, 1980.

Sullivan-Bolyai, J.Z., Nelson, D.B., Morens, D.M., and Schonberger, L.B.: Reye syndrome in children less than 1 year old: some epidemiologic observations, Pediatrics **65:**627-629, 1980.

Tanaka, K., Kean, E.A., and Johnson, B.: Jamaican vomiting sickness, N. Engl. J. Med. **295:**461-467, 1976.

Thaler, M.M.: Metabolic mechanisms in Reye syndrome Am. J. Dis. Child. **130:**241-243, 1976.

Trauner, D.A., Nyhan, W.L., and Sweetman, L.P.: Short-chain organic acidemia and Reye's syndrome, Neurology **25:**296-298, 1975.

Trauner, D.A., Brown, F., Ganz, E., and Huttenlocher, P.R.: Treatment of elevated intracranial pressure in Reye syndrome, Ann. Neurol. **4:**275-278, 1978.

Trauner, D.A., and Adams, H.: Intracranial pressure elevations during octanoate infusion in rabbits: an experimental model of Reye's syndrome, Pediatr. Res. **15:**1097-1099, 1981.

23 *Fulminant hepatic necrosis and hepatic coma*

FULMINATING HEPATIC NECROSIS

An infrequent but catastrophic form of liver disease, fulminating hepatic necrosis with its resultant hepatic coma presents a formidable challenge to the pediatric caregiver and entire health care team as well. Diagnosis is rarely difficult, but the medical support requirements in managing such patients can become extraordinarily complex.

Etiologic considerations

Fulminant hepatic necrosis may evolve as a consequence of a variety of hepatic insults. During infancy, a definitive cause can often be identified, whereas in the older child, presently available routine screening tests tend to yield negative results for known causative agents. In the first few weeks of life, fulminant hepatic necrosis occurs from disseminated herpesvirus infection, certain members of the echovirus group (types 6, 11, 14, and 19), adenovirus, and rarely the Epstein-Barr virus. Severe hepatic failure in the neonate when attributable to maternal transmission of the hepatitis B virus is usually manifest after the first 3 to 4 weeks of life. Other rare but important causes of hepatic failure in this same age group include specific inborn errors of metabolism, namely, tyrosinemia, congenital fructose intolerance, and galactosemia. Zellweger's syndrome, though an exceptional cause of liver failure in the infant, should also be considered. Severe forms of congenital heart disease, both cyanotic and acyanotic forms, have in the neonatal period been associated with massive hepatic necrosis, most likely because of a low-flow state and resultant vascular insufficiency to the organ.

In the older pediatric patient, present methods confirm a viral cause for fulminant hepatic necrosis in only 10% to 30% of cases. Screening of biologic fluids, and specific serologic determinations are routinely performed for hepatitis A and B virus, cytomegalovirus, and Epstein-Barr virus. Most cases are presumed to be caused by the non-A, non-B group of hepatotrophic viruses. When herpesvirus is responsible for severe hepatic necrosis in the older child, an underlying congenital

or acquired immunologic deficiency state most likely underlies the host's vulnerability. Hepatic failure may also supervene in the immunologically compromised individual undergoing a severe graft versus host reaction.

Occasional pediatric cases of fulminant hepatic necrosis occur after exposure to hepatotoxic drugs (acetaminophen, isoniazid, aspirin, depakene, indomethacin), halothane anesthesia, chemicals (carbon tetrachloride, phosphorus), or naturally occurring plant toxins *(Amanita phalloides)*. Isolated examples of fulminant liver necrosis have also been reported in association with Wilson's disease, acute leukemia, and the Budd-Chiari syndrome.

The incidence of fulminant hepatic necrosis is probably less than 1 in 1000 of all icteric cases of presumed viral cause. Although the rarity of secondary cases within the family is difficult to reconcile with the known behavior of other infectious agents, the rapid employment of prophylaxis with immune serum globulin to household contacts may in part be responsible for this observation. Although clustering of cases has occasionally been noted, epidemiologic studies have not been able to identify a common etiologic agent. Implicating a specific genetic vulnerability of the affected but immunologically competent host remains speculative at best.

Magnitude of problem

Fortunately, fulminant hepatic necrosis is relatively infrequent in the pediatric population because survival figures in this age group are certainly no better, and possibly worse, than those quoted for adults (Table 23-1). Early results of outcome of patients entered into the Fulminant Hepatic Failure Surveillance Study (FHFSS) in 1966 showed pediatric survival rates at 38% whereas adult figures were about 20%. Unfortunately the study did not exclude pediatric cases with Reye's syndrome, a disease with clinicopathologic findings and prognosis distinctly differing from that of fulminant hepatic necrosis. Excluding neonates, we have up to now 16 cases of histologically proved examples of fulminant hepatic

Table 23-1. Results of therapy in 17 pediatric patients with fulminant hepatic failure and hepatic coma

Treatment regimen	Number of patients	Etiology	Outcome	
			Alive	Dead
Conventional therapy alone	4	Unknown (3)	1	2
		Hepatitis B and acetylsali-cylic acid (1)		1
Conventional therapy plus				
Exchange transfusions	8	Unknown (7)		7
		Acute Wilson's disease (1)		1
Plasmapheresis with plasma exchange	3	Unknown (3)		3
Hemodialysis using polyacrylonitrite membrane	1	Unknown		1
Hemoperfusion over ac-tivated charcoal	1	Acetaminophen overdose		1

necrosis and one presumed case (without a liver biopsy being performed) from the Denver experience. The single survivor in these 17 patients is the latter case who now has clinical and biochemical evidence of cirrhosis. Specific causes or associations discovered include one case each of Wilson's disease, acetaminophen overdose, and possible hepatitis B with aspirin hepatotoxicity; all the others had unknown causes. The basic histologic lesion common to all these cases is a variable degree of massive hepatic cell necrosis with parenchymal collapse. Regenerative efforts when present are meager and limited to bile ductular proliferative changes, and small nests or nodules of hepatocytes. Undoubtedly, reversibility of this injury pattern requires more than just keeping the patient alive.

Regenerative events and subsequent restitution of normal hepatic architecture must largely be governed by the integrity of the remaining hepatocytes, the state of the reticulin framework, and the functional capability of the hepatic microcirculation. Although most patients die within 1 to 2 weeks after showing signs of hepatic failure (asterixis, fetor hepaticus, coma), a few have a more prolonged course (1 to 3 months) before succumbing, usually to a complication of the treatment. Even in this latter group, at best one sees hyporegenerative efforts (nodules or nests of hepatocytes, giant cells) at autopsy. Remarkably, some survivors have been reported to show complete restitution to normal hepatic architecture.

Generally, the favorable or fatal outcome of fulminant hepatic necrosis cannot be predicted from the initial clinical or biochemical features. Very quickly other complicating factors (cerebral edema, hemorrhage, sepsis, and so on) make their appearance and dramatically affect the prognosis. Alone, liver biopsy and quantitative assessment of the histologic damage as predictive of outcome are likewise not of consistent value.

Although the liver is known to have remarkable powers of regeneration, this is seldom observed in patients dying from fulminant hepatic necrosis. Whether hepatotrophic regenerative factors are deficient in such patients, or perhaps find unresponsive hepatocytes, remains to be determined. The lack of a suitable animal model of human fulminant hepatic failure has undoubtedly hindered progress in the understanding of the pathophysiologic mechanisms involved in this condition and in evaluation of new therapies.

Clinical features and laboratory findings

Early clues signifying an "atypical" course for viral hepatitis and suggesting that the illness is, or may become, fulminant are summarized in the list below:

1. Persistent anorexia
2. Persistent or deepening jaundice, or both
3. Relapse of initial symptoms
4. Vitamin K–resistant prolongation of prothrombin time
5. Depressed serum albumin and fibrinogen level

6. Pronounced elevation of SGOT (greater than 3000 IU)
7. Bilirubin level over 20 mg/dl
8. Rapidly shrinking liver size without clinical improvement
9. Development of ascites
10. Appearance of respiratory alkalosis
11. Neuropsychiatric changes and slowing of EEG pattern
12. Hypoglycemia
13. Low BUN
14. Leukocytosis and thrombocytopenia

Two modes of presentation of the disease have been observed with about equal frequency. In the first, the child develops the clinical features typical of benign viral hepatitis, but instead of improving during the icteric phase, the jaundice deepens in intensity, serum transaminases remain very high, the prothrombin time elongates, and neurologic symptoms become apparent. The liver, initially enlarged, suddenly begins to shrink, and progressive hepatic coma supervenes. The transaminase values often begin to decrease as massive hepatic necrosis ensues.

In the second mode of presentation, patients manifesting a typical benign course of hepatitis suddenly relapse at a time when jaundice has been decreasing and the patient was experiencing a period of relative well-being. Fever, anorexia, abdominal pain, and vomiting are most often seen during the relapse, and these symptoms parallel a sudden deterioration in liver function tests. Jaundice becomes more noticeable, transaminase levels are elevated, and changes in sensorium suggest impending hepatic coma. Coagulation studies become abnormal about this time and cannot be corrected with vitamin K given parenterally. Excessive bleeding from venipunctures, bruising at injection sites, and the appearance of gastrointestinal bleeding reflect the disturbances in coagulation. The sudden appearance of ascites carries with it a grave prognosis. Some neurologic alterations may at times be caused by cerebral edema, and sudden death may follow cerebellar or uncal herniation.

During the course of the illness, certain laboratory tests may give additional clues to ongoing liver cell destruction. Of particular worry is the precipitous rise in serum bilirubin values. Very high transaminase values that persist for over 2 weeks should cause concern. Likewise, falling transaminase levels in a deteriorating patient with a shrinking liver is also a grave finding. An ini-

tially depressed serum albumin level should suggest underlying chronic liver disease, for more commonly it is normal at the onset of the acute disease because of its long half-life (18 to 20 days) and becomes abnormal in the face of continued hepatic injury. Rarely is the prothrombin time abnormal in benign icteric hepatitis. The finding of a vitamin K–resistant prolongation of the prothrombin time strongly implies that severe hepatic cell degeneration has occurred and that little, if any, functional regeneration is taking place. Some authors have indeed used the prothrombin time as the most sensitive laboratory guide in following the healing of the hepatic lesion. A low fibrinogen level and thrombocytopenia might suggest disseminated intravascular coagulation (DIC), but assay of specific clotting factors (VII, VIII, IX, XI) and measurement of fibrin split products should reduce the diagnostic dilemma. Decreased factor VIII strongly suggests DIC. Massive hepatic necrosis predisposes to hypoglycemia, and a low blood glucose level may well explain the patient's clinical state at times. This, too, suggests a grim prognosis.

The increased respiratory rate and abnormal respiratory pattern (Kussmaul's or Biot's respiration), often present in fulminating hepatitis, result in a respiratory alkalosis seen with a partially compensated metabolic acidosis. Whether the respiratory center is stimulated by some circulating toxin normally removed by the liver or simply by the intracellular acidosis is not clear. In either case, an elevated blood pH value signifies severe-acute or chronic liver disease. Coincidentally, the serum potassium value is often depressed as hepatic coma develops and is likely caused by secondary hyperaldosteronism.

The blood urea nitrogen (BUN) level may be very low initially, since urea formation is impaired by the liver injury. Later, both the BUN and serum creatinine levels may rise to abnormal levels as renal function deteriorates and oliguria and anuria occur. Progressive hypophosphatemia may be found by serial determinations and is believed to be caused by an intracellular shift from serum, rather than by a urinary loss of the anion. Hypophosphatemia also causes a shift in the oxygen-dissociation curve and impaired oxygenation of tissues may occur, an event especially detrimental to neuronal function in fulminant hepatic failure. Acute respiratory failure may occur in hypophosphatemic states.

The blood ammonia level is often elevated in

patients with severe liver failure, but we, like others, have also noted normal blood ammonia levels in patients with fulminating hepatitis. The ammonia concentration, however, may not correlate with the state of consciousness.

The electroencephalogram may be useful in the diagnosis of the precoma state. Bilateral, slow-wave activity (2 or 3 per second) particularly in the frontal areas is the most constant abnormality.

Last, a rising white blood cell count caused by polymorphonuclear cells may indirectly reflect hepatic failure but must also be differentiated from the response to superimposed infections, a complication to which these patients are extremely susceptible. A falling white blood cell count and thrombocytopenia may indicate bone marrow failure, a dreaded complication of hepatitis.

HEPATIC COMA

Evidence of hepatic encephalopathy is a constant feature of fulminant hepatic necrosis. It can also be seen in the clinical syndrome of fulminant hepatic failure in which a sudden and severe impairment of hepatic function has occurred (Reye's syndrome). With progression, a vast range of mental and neuromuscular features may become evident, with coma and death the final outcome for most patients. The term ''hepatic encephalopathy'' is reserved for the neuropsychiatric consequences observed in acute, severe liver injury, whereas ''portal encephalopathy,'' having some similar neuropsychiatric findings, denotes a specific consequence in patients with chronic liver disease (cirrhosis) who are exposed to exogenous or endogenous precipitating factors. Portal encephalopathy may also be seen after portal-systemic shunting where prehepatic portal hypertension, an important pediatric condition, had been causative. The encephalopathy may be precipitated by gastrointestinal bleeding, excessive ingestion of proteins or amino acids, ammonia-producing substances, sedatives or tranquilizers (diazepam), excessive use of diuretics, paracentesis, electrolyte abnormalities, hypotension, hypoxia, infections, and surgical procedures, to mention the more common causes.

Clinical features, pathogenesis, and laboratory findings

Hepatic coma may be divided into four stages based on the presence of specific neurologic signs and symptoms. Staging of coma is a reliable clin-

ical means to grade the severity of the hepatic failure, but it may not reflect the severity of the histologic lesion. Serially obtained laboratory assays of hepatic synthetic function (clotting factors V, VII, fibrinogen) are the best predictors of the severity of hepatic injury. Although adults manifesting signs of advanced hepatic coma may have a considerable proportion of the hepatic parenchyma morphologically intact (functional hepatic failure), with the exception of Reye's syndrome this correlation is seldom noted in children with fulminant hepatic failure. It is uncertain whether children are less sensitive than adults to the encephalopathic actions of circulating toxins, or have other means of detoxifying these products.

Stage I hepatic coma includes those patients with a normal level of consciousness interspersed with reduced mental alertness and in whom periods of hypotonia may transiently be observed (mild asterixis). Stage II reveals drowsiness, reversal of day-night sleep pattern, confusion, especially with inappropriate use of language, palilalia, and disorientation in time and place. Agitation increases to minor stimuli, and wide swings in affect and mood are noted. In stage III, stupor and coma are now present and the patient is unresponsive to verbal commands. Response to pain exists but is usually inappropriate, with decerebrate posturing. Spasticity, hyperreflexia, and extensor plantar responses can be elicited upon examination.

Stage IV finds the patient unresponsive to painful stimuli. Sucking movements, hiccuping, and sighing respirations develop. As the depth of coma increases, reflexes disappear and seizures can be seen, followed by respiratory arrest. Mortality is at least 80% in patients reaching stage IV hepatic coma.

A most difficult clinical situation is posed by the similarity of certain neurologic features of hepatic encephalopathy and those attributable to cerebral edema, a not infrequent complication (30% to 50%) of childhood cases of fulminant hepatic failure. A sudden deterioration of the patient accompanied by a noticeable change in respiratory pattern, appearance of Cushing's sign (decreased pulse, increased blood pressure), discrepant pupil size, and lateralizing neurologic findings are indications for immediate use of hyperosmolar agents (mannitol, glycerol) to combat underlying cerebral edema.

The clinical features of hepatic encephalopathy are not difficult to recognize in the pediatric pa-

Table 23-2. Symptoms and signs of hepatic coma

Mental state	Neuromuscular state
Clouding	Incoordination
Confusion	Tremor
Restlessness	Asterixis
Irritability	Dysarthria
Inappropriate behavior	Grasping
Sullenness, paranoid be- havior, disobedience	Hiccuping
Picking at and rearranging	Deliberate move- ment
bedclothes	Cogwheel rigidity
Yawning	Masklike facies
Sucking	Dilated pupils
Crying	Roving eyes
Agitation	Muscle twitching
Disorientation	Flexion of legs
Delirium	Hyperreflexia
Drowsiness	Positive toe signs
Somnolence	Nystagmus
Lethargy	Ophthalmoplegia
Apathy	Incontinence
Stupor	
Coma	

From Zieve, L.: Arch. Intern. Med. **118**:212, 1966.

tient. A comprehensive list of changes in the mental and neuromuscular state compiled by Zieve appear in Table 23-2. In the very young child the mother will relate that the patient's behavior has changed, particularly with unexpected periods of lethargy, verbal confusion, and hypotonia (asterixis).

One should be aware of subtle changes in the respiratory pattern as an indicator of deepening coma. An apparent increase in the effort of breathing is characterized by deeper inspirations and a more obvious phase of expiration. The appearance of fetor hepaticus on the patient's breath signifies hepatic failure and usually can be detected when the patient approaches stage III coma. This odor is believed to be that of dimethylsulfide, a bacterial decomposition product of methionine. Other substances are also implicated in contributing to the odor of fetor hepaticus, including mercaptans (methanethiol). The elevation of blood mercaptan is said to correlate better than blood ammonia levels with the severity of the hepatic encephalopathy. At present fetor hepaticus is the most specific clinical sign of hepatic encephalopathy.

With deepening hepatic coma, decorticate and decerebrate posturing occur; upgoing toes, hyperreflexia, and hypotension are seen before respiratory failure occurs.

A single, satisfactory explanation for the pathogenesis of hepatic coma has been handicapped by the great number of biochemical derangements that have been identified in the tissues and body fluids of such patients. An accumulation of toxic amounts of metabolic by-products is believed to interfere with normal biologic function at all levels. An enhancement of action (synergism) by the various circulating abnormal metabolites can be demonstrated experimentally. Despite the wide range of abnormalities detected in the blood of these patients, it is remarkable that, save for cerebral edema, few pathologic changes in the target organ (brain) can be recognized in those who die in hepatic coma.

The continued impact of toxic metabolites upon brain energy metabolism is believed eventually to reduce available ATP and, in turn, lead to a breakdown in cell-membrane gradients and intracellular organelle functions. The resulting alteration in the permeability of the blood-brain barrier further contributes to this process by allowing ingress of toxic metabolites to brain tissue. Increased permeability of the blood-brain barrier substantially contributes to the cerebral edema found in many patients dying in hepatic coma.

Decreased cerebral blood flow has been documented, but the reduced oxygen consumption commonly found in hepatic coma is believed to be caused by decreased utilization of available ATP by neuronal tissue.

In hepatic failure serum and spinal fluid show an increase in all fatty acids but especially short-chain fatty acids (butyric, valeric, octanoic). Incomplete beta oxidation of long-chain fatty acids by the damaged liver probably accounts for the elevation of the short-chain group. In rats and perhaps in man, the pathologic elevation of free fatty-acids has been shown to augment the encephalopathic potential of ammonia and mercaptans.

Although short-chain fatty acids can, in the experimental animal, induce an encephalopathy with electroencephalographic changes similar to those seen in humans, their specific contribution to the clinical syndrome of hepatic coma in man remains uncertain. Other circulating "cerebral toxins" have been incriminated as possible contributors to the encephalopathy. Biogenic amines (octopamine, beta-phenylethanolamines) produced by bacterial action on ingested proteins and escaping hepatic detoxification have been found in brain tissue of patients dying with hepatic encephalopathy, as well as in the serum and urine. These substances are capable of interfering with normal synaptic impulse transmission, as do other "false neurotransmitters." Indoles and skatoles, the intestinal degradation products of tryptophan, have likewise been shown to inhibit brain respiration in vitro. Perhaps, these substances, when they escape conjugation by the diseased liver, may potentiate the toxic action of other cerebral toxins. It is still unclear as to precisely where in the brain many of

these coma-producing toxins act, but the experimental data suggest selectivity and sensitivity of the different regions of the brain.

The role of blood ammonia levels in hepatic coma remains unclear, especially in cases of acute hepatic necrosis. Susceptibility to the effects of high blood ammonia levels seems to correlate better with the presence of chronic liver disease and alkalosis. In the presence of alkalosis, impermeable NH_4^+ becomes NH_3, which penetrates into cells with relative ease and possibly exerts there its toxic effect. Although discrepancies are noted between the depth of coma and the blood level (especially on single ammonia determinations), an increased cerebral sensitivity to ammonia exists for

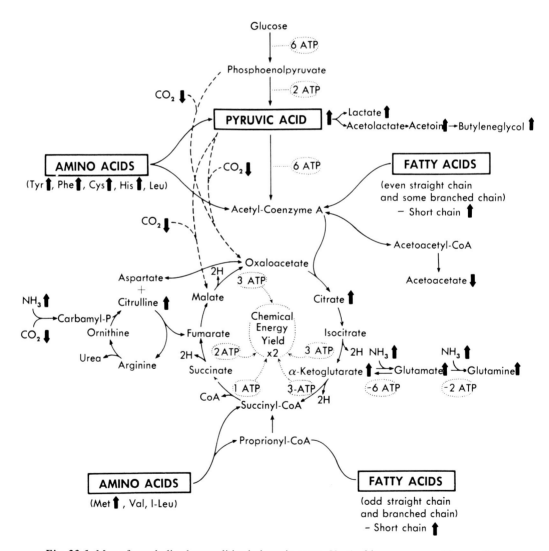

Fig. 23-1. Map of metabolic abnormalities in hepatic coma. *Vertical heavy arrows,* Abnormalities that have been observed in blood. (From Zieve, L.: Arch. Intern. Med. **118:**212, 1966.)

certain patients and for them represents the key cerebral toxin in hepatic coma. This increased cerebral sensitivity is noted especially in patients with chronic liver disease, for not infrequently minor insults (sedatives, infection, diuretics, gastrointestinal bleeding, and so on) suddenly precipitate portal-systemic encephalopathy. The experimental data infer that ammonia intoxication produces an encephalopathy by interfering with cerebral energy metabolism and thereby results in a lowering of available high-energy phosphates (ATP), especially in the infratentorial structures (brainstem). Ammonia may depress cerebral blood flow and oxygen consumption, especially in patients with evidence of portosystemic shunting. As a result of excess brain ammonia, blood and spinal fluid glutamine levels rise, a process that is energy depleting at the cellular level. It is not surprising that the close correlation between the depth of hepatic coma and the spinal-fluid glutamine levels has been consistently observed in such patients.

The derangement in acid-base metabolism certainly can be instrumental in exerting an unfavorable influence on the blood ammonia levels, organic acid levels, and cerebral blood flow. These abnormalities can be corrected during treatment of such patients, thereby counteracting the potentiating onslaught of toxic metabolites.

Raised levels of plasma amino acids are constantly found in fulminant hepatic necrosis with pronounced elevation of the aromatic amino acids and methionine compared to that of the branched chain and neutral amino acids. They probably have a role in the progression and perhaps the outcome of hepatic coma, but their specific effects are unclear.

The relationship of disturbances in cell metabolism to proposed mechanisms for the development of hepatic coma is shown in Fig. 23-1. Although hepatic coma appears to be a metabolic cerebral disorder of multifactorial origin, the exact sequence of events responsible for the encephalopathy remains to be determined. Even though the potential for irreversible injury to the brain by these toxic metabolites certainly exists (mortality over 80%), the resiliency of neurologic tissue is truly incredible because survivors from hepatic coma rarely show demonstrable neurologic deficits. This is in contrast to chronic portal encephalopathy were pathologic changes of neuronal elements can be demonstrated both clinically and histologically.

Pathology

The histopathologic lesion seen in massive hepatic necrosis is somewhat dependent on the underlying cause. In presumed hepatitis A virus or hepatitis B virus disease, the typical lesion is a widespread interlobular confluent hepatic cell necrosis and hepatic parenchymal collapse so that portal zones are found in juxtaposition to each other or to central veins. Inflammatory cells, when present, may be scattered throughout the liver, often in areas of hepatocyte fallout. The cellular response may include monocytes, polymorphonuclear cells, lymphocytes, plasma cells, and eosinophils (Fig. 23-2). Not infrequently, one is struck by the relative absence of inflammatory response in relation to the degree of hepatic necrosis.

It is not uncommon to find that recognizable liver cells in the biopsy specimen account for less than 10% of all cells present (Fig. 23-3). These may be in groups of four to six cells often arranged in a pseudoacinar or pseudoductular manner. If biopsy or autopsy material becomes available later in the disease, foci of regenerating hepatocytes may be found scattered against a background of loose mesenchyme (Figs. 23-4 and 23-5) or arranged in a more normal-appearing manner (Fig. 23-5, *C*). For some, bile ductular proliferation may be the only evidence of regenerative activity. Some regenerating hepatocytes are believed to be derived from multipotential cells lining the canals of Hering.

Some cases of drug-induced hepatic necrosis (iproniazid, acetaminophen, para-aminosalicylic acid, ethionamide, indomethacin, mercaptopurine, and others) are characterized by variable degrees of zonal necrosis with minimal inflammatory response that is sometimes distinguishable from severe virus-induced hepatic necrosis. Fulminating, halothane-associated hepatitis may be indistinguishable from severe viral hepatitis.

The histologic lesion of so-called bridging necrosis may be found in some patients progressing into hepatic coma. Characteristically, bands of hepatocyte dropout is noted to traverse portal-to-portal zones, or portal zone to the region of the central vein with focal evidence of hepatocyte injury also seen within the lobules. If the functional integrity of the remaining hepatocytes is maintained, the prognosis for survival, with or without cirrhosis, is greatly improved with this histologic lesion provided that the patient does not succumb to a potentially treatable complication of liver

Text continued on p. 668.

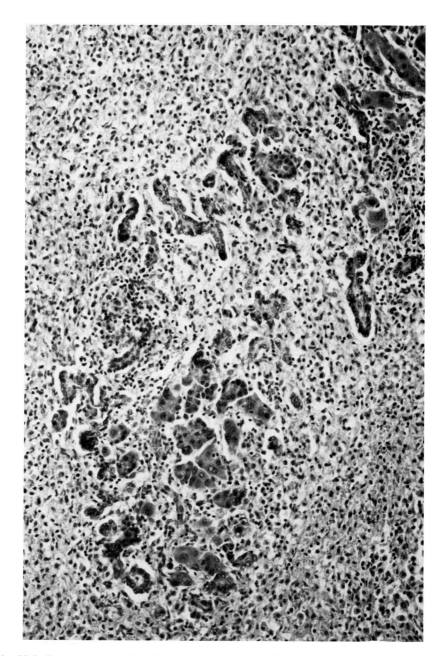

Fig. 23-2. Fulminating hepatitis. Note the severe lobular disarray, giant cells, hepatocyte necrosis, and inflammatory cellularity. A previously well 4-year-old child developed anorexia, vomiting, and jaundice leading to a diagnosis of infectious hepatitis. After transient improvement during the second week of the illness, he became progressively more jaundiced, anorexic, and disoriented. An exchange transfusion using fresh, heparinized blood was then performed to correct the coagulation abnormalities and permit percutaneous liver biopsy. Transient improvement in sensorium occurred, and two additional exchange transfusions were carried out. The child seemed to be improved, and treatment continued with a combination of therapies, including steroids, growth hormone, and chloroquine. However, jaundice never cleared, and the prothrombin time remained resistant to vitamin K administration. A respiratory alkalosis, ascites, and a mild hemolytic anemia appeared toward the end of his illness. Terminally, he developed sinusitis and pneumonia with spiking temperatures and suddenly died 63 days after the exchange transfusion.

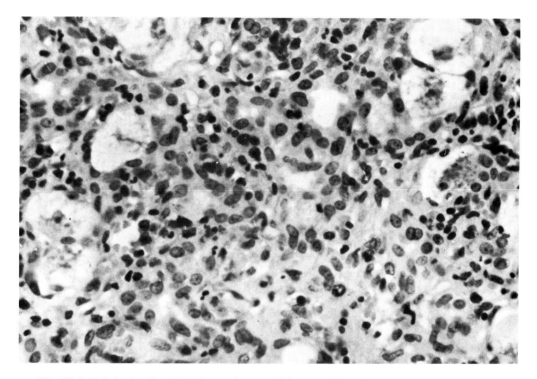

Fig. 23-3. Fulminating hepatitis. Severe hepatocellular necrosis, balloon cells, and inflammatory cellularity. An 18-month-old child developed jaundice 9 days earlier. On day of admission she became drowsy and combative. Physical examination revealed a semicomatosed, icteric child with strong fetor to the breath. The liver edge was barely palpable; serum bilirubin was 18 mg/dl, SGOT 760 IU, ammonia 116 mg/dl, albumin 2.7 gm/dl, and prothrombin time 16.8 seconds (control 12 seconds). After the first of three exchange transfusions, this liver biopsy section was obtained by the percutaneous route. Supportive medical management (steroids, chloroquine, and so on) was used for 30 days, until death occurred from *Pseudomonas* meningitis.

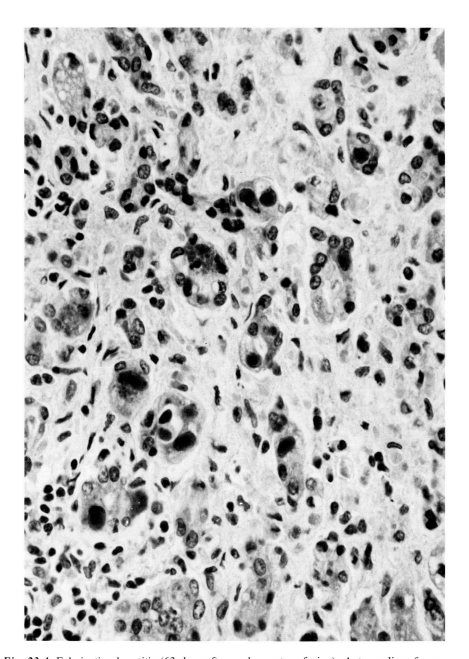

Fig. 23-4. Fulminating hepatitis (63 days after exchange transfusion). Autopsy liver from same patient described in Fig. 23-2 shows pseudoductular formation by hepatocytes lying within an amorphous matrix, associated with abundant necrotic debris. Note epithelial cells and hepatocytes with cytomegalovirus inclusions. Improvement in sensorium, awakening from coma, and temporary improvement may not be synonymous with functional hepatocyte regeneration. Cytomegalovirus inclusions were noted in lung and kidney, as well as throughout the liver parenchyma of this patient.

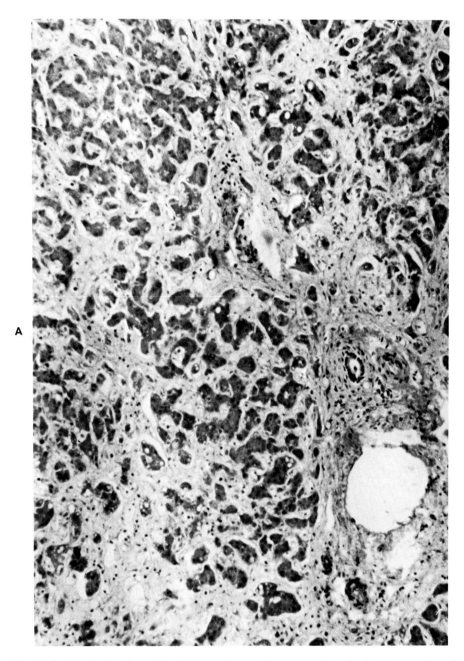

Fig. 23-5. Fulminating hepatitis (30 days after exchange transfusion). **A,** Autopsy liver from patient described in Fig. 23-3. A low-power view shows the islands of remaining hepatocytes scattered within a loose matrix of mesenchyme.   *Continued.*

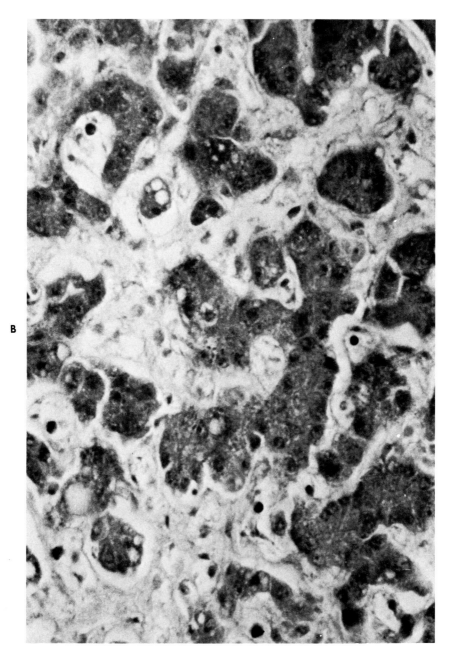

Fig. 23-5, cont'd. **B,** High-power view from **A.**

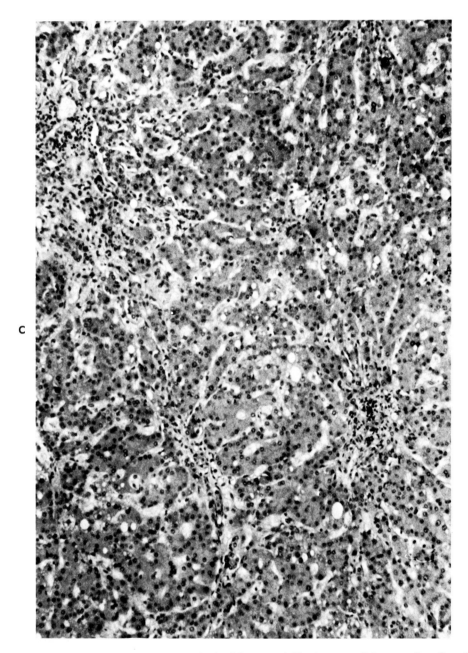

***Fig. 23-5, cont'd.* C,** Autopsy tissue obtained from a neighboring area of the same liver from **B,** demonstrating the pronounced regeneration with considerably less distortion than other neighboring zones had.

failure (sepsis, cerebral edema, hemorrhage). Estimated hepatic cell–volume fraction in biopsy specimens revealing ''bridging'' necrosis is usually over 50%.

Fulminating hepatitis with submassive necrosis may be superimposed on chronic liver disease, with features of acute necrosis found alongside areas of cirrhosis (regenerating nodules and fibrosis). This, too, may be triggered by a viral hepatitis as well as a drug-induced hepatitis.

It is not uncommon to find histopathologic alterations in other organs (pancreas, kidneys, brain, lung), especially when fulminant hepatic necrosis has been the result of hepatitis A or B virus disease. The multiorgan involvement of the hepatitis A and B viruses has been previously noted even in nonfatal cases (Chapter 21).

Treatment

There is no evidence to suggest that any of the therapeutic regimens presently employed directly aid the underlying liver disease. Attempts at removing, or at least reducing the levels of, endogenously accumulated circulating toxins may be of greater benefit to extrahepatic organ function (brain) than to the liver itself. In vivo evidence that shows the hepatotoxic effect of serum taken from patients in hepatic coma is lacking.

The poor therapeutic results, obtained in presumed viral fulminant hepatic necrosis, may paradoxically be attributable to the large functional reserve capacity of the liver; one that allows for massive injury to occur before the appearance of a commensurate clinical and laboratory expression of ongoing severe injury. With the exception of cytomegalovirus, or herpesvirus, direct evidence of viral hepatocyte infection is seldom confirmed from either electron microscopic study, or routine viral culture of liver tissue that is obtained early in the clinical course. It is not surprising therefore that the use of active or passive forms of immunoprophylaxis has not proved a beneficial treatment modality in these suspected, virus-induced cases. Another approach receiving research attention involves the study of hepatotropic factors and their potential in facilitating hepatic regeneration. Unfortunately, the specific initiating factor or factors of liver-cell regeneration remains unknown though glucagon and insulin are important in this process. The use of such substances in fulminant hepatic necrosis has great attractiveness, but it also remains to be seen whether the surviving hepatocytes can be turned on by the proper regenerative stimulus. Uncertainty also exists as to whether such treatment regimens can restore the functional integrity of the hepatocyte's microcirculation unit, a fundamental requirement for sustained hepatocyte regeneration. Since there is no specific therapy for the fulminating form of hepatitis, a host of supportive and temporizing therapies are employed, directed primarily at the prevention and treatment of the complications of liver failure.

Although perhaps overstated in cases of fulminant hepatic failure, vigorous supportive treatment is predicated on the observation that the liver has an enormous capacity to withstand injury and is capable of regenerating a normal structure; therefore one employs the heroics to buy time while awaiting regeneration and ultimate survival. The literature abounds with a variety of heroic supportive therapeutic modalities that may be employed in the treatment of patients with fulminant hepatic failure. The clinician will find it tempting to utilize the most recently acclaimed treatment modality because outcome results using older modalities in previous cases have been so disappointing. It still remains to be proved that any of the so-called heroic forms of therapy yield a greater survival rate than a control group treated by standard treatment measures. Our experience has led us to be more selective in the kind of therapy to be used. Obviously, conservative standard therapy can be initiated in all cases. The decision to employ more complicated forms of treatment should depend upon the cause of the hepatic failure, presence of underlying chronic liver disease, and, most importantly in our opinion, the remaining percentage (or volume) of presumed-viable hepatocytes. In addition, one must be certain that medical, surgical, nursing, laboratory, radiologic, and blood bank personnel are continuously available to assist in carrying out these demanding treatment measures. It is also important to consider and establish early into therapy those guidelines that will dictate the need to continue or to discontinue the treatment measures.

In a previously well child in whom a drug- or poison-induced hepatic necrosis is suspected as the underlying cause, vigorous and heroic measures are usually justified.

As soon as clinical and laboratory assessment confirms the diagnosis of fulminant hepatic failure, the patient should be readied for a percutaneous liver biopsy. Normal, or near-normal, clotting studies can be obtained with the use of fresh frozen plasma (10 ml/kg) and with platelet transfusion, if needed. In cases with more severe derangement of hemostasis, either a two-volume exchange transfusion using fresh heparinized blood (followed by protamine) or plasmapheresis and plasma exchange should be utilized to correct the coagulation abnormality. Early in the disease, while hepatomegaly is still present and ascites is absent, a successful liver biopsy can be performed with reasonable safety, provided that the patient's clotting status has been normalized.

The interpretation of the hepatic histopathologic appearance is used as follows. If the lesion is suggestive of a drug- or toxin-induced injury pattern, or shows ''bridging'' or zonal necrosis, maximum therapeutic measures are employed until the patient either recovers or dies. If the estimate of surviving hepatocyte volume is less than a range of 15% to 25%, maximal treatment measures are planned for 2 weeks. Evidence of progressive liver necrosis and failure of regenerative efforts (persistent clotting factor V or VII assays less than 10%, failure to demonstrate any hepatic uptake by DIDA scintiscan, and progressively shrinking liver size) after this time period is an indication to cease, if not all, then certainly any ongoing heroic measures of support. Naturally, liver biopsy specimens that show a substantial amount of healthy-appearing hepatocytes is an indication for maximum support while one simultaneously monitors the disease process.

Standard medical management. During the precoma period (stages I and II) a normal amount of calories is offered. The *diet* should be low in salt (10 mEq/m^2/day of Na$^+$) and protein (0.5 gm/kg) and high in carbohydrate.

A specially formulated product for patients with marginal liver function has recently been marketed. Hepatic-Aid, is a suspendable powder in which the amino acid composition is high in branched-chain amino acid and low in aromatic amino aids, a formulation considered beneficial to such patients. Up to now there has been no experience with this product in pediatric patients.

Maintenance fluid needs can be calculated (1500 ml/m^2/day) and adjustments made as indicated from input-output data and results of daily weighing. Ascites may appear with surprising rapidity if fluid volume is not carefully monitored. That many sweetened fluids preferred by children are unfortunately high in salt content should be kept in mind.

When intravenous fluids are required (stages III and VI, coma), maintenance volumes are again employed using 5% to 10% dextrose solutions with added sodium and potassium (1 to 2 mEq/kg/day). Hypophosphatemia should be corrected as soon as possible because of its detrimental effect upon the oxyhemoglobin dissociation curve, and hypoglycemia should be guarded against. Close attention to blood glucose and electrolyte concentrations is mandatory.

Protective isolation should be immediately instituted, with strict attention to proper use of gloves, mask, and gown by the health care team.

Neurologic assessment should be frequently performed and recorded every 4 to 6 hours as indicated. Changes in sensorium, responsiveness, pupil size, reflexes, and so on may indicate deepening of coma or the appearance of cerebral edema, the latter requiring immediate intervention with a hyperosomolar agent (mannitol, 1 gm/kg over 30 minutes).

Early *placement of arterial and jugular lines* permits nontraumatic blood sampling, and constant recording of central venous and arterial pressures. Hypotension and hypoxia are poorly tolerated by patients in fulminant hepatic failure.

Continued *correction of deranged clotting factors* with fresh-frozen plasma (10 mg/kg) is necessary for 12 to 24 hours after completion of the liver biopsy. Hematologic consultation should be obtained to help guide replacement therapy with clotting factors and platelets and to assist in monitoring laboratory signs of liver regenerative activity by specific clotting-factor assay analysis of either factor V or factor VII.

Attempts at *bowel sterilization* can be achieved with cleansing enemas (Fleet), cathartics (magnesium sulfate), and oral antibiotics (neomycin sulfate or colistin). With the recent popularity of lactulose syrup (Duphalac), whose action is in large part dependent on colonic bacteria, sterilization of the bowel with oral antibiotics has fallen into disfavor. A *cathartic action* is rapidly obtained with lactulose syrup, a result of highly osmolar metabolites produced by the bacterial degradation of this synthetic sugar. The fermentation products, being acidic in nature (lactic and acetic acids) prevent ammonigenesis in the lumen, the conversion of NH_4 into the absorbable NH_3, and favor the movement of blood ammonia into the lumen of the large bowel where it remains primarily as the ammonium ion until expelled by the cathartic ation. A dosage of 15 to 30 ml given every 4 to 6 hours will usually produce a laxative effect in children. The drug is contraindicated in infant cases of fulminant hepatic failure where galactosemia is a consideration. This agent is probably more valuable in cases of portal encephalopathy associated with underlying chronic liver disease and portal-systemic shunting.

Endotracheal intubation and *assisted ventilation* may become necessary as the coma progresses. When cerebral edema is suspected, respirator settings should be adjusted to achieve arterial $Paco_2$ values of not lower than 25 mm Hg. Many patients have a respiratory alkalosis, and great care in monitoring blood gases is needed, lest cerebral blood flow, already somewhat reduced in patients with fulminant hepatic failure, be further compromised.

Prophylactic use of *antibiotics* should be used whenever superimposed infection is suspected. A regimen of ampicillin (200 mg/kg/day) given every 4 hours and gentamicin (6 to 7 mg/kg/day) given every 8 to 12 hours is started until specific identification of the organism and its antibiotic sensitivity is available from culture results. Patients placed on ventilators are particularly prone to bronchopneumonia and simultaneously can be started on antibiotics.

The efficacy of *corticosteroid therapy* in fulminant hepatic necrosis was not demonstrated in a recently completed multicenter cooperative study. A double-blinded evaluation using hydrocortisone 400 mg/day, hydrocortisone up to 30 mg/kg/day, or placebo, yielded survival figures of 22%, 26%, and 25%, respectively. Another independent study using methylprednisolone versus placebo therapy again showed no enhancement of survival figures and perhaps a detrimental effect.

The role of steroids (dexamethasone, Decadron) in the control of cerebral edema that occurs in fulminant hepatic failure has not been specifically studied. In the experimental model, using a hepatic devascularization technique in pigs, intracranial hypertension could be prevented, but only when methylprednisolone was given immediately before or within 4 hours after the surgery. The indications for the use of Decadron in childhood cases of hepatic failure could be argued on the evidence that cerebral edema is much more common in this age group, once signs of hepatic en-

cephalopathy develop. Neurosurgical doses of Decadron, in the order of 0.5 mg/kg given every 6 to 8 hours, can be started as soon as the suspicion of increased intracranial pressure exists.

A variety of mechanisms may be responsible for the observed beneficial actions of L-dopa. Increasing the concentration of dopamine and norepinephrine in the brain (normal precursors) displaces accumulated false neurochemical transmitters from the synaptosomes. As with many other modalities a recent prospective controlled study found L-dopa ineffective in the treatment of cirrhotic hepatic encephalopathy. Those patients who awaken from hepatic coma and show improvement in sensorium do so without improvement of hepatic function. This agent has no obvious effect upon survival figures.

Hyperimmune anti-HBsAg gamma globulin has not been of benefit when administered to patients presenting with hepatitis B fulminant liver disease.

Heroic therapeutic modalities. The ever growing list of treatment modalities used in fulminant hepatic failure reflects the continued frustration in adequately dealing with this disease condition. Note list below:

"Heroic" modalities used in treating fulminant hepatic failure with coma

> Two-volume blood exchange
> Peritoneal dialysis
> Hemodialysis
> Plasmapheresis-plasma exchange
> Hemoperfusion over activated-charcoal columns
> Total body washout with hypothermia
> Cross-circulation with human volunteers
> Cross-circulation with baboons
> Hyperbaric oxygenation
> Heterotropic liver transplantation
> Orthotopic liver transplantation
> Heterotropic substances (insulin, glucagon, and
>   others)

Most methods are attempts at providing some reasonable degree of homeostasis for the patient while awaiting functional restitution of the incompetent liver. Other efforts have been directed at stimulating a regenerative response by the damaged organ.

With the availability of pediatric-sized Scribner shunts or other modifications that allow easier access to larger blood vessels, the most frequently employed therapeutic measures are two-volume blood exchanges, *plasmapheresis with plasma exchange,* and *hemodialysis using a high permeability membrane* (polyacrylonitrile). What is common to all these forms of therapy is the high likelihood of recovery of consciousness (35% to 60% versus 20% to 25% without extracorporeal assistance), which may be partial, complete, or transient. Unfortunately, survival rates at the present time, whenever any of these more complicated therapeutic modalities are used, are no better than conventional supportive treatment is.

Our dismal results with exchange transfusions in children with fulminant hepatic necrosis (8 patients, no long-term survivors) prompted a trial of hemoperfusion over charcoal (1), polyacrylonitrile-membrane hemodialysis (1), and plasmapheresis-plasma exchange (3) in the most recent cases. Technically, the procedures went well, and hypotension was avoided by strict attention to volume fluctuations during the dialysis period. Unfortunately, all patients eventually succumbed, none showing signs of liver regenerative activity.

Enthusiasm for using *hemoperfusion over activated charcoal* quickly diminished when a number of important adverse side effects were recognized. Specifically, hypotension develops in association with the appearance of platelet aggregates in the patient's blood. This latter phenomenon was believed directly related to the screen-filtration pressures required, and since thrombasthenia has been noted in patients with fulminant hepatic failure, their platelets are predisposed to further damage during passage through the charcoal column. The release of vasoactive substances from the damaged platelets is postulated as the mechanism for the observed hypotension. Hemodialysis should be considered only if pediatric nephrologic support is available. In addition, plasmapheresis-plasma exchange will require blood banking and hematology support as well.

Direct measurement of intracranial pressure by epidural or subdural monitors would be most beneficial in management of these complicated patients provided that hemostasis can be ensured. The newly developed Ladd 1900 intracranial pressure monitor, which can be placed in the epidural space, has greater appeal than other devices that record intracranial pressures from the subdural space or ventricular system. Otherwise, indirect assessment of cerebral edema may be obtained from computerized tomography (CT scan) based upon brain density and ventricular size.

The beneficial effect of *insulin* and *glucagon* upon the liver morphology and cell division has been shown in various experimental animal models (devascularization studies, fulminant murine hepatitis). The use of these hepatotropic substances in humans with fulminant hepatic failure has not been reported. In view of the known complexity of action of these hormones, capable of stimulating both synergistic and antagonistic events at the cellular level, clarification of the possible role of such agents must await results of additional experimental studies in other models of liver injury. The role of extrapancreatic and extraportal hepatotropic substances in hepatic regeneration also needs further clarification. Titration of the proper amounts of norepinephrine, somatomedin, intestinal glucagon, growth hormone, and probably others, to achieve a positive metabolic result that facilitates the recovery of damaged hepatocytes, remains a challenge of some magnitude.

Heterotopic liver transplantation as a means of providing temporary support while one awaits liver regeneration has had limited application. *Orthotopic liver replacement* in the face of fulminant hepatic failure is probably contraindicated for many reasons, but especially in the face of suspected virus-induced disease where the risk of infection to the transplanted organ might still exist.

Results of therapy and prognosis. A scarcity of reports dealing with fulminant hepatic necrosis in pediatric-age patients attests to the relative infrequency of this condition in children. However, the available data would challenge impressions that outcome results are better for children than adults. A French group reported 21 cases of proved, or presumed, virus-induced hepatic failure in very young children, with seven having complete recovery. Five of the survivors had hepatitis B virus infection, and all patients were treated with standard, conservative means. A British group reported nine of 31 children (38%) survived an episode of fulminant hepatic failure, but only 6% of those reaching stage IV coma. Similarly, a 33% survival figure is also reported in some adult series, and occasionally higher survival figures. These are perhaps attributable to a different cause (acetaminophen poisonings) from that usually encountered in the pediatric population. Other British workers reported a 42% survival rate using charcoal-column hemoperfusion and a 30.8% survival rate using polyacrylonitrite membrane hemodialysis, compared to their previous 13% survival rate when using conventional medical treatment. Another French group, with a very large adult experience in treatment of fulminant hepatic failure, could not demonstrate a significant change in survival figures (23% versus 18%) between a similar hemodialysis technique and standard supportive therapy. Our experience with 17 cases of fulminant hepatic necrosis has been very dismal, with only a single survivor (conservative treatment) of those reaching stage III-IV hepatic coma.

Prognosis is probably not always directly related to the severity of the liver injury; rather, it is also influenced by multifactorial events including the specific cause, host response, age of patient, and presence or absence of underlying liver disease. However, differences in outcome results are also related to prevention or treatment of intercurrent complications of acute hepatic failure, such as cerebral edema, hemorrhage, and infection. Any of these complications may occur in the face of improving liver function, with histologic evidence of reasonable hepatocyte volume fraction.

A recent adult experience (Acute Hepatic Failure Study Group, University of Southern California), in regard to etiology and prognosis, had better survival rates in younger patients (15 to 44 years) with hepatic B disease (37%) than those in non-A, non-B disease (13%). As expected, patients over 45 years of age did poorly, regardless of cause, with survival of 13% versus 17% for hepatitis B and non-A, non-B causes respectively.

Generally speaking, the young adult with acute hepatic failure from acetaminophen (Tylenol) overdosage has a better chance for survival. The main factors responsible for death in these patients are usually ones that are potentially preventable or treatable. Perhaps only 25% of patients with massive hepatic necrosis die without other complicating events and instead succumb to the direct toxic effects of circulating metabolites that accumulate in the face of incompetent liver function.

Significant cerebral edema develops in probably 50% or more of patients reaching coma of stages III and IV, with autopsy evidence of herniation of the temporal lobe, cerebellar tonsils, or brainstem being found in up to one third of cases. This finding may be present despite astute management of fluid and electrolyte therapy, careful attention to neurologic scores, and early intervention with anticerebral edema therapy.

Potential fatal *hemorrhage* becomes an important consideration in the face of thrombocytopenia. As a group, the prolongation of prothrombin and partial thromboplastin times does not correlate with the likelihood of major hemorrhage. The decline in platelets may be explained by bone-marrow hypofunction in some, by disseminated intravascular coagulation (DIC) in others, or by both. Efforts should be made to keep the platelet count above $50,000/mm^3$ while treating or eliminating the cause or causes of DIC wherever applicable.

Infection with resulting sepsis and endotoxemia accounts for the terminal event in 25% or more of patients, particularly those in whom heroic measures are responsible for prolonged survival. Ventilator support predisposes to bronchopulmonary infections, especially in patients predisposed to pulmonary edema from central causes.

Renal failure develops frequently in patients with fulminant hepatic necrosis and may have different causes. Prerenal failure can be prevented by detailed attention to fluid management and monitoring of central venous pressure. Acute tubular necrosis and oliguric renal failure may complicate the clinical picture of patients ingesting hepatonephrotoxic substances, but they have also been noted in virus-caused (hepatitis B) fulminant failure. Most commonly this complication occurs after a hypotensive episode from hemorrhage or septic shock. So-called functional renal failure (hepatorenal failure), characterized by low urine sodium concentration (less than 20 mEq/L), normal urine sediment, and urine–plasma urea ratio of less than 10, is believed to be caused by hemodynamic alterations found in fulminant hepatic failure. This renal disorder manifests itself particularly in those patients with a prolonged course and carries a poor prognosis. As a result of renal failure, the cumulative impact of toxic metabolites upon cellular function can easily be appreciated.

A few studies have examined liver biopsy material taken during hepatic coma, or soon after recovery, or immediately after death, as a possible predictor of outcome. One must remember that histologic assessment of the remaining hepatocytes in fulminant hepatic necrosis may not correlate with the functional capabilities of these same cells. In general, patients with less than 15% estimated hepatocyte volume fraction (HVF) seem to have little, if any, chance of surviving. Patients found to have over 25% HVF may survive, provided that they are not victims of the other aforementioned complications. Those that survive longer because of the use of heroic measures are at added risk to incur a complication of treatment. Chances of these complications are enhanced in those patients without evidence of liver regenerative function (improving coagulation studies, elevated alpha-fetoprotein levels) and kept alive by heroic means, but they have unfortunately been noted in patients in whom liver function has improved and histologic evidence of regeneration was present at autopsy.

The importance of obtaining histologic tissue whenever possible from patients with fulminant hepatic failure is emphasized by the observation (certainly in adults) that a poor correlation exists between the serverity of illness, as assessed by staging of coma, and the histologic lesion. Hepatic coma may supervene in selectively sensitive patients in the face of substantive amounts of morphologically intact hepatic tissue.

REFERENCES

Adler, R., Mahnovski, V., Heuser, E.T.,.and others: Fulminant hepatitis, Am. J. Dis. Child. **131**:870-872, 1977.

Auslander, M.O., and Gitnick, G.L.: Vigorous medical management of acute fulminant hepatitis, Arch. Intern. Med. **137**:599-601, 1977.

Conomy, J.P., and Swash, M.: Reversible decerebrate and decorticate postures in hepatic coma, N. Engl. J. Med. **278**:875-879, 1978.

Denis, J., Poplon, P., Nusinovici, V., and others: Treatment of encephalopathy during fulminant hepatic failure by hemodialysis with high permeability membrane, Gut **19**:787-793, 1978.

Dupuy, J.M., Frommel, D., and Alagille, D.: Severe viral hepatitis type B in infancy, Lancet **1**:191-194, 1975.

Dupuy, J.M., Dulac, O., Dupuy, C., and Alagille, D.: Severe hyporegenerative viral hepatitis in children, Proc. R. Soc. Med. **70**:228-232, 1977.

Farivar, M., Wands, J.R., Isselbacher, K.J., and Bucher, N.L.R.: Effect of insulin and glucagon on fulminant murine hepatitis, N. Engl. J. Med. **295**:1517-1519, 1976.

Fischer, J.E., Rosen, H.M., Ebeid, A.M., and others: The effect of normalization of plasma amino acids on hepatic encephalopathy in man, Surgery **80**:77-91, 1976.

Fischer, J.E., Funovics, J.M., Falcao, H.A., and Wesdorp, R.I.C.: L-Dopa in hepatic coma, Ann. Surg. **183**:386-391, 1976.

Gazzard, B.G., Henderson, J.M., and Williams, R.: Factor VII levels as a guide to prognosis in fulminant hepatic failure, Gut **17**:489-491, 1976.

Gazzard, B.G., Portmann, B., Murray-Lyon, I.M., and Williams, R.: Causes of death in fulminant hepatic failure and relationship to quantitative histological assessment of parenchymal damage, Q. J. Med., new ser. **46**(176):615-626, Oct. 1975.

Gregory, P.B., Knauer, C.M., Kempson, R.L., and Miller, R.: Steroid therapy in severe viral hepatitis, N. Engl. J. Med. **294**:681-687, 1976.

Hanid, M.A., MacKenzie, R.L., Jenner, R.E., and others: Intracranial pressure in pigs with surgically induced acute liver failure, Gastroenterology **76**:123-131, 1979.

Horney, J.T., and Galambos, J.T.: The liver during and after fulminant hepatitis, Gastroenterology **73**:639-645, 1977.

Hoyumpa, A.M., Jr., Desmond, P.V., Avant, G.R., and others: Hepatic encephalopathy, Gastroenterology **76**:184-195, 1979.

James, J.H., Ziparo, V., Jeppsson, B., and Fisher, J.E.: Hyperammonaemia, plasma aminoacid imbalance, and blood-brain aminoacid transport: a unified theory of portal-systemic encephalopathy, Lancet **2**:772-775, 1979.

Kalk, H.: Biopsy findings during and after hepatic coma and after acute necrosis of the liver, Gastroenterology **36**:214-218, 1959.

Karvountzis, G.G., Redeker, A.G., and Peters, R.L.: Long term follow-up studies of patients surviving fulminant viral hepatitis, Gastroenterology **67**:870-877, 1974.

Kaymakcalan, H., Dourdourekas, D., Szanto, P.B., and Steigmann, F.: Congestive heart failure as cause of fulminant hepatic failure, Am. J. Med. **65**:384-388, 1978.

Lepore, M.J., Stutman, L.J., Bonanno, C.A., and others: Plasmapheresis with plasma exchange in hepatic coma. 2. Fulminant viral hepatitis as a systemic disease, Arch. Intern. Med. **129**:900-907, 1972.

Michel, H., Solere, M., Granier, P., and others: Treatment of cirrhotic hepatic encephalopathy with L-dopa: a controlled trial, Gastroenterology **79**:207-222, 1980.

Murray-Lyon, I.M., Orr, A.H., Gazzard, B., and others: Prognostic value of serum alpha-fetoprotein in fulminant hepatic failure including patients treated by charcoal haemoperfusion, Gut **17**:576-580, 1976.

Popper, H.: Implications of portal hepatotrophic factors in hepatology, Gastroenterology **66**:1227-1233, 1974.

Psacharopoulos, H.T., Mowat, A.P., Davies, M., and others: Fulminant hepatic failure in childhood, Arch. Dis. Child. **55**:252-258, 1980.

Rakela, J.: A double-blinded, randomized trial of hydrocortisone in acute hepatic failure, Gastroenterology **76**:1297, 1979 (Abstract).

Rakela, J.: Etiology and prognosis in fulminant hepatitis, Gastroenterology **77**:A33, 1979 (Abstract).

Redeker, A.G., and Yamahiro, H.S.: Controlled trial of exchange transfusions therapy in fulminant hepatitis, Lancet **1**:3-6, 1973.

Rueff, B., and Benhamon, J.P.: Acute hepatic necrosis and fulminant hepatic failure, Gut **14**:805-815, 1973.

Schenker, S., Breen, K.J., and Hoyumpa, A.M., Jr.: Hepatic encephalopathy: current status, Gastroenterology **66**:121-151, 1974.

Sheinbaum, A.J., Damus, K.H., Michael, T.D., and Gitnick G.L.: Acute fulminant hepatitis: a clustering of cases, Arch. Intern. Med. **134**:1093-1094, 1974.

Scotto, J., Opolon, P., Eteve, J., and others: Liver biopsy and prognosis in acute liver failure, Gut **14**:927-933, 1973.

Silk, D.B.A., Hanid, M.A., Trewby, P.N., and others: Treatment of fulminant hepatic failure by polyacrylonitrile-membrane haemodialysis, Lancet **2**:1-3, 1977.

Terblanche, J., and Starzl, T.E.: Hepatic regeneration, Int. J. Artif. Organs **2**(2):49-52, 1979.

Teutsch, C., and Brennan, R.W.: *Amanita* mushroom poisoning with recovery from coma: a case report, Ann. Neurol. **3:**177-179, 1978.

Trewby, P.B., Warren, R., Contini, S., and others: Incidence and pathophysiology of pulmonary edema in fulminant hepatic failure, Gastroenterology **74:**859-865, 1978.

Ware, A.J., D'Agostino, A.N., and Combes, B.: Cerebral edema: a major complication of massive hepatic necrosis, Gastroenterology **61:**877-884, 1971.

Ware, A.J., Jones, R.E., Shorey, J.W., and Combes, B.: A controlled trial of steroid therapy in massive hepatic necrosis, Am. J. Gastroenterol. **62:**130-133, 1974.

Williams, R.: Fulminant viral hepatitis, Clin. Gastroenterol. **3:**419-436, 1974.

Williams, R.: Hepatic failure and development of artificial liver support system. In Popper, H., and Schaffner, F., editors: Progress in liver diseases, vol. 5, New York, 1976, Grune & Stratton, Inc.

Wilkinson, S.P., Blendis, L.M., and Williams, R.: Frequency and type of renal and electrolyte disorders in fulminant hepatic failure, Br. Med. J. **1:**186-189, 1974.

Zafrani, E.S., Pinaudeau, Y., LeCudonnec, B., and others: Focal hemorrhagic necrosis of the liver, Gastroenterology **79:**1295-1299, 1980.

Zieve, L., and Nicoloff, D.M.: Pathogenesis of hepatic coma, Ann. Rev. Med. **26:**143-151, 1975.

Zieve, L.: Hepatic encephalopathy: summary of present knowledge with an elaboration on recent developments. In Popper, H., and Schaffner, F., editors, Progress in liver diseases, vol. 6, New York, 1979, Grune & Stratton, Inc.

24 *Chronic liver disease*

CHRONIC HEPATITIS

Chronic hepatitis is defined as ongoing inflammation within the liver sustained beyond the expected time of resolution. For most adult hepatologists up to 6 months is considered an acceptable time to allow for clearing of an acute liver insult before specialized laboratory investigations or invasive studies are considered. A somewhat shorter time (3 months) is utilized by physicians involved in evaluating liver disease in children. An important reason offered for this "pediatric" deviation is that the sooner one can separate out those treatable forms of chronic hepatitis, the better the long-term prognosis will be for the child and occasionally for affected but asymptomatic siblings. This is especially true for Wilson's disease and may likewise be applicable to chronic active hepatitis. In addition, early recognition of some forms of liver disease permits prompt genetic counseling to the young parents considering large families.

Since many important liver diseases may not distinguish themselves by early expression of underlying liver injury, only a high degree of awareness will allow for their identification. Not infrequently the diagnosis of chronic hepatitis may rest on a specific pathologic lesion or biochemical data, particularly when the onset has been insidious and the real duration of illness unknown. A perplexing feature of chronic (and sometimes acute) hepatitis is lack of specificity, for clinical and biochemical evidence of ongoing liver disease may persist for varying lengths of time regardless of its cause. Variation in the clinical patterns may be seen in patients with chronic hepatitis having a similar histologic lesion. At other times clinical features and biochemical abnormalities are similar, though the cause is different. It would appear that both duration of hepatic injury and type of histologic lesion that follows liver injury are attributable to multiple influences. The specific inciting agent, persistence of the agent, underlying metabolic deficiency state, host response, and probably other factors as yet unknown are involved in these permutations.

In contrast to those of adults, most pediatric cases of chronic hepatitis have a clinically recognizable onset of disease and the diagnosis is entertained when jaundice persists, hepatitis B virus remains present, or biochemical parameters of liver injury fail to resolve when expected. Careful follow-up study of patients with acute liver disease of any cause is needed to recognize those patients in whom known hepatic disease is not resolving as expected. In such cases additional screening laboratory studies are necessary, as outlined in Fig. 21-6. In cases with an insidious presentation of unknown duration, prompt investigation to rule out treatable conditions is likewise imperative. The situation is more difficult in cases with an insidious onset, where clinical jaundice is usually lacking and other complaints may be quite nonspecific. Here the diagnosis of underlying liver disease is seldom suspected, and more likely it becomes apparent after the serendipitous results of screening laboratory studies reveal liver dysfunction. It is worthwhile to emphasize again that proper attention to details of the physical examination often yields information indicating chronic liver disease (p. 740).

Notwithstanding the well-known potential shortcoming of diagnostic liver biopsy, that of sampling error, the adage holds that *when liver disease persists, examination of liver tissue is most important:* (1) Prognosis seems to correlate better with the pathologic nature of the lesion than with the clinical and biochemical aspects of the disease, and (2) the decision to institute specific treatment for chronic hepatitis can best be made after identification and characterization of the histologic lesion in the liver. That some patients with persisting biochemical disease eventually recover completely, even after many months or years of active disease, has been documented by serial liver biopsies. Others have biochemical relapses, suggesting disease activity after having been seemingly well. When these patients are subjected to liver biopsy, the so-called benign lesion of acute or persisting hepatitis may again be apparent. Although the presence of recurrent clinical disease and prolonged disease suggests chronicity, the clinician cannot be sure of the proper diagnosis until tissue is available for examination.

Pathologic lesions

Hepatologists have been striving for an agreement of a workable classification of chronic hepatitis based on the pathologic characteristics of the liver. Two major categories of chronic hepatitis have been distinguished from pathologic specimens and are based on the location of the inflammatory lesion within the liver. Within certain limits these two groups also have clinical and biochemical correlates, which together with the histologic lesion can suggest the need for treatment, as well as the eventual prognosis. This should not suggest that each group is a distinct disease entity but rather a disease process that may have varied causes. In fact, a number of disease conditions can produce either of these histologic lesions. In other cases, features of both lesions may be present in the same biopsy material. Furthermore, the histologic lesion may change from one category to another and back again, dictated by the natural history of the disease or as influenced by therapy. These observations only serve to emphasize the importance of correlating the clinical, biochemical, and pathologic data with each individual case of chronic hepatitis before one decides upon treatment or offers a final prognosis.

If the biopsy specimen shows definite features of cirrhosis (fibrosis and regenerating nodules), it is excluded from the classification of chronic hepatitis, though both lesions often are found simultaneously.

Chronic persistent hepatitis is a pathologic diagnosis suggested by the biopsy specimen that shows sustained hepatic inflammation primarily within the portal tracts. The portal inflammatory reaction consists of lymphocytes, plasma cells, and macrophages. Basically the lobular architecture is preserved with little or no fibrosis. Features of acute hepatitis may be present, with areas of spotty hepatocellular necrosis seen in the lobules (Figs. 24-1 and 24-2). Occasionally, polymorphonuclear cells and eosinophils may also be seen in association with small interlobular bile ducts. The perilobular zone is minimally infiltrated, and the limiting plate of the lobules is intact.

This is the characteristic lesion that accompanies slowly resolving ("prolonged") viral hepatitis, is often present when persisting antigenemia (HBsAg) exists, and will be found during episodes of "relapsing" or "two-phase" hepatitis. Some variation of this basic pathologic lesion is common in systemic diseases that have a hepatic component and is referred to as non-specific reactive hepatitis. Toxic and drug causes often produce a similar histologic lesion, and metabolic liver disease also deserves special consideration, including Wilson's disease and alpha-1-antitrypsin deficiency. Specific etiologic markers are not always apparent in liver biopsy specimens. A ground-glass appearance to cytoplasm that stains positively with orcein should suggest HBV disease (Fig. 24-3). Cytoplasmic globular deposits that are PAS positive and diastase negative indicate alpha-1-antitrypsin–deficiency disease. A combination of mild steatosis, glycogen nuclei, and perilobular fibrosis is suggestive of Wilson's disease. Infiltrations of the liver by proliferative lymphoreticular diseases may look very much like chronic persistent hepatitis. Resolving neonatal hepatitis may at times yield a pathologic lesion suggesting chronic persistent hepatitis. Finally, the lesion of chronic persistent hepatitis may be the "quiescent" stage of chronic aggressive hepatitis either from spontaneous natural evolution of the disease or as a result of steroid treatment.

Chronic aggressive hepatitis categorizes another pathologic lesion found in some patients with chronic hepatitis. Here the inflammatory lesion is not restricted to the portal zone but is found around and within the lobule. Extensions of the inflammatory process from the periportal zone into the lobule destroy neighboring hepatic cells (piecemeal necrosis) and form intralobular septa. The necrosis of hepatic cells along the limiting plate of the lobule is a prime feature of this category and is said to reflect the aggressiveness of the process (Fig. 24-4). The location and nature of the inflammatory process often disturb the lobular architecture. Liver cells are swollen and may assume pseudoglandular or pseudoductular arrangements. The cellular response is impressive, with plasma cells and lymphocytes again predominating. These cells may arrange themselves as a lymphoid follicle within the inflammatory zone. Acute inflammatory cells may be found scattered within the portal zone and the lobule as well. At times features of streaklike necrosis of hepatocytes mixed with a similar inflammatory reaction bridging portal tracts or portal zones to central veins can be seen (Fig. 21-5). Fibroblasts in association with increased collagen deposition may be prominent in the zones of necrosis.

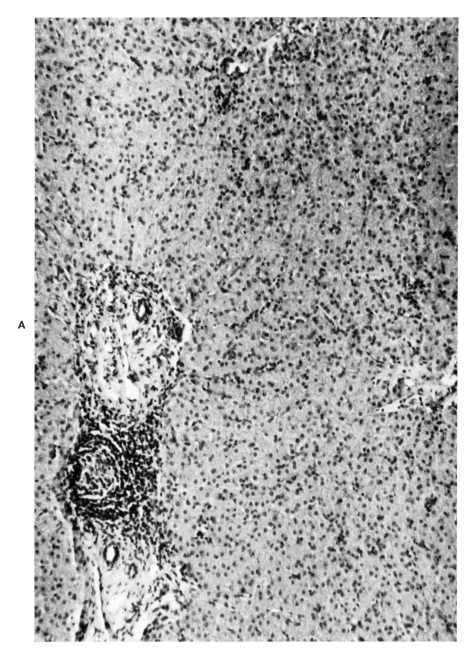

Fig. 24-1. Chronic persistent hepatitis. **A,** The biopsy specimen shows mild inflammation in the hepatic lobules and follicle formation in the portal region. Note the preservation of the basic architecture with distinct definition of the limiting plate. The liver biopsy specimen was obtained from a 3-year-old child with persistent jaundice of 2 months' duration. The initial illness was characterized by signs and symptoms believed to be compatible with hepatitis virus A disease, but the jaundice failed to resolve. Subsequent clearing did occur, and the child is now completely well. *Continued.*

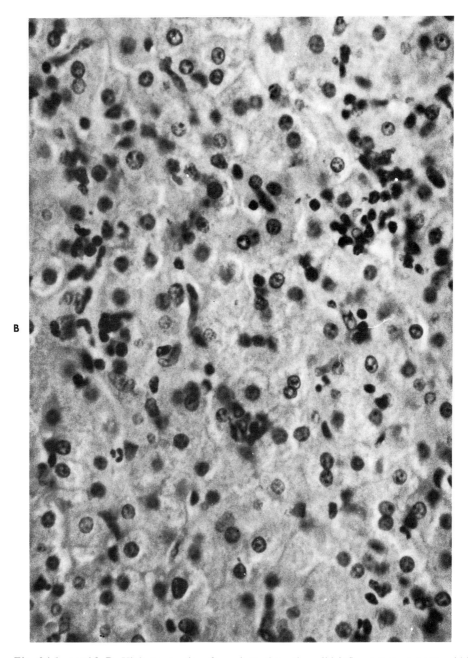

Fig. 24-1, cont'd. **B,** High-power view from **A** to show the mild inflammatory process within the lobule.

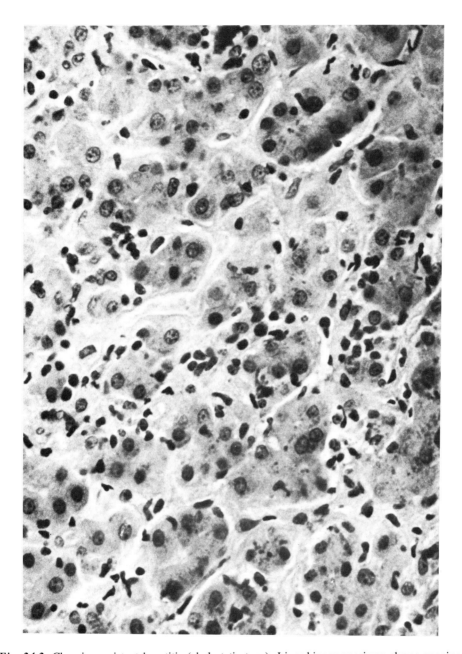

Fig. 24-2. Chronic persistent hepatitis (cholestatic type). Liver biopsy specimen shows ongoing inflammation, hepatocyte enlargement, and retention of cytoplasmic and canalicular pigment. This percutaneous needle biopsy specimen is from a 14-year-old girl with persistent jaundice of 6 weeks' duration. The initial illness was characterized by features compatible with acute hepatitis virus A disease and biochemical abnormalities consistent with this diagnosis. However, jaundice and intermittent pruritus persisted, and a modest elevation of the SGOT remained. Without further treatment, jaundice subsequently remitted within a 3-month period. Repeat liver function tests have been completely normal.

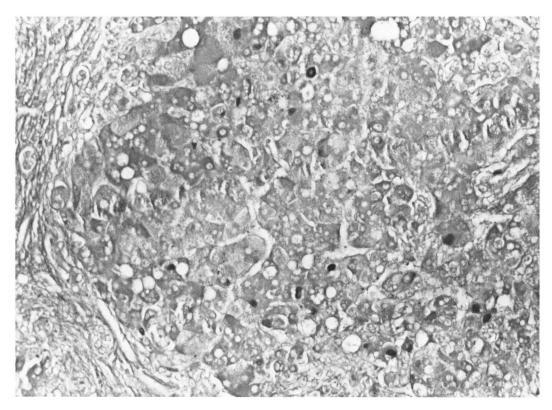

Fig. 24-3. Hepatitis B antigen. Dark cytoplasmic material indicates orcein staining of hepatitis B viral material in liver cells. (× 100.)

Again, by definition, nodular regeneration and connective tissue septa should be absent to permit inclusion of this lesion within the chronic hepatitis group. The absence of these changes may be factitious because material obtained by percutaneous or even open-liver biopsy may not provide representative sampling. Indeed, the lesion of chronic aggressive hepatitis may vary microscopically from lobule to lobule, and variations in ultrastructure may be noted from one liver cell to another when the tissue is examined by electron microscopy. It is suggested that chronic aggressive hepatitis remain a distinct pathologic classification rather than a synonym of the clinical syndrome known as chronic active hepatitis. Although most patients with the clinical features of chronic active hepatitis have this particular histologic lesion, the reverse may also occur. The lesion of chronic aggressive hepatitis may be found even though there are no clinical, biochemical, or immunochemical data suggestive of the syndrome of chronic active hepatitis (Fig. 24-5). It may simply be a more severe pathologic expression of viral hepatitis A, B, or non-A non-B. Other diagnostic possibilities should include drug hepatitis (isoniazid, L-dopa, propylthiouracil, or oxyphenisatin-containing laxatives) and underlying inflammatory bowel disease particularly chronic ulcerative colitis. Chronic aggressive hepatitis may be a rare histologic expression of Wilson's disease.

A biopsy specimen that shows chronic aggressive hepatitis generally carries a poor prognostic connotation. Reversibility of this lesion is possible, however, and it may evolve to persistent hepatitis and eventually to normal. Unfortunately, it frequently progresses to postnecrotic cirrhosis, presumably by some combination of the mechanisms proposed for self-perpetuation (see the discussion of pathogenesis on p. 682). Lobular destruction, piecemeal necrosis, and septum formation eventually result in cirrhosis of the liver.

Attempts to control the deposition of fibrous tissue by reduction of the inflammatory response with corticosteroids or inhibition of the immunologic process with azathioprine (Imuran) have been encouraging. Drug treatment, however, is not recommended in the face of chronic antigenemia. If

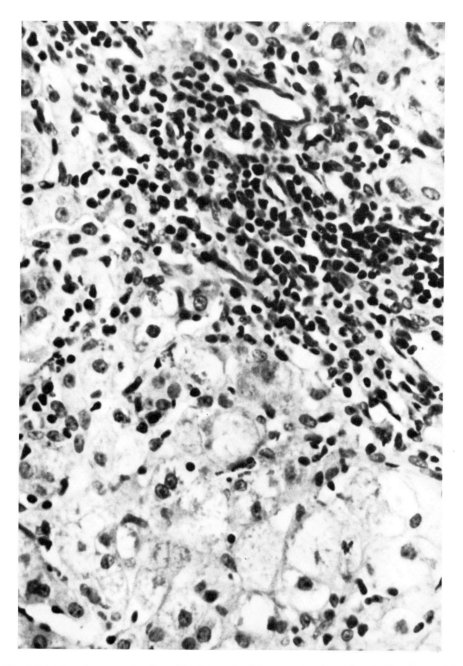

Fig. 24-4. Chronic aggressive hepatitis. Necrosis of hepatocytes along the limiting plate of the lobule is seen. The portal region contains a dense chronic inflammatory process that can be seen extending into the lobule. Persistent jaundice (3 months) was found in a 5-year-old boy who otherwise seemed well. Nontender yet moderate hepatosplenomegaly was present. Elevated gamma globulins and antinuclear antibodies were detected, in addition to abnormalities in serum bilirubin and transaminases. An open liver biopsy was done, a diagnosis of chronic active hepatitis was made, and drug therapy was then instituted.

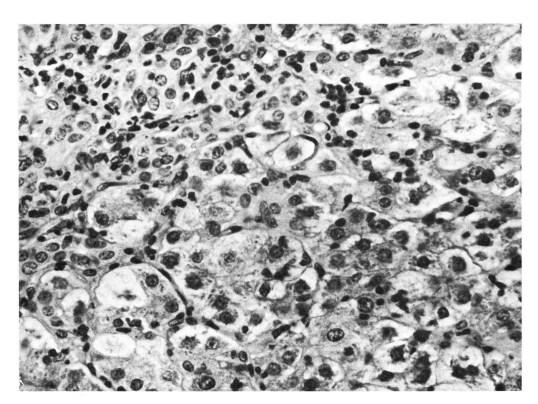

Fig. 24-5. Chronic aggressive hepatitis. Liver biopsy specimen shows loss of the limiting plate and hepatocyte necrosis along the margin of a portal zone (upper left). Lobular inflammation can also be seen. A 3-year-old child was admitted with persistent jaundice (2 months) after an illness believed to be acute viral hepatitis. Serum bilirubin and transaminase values were elevated, but other biochemical features to suggest chronic active hepatitis were lacking. No specific therapy was used, and gradual biochemical improvement was seen.

the pathologic lesion of chronic aggressive hepatitis is found in association with specific biochemical and immunologic abnormalities consistent with the syndrome of chronic active hepatitis, the use of steroids with or without immunosuppressive drugs is indicated. However, the benefits derived from these same drugs are not impressive in patients having this same lesion but not the clinical, biochemical, or immunologic features of chronic active hepatitis. In contrast to chronic persistent hepatitis, which has both pathologic and clinical specificity, chronic aggressive hepatitis refers only to a particular histologic entity. Furthermore, the clinical syndrome may evolve in a patient whose biopsy was originally believed to reflect acute hepatitis, especially when features of subacute hepatic necrosis are present. Even less severe degrees of chronic persistent hepatitis may merge imperceptibly with pathologic features of chronic aggressive hepatitis without development of clin-ical symptoms suggestive of chronic active hepatitis.

Pathogenesis

The mechanisms by which chronicity in hepatitis is established and sustained are clear for those cases in which viral hepatitis initiates the disease and continued viral infection is responsible for chronicity. Specifically the identification of hepatitis B virus surface antigen (HBsAg) in the serum of some patients with chronic hepatitis, coupled with the persistence of antigen after an acute illness that parallels clinically and histochemically active liver disease, have been taken as evidence that persistence of virus is partly responsible for chronicity in these cases.

On the other hand, the infrequent incidence of chronic hepatitis caused by type B disease in North American children has suggested to some that a different virus is more often responsible. Hepatitis

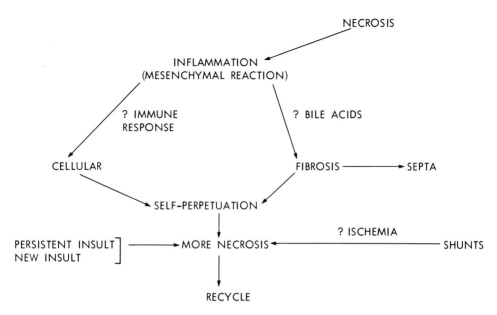

Fig. 24-6. Schematic proposal showing interrelated mechanisms for the self-perpetuation of liver disease. (From Appelman, H.D.: Am. J. Dig. Dis. **17:**463-472, 1972.)

A virus does not seem to be a likely candidate. The virus has not been recovered from stool or liver tissue of patients with chronic hepatitis or chronic active hepatitis. This is in keeping with our observations that examples of chronic active hepatitis tend to occur sporadically and a history of exposure to contacts is usually lacking. Other yet unidentified viruses (non-A, non-B group) have been found to be responsible for some examples of chronic liver disease.

Even if persistence of virus is found to be more commonly associated with chronic hepatitis than presently appreciated, host factors rather than specific causes (viral properties) may be important in perpetuation of the disease process.

Of particular importance is the heightened immunologic reactivity present in some persons to both autoantigens and foreign (viral) determinants. Some workers believe that the HLA-B8 phenotype may be a marker for this vulnerability. This may be shown after liver injury by both serologic testing and in vitro studies. Elevated levels of gamma globulins and the presence of antinuclear antibodies are taken as evidence of heightened immunologic reactivity in such persons. In addition, smooth muscle and antimitochondrial antibodies are commonly found. The persistence of high titers of antibodies to liver-specific membrane lipoprotein (anti-LSP) in patients with chronic

active liver disease especially suggests a host defect in the regulation of the activity of suppressor T-cell function. An immunologic defect in the host most likely explains the finding of HBsAg-positive chronic persistent hepatitis.

The blastic transformation of cultured lymphocytes that occurs after the addition of autologous liver homogenates from patients with chronic hepatitis indicates altered immunologic reactivity. Serum from patients with elevated titers of anti-LSP can induce in vitro normal K cells to become cytolytic to rabbit hepatocytes. In many cases of chronic liver disease it is still unclear whether the activated mesenchyme is directly responsible for the aggression or is a nonspecific, mediated response to ongoing hepatocellular injury, because of yet-undiscovered factors.

Self-perpetuation of liver disease (Fig. 24-6) has been suspected for years based on the fact that an activated mesenchyme can develop as a specific type of response to hepatic injury. The nature of the cellular response (plasma cells, lymphocytes, fibroblasts, and macrophages) is probably host-dependent but may also correlate with the severity of the initiating lesion. Mild cellular injury is associated with fewer macrophages and lymphocytes and less fibroblastic proliferation. In chronic aggressive hepatitis, it is common to see lymphocytes or plasma cells close to single liver cells or around groups of them. This association is believed to be caused by a cell-bound immunity of damaged hepatic cell membrane because specific, circulating antibodies to this structure has been recently demonstrated.

Previous studies suggested that perpetuation of hepatocellular injury in certain examples of chronic liver disease may be the result of alterations in the microcirculation of liver cells with impairment of cellular nutrition. Some alterations in blood flow are the consequence of the initial insult, but further changes result from deposition of collagen fibers by proliferating fibroblasts. Alteration in the direction of the blood flow to individual hepatic cells and impairment of cellular exchanges of nutrients and toxic products can produce cellular damage. An additional fibroblast response occurs after hepatocellular injury, and a self-perpetuation cycle develops. Failure of the reparative process to counter this response to hepatocellular injury may play a definite role in self-perpetuation in chronic hepatitis. Resorption of the pericellular and periductular framework of fibers involves, largely, the same cells (fibroblasts) that are responsible for collagen deposition. The vigor of the reparative process can be upset by host factors, the severity of the original injury, persistence of the initiating agent, nutritional status, or any combination of these. Release of specific collagenases, lysosomal hyaluronidases, and nonspecific proteolytic enzymes and the appearance of soluble collagen are events that appear necessary for removal of the scaffolding onto which collagen fibers are deposited. The inability of the host to catabolize these fibers and restore the microcirculation to the hepatic cells is now believed to be the forerunner of irreversible cirrhosis.

The role of circulating, soluble, antigen-antibody complexes arising from other tissue sites may also be important in some examples of chronic liver disease. Such a mechanism may explain the chronic liver disease seen in inflammatory bowel disease. That antigen-antibody complexes (not necessarily hepatic in origin) are taken up by hepatic cells is possible after saturation of the reticuloendothelial cells (Kupffer's cells). Fixation of these complexes in liver cells may result in injury. A pathologic lesion similar to that of chronic aggressive hepatitis can be produced experimentally by the administration of foreign protein that leads to the formation of soluble antigen-antibody complexes.

In summary, our understanding of the pathogenesis of self-perpetuation in chronic hepatitis is incomplete but the process seems to depend on an interrelationship between the host's response and the severity of the hepatocellular injury, whether the initiating agent remains. The nature of the host's response to injury is probably genetically determined; it accounts for the type of cellular response and perhaps for the balance that can be established between hepatic damage (initial and ongoing) and the reparative process.

CHRONIC PERSISTENT HEPATITIS

Chronic persistent hepatitis is also a recognized clinical syndrome that by definition includes the previously described pathologic lesion. The clinical story usually includes a previous hepatitis illness with slowly resolving biochemical parameters (and sometimes clinical features) for over 3 to 6 months, or a relapse in clinical and biochemical abnormalities after apparent resolution of the disease. Physical complaints are not particularly striking though lassitude or mild anorexia may be present. At other times, the onset of symptoms may be insidious and the diagnosis only entertained after the abnormal results of screening laboratory studies are noted. Clinical jaundice is rarely present, but the liver may be slightly enlarged. Splenomegaly is not common. The major biochemical abnormality is in elevation of serum transaminases of two- to fivefold, with the bilirubin, alkaline phosphatase, gamma glutamyl transpeptidase, and gamma globulin fraction within the normal range. All such patients should be screened for HBsAg, Wilson's disease, and alpha-1-antitrypsin deficiency. Exceptional examples may have mild hyperbilirubinemia, sometimes predominantly of the indirect fraction. Lowered levels of UDP-glucuronyl transferase have been found on liver biopsy material. This may be a consequence of chronic liver disease or, for others, a finding consistent with previously unsuspected Gilbert's disease.

Treatment and prognosis

Chronic persistent hepatitis is considered by most hepatologists to be a self-limited condition that seldom if ever requires treatment. In some patients the pathologic lesion and biochemical abnormalities may persist for years, but as long as neither significant fibrosis nor progression (aggression) occur, the prognosis remains excellent. Portal inflammation may remain as long as focal lobular injury is present. Eventual clearing is the rule, but continued follow-up study is recommended until all biochemical studies become normal. At least in children only rarely does the lesion of chronic persistent hepatitis progress to chronic aggressive hepatitis. In such cases, a sampling error in the original biopsy is the most likely explanation. Again, reevaluation of the patient's clinical course, combined with follow-up results of biochemical and immunological tests, should precede the decision to institute any form of treatment.

The prognosis for patients with chronic hepatitis and persistent antigenemia (HBsAg) is somewhat more worrisome, even when the biopsy shows classic features of chronic persistent hepatitis. Progression to chronic aggressive hepatitis, or slowly to cirrhosis, occurs in adults but fortunately is rare in North American children. A retrospective study of patients with chronic active hepatitis has shown positive results for hepatitis B virus in none to 25% of cases. It is not always possible to be certain that the presence of HBsAg in patients with chronic-active hepatitis represents cause and effect. Be that as it may, present evidence suggests that steroid treatment in HBsAg-positive patients is contraindicated.

REFERENCES

Alagille, D., Gautier, M., Herouin, C. and Hadchouel, M.: Chronic hepatitis in children, Acta. Paediatr. Scand. **62**:566-570, 1973.

Appleman, H.D.: Cirrhosis: morphologic dynamics for the non-morphologist, Am. J. Dig. Dis. **17**:463-472, 1972.

Becker, M.D., Baptista, A., Scheuer, P.J., and Sherlock, S.: Prognosis of chronic persistent hepatitis, Lancet **1**:53-57, 1970.

Boyer, J.L.: Chronic hepatitis: a perspective of classification and determinants of prognosis, Gastroenterology **70**:1161-1171, 1976.

Felsher, B.F., and Carpio, N.M.: Chronic persistent hepatitis and unconjugated hyperbilirubinemia, Gastroenterology **76**:248-252, 1979.

Popper, H.: What is chronic hepatitis? Gastroenterology **50**:444-448, 1966.

Popper, H., and Schaffner, F.: The vocabulary of chronic hepatitis, N. Engl. J. Med. **284**:1154-1156, 1971.

Redeker, A.G.: Chronic hepatitis, Med. Clin. North Am. **59**:863-867, 1975.

Sherlock, S.: Progress report: chronic hepatitis, Gut **15**:581-597, 1974.

CHRONIC ACTIVE HEPATITIS

After the first few months of life, when liver disease is primarily caused by neonatal hepatitis or anatomic aberrations of the biliary system, the leading cause of persistent jaundice and chronic liver disease in the pediatric population is chronic active hepatitis. Over the years, many names have been employed in an attempt to describe specific aspects of the clinical, laboratory, or histologic features of chronic active hepatitis: lupoid hepatitis, active juvenile cirrhosis, plasma cell hepatitis, subacute hepatitis, subacute hepatic necrosis, chronic liver disease in young people, and chronic aggressive hepatitis.

The cause of this clinicopathologic entity remains unknown. Recent evidence indicates that different inciting agents may indeed be responsible for the initial insult, whereas the disease itself most likely represents a specific kind of response to hepatic injury that becomes manifest only in certain susceptible individuals. Known causes include HBV, alpha-methyldopa, isoniazid, nitrofurantoin, and oxyphenisatin-containing laxatives. It may also be a complication of other prominent immunologic disturbances such as ulcerative colitis and Sjögren's syndrome. The hepatic lesion may at times be seen in severe viral hepatitis, Wilson's disease, and less often alpha-1-antitrypsin–deficiency disease.

There is little doubt that in some patients chronic active hepatitis may evolve as a consequence of hepatitis B virus, whereas hepatitis A virus has not been incriminated as causative. However, serial liver biopsies and laboratory tests have shown that an illness indistinguishable from acute viral hepatitis type A can become chronic active hepatitis. This progression may be very rapid (3 or 4 weeks), especially in cases with subacute hepatic necrosis, or may evolve slowly (months to years) from a lesion consistent with chronic persistent hepatitis. Although most of our cases have an abrupt onset, with a clinical syndrome similar to that of hepatitis A virus disease, documentation of exposure to or contact with usual suspected sources of hepatitis has been lacking. Secondary cases in the patient's household have similarly been extremely rare. Not surprisingly anti-HAV has also been absent in our more recent cases. Evidence for HBV-caused disease has been consistently absent in our pediatric patients with chronic active hepatitis. This latter observation is in keeping with some published reports, but it is at odds with those reporting a 3% to 50% incidence of recovery of that antigen from serums of similar patients. A viral cause remains most likely in our group of patients, and perhaps the non-A, non-B group is responsible.

When chronic hepatitis develops as a sequel to acute hepatitis B virus disease (10%), a significant number of these patients will eventually develop the clinical, biochemical, and histopathologic manifestations of chronic active hepatitis. The presence of antigen (HBsAg) in the serum of some patients with chronic liver disease has been taken as evidence that the original injury was viral in nature and that chronicity is indeed caused by persistence of this agent. Incidence figures seem quite variable at present, but there is no doubt that chronic active hepatitis evolves as a consequence of this etiologic agent in a certain number of patients. Although many cases of hepatitis B virus disease are insidious in onset, a history positive for exposure is found in 15% to 20% of adult cases.

There probably are other causes of chronic active hepatitis, and this term represents a syndrome arising from a broad range of diseases having in common the ability to produce the characteristic clinicopathologic picture repeatedly seen in such patients. If this is true, a disordered host-dependent immunologic response to liver injury best explains aspects of chronicity.

Both the development of the autoimmune phenomenon in patients with chronic active hepatitis and the nature of the mesenchymal response characteristic of the pathologic hepatic lesion is probably host-determined rather than specific for any particular cause. The role of autoimmune aggression if not the cause for this disease appears to be an important factor responsible for perpetuating the liver disease.

The genetic basis for the development of chronic active liver disease was suggested by several reports showing an increased incidence of the histocompatability antigen HLA-B8 in patients than in controls (60% versus 18%). This is an attractive observation, since the HLA loci are closely linked to the immune-responsiveness genes, and this phenotype is frequently found in other autoimmune diseases (celiac disease, dermatitis herpetiformis, myasthenia gravis, and systemic lupus erythematosus). This genetically determined, exaggerated immune responsiveness to both autoantigens and foreign (viral) determinants has also been found in relatives of patients with chronic active liver disease. These asymptomatic family members tend to have a high prevalence of seroimmunologic abnormalities. On the other hand, the familial occurrence of chronic active liver disease remains rare (we have seen it but once), and re-

cent studies have not confirmed the disproportionately high incidence of the HLA-B8 phenotype in this condition.

Another host-determined factor believed responsible for chronicity of injury to the liver (or other organs) is a defect in "suppressor" T-cell function. Some believe that the HLA-B8 is a marker for this specific vulnerability. This subpopulation of T lymphocytes is responsible for regulating the production of cell membrane–directed antibody produced by helper B cells. The observed unchecked autoantibody production and resulting ongoing antibody-dependent cell cytolysis through K-cell activity in patients with chronic active hepatitis could be explained by the defect in "suppressor" T-cell function to switch off this process.

Finally, the possibility exists that for some patients chronic liver disease develops as an unfortunate consequence of their genetic makeup that permits the development of self-antigens by the forbidden-clone theory.

Earlier evidence for the role of an autoimmune process in perpetuating chronic active hepatitis was an associative one and came indirectly from the findings of elevated seroimmunologic titers similar to those of other suspected autoimmune diseases. The most constant serologic abnormality is hypergammaglobulinemia (90%), but other serologic tests often yield positive results including antinuclear antibody (25% to 50%) and Coombs' testing. Circulating antibodies to smooth muscle (50% to 75%), antimitochondrial antibodies (25%), antiglomerular antibody, anti-*Salmonella* agglutinins, and antithyroid antibodies have also been demonstrated. During the course of the illness, extrahepatic manifestations often develop, indicating autoimmune reactivity possibly provoked by circulating antigen-antibody complexes. These manifestations include arthralgias and arthritis, colitis, pleurisy, thyroiditis, and glomerulonephritis. Further studies are still needed to determine whether the reported reduction in specific portions of the complement systems (C3) is caused by immune complexes, decreased synthesis, increased catabolism, or some other mechanism. On the other hand, earlier studies had demonstrated lymphocyte transformation by liver homogenates from patients with chronic active hepatitis, an indication that the altered immune state may be cell-bound rather than humoral.

Recently, IgG antibodies directed against a liver-specific membrane lipoprotein (LSP) and against a different liver membrane antigen (LMA) have been identified in the serum of patients with acute and chronic liver disease. Although the level of these antibodies diminishes greatly after acute liver injury, they persist in high titer in patients with chronic active liver disease. The respective titer seems to correlate with the assessment of histologic activity seen in liver biopsy specimens. Both antibodies, anti-LSP and anti-LMA, have been shown by immunofluorescent studies to bind to human and rabbit hepatocytes. Serum from patients containing these autoantibodies is also capable in vitro of inducing Fc receptor–bearing K cells to become cytotoxic for rabbit hepatocytes, presumably by attaching to the nonantibody (Fc) portion of membrane-bound antibody. Cytolysis of hepatocytes is presumed to occur in vivo by a similar mechanism in patients with chronic liver disease having high titers of LSP antibody. The interaction of T- and B-lymphocyte activity against persisting neoantigens (foreign determinants) on the hepatocyte surface (HBsAg) is believed to explain the continued production of anti-LSP and anti-LMA in these examples of chronic active liver disease. However, in HBsAg-negative cases of chronic liver disease, other mechanisms must be postulated for the perpetuation of anti-LSP production and subsequent antibody-dependent cell cytolysis. Again, defective function of ''suppressor'' T-cell activity may underlie this example of chronic hepatitis. Although the role of anti-LSP, and possibly anti-LMA, in the pathogenesis of hepatocytolysis is attractive, it fails to explain the mechanism by which chronic active liver disease can develop in patients with absence of immunoglobulin-forming cells (agammaglobulinemia).

Indirect evidence of the role of autoimmune mechanisms in this disease has come both from the observation that lymphocytes and plasma cells predominate in the hepatic lesion and from the positive results of immunosuppressive regimens employed in treating this disease process. This has been suggested by the beneficial response noted to such drugs as prednisone alone or in combination with azathioprine. The biochemical and histologic improvement (disappearance of the inflammatory reaction) induced by these drugs has been attributed to their ability to reduce the antigen-antibody reactions at or near cell surfaces while exerting a beneficial effect intracellularly as well. Although improvement in long-term survival certainly occurs with treatment, the progression to cirrhosis in unfortunate patients may not be dependent on either the inflammatory reaction or the cell-bound immune phenomenon.

If a host susceptibility exists, it is not age dependent. For some time, it was believed that chronic active hepatitis was a disease peculiar to young adults, particularly women. On the contrary, the number of cases affecting very young children is also quite large. The youngest patient reported up to now whose case fits the clinical, laboratory, and histologic picture of chronic active hepatitis is an 8-month-old infant. Almost half of the children we have studied with this disease were less than 12 years of age at the onset of the disease. Although girls are affected three times more than boys, no interpretation of this sex difference can be made at present.

Clinical features

Table 24-1 summarizes the clinical features of chronic active hepatitis in 38 children. As we have repeatedly observed in this disease, it more frequently affects females than males (3 to 1). An acute hepatitis–like illness is a forerunner of most cases of chronic active hepatitis. Of the clinical findings, our experience suggests that persistent jaundice is the single most consistent abnormality in pediatric patients, being noted in all 24 patients whose illness started abruptly, and frequently (9 of 14) in those whose illness was more insidious. Therefore, failure of jaundice to resolve after 4 weeks, regardless of the mode of onset, should always be viewed suspiciously. Relapsing jaundice occurring after 8 to 10 weeks after the original time of onset of disease is also cause for concern and indeed was the presenting complaint in about 50% of patients. Those patients with an insidious presentation may only manifest extrahepatic complaints, such as arthralgia and arthritis, fever, rash (erythema nodosum), or colitis. In its most subtle form, chronic active liver disease may explain the child's fatigue, lethargy, and anorexia.

In our patient group, 90% had jaundice and hepatosplenomegaly when first seen. Spider angiomas, digital clubbing, liver palms, and erythema nodosum were seen only sporadically. A history of easy bruisability with scattered petechiae over the body is sometimes present in patients with complaints suggesting underlying chronic liver disease. Endocrine manifestations of

Table 24-1. Clinical features of chronic active hepatitis in 38 children*

	Patients		
Features	Female	Male	Total
Historic			
Sex	30	8	38
Age at onset (years)			
3-11	14	3	17
12-15	16	5	21
Type of onset			
Acute			24
Insidious			14
Patterns of jaundice			
Persisting			23
Relapsing			15
Exposure or contacts			1
Secondary cases			1
(sibling)			
Physical			
Jaundice			33
Hepatomegaly			30
Splenomegaly			28
Ascites			9
Acne			6
Digital clubbing			6
Cushingoid facies			3
Gynecomastia			2

*Seen at The Children's Hospital, Denver, and University of Colorado Medical Center. Courtesy R. S. Dubois and A. Silverman.

Table 24-2. Extrahepatic manifestations in 38 children with chronic active hepatitis*

Symptom	Number of patients
Arthralgia, arthritis	9
Amenorrhea	7
Erythema nodosum	3
Colitis	3
Thyroiditis	3
Hematuria	3
Pruritus	2
Diabetes	2
Pleurisy	1

*Seen at The Children's Hospital, Denver, and University of Colorado Medical Center. Courtesy R. S. Dubois and A. Silverman.

Table 24-3. Biochemical data from 38 children with chronic active hepatitis*

Findings	Number of patients
Serum bilirubin (mg/dl)	
1.6-5	20
5.1-10	11
10.1-20	1
More than 20	6
SGOT (IU)	
60-300	7
301-999	15
1000-2000	12
More than 2000	4
Serum albumin (less than 3 gm/dl)	17
Gamma globulin (gm/dl)	
2.1-2.9	4
3.0-3.9	19
4.0-4.9	8
More than 5	7
LE cells	13/33
Antinuclear antibody factor	14/23
Positive direct Coombs' reaction	5/23
HBsAg	0/28

*Seen at The Children's Hospital, Denver, and University of Colorado Medical Center. Courtesy R.S. Dubois and A. Silverman.

hyperadrenocorticism may be seen, and they often complicated therapy. Cushingoid facies, malar flush, acne, and pigmented nipples were most representative expressions of this condition. Secondary amenorrhea in our group of patients was noted in seven of eight patients in whom menses had started before their disease. In two patients thyroiditis developed before the liver disease became clinically apparent and in one after the disease was in remission. Three patients in the original group had symptoms of colitis, and we recently have seen a fourth case present in a similar manner. Hematuria, or proteinuria, which previously has been reported in a significant number of pediatric patients, was seen infrequently in our group of patients. A summary of the extrahepatic manifestations of that group is seen in Table 24-2. Surprisingly, some patients first present for medical care with advanced features of liver failure including ascites or hepatic encephalopathy. Others appear strikingly well and free of complaints. These observations may not correlate with the severity of the underlying histologic lesion.

Laboratory findings

Representative laboratory data from 38 children with chronic active hepatitis are seen in Table 24-3. Elevated serum bilirubin values (usually less

Table 24-4. Liver in chronic active hepatitis and acute viral hepatitis

Abnormality	Chronic active hepatitis	Acute viral hepatitis
Uniformity in severity and distribution	50%	100%
Parenchymal necrosis and cell fallout	Perilobular; widespread, lobular	Focal; pericentral
Perilobular necrosis	20%	Rare
Balloon cells, parenchymal	Prominent, perilobular	Occasional, focal
Acidophilic degeneration	Various types; Councilman bodies	Typical; Councilman bodies
Inflammatory reaction	Perilobular; portal	Portal; focal; pericentral
Bile stasis	Pericentral; perilobular	Pericentral
Fibrosis	Portal; septal; intralobular	Rare
Ductular proliferation	Common	Rare
Nodular regeneration	Common	Nil
Cirrhosis	Common	Rare
Fatty infiltration	Rare	Nil

From Mistilis, S.P., and Blackburn, C.R.B.: Am. J. Med. **48:**784, 1970.

than 10 mg/dl), elevated transaminases (SGOT), 100 to 2000 IU), and hypergammablobulinemia (greater than 2 gm/dl) are invariably present. Sulfobromophthalein retention whenever measured was abnormal (more than 5%). Antinuclear antibody of the speckled type is more likely to be present than the LE cell phenomenon and occurred in about half the patients. Up to now we have not demonstrated HBsAg in any of our patients, but in other pediatric series HBsAg may be present in 15% to 25%.

Serum albumin tended to be low or low-normal in most patients (range 1.8 to 4 gm/dl, with a mean of 2.97 gm/dl). The prothrombin time was seldom below 30% of normal; however, more than half the patients (20) had a prothrombin time of less than 50% of controls. Both in the more severe cases and terminally, further abnormalities in the serum albumin and prothrombin time become apparent. In the majority of cases the rheumatoid factor, direct Coombs' reaction, or smooth muscle antibodies will be positive. Thyroglobulin antibodies should also be sought. Elevated levels of anti-*Salmonella* agglutinins have been reported as well as circulating antiglomerular antibodies. Except for the latter antibody, these tests are generally less specific, since these serologic abnormalities may be found in patients with acute viral hepatitis (10%). Cortisol levels may be elevated in 5% of patients with chronic active hepatitis, whereas few have had low serum complement values when tested.

When hematologic abnormalities are present, they usually signify the existence of portal hypertension with hypersplenism. Mild anemia, leuko-penia, and thrombocytopenia are the most usual abnormalities. The presence of an increased reticulocyte count may be caused by increased hemolysis or blood loss through the gastrointestinal tract (esophageal varices). The finding of acanthocytes (burr cells) on the peripheral smear often indicates more advanced liver disease.

Histologic lesion (chronic aggressive hepatitis)

Many attempts have been made to distill the basic abnormality reported in chronic active hepatitis to a recognizable fundamental lesion. Because the pathologic lesion of chronic aggressive hepatitis may occur without the clinical, biochemical, or immunochemical features of the syndrome of chronic active hepatitis, some prefer to reserve the heading of chronic aggressive hepatitis to describe the liver abnormality and use the term ''chronic active hepatitis'' only for those patients having both this histologic picture and the aforementioned clinical, biochemical, and immunochemical syndrome. The liver disease in this entity and in acute viral hepatitis is compared in Table 24-4.

Histologic changes signifying active, ongoing disease in chronic active hepatitis are recognized by hepatocellular necrosis and degeneration that is typically patchy and variable but most noticeable along the limiting plate of the lobule (Fig. 24-4). At times, almost entire lobules are destroyed, and portal zones can be seen very close to each other. This represents submassive collapse from subacute hepatic necrosis. This picture may dominate the biopsy specimen or be patchy, neighboring

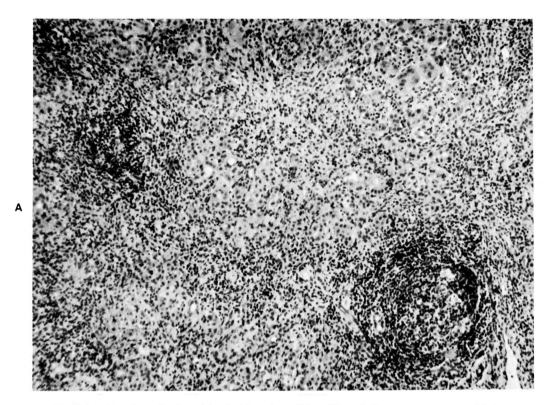

Fig. 24-7. Chronic active hepatitis. **A,** Note the striking diffuse inflammatory process with lymphoid follicle formation in the portal regions. There is associated ballooning and disorder of the liver cells with complete obliteration of the limiting plate. This liver biopsy specimen was from a 5-year-old girl with persistent jaundice of 3 months' duration. The initial illness was indistinguishable from acute viral hepatitis that failed to resolve. On physical examination 3 months later, moderate jaundice and pronounced hepatomegaly were present. Biochemical abnormalities suggesting chronic active hepatitis were found, and open biopsy was performed. Treatment with prednisone was then started. **B,** High-power view just inside a portal region from **A** to show the chronic inflammatory cells and associated degenerating hepatocytes. Note the predominance of lymphocytes and plasma cells.

lobules or zones showing much less severe changes. The hepatic cells and their nuclei vary in size and staining characteristics. Regenerating liver cells showing mitotic figures and giant multinucleated cells may be found. The inflammatory response is mainly portal and perilobular in distribution but occasionally is noted to encompass smaller groups of degenerating parenchymal cells in the manner typical of piecemeal necrosis (Fig. 24-7, *A*). The inflammatory cells are predominantly lymphocytes and plasma cells, with some polymorphonuclear leukocytes and eosinophils scattered throughout (Fig. 24-7, *B*). Macrophages are frequently seen scattered within this mesenchymal response. The inflammatory response may seem to completely replace areas in the specimen from which normal liver cells have disappeared. Actually, the hepatomegaly noted early

in this disease perhaps results from the inflammatory response rather than the hepatocellular "swelling."

Another characteristic is strands of fibrous tissue extending into lobules. These may originate from the portal zones and at times from the interlobular septum and produce piecemeal isolation of segments of a lobule, thus probably playing a significant role in the poor prognosis for patients with chronic active hepatitis.

Histologically, chronicity is indicated by the predominating type of inflammatory cell, the degree of fibrosis, and the architectural disorganization between portal zones and central veins. Activity is usually present along the limiting plate, which is distorted and irregular, and here piecemeal necrosis of small groups of liver cells can be

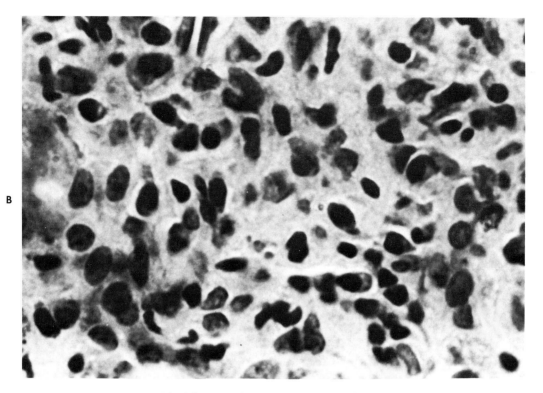

B

Fig. 24-7, cont'd. For legend see opposite page.

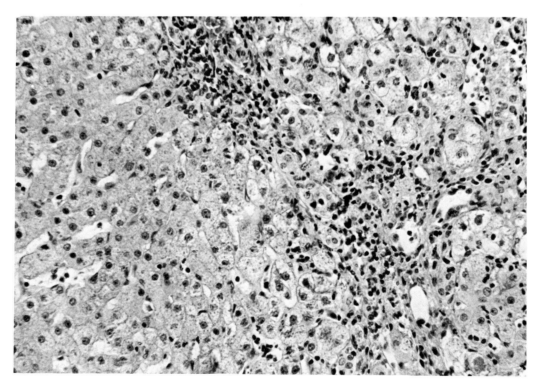

Fig. 24-8. Chronic active hepatitis. Liver biopsy specimen from an 8-year-old girl shows the lobular variation in this disease. To the left is a relatively well-preserved hepatic lobule and, to the right, one characterized by ongoing inflammatory disease. Also, note the piecemeal necrosis along the margin of the lobule.

seen. Some portal and interlobular zones may be significantly widened by fibrous connective tissue. Less active areas with features of chronicity may adjoin areas of activity but less chronicity. This variation may be present in a single biopsy specimen, but at times material from both hepatic lobes is required to appreciate this feature of the disease (Fig. 24-8).

Late in the disease, changes of cirrhosis predominate, which again may be quite spotty, with the combination of lobular collapse, nodular regeneration, and fibrosis being most typical. The cirrhosis can be either micronodular or macronodular in type, with the latter predominating. Resolution to a lesion of chronic persistent hepatitis may be seen in up to 25% of untreated cases and half of those treated. Restoration of normal architectural relationships occurs infrequently (10% to 30%) in the lesion of chronic aggressive hepatitis.

Diagnosis

The diagnosis of chronic active hepatitis should not be missed if one follows some basic rules in studying the child with jaundice, whether his disease is abrupt in onset or of an insidious nature (Fig. 21-6). One should not assume, except perhaps during epidemics of hepatitis, when definite exposure is known, that jaundice observed is actually occurring for the first time. Not infrequently preexisting liver disease, suggested only by a history of protracted asthenia, is present in the child at the time jaundice is detected. Therefore, we routinely include the serum protein electrophoresis (looking for decreased albumin and increased gamma globulin), prothrombin time, HBsAg, alpha-1-antitrypsin levels, and antinuclear antibody in the laboratory study of patients with jaundice. If chronic active hepatitis is strongly suspected, the other laboratory tests, mentioned earlier, are also done. Of course, all patients with acute or chronic liver disease should have proper studies done to rule out Wilson's disease.

With this approach to evaluating children with jaundice, we have been able to detect laboratory values consistent with chronic active hepatitis within 3 weeks of known onset of disease.

The failure of resolution of the jaundice within 3 or 4 weeks or the recurrence of jaundice after clearing should make the physician suspect chronic active hepatitis. Acute viral hepatitis may slowly improve over an 8- to 10-week period, and even when relapse occurs at this time (5% to 10%),

complete recovery should promptly follow. Elevated transaminases ("transaminitis") may remain, but the gamma globulin fraction should remain below 2 gm/dl. Although these variations may still be compatible with chronic persistent hepatitis, which may last for months with eventual complete recovery without specific treatment, laboratory clues mentioned previously and histology should be sought to clarify the problem. In addition, a rare case of subacute hepatic necrosis may have persisting jaundice as the major clinical feature before results of these laboratory tests suggest the severity and progression of the underlying lesion. The appearance of extrahepatic signs, which occur less commonly in HAV disease and usually antedate the development of icterus in HBV liver disease, should also make one suspect chronic active hepatitis. In particular, arthralgias, rashes (erythema nodosum), nephritis, cushingoid facies, acne, and colitis are most common.

Any combination of these clinical or laboratory clues that cannot resolve the diagnostic dilemma indicates the need for liver biopsy. Histologic support for specific diagnosis is mandatory before one uses potentially hazardous drugs. Liver tissue is best obtained from intraoperative biopsies or under direct vision using the laparoscope, techniques that allow sampling from nodular and internodular zones. The frequent coagulation abnormalities and the variability of this lesion not only within a biopsy specimen but also between lobes of the liver suggest that ideally direct vision biopsies are preferable. Sampling errors are especially likely to occur with the Menghini biopsy technique when cirrhosis or fibrosis is present. Laparoscopy can also be used in follow-up study for viewing changes in the liver surface while one is obtaining subsequent biopsy material. The gross morphologic evolution of the disease in response to therapy can then be correlated with the clinical and pathologic findings.

In our original patient group, liver tissue was obtained during life by either open (19) or closed (17) methods in 36 patients and at autopsy in 2 others. Severe coagulation disturbances prevented biopsy in the latter cases. Of the patients (6) with the histologic lesion of subacute hepatic necrosis with lobular collapse, high serum bilirubins and prolonged prothrombin times were the rule. Features of cirrhosis were present in 16 patients at the time of the original biopsies, a very disturbing finding. In view of the known patchy nature of the histologic lesion of chronic active hepitis and the high incidence (50%) of sampling error with percutaneous needle biopsy, the numbers of cases with cirrhotic changes may actually be higher.

That chronic active hepatitis may have other modes of presentation besides liver disease will be important to remember if this diagnosis is to be made in such cases. Unexplained joint symptoms, recurrent erythema nodosum, and colitis are the most frequent extrahepatic manifestations. In these patients, careful physical examination is so important, for low-grade icterus and hepatosplenomegaly can be detected in 90% of patients. Signs of chronic liver disease may also be present. Digital clubbing, spider nevi, liver palms (speckled palms), gynecomastia, or ascites may be detected on routine examination. The serendipity of laboratory tests by mass screening techniques has also been responsible at times for leading the physician to the right diagnosis.

In pediatrics, the differential diagnosis of chronic liver disease is not too difficult or too vast. Chronic persistent hepatitis, Wilson's disease, cystic fibrosis, and postnecrotic cirrhosis occurring after neonatal hepatitis or associated with alpha-1-antitrypsin deficiency may be considered in the differential diagnosis but can easily be distinguished by specific laboratory tests or by liver biopsy. Up to now there are no reported cases of chronic active hepatitis in children after drug therapy (methyldopa, oxyphenisatin).

A very difficult diagnostic dilemma confronts the physician when the liver disease of chronic ulcerative colitis antedates and dominates the bowel lesion. In such cases liver biopsy may be most helpful if the lesion of pericholangiolitic hepatitis is found, since this would suggest that the inflammatory bowel disease is the primary disorder.

Treatment and clinical course

The results of three controlled studies that evaluated the efficacy of drug therapy in adults with chronic active liver disease have reinforced our previous position on the value of early and vigorous treatment of this entity in the pediatric patient. All studies have shown an impressive beneficial effect when prednisone is used alone or in combination with azathioprine, but not when azathioprine is used alone. Clinical, biochemical, and immunochemical improvement can be expected in 75% to 85% of treated patients. This compares to a reported 40% mortality within 6 months in adult patients not treated with steroids. One should keep in mind that spontaneous remissions may be seen in 25% of adult patients.

As indicated, we have undertaken aggressive therapy in patients with chronic active hepatitis as soon as the clinical and laboratory diagnosis has been substantiated with histologic evidence. In a few cases confirmation of the diagnosis can be made within 6 to 8 weeks of illness.

There are several treatment protocols available for children, unfortunately, none of them controlled, provided that the patient is HBsAg negative. Our therapeutic program is to start prednisone 2 mg/kg/day up to a maximum of 60 mg daily. Once clinical and biochemical improvement is documented (usually within 2 to 4 weeks) azathioprine (Imuran) 1 mg/kg/day is added. Failure of prednisone to suppress the clinical and biochemical abnormalities within 2 to 4 weeks should prompt one to reevaluate the diagnosis of chronic active hepatitis and perhaps consider other causes of hepatocellular disease such as subacute hepatic necrosis, drug hepatitis, or severe viral hepatitis. While clinical and biochemical parameters of disease activity are monitored every 2 to 4 weeks, the prednisone dosage is reduced by 10 mg increments per week until the patient is on 20 mg daily. Thereafter, weekly reductions of 2.5 mg in a daily dose continue until the patient is off prednisone. Mild rebound elevations in transaminase may occur during weaning, at which time the prednisone dose is kept the same for 2 additional weeks and then weaning is resumed if biochemical improvement is noted. Failure of the serum transaminases to continue toward normal is an indication to raise the prednisone dose to previous levels and reevaluate the patient again in 2 to 4 weeks. An alternate-day prednisone schedule with daily azathioprine (Imuran) may sometimes be employed in patients with relapsing or persistent biochemical abnormalities during the weaning process. Azathioprine with or without daily low-dose prednisone (10 to 15 mg/day) is continued for 18 to 24 months. If possible, liver biopsy should be obtained just before the cessation of therapy. Variations in the histologic features may be noted, from a normal biopsy to quiescent cirrhosis, or more frequently the lesion of chronic persistent hepatitis is seen. A clinical and biochemical relapse may subsequently occur in up to 50% of patients with the latter lesion. Fortunately, retreatment of such individuals again leads to improvement in the clinical and biochemical features and possibly in the liver lesion as well. It has been the experience of others that patients with HBsAg-positive chronic active hepatitis are especially prone to relapse.

With this treatment regimen, the disagreeable side effects of prednisone for the pediatric age patient can be kept to a minimum. Obviating the growth-suppressive effect and undesirable cosmetic impact of prednisone is especially warranted in children. Another early side effect of prednisone occasionally reported is the appearance of ascites without peripheral edema. A decrease in dietary sodium and judicious use of diuretics is sufficient to promote diuresis. A gentle approach in therapy will prevent excessive fluid mobilization and excretion and obviate the likelihood of hypotension. Antacids and potassium supplements are occasionally needed by some patients receiving prednisone, especially early in the course of treatment. Hypertension has rarely been encountered.

Gastrointestinal upset from azathioprine may be overcome when the drug is given with meals or the dose is split. Serial white blood cell counts are needed initially though leukopenia is not likely to be severe. Up to now we have seen no other complications with azathioprine when used in this dosage. In severe liver disease the conversion of azathioprine to active 6-mercaptopurine may not occur and perhaps explains the rare cause of failure of drug therapy. How long to treat the patient with persistent biochemical parameters is best answered after reexamination of liver biopsy material. One is especially hesitant to use azathioprine indefinitely in the pediatric age group, since the long-term effect upon fertility and teratogenicity and a potential for the late development of malignancy remain uncertain in such patients. In patients with recalcitrant disease the amount of prednisone needed to achieve a clinical and reasonable biochemical remission may still produce serious side effects. In such cases, unfortunately, the use of alternate-day, high-dose steroids has been disappointing in achieving the desired response.

After discontinuation of medication, periodic follow-up study is recommended at 3-month intervals for the first year and at 6-month intervals for the next 2 to 3 years.

Another treatment program in pediatric patients uses steroids alone, also at the high dosage of 2 mg/kg/day up to a maximum of 60 mg. At monthly intervals, after clinical and biochemical remission has occurred (SGOT less than 100 IU), the same dosage is switched to alternate-day therapy and thereafter reduced by 5 mg per month, provided that satisfactory results of biochemical tests continue. Azathioprine (Imuran) is added only to refractory cases. Daily prednisone is resumed if relapses occur, followed by alternate-day steroids and subsequent weaning if the remission is sustained. Eventually all medication is discontinued (once complete remission is achieved), and the patient is followed as previously mentioned. Again a 25% to 50% relapse rate may be expected after discontinuation of medication, though patients will probably respond again if they did so initially.

The beneficial effects of the drug therapy regimen can be expected in both the very sick child and those whose disease is of more insidious onset. Even when liver biopsy shows subacute hepatic necrosis and collapse as the dominant feature, there is clinical and biochemical response to drug therapy. Freedom from extrahepatic manifestations and their respective symptoms and a definite sense of well-being can be attained in most treated patients. Despite use of both prednisone and azathioprine, a few patients will develop colitis, arthritis, and erythema nodosum. In our experience colitis will respond to sulfasalazine.

Sustained remission has been noted in most patients (14 of 15) in whom both prednisone and azathioprine could be discontinued after 18 to 24 months of therapy (clinical and biochemical). Relapse has occurred in 1 patient from the group who could be completely withdrawn from drug therapy. Histologic "cure" has been present in only 2 of 6 repeat biopsies (Fig. 24-9). Sampling errors must again be considered in a disease known to produce patchy variation throughout the liver.

Unfortunately, a significant number of patients continue to show laboratory and histologic evidence of smoldering disease despite therapy. Slightly increased SGOT and increased gamma globulin fraction suggest that a more aggressive "active" underlying histologic lesion will be found (Fig. 24-10).

This treatment "failure" group often includes those patients presenting with pronounced hyperbilirubinemia (greater than 20 mg/dl) and prothrombin time below 30% of normal. Patients with persistent or recurrent clinical and biochemical abnormalities despite therapy can be expected to have the histologic features of both ongoing liver

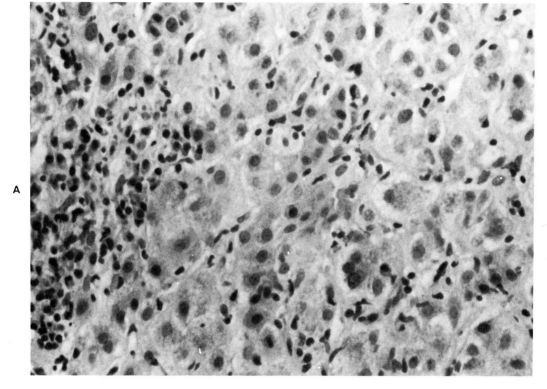

Fig. 24-9. Chronic active hepatitis. **A,** This section shows the portal inflammatory reaction characterized by acute and chronic inflammatory cells. Hepatocytes are characterized by giant cell formation; balloon cells with scattered acute inflammatory cells are noted throughout the lobule. This tissue was obtained by percutaneous needle biopsy from a 12-year-old boy with a 6-week history of persistent jaundice. His initial illness was characterized by anorexia and vomiting, with the subsequent development of jaundice. Physical examination revealed moderate jaundice, acne, and hepatosplenomegaly. Serum bilirubin was 18 mg/dl, SGOT 500 IU, and gamma globulin value 4.5 gm/dl. A lupus erythematosus preparation was positive on two occasions. Though the liver disease was less severe than that in other patients, it was believed that this boy fit the clinical-biochemical-pathologic criteria for chronic active hepatitis. A course of prednisone was begun. *Continued.*

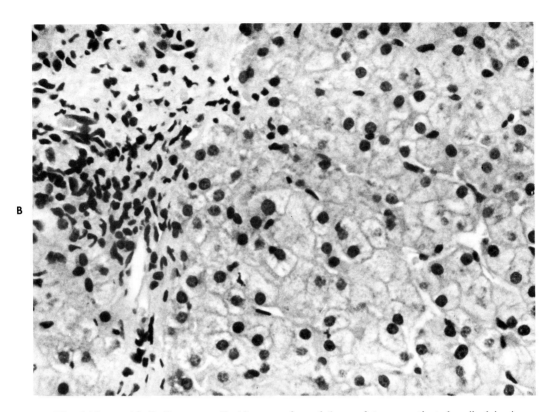

Fig. 24-9, cont'd. **B,** Repeat needle biopsy performed 1 year later on patient described in **A** shows the lobular resolution of the previous process, with persistence of mild chronic inflammatory reaction within the portal areas. After beginning prednisone therapy, the patient promptly improved biochemically but became strikingly cushingoid and developed insulin-dependent diabetes. A gradual weaning off prednisone was possible over the final 3-month period, and his diabetes also disappeared. Subsequently, he developed overt thyroiditis, became hypothyroid, and required replacement therapy. His liver disease remains quiescent.

disease and cirrhosis when subjected to follow-up biopsy.

Despite the enthusiasm for utilizing this form of drug therapy in treating chronic active hepatitis, one must be disturbed by the recent report of patients developing chronic active hepatitis after renal transplantation and while receiving both prednisone and azathioprine. Although no satisfactory explanation exists to explain this observation, one must wonder whether it indeed represents a form of hepatotoxicity to azathioprine in the immunosuppressed transplant recipient.

In untreated patients spontaneous clinical and biochemical remission may occur in 20% to 25% of cases, but features of cirrhosis may be expected in the liver biopsy. On the other hand, 90% of children can be expected to show a prompt clinical response once therapy is started, and 75%, a biochemical remission. When the disease is ac-

tive, some patients may feel ill, complaining of lethargy, anorexia, or low-grade fever. Arthralgia, pleurisy, abdominal pain, erythema nodosum, and symptoms of colitis can occur intermittently. Jaundice may or may not be present when the disease is active.

When cirrhosis is present, portal hypertension eventually develops, with congestive splenomegaly and hypersplenism. Liver failure is heralded by the late reappearance of icterus and the development of ascites. Eventually hepatic coma supervenes. Episodes of esophageal bleeding may precede the hepatic coma but are a late consequence of this disease. Hepatocarcinoma has now been reported in patients with chronic active hepatitis.

One cannot always predict the course of this disease for any one patient on the basis of etiologic, laboratory, and histologic findings present at the time of the original diagnosis. The discrep-

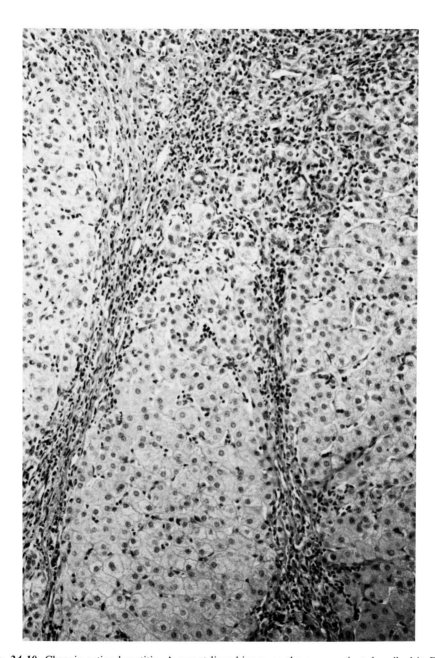

Fig. 24-10. Chronic active hepatitis. A repeat liver biopsy on the same patient described in Fig. 24-7 after 1 year of treatment with prednisone. The liver shows persistence of the inflammatory process, with proximity of portal tracts suggesting lobular collapse and piecemeal necrosis. Though serum bilirubin levels returned to normal, a modest elevation of transaminase and gamma globulin fraction persisted. Severe cushingoid changes, growth retardation, and epigastric pain complicated therapy. After the biopsy, azathioprine (Imuran) was started. This permitted reduction in the steroid dosage with biochemical suppression of the disease.

ancy between the clinical and biochemical status of the patient and the severity of the pathologic lesion seen on liver biopsy is frequent and dramatic. It appears that the subsequent course is likely to be better for those surviving the abrupt type of onset of their disease than for those in whom onset is insidious.

With the exception of teen-agers, the need for prolonged hospitalization for pediatric patients with chronic active hepatitis is apparently less than that reported for adults. Changes in drug therapy and control of ascites or bleeding will require temporary hospitalization, but the need for prolonged periods of rest in bed should be rare for the child with this entity.

Prognosis

In a single report dealing with children, a definite prolongation of life was noted in the patients receiving drug therapy; their number of survivors was double that of patients not receiving treatment in an earlier study, and double that of a mixed-age population group treated with azathioprine only.

Our early impression from an uncontrolled treatment regimen, and since substantiated by others, suggested that the prognosis in children with chronic active hepatitis was likewise more favorable than that reported for adults. Subsequently, the results of controlled clinical trials in adults have shown that they, too, can be substantially aided by proper drug therapy. Not only can one expect a prompt clinical and biochemical response to therapy, but long-term remissions in adults, after cessation of therapy may also be expected in 25% to 35% of patients.

Our own data support these prognostic expectations in treated patients (Table 24-5). Over 70% of these children receiving either long-term combination therapy (prednisone and azathioprine) or prednisone therapy alone had a complete biochemical remission. This compares favorably to the Mayo Clinic controlled studies, in which a 75% clinical and biochemical remission was noted. Although a relapse rate of 50% has been noted in adults after histologic improvement to chronic persistent hepatitis with treatment, only infrequently have we seen relapses in our children once drug therapy has been successfully withdrawn after 18 to 24 months of treatment. The reason for this difference is not certain at this time, but the absence of cases caused by chronic HBsAg dis-

Table 24-5. Clinical course of 38 children with chronic active hepatitis followed from 1968 to 1975*

Clinical course	Number of patients
Prompt clinical remission (on prescription)	33
Clinical and biochemical remission (on prescription)	25
Sustained remission (off prescription)	14/15
Deaths	9

*Seen at The Children's Hospital, Denver, and University of Colorado Medical Center. Courtesy R. S. Dubois and A. Silverman.

ease could be the reason. Even when the histologic lesion during relapse reverts to that of aggressive hepatitis, the prognosis for this group does not seem to be any worse than for those who remain in remission with the histologic lesion of chronic persistent hepatitis. Response to therapy can be anticipated in the former group. However, it would appear that a slow progression to cirrhosis occurs with equal frequency in patients manifesting a relapsing or a nonrelapsing course.

At present histologic "cures" of 18% to 20% are being reported in adults with chronic active hepatitis. Long-term follow-up study of patients whose hepatic lesions evolve to a chronic persistent lesion is suggested, since some of these will eventually normalize even in those requiring a long treatment course (5 to 10 years). Comparative data in children are not available, since few have had follow-up biopsies after cessation of therapy.

Of our 38 patients previously reported with this disease, 9 patients have died, 3 of them from the disease, the therapy, or both. Another died 1 month after starting therapy from hepatic failure and *Pseudomonas* sepsis, another in hepatic coma before therapy, and another 6 months after therapy was instituted; the fifth died of acute dysentery and shock caused by shigellosis. Three patients died after orthotopic liver transplantation. One patient died an accidental death 9 years after diagnosis and treatment.

Contrary to the experience in children, the prognosis for adults with chronic active hepatitis was unfavorably affected if the disease had an acute, hepatitis-like onset. In these adult cases hepatic coma or ascites tended to occur early, especially if cholestasis was persistent and if colitis developed. We have been unable to make this correlation in pediatric patients, though most of our cases have a hepatitis-like onset. Three patients who developed colitis while receiving immunosuppressive therapy are doing as well as the other survivors requiring continued drug therapy. No correlation with prognosis could be found in children with chronic active hepatitis by comparison of age, sex, presence of antinuclear antibodies, high gamma globulin levels, or other organ involvement. Whether the development of colitis will significantly affect survival remains to be seen.

In children and adults with chronic active hepatitis, over 70% will be alive after 5 years, with treatment. Drug therapy undoubtedly yields a greater number of survivors of the acute phase of the disease, and indeed prolongs the overall survival figures. The prognosis despite drug therapy is certainly worse if the initial lesion shows pronounced subacute hepatic necrosis or cirrhosis, or both.

REFERENCES

Arasu, T.S., Wyllie, R., Hatch, T.F., and Fitzgerald, J.F.: Management of chronic aggressive hepatitis in children and adolescents, J. Pediatr. **95:**514-522, 1979.

Cochrane, A.M.G., Moussouros, A., Smith, A., and others: Autoimmune reaction to a liver specific membrane antigen during acute viral hepatitis, Gut **17:**714-718, 1976.

Czaja, A.J., Ludwig, J., Baggenstoss, A.H., and Wolf, A.: Corticosteroid-treated chronic active hepatitis in remission, N. Engl. J. Med. **304:**5-9, 1981.

Czaja, A.J., Ammon, H.V., and Summerskill, W.H.J.: Clinical features and prognosis of severe chronic active liver disease (CALD) after corticosteroid-induced remission, Gastroenterology **78:**518-523, 1980.

De Groote, J., Fevery, J., and Lepoutre, L.: Long-term follow-up of chronic active hepatitis of moderate severity, Gut **19:**510-513, 1978.

Dubois, R.S., and Silverman, A.: Treatment of chronic active hepatitis in children, Postgrad. Med. J. **50:**386-391, 1974.

Eddleston, A.L.W.F.: Genetically determined immune hyperreactivity in human liver disease, Proc. R. Soc. Med. **70:**525-529, 1977.

Farivar, M., Wands, J.R., Genson, G.D., and others: Cryoprotein complexes and peripheral neuropathy in a patient with chronic active hepatitis, Gastroenterology **71:**490-493, 1976.

Freiberger, Z., Anuras, S., Koff, R.S., and Bonney, W.W.: Chronic active hepatitis without hepatitis B antigenemia in renal transplant recipients, Gastroenterology **66:**1187-1194, 1974.

Galbraith, R.M., Smith, M.S., Mackenzie, R.M., and others: High prevalence of seroimmunologic abnormalities in relatives of patients with active chronic hepatitis or primary biliary cirrhosis, N. Engl. J. Med. **290:**63-69, 1974.

Harris, R.C., Schaffner, F., and Tabor, E.: When is hepatitis chronic? J. Pediatr. **95:**551-552, 1979.

Holdsworth, C.D., Hall, E.W., Dawson, A.M., and Sherlock, S.: Ulcerative colitis in chronic liver disease, Q. J. Med. **34:**211-227, 1965.

Jensen, D.M., McFarlane, I.G., Portmann, B.S., and others: Detection of antibodies directed against a liver-specific membrane lipoprotein in patients with acute and chronic active hepatitis, N. Engl. J. Med. **299:**1-7, 1978.

Joske, R.A., Laurence, B.H., and Matz, L.R.: Familial active chronic hepatitis with hepatocellular carcinoma, Gastroenterology **62:**441-444, 1972.

Kawanishi, H., and MacDermott, R.P.: K-cell–mediated antibody-dependent cellular cytotoxicity in chronic active liver disease, Gastroenterology **76:**151-158, 1979.

Korman, M.G., Hofmann, A.F., and Summerskill, W.H.J.: Assessment of activity in chronic active liver disease, N. Engl. J. Med. **290:**1399-1402, 1974.

Lam, K.C., Lai, C.L., Trepo, C., and Wu, P.C.: Deleterious effect of prednisolone in HBsAg-positive chronic active hepatitis, N. Engl. J. Med. **304:**380-386, 1981.

Levy, R.L., and Hong, R.: Anti-glomerular antibody in chronic active and chronic persistent hepatitis, J. Pediatr. **85:**155-158, 1974.

Mackay, I.R., and Morris, P.J.: Association of autoimmune active chronic hepatitis with HL-A1,8, Lancet **1:**793-795, 1972.

Scott, B.B., Rajah, S.M., and Losowsky, M.S.: Histocompatibility antigens in chronic liver disease, Gastroenterology **72:**122-125, 1977.

Smith, A.L., Cochran, A.M.G., and Mowat, A.P.: Cytotoxicity to isolated rabbit hepatocytes by lymphocytes from children with liver disease, J. Pediatr. **91:**584-589, 1977.

Soloway, R.D., Baggenstoss, A.H., Schoenfield, L.J., and Summerskill, W.H.J.: Observer error and sampling variability tested in evaluation of hepatitis and cirrhosis by liver biopsy, Am. J. Dig. Dis. **16:**1082-1086, 1971.

Soloway, R.D., Summerskill, W.H.J., Baggenstoss, A.H., and others: Clinical, biochemical and histological remission of severe chronic active liver disease: a controlled study of treatment and early prognosis, Gastroenterology **63:**820-833, 1972.

Summerskill, W.H.J.: Chronic active liver disease reexamined: prognosis hopeful, Gastroenterology **66:**450-464, 1974.

Summerskill, W.H.J., Korman, M.G., Ammon, H.V., and Baggenstoss, A.H.: Prednisone for chronic active liver disease: dose titration, standard dose, and combinatin with azathioprine compared, Gut **16:**876-883, 1975.

Thomson, A.D., Cochrane, M.A.G., McFarlane, I.G., and others: Lymphocyte cytotoxicity to isolated hepatocytes in chronic active hepatitis, Nature **252:**721-722, 1974.

Ware, A.J., Cuthbert, A., Shorey, J., and others: A prospective trial of steroid therapy in severe viral hepatitis, Gastroenterology **80:**219-224, 1981.

Wiggins, R.C., and Cochrane, C.G.: Immune-complex-mediated biologic effects, N. Engl. J. Med. **304:**518-520, 1981.

Wright, E.C., Seeff, L.B., Berk, P.D., and others: Treatment of chronic active hepatitis: an analysis of three controlled trials, Gastroenterology **73:**1422-1430, 1977.

WILSON'S DISEASE

Wilson's disease (hepatolenticular degeneration), a genetic-metabolic disorder, is discussed separately as a cause of chronic liver disease in childhood for two important reasons: (1) to remind physicians caring for children that this entity frequently presents during childhood either as an insidious cirrhosis, or as a slowly resolving hepatitis with histologic and biochemical features that may mimic chronic active hepatitis or chronic persistent hepatitis; (2) in our experience it appears to be the leading cause, after chronic active hepatitis of postnecrotic cirrhosis in school-age children.

Early diagnosis can often be made if one considers Wilson's disease in the differential diagnosis of every case of pediatric liver disease occurring in the school-age child. Indeed, the opportunity for diagnosis of Wilson's disease is available during childhood since greater than 50% of all patients have symptoms before reaching 15 years of age. Over 50% manifest overt hepatic involvement. On occasion it does present as acute severe liver disease thereby requiring inclusion of this disorder in the differential diagnosis of fulminant hepatic failure. Twenty-five percent of cases of Wilson's disease are identified by screening of asymptomatic family members (homozygotes), perhaps 15% recognized because of neuropsychiatric symptoms, and the remaining few identified because of other unusual manifestations (hemolytic anemia, gallstones). It is important to seize upon this opportunity for early diagnosis in the index case, since (1) prompt and specific therapy affords a favorable prognosis for many; (2) subsequent identification and treatment of asymptomatic homozygote's siblings can be promptly undertaken; (3) genetic counseling and family planning can also be promptly undertaken.

Wilson's disease is transmitted as an autosomal recessive trait. The prevalence rate of carriers of this disease (heterozygotes) stands at 1 in 200 to 1 in 500.

The various manifestations of Wilson's disease have been attributed to the toxic effect of copper deposition in the specific organs. This is particularly true for the neurologic and hepatic lesions, the ophthalmologic findings, the renal tubular defect, and possibly the skeletal abnormalities as well, since copper is a potent inhibitor of various cell membrane and intracellular enzyme systems. The hemolytic anemia that occurs in some patients with

Wilson's disease is probably a result of rapid release of tissue copper to the plasma, with resultant red cell hemolysis. The exact site of the defect in Wilson's disease is unknown, though an abnormality in hepatic transport and storage of this metal is probably involved. Studies using ^{64}Cu have suggested a lysosomal defect in these patients that prevents the normal hepatic excretion of biliary copper and results in the hepatic accumulation of the metal.

Other postulated mechanisms for Wilson's disease include a block in the transfer of copper from the site of hepatocyte uptake to the lysosomes. This might involve a deficiency or abnormality in a copper-binding protein or enzymes required for intracellular transfer and transport of the metal. An early report indicating that an abnormal hepatic metal-binding protein with an increased affinity for copper (copper thioneine) may be synthesized by patients homozygous to Wilson's disease has, unfortunately, not been subsequently confirmed. That a block in ceruloplasmin synthesis underlies the phenomenon of copper retention can be challenged by the observation that 5% of patients with this disease have normal ceruloplasmin concentration and 10% of heterozygotes may have low ceruloplasmin levels in the absence of elevated or toxic amounts of tissue copper. Rather, defective ceruloplasmin production may be a phenomenon secondary to the diminished availability of copper to bind to its apoprotein.

The absorption of copper from the intestine into the portal blood is normal, and early in Wilson's disease, the rate of hepatic clearance of the albumin-bound metal also occurs at a normal rate. Transfer to ceruloplasmin occurs, but the secondary rise in serum levels (copper-bound ceruloplasmin) noted in normal patients does not occur in those with Wilson's disease, suggesting abnormal storage within the liver. This observation provides the basis for the diagnostic radiocopper-clearance test employed in confusing cases. It is particularly useful in distinguishing patients with Wilson's disease who have normal ceruloplasmin levels from patients with nonwilsonian liver disease (p. 704).

Whatever the underlying defect in copper metabolism is, failure to excrete lysome-bound copper into the biliary system is shown to result in a positive copper balance of 50 to 600 µg/day in patients with Wilson's disease. During the early phase of the disease and before symptoms are manifest, hepatic copper concentration gradually

Table 24-6. Clinical findings in 11 pediatric patients with Wilson's disease

Case number	Diagnosis age (year)	Age at onset of symptoms (year)	Sex	Mode of presentation	Jaundice
1	13	13	F	Hemolytic crisis	+
2	14	14	M	Asymptomatic sibling	No
3	17	14	M	Dystonia and dysarthria	No
4*	13	11	M	Tremor	No
5*	13	13	F	Asymptomatic sibling	No
6	18	16	F	Liver disease	+
7	15	15	M	Asymptomatic sibling	No
8	17½	17½	M	Asymptomatic sibling	No
9	13	11	M	Liver disease	+
10	15	11	M	Liver disease	+
11	11	6	M	Liver disease	+

Modified from Slovis, T.L., Dubois, R.S., Rodgerson, D.O., and Silverman, A: J. Pediatr. **78:**578-584, 1971.
*Identical twins.

increases to a range of 30 to 50 times above its normal concentration. As the disease progresses and the hepatic parenchyma becomes saturated, liver damage occurs, excess copper is now deposited in other organs (brain, eyes, kidney, bones), and new symptoms become manifest. The deposition of copper into extrahepatic sites is most likely the result of the elevated nonceruloplasmin copper, but binding to an abnormal tissue protein is still a possibility. This latter concept stems from studies showing that even the initial clearance of albumin-bound serum copper did not occur when the hepatic parenchyma had become saturated with copper.

Clinical features

Other than for the presence of Kayser-Fleischer rings in a noncholestatic patient, no other clinical feature in either the history or the physical examination is unique to Wilson's disease. Regarding Wilson's disease in the pediatric population, the most significant aspect is again its hepatic manifestations. It is not surprising that the dominant feature of this disease in childhood is some expression of either acute or chronic liver disease. Since the liver slowly accumulates toxic amounts of the metal, any extrahepatic involvement (neurologic, ophthalmologic, renal, and so on) does not occur until saturation and damage to the liver have resulted. Indeed, the clinical aspects in over 50% of the cases are consistent with either acute or chronic hepatitis, fulminant liver failure, or cirrhosis. In our own experience (Table 24-6), 9 of

11 children had demonstrable liver involvement when diagnosis finally was made. Four of these were asymptomatic siblings with clinical evidence of chronic liver disease. In another large pediatric series of Wilson's disease, the primary mode of presentation in 11 of 18 symptomatic patients was again liver disease; their 7 asymptomatic siblings who were homozygous for the disease were also noted to have liver involvement. From these observations it is apparent that in Wilson's disease the progression to cirrhosis is often insidious and without noticeable jaundice. In fact, the cirrhosis may be accompanied by normal results of routine liver function studies. Not until the manifestations of portal hypertension appear (bleeding esophageal varices, complications of hypersplenism) and careful physical examination reveals a small firm liver, splenomegaly, petechiae, and spider nevi, will the diagnosis of cirrhosis be suggested in many of these patients.

A few patients may have their clinical course punctuated by recurring episodes of jaundice resulting from an undiagnosed hemolytic crisis. Such unexplained episodes of hemolysis should always be regarded as a possible sign of Wilson's disease. At times acute intravascular hemolysis may accompany acute liver failure as the first manifestation of Wilson's disease. The hemolytic episodes may eventually result in gallstones, which in turn may produce symptoms.

The neurologic manifestations of Wilson's disease usually begin after 10 years of age and are the same in children as in adults, but delay in

Ascites	Splenomegaly	Varices	Gastro-intestinal bleeding	Kayser-Fleischer rings	Hepatic or neurologic symptoms
+	+	+	+	No	Hepatic coma
No	No	No	No	No	None
No	No	No	No	+	Dystonia
No	+	No	No	+	Intention tremor
No	+	No	No	+	None
+	No	No	No	+	Tremor, dysarthria, and chorea
No	No	No	No	No	None
No	No	No	No	+	None
+	+	+	No	+	None
+	+	+	+	+	None
+	+	+	+	No	Prehepatic coma

proper diagnosis occurs, again because few clinicians expect to find this disease in pediatric patients. (See chart above.)

The early subtleties of neurologic involvement are frequently reflected in a deterioration of school performance. Incoordination, particularly involving fine motor skills, is first recognized as a worsening of the patient's handwriting. An intention tremor and clumsiness are easily exacerbated by the coexisting heightened emotional lability. The personality change in these teen-agers is frequently misinterpreted as being consistent with other commonly observed psychological problems of adolescence. In severe and rapidly progressing cases a frank psychotic break may occur. In the absence of prompt diagnosis and treatment, progressive deterioration of neurologic function relentlessly evolves, including dysarthria, dystonia, chorioathetoid movements, spasticity, and even dysphasia. The parkinsonian-like stare and the slightly opened mouth with saliva pooled in the angles give a suggestive appearance. In contrast to patients with only hepatic manifestations of Wilson's disease, once neurologic involvement becomes apparent, Kayser-Fleischer rings are invariably present. Any cutaneous sign of acute or chronic liver disease should always be suspected as possibly having been caused by Wilson's disease. Brownish discoloration over the anterior tibia has been noted in some patients.

The delay in diagnosis has been repeatedly reported by us and others. Six of 7 symptomatic children in our series had a 2- to 5-year delay in diagnosis despite the presence of the clinical features mentioned in Table 23-6. Less common features in some patients include high temperatures of unknown origin and spontaneous fractures. Other historical features suggesting Wilson's disease include "familial cirrhosis" or neurologic disease in siblings, especially if consanguinity exists.

Diagnosis

Results of routine laboratory screening tests will not permit a fortuitous diagnosis of Wilson's disease. The physician must be sufficiently knowledgeable so as to request the proper laboratory tests once he entertains the possibility of this condition in his differential diagnosis, be it for children with acute or chronic liver disease or those with neuropsychiatric conditions. If a Kayser-Fleischer ring is detected at physical examination (most rare) or, more likely, during routine ophthalmologic refraction, the diagnosis is immediately established. Accumulation of copper in the lateral margin of the cornea, in Descemet's membrane, is best made visible by slit-lamp examination and, in the absence of overt cholestasis, is pathognomonic for Wilson's disease. However, Kayser-Fleischer rings may be absent even if liver disease in the child is severe. Four of 11 patients in our series did not have Kayser-Fleischer rings at the time of diagnosis.

Therefore the diagnosis for most pediatric patients is confirmed by reports of specific laboratory tests of serum, urine, and liver tissue (Table 24-7).

Copper-binding protein (serum ceruloplasmin). A low level of serum ceruloplasmin, or its absence, when serum protein values are normal, implies homozygocity or occasionally heterozygoc-

Table 24-7. Measurements of copper metabolism

Patients	Hepatic copper (μg/gm dry weight)	Urinary copper (μg/24 hours)	Ceruloplasmin (mg/dl)
Wilson's disease			
1	537	750	7
2	1360	290	10
3	1050	245	12
4	1112	2262	1
5	807	172	31
6	1195	202	31
7	411	510	20
8	600	592	2
Chronic active hepatitis			
9	46	33	41
10	168	439	7
11	297	136	20
12	205	366	65
13	50	85	76
14	67	182	64
Normal	<50	48 ± 16	22-49

From Perman, J.A., and others: J. Pediatr. **94**:564-568, 1979.

ity for this disease. In a large series of adult cases, values of less than 20 to 22 mg/dl are noted in 95% of homozygotes and in 10% of heterozygotes. That reliance upon the serum ceruloplasmin may be less certain in pediatric cases was suggested by a report finding that only 19 of 25 cases (76%) of homozygotes for Wilson's disease had ceruloplasmin levels of less than 22 mg/dl. Serum ceruloplasmin has also been found to be low in children with nonwilsonian liver disease such as chronic active hepatitis and fulminant hepatic necrosis. Other pediatric conditions that predispose to lowering of serum proteins (nephrotic syndrome, kwashiorkor, celiac disease, intestinal lymphangiectasia) may demonstrate a "positive" result (low ceruloplasmin) for Wilson's disease. On the other hand, ceruloplasmin, an alpha-2-globulin, is an acute-phase reactant and is often temporarily elevated during acute liver disease. However, a value of over 30 mg/dl is said to exclude Wilson's disease.

Copper. Values for serum copper generally parallel the level of serum ceruloplasmin yet are abnormal (less than 80 μg/dl) in only 50% to 80% of patients. Normal or high values can be found, even in homozygotes for Wilson's disease, and therefore this test is of little diagnostic usefulness.

Urine copper excretion values. The level of copper present in the urine, presumably in the form of amino acid–copper complexes, is usually high in Wilson's disease. Normal urine rarely contains more than 30 μg/24 hours of copper, and values greater than 50 μg/24 hours should be considered abnormal. Other liver disorders such as chronic active hepatitis, chronic hepatitis, biliary tract disease especially with cirrhosis, or direct contamination from the container may give false high values into the range considered typical for Wilson's disease. All symptomatic patients with Wilson's disease have urine copper excretion values of over 100 μg/24 hours with a range of 100 to 3000 μg/24 hours.

Early in the disease, even urine copper excretion may be normal, but a urine sample obtained 6 hours after D-penicillamine (500 mg orally) that yields copper values greater than 500 to 700 μg/6 hours (normal for this test is less than 300 μg/6 hours) permits proper diagnosis.

Copper quantitation of liver tissue. Since accumulation and storage of copper in the liver are basic to this disease, quantitation of hepatic copper should provide the most meaningful information. Values greater than 50 μg/gm of dry weight of liver tissue obtained by either percutaneous or open-liver biopsy are considered abnormal. Most patients with Wilson's disease will have hepatic copper levels greater than 250 μg/gm dry weight. Modest elevations, but usually less than 250 μg/gm of hepatic copper, can be found in some het-

Table 24-8. Liver copper content in normal subjects and those with Wilson's disease and other hepatic disorders

	μg/gm dry weight	M ± S.D.
Normal		
Adults	15-57	
Newborn	15-65	
Wilson's disease		
Heterozygote	39-213	117 ± 51
Asymptomatic	152-1828	983 ± 365
Symptomatic	94-1360	588 ± 304
Other liver disease		
Cirrhosis	17-136	39
Chronic active hepatitis	15-80	40 ± 22
Primary biliary cirrhosis	80-940	411 ± 261
Biliary tract lesion	120-350	203 ± 77

From Mowat, A.P.: Liver disorders in childhood, Sevenoaks, Kent, 1979, Butterworth & Co. (Pubs), Ltd.

erozygotes, as well as in children with chronic cholestatic conditions, biliary or postnecrotic cirrhosis, and rarely chronic hepatitis (Table 24-8). These values in nonwilsonian examples of liver disease can overlap with the less severe cases of Wilson's disease or those who come to early diagnosis. The dilemma is often resolved by other clinical and laboratory studies (see below).

Radiocopper ceruloplasmin incorporation test. The role of radiocopper in the diagnosis of Wilson's disease has its greatest value in those unusual circumstances where one must differentiate between nonwilsonian liver disease with increased urine and liver copper concentrations, and Wilson's disease with a normal ceruloplasmin level. After oral administration of the radioactive-labeled copper, an early rise in plasma radioactivity at 1 to 2 hours is found in both normal subjects and patients with Wilson's disease. As the radioactive copper is taken up by the liver, the plasma radioactivity rapidly decreases, but increased counts are subsequently present as the radiocopper-bound ceruloplasmin reappears in the blood. This secondary rise in plasma radioactivity peaks at 48 hours in both normal persons and those with nonwilsonian liver disease. In contrast, patients with Wilson's disease whose basic defect prevents the hepatic incorporation of radiocopper into ceruloplasmin, manifest only a meager *secondary rise* in plasma radioactivity (Figs. 24-11 and 24-12). The ratio of the radioactive copper value at 48 hours divided by the value found at 1 to 2 hours usually resolves the diagnostic dilemma (patients with Wilson's disease having normal ceruloplasmin levels distinguished from the patients with

nonwilsonian liver disease). It is believed that this test should not serve as a substitute for the important aforementioned laboratory studies except when histologic examination and hepatic copper quantitation cannot be obtained as occurs in special circumstances. The radiocopper incorporation test reinforces the impression that the ceruloplasmin level in Wilson's disease seems only to be an indirect biochemical expression of the underlying condition.

Results of other laboratory tests have been reported as abnormal at times, but none are of diagnostic value. Proximal renal tubular abnormalities are present in more advanced cases, with generalized aminoaciduria, glucosuria, proteinuria, phosphaturia, uricosuria, and loss of renal acidifying mechanisms all being reported. Low serum phosphate and urate concentration has also been found.

Abnormalities of liver function are nonspecific early in the disease and cannot be distinguished from the laboratory abnormalities seen in viral hepatitis. The hypergammaglobulinemia that may occur in patients with Wilson's disease having the hepatic lesion of chronic aggressive hepatitis can cause difficulty when one tries to rule out the syndrome of chronic active hepatitis. Later in the disease, when cirrhosis is suspected, prolonged sulfobromophthalein retention and depressed serum albumin levels are more commonly found but likewise are nonspecific. At this point in time serum bilirubin and even transaminase levels may be perfectly normal.

Laboratory evidence of hypersplenism (thrombocytopenia, leukopenia) should suggest portal

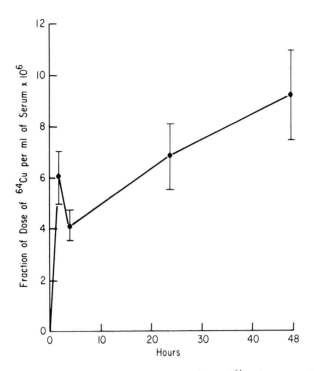

Fig. 24-11. Mean ($\pm$ standard error of mean) concentrations of ^{64}Cu in serum of 11 patients with miscellaneous liver diseases at various times after ingestion of a 2 mg dose of radiocopper. (From Sternlieb, I., and Scheinberg, I.H.: Gastroenterology **77:**138-142, 1979.)

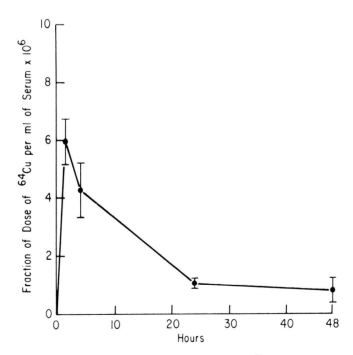

Fig. 24-12. Mean ($\pm$ standard error of mean) concentrations of ^{64}Cu in serum of 11 patients with Wilson's disease at various times after the ingestion of a 2 mg dose of radiocopper. (From Sternlieb, I., and Scheinberg, I.H.: Gastroenterology **77:**138-142, 1979.)

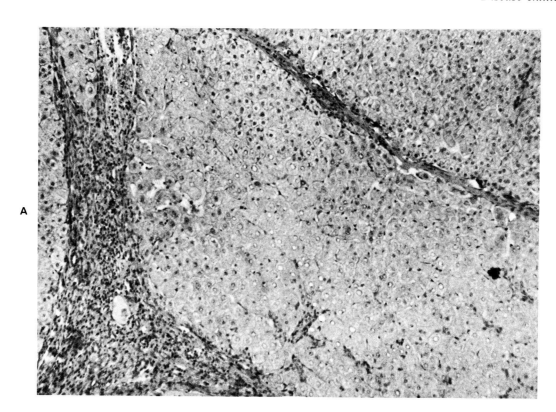

Fig. 24-13. Wilson's disease. **A,** Liver biopsy section showing masses of hepatic cells separated by coarse and cellular fibrous bands characterizing a coarsely nodular cirrhosis. This specimen is from a 13-year-old girl with a 2-year history of fine tremors of the hand exacerbated by emotional stress. Difficulties in school were believed to result from psychologic problems, but her symptoms progressed despite supportive therapy. She was admitted to the hospital for psychologic testing when splenomegaly was noted on physical examination. In addition, Kayser-Fleischer rings were apparent on examination of her eyes. Subsequent laboratory investigation confirmed the diagnosis of Wilson's disease. At the time of liver biopsy the only biochemical abnormality suggesting chronic liver disease was a modest elevation of the BSP (6.5%) and hematologic abnormalities suggesting hypersplenism. In addition, this girl has an identical twin sister who was completely asymptomatic. On physical examination of the sibling, splenomegaly and Kayser-Fleischer rings were also found. Laboratory investigations and liver biopsy then confirmed the presence of Wilson's disease. **B,** High-power view of the lobule from **A** showing the nucleomegaly and glycogenization.

hypertension as possibly arising from intrahepatic causes, and Wilson's disease should automatically be included in the ensuing differential diagnosis.

Evidence of hemolysis may be reflected by red blood cell indices that show a nonspherocytic anemia in the face of an elevated reticulocyte count. During active hemolysis, decreased haptoglobin levels with hemoglobinemia and hemoglobinuria can be found.

Liver pathology

The histologic appearance of the liver may at times seem to indicate the diagnosis of Wilson's disease to the pathologist, but confirmation must await the results of laboratory tests described. Suspicious but not diagnostic clues in the liver biopsy specimen include fatty vacuolization in degenerating liver cells, glycogen nuclei, and cytoplasmic alcoholic hyalin (Mallory bodies). Mallory bodies are rarely found in hepatic tissue from children and should indicate to the pathologist the acute form of Wilson's disease. Otherwise, the histologic appearance of the liver is that of macrolobular or postnecrotic cirrhosis (Figs. 24-13 and 24-14).

The fibrotic reaction consists of fine bands sep-

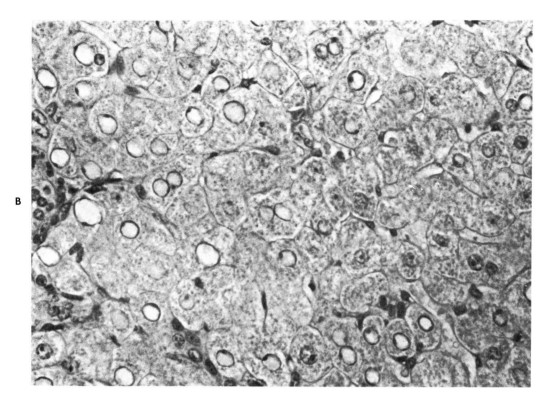

B

Fig. 24-13, cont'd. For legend see opposite page.

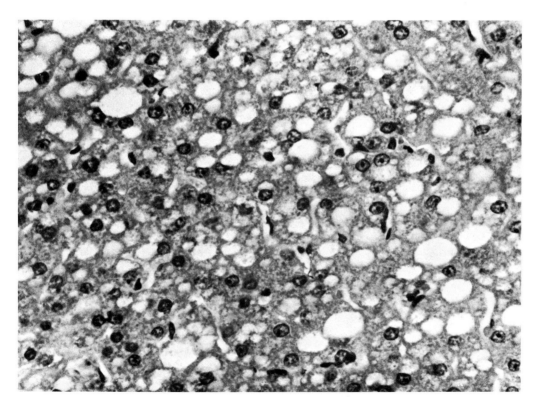

Fig. 24-14. Wilson's disease. Liver biopsy specimen taken from an asymptomatic 14-year-old sibling of another child with proved Wilson's disease shows the moderate hepatic steatosis often characteristic of this disease.

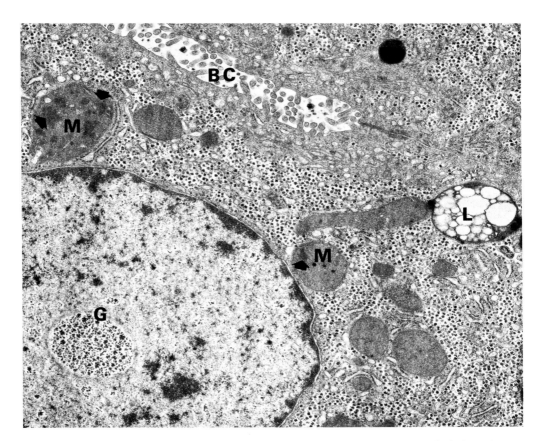

Fig. 24-15. Wilson's disease. Electron micrograph showing intranuclear glycogen inclusion *(G)*, dense clusters of paracrystalline inclusions, *arrows,* within mitochondria *(M)*, and round multivacuolated type of lysosomal granule *(L)* located near a bile canaliculus *(BC)* and believed to store copper. (×24,000.) (Courtesy G. Mierau, research technologist, The Children's Hospital, Denver.)

arating nodules of different size. At times a portal lymphocytic infiltration may mimic the lesion of chronic persistent hepatitis, though periportal and perilobular necrosis may be found to suggest chronic active hepatitis. Ultrastructural changes in Wilson's disease are not diagnostic, but mitochondrial pleomorphism is noted as is the presence of paracrystallin granules within enlarged peroxisomes. A multivacuolated type of lysosomal granule is often found in the liver tissue (Fig. 24-15), although special stains for copper (rubianic acid) early in the disease reveal it to be diffusely scattered throughout the cytoplasm. Later in the disease, especially when cirrhosis is present, most of the copper is concentrated in lysosomes lying close to the bile canaliculi. The hepatic abnormalities found in our cases are listed in Table 24-9. No matter how certain the pathologist is about the diagnosis, quantitative determination of hepatic copper is required for ultimate confirmation.

Once diagnosis is established, all members of the family should be properly screened for the disease. Examination of liver tissue and quantitation of hepatic copper will be necessary for those unusual persons heterozygote for Wilson's disease but having a low ceruloplasmin level (10%). Early detection of asymptomatic homozygote patients and institution of therapy are most important to their well-being and longevity.

Treatment

The goals of therapy are to lower tissue copper concentration and thereby reverse the symptoms and restore normal function to affected organs. Unfortunately, delayed diagnosis has been responsible for the many treatment failures, an observation of considerable importance, since re-

Table 24-9. Pathologic findings in 11 pediatric patients with Wilson's disease

Case number	Histologic findings in liver biopsy
1	Advanced postnecrotic cirrhosis
2	Postnecrotic cirrhosis
3	Normal liver
4*	Postnecrotic cirrhosis
5*	Postnecrotic cirrhosis
6	Postnecrotic cirrhosis with mild chronic hepatitis
7	Inadequate sample
8	Normal liver
9	Postnecrotic cirrhosis
10	Postnecrotic cirrhosis, periportal fibrosis
11	Postnecrotic cirrhosis, Mallory bodies; proliferation of bile ducts

Modified from Slovis, T.L., Dubois R.S., Rodgerson, D.O., and Silverman, A.: J. Pediatr. **78:**578-584, 1971.
*Identical twins.

versibility of the hepatic lesion is possible when therapy is begun early in the disease. At present, therapy is most effective in preventing symptoms in precirrhotic asymptomatic siblings homozygous for the recessive gene.

D-Penicillamine (Cuprimine) is the drug of choice. A low starting dose of 250 mg/day is recommended, since rapid mobilization of copper from tissue stores may cause acute hemolysis or deterioration of neurologic functions. Thereafter, 250 mg increments per week may be added until the patient is on 1000 to 1250 mg/day. This drug is generally well tolerated orally and can be expected to promote a prompt cupruresis in affected patients. The magnitude and duration of this chelating effect will obviously depend on the tissue saturation at the time of diagnosis and on the daily upper intake.

The quantitative daily urine copper excretion values are generally one third or less of the pretreatment values after 6 to 12 months of treatment. Daily urine copper excretion values that remain at pretreatment levels should make one suspicious of noncompliance. The Kayser-Fleischer rings gradually disappear in most patients after 1 to 2 years. Clinical improvement of part of all of the neuropsychiatric manifestations is most gratifying. Routine hepatic function studies likewise can be expected to improve toward normal. Examples of reversibility of the early cirrhotic lesion

exist when penicillamine therapy is instituted early in the disease course. This has been attributed to the ability of penicillamine (in addition to its copper-binding property) to inhibit the maturation of collagen fibers, thereby prolonging the time during which continued enzymatic degradation of fibrous tissue by collagenase, hyaluronidase, and so on may occur.

Toxic side effects related to the use of this drug do occur and need to be closely watched for. Leukopenia is most frequent and troublesome; less often, lymphadenopathy, glossitis, cheilosis, rash, fever, and the nephrotic syndrome may also develop. A lupuslike syndrome with polyarthralgia, pericarditis, pleurisy, fever, and aortic regurgitation has been reported in a patient being treated for Wilson's disease with D-penicillamine. This drug has also been implicated in causing Goodpasture's syndrome in a few patients. These unusual symptoms usually respond to reduction of the dose or discontinuance of D-penicillamine therapy and employment of a short course of prednisone. With resolution of symptoms, the D-penicillamine may be reinstituted at a lower dosage, and several weeks later prednisone may be stopped. Membranous glomerulonephritis has been noted on renal biopsy specimens from patients taking D-penicillamine for rheumatoid arthritis. Drug-induced optic neuritis may be prevented by vitamin B_6 (pyridoxine) supplementation, 5 to 10 mg/24 hours.

Excessive decoppering of the patient may be responsible for leukopenia and occasionally thrombocytopenia. Obviously these findings will have to be cautiously interpreted if portal hypertension and hypersplenism coexist. The known effect of this drug in producing defective collagen synthesis may pose added risks to the fetus when it is taken during pregnancy. An infant with physical features suggesting a congenital connective tissue defect has been reported in such a situation.

If the patient has a severe toxic reaction to penicillamine, cessation of therapy may be required. For the rare patient who cannot tolerate D-penicillamine, the chelating agent triethylene tetramine hydrochloride (trien-2HCl, TETA), 800 mg taken twice daily, has been used successfully. This drug remains in limited supply and has not been approved by the Food and Drug Administration.

Avoidance of certain foods known to contain high levels of cooper is reasonable, and an attempt should be made to keep dietary copper intake at 1 mg per day. Chocolate, nuts, and dried

Table 24-10. Results of treatment in 11 patients with Wilson's disease

Case number	Age (years)	Years of follow-up after diagnosis	Treatment	Clinical course
1	13	—	Penicillamine	Died
2	14	2	Penicillamine	Unchanged
3	17	2/12	Penicillamine	Unchanged
4	13	1	Penicillamine	Tremor resolved
5	13	1	Penicillamine	Unchanged
6	18	3	Penicillamine, dimercaprol	Improved
7	15	3	Penicillamine	Unchanged
8	17½	3/12	Penicillamine	Unchanged
9	13	3/12	Penicillamine, TETA	Unchanged
10	15	4	Penicillamine	Improved
11	11	6/12	Liver transplant	Improved

Modified from Slovis, T.L., Dubois, R.S., Rodgerson, D.O., and Silverman, A.: J. Pediatr. **78:**578-584, 1971.

fruits, high in copper content, are favorites of young children but should be avoided. Shellfish, mushrooms, beer, and some whiskey also contain substantial amounts of copper. Copper water pipes in most modern homes may at times be a problem. The addition of potassium sulfide (Carbo-Resin), 30 to 40 mg three times a day, can be helpful because it binds copper in the intestinal tract. Except for the complaint of body odor, no deleterious side effects to potassium sulfide therapy have been reported.

In Wilson's disease surgical treatment of the deleterious consequences of portal hypertension (bleeding esophageal varices, severe hypersplenism) carries with it a high likelihood of inducing hepatic decompensation and severe portal encephalopathy. If surgical decompression of portal hypertension becomes a necessity (recurrent or uncontrolled variceal bleeding), it is always best carried out after a course of decoppering with D-penicillamine. If this is not possible, ligation or sclerosing of the esophageal varices is the preferred, though temporary, treatment of choice.

The patient with Wilson's disease must receive drug therapy throughout life. Periodic checks of basal urine copper excretion are worthwhile. One can do an occasional evaluation of the effectiveness of therapy by collecting urine for copper after temporarily increasing the dose of D-penicillamine. This verifies not only that therapy is effective but also that the patient is taking the drug as prescribed. The results of treatment in our group of patients are summarized in Table 24-10.

Prognosis

Untreated, all patients invariably die of liver disease or from complications of the neurologic disease. A few patients die during the initial hepatic insult, with a clinical picture of fulminating hepatitis. The prognosis appears to be best in the patient affected, but free of symptoms and without serious liver involvement (cirrhosis), who continues to receive therapy. In such cases subsequent clinical manifestations will be prevented. The functional impairment derived from lesser degrees of liver injury can likewise be reversed with therapy. That the morphologic hepatic lesion can be dramatically improved has been shown on serial biopsy, but essentially it is limited to patients in the precirrhotic state. On the other hand, for those patients whose original liver biopsy revealed histologic features of both active and chronic disease, the long-term prognosis is less certain. The improvement in laboratory studies seen with treatment in this latter group cannot be equated with histologic evidence of healing without reexamination of liver tissue.

However, even in the presence of postnecrotic cirrhosis, survival can be prolonged with therapy. Eventually signs of liver failure will appear and include ascites and portal encephalopathy. Bleeding from esophageal varices portends a very grim prognosis with survival thereafter seldom longer than 1 to 2 years. Some reversal of neurologic signs can be accomplished with therapy, and this seems to be an individual effect.

Orthotopic hepatic transplantation has been performed on two patients with Wilson's disease, one with liver failure and the other with a deteriorating neurologic status despite D-penicillamine therapy. Subsequent homograft biopsy specimens showed normal hepatic copper levels and normal serum ceruloplasmin levels, but mild cupruresis, persistence of Kayser-Fleischer rings (one patient), and slow partial resolution of neurologic symptoms (in the other). One patient died; the other was still alive at last report. These interesting observations serve to further emphasize the need for early diagnosis and treatment, since complete removal of extrahepatic copper stores may not be possible in advanced cases.

Clearly, the emphasis in this disease must be placed on early diagnosis, family screening, and adequate and effective institution of specific therapy if the prognosis of this dreadful but treatable disease is to be further improved.

REFERENCES

Adler, R., Mahnovski, V., Heuser, E.T., and others: Fulminant hepatitis: a presentation of Wilson's disease, Am. J. Dis. Child. **131:**870-872, 1977.

Buchanan, G.R.: Acute hemolytic anemia as a presenting manifestation of Wilson's disease, J. Pediatr. **86:**245-247, 1975.

Cartwright, G.E.: Diagnosis of treatable Wilson's disease, N. Engl. J. Med. **298:**1347-1350, 1978.

Epstein, O., and Sherlock, S.: Is Wilson's disease caused by a controller gene mutation resulting in perpetuation of the fetal mode of copper metabolism into childhood, Lancet **1:**303-305, 1981.

Evans, J., Newman, S., and Sherlock, S.: Liver copper levels in intrahepatic cholestasis of childhood, Gastroenterology **75:**875-878, 1978.

Frommer, D.J.: Defective biliary excretion of copper in Wilson's disease, Gut **15:**125-129, 1974.

Frommer, D., Morris, J., Sherlock, S., and others: Kayser-Fleischer-like rings in patients without Wilson's disease, Gastroenterology **72:**1331-1335, 1977.

Gibbs, K., and Walshe, J.M.: Biliary excretion of copper in Wilson's disease, Lancet **2:**538-539, 1980.

Grand, R.J., and Vawter, G.F.: Juvenile Wilson disease: histologic and functional studies during penicillamine therapy, J. Pediatr. **87:**1161-1170, 1975.

Groth, C.G., Dubois, R.S., Corman, J., and others: Hepatic transplantation in Wilson's disease, Birth Defects **9:**106-108, 1973.

Kaplinsky, C., Sternlieb, I., Javitt, N., and Rotem, Y.: Familial cholestatic cirrhosis associated with Kayser-Fleischer rings, Pediatrics **65:**782-788, 1980.

LaRusso, N.F., Summerskill, W.H.J., and McCall, J.T.: Abnormalities of chemical tests for copper metabolism in chronic active liver disease: differentiation from Wilson's disease, Gastroenterology **70:**653-655, 1976.

Perman, J.A., Werlin, S.L., Grand, R.J., and Watkins, J.B.: Laboratory measures of copper metabolism in the differentiation of chronic active hepatitis and Wilson disease in children, J. Pediatr. **94:**564-568, 1979.

Roche-Sicot, J., and Benhamou, J.P.: Acute intravascular hemolysis and acute liver failure associated as a first manifestation of Wilson's disease, Ann. Intern. Med. **86:**301-303, 1977.

Rosenfield, N., Grand, R.J., Watkins, J.B., and others: Cholelithiasis and Wilson disease, J. Pediatr. **92:**210-213, 1978.

Scott, J., Gollan, J.L., Samourian, S., and Sherlock, S.: Wilson's disease, presenting as chronic active hepatitis, Gastroenterology **74:**645-651, 1978.

Spechler, S.J., and Koff, R.S.: Wilson's disease: diagnostic difficulties in the patient with chronic hepatitis and hypoceruloplasminemia, Gastroenterology **78:**803-806, 1980.

Sternlieb, I., and Scheinberg, I.H.: Chronic hepatitis as a first manifestation of Wilson's disease, Ann. Intern. Med. **76:**59-64, 1972.

Sternlieb, I., Scheinberg, I.H., and Walshe, J.M.: Bleeding esophageal varices in patients with Wilson's disease, Lancet **1:**638-641, 1970.

Sternlieb, I., and Scheinberg, I.H.: The role if radiocopper in the diagnosis of Wilson's disease, Gastroenterology **77:**138-142, 1979.

Sternlieb, I., van den Hamer, C.J.A., Morrell, A.G., and others: Lysosomal defect of hepatic copper excretion in Wilson's disease (hepatolenticular degeneration), Gastroenterology **64:**99-105, 1973.

Walshe, J.M.: Copper chelation in patients with Wilson's disease, Q. J. Med. **42:**441-452, 1973.

Werlin, S.L., Grand, R.J.., Perman, J.A., and Watkins, J.B.: Diagnostic dilemma of Wilson's disease: diagnosis and treatment, Pediatrics **62:**47-51, 1978.

Wilson's disease and copper-associated protein, Lancet **1:**644-646, 1981 (Editorial).

ALPHA-1-ANTITRYPSIN DEFICIENCY DISEASE

In 1969, Sharp and colleagues first pointed out the clear association of juvenile cirrhosis with alpha-1-antitrypsin (α_1-AT) deficiency.

It soon became apparent that in this condition liver disease may (1) become manifest in the neonate as a "cholestatic syndrome," (2) serendipitously be discovered from biochemical and histologic studies obtained later in infancy when one is evaluating hepatomegaly or failure to thrive, or finally (3) progress insidiously by anicteric hepatitis to cirrhosis. In fact, from 5% to 35% of pediatric liver disease cases are now believed to be caused by alpha-1-antitrypsin deficiency.

Subsequently, large neonatal screening programs in Sweden (200,000 infants) and in the United States (107,038 infants) found the incidence of α_1-AT deficiency associated with PiZZ phenotype in 1 in 1714 and 1 in 5000 births, respectively. Of these homozygote-deficient individuals, 11% in the Swedish group (with three progressing to cirrhosis) and 5% in the United States group manifested a neonatal cholestatic condition. Equally important was the observation that 50% in the Swedish and 28% in the United States' study of patients with PiZZ continued to show either clinical or biochemical abnormalities of liver function suggesting hepatic damage. The eventual significance of these observations must await the results of long-term follow-up studies. This important data should serve to confirm or refute the previous clinical impression that individuals with α_1-AT who acquire liver disease rarely make a full recovery, including normalization of the histopathologic appearance, despite the resolution of the early jaundice.

Alpha-1-antitrypsin is an important biologic glycoprotein (alpha-1-globulin) produced by the hepatocytes under the influence of two autosomally inherited codominant alleles. Each allele appears to control the production of its own kind of α_1-AT molecule. The physicochemical properties of the respective molecule in turn seem to influence the serum level of this protein. The major function of α_1-AT is in its role as a proteolytic enzyme inhibitor (trypsin, pancreatic elastase) and an inhibitor of neutral proteases of polymorphonuclear leukocytes and acid proteases of alveolar macrophages. Up to now 26 different alleles of this protease-inhibitor (Pi) system have been reported. The alleles are lettered (named) according to their electrophoretic mobility.

The *PiM* allele is most common in the general population, with a frequency of 0.87, and the so-called normal individual has the phenotype *PiMM*. The *PiZZ* phenotype is associated with virtual or complete deficiency of plasma α_1-AT (10% to 15% of normal). The *PiMZ* phenotype, considered the heterozygote state of α_1-AT deficiency, has intermediate levels of α_1-AT (50% of normal) and is said to be present in 2.2% to 3% of the population, being higher in northern Europeans. An increased prevalence of this phenotype (PiMZ) is present in patients with cryptogenic cirrhosis and non-HBV chronic active hepatitis. The phenotype *PiSZ* may also be important in predisposing to liver disease.

Probably 10% to 20% of patients with α_1-AT deficiency eventually will develop liver disease. It remains unclear why some phenotypically similar individuals escape without apparent hepatic damage despite both low circulating α_1-AT levels and α_1-AT deposits in their hepatocytes. The exact pathogenesis of α_1-AT liver disease remains to be elucidated. It appears that the hepatocytes are unable to secrete the glycoprotein manufactured by the controlling PiZ allele because of the abnormal structure of the molecule. Several abnormalities of the glycoprotein have been identified including excess mannose and a deficiency of sialic acid residues, both of which appear to predispose the molecule to excessive aggregation. Such aggregation apparently prevents the molecule from successfully migrating from rough to smooth endoplasmic reticulum and eventually to the Golgi apparatus before excretion. Although the accumulated α_1-AT material is believed to be important in the evolving liver pathologic condition, apparently it is not an absolute requirement. Indeed, all patients with the Z allele, be it in the homozygote or heterozygote state, accumulate α_1-AT in their hepatocytes, but liver damage may not be present. Many PiZZ neonates show hepatic injury by 6 to 12 weeks of age, usually as part of a cholestatic condition, but α_1-AT deposits are infrequently observed in their hepatocytes before 8 to 10 weeks of life.

The variable clinical expression of α_1-AT deficiency indicates that other factors (genetic, environmental, infectious, chemical, toxin, and still others) may play a primary role in "stressing" the vulnerable α_1-AT deficient host to develop permanent liver (and lung) damage. One unproved hypothesis implicates excess circulating elastases, or proteases, especially those released from intestinal flora that are normally neutralized by α_1-AT. They are purported to overwhelm the reticuloendothelial system of the liver and in turn produce injury to the hepatocytes. However, this hypothesis is much more plausible for the lung disease in view of the lung's large concentration of elastin. Just how α_1-AT and the accumulated glycoprotein increases the liver's susceptibility to injury is unknown. It is intriguing to consider another genetic susceptibility, perhaps colinked to the PiZ allele that predisposes to the development of chronic liver disease once hepatic injury occurs.

The previously known association between α_1-AT deficiency and early adulthood emphysema may also have significance for the pediatric patient. Indeed, the onset of chronic lung disease (recurrent bronchitis, pneumonia, reactive airway disease) in such patient may commence in childhood, with or without concurrent liver disease.

Clinical features

The hepatic involvement in alpla-1-antitrypsin deficiency disease lacks specific clinical features. In the neonate, the "triggering" even that results in liver damage probably occurs in utero, and up to 45% of these affected newborns are small for gestational age. Thereafter, a history of poor feeding, mild failure to thrive, irritability, and lethargy are common symptoms that accompany the discovery of icterus at 3 to 12 weeks. Jaundice may be noted earlier or later in some cases. Clinically, the jaundice is of the cholestatic type, which one can surmise from observing the dark urine that stains the diaper and sometimes from the pale- to acholic-appearing stools. Physical examination is not specific. The infant looks a bit undernourished, whereas the abdominal exam frequently reveals a smooth but firm quality to the hepatomegaly. Slight enlargement of the spleen is typical. It is axiomatic that when confronted with features of cholestasis in an unwell, nonthriving infant, the possibility that a genetic-metabolic defect underlies the condition should always be seriously considered. Serum quantitative levels of α_1-AT are mandatory in all such cases.

When α_1-AT deficiency is responsible for the neonatal cholestatic syndrome, many of these infants (50% to 75%) will show slow resolution of jaundice over 6 to 8 months. In those examples with persistent (3 to 4 months) clinical and laboratory features of "complete" cholestasis, including acholic stools and failure of observing hepatic excretion of radioisotope-labeled material into the intestines, differentiation from biliary atresia may be extremely difficult and eventually require laparotomy and operative cholangiography to resolve the diagnostic dilemma. Both hypoplasia and atresia of the extrahepatic biliary system has on occasion been noted in association with α_1-AT deficiency. Thereafter hepatomegaly and often biochemical abnormalities continue to persist for several years. Finally the liver size slowly recedes as cirrhosis relentlessly evolves in many unfortunate cases. Splenomegaly may now reappear, as will cutaneous signs indicative of chronic liver disease.

After the neonatal and early infancy period, failure to thrive and isolated hepatomegaly may be found during routine well-child care visits and should suggest underlying liver disease. A previous history of jaundice (neonatal) may be lacking, but the abnormal results of screening routine liver function tests should prompt one to consider α_1-AT deficiency as the possible cause.

When signs of chronic liver disease are found in some unfortunate infants, that is, an enlarged hard liver, splenomegaly, prominent abdominal veins, ascites, digital clubbing, and so on, a positive history of neonatal jaundice can usually be elicited. In the older child or adolescent, a somewhat similar clustering of physical findings indicating chronic liver disease may be noted except that the total liver size is suspiciously small by percussion whereas splenomegaly may be striking. Cutaneous manifestations including "liver palms," spider angiomas, signs of pruritus, bruising, and petechiae are also found more commonly. In contrast to that of younger infants and children, growth and nutrition may appear reasonably good. At times, the complications of portal hypertension (hematemesis from esophageal varices) may initiate the discovery of underlying chronic liver disease in α_1-AT patients. Temporary diagnostic confusion is not surprising especially when a history of early (neonatal) liver disease is lacking.

In unusual cases, evidence of renal disease suggesting nephritis (hematuria, casts, proteinuria) may incidentally be found in association with α_1-AT liver disease. Some cases progress to renal failure.

Lastly, the presence of liver disease should be considered in the rare child presenting in early life with recurrent pulmonary symptoms (bronchitis, pneumonia) caused by α_1-AT deficiency.

Routine laboratory diagnosis

The diagnosis is made by quantitation of circulating α_1-AT levels using an immunoprecipitation method. Normal values of PiMM phenotype range from 200 to 300 mg/dl. PiZZ values are very low, being 10% to 15% of normal but not above 100 mg/dl. Heterozygotes with phenotype PiMZ, PiSZ, or PiMS have intermediate levels (100 to 200 mg/dl). Since α_1-AT is an acute-phase reactant, elevated (false-negative) values may occasionally be the result of intercurrent infections, neoplastic disease, or pregnancy or in an individual taking estrogen-containing products. However, this situation is seen more frequently in heterozygote persons with moderate, rather than severe, deficiency of α_1-AT. The homozygotes are incapable of raising their levels in response to such stimuli.

Only phenotypes PiZZ, PiNull and rarely PiSZ have been definitely associated with liver disease. It is imperative that phenotype determination be performed to confirm the association of α_1-AT deficiency and the patient's clinical condition. Protease-inhibitor (Pi) typing is a specialized study that requires a combination of acid starch–gel electrophoresis and antigen-antibody cross-electrophoresis in agarose. Since α_1-AT accounts for about 90% of the circulating alpha-1-globulin fraction, at times a suspicion of α_1-AT deficiency may be gleaned when one observes an absent or very low (less than 0.2 gm/dl) concentration of the alpha-1-globulin level in the serum-protein electrophoretic pattern obtained in biochemical screening of patients with liver disease.

Results of standard liver function tests are variable, indicating nonspecific hepatocellular injury during the icteric phase, with inconstant abnormalities in the aminotransferase and alkaline phosphatase levels. During the so-called quiescent period or during the cirrhotic stage of the disease, the sulfobromophthalein test may show prolonged retention in the face of normal or near-normal aminotransferase values.

Liver pathology

The characteristic finding in liver tissue, whenever it is obtained from individuals with a PiZ gene for α_1-AT, is the presence of eosinophil-appearing cytoplasmic granules and hyaline masses observed in sections stained with hematoxylin and eosin (Fig. 24-16). Occasionally this material may be seen in the nucleus of some hepatocytes. This material is diastase-fast, stains intensely with periodic acid–Schiff (PAS) stain, and is concentrated in cells, particularly in periportal zones (Fig. 24-17). The amount of this material varies from cell to cell, and many hepatocytes have none. Immunofluorescence studies have shown that this amorphous material reacts with antibodies against α_1-AT, and electron microscopy shows that the accumulations reside primarily in the smooth endoplasmic reticulum, but some also is present in the rough endoplasmic reticulum of the hepatocytes.

Liver biopsy material obtained from symptomatic patients during the neonatal period shows some combination of disturbed lobular architecture (giant cells, pseudoacinar formation, spotty necrosis), interlobular bile ductular alterations, and portal fibrosis. Cholestasis is almost always confined to the hepatocytes. Variable steatosis occurs and in this age group should suggest underlying metabolic liver disease. The inflammatory response is not significant, being portal in location and predominantly monocytic in nature (see Fig. 19-5).

It has been suggested that the subsequent disease course and perhaps the eventual prognosis can

Fig. 24-16. Cirrhosis associated with alpha-1-antitrypsin deficiency. **A,** Tissue obtained at surgery from a 13-year-old girl who had neonatal hepatitis. This biopsy section demonstrates extension of the portal cellularity and lobular change. Portions of the specimen contain fatty changes with some variation in the character of the hepatocytes. Hyaline concretions can be seen, especially in the lower right-hand portion of the specimen. After spontaneous resolution of the neonatal illness, this girl was completely well until 13 years of age, when she suddenly complained of abdominal pain and nausea and then vomited approximately 2 cups of bright red blood and passed a tarry stool. Hospitalization was required for treatment of the gastrointestinal bleeding, and physical examination revealed signs of chronic liver disease. The liver was small to palpation and percussion, and the spleen was enlarged to 3 cm. An elevated BSP retention (10%) and depressed serum albumin level (2.5 gm/dl) were found to support this impression. An esophagogram revealed large varices in the distal portion of the esophagus. A splenoportogram suggested a block in the extrahepatic portion of the portal vein. At surgery a small, shrunken, mildly nodular liver was noted, and the portal pressure was elevated at 36 cm H_2O. The portal vein felt woody and fibrotic, and a mesocaval shunt and needle biopsy of the liver were performed. **B,** High-power view of the liver in **A** demonstrates the presence of cytoplasmic hyalin, fatty change, and delicate fibrous tissue bands. The finding of cytoplasmic hyalin is extremely rare in children and can occur in acute Wilson's disease and alpha-1-antitrypsin deficiency disease. The patient was subsequently found to have alpha-1-antitrypsin deficiency disease. The patient was subsequently found to have alpha-1-antitrypsin deficiency. A screen of the family members revealed two siblings with homozygote levels and one parent in the heterozygote range for alpha-1-antitrypsin.

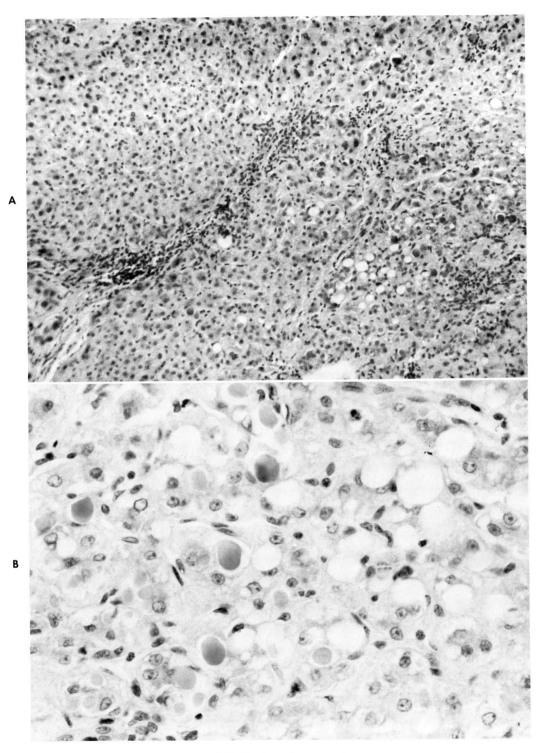

Fig. 24-16. For legend see opposite page.

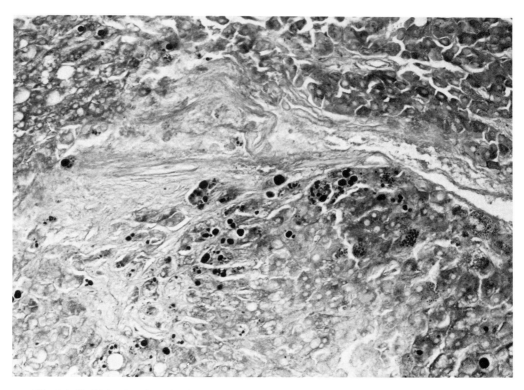

Fig. 24-17. Alpha-1-antitrypsin deficiency and cirrhosis. This histologic section shows the intense staining of this material with periodic acid–Schiff (PAS) stain. The stained material is diastase resistant and tends to be most prevalent in the periportal zone.

be predicted from the histologic injury pattern. When the disturbance in lobular architecture, rather than changes in the portal zones, dominates the histologic lesion, the prognosis seems more favorable. Subsequent clearing of jaundice, regression of hepatomegaly, and either absence or very slow evolution of portal hypertension can be anticipated. A biopsy specimen showing predominant portal fibrosis and neoductualar proliferation, a feature that closely resembles the histologic lesion of biliary atresia, generally connotes a poor prognosis. Even with clinical resolution of icterus, which is often delayed (8 to 12 months), progression to cirrhosis seems to be almost a certainty. Lastly, a biopsy that reveals abnormal-appearing or reduced numbers of interlobular bile ducts, is predictive of a long cholestatic phase, persistent hepatomegaly, and eventual portal hypertension in most.

Later in life, features of postnecrotic cirrhosis (micronodular) predominate. Regenerating lobules are surrounded by slender bands of collagen, with few inflammatory cells noted. Periportal hepatocytes reveal the eosinophilic inclusions, and a mild amount of steatosis can also be found (Fig.

24-16). Cholestasis is not present except in the advanced stages of liver failure, and numbers of interlobular bile ducts vary from one portion of the liver to the other, where they may be either proliferative or absent.

It is important to note that the typical inclusion bodies (PAS positive, diastase resistant) may be found in all α_1-AT–deficient livers, with or without overt liver disease. Furthermore, these inclusion bodies have also been noted in the cirrhotic liver of a patient heterozygous for α_1-AT. Unless looked for specifically, the granules may be easily missed in the neonate, since they are usually smaller and fewer in number than those later in life.

Treatment

Unfortunately, there is no specific treatment for this condition. The usual measures for medical management of the neonate with cholestatic jaundice applies when the diagnosis can be established early in life. In particular, cholestyramine, phenobarbital, medium-chain triglyceride formula, and water-miscible vitamins are desirable adjuvants as described in Chapter 19.

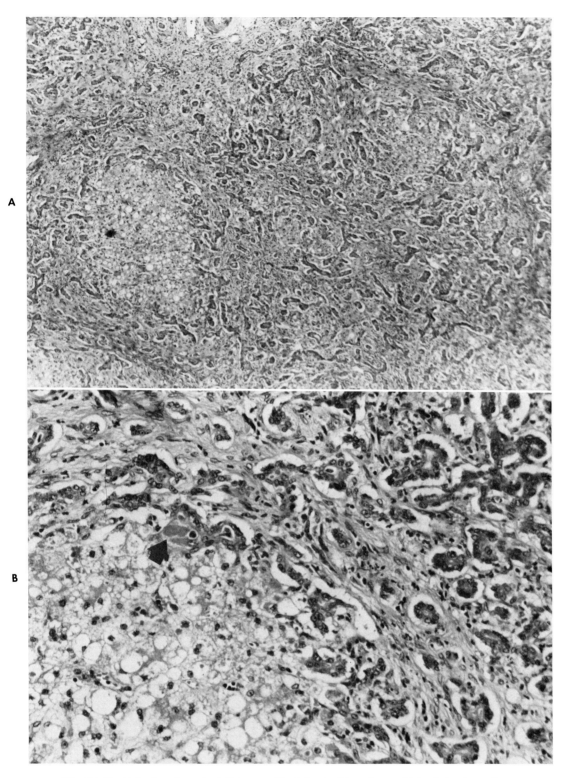

Fig. 24-18. Alpha-1-antitrypsin deficiency with cirrhosis. Liver tissue obtained at autopsy from a 9-month-old child dying of liver failure. Cholestatic jaundice has persisted from 3 weeks of age. **A,** The cirrhosis is associated with exuberant neoductular proliferation and moderate steatosis. **B,** High-power view of a portion of the steatotic nodule to the left of center showing cytoplasic accumulation of alpha-1-antitrypsin in hepatocytes, *arrow*. (**A,** ×45; **B,** ×100.)

The complications of chronic liver disease should be treated in a manner consistent with maintaining the best quality of life for these patients. Bleeding esophageal varices may require endosclerosis, rarely portacaval anastomosis. Gentle use of diuretics and sodium restriction are often required for the alleviation of ascites. The late appearance of jaundice is a grave prognostic sign, though temporary improvement may be obtained with cholestryramine or phenobarbital therapy, or both.

Perhaps prevention of exposure to hepatotoxins (by alcohol, transfusion of blood products, hydrocarbons, and so on) should be emphasized once the diagnosis is established. The avoidance of unnecessary exposure to respiratory viruses and, obviously, of smoking needs to be encouraged. Prevention through genetic counseling may become a reality, since heterozygotes (PiMZ) can be suspected by simple laboratory testing. Recently, prenatal diagnosis of α_1-AT deficiency has been made by analysis of fetal blood obtained at fetoscopy.

Up to now, liver transplantation has been employed for treatment of the advanced liver disease in seven patients with α_1-AT deficiency. It would appear that the metabolic defect can be permanently corrected in patients surviving the procedure; the phenotypes of the recipients become those of the donor, and α_1-AT levels return to normal. At the present time, orthotopic liver transplantation remains the only hope for cure, but, unfortunately, the long-term survival figures continue to be disappointing. Replacement of the protein by transfusion therapy is handicapped by its short half-life (4 to 6 days).

Prognosis

Although not all persons with α_1-AT deficiency will develop concomitant liver disease (or early emphysema), those who do are at significant risk of progressing to cirrhosis and eventually succumbing to liver failure. The prognosis is probably worse if the liver disease begins in the neonatal period, with cirrhosis expected in over 60% of survivors. For unknown reasons the liver disease in some neonates runs a malignant course, with hepatic failure occurring before the infant reaches his first birthday (Fig. 24-18). One would surmise that the likelihood of developing asymptomatic chronic liver disease would increase for those persons with α_1-AT as they survive into adulthood. However, some large surveys indicate that α_1-AT deficiency is not an important determinant of acute or chronic liver or biliary disease in adults. In one large series only 1% of the adult patients with liver disease were found to be homozygous for the PiZZ phenotype and all had a history of neonatal liver disease. One would hope that the long-term follow-up study of children recently identified by neonatal screening for α_1-AT deficiency will provide an accurate assessment of prognosis for all such persons. Last, the risk of subsequently developing hepatic carcinoma seems to be very much increased in these patients.

REFERENCES

Brand, B., Bezahler, G.H., and Gould, R.: Cirrhosis and heterozygous antitrypsin deficiency in an adult, Gastroenterology **66**:264-268, 1974.

Cottrall, K., Cook, P.J.L., and Mowat, A.P.: Neonatal hepatitis syndrome and alpha-1-antitrypsin deficiency: an epidemiological study in southeast England, Postgrad. Med. J. **50**:376-380, 1974.

Feldmann, G., Bignon, J., Chahinian, P., and others: Hepatocyte ultrastructural changes in alpha-1-antitrypsin deficiency, Gastroenterology **67**:1214-1224, 1971.

Fisher, R.L., Taylor, L., and Sherlock, S.: Alpha-1-antitrypsin deficiency in liver disease: the extent of the problem, Gastroenterology **71**:646-651, 1976.

Glasgow, J.J.F., Lynch, M.J., Hercz, A., and others: Alpha-1-antitrypsin deficiency in association with both cirrhosis and chronic obstructive lung disease in two sibs, Am. J. Med. **54**:181-194, 1973.

Hadchouel, M., and Gautier, M.: Histopathologic study of the liver in the early cholestatic phase of alpha-1-antitrypsin deficiency, J. Pediatr. **89**:211-215, 1976.

Hercz, A., Katona, E., Cutz, E., and others: Alpha-1-antitrypsin: the presence of excess mannose in the Z variant isolated from liver, Science **201**:1229-1232, 1978.

Hodges, J.R., Millward-Sadler, G.H., Barbatis, C., and Wright, R.: Heterozygous MZ alpha-1-antitrypsin deficiency in adults with chronic active hepatitis and cryptogenic cirrhosis, N. Engl. J. Med. **304**(10):557-560, 1981.

Hood, J.M., Koep, L.J., Peters, R.L., and others: Liver transplantation for advanced liver disease with alpha-1-antitrypsin deficiency, N. Engl. J. Med. **302**:272-275, 1980.

Jeppsson, J.O., Larsson, C., and Eriksson, S.: Characterization of alpha-1-antitrypsin in the inclusion bodies from the liver in alpha-1-antitrypsin deficiency, N. Engl. J. Med. **293**:576-579, 1975.

Jeppsson, J.O., Cordesius, E., Gustavill, B., and others: Prenatal diagnosis of alpha-1-antitrypsin deficiency by analysis of fetal blood obtained at fetoscopy, Pediatr. Res. **15**:254-256, 1981.

Morin, T., Martin, J.P., and Feldmann, G.: Heterozygous alpha-1-antitrypsin deficiency and cirrhosis in adults: a fortuitous association, Lancet **1**:250-251, 1975.

Moroz, S.P., Cutz, E., Balfe, J.W., and Sass-Kortsak, A.: Membranoproliferative glomerulonephritis in childhood cirrhosis associated with alpha-1-antitrypsin deficiency, Pediatrics **57**:232-238, 1976.

Morse, J.O.: Alpha-1-antitrypsin deficiency. Parts I and II, N. Engl. J. Med. **299:**1045-1048, 1099-1105, 1978.

O'Brien, M.L., Buist, N.R.M., and Murphey, W.H.: Neonatal screening for alpha-1-antitrypsin deficiency, J. Pediatr. **92:**1006-1010, 1978.

Odièvre, M., Martin, J.P., Hadchouel, M., and Alagille, D.: Alpha-1-antitrypsin deficiency and liver disease in children: phenotypes, manifestations and prognosis, Pediatrics **57:**226-231, 1976.

Psacharopoulos, H.T., Mowat, A.P., Portmann, B.T., and Williams, R.: The prognosis in childhood of liver disease associated with alpha-1-antitrypsin deficiency (PiZZ). In Japanese Medical Research Foundation, editors: Cholestasis in infancy: its pathogenesis, diagnosis, and treatment, Tokyo, 1980, University of Tokyo Press.

Scully, R.E., Baldabini, J.J., and McNeely, B.U.: Alpha-1-antitrypsin deficiency and hypoplasia of extrahepatic ducts, N. Engl. J. Med. **302:**1405-1413, 1980.

Sharp, H.L., Bridges, R.A., Krivit, W., and Frier, E.F.: Cirrhosis associated with alpha-1-antitrypsin deficiency: a previously unrecognized inherited disorder, J. Lab. Clin. Med. **73:**934-939, 1969.

Sveger, T.: Liver disease in alpha-1-antitrypsin deficiency detected by screening of 200,000 infants, N. Engl. J. Med. **294:**1316-1321, 1976.

Sveger, T.: Alpha-1-antitrypsin deficiency in early childhood, Pediatrics **62:**22-25, 1978.

Talamo, R.C., and Feingold, M.: Infantile cirrhosis with hereditary alpha-1-antitrypsin deficiency, Am. J. Dis. Child. **125:**845-847, 1973.

Talamo, R.C.: Basic and clinical aspects of alpha-1-antitrypsin, Pediatrics **56:**91-99, 1975.

Wilkinson, E.J., Raab, K., Browning, C.A., and Hosty, T.A.: Familial hepatic cirrhosis in infants associated with alpha-1-antitrypsin SZ phenotype, J. Pediatr. **85:**159-164, 1974.

OTHER METABOLIC LIVER DISEASE
Galactosemia

Galactosemia is an inherited defect transmitted as an autosomal recessive trait in which the enzyme galactose-1-phosphate uridyl transferase is absent in the homozygote state. It is an uncommon genetic condition with an incidence of about 1 in 40,000, and the carrier frequency put at 1 in 100. Several variants have now been described and may be associated with symptoms (Rennes, Indiana), with others being asymptomatic (Duarte, Los Angeles). The deficiency of galactose-1-phosphate uridyl transferase allows for the excess accumulation of galactose, galactose-1-phosphate, and galactitol in the body tissues (especially liver, kidneys, eyes, and central nervous system) where they produce toxic damage.

Clinical symptoms caused by this inborn error of metabolism begins in the homozygote neonate within 2 weeks after ingestion of lactose-containing milk products (breast, cow's, goat's, and cow's milk–derived formulas). These manifestations most commonly include anorexia, lethargy, vomiting, and poor initial weight gain. Signs of liver disease appear as jaundice and hepatomegaly. The liver may be surprisingly firm. Elevated bilirubin is usually of the "mixed" type (though rarely may be predominantly unconjugated), resulting in dark-colored urine that stains the diaper and stools that are normal to partially colored. Symptoms of bacterial sepsis may be present. Cataracts begin to form early and can be seen postnatally by slit-lamp examination within the first week or two. Rapid progression of the liver injury is indicated by the appearance of spontaneous hemorrhages and the finding of abnormal results of coagulation studies. Ascites, associated with early cirrhosis, may be present within 3 months in undiagnosed cases even in the absence of the "typical" clinical picture. A delay in motor milestones is frequently reported. Incomplete forms of galactosemia also exist, expressing isolated clinical findings such as mental retardation or cataracts, but rarely cirrhosis.

Laboratory findings include mild acidosis, hypoglycemia, mixed hyperbilirubinemia, elevated transaminases, and prolonged clotting studies. Urine findings suggesting renal tubular dysfunction include the presence of reducing sugar (galactosuria) and proteinuria. The generalized aminoaciduria and organic aciduria are found by urine chromotography.

Diagnosis is made by direct measurement of enzyme activity of galactose-1-phosphate uridyl transferase in red blood cells. In most states the routine neonatal screening test includes this diagnostic possibility.

The *pathohistologic appearance* of the liver is suggestive of underlying metabolic disease. Cholestasis is striking. Prominent canalicular bile plugs are often surrounded by the pseudoacinar arrangement of hepatocytes. The liver cells show mild to moderate steatosis and spotty cellular necrosis; the overall appearance is that of lobular disarray. Surprisingly, inflammation is lacking, even when significant portal and perilobular fibrosis is common. Histologic features of early cirrhosis are noted in severe cases within 2 to 3 months of life (Fig. 24-19).

The differential diagnosis of an ill neonate with cholestatic features should also include other inborn errors of metabolism, such as congenital fructose intolerance and tyrosinemia. Neonatal hepatitis caused by infection needs to be ruled out

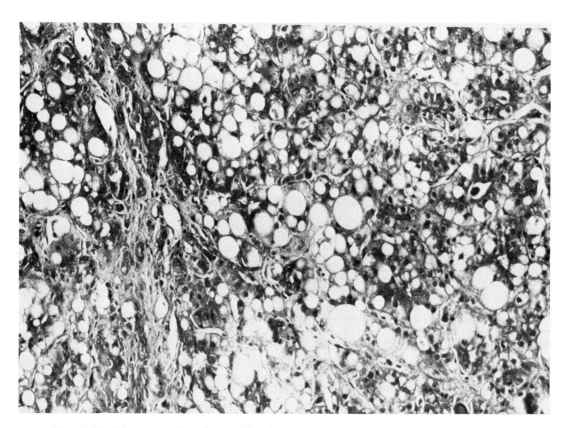

Fig. 24-19. Galactosemic liver disease. Liver biopsy section from a 10-week-old infant presenting with jaundice, failure to thrive, vomiting, and seizures. In addition, hepatomegaly and ascites were noted on examination. The urine contained reducing sugars, and galactose-1-phosphate uridyl transferase was not detectable in the patient's red blood cells. The biopsy section shows classic features of metabolic liver disease including steatosis, lobular disarray, pseudogland formation, canalicular cholestasis, perilobular fibrosis, and insignificant inflammatory response (Trichrome, $\times 100$). Follow-up biopsy after 2 years of treatment showed restoration of normal liver architecture, but the child was both mentally and developmentally delayed.

as well. Congenital fructose intolerance can be considered only if fructose has been fed, whereas tyrosinemia may be a diagnosis of exclusion. The early onset of symptoms attributed to galactosemia in a neonate ingesting galactose-containing milk demands red blood cell quantitative analysis of the enzyme galactose-1-phosphate uridyl transferase. Routine urine testing cannot be relied upon early in the disease because the patient's urine may not contain sufficient concentration of the reducing sugar to be detected by Clinitest. Other entities that produce metabolic or toxic liver disease can usually be eliminated by history taking and physical examination.

Treatment of galactosemia is prompt withdrawal of galactose from the diet. Substitution of other milk formulas, free of galactose is easily accomplished using soy-based formula, Nutrami-

gen, or Pregestimil, and improvement follows in 5 to 7 days. Jaundice disappears, and hepatomegaly slowly recedes over 6 to 18 months. A galactose-free diet is recommended for 5 to 8 years, but whether it is necessary to remain on the diet for a lifetime is still controversial. Serial determinations of galactose-1-phosphate levels assure that dietary compliance is being achieved.

Prognosis is excellent for those coming to diagnosis and treatment early in the evolution of the disease. Reversibility of the liver disease is common even in the face of more severe hepatic involvement. Although residual portal or perilobular fibrosis is not uncommon, cirrhosis is most unusual in cases treated early. This is supported by the results of galactosemia screening in adults with cirrhosis, and few indeed are positive. If significant neonatal hypoglycemia was present, residual neurologic sequelae (mental and developmental retardation) may unfortunately be found.

The heterozygote pregnant mother should be on a galactose-free diet throughout gestation. One can make a prenatal diagnosis in the affected fetus by demonstrating the enzyme deficiency in cells obtained from amniotic fluid, thereby permitting the proper selection of a substitute milk product to be fed after the infant is born.

Congenital (hereditary) fructose intolerance

Congenital fructose intolerance is another inherited defect transmitted as an autosomal recessive trait. In the homozygote state the enzyme fructose-1-phosphate aldolase is severely reduced. Fructose-1,6-diphosphate aldolase is also reduced but to a lesser degree. The incidence of this disease is about the same as that reported for galactosemia (1 in 40,000). The deficiency of fructose-1-aldolase allows for the accumulation in body tissues of excess quantities of fructose and fructose-1-phosphate, which in turn are believed responsible for the resulting damage. Liver cells seem most affected by these incompletely metabolized substances because pathways for both gluconeogenesis and glycogenolysis are inhibited, a condition leading to reduced levels of hepatic ATP and inorganic phosphorus.

The *clinical picture* is similar to that seen in galactosemic infants and symptoms begin shortly after sucrose-containing formulas (soy-based formula, Nutramigen) or foods (fruits) are introduced into the diet. Vomiting and hepatomegaly are almost constant findings. Pallor, lethargy, jaundice, and seizures can be noted. Cataracts, however, are not present. Stools are partially acholic to normal in color; urine is typically dark. Milder forms of the disease that manifest these symptoms later in life are reported. A natural aversion to sweets may be the only historical clue to the underlying condition.

Laboratory findings that confirm the liver disturbance include a mixed hyperbilirubinemia, elevated transaminases, prolonged clotting studies, and hypoalbuminemia. Hypophosphatemia and hypoglycemia are occasionally present. Acidosis may be found, especially when dehydration and shock accompany the presentation. Renal tubular dysfunction (fructosuria and proteinuria) and urine amino and organic acid patterns are also suggestive of underlying metabolic disease.

Histologic findings on liver biopsy are indistin-guishable from those described for galactosemia (see Fig. 19-4). Serious fibrosis or cirrhosis will be found as long as fructose is consumed in the diet.

Whenever neonatal cholestasis is noted with generalized systemic symptoms, the differential diagnosis is similar to that described for galactosemia. In the absence of cholestasis, septic causes, gastrointestinal and anatomic lesions, and other inborn errors (glycogen-storage disease) should be considered because vomiting dominates the early clinical abnormality.

The *diagnosis* is confirmed by the response to withdrawal of fructose from the diet, a carefully performed fructose tolerance test several weeks later, or measurement of fructose-1-aldolase activity in liver tissue obtained after coagulation studies have returned to normal.

With dutiful commitment to avoid fructose in the diet, the *prognosis* is excellent. The liver may remain firm and enlarged for several years. Follow-up biopsy often shows residual fibrosis and periportal hepatocyte steatosis, even when the patient is maintained on a complete fructose-elimination diet. If significant hypoglycemia was present in the neonatal period, neurologic sequelae and developmental delays may persist. In milder cases, failure to thrive or rarely the signs of chronic liver disease (cirrhosis) will be recognized clinically and eventually lead to the specific diagnosis. Newborns in a family with an affected sibling should be on a fructose-free diet until 3 to 6 months of age when a diagnostic fructose-tolerance test can be performed. It is recommended that the pregnant heterozygote mother be placed on a low-fructose diet during gestation.

Hereditary tyrosinemia

Tyrosinemia has a number of different clinical forms, all of which seem to have transient or permanent deficiency of *p*-hydroxyphenylpyruvic acid oxidase. The disease is transmitted as an autosomal recessive trait and is more commonly reported from Quebec province and Scandinavia as a rare cause of severe neonatal liver disease. The clinical features are strikingly similar to that of galactosemia and congenital fructose intolerance. Although renal and pancreatic involvement may also occur, signs of hepatic failure often dominate the clinical picture.

A variant of this disorder with slower progression eventually leads to cirrhosis, renal tubular abnormalities, and vitamin D–resistant rickets in the older child. Not infrequently, hepatoma develops in the cirrhotic liver.

Although tyrosine and methionine metabolism is abnormal, the hepatic toxic substance is not clearly known. Nonspecific (especially in severe liver disease) hyperaminoacidemia is believed to reflect both the abnormal metabolism of these amino acids and the effects of severe hepatocyte injury. In the neonate with severe liver disease, an elevated alpha-fetoprotein level, coupled with failure to respond to a galactose-free diet or, if applicable, a fructose-free diet favor the diagnosis of hereditary tyrosinemia.

The liver histologic appearance shows significant necrosis, architectural disarray, and fibrosis, as well as "toxic" features of metabolic liver disease described in galactosemia and congenital fructose intolerance.

Despite the use of low tyrosine and methionine diets, the immediate prognosis is grim. For most surviving the early hepatic consequences, progressive cirrhosis is the rule despite therapy. Hepatic decompensation is often noted within the first few years of life. In the incomplete form found in older children (greater than 6 months) nodular cirrhosis develops and death is caused by either liver failure or hepatoma before adulthood.

Glycogen storage disease

The hepatic abnormality in this complex group of enzymatic deficiencies in either glycogen synthesis or degradation varies from uncomplicated hepatomegaly to modest portal and septal fibrosis to cirrhosis. Hepatic adenoma and even hepatoma may eventually develop. Other than type IV and rarely type III disease, the hepatic involvement is not a primary determinant of the patient's prognosis and eventual outcome. Hepatomegaly is impressive in most glycogenoses, and therefore these conditions are usually included in the differential diagnosis that, one would hope, will explain this physical finding. Obviously, the presence or absence of other important clinical and laboratory features will help in the initial sorting process (Table 24-11).

Type I glycogenosis (von Gierke's disease), caused by glucose-6-phosphatase deficiency and pseudo–type I, with normal glucose-6-phosphatase activity, almost always presents early in life (the first 3 to 6 months) with failure to thrive, seizures (hypoglycemia), and developmental delays. Diagnosis is suggested from the physical

findings of "cherublike" facies, prominent abdomen, and massive hepatomegaly (but without splenomegaly), renomegaly, and wasted extremities. Jaundice is absent. Important laboratory studies reveal fasting (3- to 4-hour) hypoglycemia, lactic acidosis, hyperlipidemia, hyperuricemia, elevated transaminases, and thrombocytosis but with thrombasthenia. The liver histologic appearance shows large, pale hepatocytes filled with glycogen of normal structure (periodic acid–Schiff stain positive, diastase positive). Steatosis is usually present. The diagnosis is made by measurement of glucose-6-phosphatase activity in liver tissue, which will be low to absent in type I disease and normal in pseudo–type I. Significant long-term dietary problems attending the management of these children are common and may require frequent small feedings or continuous nighttime nasogastric feedings. Results obtained after surgical creation of a portacaval shunt in those difficult and refractory cases have been encouraging, with reversal of the persistent failure to thrive, lactic acidosis, and recurrent hypoglycemic episodes reported. The long-term prognosis is not particularly favorable, however, because all the children seem to be at risk to developing either renal failure, hepatic adenoma, or hepatoma, or all three.

Type III glycogenosis is caused by a deficiency of the debrancher enzyme amylo-1,6-glucosidase. Most cases present in the first year of life with hypoglycemic seizures and massive hepatomegaly. In these children, unless one is careful to palpate the abdomen from the groin upward, the liver edge may easily be missed. A history of delay in motor milestones may be reported, and hypotonia is found on physical examination. Short stature is likewise common. The important laboratory finding is fasting (6- to 8-hour) hypoglycemia usually without acidosis. Most do not demonstrate elevation in blood lactic acid or uric acid, or the presence of hyperlipidemia, abnormalities that are very constant in type I glycogenosis. Lactic acid levels may rise after a glucose load, a finding also noted to occur in type IX disease. Mildly elevated transaminases are found while the bilirubin is normal. The liver histologic appearance is similar to that of type I disease, except that the stored glycogen is abnormal (limit dextrin) and fails to be completely digested with diastase. Fibrous tissue is not unusual, being portal, central, or even intralobular at times (Fig. 24-20). Generally, the prognosis for these children is much better than that for type

Table 24-11. Glycogen storage disease with important liver involvement

Types	I	III	IV	VI	IX
Enzyme deficiency	Glucose-6-phosphatase	Amylo-1,6-glucosidase	Amylo-1,4-1,6 transglucosidase	Phosphorylase	Phosphorylase kinase
Hepatomegaly	4+	4+	3-4+	1-3+	1-3+
Splenomegaly	—	—	2-3+	—	—
Failure to thrive	4+	2-4+	4+	0-1+	0-1+
Hypoglycemia	4+	2-4+	—	0-1+	0-1+
Developmental delays	4+	2-4+	2+	0-1+	0-1+
Lactic acidemia	4+	1-2+	—	—	—
Hyperlipidemia	4+	1-2+	—	—	—
Abnormal liver function tests					
Transaminase	2-3+	2-3+	4+	—	—
Bilirubin	—	—	1-2+	—	—
Hepatic fibrosis	—	2+	4+	—	—
Cirrhosis	—	Rare	4+	—	—
Adenoma	+	+	—	—	—
Hepatoma	+	+	—	—	—
Tissue for diagnosis of enzyme deficiency	Liver	Liver, white blood cells	Liver, white blood cells	Liver, white blood cells	Liver, red blood cells

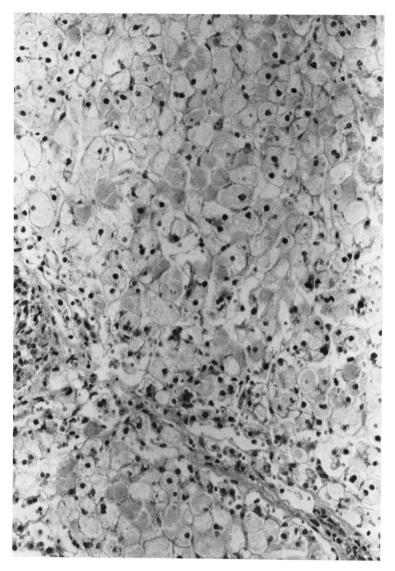

Fig. 24-20. Type III glycogenosis. Liver biopsy section from a 19-month-old infant with recurrent hypoglycemic seizures and huge hepatomegaly. The distended hepatocytes contain poorly staining homogeneous cytoplasmic material giving them an "empty" appearance. Minimal perilobular fibrosis was also present. (× 100.)

I. Spontaneous improvement often occurs just before or during adolescence. Rare refractory cases may benefit from a portacaval shunt procedure. Progression of the liver disease to cirrhosis is extremely rare, but hepatic adenoma formation has been reported. Diagnosis is best made by measurement of glycogen content in red blood cells and enzyme activity in leukocytes, liver, or muscle tissue.

Type IV glycogenosis, strictly speaking, is not a glycogenosis. The deficiency of the glycogen forming enzyme amylo-1,4-1,6-transglucosidase

(branching enzyme) leads to the accumulation of an abnormal polysaccharide material in the hepatocytes and other tissues. This amylopectin-like glycogen is believed to be responsible for the hepatic damage that rapidly progresses to cirrhosis and liver failure. It is an extremely rare form of liver disease, with only a few cases being reported in the world literature. Manifestations appear early in life as poor feeding, vomiting, and failure to thrive. Delay in motor milestones with accompanying hypotonia has been observed. Not only is firm hepatomegaly present but splenomegaly too, suggesting underlying cirrhosis with portal hypertension. In this glycogenesis, liver function tests are conspicuously abnormal with increased transaminases and probably bilirubin. Neither fasting hypoglycemia nor acidosis is likely to be found. Liver biopsy material shows cytoplasmic glycogen deposits, perilobular and intralobular fibrosis, and a micronodular cirrhosis. The histologic lesion may easily be confused with that of alpha-1-antitrypsin–deficiency disease because the intracytoplasmic deposits are likewise PAS positive and diastase resistant. The deposits, whether in liver or other tissues (heart and skeletal muscle, brain), can be digested with pectinase. Of course, quantitative alpha-1-antitrypsin levels should be normal in type IV disease. The correct diagnosis is confirmed by demonstration of deficient activity of the brancher enzyme either in leukocytes or liver tissue. No treatment exists for this fatal disease.

In *type VIa glycogenosis* the deficiency in liver phosphorylase results in hepatomegaly, but this finding varies when the liver fluctuates in size, being enlarged during periods of well-being, and of normal size to only slightly enlarged during intercurrent illnesses. Failure to thrive is absent or minimal in most. Fasting (12-hour) hypoglycemia and ketonuria may be found. Liver function tests are usually normal. The liver histologic appearance shows typically large, pale hepatocytes with structurally normal glycogen. The diagnosis can be made by measurement of the phosphorylase system in red blood cells or white blood cells. Prognosis is excellent, with spontaneous resolution of the hepatomegaly and catch-up growth occurring during adolescence.

Type IX glycogenosis is associated with phosphorylase kinase deficiency and gives rise to a clinical and pathologic picture very similar to that in type VIa. A sex-linked mode of transmission has been noted and most cases are males.

There are *other glycogenoses*. Variable degrees of hepatomegaly are a constant feature in the remaining rare disorders of glycogen metabolism; however, the important clinical manifestations emanate from affected organs other than the liver. For example, type II glycogenosis (Pompe's disease) characterized by the lysosomal deficiency of alpha-1,4-glucosidase (acid maltase) primarily affects heart and muscle. A hepatic glycogenosis with predominantly renal tubular dysfunction may oc-

cur, but the enzyme defect has not been identified. A rare form of hepatic glycogenosis with multiple glycolytic enzyme deficiencies (glucose-6-phosphatase, debrancher enzyme, and phosphorylase) has also been reported.

Lysosomal diseases

Disorders of lysosomal function gives rise to a group of conditions categorized as either lipidoses, mucopolysaccharidoses, or mucolipidoses, most of which are associated with hepatomegaly and occasionally terminate with cirrhosis.

Sphingolipidoses

Niemann-Pick disease. The infantile, acute neuropathic form of Niemann-Pick disease has a predilection for individuals of Eastern European Jewish ancestry. The disease may present as a cholestatic syndrome at 2 to 3 months of age with jaundice and hepatosplenomegaly. A cherry-red spot may be seen in the retina. The deficiency of lysosomal sphingomyelinase in reticuloendothelial cells is believed responsible for the accumulation of sphingomyelin in the liver, spleen, bone marrow, and central nervous system. Cirrhosis, though rare, may be found in autopsy cases. Diagnosis can be suspected from the appearance of "foam cells" in the bone marrow, liver biopsy specimen, spleen, and lymph nodes (see Fig. 19-9). Vacuolated lymphocytes are commonly seen in the peripheral smear. Diagnosis is confirmed when one finds decreased sphingomyelinase activity by lipid analysis in peripheral white blood cells or liver and spleen tissue.

Variants of Niemann-Pick disease do exist, usually occurring in non-Jews. Signs and symptoms tend to have a delayed appearance. One juvenile variant of Niemann-Pick disease is associated with a history of prolonged neonatal jaundice, hepatosplenomegaly, paralysis of upward gaze and, later in life, the finding of "foamy" and sea-blue macrophages in the bone marrow. Most of these cases have occurred in children of Spanish-American ancestry. Another variety, the type D variant (Nova Scotia) of Niemann-Pick disease, is associated with a high incidence of cirrhosis.

Gaucher's disease. Gaucher's disease results in intracellular accumulation of glucocerebroside and causes a greater degree of structural damage to the liver than that seen in Niemann-Pick disease. Three forms of Gaucher's disease are now recognized, and each can be distinguished when the age

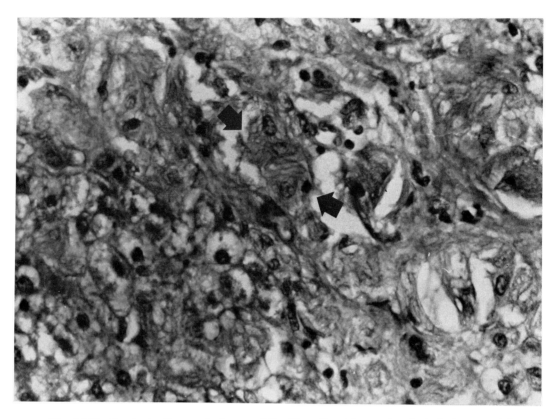

Fig. 24-21. Gaucher's disease. A cluster of Kupffer cells with cytoplasmic inclusion material presenting a wrinkled look, *arrows.* Liver tissue obtained from a 1-year-old developmentally delayed child with hepatosplenomegaly born of consanguineous parents. Histologic features of cirrhosis were not found. (× 250.)

of onset and the dominant clinical manifestations are considered. A primary neuropathic form starts early in infancy, and death usually occurs by 2 to 3 years. Another variety also begins early in life but shows predominantly visceral features including hepatosplenomegaly, bone pain, and skeletal deformities. Neurologic manifestations eventually develop before 10 years of age. Thereafter the disease process is slow and progressive, with death occurring in adulthood. A predominantly visceral form without neurologic involvement may become manifest at any age and is characterized by a slow progression to cirrhosis. Liver function studies in most varieties are only modestly abnormal with elevated transaminases and alkaline phosphatase. The diagnosis is usually suspected from the bone marrow (or liver biopsy) examination by the presence of foam cells, with a "wrinkled" look to the cytoplasm (Fig. 24-21). Bone marrow biopsy may provide a higher yield of Gaucher's cells than that obtained from a marrow

aspirate alone. The presence of vacuolated lymphocytes in the peripheral smear, roentgenologic abnormalities especially in the long bones, and increased acid phosphatase levels are all highly suspicious of Gaucher's disease. Diagnosis is confirmed by lipid enzyme studies using peripheral leukocytes.

Mucopolysaccharidoses

Hurler's syndrome, type I is an autosomal recessive disease caused by the absence of alpha-iduronidase in lysosomes, leading to the accumulation of an abnormal mucopolysaccharide, which in turn produces the various manifestations noted in this condition including hepatic damage. Features of cirrhosis may eventually develop in long-standing cases. Diagnosis of Hurler's disease is usually made before serious liver damage from clinical assessment of the characteristic physical features. The coarse facies, hepatosplenomegaly and umbilical hernia, stiff finger joints, corneal clouding, and a gibbus are essentially diagnostic in the retarded child. The excess quantities of mucopolysaccharides excreted in the urine are predominantly dermatan sulfate and heparatin sulfate. The disease for most is rapidly progressive, with death occurring by 10 years of age.

Hunter's syndrome is a sex-linked recessive inherited disease in which a severe form has hepatosplenomegaly, but without corneal clouding or gibbus formation. Mental retardation is not so striking as in Hurler's syndrome. The lysosomal hydrolase sulfoiduronate sulfatase is deficient. The urinary mucopolysaccharide excretion pattern is similar to that in Hurler's disease.

Other mucopolysaccharidases have inconstant visceromegaly including, Sanfilippo syndrome (sulfamidase deficiency), Maroteaux-Lamy syndrome (arylsulfatase B deficiency), beta-glucuronidase–deficiency disease. The diagnosis of these conditions is generally made from specific clinical features, roentgenologic studies, and chromatographic analysis of the mucopolysaccharide pattern in urine.

Mucolipidoses

Type II (I-cell disease) is a rapidly progressive condition with onset in infancy and death within the first year of life. Many clinical features are similar to those found in Hurler's disease, including hepatosplenomegaly. Diagnosis is usually confirmed when one finds a generalized decrease in several lysosomal hydrolases including beta-glucuronidase, hexosaminidase, and arylsulfatase in cultured fibroblasts. The hepatic architecture is not seriously altered. Hepatocytes are distended and pale; refractile inclusions may be identified in the cytoplasm. Microvesicular steatosis is also present.

Type I mucolipidosis is a less severe condition beginning later in childhood evidenced by mental retardation, coarse facies, and skeletal abnormalities (dysostosis multiplex). Neurologic features besides moderate dementia include a peripheral neuropathy and nerve deafness. The diagnosis sometimes can be suspected from the features in liver biopsy material showing vacuolated hepatocytes and Kupffer cells. Increased hepatic beta-galactosidase is found in some patients.

The infantile form of *GM_1 gangliosidosis,* caused by beta-galactosidase deficiency, is a generalized severe condition in which hepatomegaly is common. In addition, downy hirsutism, umbilical and inguinal hernias, retinal cherry-red spot, and bony changes accompany the severe dementia. Seizures are frequent and most will die before 2 years of age.

Mannosidosis (alpha-mannosidase deficiency) and *fucosidosis* (alpha-L-fucosidase deficiency) are additional examples of mucolipidoses that may have visceromegaly.

The diagnosis of all these lysosomal hydrolase–deficiency states is generally made by specific enzyme analysis in cultured skin fibroblasts or peripheral leukocytes and, where applicable, from the results of specific enzyme analysis in serum. One can also diagnose many of these disorders in utero using amniotic cells for the enzyme assays.

Cystinosis

Cystinosis, a rare defect, is inherited as an autosomal recessive trait. Three types of cystinosis have been identified: infantile, adolescent, and adult. The first one is not only the most common type but also the most severe. Cystine is found in virtually all body tissues and especially localized to the lysosomes. A deficiency or structural abnormality in lysosomal cystine reductase has been postulated as the underlying defect in this disease. The accumulated crystals gradually result in cell injury and cell death, with the kidneys being most susceptible. Slit-lamp examination of the cornea reveals the pathognomonic ground-glass ''dazzle'' appearance because of the presence of cystine crystals. With prolonged survival of these infants (chronic dialysis program), hepatic involvement becomes manifest by hepatomegaly. The cystine deposits are usually present within the reticuloendothelial cells of the liver but have also been described in the parenchymal cells. Here they cause local inflammation and hepatic cell cytolysis and stimulate fibrous deposition, especially in portal zones. Although renal transplantation is beneficial for relieving severe kidney failure, its effect upon other organ involvement has not been determined.

Lysosomal lipid storage disease

Wolman's disease is caused by the deficiency of lysosomal acid esterase activity, which allows for the rapid accumulation of cholesterol esters and triglycerides, particularly in liver, gastrointestinal mucosa, and adrenal glands. Gastrointestinal symptoms, characterized by vomiting and diarrhea, appear within the first month or two of life and the infant fails to thrive. Hepatosplenomegaly gradually develops over the next several months. Diagnosis can be immediately suspected in these infants if calcium deposits in the area of the adrenal glands are recognized on plain abdominal films. Vacuolated peripheral lymphocytes are common, and "foam cells" are present in bone marrow aspirate. The overall liver histologic picture reveals disruption of the normal architecture with portal fibrosis. The hepatocytes are distended with vacuoles, and clusters of foamy histiocytes may be noted in portal and periportal areas. Portal fibrosis progressing to cirrhosis may occur within 2 to 6 months of age. The specific enzymatic defect can be determined from analysis of either blood lymphocytes or skin fibroblasts. A variant with delayed onset and slower progression has also been described.

Cholesterol ester storage disease is featured clinically mostly as hepatomegaly, which may evolve at any age, from infancy to adulthood. A deficiency of lysosomal acid lipase is believed responsible for the hepatic accumulation of cholesterol esters. Surprisingly, hyperlipidemia is not a constant finding. Material obtained by liver biopsy is strikingly butter yellow in appearance. The hepatocytes are enlarged and contain numerous lipid droplets (cholesterol esters) that stain positive for fat. Variable degrees of fibrosis have been reported. The long-term prognosis is uncertain but seems to be good.

Hepatocerebral degeneration

Hepatocerebral degeneration is a rare disorder of unknown cause that is usually fatal by 3 years of age. The condition is probably inherited as an autosomal recessive trait for the disease has frequently occured in siblings of asymptomatic parents. Clinical findings include a rapid onset, severe seizure disorder superimposed upon mild to moderate developmental delays, and hypotonia. The seizures become multifocal and are usually refractory to treatment. Progressive stupor, coma, cortical blindness, and optic atrophy are seen before death. Evidence of hepatic disease is more subtle during life with modestly elevated transaminases present. Before death, however, jaundice and ascites may develop. In other examples, underlying severe liver disease may first be recognized at surgery for other reasons, or at autopsy. Microscopically the liver shows portal fi-

brosis, a micronodular cirrhosis, mild to moderate microvesicular and macrovesicular fatty changes, collapse of the reticulin framework, and parenchymal cytolysis without a significant inflammatory response (lymphocytes). Zones of hepatocyte necrosis may bridge portal areas together. The cytoplasm in the dying hepatocytes has a fine granular appearance that stains more intensely with eosin (Fig. 24-22). The brain disease includes loss of cortical neurons and Purkinje cells. Foci of demyelination and Alzheimer type II cells can be found in some cases. Although this entity clinically mimics that of other known inborn errors of metabolism (see discussion under Reye's syndrome, pp. 633 to 635), neither an enzyme deficiency nor abnormal storage material has been identified up to now.

Lipoprotein-deficiency syndromes

Tangier's disease (familial alpha-lipoprotein deficiency) is a rare autosomal recessive condition that results in the accumulation of cholesterol esters in many organs including the liver. The deficiency of the lipid-packaging alpha-apoproteins, both high-density lipoprotein (HDL) and very low density lipoprotein (VLDL) are believed responsible for accumulation of the lipid. Plasma cholesterol levels are also abnormally low. The yellow-orange color of the enlarged tonsils is said to be diagnostic. The liver histologic condition shows an intralobular accumulation of "foam cells" without disruption of the hepatic architecture. Prognosis is apparently not governed by the liver findings.

Abetalipoproteinemia (Bassen-Kornsweig) is a syndrome usually suspected in the first year or two of life from symptoms of chronic diarrhea, steatorrhea, failure to thrive, spinocerebellar ataxia and retinitis pigmentosa. Mild to moderate hepatomegaly occurs because of fatty metamorphosis of the nutritional type. However, a child showing progression of the liver disease to micronodular cirrhosis has now been reported. The diagnosis is confirmed by lipoprotein electrophoresis that reveals an absence of beta-lipoprotein. In addition, low cholesterol and phospholipid levels are constant, as is acanthocytosis of red blood cells noted in the peripheral blood smear. The use of a medium-chain triglyceride diet is beneficial in regard to the gastrointestinal component, but it may not prevent the progression of the neurologic or he-

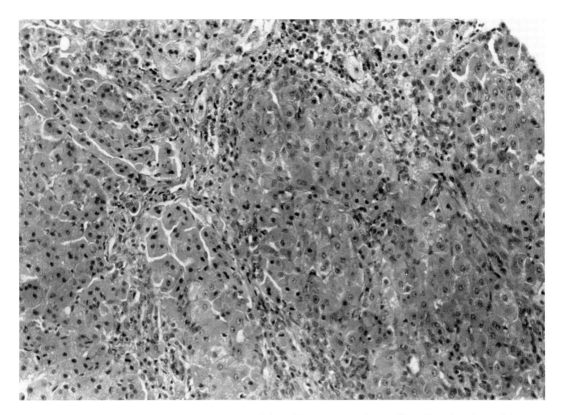

Fig. 24-22. Hepatocerebral syndrome. Nodules of hepatocytes show cells with pyknotic nuclei that occasionally demonstrate pseudoacinar development. Other hepatocytes appear normal (× 100). This liver biopsy specimen was obtained from a 12-month-old infant with seizures and severe mental and developmental retardation. At time of gastrostomy the liver was noted to be small and finely nodular. Liver-function studies revealed elevated aminotransferases but normal serum bilirubin. An older sibling had died with the same clinical pathologic picture.

patic disease. However, maintaining normal serum levels of vitamin E may benefit the neurologic consequences of this entity.

Iron-overload liver conditions

Hemoglobinopathies take many forms. Hepatic involvement is common in both sickle-cell disease and beta-thalassemia. In *sickle-cell disease,* the hepatomegaly is attributable primarily to congestion within the sinusoids of sickled red blood cells. In some patients central venous congestion caused by chronic anemia and at times right-sided heart failure may also contribute to the hepatomegaly. When hepatocytes are impeded in the microcirculation, local hypoxia results, an event believed responsible for initiating fibrogenesis. When features of chronic persistent hepatitis or postnecrotic cirrhosis are found on biopsy, transfusion hepatitis (HBV, non-A non-B, CMV) is most likely the cause. Iron overload by itself is seldom a cause of significant hepatic injury in sickle-cell disease.

However, in *beta-thalassemia* the severity of the anemia and necessity of frequent blood transfusion result in extreme iron overload, and hemosiderosis occurs in most tissues. After saturation of the reticuloendothelial cells, excess iron is deposited in hepatocytes and results in cell injury. Either hepatic fibrosis or features of cirrhosis are commonly found at autopsy. As in sickle-cell disease, the role of chronic right-sided heart failure, anemia, or transfusion-acquired liver disease needs to be carefully considered. Most patients succumb to complications of infection or heart failure before young adulthood.

Hemochromatosis is caused by congenital transferrin deficiency and is a rare cause of hepatomegaly in the young child. Laboratory clues for diagnosis come from finding a high serum ferritin concentration in the face of a microcytic, hypochromic anemia. *Idiopathic hemochromatosis,* an autosomal recessive disorder, seldom produces clinical symptoms in the pediatric-age group. In adults, however, it leads to excessive iron overload, hepatic fibrosis, or often cirrhosis, with the eventual malfunction of other organs including the heart, pancreas, and endocrine glands. Serum ferritin levels may be normal or only slightly elevated early in this disease.

Zellweger's syndrome (cerebrohepatorenal syndrome) is a rare but serious condition leading to death within the first few months of life. The hepatic involvement may be mild to severe. It becomes evident in the neonatal period either as a cholestatic condition or with features suggesting massive hepatic necrosis (Fig. 19-10). Evidence of chronic liver disease (fibrosis and cirrhosis) may be present at autopsy. The biochemical defect is unknown, but striking hemosiderosis of the liver and other organs has been reported. When studied, serum ferritin in that syndrome has been significantly elevated. In addition, elevated levels of pipecolic acid are reported in blood and urine of these patients.

Hepatic porphyrias are a complicated group of metabolic disorders in which the biosynthesis of heme, in either the bone marrow or liver, leads to an overproduction of porphyrins or their precursors. The disorders are rarely of concern to the pediatrician, but occasionally symptoms may develop in teen-age children manifested by skin photosensitivity and mild anemia. Biochemical evidence of hepatic dysfunction may likewise be detected, but the significance of these findings will be dictated by the specific variety of porphyria.

Mild hepatic damage (fatty infiltration, focal necrosis, hepatic siderosis) occurs in *porphyria cutanea tarda,* whereas more important hepatic structural changes can be seen in *protoporphyria* including fibrosis or cirrhosis. The birefringent protoporphyrin pigment deposits are present in hepatocytes, Kupffer cells, and bile canaliculi. In porphyria cutanea tarda an increase in urinary excretion of uroporphyrins occurs, whereas in protoporphyria the principal biochemical abnormality is an increase in protoporphyrin in red blood cells and in the feces. Patients with these conditions should avoid porphyrin-stimulating agents such as estrogen-containing oral contraceptives, chloro-

quine, griseofulvin, iron compounds, and alcohol. Since protoporphyrins are excreted only into the bile and then into the intestinal lumen, the organic acid-binding resin cholestyramine has been utilized to reduce the protoporphyrin pool and thereby halt the progression of the liver disease or even reverse the process.

Diabetic liver disease

Hepatomegaly is found in up to 30% of juvenile diabetics, especially those poorly controlled. Liver biopsy usually reveals excess accumulation of hepatic lipid in 15% to 50% of such cases. The mechanism is believed to be caused by the lack of insulin, which favors increased lipolysis and resulting hyperlipidemia and hepatic steatosis. In addition, insulinopenia causes decreased hepatocyte lipoprotein synthesis, resulting in deficient removal of lipid from the plasma and inadequate secretion from hepatocytes. Painful hepatomegaly occurs during episodes of ketoacidosis, and biopsy tissue obtained during "attacks" show increased glycogen stores in the nucleus as well as cytoplasm. Fatty change may or may not be present. However, the hepatomegaly often persists after correction of the ketoacidosis. Liver function abnormalities are characterized by mildly elevated transaminase values, and sulfobromophthalein (BSP) retention is prolonged in up to 40% of cases. That the hepatic findings in juvenile diabetes will progress from those of fatty liver to cirrhosis has not been clearly established.

The association of dwarfism, truncal obesity, moon facies, and hepatomegaly constitutes *Mauriac's syndrome* and is seen in poorly controlled "brittle" diabetics. Liver biopsy specimens obtained from these patients show either or both increased fat and glycogen deposits, but seldom fibrosis or inflammatory changes. Preventing the wide fluctuations in blood glucose levels and episodes of ketoacidosis with long-acting insulin may alleviate this syndrome.

Fatty liver

Excessive steatosis within the liver can be responsible for striking hepatomegaly and often gives to the liver a smooth but firm quality to palpation. This condition may be first appreciated fortuitously by the radiologist who recognizes the abnormal radiolucency of the liver. Except for liver tenderness to palpation, any associated symptoms will depend on the underlying cause responsible for the accumulation of intrahepatic lipid. The biochemical abnormalities of routine liver function tests do not correlate well with the severity of the steatosis. The BSP-clearance test is the most sensitive indicator of underlying hepatic steatosis. Transaminases are slightly elevated, and jaundice is rarely observed.

The accumulation of hepatocyte lipid is the result of interruption of one or more of the complex interdependent pathways that control lipid metabolism (Fig. 24-23). Excessive quantities of free fatty acids may reach the liver from exogenous dietary sources, or endogenously, as the result of lipolysis occurring in adipose stores. In addition,

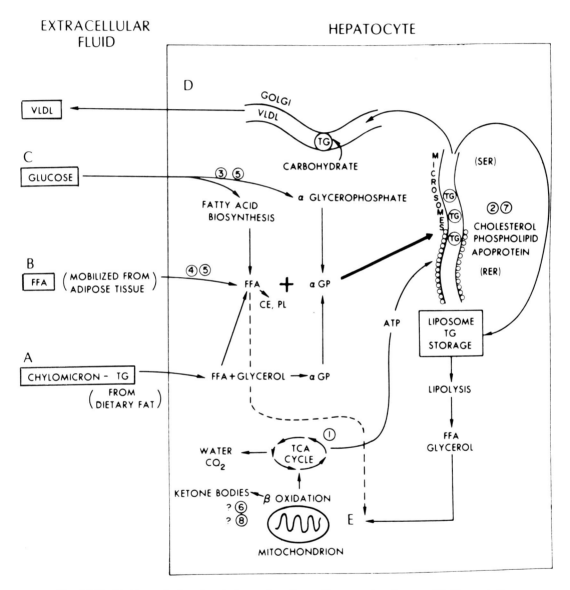

Fig. 24-23. Lipid metabolism in relation to fatty liver. The normal pathways of lipid metabolism are designated by the letters *A* to *E* and the presumed primary abnormalities in the different types of fatty liver are shown by the numbers *1* to *8*. *1*, Alcohol induced; *2*, kwashiorkor; *3*, obesity; *4*, postjejunal bypass; *5*, diabetes; *6*, idiopathic fatty liver of pregnancy) *7*, tetracycline; *8*, Reye's syndrome. α*GP*, Alpha glycerophosphate; *ATP*, adenosine triphosphate; *CE*, cholesterol ester; *FFA*, free fatty acid; *PL*, phospholipid; *RER*, rough endoplasmic reticulum; *SER*, smooth endoplasmic reticulum; *TCA cycle*, tricarboxylic acid cycle; *TG*, triglyceride; *VLDL*, very low density lipiprotein. (From Hoyumpa, A.M., Jr., et al.: Am. J. Dig. Dis. **20**:1142-1170, 1975.)

intrahepatic synthesis of free fatty acids can be stimulated by excess dietary intake of carbohydrates and further contributes to the total lipid load to be processed by the hepatocytes. The disposition of hepatic free-fatty acids depends on the mechanisms that allow for (1) their esterification to triglycerides, followed by (2) coupling to apoprotein B to form very low density lipoprotein (VLDL) particles, and (3) their release from the hepatocyte into the circulation. In addition, the integrity of the hepatic pathways involved in free fatty acid oxidation also dictates the outcome of intrahepatocytic lipids. Fatty acid oxidation is governed primarily by insulin levels and the availability of alpha-glycerophosphate. When the levels of these substances are high, free fatty acids are preferentially esterified into triglycerides. When either or both are low, lipolysis is encouraged and the rate of free fatty oxidation is increased.

Most examples of fatty liver can be explained by identification of the condition or conditions that result in (1) increased delivery of fatty acids (dietary or adipose stores), (2) increased synthesis of fatty acids within the hepatocytes, (3) decreased hepatic oxidation of fatty acids, and (4) impaired release of the hepatic triglyceride as VLDL particles. A comprehensive list of pediatric disorders associated with fatty liver appears below.

Major causes of fatty liver in children*

Systemic diseases
  Acute dehydration
  Severe infection
  Acidosis
  Fasting
  Intoxication
    Tetracycline
    Orotic acid
    Vitamin A
  Malnutrition
    Pancreatic insufficiency
    Cystic fibrosis
    Geophagia
Metabolic diseases
  Diabetes mellitus
  Obesity
  Hypercorticism
    Cushing's syndrome
    Iatrogenic
  Nephrotic syndrome
  Lipoatrophic diabetes

Enzyme deficiency syndromes
  Glycogenoses
  Deficiency of gluconeogenesis
  Abetalipoproteinemia
  Hyperlipidemia
  Wolman's disease
  Cholesterol ester storage disease
  Triglyceride storage disease
  Galactosemia
  Hereditary fructose intolerance
  Hereditary tyrosinemia
  Wilson's disease
  Alpha-1-antitrypsin deficiency
  Disorders of the urea cycle
  Reye's syndrome
  Intolerance to dibasic amino acids
  Congenital lactic acidosis
  Methylmalonic aciduria
  Homocystinuria
Other causes
  Prolonged parenteral nutrition
  Liver regeneration

Kwashiorkor. The hepatic lesion in this extreme expression of protein-calorie malnutrition appears early in its evolution. The fat deposits are typically periportal in distribution. The mechanism is believed to be caused by a combination of increased peripheral mobilization of free fatty acids from adipose stores, which in turn overwhelms the hepatocyte's ability to remove the triglyceride since the protein depleted host has insufficient quantities of apoprotein B needed to form VLDL. In time, the entire liver lobule shows large-droplet fat deposits, which displace the nucleus to the periphery of the cell. Increasing fibrous tissue deposition widens the portal zones, which may also contain a mild cellular inflammatory response. The morphologic findings are believed to be completely reversible, though it may take weeks to months once renutrition has begun.

Cystic fibrosis. The underlying pancreatic insufficiency in up to 80% of infants with this disease results in protein-calorie malnutrition. Not unexpectedly, the most common hepatic lesion is moderate to severe steatosis (Fig. 19-7). The basic mechanism is believed to be similar to that in kwashiorkor; the low levels of low-density lipoproteins suggest that there may be insufficient apoprotein B to excrete fat out of the liver. Other unknown factors are also probably involved, since the steatosis, though to a lesser degree, remains after adequate (presumed) pancreatic enzyme replacement has been employed. The fatty liver may

*From Alagille, D., and Odièvre, M.: Liver and biliary tract disease in children, New York, 1978, John Wiley & Sons.

be especially striking in infants with cystic fibrosis fed either a soybean-based formula or exclusively breast milk. In addition, hypoproteinemia and anemia are often present in such cases.

Morbid obesity. Undoubtedly the result of excessive dietary intake of free fatty acids and overall increased body stores, the hepatic accumulation of fat in this condition tends to be centrilobular rather than periportal, as seen early in protein-calorie malnutrition. Liver-function abnormalities are seldom identified. Progression to a more severe hepatic lesion does not occur unless the condition is complicated by predisposing circumstances such as intestinojejunal bypass surgery, hepatitis, or alcoholism.

Ethanol-induced fatty liver. Fortunately, this problem is seldom encountered in pediatric patients but occasionally will require consideration in the adolescent with hepatomegaly, a history of qualitatively inadequate diet, and abnormal liver function tests. Alcohol exerts a toxic-like effect by causing an increase in the ratio of NADH/NAD. This shift in redox potential in turn inhibits mitochondrial function at the level of the citric-acid cycle, thereby preventing free fatty acid oxidation from occurring. As a result, acyl-CoA derivatives accumulate, and the accumulation in turn further interferes with mitochondrial energy production (ATP) and cell damage results. For unknown reasons, collagen synthesis is increased early in alcoholic liver disease, but significant fibrosis seems to depend on other hepatototxic events.

Parenteral hyperalimentation. Fatty liver may be a striking complication of prolonged parenteral hyperalimentation, though the exact mechanism remains unclear. The toxic effect may be attributable to improper formulation of the amino acid solution or to the presence of additives used to stabilize the solution. The fatty changes in the liver are said to occur more frequently when one does not use fat given intravenously (Fig. 24-24). This observation suggests that some forms of TPN-re-

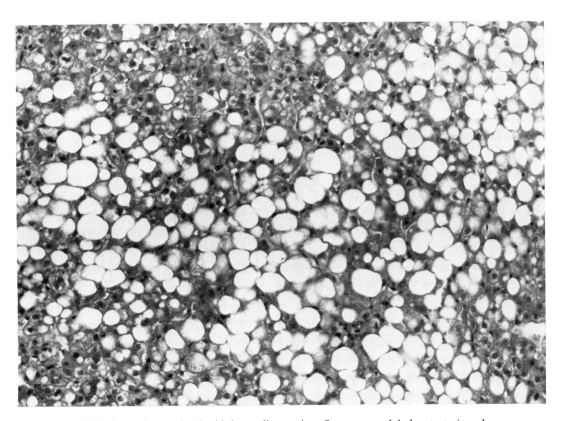

Fig. 24-24. Steatosis associated with hyperalimentation. Serve macroglobular steatosis and pseudogland formation were found on liver biopsy section obtained from a 12-year-old patient (×100). After 4 weeks of total parenteral hyperalimentation, firm hepatomegaly gradually appeared. The serum aminotransferases were modestly elevated but bilirubin remained normal.

lated steatosis are a manifestation of essential fatty acid deficiency. The lesion is usually reversible, but significant portal fibrosis may remain. Cirrhosis is rarely found.

Hereditary hemorrhagic telangiectasis (Rendu-Osler-Weber disease)

This telangiectasia may produce a variety of hepatic lesions, including hepatic fibrosis or changes indistinguishable for postnecrotic cirrhosis. The arteriovenous shunting of blood and resultant nutritional deprivation of hepatic cells trigger fibroblast activity, and collagen formation and deposition follow.

Histiocytosis X

In histiocytosis X proliferation of macrophages in the subgroup called reticuloendotheliosis causes enlargement of the liver, hepatocellular injury, and occasionally cirrhosis in severe cases.

REFERENCES

Applebaum, M.N., and Thaler, M.M.: Reversibility of extensive liver damage in galactosemia, Gastroenterology 69:469-502, 1975.

Aylsworth, A.S., Thomas, G.H., Hood, J.L., and others: A severe infantile sialidosis: clinical, biochemical and microscopic features, J. Pediatr. 96:662-668, 1980.

Beaumont, C., Simon, M., Smith, P.M., and Worwood, M.: Hepatic and serum ferritin concentrations in patients with idiopathic hemochromatosis, Gastroenterology 79:877-883, 1980.

Bloomer, J.R.: The hepatic porphyrias: pathogenesis, manifestations and management, Gastroenterology 71:689-701, 1976.

Burton, B.K., and Nadler, H.L.: Clinical diagnosis of the inborn errors of metabolism in the neonatal period, Pediatrics 61:398-405, 1978.

Chase, H.P., Kumar, V., Caldwell, R.T., and O'Brien, D.: Kwashiorkor in the United States, Pediatrics 66:972-976, 1980.

Herbert R.N., Gotto, A.M., and Frederickson, D.S.: Familial lipoprotein deficiency (abetalipoproteinemia, hypobetalipoproteinemia, and Tangier disease). In Stanbury, J.B., Wyngaarden, J.B., and Frederickson, D.S., editors: The metabolic basis of inherited disease, ed. 4, New York, 1978, The McGraw-Hill Book Co.

Howell, R.R.: The glycogen storage diseases. In Stanbury, J.B., Wyngaarden, J.B., and Fredrickson, D.S., editors: The metabolic basis of inherited disease, ed. 4, New York, 1978, The McGraw-Hill Book Co.

Hoyumpa, A.M., Jr., Greene, H.L., Dunn, G.D., and Schenker, S.: Fatty liver: biochemical and clinical considerations, Am. J. Dig. Dis. 20:1142-1170, 1975.

Huttenlocher, P.R., Solitare, G.B., and Adams, G.: Infantile diffuse cerebral degeneration with hepatic cirrhosis, Arch. Neurol. 33:186-192, 1976.

James, S.P., Stromeyer, F.W., Chang, C., and Barranger, J.A.: Liver abnormalities in patients with Gaucher's disease, Gastroenterology 80:126-133, 1981.

Karayalcin, G., Rosner, F., Kim, K.Y., and others: Sickle cell anemia: clinical manifestations in 100 patients and review of the literature, Am. J. Med. Sci. 269:51-68, 1975.

Larochelle, J., Mortezai, A., Belanger, M., and others: Experience with 37 infants with tyrosinemia, Can. Med. Assoc. J. 97:1051-1055, 1967.

Leblanc, A., Hadchouel, M., Jehan, P., and others: Obstructive jaundice in children with histiocytosis X, Gastroenterology 80:134-139, 1981.

Levy, H.L., and Hammersen, G.: Newborn screening for galactosemia and other galactose metabolic deffects, J. Pediatr. 92:871-877, 1978.

Levy, H.L., Sepe, S.J., Shih, V.E., and others: Sepsis due to Escherichia coli in neonates with galactosemia, N. Engl. J. Med. 297:823-825, 1977.

Lough, J., Fawcett, J., and Wiegensberg, B.: Wolman's disease: an electronmicroscopic, histochemical and biochemical study, Arch. Pathol. 89:103-110, 1970.

Malone, H.J.: The cerebral lipidoses, Pediatr. Clin. North Am. 23:303-326, 1976.

McKusick, V.A.: Heritable disorders of connective tissue, ed. 4, St. Louis, 1972, The C.V. Mosby Co.

Mezey, E.: Ethanol: metabolism and adverse effects, Viewpoints Dig. Dis., vol. 2, no. 2, March 1979.

Monk, A.M., Mitchell, A.J.H., Milligan, D.W.A., and Holton, J.B.: Diagnosis of classical galactosaemia, Arch. Dis. Child. 52:943-946, 1977.

Najjar, S., and Ayash, M.A.: The Mauriac syndrome, Clin. Pediatr. 13:723-725, 1974.

Odièvre, M., Beutil, C., Gautier, M., and Alagille, D.: Hereditary fructose intolerance in childhood, Am. J. Dis. Child. 132:605-608, 1978.

Partin, J.S., Partin, J.C., Schubert, W.K., and McAdams, A.J.: Liver ultrastructure in abetalipoproteinemia: evolution of micronodular cirrhosis, Gastroenterology 67:107-118, 1974.

Roy, C.C., Weber, A.M., Morin, C.L., and others: The role of liver function in cystic fibrosis. In Rosi, E., editor: Monographs in paediatrics, Berne, Switzerland, 1981, S. Karger AG.

Schneider, J.A.: Cystinosis: a review, Metabolism 26:817-839, 1977.

Sheehy, J.W.: Sickle cell hepatopathy, South. Med. J. 70:533-538, 1977.

Spritz, R.A., Doughty, R.A., Spackman T.J., and others: Neonatal presentation of I-cell disease, J. Pediatr. 93:954-958, 1978.

Sterns, R.C., Stevens, D.P., Boat, T.F., and others: Symptomatic hepatic disease in cystic fibrosis: incidence, course and outcome of portal systemic shunting, Gastroenterology 70:645-649, 1976.

Wenger, D.A., Barth, G., and Githens, J.H.: Nine cases of sphingomyelin lipidosis: a new variant in Spanish-American children, Am. J. Dis. Child. 131:955-961, 1977.

Wilroy, R.S., Jr., Crawford, S.E., and Johnson, W.W.: Cystic fibrosis with extensive fat replacement of the liver, J. Pediatr. 68:67-73, 1966.

Zelman, S.: Liver fibrosis in hereditary hemorrhagic telangiectasia, Arch. Pathol. 74:66-72, 1962.

CIRRHOSIS

Cirrhosis is a clinicopathologic condition representing the end stage of chronic liver disease. It may exist in a compensated or decompensated state, whereas the causative process may be active or inactive.

Pediatric caregivers are infrequently called upon to care for a child with cirrhosis; this condition is not among the 10 leading causes of death in the 0 to 14-years-of-age group. Not unexpectedly, it may therefore pose difficulty in diagnosis, management, or both, when it occurs in a child. However, cirrhosis appears as an important health problem in the next older age bracket (15 to 34 years) where it ranks sixth as a cause of death.

This sudden ascendency of significant numbers of end-stage liver disease in the teen-age and young adult population is probably multifactorial in origin. (1) Delayed recognition is an important component. Cirrhosis, even when acquired at an early age, may not be recognized during childhood in either the stable form or when slowly progressive, since cirrhosis is often compatible with normal growth and development for many years. (2) Infectious causes (hepatitis A and B virus) occur with greater frequency in the school-age population, and thereafter some develop cirrhosis as a consequence. This slightly older age group also seems at added risk to develop chronic active liver disease, a forerunner of cirrhosis in many cases. (3) Several genetometabolic conditions are associated with a slowly progressive but significant liver disease as part of their complete expression. Although the clinical onset of liver involvement may occur early in childhood, these conditions are compatible with long-term survival, at least into adolescence and early adulthood when the complications of chronic liver disease again dominate the clinical picture. This especially applies to conditions such as Wilson's disease, alpha-1-antitrypsin deficiency, and cystic fibrosis. (4) Both genetic and nonfamilial causes of intrahepatic and extrahepatic anatomic abnormalities of the biliary system may first become recognized in the older school-age and adolescent child, evidenced as biliary cirrhosis. Also, an increasing number of older children surviving with biliary cirrhosis are the result of the present surgical "success" in over 30% of infants with previously considered "noncorrectable" biliary atresia. Undoubtedly, earlier surgical intervention (at 6 to 8 weeks), effective antibiotic treatment of episodes of ascending cholangitis, and detailed attention to nutritional needs have also contributed to their prolonged survival.

As previously mentioned, the diagnosis of cirrhosis may provide the earliest clue to a familial disorder such as Wilson's disease, alpha-1-antitrypsin deficiency or cystic fibrosis. Although delayed diagnosis and treatment may not substantially benefit these individual patients, identification of the index case obviously has importance in genetic counseling, family planning, or, where applicable, institution of specific therapy for affected siblings who are asymptomatic. Whenever possible, prevention and elimination of causative factors and treatment of the complications of cirrhosis continue to dominate the caregiver's involvement in this expression of end-stage liver disease. Meanwhile, the hope continues that orthotopic liver transplantation may eventually become a satisfactory treatment modality for some if not all of these patients.

Pathogenesis of the lesion

Cirrhosis is defined by the morphologic appearance of the liver, in which regenerating nodules devoid of central veins are surrounded by variable amounts of connective tissue that distorts the normal architectural appearance. The process may be active, with ongoing cell necrosis and portal or intralobular inflammation, or it may be seemingly quiescent. In either situation, the characteristic lesion of cirrhosis is present and easily recognized. Evidence suggesting a specific cause may be recognizable even in advanced hepatic cirrhosis, but usually only two general classifications can be made in pediatric patients: biliary cirrhosis and postnecrotic cirrhosis (Figs. 24-25 and 24-26). In either group, the normal hepatic architecture is sufficiently distorted to disturb hepatic circulation and hepatic cellular function, which in turn is responsible for the many complications associated with cirrhosis of the liver. Increased resistance to blood flow through the organ results in portal hypertension while portal-systemic shunting of blood occurs both within and outside the liver. The resulting vascular deprivation to hepatocytes, especially within the regenerating nodules, precludes their usefulness in sustaining adequate hepatic function.

The development of cirrhosis after liver injury from whatever cause was believed to depend primarily on the severity of the initial insult, the persistence of the offending agent, and the nature of

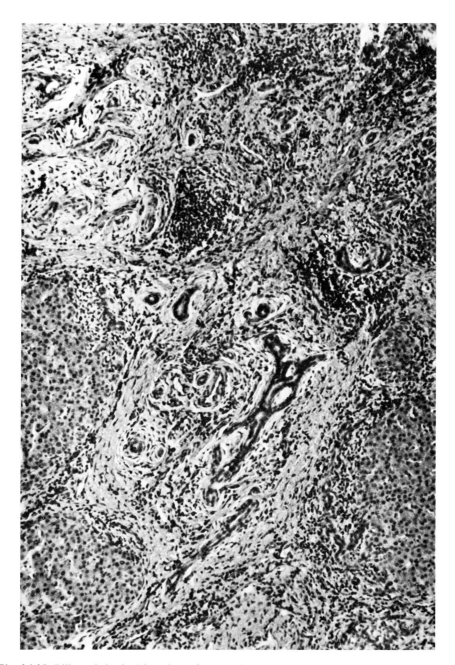

Fig. 24-25. Biliary cirrhosis. Liver tissue from a 16-month-old child dying of cirrhosis caused by extrahepatic biliary atresia. Note the broad bands of fibrous tissue and bile duct proliferation surrounding island of regenerating nodules.

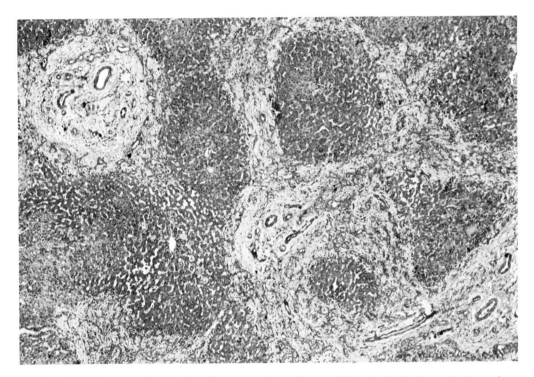

Fig. 24-26. Postnecrotic cirrhosis. Autopsy specimen from a child who died of complications of chronic liver disease. Broad bands of fibrous tissue surround regenerating nodules of hepatocytes without obvious inflammation.

the hepatocellular regeneration. Bands of fibrous septa were believed to represent the effect of compression of preexisting collagen by the regenerating nodules formed in response to hepatic cell necrosis. Present data suggests that hepatocellular injury (with or without inflammation) activates fibroblasts that respond by synthesizing collagen, thus forming fibrous tissue. The neoductular response that follows intrahepatic and extrahepatic injury directed at the biliary system is also believed to provide a template that encourages the deposition of fibrous tissue at this location. The balance between synthesis of collagen fibers and their catabolism and removal appears to determine the degree of hepatic fibrosis and the eventual outcome. Once mature fibrous septa are formed, reversibility is unlikely, and a vicious cycle may ensue. Vascular canalization of these fibrous septa provide anastomoses that deprive hepatocytes of their afferent blood supply. Additional cell necrosis, inflammation, and local hypoxia stimulate additional fibroblastic activity and fibrogenesis. One can see how self-perpetuation of this process leading to cirrhosis may occur long after the initiating offender has been removed (Fig. 24-6).

The distribution of fibrous tissue within the parenchyma apparently depends on the original cause. Drug-induced hepatitis, viral hepatitis, and chronic active hepatitis primarily produce periductular and pericellular fibrosis. On the other hand, abnormalities of biliary drainage result in deposition of fibrous tissue that is predominantly periportal and perilobular. In some instances of massive hepatic injury, septal bridging may be found between central vein and portal zone, whereas central vein–to–central vein bridging may indicate passive venous congestion as a possible cause.

The role given to fibroblast activation in the development of cirrhosis has therapeutic implications that are more critical during the acute injury, when reversal of fibrogenesis is still possible, than later when the collagen matures.

Etiology

The causes capable of producing cirrhosis are legion, and a list is included in the outline on the next page. The major categories of biliary cirrhosis and postnecrotic cirrhosis easily apply in most instances to their respective causes, but at other times the cause and effect are less distinct.

Causes of cirrhosis in children

I. Biliary cirrhosis
   A. Extrahepatic biliary atresia
   B. Paucity of the interlobular bile ducts
   C. Choledochus cysts
   D. Bile duct stenosis
   E. Cystic fibrosis
   F. Ascending cholangitis
      1. Postoperative, portoenterostomy
      2. Cholecystitis, cholelithiasis
      3. Tumors of biliary tree
      4. Strictures
      5. Parasites (*Clonorchis, Fasciola, Ascaris*)
   G. Drugs—phenytoin (Dilantin), chlordiazepoxide (Librium), imipramine (Tofranil), chlorpromazines, thiouracil
   H. Familial intrahepatic cholestasis (Byler's disease, North American Indian cirrhosis)
   I. Ulcerative colitis
   J. Neonatal hepatitis (?cytomegalovirus)
II. Postnecrotic cirrhosis
   A. Hepatitis A virus disease, severe
   B. Hepatitis B virus disease (severe-acute, chronic)
   C. Non-A, non-B virus
   D. Neonatal hepatitis
      1. Rubella (rare)
      2. Toxoplasmosis (rare)
      3. Cytomegalovirus
      4. Syphilis
      5. Enteroviruses
      6. Herpesvirus
      7. Idiopathic (giant-cell type)
   E. Chronic active hepatitis (chronic aggressive hepatitis)
   F. Genetometabolic
      1. Wilson's disease
      2. Alpha-1-antitrypsin–deficiency cirrhosis
      3. Glycogen storage, type 4, ?type 3
      4. Galactosemia
      5. Tyrosinemia
      6. Cystinosis
      7. Rendu-Osler-Weber disease
      8. Porphyria hepatica
      9. Fructose intolerance
      10. Niemann-Pick disease and variants
      11. Gaucher's disease
      12. Hurler's syndrome
      13. Histiocytosis X
      14. Sickle-cell disease
      15. Zellweger's syndrome
      16. Cholesterol ester storage disease
      17. Abetalipoproteinemia
      18. Hemachromatosis
      19. Hepatic cirrhosis with infantile diffuse cerebral degeneration
      20. Wolman's disease
      21. Thalassemia major, hemoglobin-S thalassemia
      22. Severe Rh isoimmunization
   G. Ulcerative colitis
   H. Passive venous congestion, severe, late
      1. Constrictive pericarditis
      2. Ebstein's anomaly
      3. Pulmonary hypertension
      4. Severe anemia
      5. Protein malnutrition
      6. Budd-Chiari syndrome, severe
         a. Congenital abnormality of hepatic veins
         b. Tumor-occlusion of hepatic veins
         c. Idiopathic occlusion of hepatic veins
   I. Hemangioendothelioma
   J. Veno-occlusive disease, Jamaican
   K. Indian childhood cirrhosis
   L. Egyptian childhood cirrhosis
   M. South African childhood cirrhosis
   N. Kwashiorkor
   O. Drugs, toxins, poisons
   P. Radiation therapy

Each causes hepatocellular injury with or without inflammation. Once triggered, the balance achieved between response to injury (fibrogenesis) and repair (regeneration and fiber removal) depends on many known and unknown factors.

When a specific cause of the initial lesion can be identified and removed, the prognosis is generally favorable. The mechanism by which some of these agents produce liver injury is not completely understood. The most common entities and proposed pathogenetic mechanisms are previously discussed in this chapter.

Clinical aspects

Clinical aberrations are primarily the result of disturbed hepatocellular function and increased resistance to intrahepatic blood flow (portal hypertension), and although they may vary somewhat according to the underlying cause, many features of cirrhosis are strikingly consistent for all causes.

The major manifestations applicable to both large categories of cirrhosis (biliary cirrhosis, postnecrotic cirrhosis) are the consequences of portal hypertension, that is, esophageal varices, ascites, and hypersplenism. Although uncommon in children, portal encephalopathy, a consequence of portal-systemic shunting in the presence of portal hypertension, may cause distressing symptoms. Minor manifestations common to both groups include anemia, hemodynamic adjustments, digital clubbing, steatorrhea, fatigue, and anorexia.

Biliary cirrhosis. In most children with biliary cirrhosis, the disease is caused by an obstruction of bile flow; therefore jaundice is almost always detected early in the course of the illness. In subtle cases, cholestasis from chronic liver disease may be suspected when recalcitrant pruritus is reported, or skin lesions (xanthoma) are noted. For those lesions not correctable by surgery, progressive hepatic damage ensues, eventually culminating in biliary cirrhosis. This group of conditions is represented by patients with extrahepatic biliary atresia, congenital or acquired strictures of the biliary system, and choledochal cysts. Medical conditions that can progress to biliary cirrhosis include familial cholestatic syndromes (Byler's disease), the entity of paucity of the interlobular bile ducts, and cystic fibrosis. In the last two conditions, clinical jaundice may be absent in the face of underlying cirrhosis. A more complete list of conditions that may result in biliary cirrhosis appears on p. 738.

Besides pruritus and xanthomas, other clinical features of progressive biliary cirrhosis are usually secondary to the gastrointestinal manifestations and nutritional consequences. Relative degrees of fat malabsorption affect normal weight gain and growth of the infant, resulting in mild to moderate failure to thrive. This is especially noticeable after 6 to 12 months of progressive disease. Signs and symptoms that reflect a specific fat soluble vitamin–deficiency state of A, D, K, and E may be present. In fact, hemorrhagic manifestations from vitamin K deficiency sometimes

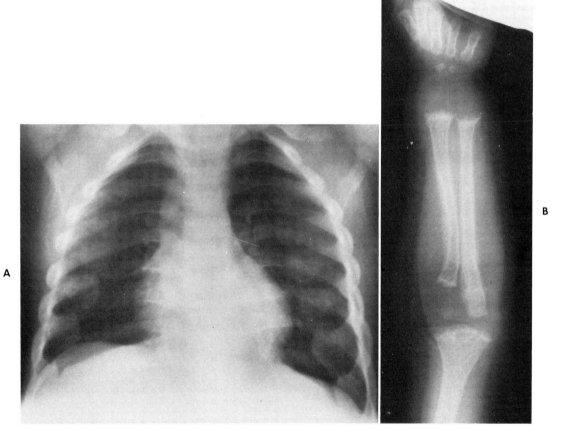

Fig. 24-27. Rickets. Despite minimal icterus, this 18-month-old child with persistent cholestatic syndrome since the neonatal period developed a rachitic rosary and widening of the epiphyses at the wrists and ankles. **A,** Roentgenogram of the chest, showing "clubbing" of the rib ends. **B,** Bone film of the patient's arm, showing loss of density (osteomalacia), cupping, and fraying of the distal ends of both radius and ulna. Large doses (5000 to 10,000 IU) of vitamin D were required to correct this abnormality.

dominate the clinical picture. So-called hepatic, or biliary, rickets seldom causes difficulty, but widening of the epiphyses or a rachitic rosary may produce striking clinical signs in some patients (Fig. 24-27).

Dark urine and pale to acholic-appearing stools are found in most. Steatorrhea is suggested by the excessively foul odor to the stool. Recurrent fevers and abdominal pain with relapsing jaundice may be reported, especially when biliary infections complicate the obstructive process.

Progressive biliary cirrhosis eventually leads to the complicating events of ascites and bleeding from esophageal varices. Susceptibility to respiratory infections, especially bronchitis and pneumonia, increases at this stage of the disease and is frequently the cause of death. Death from hemorrhage of esophageal varices or hepatic decompensation is less common than from metabolic derangements accompanying terminal infection.

Postnecrotic cirrhosis. Contrary to the adult experience, a definite history of previous hepatic insult or the presence of ongoing disease (active cirrhosis) is frequently present in children with *postnecrotic cirrhosis*. Indeed, a specific diagnosis can usually be made by application of proper investigative techniques. Excluding biliary cirrhosis caused by congenital obstructive defects or by cystic fibrosis, cirrhosis in children is most likely the result of neonatal hepatitis, chronic active hepatitis, genetometabolic entities, such as Wilson's disease, alpha-1-antitrypsin deficiency, and hereditary tyrosinemia. In cases of chronic active hepatitis, intermittent episodes of jaundice, lethargy, joint swellings, and so forth may punctuate the progression to cirrhosis. Wilson's disease may have a definite transient episode of identifiable liver involvement and then insidiously progress to postnecrotic cirrhosis. A comparable number of pediatric patients with Wilson's disease never have a documented episode of jaundice (Fig. 24-28). The presence of cirrhosis may first be suspected clinically by the finding of splenomegaly. When Wilson's disease is diagnosed by other findings (Kayser-Fleischer rings, neurologic symptoms), cirrhosis is invariably present and will be recognized by proper investigations. Survival of the child with fulminating hepatitis is so rare that postnecrotic cirrhosis attributable to this entity is an infrequent cause in our experience (Chapter 23). Idiopathic or so-called cryptogenic cirrhosis, for which no cause can be detected, is still responsible for a

sizable number of pediatric cases of cirrhosis, especially in underdeveloped countries of the world. Insidious progression to cirrhosis may also occur with some to these same conditions, such as Wilson's disease, alpha-1-antitrypsin–deficiency cirrhosis, and certain in utero infections (cytomegalovirus disease, HBV disease) before significant clinical manifestations of end-stage liver disease are apparent.

The nutritional impact on children with insidious postnecrotic cirrhosis is not severe, and failure to thrive is not likely to be noted. Susceptibility to pulmonary infections is likewise less common in postnecrotic cirrhosis than in biliary cirrhosis. Signs and symptoms of bacterial peritonitis may develop in the presence of ascites. It is especially common in infants and children with end-stage liver disease secondary to biliary atresia. Generally speaking, the physical findings rather than the vague symptoms often lead to proper diagnosis. Such complaints as recurrent abdominal pain, intermittent anorexia, easy fatigability, and tiredness may not be immediately recognized as caused by chronic liver disease unless they are accompanied by failure to thrive or a history of jaundice.

Physical findings

The major physical findings indicative of chronic liver disease are present in the skin, cardiovascular system, and abdomen.

Icterus, cutaneous or scleral, is present in almost all cases of biliary cirrhosis, except for those patients with paucity of the intrahepatic bile ducts, congenital stricture of the common hepatic bile duct, and cystic fibrosis. Jaundice is usually a terminal event in biliary cirrhosis caused by cystic fibrosis, and it may be absent or of very low grade in the intrahepatic bile duct hypoplasia group. On the other hand, jaundice is often fluctuating or absent in postnecrotic cirrhosis. Pruritus, excoriations, and xanthomas are often present in biliary but not in postnecrotic cirrhosis. The significance of spider angiomas (''arterioectasias'') in children is difficult to evaluate because lesions on the face, hands, and arms occasionally occur, especially in girls. However, angiomas on the chest and back are always significant. Telangiectasias (venectasias) may be prominent in the same locations. Palmar erythema (liver palms) is also difficult to evaluate because of peripheral vasomotor instability in many children. ''Speckled palms'' seems to

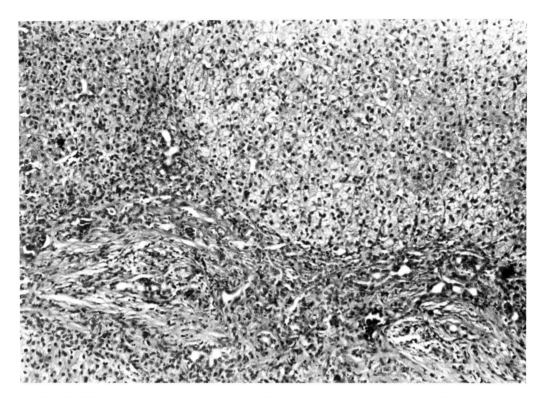

Fig. 24-28. Postnecrotic cirrhosis caused by Wilson's disease. Autopsy specimen from a small, coarsely nodular liver. The microscopic features shown demonstrate severe postnecrotic cirrhosis with regenerating nodules and broad bands of connective tissue. The 13-year-old girl was believed to be in excellent health until 1 month before admission, when she became jaundiced. Abnormal liver function tests and hemolytic anemia were found. Rapid deterioration occurred, and the girl became comatose; two exchange transfusions did not improve her clinical condition. On the basis of an unknown hemolytic state and liver disease, the diagnosis of Wilson's disease was entertained and confirmed biochemically. The patient subsequently died, and hepatic copper was found elevated (203 mg/gm of wet weight tissue). An asymptomatic 14-year-old brother was detected on screening of the family.

be a better description of this physical finding in chronic liver disease, though diffuse erythema may also be seen. That the skin is often warm and the patient may look flushed (malar erythema) though fever is absent probably reflects decreased peripheral vascular resistance frequently accompanying chronic liver disease. The exposed areas of skin may show increased pigmentation from melanin deposits.

Digital clubbing is present in 10% to 25% of children with biliary cirrhosis (Fig. 24-29). Variable degrees of cyanosis may be noted in the nail beds, especially if clubbing is present. Other cutaneous findings of significance may also be noted. Signs of hypersplenism may be manifested by petechiae and ecchymoses caused by thrombocytopenia, whereas some degree of pallor is seen as the result of the anemia of cirrhosis.

The cardiovascular system undergoes certain adjustments in chronic liver disease, with augmented cardiac output a usual consequence. The pulse is full and bounding, and not infrequently a high-output murmur can be heard. Murmurs indicating pulmonary artery stenosis or peripheral pulmonic stenosis can be frequently heard especially in the syndromic form of paucity of the intrahepatic bile ducts. Bruits, believed to originate from bronchopulmonary shunts, can be heard over the chest and may radiate into the neck and head. Increased circulating estrogens may lead to feminization in males, resulting in gynecomastia or deeply pigmented nipples.

The abdominal findings are variable and depend on the underlying disease. Distention of the

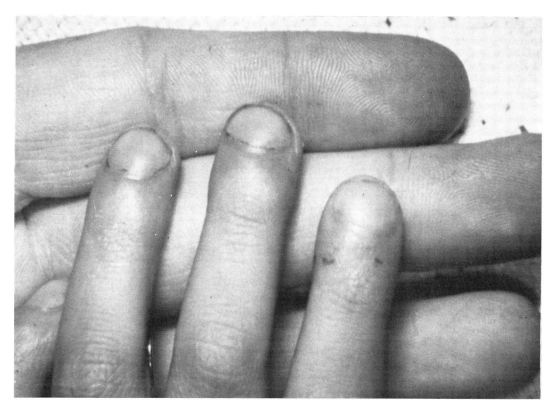

Fig. 24-29. Digital clubbing in a 3-year-old girl with postnecrotic cirrhosis. Moderate arterial desaturation also was present and her nail beds are cyanotic as well.

abdominal wall is usually caused by hepatosplenomegaly, especially in biliary cirrhosis. Ascites occurs earlier in the course of biliary cirrhosis than in that of postnecrotic cirrhosis and is always a grim prognostic finding. The liver may actually be small, and percussion dullness over the right anterolateral side of the chest may be absent or found in only a small area. The inferior edge of the liver may not be palpable in such cases. If the liver is enlarged, it may feel firm to hard and the inferior edge reveals an irregular contour. Even small (0.5 to 1 cm) regenerating macronodules can be palpated in some cases. At times the left lobe of the liver undergoes a striking compensatory hypertrophy while the right lobe is discrepantly small. Palpation of the spleen in children requires a light touch, with finger ballottement during inspiration being the best technique. Fluid, if present, is best detected by demonstration of shifting dullness rather than a fluid wave. The late appearance of an umbilical hernia usually indicates the presence of ascites. Prominence of the superficial abdominal veins may be noted in advanced cases of cirrhosis when

portal hypertension is severe. Reversal of flow in the veins below the umbilicus may be demonstrated.

Hemorrhoids, rare in children, can be the result of portal hypertension but more often have other causes (such as Crohn's disease).

Laboratory findings

Results of isolated laboratory tests may not be helpful, whereas results of a group of liver function tests may indicate chronic liver disease. The most useful tests are sulfobromophthalein retention (normal if less than 5% within 45 minutes) and serum protein electrophoresis. The presence of a low albumin level with normal or increased gamma globulins is the frequent pattern in cirrhosis. One should keep in mind the reciprocal relation that exists between the plasma albumin level and the hepatic sulfobromophthalein removal so as to not misinterpret low retention values of the dye. If elevated, the serum bilirubin shows variable degrees of elevation and is of the "mixed" type. Depending on the degree of ongoing liver disease, transaminases and lactic dehydrogenase activity can also be increased. Alkaline phosphatase, gamma glutamyl transpeptidase (GGT), and cholesterol are often greatly increased in most cases of biliary cirrhosis.

Prolongation of the prothrombin time, which is corrected by intramuscular administration of vitamin K in a child with chronic liver disease, points to a biliary type of cirrhosis. Elevation of the serum bile acids is commonly found in biliary tract disease even if pruritus is absent; the relationship between serum bile acids and pruritus is poor. The red blood smear shows an increased number of acanthocytes and fragmented forms that may be stiff and less pliable than normal cells. Modest anemia, leukopenia, and thrombocytopenia are common when splenomegaly is present. Measurement of serum pH and blood gases often shows a respiratory alkalosis in chronic liver disease. Hyperaldosteronism with further depletion of potassium can accentuate the alkalosis.

Ceruloplasmin and urine copper excretion of all pediatric patients with unexplained cirrhosis should routinely by measured. In addition, hepatitis B virus surface antigen (HBsAg) should be sought, alpha-1-antitrypsin level quantitated, sweat chlorides checked, and urine screened for reducing substances and amino and organic acids. Other diagnostic laboratory testing will be better dictated by the clinical story and physical findings.

Roentgenographic studies are helpful in detecting esophageal varices or, at times, may suggest the presence of abdominal fluid. Evaluation of liver size from roentgenographic studies is at best unrealiable. Abdominal ultrasound examination is extremely sensitive in detecting small amounts of free abdominal fluid. When biliary obstructive disease is suspected, ultrasonography of the extrahepatic biliary system may be most instructive in allowing prediction of the underlying cause and in suggesting the subsequent investigative approach. Transhepatic cholangiography can be successfully employed in children if the intrahepatic bile ducts are dilated. Evaluation of the hepatobiliary system with radiopharmaceuticals (^{99m}Tc-DIDA or ^{99m}Tc-PIPIDA) is gaining in popularity as a technique useful in the evaluation of diseases of the medium and large bile ducts. Retrograde cholangiography by endoscopy is seldom employed in the pediatric-age group. Sulfur-colloid scintiscan is infrequently needed for the diagnosis of chronic liver disease. Likewise, special angiographic studies through the splenic or superior mesenteric artery or by splenoportography are more useful in assessment of hemodynamic aspects of hepatic arterial and portal blood flow than about the disease within the liver.

Diagnosis

From the foregoing, it would appear that the diagnosis of cirrhosis may be easily made in some circumstances and may be extremely difficult in others. Acute awareness is required if diagnosis is to be established early in the insidious forms of cirrhosis. Sometimes early and accurate diagnosis may prolong life when the inciting cause can be removed or altered by specific medical therapy, such as that with Wilson's disease, galactosemia, fructose intolerance, tyrosinemia, and cystinosis.

Ultimate confirmation of cirrhosis requires histologic examination of the liver. Tissue obtained by open biopsy or under direct vision during laparoscopy is more likely to obviate the high degree of sampling error (50%) that accompanies the "blind" percutaneous biopsy in patients with cirrhosis (Fig. 24-30). Exploratory "minilaparotomy" is indicated in almost all cases of biliary cirrhosis when the underlying cause has not been previously determined. In advanced liver disease the initial lesion, which might have been specific and identifiable, is replaced by the nonspecific findings of fibrosis, regenerating lobules, and distorted hepatic architecture, with or without bile duct proliferation. When esophageal varices are suspected, direct visualization of these lesions should be sought by use of a pediatric fiberoptic endoscope. The presence of esophageal varices can be taken to imply significant portal hypertension and is of utmost importance in the long-term management of patients with cirrhosis. When portal hypertension dominates the signs and symptoms of a patient without other features of cirrhosis, considerations in diagnosis must include those causes of portal hypertension that may exist in the absence of cirrhosis (congenital hepatic fibrosis, prehepatic portal hypertension). The organized approach to this diagnostic dilemma is discussed in detail in Chapter 25.

Complications and management

Except for those causes of cirrhosis amendable by specific therapy, treatment is usually directed toward the complications of chronic liver disease. The major complications seen in children with

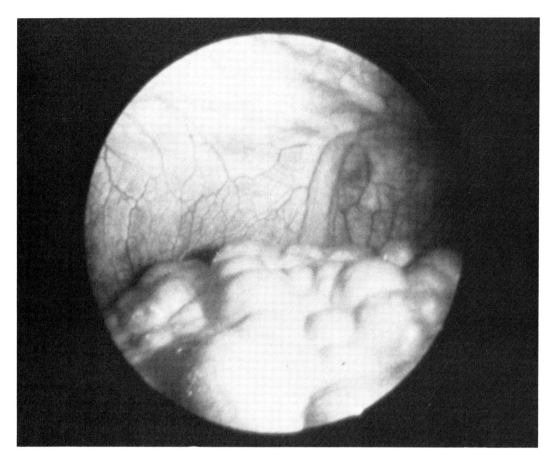

Fig. 24-30. Macronodular cirrhosis as seen through the laparoscope. "Blind" percutaneous needle biopsy of such a liver often obtains inadequate amount of tissue or samples a histologically nonrepresentative segment of liver (large regenerating nodules with few if any portal zones).

chronic liver disease have the same pathogenic mechanisms as in adults and basically require the same therapeutic approaches. A greater interest in the nutritional needs of these children is vital if the quality of the longevity is to be improved.

Malabsorption in chronic liver disease. About 50% of the adults and most of the children with cirrhosis exhibit steatorrhea. A relative degree of exocrine pancreatic insufficiency and pancreatic morphologic changes has been described in adult cirrhotic patients, but in our experience with children, pancreatic function and structure are normal; there is no evidence of intestinal mucosal disease, and the D-xylose absorption is normal.

In general, there is poor correlation between the degree of biliary obstruction and the amount of fat excreted in the stools. It is likely that even if biliary obstruction is absent, intestinal bile salts are well below the so-called critical micellar concentration, so that intraluminal products of lipolysis cannot form micellar solutions. Hypoprothrombinemia is almost always present and responds to vitamin K until other signs of hepatic decompensation set in. With progression of the cirrhotic process, anorexia, failure to thrive, ascites, and hypoprothrombinemia not responding to parenterally given vitamin K are the rule; concomitantly, there is a significant increase in steatorrhea. When biliary cirrhosis has been accompanied by longstanding cholestatis, chronic vitamin E deficiency may result in neurologic abnormalities including areflexia, selective ophthalmoplegia, and disturbances in balance and gait. Hypocalcemia with striking roentgenographic features of rickets, osteomalacia, and bone deformities may develop in younger children.

Management. A nutritionist sympathetic to the dietary idiosyncrasies of children should be called upon to construct a diet that remains palatable and yet of adequate caloric value. This is not a simple matter when one considers the restraints imposed by end-stage liver disease, especially in regard to the marginal tolerance of such patients when ingesting long-chain dietary fats and excessive protein and sodium. The prevailing degree of anorexia and lassitude may in the final analysis dictate the qualitative and quantitative alterations that are possible in the child's diet.

Use of a low-fat diet supplemented with medium-chain triglycerides (Pregestimil or Portagen) decreases the degree of steatorrhea and improves the nutritional status of the patient. However, once the decompensated stage has been reached, the dietary changes just described have no effect whatever on the failure to thrive even though the steatorrhea is decreased. The experience accumulated with extrahepatic biliary atresia is that failure to thrive and a rapid downhill course are invariable once there are signs of hepatic decompensation. In cases of paucity of the interlobular bile ducts, the use of cholestyramine (Questran, Cuemid), 4 to 16 gm/24 hr, in conjunction with a low-fat diet supplemented with medium-chain fatty acids can dramatically improve not only pruritus and nutrition but also liver function. This therapeutic approach is also recommended in cases of postnecrotic cirrhosis because signs of decompensated liver disease may respond in a dramatic fashion (weight gain, disappearance of ascites, normal prothrombin time).

Because of the malabsorption of the fat-soluble vitamins, a double daily dose of a water-dispersible preparation of vitamins A, D, and E is suggested. A daily oral 5 mg tablet of vitamin K can at times correct the hypoprothrombinemia associated with fat malabsorption. In other cases, a weekly injection of vitamin K is necessary. In cases with neurologic manifestations, large doses (50 to 100 mg/kg/day) of vitamin E can be tried.

Large doses of vitamin D supplements (5000 to 20,000 IU) may at times be needed to correct osteomalacia (rickets), especially in prolonged cases of cholestatic jaundice. Oral supplementation with 1,25-dihydroxy-vitamin D_3 (0.2 μg/kg/day) is also recommended.

Ascites in chronic liver disease

Mechanisms. The development of ascites is a late complication of liver disease and signifies a poor prognosis. It seems to occur earlier in the course of biliary cirrhosis than in postnecrotic cir-

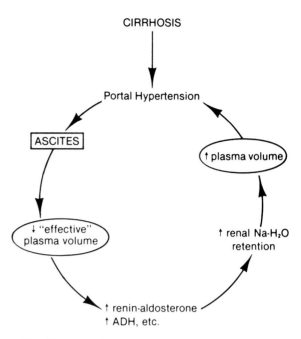

Fig. 24-31. Traditional theory of ascites formation in hepatic cirrhosis. (From Witte, C.L., Witte, M.L., and Dumont, A.E.: Gastroenterology **78:**1059-1068, 1970, by permission.)

rhosis. In the most simplistic of terms, fluid accumulates in the peritoneal cavity of cirrhotic patients because of alterations in the physiologic equilibrium between hydrostatic and osmotic forces (Starling's law). Although one finds an increase in hydrostatic pressure (portal hypertension) and a decrease in osmotic forces (hypoalbuminemia) in patients with chronic liver disease and cirrhosis, not all such patients have ascites. The problem appears to be more complex, with other factors involved in its development.

Although many mechanisms have been implicated in the production of liver ascites, a unifying principle has not been found. Up to now, three basic theories have been popularized (Figs. 24-31 to 24-33). The first or so-called *classic theory* relegates the changes associated with chronic liver disease that distort the hepatic architecture and produce an increased resistance to blood flow within the organ as the primary driving force in the development of ascites. The resulting maldistribution of extravascular and intravascular fluid leads to a decrease in the ''effective'' plasma volume, which in turn triggers the renin-aldosterone pathway and the release of antidiuretic hormone (ADH). These latter events cuse increased renal

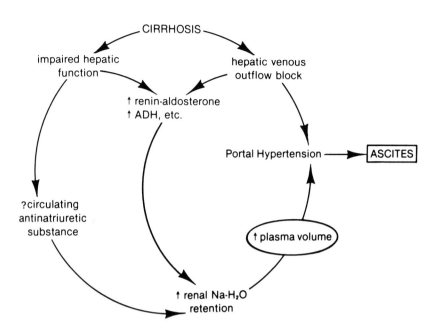

Fig. 24-32. Schematic diagram of the overflow theory of ascites formation in hepatic cirrhosis. (From Witte, C.L., Witte, M.L., and Dumont, A.E.: Gastroenterology **78:**1059-1068, 1970, by permission.)

sodium and water retention, with expansion of plasma volume. Unfortunately, this further contributes to the portal hypertension and more ascitic fluid is produced, so that there is a perpetuating of the process initiated by the evolving cirrhosis.

The second or *"overflow" theory* suggests that ascites develops after renal responses to hepatic damage produce an increase in plasma volume, and fluid (ascites) "overflows" then from the congested portal system. This theory implicates a circulating humoral substance with antinatriuretic activity that is either elaborated or not adequately detoxified by damaged liver, but supposedly independent from aldosterone and ADH. The third proposal is the so-called *lymph imbalance theory,* which suggests that ascites forms after all reserve mechanisms, including augmented lymph flow, have been encroached upon, when finally lymph reabsorption fails to keep up with lymph formation. Only when this balance fails does the abnormal distribution of fluid between the extravascular and vascular space lead to ascites. Again, this in turn triggers the homeostatic renal-endocrine responses previously mentioned. Thereafter, a self-perpetuating process of lymph formation evolves with continued accumulation of large amounts of ascites. The reduced intracapillary oncotic pres-

sure from hypoalbuminemia is counteracted by mechanisms that increase both the transsinusoid hepatic and splanchnic transcapillary oncotic gradients.

The accumulation of the protein-rich transudate (from hepatic lymph and capillaries) in the abdominal cavity itself exerts an osmotic pull in the direction of the peritoneal cavity. The accumulation of ascites in this location ("fourth space") is also favored by several factors that evolve in portal hypertension including increased splanchnic capillary pressure and increased splanchnic blood flow. The role of the low serum albumin level is still debated. This disease-developed "fourth space" has some unique peculiarities. Studies have shown that egress of accumulated ascitic fluid occurs at a slower rate than ingress into the peritoneal cavity. This phenomenon is responsible for failures noted in the medical treatment of ascites. Whether this discrepancy of water and electrolyte transfer (and perhaps proteins) across the peritoneal membrane develops as a consequence of liver disease or is a normal phenomenon in this distinct compartment of the extracellular space is not completely clear.

Inability of cirrhotic patients to excrete a water load has been attributed to an excess of circulating antidiuretic hormone, which adds further to

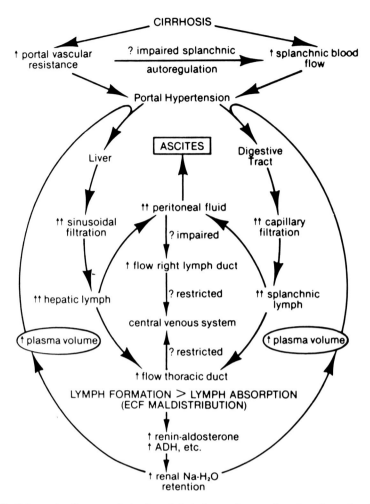

Fig. 24-33. Schematic diagram of the lymph-imbalance theory of ascites formation in hepatic cirrhosis. (From Witte, C.L., Witte, M.L., and Dumont, A.E.: Gastroenterology **78**:1059-1068, 1970, by permission.)

the problem. There is some evidence to suggest that another natriuretic hormone (the "third" factor) may be responsible for the disproportionate fractional reabsorption of sodium and water in the proximal tubules that occurs even when effective renal plasma flow has been achieved.

Medical treatment. In the face of cirrhosis most children develop ascites at a slow, insidious rate, paralleled by hemodynamic adjustments. Rapid development of ascites occasionally follows gastrointestinal hemorrhage with further hepatic decompensation, infections, dietary indiscretions, or fulminating hepatic necrosis. However, changes that have developed slowly are usually well compensated for by the patient, and the approach to alter this new equilibrium should be gentle. Because treatment of ascites does not substantially

affect the underlying liver disease or necessarily prolong survival, instituting medical measures should be dictated by the degree of discomfort produced by the fluid that limits the patient's enjoyment of life while also one keeps in mind the fact that other complications may develop in its presence.

Not infrequently, the treatment may make management of the patient's condition more difficult because complications of therapy are frequent. The positive response to therapy (diuresis) may have prognostic value, often signifying at least 1 more year of life. It is substantially better than if no response is achieved.

DIET. Strict observance of dietary sodium restriction is the key to an effective diuretic program in children as well as adults. For food to be palatable, some sodium must be present or the child will simply not eat the food. Between 1 and 2 mEq/kg/day (10 and 20 mEq/m^2) should be an adequate amount to effect diuresis but hardly makes the food edible. The laboratory determination of urinary sodium losses is frequently needed to ascertain the effectiveness of the dietary sodium restrictions and diuretic program in producing the negative balance of sodium. One can assume that a negative balance of 130 to 140 mEq of sodium will result in a loss of approximately 1 liter of water. Protein intake may need to be limited if impending coma exists, but adequate calories, proteins, carbohydrates, and vitamins are essential. Unfortunately, only about 10% to 20% of these patients experience diuresis with salt restriction alone.

DIURETICS. The availability of new and potent agents has improved the effectiveness of diuresis in a greater number of patients. Although complications have been reported with all forms of diuretics, attention to certain basic principles should keep them to a minimum. The patient's physical signs should be carefully observed, particularly for determination of whether peripheral edema is present. Caution in diuresis should be employed when ascites is present without obvious peripheral edema. Based on studies of ingress and egress of ascitic fluid after diuresis in the absence of edema, one can expect further reduction of "effective" plasma volume because mobilization of ascites into the vascular space is limited (800 to 900 ml/24 hr in adults). The reduced renal plasma flow that follows may further stimulate release of sodium-retaining hormone. Therefore, the recommendation has been made to limit diuresis in such patients to achieve a weight loss of 200 to 300 gm/24 hr. When peripheral edema is present, circulatory adjustments occur more readily, and loss of 500 to 1000 gm/24 hr can be well tolerated. Excessive fluid loss can cause shock, and the resultant hypoxia and acidosis further aggravate the liver condition.

Attention must be paid to potassium losses in the urine during diuresis. Hypokalemia is frequent with the chlorothiazides, but it also occurs with furosemide and ethacrynic acid. Hypokalemic alkalosis may favor the conversion of ammonium to highly permeable ammonia and precipitate hepatic coma. Hyponatremia is the most common electrolyte abnormality that develops during diuretic therapy. It carries a poor prognosis if seen with hypokalemia, hypochloremia, and elevated serum bicarbonate level. It is frequently seen in the terminal state of chronic liver disease, especially when the newer diuretics are employed.

Other complications of diuretic therapy are less common and include azotemia and hypochloremic alkalosis. They are more likely with the use of furosemide and ethacrynic acid. Lysine monochloride, 50 to 100 mEq/24 hr, may be used to combat hypochloremic alkalosis. Ammonium chloride or acetazolamide are contraindicated. Specific signs of drug toxicity such as abdominal pain, nausea, rashes, and leukopenia need to be watched for. Acute pancreatitis may be a complication of the thiazides.

The use of combination diuretic therapy acting on different sites of the nephron has physiologic merit in cases of cirrhotic ascites, though this has been contested in at least one adult study. The reduced filtered load of sodium common to these patients can be improved on by the use of a drug that can act on the proximal nephron. Concurrently, a drug whose site of action is the more distal nephron can influence the sequential nature of sodium reabsorption. Our most effective combination has been furosemide (Lasix), 100 mg/1.73m^2 given daily orally in two divided doses, and spironolactone (Aldactone), 200 to 400 mg/1.73m^2 in four divided doses. This combination of drug therapy is generally reserved for refractory cases associated with end-stage liver disease. The infusion of salt-poor albumin (1 gm/kg) for 30 to 60 minutes before and during the intravenous administration of furosemide has been a useful adjunct in otherwise refractory cases of ascites. The initial regimen employs the daily administration of aldactone (200 mg/1.73m^2). This drug generally requires 3 to 4 days of administration before any therapeutic effect can be noted, as reflected by the increased urine sodium content and accompanying weight loss. Lack of response is a signal to double the dose of aldactone (400 mg/1.73 m^2). Should this fail, hydrochlorothiazide (130 mg/1.73 m^2/day) can be added. Potassium supplements are mandatory, except in cases where aldactone alone is used. Potassium chloride (3 to 5 mEq/kg) is the only acceptable potassium salt.

As mentioned above, the intravenous administration of furosemide (1 to 3 mg/kg) can be used at times when the oral route is contraindicated or when respiratory distress creates a life-threatening situation calling for immediate diuresis. Close monitoring of serum and urine electrolytes, input and output balance sheet, and vital signs is mandatory.

Dosages of diuretics need to be tailored so that the smallest effective dose is eventually employed, with the physician resisting the temptation of completely clearing up the ascites, particularly in the final stages of decompensated cirrhosis. One should remember that surprisingly large doses of diuretics may be required in some patients. The expanded extravascular space provides a much larger volume of distribution for the diuretic agent, and pharmokinetic studies may be required to define precisely the correct drug dosage and frequency of administration in confusing or refractory cases. In rare patients hyperglycemia and hyperuricemia may develop while furosemide is being used.

BED REST. Although the recumbent position is said to increase renal blood flow and promote a diuretic effect in normal individuals, it has never been proved effective in managing the ascitic patient. The difficulty of keeping a very young patient in this position is often monumental, even when good reasons exist for enforcing this posture.

FLUID RESTRICTION. Rather than setting firm figures for fluid intake, one is best guided by the clinical and laboratory responses to the overall program. If hyponatremia and inappropriate fluid retention fail to develop while ad libitum access to fluids is allowed, there is obviously no need for water restriction. If evidence for inappropriate retention exists (increasing weight, falling serum sodium), limiting the fluid intake to 1000 ml/m^2 is suggested. One must be careful to avoid further compromise of renal function by water restriction.

Surgical treatment. The surgical technique most frequently used for removal of ascitic fluid has been paracentesis. We rarely use this procedure unless abdominal pain and respiratory distress is present or the patient has reached end-stage liver disease accompanied by drug-resistant ascites. Not uncommonly, an oliguric reaction is noted after this procedure, especially in patients with tense ascites but without peripheral edema. The mechanism, again, is probably similar to that discussed previously whereby the rapid reaccumulation of ascites without compensatory adjustments to the contracted plasma volume occurs and renal perfusion is reduced. If peripheral edema is present, paracentesis is accompanied by increased venous return and cardiac output. To avoid sudden hemodynamic consequences, paracentesis should remove only sufficient fluid to improve the patient's comfort, and the volume removed should be limited to less than 1 to 2 L/24 hr, depending on the child's size. Bleeding and infection are definite risks attending this procedure.

The combined use of venous reinfusion of ascitic fluid obtained by paracentesis and diuretic drugs has been a successful form of treatment in refractory cases. Caution about rapid overexpansion of the vascular space in cirrhotic patients is required, since it may increase hepatic sinusoid pressure as well as precipitate variceal hemorrhage. Before reinfusion, ultrafiltration of the ascitic fluid allows removal and concentration of the protein content and thereby reduces the risk to rapid hyperexpansion of the vascular space. The protein must be returned, lest its rapid depletion quickly limit the usefulness of this modality of treatment. Following this therapeutic regimen there may be a surprising amelioration of ascites, which may be sustained for weeks to months.

A similar beneficial effect can be obtained, but without need for supplemental diuretic drugs, by surgical introduction of a peritoneojugular venous shunt (LeVeen). The low-pressure, one-way, sensitive valuve is connected with silicone rubber tubing to the jugular vein and serves as a "megalymphatic" between the abdominal cavity and the bloodstream. The normal diaphragmatic excursion in respiration is sufficient to activate the valve and propel fluid cephalad, but breathing exercises should be employed for maximal benefit of shunt function. The device has had limited application in the pediatric-age group, but there is an extensive experience in the adult population. Adults crippled by intractable ascites have responded with mobilization of ascites, a simultaneous increase in renal blood flow, and dramatic renal excretion of salt and water. Complications, unfortunately, are common with the use of the LeVeen shunt and have recently tempered the initial enthusiasm. These include consumption coagulopathy, fever, shunt occlusion and embolism, hypokalemia, and infection. Its value in reversing the hepatorenal syndrome, a seldom observed consequence of prolonged intractable ascites in children, remains to be proved.

Finally, portal-systemic shunting to treat intractable ascites has been employed reluctantly because it represents a large undertaking in a chronically ill patient and carries a high operative mortality (40%). The shunt of choice for ascites is said to be a side-to-side portacaval anastomosis. In this anastomosis, retrograde flow via the portal vein is possible and therefore accomplishes decompression of both the postsinusoid and presinusoid portal hypertension.

Complications. The presence of a sizable accumulation ascites itself predisposes the patient to certain complications, the major ones being abdominal distention and upward displacement of the diaphragm, causing respiratory distress. Basilar atelectasis is common and may invite pneumonitis, hypoventilation, and hypoxemia as well. Pleural effusions may further contribute to the respiratory embarrassment. Pulmonary arteriovenous shunting and hypoxia develop, which may also be injurious to the compromised liver. Umbilical and inguinal hernias are frequently noted in children with tense ascites but seldom cause difficulty from incarceration. Decreased mobility, anorexia and lassitude are commonly noted.

The increased abdominal pressure created by ascites can impair the function of the cardioesophageal junction and permit gastroesophageal reflux. The potential exists for erosion of esophageal varices and resultant hemorrhage. The risk of variceal bleeding is therefore strikingly increased in the presence of tense ascites.

Bacterial contamination of the ascitic fluid, particularly with pneumococcus and *Escherichia coli,* may produce peritonitis. Sudden onset of fever, leukocytosis, chills, and peritoneal signs herald this complication of ascites, and organisms are frequently recovered from the peritoneal fluid and blood. One must be alert to signs of bacterial contamination because medical management with antibiotics is curative, whereas operative intervention can be catastrophic.

Many believe that renal failure occurring terminally in most patients with cirrhosis may reflect a complication of diuretic therapy rather than the effects of ascites and chronic liver disease. However, the presence of ascites can increase intraabdominal pressure and cause a decrease in renal blood flow, perpetuating the sequence of events that leads to aldosterone secretion. Furthermore, azotemia and the appearance of the "hepatorenal syndrome" are rarely seen in the absence of ascites. Terminally, about 50% of the patients with cirrhosis have progressive oliguria, anuria, and azotemia. Undoubtedly, a number of these patients will have terminal renal failure as a result of iatrogenic causes, most notably the vigorous and misdirected use of diuretic drugs.

Prognosis. Development of ascites is a grave finding and carries a poor prognosis. Few patients, if any, survive beyond 1 year if diuresis cannot be achieved and sustained. Keep in mind that the treatment of ascites by any method does not alter the underlying hepatic disease, and surgical treatment can immediately worsen the process in unfortunate patients. Death is likely from hepatic failure with coma or from gastrointestinal hemorrhage and not from the ascites itself. The patients with transient ascites do better than those whose fluid is controlled but chronically present. The prognosis is also said to be grave if such complications of diuretic therapy as hyponatremia, hypochloremic alkalosis, and azotemia develop.

Esophageal varices and gastrointestinal bleeding. These complications of chronic liver disease are discussed in Chapter 25.

Hepatic encephalopathy. The appearance of neuropsychiatric signs and symptoms may be the result of intrahepatic or extrahepatic events that further stress the marginally compromised host. A sudden additional deterioration in the liver's "detoxifying" function may occur during exacerbations of the underlying disease process or, not infrequently, after unexplained infarction of hepatic tissue. More commonly, the encephalopathy is precipitated by dietary indiscretions, increased protein intake, gastrointestinal bleeding, overzealous diuretic therapy, intercurrent infection, improper selection of sedatives (especially diazepam), surgical procedures (paracentesis, portacaval shunting) or renal failure.

Although many biologic derangements are seen in the face of the hepatic encephalopathy, the major candidates implicated in the neuropsychiatric disturbance are elevated blood ammonia, free fatty acids, false neurotransmitters (octopamine), and mercaptans. Clinical features in children include peculiar behavior, loss of recent memory, abnormal sleep patterns, dysarthria, and a "babbling" speech. Hyperreflexia, incoordination of fine motor movements, and eventually the "flapping tremor" (asterixis) characteristic of hepatic encephalopathy appear. Deepening of coma and cardiorespiratory arrest may occur before detection of *fector hepaticus,* a finding typically observed in fulminant hepatic necrosis associated with other features of hepatic encephalopathy. Additional signs and symptoms and the mechanism of action in hepatic encephalopathy are discussed in greater detail in Chapter 23.

A precipitating cause should be sought and, wherever possible, eliminated by specific treatment. Infections of the blood, peritoneal cavity, lungs, and urinary tract should be considered and appropriate cultures taken. If suspicion of infection is high, antibiotics should be started at once. Electrolyte abnormalities may need correction, especially potassium depletion, followed then by proper adjustment in diuretic drug dosage. Gastrointestinal bleeding is usually from esophageal varices or at times from peptic disease and should be confirmed endoscopically and treated appropriately (Chapters 7 and 25). Since gastrointestinal bleeding can provide significant amounts of substrate (protein) for ammonia production by bacterial action, it should be promptly eliminated by use of nasogastric suction, cathartics (magnesium sulfate, lactulose), and enemas. Intestinal ammonia can be "trapped" when the intraluminal pH is reduced to 5.5 or less by the use of lactulose. In this acidic environment, ammonia is changed to the nonabsorbable ammonium anion. Lactulose also has a cathartic action (hyperosmolar), which hastens the elimination of the "trapped" ammonia. Since the actions of this drug are dependent on bacterial fermentation, it should be used in place of neomycin. If lactulose cannot be employed, the bacterial flora can be reduced by oral administration of neomycin, 500 mg four times daily.

A reduction in dietary protein (0.5 to 1 gm/kg/day) may correct the prodromal signs of hepatic encephalopathy Slightly higher levels of dietary protein may be offered along with chronic lactulose use. Patients previously showing clinical features of hepatic encephalopathy can be expected to deteriorate rapidly if subjected to a portacaval shunt. In the absence of an identifiable precipitating cause for the hepatic encephalopathy the prognosis is extremely grave no matter what procedures or treatments are employed.

Hemodynamic adjustment in cirrhosis. The ability of the diseased liver to affect the systemic circulatory system has been observed repeatedly. Most patients studied have been adults, but children, too, can suffer the gamut of circulatory adjustments attending liver disease, listed in the next column.

Systemic circulatory changes in liver disease

1. Venous distention (abdomen and chest)
2. Spider angiomas and "white spots"
3. "Liver" palms
4. Rapid pulse
5. Wide pulse pressure
6. Warm skin
7. Expanded blood volume
8. Augmented aortic blood flow
9. Decreased peripheral vascular resistance
10. Cyanosis
11. Digital clubbing
12. Arterial desaturation
13. Decreased circulation time

In 10% to 25% of children with biliary cirrhosis, digital clubbing (Fig. 24-29) can be noted. Arterial desaturation is likewise present in these children, and cyanosis of the nail beds can be detected clinically. It is most likely that pulmonary, precapillary shunts are responsible for the arterial desaturation. The mechanisms by which these potential, nonfunctioning shunts are made to open is not clear, but a circulating humoral substance (reduced ferritin) released by the damaged liver has been implicated. Pulmonary infections causing local irritation and initiating blood flow through potential arteriovenous anastomosis have also been implicated as an inciting factor. During life, extracardiac right-to-left shunting may also be demonstrated by peripheral venous contrast echocardiography and further identified by pulmonary angiography.

Dye-injection studies of lungs of patients dying of cirrhosis and manifesting the cyanosis–digital clubbing syndrome have shown these small arteriovenous anastomoses (Fig. 24-34). During life, the failure of the arterial desaturation to be fully corrected after the patient breathes 100% oxygen constitutes evidence of pulmonary arteriovenous shunting. Although most patients demonstrating cyanosis and digital clubbing have advanced cirrhosis, this syndrome has beset patients with acute liver disease as well and seems to be reversible when the injured liver returns to normal.

The elevated cardiac output in patients with cirrhosis cannot be explained simply by the presence of pulmonary arteriovenous anastomosis or even the portal-pulmonary shunts that have also been demonstrated by cast-erosion studies. Although the matter remains unsettled, the augmented aortic output in patients with cirrhosis is probably produced by decreased peripheral vascular resistance

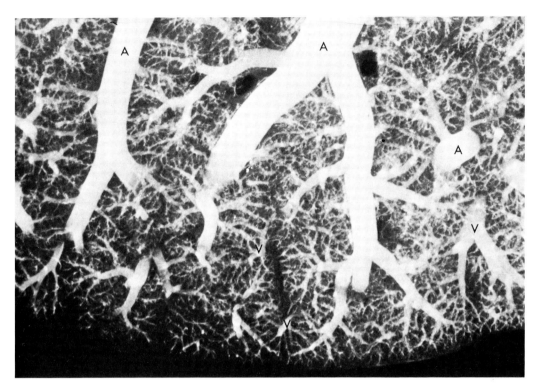

Fig. 24-34. Pulmonary arteriovenous shunts. A 4-year-old girl died of chronic liver disease, with digital clubbing and cyanosis; a sagittal section of lung was taken after postmortem barium sulfate injection into the pulmonary artery. Arterial branches, *A,* and three veins, *V* (lower center and lower right of illustration) are both visualized. (From Silverman, A., Cooper, M.D., Moller, J.H., and Good, R.A.: J. Pediatr. **72:**70-80, 1968.)

and increased flow into these regions. Reduced arteriovenous differences are common, and, again, peripheral precapillary arteriovenous shunts may be operative. These observations have been taken to explain the clinical findings of rapid pulse, wide pulse pressure, shortened circulation time, warm skin, and high-output murmurs.

Anemia in cirrhosis. Eventually, about half of patients with chronic liver disease suffer mild or moderate degrees of anemia. Severe hemolytic disease, both Coombs' positive and Coombs' negative, may be one of the initial manifestations of acute liver disease. It may occur rarely with neonatal hepatitis, chronic active hepatitis, and Wilson's disease. Within a few years (or sooner), most children with cirrhosis have a type of anemia usually refractory to standard therapy measures. Several possible causes have been postulated, and, indeed, it is not unusual for more than one factor to be responsible for the anemia in cirrhosis. The obvious considerations include excessive blood loss via the gastrointestinal tract, expanded blood vol-

ume, shortened red blood cell survival (intravascular hemolysis or splenic sequestration), decreased bone marrow production, and high circulating levels of bile salts.

The unreliability of hematocrit and hemoglobin determinations in establishing the presence of anemia in patients with cirrhosis has been emphasized by figures obtained from studies of the red blood cell mass and total blood volume. A normal but diluted circulating red blood cell mass can be found in the expanded plasma space of some patients suspected of being anemic solely on the basis of hemoglobin or hematocrit values.

Careful, repetitive stool examination for blood loss through the intestinal tract is essential in these anemic children. The major sources of blood loss can be expected to arise from esophageal and gastric varices or a duodenal ulcer, but associated thrombocytopenia and other abnormalities in coagulation factors may be responsible for mild degrees of blood loss. Alterations in intestinal capillary wall integrity and permeability are likely to

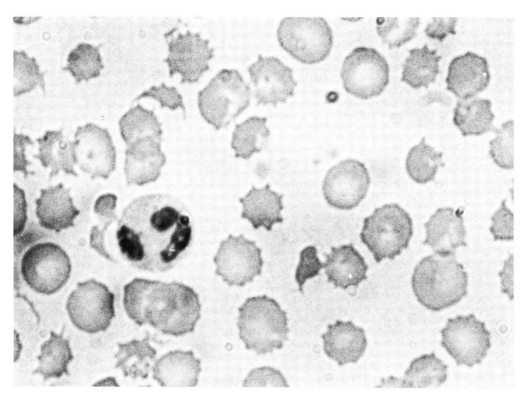

Fig. 24-35. ''Burr'' cells in cirrhosis. A peripheral blood smear from a patient with terminal liver disease, showing severe burr cell formation of the red blood cells.

occur in cirrhosis, especially if portal hypertension is severe and ascites is present, events that contribute to a loss of both protein and red blood cells.

Shortened red blood cell survival has been demonstrated in about half the patients with cirrhosis. Certainly, the greatest factor is the presence of the large, congested spleen in which slow-moving red blood cells are sequestered and removed by this organ. Some patients respond to portacaval shunts, splenectomy, or both, with a rise in the red blood cell mass and fall in indirect-reacting serum bilirubin levels. Attention has been given to alterations in the red blood cell membrane that predispose the spleen to early sequestration of these cells. The process of red cell destruction in chronic liver disease is dependent on two separate and sequential alterations in red cell membrane. The first step is the selective acquisition of cholesterol within the red cell membrane, which produces a change in surface area when the cell assumes a scalloped contour. The next step is characterized by the splenic transformation (conditioning) of the cell to a spiculated contour, fur-

ther loss of the cell's surface area and lipid content, and increased susceptibility to osmotic threat. This latter phase seems responsible for the hemolytic effect. The distortions seen in some of the erythrocytes are not specific for cirrhosis, but burr cells (acanthocytes) and other peculiarly shaped red blood cells are frequently seen, especially terminally (Fig. 24-35). Other red cells that appear normal in these patients have been noted to be ''stiff'' by tests measuring the deformability of the cell. Unfortunately, this observation has not been consistently demonstrated by other techniques. The serum of such patients can induce this change in normal red blood cells in vitro, and normal red blood cells that are transfused into patients with cirrhosis have a shortened half-life as well. On the other hand, incubation with normal serum does diminish the so-called stiffness of washed red blood cells from cirrhotic patients. The addition of glucose to the system does not alter the membrane property nor does the addition of vitamin E. However, infants and very young children with biliary cirrhosis may have a profound deficiency of this vitamin, and subsequent correction of this condition sometimes lessens the degree of anemia.

The presence of low levels of reduced glutathione in the red blood cells of some patients with cirrhosis is also believed to play a role in increased susceptibility to hemolysis. The reason for the diminished levels of reduced glutathione is unclear, since intracellular mechanisms for its reduction are supposedly intact.

Finally, decreased bone marrow production may be a factor in some cases of anemia in cirrhosis. The inability of some patient's marrow to compensate for a mild hemolytic anemia by increasing red blood cell output from the marrow has been taken as evidence of decreased production. At times, this inability is simply caused by decreased iron stores in the marrow from several causes. Excessive blood loss, poor absorption at the intestinal level, and decreased carrier-protein (transferrin) are all found in cirrhosis. When these possibilities are eliminated, a circulating inhibitor to red blood cell production and release from the bone marrow has been implicated.

Oral iron preparations are indicated only if the serum iron level is low in the face of anemia. Steroids have also been used with some success in decreasing the rate of hemolysis in cases of chronic liver disease showing positive results of Coombs' test.

Thrombocytopenia in cirrhosis. Decreased numbers of circulating platelets is an indication of hypersplenism. Raised splenic pulp pressure, a natural consequence of portal hypertension, leads to increased sequestration of platelets as a result of their prolonged transit through this organ. Thrombocytopenia seldom increases the risk to serious bleeding unless the count is below 50,000 or there is platelet dysfunction (from salicylates) and the bleeding time is prolonged. Another cause of thrombocytopenia is consumptive coagulopathy, which may develop during an intercurrent infection, or terminally in the face of acid-base and electrolyte disturbances. Emergency splenectomy is occasionally indicated during a so-called splenic crisis, but if at all possible it should be combined with a portal decompression shunting procedure. Unfortunately, the mortality in such instances is extremely high even with the administration of platelet transfusions and clotting factors to restore normal coagulation.

Endocrine abnormalities in cirrhosis. Since alcohol-induced cirrhosis is essentially nonexistent in the pediatric population, important manifestations of disturbances in the hypothalamic-pituitary-gonadal axis are seldom seen. A substantial body of accumulated evidence suggests that alcohol abuse in itself can produce dysfunction in this endocrine axis even in the absence of liver disease. Recent studies in nonalcoholic and presumed virus-induced (postnecrotic) cirrhotic adult males found absence of gonadal defects in either the reproductive (spermatogenesis) or endocrine (testosterone) cell function. Indeed, the feminizing effects of excess estrogen (gynecomastia, female escutcheon, broad hips) are an exceptional finding in teen-age males with chronic liver disease. Furthermore, growth-hormone levels are normal as is the hypothalamic-pituitary-axis of thyroid function. In teen-age girls delayed menses, abnormal periods, "excess acne," and the early appearance of striae have previously been taken as evidence of malfunction in the hypothalamic-pituitary-ovarian axis. Control data that implicates either excessive blood estrogen levels or heightened estrogen-responsive tissue is not available for these nonalcohol-induced cases.

Delayed pubescence and menarche are most often seen in the face of long-standing cirrhosis associated with marginal caloric intake. Persons with chronic liver disease often gain and grow slowly and therefore fail to achieve the critical body mass needed to initiate these hormonal events until later into adolescence. Physicians should be alerted to the social and psychological impact that accompanies significant delays in growth and pubescence and be prepared to deal with it directly or with the use of other professionals (school counselors, social workers, psychologists, and so on). Making an effort to increase the caloric intake is sometimes indicated, but specific measures are not available for altering the presumed disturbances in endocrine function.

Prognosis

In general the prognosis for prolonged survival is extremely poor in cirrhosis affecting children, though the duration and quality of life will vary not only with the severity of the histologic lesion but often directly with the underlying cause. Save for a few rare and unusual genetometabolic defects amenable to specific therapy, only orthotopic liver transplantation offers a remote but possible chance of a permanent cure. Management of the patient with cirrhosis really involves prevention and treatment of the complications of chronic liver disease, since the complications often determine the eventual fate of the patient.

The majority of infants and children with biliary cirrhosis caused by congenital biliary atresia of the extrahepatic ducts do poorly. Of those infants with biliary atresia undergoing surgery (Kasai's procedure) over 25% are alive after 2 years, but many of these survivors have clinical and histologic evidence of biliary cirrhosis. The long-term prognosis for this select group of survivors remains to be determined. Death is frequently caused by intercurrent infections, electrolyte disturbances, pulmonary complications as ascites, or hepatic decompensation.

Once complications of cirrhosis such as ascites, hemorrhage from varices, renal failure, and so forth, develop, the survival time is predictably shortened. Few of these patients live more than from 6 months to 3 years, depending on the response to additional therapy measures. Failure to respond to diuretics and further hepatic decompensation after hemorrhage and progressive oliguria all carry a grim prognosis, and survival is rare even for 3 months.

The results of even the most knowledgeable application of medical and surgical therapy measures in children with cirrhosis from all causes are disappointing. Early detection of some causes, as well as institution of specific therapy, does prevent cirrhosis from developing. D-Penicillamine, besides its known beneficial action in Wilson's disease, has recently been shown to improve survival when given late in the course to adults with primary biliary cirrhosis. Since the drug, which experimentally has antifibrotic properties, did not prevent on-going fibrosis, its beneficial effect has been attributed to the known copper-chelating and immunologic actions. The potential application of this agent to pediatric patients with other forms of chronic cholestatic liver disease and cirrhosis needs to be determined.

Obviously, prevention would best improve the prognosis of childhood cirrhosis. Genetic counseling would reduce the numbers of cases produced by the many genetometabolic causes. Development of specific vaccines (Heptavax·B) and improvement in public health measures might reduce the numbers of cases of hepatitis and lower the contribution made by this growing group going on to cirrhosis. The possibility that even biliary atresia may represent the final consequence of an in utero infection therefore has preventive implications.

REFERENCES

Appelman, H.D.: Cirrhosis: morphologic dynamics for the non-morphologist, Am. J. Dig. Dis. **17**:463-472, 1972.

August, C., and Gross, G.: Burr cell hemolysis in childhood liver disease, Clin. Res. **19**:207, 1971.

Baggenstoss, A.H.: Morphologic features: their usefulness in the diagnosis, prognosis and management of cirrhosis. In Popper, H., editor: Cirrhosis, Clin. Gastroenterol. **4**:227-246, 1975.

Cooper, R.A., Kimball, D.B., and Durocher, J.R.: Role of the spleen in membrane conditioning and hemolysis of spur cells in liver disease, N. Engl. J. Med. **290**:1279-1284, 1974.

Conn, H.O.: The rational management of ascites. In Popper, H., and Schaffner, F., editors: Progress in liver diseases, vol. 4, New York, 1972, Grune & Stratton, Inc.

Craig, J.M., Gellis, S.S., and Hsia, D.Y.: Cirrhosis of liver in infants and children, Am. J. Dis. Child. **90**:299-322, 1955.

Czaja, A.J., Wolf, A.M., and Baggenstoss, A.H.: Clinical assessment of cirrhosis in severe chronic active liver disease, Mayo. Clin. Proc. **55**:360-364, 1980.

Eknoyan, G., Martinez-Maldonado, M., and Yium, J.J.: Combined ascitic-fluid and furosemide in fusion in the management of ascites, N. Engl. J. Med. **282**:713-717, 1970.

Epstein, M.: The LeVeen shunt for ascites and hepatorenal syndrome, N. Engl. J. Med. **302**:628-630, 1980.

Epstein, M., Calia, F.M., and Gabuzda, G.J.: Pneumococcal peritonitis in patients with postnecrotic cirrhosis, N. Engl. J. Med. **279**:69-73, 1968.

Felsher, B.F., Redeker, A.G., Reynolds, T.B.: Indirect-reacting hyperbilirubinemia in cirrhosis: its relation to red cell survival, Am. J. Dig. Dis. **13**:598-607, 1968.

Frazier, H.S., and Yager, H.: The clinical use of diuretics, N. Engl. J. Med. **288**:246-249, 455-457, 1973.

LeVeen, H.H., Christoudias, G., Moon, I.P., and others: Peritoneovenous shunting for ascites, Ann. Surg. **180**:580-591, 1974.

Linscheer, W.G.: Malabsorption in cirrhosis, Am. J. Clin. Nutr. **23**:488-492, 1970.

Martini, G.A.: Extrahepatic manifestations of cirrhosis, Clin. Gastroenterol. **4**:439-460, 1975.

Popper, H., and Udenfriend, S.: Hepatic fibrosis: correlation of biochemical and morphological investigations, Am. J. Med. **49**:707-721, 1970.

Ruggieri, B.A., Baggenstoss, A.H., and Logan, G.B.: Juvenile cirrhosis: a clinico-pathologic study of 27 cases, Am. J. Dis. Child. **94**:64-76, 1957.

Schenker, S., Breen, K.J., and Hoyumpa, M., Jr.: Hepatic encephalopathy: current status, Gastroenterology **66**:121-151, 1974.

Shear, L., Ching, S., and Gabuzda, G.J.: Compartmentalization of ascites and edema in patients with hepatic cirrhosis, N. Engl. J. Med. **282**:1391-1396, 1970.

Sheehy, T.W., and Berman, A.: The anemia of cirrhosis, J. Lab. Clin. Med. **56**:72-82, 1960.

Sherlock, S.: Nutritional complication of biliary cirrhosis: chronic cholestasis, Am. J. Clin. Nutr. **23**:640-644, 1970.

Sherlock, S., Walker, J.G., Senewiratne, B., and Acott, A.: The complication of diuretic therapy in patients with cirrhosis, Ann. N.Y. Acad. Sci. **139**:497-505, 1966.

Sherlock, S.: Viral hepatitis and cirrhosis. In Popper, H., editor: Cirrhosis, Clin. Gastroenterol. **4**:281-296, 1975.

Silber, R., Amorosi, E., Lhowe, J., and Kayden, H.J.: Spur-shaped erythrocytes in Laennec's cirrrhosis, N. Engl. J. Med. **275:**639-643, 1966.

Silverman, A., Cooper, M.D., Moller, J.H., and Good, R.A.: Syndrome of cyanosis, digital clubbing and hepatic disease in siblings, J. Pediatr. **72:**70-80, 1968.

Spagnolo, S.V.: Cyanosis of cirrhosis, Med. Clin. North Am. **59:**938-987, 1975.

Summerskill, W.H.J.: Acites: the kidney in liver disease. In Schiff, L., editor: Disease of the liver, ed. 3, Philadelphia, 1969, J. B. Lippincott Co.

Van Thiel, D.H., and Lester, R.: Hypothalamic-pituitary-gonadal function in liver disease, Viewpoints Dig. Dis. **12:**13-16, 1980.

Weber, A., and Roy, C.C.: Malabsorption et traitement médical des affections hépatiques chroniques de l'enfant, Union Med. Can. **100:**1171-1175, 1971.

Witte, C.L., Witte, M.H., and Dumont, A.E.: Lymph imbalance in the genesis and perpetuation of the ascites syndrome in hepatic cirrhosis, Gastroenterology **78:**1059-1068, 1980.

Wyllie, R., Arasu, T.S., and Fitzgerald, J.F.: Ascites: pathophysiology and management, J. Pediatr. **97:**167-176, 1980.

25 *Portal hypertension*

By definition portal hypertension exists when the measured pressure in this venous system is greater than 10 to 12 mm Hg, or 17 to 20 cm H_2O. For practical purposes an increase in portal pressure is caused mostly by conditions that impede the normal flow of blood through this system. Three anatomic levels of obstruction have been recognized: (1) *prehepatic,* where obstruction to venous flow is caused by a structural abnormality of the extrahepatic portal vein (congenital or acquired) or one of its immediate tributaries; (2) *intrahepatic,* from conditions that produce an increase in vascular resistance within the liver, with or without cirrhosis; and (3) *suprahepatic,* where obstruction to hepatic venous outflow exists. Rarely is portal hypertension caused by an increase in blood flow to the liver (''forward flow''); for example, arteriovenous fistulas may be the cause. In other cases increased splenic blood flow associated with nonhepatic diseases, such as myeloproliferative disorders, leukemia, Hodgkin's disease, splenic hemangiomas, systemic mastocytosis, and osteopetrosis, may result in forward-flow portal hypertension. Localizing the anatomic level and thereby the source of origin for the portal hypertension reduces the diagnostic possibilities and can dictate proper therapy. Obtainment of this information will require an organized and selective investigative approach.

GENERAL CONSIDERATIONS

The consequences and clinical manifestations of elevated portal venous pressure are similar for children and adults. However, the modes of presentation, cause, diagnostic considerations, investigations, and treatment may vary considerably between the two groups. Failure to appreciate the differences may in part be responsible for the previously noted high morbidity and mortality figures reported for children with portal hypertension. A number of factors may be responsible for such events: (1) Incomplete investigation may result in erroneous diagnosis, which can deprive the patient of proper treatment. (2) Certain liver diseases capable of producing portal hypertension need specific and early diagnosis because delay permits

continuing deterioration of the liver disease when one does not employ specific therapy that may arrest or even improve the underlying condition (Wilson's disease, chronic active hepatitis). Equally concerning would be the missed opportunity for diagnosis and treatment of asymptomatic siblings of the index case, especially in genetometabolic causes of liver disease. (3) Furthermore, incomplete investigations may result in inappropriate management decisions for some patients, which in turn contribute to additional morbidity, if not mortality. This can include hasty surgical intervention that results in splenectomy without creation of a decompressing vascular shunt, or the improper selection of vessels to be used in the shunting procedure. Both ill-advised decisions have the potential to increase the frequency and worsen the severity of variceal hemorrhage.

MAJOR CLINICAL MANIFESTATIONS AND DIAGNOSTIC CONSIDERATIONS

The hemodynamic consequences of increased portal venous pressure is the common denominator that underlies the observed clinical manifestations, be it splenomegaly, esophageal varices, ascites, portal encephalopathy, hemorrhoids, or the prominent abdominal venous pattern. Suggestions for evaluating these findings in relation to underlying portal hypertension are detailed below.

Splenomegaly

That the spleen should rapidly reflect the consequences of portal hypertension is not surprising, since the splenic vein draining this organ is relatively large and communicates directly with the portal vein. In fact, the splenic vein after entrance of the inferior mesenteric vein merges distally with the superior mesenteric vein, to make the origin of the portal vein (Fig. 25-1).

Splenomegaly then is often the first clinical finding that will suggest portal hypertension. Its recognition, however, almost always depends on physical examination, since the enlargement is painless and early in its evolution may not lead to noticeable change in abdominal girth. Since care-

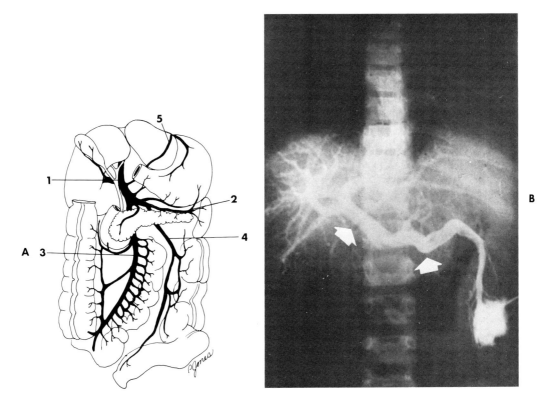

Fig. 25-1. A, Prehepatic portal venous drainage system. *1,* Portal vein; *2,* splenic vein; *3,* superior mesenteric vein; *4,* inferior mesenteric vein; *5,* coronary vein. **B,** Normal portal venous system shown by splenoportography. The contrast material immediately opacifies the splenic and portal veins, *arrows.* The intraheptic branches of the portal system are also well visualized.

ful abdominal examination is included as part of the routine follow-up evaluation of patients with known liver disease, splenomegaly is not likely to be missed in such cases. However, in the absence of a history suggesting previous liver disease, splenomegaly is likely to be discovered only if the examination of the abdomen is routinely included in the physical assessment during well- and sick-child encounters (Chapter 2). Occasionally the splenic enlargement may be discovered by chance from abdominal roentgenograms obtained for other reasons. It may also be revealed intraoperatively when abdominal trauma has led to splenic rupture requiring surgery.

Although splenomegaly is the most consistent early finding in evolving portal hypertension, a causative relation may neither be appreciated nor properly pursued. That the cause may be attributable to portal hypertension can be immediately suggested by the history of previous liver disease. If ascites is absent, splenic enlargement from por-

tal hypertension is unlikely to be suprahepatic in origin. When obstruction to portal venous flow is intrahepatic and associated with cirrhosis, additional evidence of chronic liver disease is usually identified (Chapter 24). Prehepatic portal hypertension as a cause of splenomegaly can be suspected from some of the additional clues discussed on p. 770.

Obviously, when splenomegaly cannot be immediately explained with certainty, a search for its cause must be pursued. Most often, a combination of history, physical examination, and minimal office laboratory data is likely to be of immediate help, especially if portal hypertension is *not* causative. In these examples splenomegaly is usually caused by acute infections (streptococci, infectious mononucleosis, fungal diseases, tuberculosis, hepatitis), hematologic causes (iron-deficiency anemia, congenital hemolytic anemia, hemoglobinopathies, leukemia, lymphoma), or storage diseases (Gaucher's, Niemann-Pick, mucopolysaccharidosis, histiocytosis X). Hyperexpansion of the lungs with resultant depression of the diaphragm occurs in bronchiolitis and asthma and may produce "factitious" splenomegaly. Failure to satisfactorily explain the finding of splenomegaly after the above considerations should prompt the physician to order the following investigative studies. A bone-marrow examination should be performed and, if consistent with hypersplenism, roentgenography or an endoscopic search for esophageal varices should be undertaken (see below); finally, use of radioisotope liver-spleen scan or ultrasound study of the spleen may be needed to reveal rare causes of splenomegaly, such as splenic cyst.

Hematemesis, melena, or both

An alarming and important manifestation of portal hypertension is hemorrhage from esophageal varices. This event usually results in hematemesis, since the amount of blood presented to the stomach is large, causing nausea and gastric distress. Melena is often noted simultaneously or shortly thereafter. As a rule, if small quantities of blood are lost from esophageal varices, melena without hematemesis may be reported. Occasionally, however, a significant esophageal hemorrhage can present as melena but without associated hematemesis.

Bleeding from esophageal varices, with only rare exceptions, is a direct consequence of increased portal venous pressure and accounts for 5% to 8% of all causes of gastrointestinal bleeding in children. Increased resistance to portal flow leads to hemodynamic alterations that redirect the flow of blood away from the liver (hepatofugal flow). As a result, both a reversal of venous blood flow that normally drains into the portal vein and the reopening of preexisting but nonfunctioning collateral communications occur. The redirection of blood flow through gastroesophageal connections (coronary vein) is primarily responsible for the enlargement of submucosal (varices) and periesophageal veins in the distal esophagus. A large volume of blood may be redirected through this system, especially in the face of intrahepatic or suprahepatic obstruction, with blood flowing from the existing portal vein into the coronary vein and then to the esophageal veins. This drainage system is further stressed by the contribution of other collateral communications draining venous blood from the stomach and spleen. If the portal vein is obliterated as occurs in prehepatic portal hypertension, the coronary vein may or may not be present, but other collateral communications emptying into the gastroesophageal system can be demonstrated.

Although portal hypertension results in the establishment of a number of collateral circulations, only the impact upon the gastroesophageal drainage system places the patient at significant risk to hemorrhage. A collateral circulation by way of the hemorrhoidal veins also develops and serves to decompress the inferior mesenteric venous drainage system by way of the hypogastric veins. When present, hemorrhoids from portal hypertension are seldom symptomatic in children.

The differential diagnosis of hematemesis is discussed in Chapter 2. The diagnosis of esophageal varices as a cause of upper gastrointestinal bleeding may be strongly suspected if evidence of underlying chronic liver disease can be documented in either the history or physical examination of the patient. The presence of splenomegaly in a person suspected of having an upper gastrointestinal hemorrhage, even without a history of previous liver disease, should make one suspect portal hypertension and esophageal varices as causative. One should keep in mind that gastrointestinal bleeding may result in contraction of the vascular space; therefore the spleen may not be palpable during the initial physical examination. Hemorrhage from esophageal varices when caused by a "congenital" abnormality in the gastroesophageal venous drainage system may occur in the absence of splenomegaly with or without demonstrable portal hypertension (Fig. 25-2).

As a rule, if bleeding from esophageal varices is the first indication of portal hypertension, the site of origin is more likely to be prehepatic or intrahepatic, rather than suprahepatic. The disease conditions responsible for the latter form of portal hypertension result in other important clinical manifestations (ascites, deterioration of liver function, and so forth) before the patient demonstrates complications of esophageal varices.

Presently, fiberoptic endoscopy performed after stabilization of the child is the most accurate means of diagnosing the cause of acute upper gastrointestinal bleeding. In experienced hands this technique is relatively easy to perform, requiring light sedation though occasionally a general anesthetic is necessary. Numerous studies have shown this technique capable of identifying the cause of

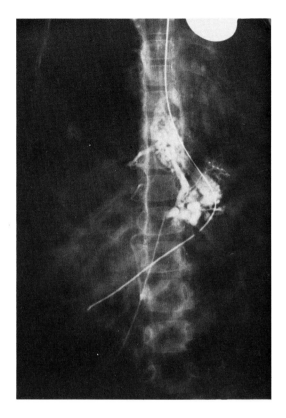

Fig. 25-2. Esophageal varices demonstrated by intraoperative contrast injection of an omental vein. Patient was a 4-year-old child presenting after several episodes of hematemesis. Endoscopy revealed distal esophageal varices, but the absence of splenomegaly was confusing. Intraoperative studies revealed elevated portal pressure and abnormal collateral circulation. The spleen was of normal size; liver biopsy study likewise showed normal results.

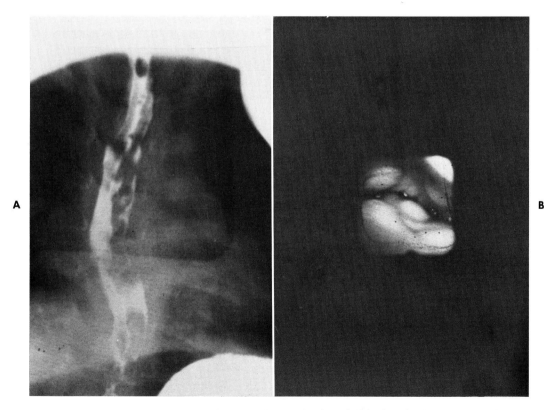

Fig. 25-3. A, Huge esophageal varices extend up to the thoracic inlet in this 12-month-old child. History revealed that an umbilical vein catheter used for exchange transfusions in the neonatal period was left in situ for 7 days. Splenomegaly was noted at 4 months of age. First large variceal hemorrhage occurred at age 2. **B,** Endoscopic view of the varices seen in **A.** Irregular-shaped cobblestone masses are dilated veins.

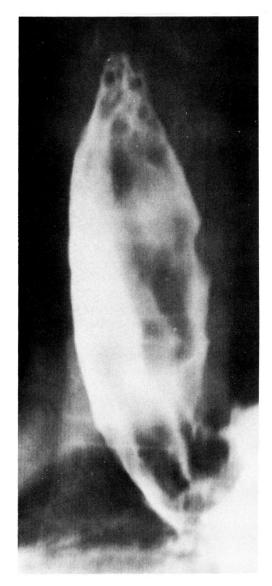

Fig. 25-4. Large esophageal varices in a 15-year-old girl with extrahepatic portal hypertension caused by "idiopathic" thrombosis of the portal vein.

bleeding in up to 90% of cases. Through the endoscope the esophageal varices appear as whitish, blue gray, or pink irregular elevations in the distal esophagus that fail to efface with insufflation of air. In advanced cases they may extend up into the body of the esophagus and reveal a striking cobblestone appearance (Fig. 25-3). In subtle cases they may be confused with distal longitudinal esophageal folds but differentiated when one uses air insufflation, since varices remain visible whereas mucosal folds will be completely effaced.

Using a thick barium medium, one can demonstrate esophageal varices roentgenographically in up to 80% of cases. A slightly lower figure may be reported if examination is done before restoration of blood volume. When present, the irregular cobblestone-like filling defects of the lower part of the esophagus are characteristic (Fig. 25-4). The problem lies in obtaining films that make the lesions visible. The older patient can be told to hold his breath and strain, but the infant has to be filmed while crying; tricks such as having the patient blow through a straw or placing the hand over the nose and mouth of the crying infant may be helpful. Roentgenographic visualization of esophageal varices may also be enhanced by the intramuscular injection of anticholinergic drugs just before the examination. Both propantheline bromide (Pro-Banthine) and atropine sulfate have been employed in the older child.

The event initiating bleeding from varices is unknown. That gastric acid has an erosive effect on these vessels has little firm support, since bleeding from varices has occurred in patients with achlorhydria. The onset of variceal bleeding has been repeatedly noted in association with intercurrent infections of the respiratory tract especially when cough is present, an observation suggesting that sudden increases in pressure may be responsible. However, attempts to explain the onset of bleeding from physiologic data have not been possible. Lack of correlation exists between the wedged hepatic vein pressure or portal vein pressure with onset of bleeding from varices. This apparently is true in all forms (causes) of portal hypertension. In fact, examples of bleeding from esophageal varices have been reported in the face of normal portal pressure. It is unclear if this also applies to children with portal hypertension because measurements are infrequently obtained in this age group before the onset of bleeding. Some believe that hemorrhage from varices is related to their size, yet variceal size correlates poorly with portal pressure. It would appear that the risk of bleeding is increased in the face of ascites. Salicylates, by interfering with platelet function, are more likely to worsen the severity of hemorrhage rather than induce bleeding.

The clinical impact of a single upper gastrointestinal bleed from esophageal varices will depend on (1) the volume of blood lost, (2) the rapidity with which vascular volume can be replaced, (3) the ability to control ongoing bleeding, and (4) the presence or absence of underlying liver disease.

In patients with prehepatic portal hypertension, death from exsanguination is possible but, fortunately, extremely rare. The spontaneous cessation of the bleeding is commonly confirmed at endoscopy performed in the first 24 hours. When esophageal bleeding from intrahepatic causes of portal hypertension is associated with cirrhosis, the immediate prognosis is less certain. Deterioration of liver function, portal-systemic encephalopathy, ascites, and electrolyte imbalance may occur, further complicating the immediate clinical course and needs of the patient, events likely to increase morbidity.

The clinical impact caused by discovery of esophageal varices in a patient with portal hypertension is significant for most subsequent management decisions in the patient will be influenced by this new finding.

Ascites and abdominal enlargement

Statistically, most patients with ascites have portal hypertension associated with cirrhosis (intrahepatic ''block''), and the fluid accumulates as a result of complex interactions involving vascular, renal, and endocrine mechanisms described in detail in Chapter 24. The appearance of ascites is usually a late phenomenon in the evolution of chronic liver disease but may be precipitated at an earlier time by events that upset the patient's water and electrolyte balance, or the vascular volume (hemorrhage). Although suprahepatic causes of portal hypertension are uncommon in children, 95% of these patients will have rapid abdominal enlargement because of a combination of significant ascitic fluid accumulation and hepatomegaly. Ascites from prehepatic portal hypertension does occur in 10% to 30% of cases, and here the fluid produces transient episodes of painless abdominal enlargement and regresses spontaneously. Most often no precipitating cause of the ascites is found in this latter example of portal hypertension, but it may predictably follow an acute, brief gastrointestinal bleed. Only rarely is the volume of ascites significant in patients with prehepatic portal hypertension. The mechanism for ascites formation in these patients is not entirely clear, but alterations in the flow dynamics of interstitial-lymph fluid, in both the intestinal tract and mesentery, are believed to be causative. At times hypoalbuminemia, which can occur after a variceal bleed,

may precipitate ascites accumulation in this particular group of patients.

The clinical detection of ascites is best accomplished when shifting dullness is demonstrated. A succussion splash may be obtained when large amounts of fluid are present. That the fluid is indeed free within the peritoneal cavity can be appreciated on plane abdominal films showing centrally located air-filled loops of intestine. Abdominal ultrasound examination is a very sensitive technique in the diagnosis of free abdominal fluid, detecting as little as 100 ml of fluid. Ultrasound is also particularly useful in differentiating free fluid from a fluid-filled cyst (mesenteric, omental, ovarian).

That the ascitic fluid is the result of portal hypertension may be suspected from clinical history and physical examintaion, especially if evidence of cardiac or liver disease is discovered. At times other etiologic explanations for the abdominal fluid need to be ruled out, and this can be expedited from the results of a diagnostic paracentesis. Entities including chylous ascites, pancreatic ascites, peritoneal tumors (primary or metastatic), miliary Crohn's disease, or tuberculosis may be identified from the appearance and laboratory analysis of the ascitic fluid. So-called liver ascites from suprahepatic or intrahepatic causes is relatively rich in protein content, often being greater than 2 gm/dl, whereas prehepatic ascitic fluid tends to have a lower protein content (1 gm/dl or less).

Portal-systemic encephalopathy

The evolution of hepatofugal venous flow involving portal-systemic shunting is a basic prerequisite for portal-systemic encephalopathy. By way of these collaterals, a substantial fraction of splanchnic blood flow bypasses the liver and fails to avail itself (at least initially) of the liver's detoxifying function. Precipitating causes may be products of digested dietary proteins, gastrointestinal bleeding, ammonia derived from intestinal flora, endotoxins, medications, tranquilizers (diazepam), and other substances not yet identified.

The impact of portal-systemic shunting upon the central nervous system seems greatest if underlying liver disease is present, since major neuropsychiatric manifestations (coma, extrapyramidal signs) are not seen in children with prehepatic portal hypertension, at least before surgical creation of a portal-systemic shunt. A growing concern that chronic or minimal portal encephalopathy (either presurgical or postsurgical shunting) may have more subtle expressions in children, especially in perceptual and cognitive learning skills, needs to be answered by future studies.

OTHER CLINICAL MANIFESTATIONS OF COLLATERAL CIRCULATION

The *presence of dilated venous channels on the abdomen of a child* should make one suspect portal hypertension. Increased portal vein pressure may cause the fetal umbilical vein–epigastric vein anastomosis to reopen. A Cruveilhier-Baumgarten murmur may be heard over this area, but it develops only when portal hypertension is intrahepatic, since in prehepatic portal hypertension the block is proximal to the junction of the left branch of the portal vein and umbilical vein.

Hemorrhoids, rare in children, can be quite troublesome but infrequently are caused by portal hypertension. Communications exist between the hemorrhoidal venous system, the inferior mesenteric vein, and the hypogastric vein, and as a consequence of portal hypertension, dilatation of this venous system develops. Both internal and external hemorrhoids may be found, but they are very rare in prehepatic portal hypertension and are more likely to be seen in cirrhosis.

Progressive pulmonary hypertension leading to cardiac decompensation has been seen in children in the face of portal hypertension. The portal-systemic or portopulmonary collateral circulation that develops in the face of portal hypertension may allow pulmonary vasoconstrictive humoral substances to escape hepatic detoxification and thereby exert their effect upon the pulmonary artery circulation.

Splanchnic and pelvic venous collateral communications with the paravertebral venous systems (veins of Batson) may predispose an unfortunate patient with portal hypertension to brain abscess.

INVESTIGATION OF PORTAL HYPERTENSION
Goals

These efforts should result in (1) confirmation of the diagnosis, thereby providing a satisfactory explanation for the clinical manifestations previously discussed; (2) localize the site of portal hypertension as either prehepatic, intrahepatic, or suprahepatic; (3) identify the cause responsible for the portal hypertension; and (4) when indicated,

dictate further specialized studies that will influence decisions regarding surgical alleviation of the portal hypertension.

The confirmation of the diagnosis of portal hypertension may ultimately come from the measurement of splenic pulp pressure or from a vein known to reflect portal venous pressure. However, contraindications to some, or all, of the procedures required for obtainment of this information may exist, and therefore direct pressure measurement will not always be possible. Nor is direct pressure measurement always required for the confirmation of the diagnosis of portal hypertension. Often the accumulated evidence from a systematic and thorough investigation of the patient's clinical manifestations provide sufficient, though circumstantial, data to make the diagnosis of portal hypertension. Furthermore, since direct confirmation of increased portal pressure requires an invasive procedure, the prior work-up can help to clearly define the indications and selection of the investigative procedure of choice. The order of inquiry should be dictated by the patient's clinical presentation and associated historical and physical findings.

Screening tests

Investigative laboratory studies for splenomegaly
1. Complete blood count and red blood cell indices
2. Platelet count
3. Reticulocyte count
4. Mononucleosis spot test
5. Bone marrow examination
6. Liver-spleen scan
7. Ultrasound of the spleen (for tumors, cysts)

If the results of these studies are consistent with congestive splenomegaly that is, thrombocytopenia, slightly low granulocyte count, reactive hyperplasia in the bone marrow, and so on, portal hypertension must be seriously considered and additional investigations undertaken to determine the site and cause of this finding.

Investigative laboratory studies regarding chronic liver disease
1. Routine liver function tests
2. HBsAg
3. Serum protein electrophoresis
4. Prothrombin time
5. BSP clearance test
6. Quantitative serum alpha-1-antitrypsin level

7. Ceruloplasmin
8. Sweat chlorides
9. Urine for reducing sugar and organic acids

Invasive tests

One should make investigative studies to (1) *establish the site of origin of portal hypertension,* (2) *obtain portal vein pressure,* and (3) *identify the collateral circulation.* These investigations all require invasive procedures and therefore indications for their employment should be established from the aforementioned screening tests. The sequence of selected studies should be dictated by the likely diagnosis based on the assessment of previous data.

Liver biopsy. Details of this procedure are discussed in Chapter 32. The indication for liver biopsy in patients with portal hypertension should include a positive history or physical findings of liver disease, abnormal liver function studies, and specific liver disease (Wilson's disease, alpha-1-antitrypsin deficiency, cystic fibrosis) identified from diagnostic studies.

Liver biopsy is also indicated if esophageal varices are present in a patient with normal or near normal liver function studies, or if the splenoportogram demonstrates an intrahepatic portal venous pattern suggestive of congenital hepatic fibrosis (p. 789). Contraindications to a surgical liver biopsy include a coagulation defect that cannot be corrected by standard means (vitamin K, fresh-frozen plasma) and impending liver failure. Percutaneous needle liver biopsy is contraindicated if suprahepatic portal hypertension is suspected, or if ascites is present. When portal hypertension is strongly suspected, our preference is to perform an operative biopsy (minilaparotomy) for several additional reasons. Intraoperative measurement of portal pressure and a contrast venous roentgenogram of the portal circulation can often be obtained with only slight prolongation of the operative procedure. This immediately localizes the site of obstruction and, to a reasonable degree, demonstrates the extent of the collateral circulation. Furthermore, sampling error is greatly reduced when tissue is obtained at surgery, especially if both wedge and deep needle biopsy specimens are taken. When indicated, specialized studies involving chemical or enzymatic determinations generally necessitate a larger sample of liver tissue, which is obtainable only by open biopsy.

Splenoportography. Provided that experienced personnel ("procedure" radiologist, angiographer, pediatric surgeon) and equipment are available and no contraindications exist (bleeding disorder, ascites, percutaneous liver biopsy done in the past 24 hours), a number of potential benefits may be derived from this procedure, which is described as follows.

Measurement of splenic pulp pressure. Within certain limits, measurement of splenic pulp pressure reflects portal vein pressure, and values greater than 20 to 23 cm H_2O are to be considered abnormal. When simultaneous pressure readings are taken from the portal vein and spleen, small differences are found. This discrepancy is magnified when splenic pulp pressure is only slightly elevated. When one is measuring splenic pulp pressure, it is important to confirm fluoroscopically that the recording catheter tip is as close to the hilum of the spleen as possible, especially if cardiac pulsations are not transmitted to the manometer. Also, the lower portion of the manometer should be held at the midaxillary line and the system filled with sterile saline solution, which ensures catheter patency. Failure to obtain satisfactory pressure results is usually attributable to improper intrasplenic positioning of the catheter or clotted blood in the tubing.

Contrast injection studies. Contrast injection studies from this site may yield the following important information: (1) precise location of the site of venous obstruction, (2) establishment of patency and size of the splenic vein, (3) establishment of patency and size of the portal vein if present, (4) identification of major collateral circulation (portal-systemic, portal-pulmonary), and (5) indication of intrahepatic disease (cirrhosis, congenital hepatic fibrosis).

Although the safety of splenoportography has been greatly improved with the availability of flexible Teflon catheters, a 5% to 10% morbidity, including subcapsular hemorrhage, intraperitoneal hemorrhage, and shoulder pain, remains. The procedure does require a general anesthetic, which in itself carries a small but definite risk. The age of the patient is not in itself a contraindication, though adjustments in selection of needle and catheter size and volume of contrast employed should be modified accordingly. The major objection of splenoportography in the very young patient (less than 3 years) applies to the rare situation (perhaps less than 1%) of traumatic splenic rupture and significant hemorrhage, requiring emergency surgery and possible splenectomy. Since the likelihood of establishing a vascular shunt (splenorenal, mesocaval) that will remain patent is remote in this age group (even with improvements in microvascular surgical techniques and intraoperative heparinization), careful consideration to indications for splenoportography are mandatory. Splenectomy without accomplishing a successful shunt anastomosis is often followed by both increased frequency and severity of esophageal hemorrhage.

Another shortcoming of splenoportography is its inability to visualize patency of other venous channels that might be available for shunt surgery, that is, superior mesenteric vein, inferior mesenteric vein, proximal portion of the portal vein, and renal vein. Visualization of these venous drainage systems is best obtained by a selective splanchnic angiography.

On the other hand, much better visualization of the splenic vein and the collateral flow is obtained by splenoportography over that obtained from selective angiography, especially if pronounced splenomegaly is present. In addition, contrast visualization of the portal vein (when one exists) may be equal to or better than that obtained during the venous phase of superior mesenteric artery or celiac artery injection. In exceptional cases significant hepatofugal flow attributable to supra- and intrahepatic causes of portal hypertension can make the assessment of portal vein patency by angiographic studies quite difficult. On the other hand, if a large portal-systemic shunt is present, the portal vein, though patent, may not be visualized by splenoportography. Whenever patency of the portal vein remains in doubt, selective angiography through the superior mesenteric artery should be carried out.

Selective splanchnic angiography. Rapid-sequence films taken immediately after the arterial injection of contrast material provides information about that segment of the portal venous drainage system not adequately revealed by splenoportography. Injection of contrast into the superior mesenteric artery will determine the patency of the superior mesenteric vein, an important point in later surgical considerations. The portal vein (if one exists) is well visualized except in unusual circumstances, when increased hepatofugal flow develops from suprahepatic or intrahepatic causes of portal hypertension. In prehepatic portal hypertension a tortuous conglomeration of vessels may be seen close to the hilum of the liver and constitutes the "cavernomatous transformation" (Fig. 25-5). A large neoportal vein showing hepatopetal flow may easily be misinterpreted as the normal vessel unless attention is paid to the tortuosity and reversal of caliber size of that normally encountered in the portal vein (Fig. 25-6). The portal-systemic collateral circulation through the coronary gastroesophageal drainage system is usually well visualized by angiography, though better films of

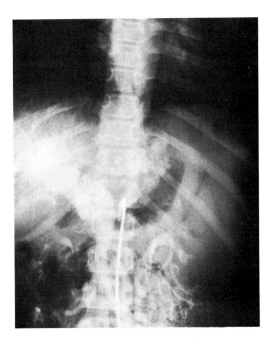

Fig. 25-5. Cavernomatous transformation of the portal vein. Venous phase of injection into the superior mesenteric artery of a 7-year-old girl suspected of having extrahepatic portal hypertension. Note the tortuous agglomeration of vessels at the hilum of the liver, with retrograde filling of the coronary-gastroesophageal collaterals. This child had an unexplained episode of hematemesis at 1 year of age. Splenomegaly was detected at 5 years of age, and she rebled at 6 years of age. An exploratory laparotomy revealed some ascites but no cause for the bleeding. Anemia and esophageal varices were noted at 7 years of age. Physical examination revealed a seemingly healthy child, with splenomegaly being the only positive finding. Liver function tests were normal, as was the wedged hepatic vein pressure (8 mm Hg).

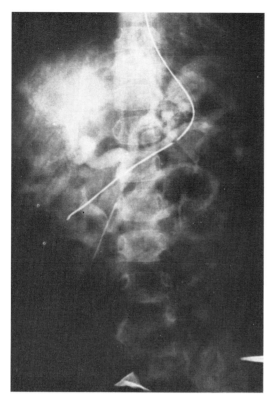

Fig. 25-6. "Neoportal" vein opacified by contrast medium injected into a large mesenteric vein during laparotomy. The location suggests a portal vein, but the tortuous course before reaching the liver hilum and the abnormal intrahepatic venous pattern indicate this structure to be a neocollateral vessel. Also note filling of coronary vein and gastroesophageal drainage system.

this circulation can be obtained by splenoportography.

Selective catheterization of the splenic and hepatic arteries is possible through the celiac artery, and studies obtained from these arterial sites may be useful in ruling out arteriovenous fistulas or other causes of "forward-flow" portal hypertension. The hepatic vascular architecture can also be evaluated from films taken during the sinusoid and venous phase after hepatic artery injection and provide clues as to intrahepatic disease conditions. In the face of substantial splenomegaly, intrasplenic dilution of the contrast material after splenic artery injection often negates the usefulness of this particular study in the evaluation of splenic or portal vein anatomy.

An incidental yield from arteriography performed from any of these sites is information about

the anatomy and vascular supply of the kidneys, again important when surgery is being discussed.

The major complication attending selective angiography is that it requires a femoral arterial puncture. Arterial spasm and vessel thrombosis produces ischemia to the extremity and is a most worrisome event. The risk is greatest in the younger patient (less than 3 years), but even here they can be substantially reduced when the catheterization skills of the pediatric cardiologist are employed.

Wedged hepatic vein pressure. Depending on the age of the child, the hepatic vein is reached by catheterization of either the brachial or the cephalic vein in the arm or the femoral vein in the groin. When the catheter tip is wedged into the hepatic vein (a procedure usually requiring confirmation by a small injection of contrast material), the pressure recorded corresponds to the postsinusoid or sinusoid pressure. In cirrhosis, intrahepatic anastomoses develop, and the wedged hepatic pressure reflects portal vein pressure. The catheter is then withdrawn slightly, and free hepatic vein pressure (normal: 1 to 5 mm Hg) or inferior vena cava pressure is obtained as a reference point. The difference between the wedged and free hepatic vein pressures should be less than 5 mm Hg in normal individuals.

Portal hypertension with normal wedged pressure is indicative of a presinusoidal problem, which may be intrahepatic or extrahepatic in location. Conditions such as congenital hepatic fibrosis, some cases of Wilson's disease, nodular noncirrhotic regenerative hyperplasia, and hepatic schistosomiasis are examples of intrahepatic lesions that result in normal wedged pressure measurements. In these conditions the development of anastomotic connections between small vascular units are such that the wedged catheter does not produce a sufficient degree of venous stasis and therefore fails to appreciate the increased pressure in the portal system. Since the "block" in prehepatic portal hypertension is presinusoidal, both the wedged and free hepatic vein pressure measurement should be normal.

Elevated pressure in the right atrium or supradiaphragmatic or infradiaphragmatic portion of the vena cava, or when the catheter is in the free hepatic vein position, is compatible with suprahepatic portal hypertension. If not previously done, an electrocardiogram and echocardiogram are cer-

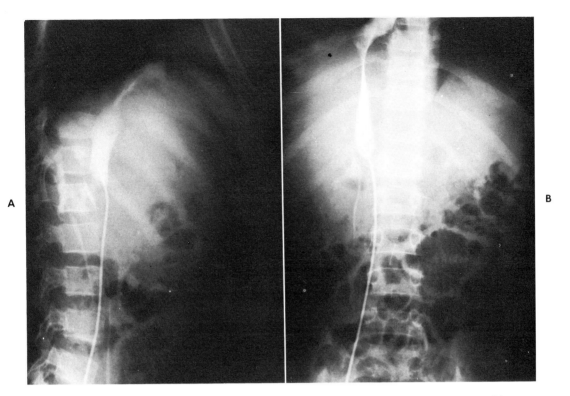

Fig. 25-7. Venacavogram showing infradiaphragmatic compression of the vena cava caused by ascites. **A,** Anteroposterior view. **B,** Lateral projection.

tainly indicated in such cases. Measurement of wedged hepatic vein pressure carries a very low risk, whereas the same cannot be said of a percutaneous liver biopsy when done in the face of suprahepatic portal hypertension. In the absence of ascites, which can produce false-high values, a normal free hepatic vein but elevated wedged hepatic vein pressure should alert the physician to intrahepatic causes of portal hypertension, that is, cirrhosis. Normal vena cava pressure with elevated free hepatic vein and wedged hepatic pressure signifies veno-occlusive disease.

Other roentgenographic investigations

Saphenous venography will allow visualization of the inferior vena cava and any attending pathologic condition. The inferior vena cava may be occluded by an intraluminal web or diaphragm, thrombosis, tumor, or other abnormality, and be responsible for examples of suprahepatic portal hypertension (Budd-Chiari syndrome). The vena cava may also be externally compressed from neighboring tumor growth, hepatic lobar hypertrophy, or ascites, especially at the diaphragmatic

hiatus (Fig. 25-7). Both the presence and patency of the vena cava need ascertainment when a portacaval shunt procedure is being considered. This is especially crucial in cases of extrahepatic biliary atresia requiring shunt surgery, since congenital absence of the infradiaphragmatic portion of the inferior vena cava may coexist.

Percutaneous transhepatic portography using the "skinny needle" has had very limited application in the pediatric age group, and only recently it has been popularized in the evaluation of the adult with portal hypertension. An interesting application of this technique is the treatment of bleeding esophageal varices by selective catheterization of the coronary vein, followed by injection into the vessel of small beads or strips of gel-foam soaked in sodium tetradecyl sulfate.

PREHEPATIC (EXTRAHEPATIC) PORTAL HYPERTENSION

Defect. In prehepatic portal hypertension the obstruction to portal blood flow lies somewhere between the hilum of the liver and the hilum of the spleen. The portal vein may be a fibrous remnant, contain an organized thrombus, be stenotic, contain webs or diaphragms, or be replaced by a multiple collection of small portoportal recanalized collaterals called a "cavernous transformation." Also, in rare cases the obstruction may be caused by external compression from neighboring hyperplastic nodes or neoplastic tissue.

Etiology. The cause of this condition remains obscure in over half the cases. The finding of other anomalies in over 40% of these "idiopathic" cases is suggestive that the portal vein aberration is part of a more widespread *congenital* developmental insult. On the other hand, that portal vein abnormalities and prehepatic portal hypertension are the result of an *acquired* postnatal event, is supported by the observation that this entity is not found in newborn or stillborn infants dying from other causes. Furthermore, the experimental data obtained with animals indicates that the process develops slowly and insidiously, as it does in most pediatric cases, and the entire process cannot be reproduced by simple ligation of the portal vein. If congenital causes were indeed at fault, evidence of portal hypertension should become apparent (at least splenomegaly) within the first year of life, and be detected with greater frequency than that reported in this age group. In fact, the opposite is true; few cases are identified before 1 year, despite the fact that routine child care visits are more frequent during this time.

Specific neonatal events superimposed upon the physiologic process of closure of the umbilical vein and ductus venosus may be responsible for initiating the obliterative process. It is possible that incomplete or segmental closure of the umbilical vein–portal vein–ductus venosus channel might temporarily slow the venous flow, with stasis or sludging of blood within this system. This, in turn, could predispose this area to entrapment of noxious substances, possibly bacteria, which then initiate local endophlebitis, phlebosclerosis, or frank thrombosis of the vessel. In fact, over one third of the cases of prehepatic portal hypertension are believed to be caused by documented neonatal predisposing conditions. Neonatal infections, whether directly involving the umbilical area (omphalitis, peritonitis) or arising from some distant site (sepsis, diarrhea, and dehydration), or the events surrounding the use of umbilical vein catheters have been the most common reported circumstances believed to be responsible for initiating portal vein thrombosis. Although the associa-

tion between indwelling umbilical vein catheters and prehepatic portal hypertension cannot be underestimated, the risk of developing this complication may be dependent on other clinical variables that dictate the need for the use of the catheter. Indeed, in uncomplicated neonates umbilical vein catheterization in the hands of experienced newborn personnel carries a very low risk to the subsequent development of portal hypertension. However, it is not difficult to envision how an umbilical vein catheter may initiate thrombosis or the obliteration process of the portal vein.

First, catheter insertion and passage to the desired location may be difficult, and even relatively gentle forces often cause injury to the endothelial lining of the vessels which in turn may initiate thrombus formation.

Second, the length of time that the catheter remains in place is very important, since thrombi can be identified on the tip of the catheter usually within 12 hours and are always present after 24 hours of constant use. Historically the need for prolonged catheter placement occurs when (1) multiple exchange transfusions in severe hemolytic disease are anticipated, (2) initial difficulty is met in passing the catheter, (3) neonatal conditions requiring a "central line" when umbilical artery or peripheral intravenous sites are not available.

Third, thrombus formation in the main portal vein may occur if the catheter tip resides directly in this undesirable location or from a retrograde process beginning at the junction of the umbilical vein and left portal vein. The likelihood of an umbilical venous catheter lying in the portal venous system rather than in the superior vena cava is enhanced by several factors. Since the umbilical vein outlet and the ductus venosus inlet are frequently offset (the latter to the right) in their alignment, misdirection of the catheter into the left portal vein may occur (Fig. 25-8). In addition, difficulty in gaining entrance into the ductus venosus is attributable to both narrowing and early closure of the proximal end of this structure immediately after birth. To ensure proper placement of the catheter tip, one must obtain a lateral film of the thoracoabdominal anatomy. An anteroposterior film alone cannot be relied on to accurately determine catheter position.

Fourth, also needing consideration in initiating portal vein obliteration is the administration of "high-risk" fluids through the catheter, especially

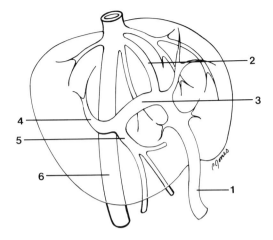

Fig. 25-8. The liver circulation in the human fetus. Note that the umbilical vein is continuous with the left branch of the portal vein. In the fetus, most blood flowing through this system bypasses the liver through the ductus venosus to reach the right side of the heart. Since the ductus venosus is somewhat offset from the line of entry of the umbilical vein, it is not surprising that an umbilical vein catheter can reach the main portal vein. *1,* Umbilical vein; *2,* ductus venosus; *3,* left portal vein; *4,* right portal vein; *5,* main portal vein; *6,* inferior vena cava.

Table 25-1. Experience with 29 cases of extrahepatic portal hypertension*

Clinical features	Number of patients
Sex	
Females	16
Males	13
Age at onset of symptoms	
Under 1 year	5
1 to 5 years	20
Over 5 years	4
Mode of presentation	
Splenomegaly (with or without anemia)	9
Hematemesis and melena	15
Splenomegaly, hematemesis, and melena	5
Neonatal history	
Not remarkable	17
Umbilical vein catheters	
For exchanges	4
For respiratory distress syndrome	4
Gastroenteritis, viral illness, omphalitis	4

*From The Children's Hospital, Denver, University of Colorado Medical Center, and Denver General Hospital.

when the tip is lying in the main portal vein. Hyperosmolar solutions of hypertonic glucose, sodium bicarbonate, calcium gluconate, calcium chloride, antibiotics, and so on may add to the risk of thromboses at this vulnerable site.

Fifth, the relationship between in-dwelling umbilical vein catheters and necrotizing enterocolitis is recognized as cause and effect in some neonates. Perhaps by a somewhat similar mechanism the in-dwelling umbilical catheter lying near the origin of the portal vein causes increased pressure in the splanchnic venous system, which in turn focally disrupts the mucosal integrity in the small and large intestine. A break in the mucosal barrier might result in portal bacteremia, endotoxemia, or other conditions. These toxic products, upon reaching the area of stagnant or altered blood flow, can become ''trapped'' and initiate the process of endophlebitis or frank thrombosis.

One wonders if many of the so-called ''idiopathic'' examples of prehepatic portal hypertension are not in fact the result of one of the mechanisms described in the last example, occurring during the neonatal period but in an unsuspected ''subclinical'' state not requiring umbilical vein catheterization.

These ''idiopathic'' examples of prehepatic portal hypertension are not to be taken lightly, since the strong possibility exists that an underlying congenital anomaly will also be present. Lesions that can influence the patient's subsequent prognosis and future decisions for surgical intervention are not infrequently identified during the course of additional investigations. In particular, congenital heart defects, renal agenesis and vascular anomalies of the vena cava are the most frequently encountered anomalies.

Causes of prehepatic portal hypertension in older children are easier to identify and are caused by such events as abdominal trauma, duodenal ulcer, pancreatitis, parasitic infestation, and localized lymphadenopathy leading to portal venous obstruction.

Clinical features. Most children with prehepatic portal hypertension manifest signs of their disease before 5 years of age. A few are detected before 1 year of age (our youngest was 4 months), but most are between 3 and 5 years of age (Table 25-1). A positive history of neonatal umbilical vein catheterization is frequently obtained when signs develop before 1 year of age.

The major mode of presentation for prehepatic

portal hypertension is either (1) splenomegaly, (2) hematemesis and melena from esophageal varices, or (3) abdominal enlargement from ascites.

Splenomegaly

In prehepatic portal hypertension, splenomegaly is usually discovered during the routine physical examination performed in the course of well-child care. The splenic enlargement is not difficult to detect during careful abdominal examination. However, massive splenomegaly is seldom encountered. Investigative laboratory studies for splenomegaly have been previously described (pp. 757 and 763). Additional clues to the correct diagnosis of prehepatic portal hypertension in the patient with splenomegaly may be gathered from the following historical and physical features: (1) The child looks well. (2) Growth and weight are not severely disturbed. (3) No history of liver disease or jaundice is obtained. (4) There is a history of neonatal illness (omphalitis, sepsis, or dehydration) in 30%. (5) A history of umbilical vein catheterization for exchange transfusion or respiratory distress syndrome is obtained. (6) Physical signs of chronic liver disease are lacking. (7) A history of unexplained, intermittent abdominal distention is found, or the presence of some ascites is detected. (8) There is no family history of liver or kidney disease.

These points are useful in prediction of the location of portal venous obstruction, but some overlap does exist with other causes of portal hypertension.

Hematemesis, melena, or both

Hematemesis may be the first clinical manifestation of prehepatic portal hypertension, or may follow by 1 to 3 years the finding of splenomegaly when it has the same cause. In fact, most cases of prehepatic portal hypertension present with hematemesis or melena for the following reasons. (1) Because most cases are "idiopathic" and neonatal clues are lacking, there is no reason for the physician to suspect evolving portal hypertension. (2) Abdominal palpation may not always be part of the routine examination of infants and children, and the skills of caregivers to detect early enlargement of the spleen may not be sufficiently developed. (3) Marginal splenomegaly, when discovered, may be incompletely investigated or assigned an incorrect cause.

The presentation of hematemesis is usually dramatic. The previously well child suddenly complains of abdominal pain, looks surprisingly pale, and vomits a large amount of bright red blood with clots. Melena is often noted simultaneously or shortly thereafter. About 50% of the time the onset of hematemesis may coincide with an intercurrent upper respiratory infection or bronchitis for which antitussives and salicylate-containing medications have been consumed. The child may become lethargic, show signs of orthostatic hypotension, and is rapidly brought to the attention of those who give medical care. Physical examination of the child with this mode of presentation of prehepatic portal hypertension may be as unremarkable as the past medical history of the patient. If the hemorrhage has been significant, pallor, tachycardia, and even hypotension may be noted. In fact, unless a palpable spleen is present (it may not be detectable immediately after the hemorrhage) or a history of salicylate intake is obtained, the differential diagnosis is really that of an upper gastointestinal bleed. However, if splenomegaly is present, the cause of the upper gastrointestinal bleed in a child is most certainly esophageal varices. That esophageal varices are the source of the present hemorrhage can sometimes be suspected by the large volume of blood contained in the vomitus and the suddenness of the complaint, whereas prehepatic portal hypertension as the underlying cause may be strongly considered from similar queries enumerated for splenomegaly (p. 770).

The necessary investigative studies that will establish esophageal varices as the cause of upper gastrointestinal hemorrhage have been discussed previously (p. 759). Another important observation consistent with prehepatic causes is the absence of signs of encephalopathy, both during and after the gastrointestinal hemorrhage.

Abdominal enlargement (ascites)

The frequency with which abdominal enlargement is the mode of presentation of prehepatic portal hypertention in children is difficult to assess. We continue to observe this clinical clue in up to 30% of cases. When present, a history of transient abdominal enlargement is most frequently reported, though occasionally significant and persistent ascites has been present. This manifestation of prehepatic portal hypertension seems more common in the older child and is seldom noted in the group under 2 to 3 years of age. We and others have noted that transient ascites of moderate degree can follow esophageal hemorrhage and may also occur as a postoperative event.

The clinical detection of abdominal fluid and mechanisms of formation have been previously discussed (pp. 645 and 762).

Generally speaking, when portal hypertension presents as ascites, intrahepatic or suprahepatic causes are much more likely than a prehepatic "block" is.

Laboratory and procedural investigations in prehepatic portal hypertention

Complete blood count and platelet count. Taking these counts will reveal the magnitude of the recent hemorrhage and severity of hypersplenism. Recall, however, that thrombocytosis may follow an acute hemorrhage.

Coagulation studies and bleeding time. The prothrombin time and partial thromboplastin time should be normal. The bleeding time may be prolonged if the patient has been on salicylate-containing products or if the platelet count is severely depressed.

Routine liver function tests. These tests are most often obtained if splenomegaly is present. They generally show normal or minimal elevation of aminotransferase levels.

Total serum protein and albumin-globulin (A/G) ratio. Serum albumin may be low if the variceal hemorrhage has been large.

Fiberoptic endoscopy. Fiberoptic endoscopy should be performed within 24 hours after an unexplained upper esophageal hemorrhage and will identify the source of the bleeding in up to 95% of cases.

Barium contrast esophagram and upper gastrointestinal series. Large varices or a peptic ulcer can be detected by this study. Anterior displacement of the second portion of the duodenum suggesting retroperitoneal edema is noted in prehepatic portal hypertension (Clatworthy's sign) and may be extremely useful information (Fig. 25-9).

Electrocardiogram and echocardiogram. These records should be routinely obtained when unexplained ascites and hepatomegaly are encountered. Specific causes of superhepatic portal hypertension may be identified by these techniques (see p. 791).

Liver biopsy. Liver biopsy is indicated in confusing cases or, at times, to rule out other intra-

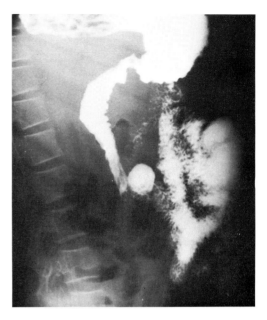

Fig. 25-9. Pronounced retroperitoneal edema (Clatworthy's sign) seen displacing the duodenum anteriorly. This patient is a 15-year-old girl with prehepatic portal hypertension.

hepatic causes of portal hypertension. Histologically the liver is generally normal in prehepatic portal hypertension, but occasionally shows mild portal fibrosis or stellate scars extending in a perilobular manner. Intralobular changes, if present, are subtle and more commonly reported in the "idiopathic" variety of prehepatic portal hypertension.

Splenoportography. If the child has not bled, it is best to wait until he is 3 years of age or older before this procedure is performed. When other compelling reasons exist, splenoportography can be undertaken at an earlier age to confirm the diagnosis and, equally as important, to aid in formulating the proper decisions regarding future treatment of the condition (Fig. 25-10).

Selective arterial angiography. As with splenoportography, this procedure is relatively safe in children over 3 years of age and is crucial before surgery is planned. It will determine patency of the superior mesenteric vein, the presence and extent of involvement of the portal vein, and, by retrograde flow, patency of the splenic vein in selected cases (Fig. 25-11).

Wedged hepatic vein pressures. This study is particularly useful when both above procedures are contraindicated, perhaps because of the patient's

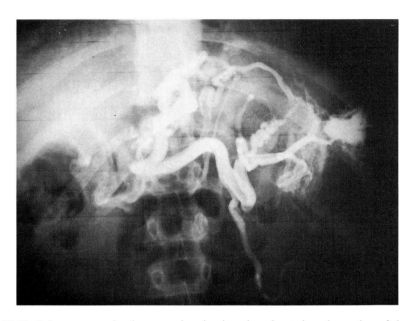

Fig. 25-10. Splenoportography demonstrating the thrombosed extrahepatic portion of the portal vein. Note the exceptional collaterals on the capsule of the spleen and the large coronary-gastric collateral vessel.

young age. Wedged hepatic vein pressures should be sought when suprahepatic causes of portal hypertension are considered as diagnostic possibilities.

Additional comments concerning investigative work-up

Liver function tests. Few reports document slightly elevated bilirubin or dye retention values (BSP test). Serum albumin may be mildly depressed. On rare occasions and later in child's life (some 10 to 15 years into the disease), further deterioration may be reflected both by worsening liver function tests and liver histologic appearance. For unknown reasons, this event is more frequently encountered in the "idiopathic" variety of prehepatic portal hypertension. Transient alteration in results of liver function tests (transaminases) is not unusual after an acute episode of bleeding from esophageal varices. Blood ammonia levels remain normal.

Barium esophagography and upper gastrointestinal series. As mentioned previously, demonstration of varices is dependent on the experience of the radiologist and his familiarity with various maneuvers that make visible the desired structures (thick barium, blowing through a straw, Valsalva maneuver, and so forth). Fifteen percent to 20% of esophageal varices may not be demonstrated by esophagography. If this examination is done dur-

ing or shortly after acute hemorrhage, varices may not be visualized because of contraction of the vascular space. It is important that other causes of upper gastrointestinal tract bleeding be considered by both the physician and the radiologist. Hiatal hernia and a duplication cyst of the esophagus may be found by the esophagogram, but rarely will either be responsible for bleeding of a magnitude similar to that occurring when portal hypertension is present. Whether or not esophageal varices are present, roentgenographic studies should always include careful fluoroscopic examination of the stomach and duodenum. Varices in the cardia of the stomach are not uncommon in this condition and indeed may be more troublesome for some patients than varices in the esophagus. The duodenum should be carefully observed for evidence of peptic disease. Retroperitoneal edema (Clatworthy's sign) should be looked for (Fig. 25-9). This striking finding, which displaces the duodenum anteriorly, is very suggestive of prehepatic portal hypertension. Its presence should alert the surgeon to possible difficulties if a surgical procedure is contemplated.

Clinical course of splenomegaly

Most patients with prehepatic portal hypertension continue to grow and develop normally. The spleen continues to enlarge but is seldom voluminous. Significant complications of splenomeg-

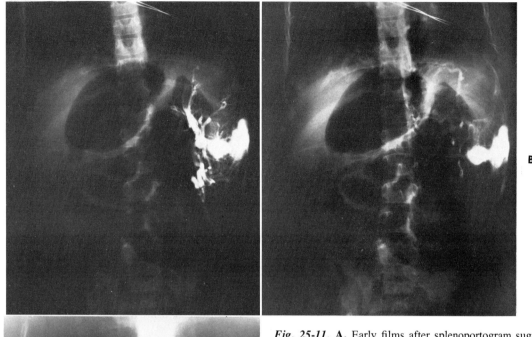

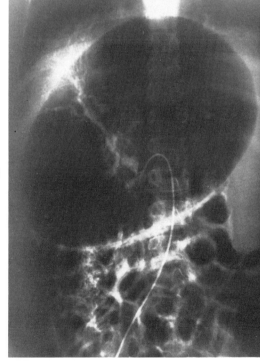

Fig. 25-11. **A,** Early films after splenoportogram suggest a splenic vein occlusion at the hilum of the spleen. **B,** Delayed films show splenogastroesophageal collateral drainage. **C,** Venous phase of selective arteriography (superior mesenteric artery) revealed the cavernomatous transformation of the portal vein but failed to fill the splenic or coronary vein in retrograde fashion. The splenic vein is presumably occluded in its entirety and not suitable in future shunt considerations.

aly are usually a result of direct trauma to the organ with subcapsular or intra-abdominal hemorrhage. Progressive evidence of hypersplenism is noted in follow-up laboratory evaluations, but clinically important symptoms are infrequent. Anemia is seldom striking and not incapacitating, and the leukopenia does not predispose the patient to increased numbers of infections. Thrombocytopenia does not correlate with increased episodes of spontaneous hemorrhage. Cessation of bleeding, however, may be influenced by thrombocyte counts that are less than 50,000/mm^3.

Management of splenomegaly

Most patients require no special care. A regular diet and full activity is allowed, but contact sports are to be avoided in the older school-age child. All patients should be provided with a list of aspirin-containing products to be assiduously avoided (see list below). During the first 10 years of life, neither the enlargement of the spleen nor laboratory evidence of hypersplenism should be taken as indication for splenectomy. As the child becomes older (a teen-ager), indications for surgical intervention may now include the psychologic impact of abdominal enlargement or restricting the child's activity to noncontact sports. Significant platelet count depression (less than 50,000/mm^3), especially when associated with frequent and severe bleeding episodes, or a splenic "crisis" with a sudden reduction in circulating blood elements, are clear-cut indications for splenectomy combined with decompression shunt surgery.

Preparations containing aspirin

A.S.A. (Lilly)
A.S.A. Compound (Lilly)
Alka-Seltzer (Miles)
Alprine Bi Tabs (Ulmer)
*Anacin (Whitehall)
Anodynos-DHC Tablets (Tilden-Yates)
Ascodeen-30 (Burroughs-Wellcome)
Ascriptin (Rorer)
Aspirin
Bayer Aspirin (Glenbrook)
Buff-A Comp (Mayrand)
*Bufferin (Bristol-Myers)
Cirin (Zommer)
Codempiral (Burroughs-Wellcome)
Cope (Glenbrook)

Cordex preparations (Upjohn)
*Coricidin preparations (Schering)
Covangesic (Mallinckrodt)
Daprisal (Smith, Kline and French)
Daragesic (Meyer)
*Darvon Compound (Lilly)
Darvon w/A.S.A. (Lilly)
Demerol w/A.P.C. (Winthrop)
*Dristan (Whithall)
Drocogesic No. 3 (Carrtone)
Ecotrin (Smith, Kline and French)
Empirin preparations (Burroughs-Wellcome)
Emprazil preparations (Burroughs-Wellcome)
Equagesic (Wyeth)
*Excedrin (Bristol-Myers)
*Fiorinal preparations (Sandoz)
Monacet preparations (Rexall)
Nemu-gesic (Abbott)
Norgesic (Riker)
Novahistine w/A.P.C. (Pitman-Moore)
Pabirin Buffered Tablets (Dorsey)
Pentagesic (Kremers-Urban)
Percobarb preparations (Endo)
*Percodan preparations (Endo)
Persistin (Copper)
Phenaphen preparations (Robins)
Phenodyne preparations (Blue Line)
Predisal (Mallard)
Pyrroxate (Upjohn)
Robaxisal preparations (Robins)
Sigmagen (Schering)
Stero Darvon w/A.S.A. (Lilly)
Supac (Mission)
Synalgos preparations (Ives)
Synirin (Poythress)
Tetrex A.P.C. w/Bristamin (Bristol)
Trancogesic (Winthrop)
Vanquish (Glenbrook)
Vingesic (Amid)
Zactirin Compound-100 (Wyeth)

Premature splenectomy with or without shunt surgery often proves to be a disservice to the patient for the following reasons: Failure to use the splenic vein to create a shunt at the time of splenectomy eliminates its future use forever. Except in the most experienced hands, sustained patency of the splenorenal shunt when performed in the patient less than 5 to 8 years is unlikely to be achieved because of small vessel size and resulting thrombosis (Table 25-2). In addition, splenectomy severs those "safe" collaterals that originate from the splenic capsule and bypass the coronary esophageal drainage system, delivering venous blood to the right side of the heart through

*Preparations in common use, whose aspirin content is not widely known.

Table 25-2. Medicosurgical history of 19 cases of prehepatic portal hypertension at The Children's Hospital, Denver, and University of Colorado Medical Center (1965–1975)

Initial surgery	Age at initial surgery (year)	Subsequent course	Type of subsequent operation	Status through 1975
Splenectomy with sple- norenal shunt (9 cases)	7	Bleeding*	Colon interposition	Bleeding × 1
	3	Bleeding	Colon interposition	Dysphagia
	3	Bleeding ⎤	Stripping varices, ligation varices, transection var- ices (esophagus, stom- ach)	Bleeding × 1, hepatitis
	4	Bleeding ⎦		Bleeding × 4, varices
	6	Bleeding	Mesocaval shunt	No bleeding, varices
	10	Bleeding	Mesocaval shunt	No bleeding, no varices
	7	Bleeding	Mesocaval shunt	Bleeding × 1, varices
	12	None		No bleeding, varices
	10	None		No bleeding
Splenectomy without shunt; severe retro- peritoneal edema and ascites (2 cases)	4/12	Sepsis		Died, age 6 months
	7	Bleeding	Mesocaval shunt	Bleeding × 2, varices
Diagnostic laparotomy (with or without liver biopsy) (8 cases)	9/12			No further bleeding (5 years); has sponta- neous shunt
	7	Rebleeding × 3	Mesocaval shunt	No bleeding (4 years)
	10/12	Rebleeding × 1 (3½ yr)		Well
	7	Rebleeding × 2	Splenorenal (side to side) without splenectomy	No bleeding (2 years)
	4	Rebleeding × 2	Laparotomy only (15 years) because of severe retroperitoneal edema	Stable
	5	Transient ascites		Well
	1¼	Rebleeding × 1		Well
	8	Rebleeding × 3		Well

*Episodes refer to gastrointestinal bleeding as either hematemesis or melena.

diaphragmatic-azygous-pulmonary vein anastomoses. Other perisplenic collaterals empty into veins in the retroperitoneal space and then into the inferior vena cava. Venous blood reaching both these venous drainage systems may be derived from the mesenteric venous system. By removal of the spleen and in the absence of successful shunt surgery, this large volume of venous blood flow is then directed into the coronary-esophageal system. It is not surprising therefore that patients having splenectomy but without successful shunt surgery not only bleed more frequently from varices but also with greater severity. Finally, fatal bacterial sepsis is more frequent in splenectomized young children (less than 5 years of age).

Clinical course of acute bleeding episode (see also p. 770)

A curious yet important observation concerning hemorrhage from esophageal varices that seems unique to prehepatic causes of portal hypertension is the frequency with which the initial bleeding episode stops spontaneously or after use of minimal conservative measures. Subsequent bleeding episodes, however, do have a tendency to be more severe. That the bleeding episodes are sporadic and cease spontaneously often contributes to delay in proper diagnosis, particularly if hematemesis is absent. A clustering of bleeding episodes is not infrequently noted during episodes of respiratory illness. This same patient may then experience a prolonged asymptomatic period without

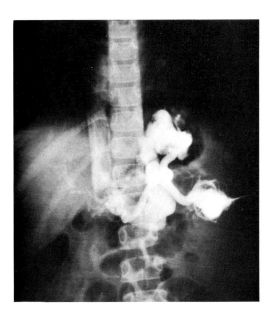

Fig. 25-12. Splenoportography demonstrating a large natural shunt that promptly fills the inferior vena cava, presumably through the left adrenal-renal vein. The portal vein is not visualized. This boy had an episode of severe gastroenteritis in the newborn period with moderate dehydration. At age 9 months he passed tarry stools. Exploratory laparotomy was nonrevealing. Liver biopsy results were normal. At 14 months he rebled, and splenomegaly appeared at 5 years of age. A rebleed occurred at age 7, and esophageal varices were noted. Further surgery is not contemplated.

signs of esophageal bleeding. Occasionally a patient has spontaneous regression of varices in his late teens, probably the result of important neocollateral formation (Fig. 25-12). That patients with prehepatic portal hypertension tolerate bleeding from esophageal varices undoubtedly is best explained by the absence of underlying liver disease. Signs of portal encephalopathy are absent, and only mild transient disturbances of liver function tests appear after the bleeding episodes. Some cases are quite concerning, especially when immediate cessation of bleeding does not occur and thrombocytopenia is present. With recurrent hemorrhage the increased risk to posttransfusion hepatitis, transfusion reactions, and the morbidity associated with even conservative measures to halt the bleeding, including psychologic factors, become dominant. These and other risk factors eventually influence the subsequent discussions regarding surgical management of patients with prehepatic portal hypertension.

Management of acute bleeding episode

One can quickly assess the severity of the hemorrhage by determining the presence or absence of erythema within the palmar creases when the fingers are hyperextended. In the absence of anemia and even in the presence of shock, the palmar creases are bright red in color. Not until the circulating volume of hemoglobin is less than 50% of normal is this sign lost. Tachycardia and systemic hypotension are late signs and indicate shock. Obviously, close monitoring of vital signs and obtainment of serial hematocrit determinations are mandatory once the diagnosis of upper gastrointestinal hemorrhage is considered.

The children are best cared for in an intensive care unit that allows for attentive monitoring of all needed parameters. Blood should also be drawn for type and cross match of 1 to 2 units of fresh whole blood and 1 unit of packed red blood cells. In addition, platelet count should be obtained, as well as coagulation studies and a bleeding time. A large-bore orogastric tube (28 to 32 F Ewald tube) should be placed into the stomach so that irrigations using iced water or half-normal saline solution may be carried out over 20 to 30 minutes. In a slightly older child with a clear sensorium, spraying the posterior pharynx with a local anesthetic (Cetacaine) before insertion of the orogastric or nasogastric tube can prevent gagging and retching, protective reflexes that can enhance the likelihood of rebleeding. In addition, the patient should be kept at at least a 45-degree angle while the tube is in place to prevent cardioesophageal reflux. It is advisable to allow the irrigation fluid to empty by gravity or gentle suction to avoid mucosal injury. If bloody return continues after 30 to 45 minutes of irrigation, this modality can be considered useless and other forms of treatment instituted. Simultaneously, the largest-gauge needle should be placed in the largest accessible peripheral vessel and initial expansion of the vascular space accomplished with normal saline at 10 to 20 ml/kg given over 1 hour. When replacement blood becomes available, this should be given, but care should be exercised to avoid overexpansion of the vascular space because bleeding may recur. A hematocrit of 30 vol% is sufficient. The nasogastric tube should remain in place for 24 hours after bleeding has ceased.

If melena without hematemesis was reported, passage of a smaller-sized nasogastric tube (16 to 18 F) into the stomach for sampling the gastric contents is advisable. If gastric contents are devoid of blood, the site of origin for the gastrointestinal bleeding may be difficult to localize without endoscopic evaluation.

Should severe thrombocytopenia be present, platelet transfusions may be required to stop the bleeding by improving clot retraction. Once the patient is in a stable condition, preparations to examine the patient with a fiberoptic flexible endoscope should be made. Panendoscopy will allow identification of the lesion or lesions that are still actively bleeding or oozing and, one would hope, identification of any other possible conditions that might explain the hemorrhage.

If, after the above measures, the upper gastrointestinal bleeding remains significant, that is, requiring more than a range of 10 to 15 ml/kg of blood during the first 8 hours, a central venous catheter should be inserted (if not previously done) and the surgical team should be alerted to the possibility that a surgical procedure may have to be done. Vasopressin (Pitressin) administered by slow intravenous infusion at a dose of 0.2 to 0.4 unit/1.73 m^2/min often leads to a slowing or cessation of the bleeding within 20 to 40 minutes in patients with prehepatic portal hypertension. Present data fails to show any advantage to the infusion of vasopressin through the superior mesenteric artery over its administration by a peripheral vein. Vasopressin causes a decrease in splanchnic-bed arterial flow, and a dramatic lowering of portal pressure follows. However, undesirable side effects include hypertension, bradycardia, arrhythmias, hyponatremia, and seizures from significant water retention: therefore patients need to be closely monitored.

Failure of intravenously administered vasopressin to control the esophageal hemorrhage, or complications precluding its continued use, is an indication that balloon tamponade with a pediatric Sengstaken-Blakemore (SB) tube should be attempted. The successful application of this therapeutic measure requires selection of the proper tube size, previous experience with the device, and diligent nursing care. The SB tube is a triple-lumen tube to which an esophageal and gastric balloon are attached. These can be individually inflated and their volumes checked before passage. The third lumen opens as side holes at the distal end of the tube permitting aspiration of intragastric contents (Fig. 25-13). The tube should be passed through the mouth and into the stomach, wherein

the gastric balloon is inflated, depending on its size, with 25 to 100 cc of air and gently withdrawn until resistance is encountered at the gastroesophageal junction. This can also be ascertained by fluroscopic control. The esophageal balloon is then slowly inflated by use of an airtight blood pressure manometer system to a range of 30 to 40 mm Hg (adults use 40 to 60 mm Hg). This should be done slowly so as to avoid further mucosal injury overlying the varices. The intragastric portion of the tube should be connected to a system that drains by gravity rather than by negative pressure. The passage of an additional small-size tube located just proximal to the esophageal balloon allows swallowed secretions to be aspirated. The SB tube, when correctly selected for patient size and properly deployed, is most effective in stopping esophageal bleeding (85% of cases) in patients with prehepatic portal hypertension. Complications in the use of this device can be life threatening and almost always are attributable to malpositioning of the tube and balloons causing upper airway obstruction. Traction upon the tube should be avoided because migration of the esophageal balloon portion of the tube into the hypopharynx may occur. This may also happen should the gastric balloon fail to remain inflated. Furthermore, both increased discomfort and secretions invariably accompany traction on the SB tube. Care should be taken to avoid abrupt changes or excessive esophageal pressures, either of which may result in esophageal perforation or restart the hemorrhage. Failure to properly take care of the upper esophagus and hypopharynx invariably results in aspiration of swallowed secretions, increased cough, and respiratory distress.

Continued bleeding in the face of a well-positioned inflated esophageal balloon suggests gastric varices as the likely source. The SB tube is usually ineffective in stopping bleeding from this site because of the small size of the gastric balloon volume and the lack of traction. The Linton-Nachlas tube is better suited for treating gastric varices, at least in adults, since the balloon volume is close to 600 cc and traction may be utilized.

The esophageal balloon is decompressed every 12 to 24 hours and the stomach is gently irrigated through the intragastric portion of the tube for checking signs of rebleeding. Should this occur, the esophageal balloon is once again reinflated for an additional 6 to 8 hour time period. The lowest

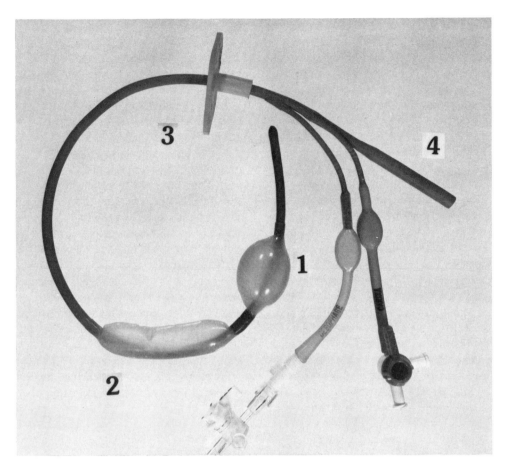

Fig. 25-13. Sengstaken-Blakemore tube for pediatric use. *1*, Gastric balloon; *2*, esophageal balloon; *3*, mouth guard; *4*, proximal end of gastric tube. The gastric and esophageal pressures can be continuously monitored when the stopcock attachments are connected to a pressure transducer recording system.

esophageal balloon pressure that is required to obtain cessation of bleeding should be employed. Up to 24 hours of occlusion time may be tolerated without significant damage to the esophageal mucosa. A greater problem is lack of compliance and patient cooperation with this very uncomfortable specialized tube. Sedation with intravenously administered diazepam or morphine is helpful but is not without risk. As a precaution, the deflated tube should remain in place for an additional 12 to 24 hours after bleeding has ceased.

Treatment of any associated respiratory infection and attendant symptoms is important to reduce the chances of bleeding. Codeine can be used to suppress the cough.

The direct obliteration of the bleeding varix using a sclerosing solution (sodium moruate, ethanolamine oleate) is indicated in the emergency treatment of refractory bleeding. The procedure is also beneficial in special instances as a prophylactic treatment measure. This technique (endosclerosis) requires a specially constructed, slightly oversized rigid pediatric esophagoscope that allows isolation of the varix in the slotted portion of the esophagoscope. While prolapsed into the lumen of the instrument, the varix is accessible for injection by use of a long specialized needle with the sclerosing solution (Fig. 25-14). Only those varices at the gastroesophageal junction need be injected, and the procedure can be repeated every 2 to 4 weeks until all varices at this location are obliterated. An unfortunate complication with this technique is esophageal stricture, which may require gentle dilatation, but not until all remaining varices have been sclerosed. Endosclerosis has been extremely effective in controlling esophageal

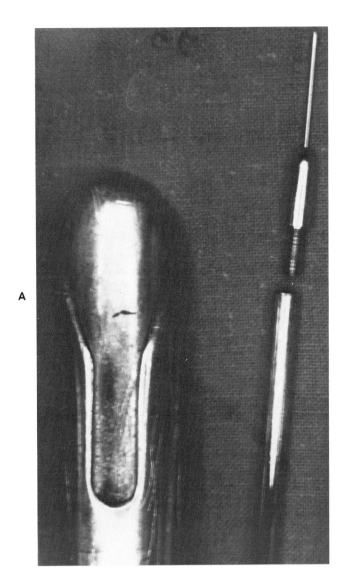

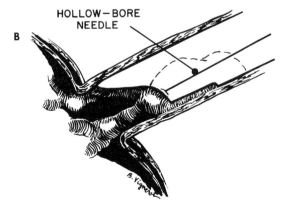

Fig. 25-14. **A,** Specially slotted rigid esophagoscope and hollow-bore needle holder and needle used in sclerotherapy. **B,** Diagrammatic in situ visualization of an esophageal varix "trapped" in the slot of the esophagoscope and being injected.

hemorrhage when other modalities have failed. Recent prospective controlled trials in adults using the flexible fiberoptic endoscope have reported favorable results.

In desperate situations direct variceal ligation may be necessary. Although providing only temporary benefit, this mode of therapy is preferable to emergency splenectomy and attempted shunt surgery in the child under 3 years of age. The percutaneous transhepatic portal vein catheterization technique under radiologic control can be used to deliver fibrin or Gelfoam pellets soaked in sodium tetradecylsulfate into the coronary-gastroesophageal drainage system, and this technique has application only if this communication exists, an unlikely event in prehepatic portal hypertension. Although of unproved value in esophageal hemorrhage because of varices, cimetidine, which does reduce hepatic blood flow and gastric acidity, may be used in this form of bleeding. Somatostatin and propranolol are currently being evaluated in adults as other modalities to lower portal pressures in the face of esophageal hemorrhage.

Clinical course and management of ascites

Most often the appearance of ascites in patients with prehepatic portal hypertension is a transient event occurring before or after esophageal bleeding. In those individuals in which the ascites seems more persistent, a reduction in dietary sodium intake and the use of either hydrochlorothiazine (Hydrodiuril) at a dose of 130 mg/1.73 m^2 or furosemide (Lasix) at a dose of 1 to 2 mg/kg is usually effective in mobilizing the fluid. Unusually severe cases may require paracentesis especially if respiratory distress exists. There appears to be no positive correlation between the development of ascites and deterioration of liver function in patients with prehepatic portal hypertension.

Indications for surgical shunt procedures in prehepatic portal hypertension

One starts with the assumption that for many patients with prehepatic portal hypertension the use of conservative measures in the management of the bleeding episodes is consistent with a long-term prognosis that is usually very good. Therefore only compelling indications for surgery should be admissible in the discussion of definitive shunt procedures. The natural history of the bleeding episodes from esophageal varices in prehepatic portal hypertension gives support to the antici-

pated favorable outcome for many patients. That the patients have decreasing episodes of bleeding as they get older has been repeatedly observed. Most patients in fact never rebleed after reaching 18 to 20 years of age. Not only may bleeding episodes eventually diminish, but also spontaneous cessation of bleeding from varices is common, and death from exsanguination is quite unusual. Over the past 15 years we have not had a single death attributed to esophageal hemorrhage in patients with prehepatic portal hypertension. Provided that the bleeding stops, they tolerate the episode reasonably well. Encephalopathy does not occur since liver function is basically intact.

Any serious discussion of shunt surgery seems inappropriate at least until after the first bleed. Even then, a palliative surgical procedure (sclerotherapy) may be appropriately considered, especially in the younger child. Following are important indications that may determine early surgical intervention in patients: (1) Recurrent life-threatening hemorrhage because of (proved) esophageal varices. (2) Geographic considerations for those living great distances from primary emergency services or in areas underserved by emergency medical services, so that concern about early stabilization of the patient or lack of blood banking facilities exists; the unavailability of an organized rapid-transport system may be an important factor. (3) When splenectomy is being contemplated, be it for severe thrombocytopenia or traumatic rupture, or in an older child for prophylactic prevention of this occurrence, a portal-systemic shunt should be planned to be carried out simultaneously. (4) If the patient has a rare blood type, difficulty in cross-matching because of previous sensitization, or transfusion reactions are frequent, early surgical intervention becomes pressing.

However, shunt surgery should not be considered unless one is completely confident about the competency, experience, and previous results of the person delegated the task of performing this highly technical microvascular surgery. Referral to a regional pediatric center for such surgery is usually necessary. As often occurs, the patient with prehepatic portal hypertension has a limited number of available vessels that can be successfully used to construct a portal-systemic shunt. Wastage of any of these options by inadequate surgical skills should be assiduously avoided. Small vessel size (less than 1 cm in diameter), previously associated with a high likelihood of thrombosis and shunt closure, is presently a less compelling contraindication when surgery is performed by experienced and competent personnel. Finally, shunt surgery should not be undertaken until the patient has been completely investigated as previously discussed. Emergency surgical shunt procedures carry with them a high morbidity and mortality figure, and it is better to consider palliative but temporary stopgap measures in these unusual circumstances.

The selection of the specific shunt procedure will depend on the caliber of available veins that drain the portal venous system, the presence or absence of the left kidney, the presence or absence of significant retroperitoneal edema, consequences of previous surgical attempts in alleviating this condition, and again the experience of the surgical team. Previously, various procedures, conventional or makeshift, have been employed with overall poor results. Only recently the combination of microvascular surgery, intraoperative heparinization (a controversial point), and confirmation of the patency of the shunt before the abdomen is closed have resulted in a high likelihood of shunt patency. Some surgeons prefer to continue heparinization of the patient for up to 1 week postoperatively either intravenously or subcutaneously. Shunt patency is better evaluated during the operation by angiography rather than by measurment of pressure gradients across the anastomotic site. When small vessels have been employed in the creation of the shunt, significant differences in pressure may not be appreciated immediately thereafter. The group from Bicêtre (near Paris) reported that, of 26 children subjected to a splenorenal shunt (21 under 10 years of age), shunt occlusion rate was only 15%. Amazingly a number of the children were under 4 years of age, and splenic vein size in many measured only 3 to 5 mm in diameter. From this data it appears that age itself may become less important a determining factor in influencing the timing of surgical decisions. Unfortunately these good results have not been duplicated by other surgical teams. The frequency of thrombosis in splenorenal shunts, for example, is reported at 50% to 80% in most reports.

The mesocaval shunt (Clatworthy-Marion) remains popular in many United States centers. Before undertaking this procedure, results of superior mesenteric angiography must be available to ensure patency of the superior mesenteric vein.

On occasion the original thrombus or obliterative process in the area of the portal vein extends retrograde down into the superior mesenteric vein. In this procedure the superior mesenteric vein is then anastomosed to the inferior vena cana with the spleen being left in situ. The presence of retroperitoneal edema (Clatworthy's sign) often contraindicates use of this operative procedure, since "strangulation" of the shunt may occur. Varicosities of the lower extremities with mild pedal edema infrequently follows the mesocaval shunt. The interposition mesocaval shunt has been advocated by some groups using either a Teflon or knitted Dacron graft to bridge the vessels. More recently a segment of external jugular vein has been a better choice for the interposition graft material. Some surgeons prefer the mesocaval technique as the primary shunt procedure, whereas others reserve its use when other anastomoses cannot be successfully created.

A portacaval shunt, if at all possible, would certainly be the procedure of choice. Unfortunately, most patients with prehepatic portal hypertension have blockage of the portal vein, and this vessel is unavailable for the usual shunting procedures. On rare occasion a "neoportal" vessel of large size may be connected into the vena cava.

Finally, the distal splenorenal shunt (Warren's procedure), which has the advantage of leaving the spleen intact, has not gained much popularity in the pediatric age patient with portal hypertension.

Postoperatively, patency of the shunt can be assumed by the absence of esophageal bleeding and confirmed by fiberoptic endoscopy, which shows reduction in variceal size or their disappearance. It is helpful to document these observations by photography. Selective angiography from the superior mesenteric artery will positively confirm the patency of a splenorenal shunt by retrograde filling during the venous phase. A mesocaval shunt can be assessed for patency by a splenoportogram if this organ is still available.

Esophagogastrectomy, with or without colonic interposition (Sugiura's precedure), and variceal ligation are again considered stopgap measures at best, and bleeding commonly recurs. It is postulated that similar short-term benefits can be expected from the simpler procedure of endosclerosis of the varices. The long-term likelihood of recurrence of hemorrhage is often dictated as much by the natural history of variceal hemorrhage in prehepatic portal hypertension as by the particular surgical procedure selected.

Protein restriction is seldom necessary after creation of a portal systemic shunt in patients with prehepatic portal hypertension. Because an acute portal encephalopathy may follow large protein dietary indiscretions, caution should be exercised to prevent an excessive intake of this food substance.

REFERENCES

Batson, O.V.: The function of the vertebral veins and their role in the spread of metastases, Ann. Surg. **112:**138-149, 1940.

Bismuth, H., and Franco, D.: Portal diversion for portal hypertension in early childhood, Ann. Surg. **183:**439-447, 1976.

Bosch, J., Kravetz, D., and Rodes, J.: Effects of somatostatin on hepatic and systemic hemodynamics in patients with cirrhosis of the liver: comparison with vasopressin, Gastroenterology **80:**518-525, 1981.

Burchell, A.R., Moreno, A.H., Panke, W.F., and Nealon, T.F., Jr.: Hemodynamic variables and prognosis following portacaval shunts, Surg. Gynecol. Obstet. **138:**359-369, 1974.

Denison, E.K., Peters, R.L., and Reynolds, T.B.: Portal hypertension in a patient with osteopetrosis, Arch. Intern. Med. **128:**279-283, 1971.

Donovan, A.J., Reynolds, T.B., Mikkelsen, W.P., and Peters, R.L.: Systemic-portal arteriovenous fistulas: pathological and hemodynamic observations in two patients, Surgery **66:**474-482, 1969.

Drapanas, T.: Interposition mesocaval shunt for treatment of portal hypertension, Ann. Surg. **176:**435-448, 1972.

Ehrlich, F., Pipatanagul, S., Sieber, W.K., and Kiesewetter, W.B.: Portal hypertension: surgical management in infants and children, J. Pediatr. Surg. **9:**283-287, 1974.

Fonkalsrud, E.W., and Longmire, W.P.: Reassessment of operative procedures for portal hypertension in infants and children, Am. J. Surg. **118:**148-156, 1969.

Gleason, W.A., Jr., Tedesco, F.J., Keating, J.P., and Goldstein, P.D.: Fiberoptic gastrointestinal endoscopy in infants and children, J. Pediatr. **85:**810-813, 1974.

Grundfest, S., Cooperman, A.M., Ferguson, R., and Benjamin, S.: Portal hypertension associated with systemic mastocytosis and splenomegaly, Gastrointerology **78:**370-373, 1980.

Helikson, M.A., Shapiro, D.L., and Seashore, J.H.: Hepatoportal arteriovenous fistula and portal hypertension in an infant, Pediatrics **60:**921-924, 1977.

Johnson, A.O., Obisesan, A.O., and Williams, A.O.: Extrahepatic portal hypertension due to congenital obstruction of the portal vein and associated gross hepatic lobulation, Clin. Pediatr. **18:**619-621, 1979.

Johnson, W.C., Widrich, W.C., Ansell, J.E., and others: Control of bleeding varices by vasopressin: a prospective randomized study, Ann. Surg. **186:**369-376, 1977.

Johnston, G.W., and Gibson, J.B.: Portal hypertension resulting from splenic arteriovenous fistulae, Gut **6:**500-502, 1965.

Lauridsen, U.B., Enk, B., and Gammeltoft, A.: Oesophageal varices as a late complication to neonatal umbilical vein catheterization, Acta Paediatr. Scand. **67:**633-636, 1978.

Levine, O.R., Harris, R.C., Blanc, W.A., and Mellins, R.B.: Progressive pulmonary hypertension in children with portal hypertension, J. Pediatr. **83:**964-972, 1973.

Lilly, J.R.: Endoscopic sclerosis of esophageal varices, Surgery **152:**513-514, 1981.

Malt, R.A., Nabseth, D.C., Orloff, M.J., and Stipa, S.: Portal hypertension—1979, N. Engl. J. Med. **301:**617-618, 1979.

Martin, L.W.: Changing concepts of management of portal hypertension in children, J. Pediatr. Surg. **7:**559-564, 1972.

Martin, L.W.: A different approach permitting portal-systemic shunt for extrahepatic portal thrombosis, Aust. N.Z. J. Surg. **42:**123-125, 1972.

Melhem, R.E., and Rizk, G.K.: Splenoportographic evaluation of portal hypertension in children, J. Pediatr. Surg. **5:**522-526, 1970.

Odièvre, M., Pige, G., and Alagille, D.: Congenital abnormalities associated with extrahepatic portal hypertension, Arch. Dis. Child. **52:**383-385, 1977.

Odom, L.F., and Tubergen, D.G.: Splenomegaly in children: identifying the cause, Postgrad. Med. **65:**191-200, 1979.

Pitlik, S., Cohen, L., Hadar, H., and others: Portal hypertension and esophageal varices in hemangiomatosis of the spleen, Gastroenterology **72:**937-940, 1977.

Reynolds, R.G.F.: Occlusion of the hepatic veins in man, Medicine **38:**369-402, 1959.

Reynolds, T.B.: Interrelationships of portal pressure, variceal size and upper gastrointestinal bleeding, Gastroenterology **79:**1332-1339, 1980.

Rosch, J., and Dotter, C.T.: Extrahepatic portal obstruction in childhood and its angiographic diagnosis, Am. J. Roentgenol. **112:**143-149, 1971.

Rosen, M.S., and Reich, S.B.: Umbilical venous catheterization in the newborn: identification of correct positioning, Radiology **95:**335-340, 1970.

Schaefer, J, Bramschreiber, J., Mistilis, S., and Schiff, L.: Gastroesophageal variceal bleeding in the absence of hepatic cirrhosis or portal hypertension, Gastroenterology **46:**583-588, 1964.

Smith-Laing, G., Camilo, M.E., Dick, R., and Sherlock, S.: Percutaneous transhepatic portography in the assessment of portal hypertension, Gastroenterology **78:**197-205, 1980.

Sonnenberg, G.E., Keller, U., Perruchoud, A., and others: Effect of somatostatin on splanchnic hemodynamics in patients with cirrhosis of the liver and in normal subjects, Gastroenterology **80:**526-532, 1981.

Sugiura, M., and Futagawa, S.: Further evaluation of the Sugiura procedure in the treatment of esophageal varices, Arch. Surg. **112:**1317-1321, 1977.

Sullivan, A., Rheinlander, H., and Weintraub, L.R.: Esophageal varices in agnogenic myeloid metaplasia: disappearance after splenectomy, Gastroenterology **66:**429-432, 1974.

Symansky, M.R., and Fox, H.A.: Umbilical vessel catheterization: indications, management and evaluation of the technique, J. Pediatr. **80:**820-826, 1972.

Terblanche, J., Northover, J.M.A., Bornman, P., and others: A prospective evaluation of injection sclerotherapy in the treatment of acute bleeding from esophageal varices, Surgery **85:**239-245, 1979.

Teres, J., Cecilia, A., Bordas, J.M., and others: Esophageal tamponade for bleeding varices, Gastroenterology **75:**566-569, 1978.

Witte, C.L., Cung, Y.C., Witte, M.H., and others: Observations on the origin of ascites from experimental extrahepatic portal congestion, Ann. Surg. **170:**1002-1015, 1969.

Witte, M.H., Witte, C.L., and Dumont, A.E.: Estimated net transcapillary water and protein flux in the liver and intestine of patients with portal hypertension from hepatic cirrhosis, Gastroenterology **80:**265-272, 1981.

INTRAHEPATIC PORTAL HYPERTENSION (PERISINUSOIDAL)

The discussion of intraheptic causes of portal hypertension includes the categories of disease that alter resistance to vascular flow principally at the sinusoidal or immediate postsinusoidal level. It includes almost all forms of cirrhosis, as well as intrahepatic conditions that primarily affect presinusoidal blood flow. Those intrahepatic but postsinusoidal causes of portal hypertension (veno-occlusive disease) are traditionally assigned to the larger category of ''suprahepatic'' causes.

The major challenges presented by intrahepatic causes of portal hypertension emanate from those examples of cirrhosis having an insidious evolution and from presinusoidal conditions wherein the underlying liver disease is seldom suspected before manifestations of portal hypertension. Clues that intrahepatic liver disease exists are sometimes obtained from detailed history taking appropriate for the specific mode of presentation of portal hypertension (see the discussion of clinical manifestations of portal hypertension, p. 757). Underlying familial liver disease may be suggested when similar disease exists in another family member, or if consanguinity is present. Most often the carefully performed physical examination reveals important findings to suggest cirrhosis, even when the liver disease has been insidiously progressive. This is especially true if signs of portal hypertension are present.

In contrast, presinusoidal causes are classically noncirrhotic and therefore extrahepatic manifestations of cirrhosis are absent on physical examination. However, careful palpation of the liver often reveals some degree of hepatomegaly, an important finding that suggests an abnormality within the liver parenchyma.

When intrahepatic liver disease cannot be appreciated from history taking and physical examination, the selection and sequence of the investigative studies required to elucidate the cause of portal hypertension, as well as to localize the site of the ''block,'' should follow the discussion starting on p. 763. Even if results of preliminary studies confirm the existence of portal hypertension and establish that the site of the block is within the liver, one cannot assume that cirrhosis exists. The diagnosis must be confirmed by a surgical liver biopsy whenever possible.

The importance of making an accurate diagnosis stems from the different clinical course and long-term prognosis that pertains to cirrhotic and noncirrhotic conditions. Furthermore, decisions about surgical treatment of portal hypertension, when it has intrahepatic causes, will be strongly influenced by the specific disease condition. In general, the clinical approach will also be totally different if signs of portal hypertension develop in a child with known and progressive liver disease. The challenge in these patients is rather identifying a cause, especially those with genetic impact, instituting proper therapy whenever possible for both the patient and affected but asymptomatic siblings, treating episodes of upper gastrointestinal bleeding (from varices), and managing ascites. Since the site of the ''block'' is usually obvious in patients with cirrhosis, specific studies to further localize it are seldom necessary. A great problem in this group of patients involves the place of surgery as a means of treating severe *symptoms* of portal hypertension. In children with presinusoidal intrahepatic liver disease, the major problems are those of treating the acute bleeding episodes and timing of the eventual shunt surgery.

Portal hypertension with cirrhosis

Development of portal hypertension with its attendant signs of splenomegaly, esophageal varices, and ascites is a regular feature that eventually complicates the course of cirrhosis of the liver. The process of cirrhosis results in disruption of the normal hepatic architecture by the combination of fibrosis and lobular regeneration, scarring and collapse, events that distort the intrahepatic vasculature and thereby increase vascular resistance within the liver. Elevated wedged hepatic vein pressure has been taken as evidence that the vascular consequence of cirrhosis is felt more at the sinusoidal level than at the presinusoidal level, but the observed pressure elevation in these cases also reflects portal vein pressure. Indeed, simultaneous measurements of wedged hepatic vein pressure and portal pressure yield similar values in most forms of cirrhosis (postnecrotic, alcoholic, and so-called cryptogenic).

Of pediatric patients with portal hypertension, 75% to 90%, have cirrhosis of the liver as the primary cause. Of these, the majority have a positive history that aids in specific diagnosis, that is, neonatal hepatitis, extrahepatic biliary atresia, severe viral hepatitis, Wilson's disease, cystic fibrosis, and other metabolic causes of cirrhosis. With the exception of cystic fibrosis and some examples of Wilson's disease, each of these entities is usually recognized during its active phase. However, one needs to recall that certain liver diseases may have a subclinical course and progress insidiously, and patients with such diseases are devoid of symptoms. The first clue that an underlying intrahepatic problem exists comes late in the illness when the signs of portal hypertension (splenomegaly, esophageal varices, ascites, or a combination of these) become manifest. Cirrhosis associated with alpha-1-antitrypsin disease, hepatitis B virus disease, Wilson's disease, and cystic fibrosis typifies this group. A more complete discussion of chronic liver disease associated with cirrhosis is discussed in Chapter 24.

Diagnosis. By definition, cirrhosis of the liver is a pathologic condition characteristic of end-stage liver disease. It follows therefore that liver tissue, preferably obtained by surgery, should be available for final diagnosis. Obviously, when signs of portal hypertension develop in a patient being followed with known liver disease, in either the active or inactive phase of its progression, cause and effect can be correctly assigned with little hesitation. If findings of portal hypertension antedate the diagnosis of cirrhosis, careful attention to details of the history and physical examination usually reveals evidence that underlying liver disease exists (see Chapter 24). Cirrhosis may be strongly suspected if signs of hepatic or portal encephalopathy are observed, especially after an upper gastrointestinal hemorrhage.

Nonspecific but abnormal laboratory studies suggestive of cirrhosis include prolonged retention of the sulfobromophthalein, especially in conjunction with low serum albumin levels and a prolonged prothrombin time. Mild elevations of transaminases are not unusual, whereas the serum bilirubin may be normal. The finding of an elevated 2-hour postprandial serum bile acid level has been taken as evidence of underlying chronic liver disease. Where appropriate, specific laboratory studies to rule out insidious causes of cirrhosis should be obtained. Tests or determinations of serum ceruloplasmin, alpha-1-antitrypsin level, HBsAg, sweat chloride, and 24-hour quantitative urine copper are helpful in this regard.

Results of investigative studies for portal hypertension highly suggestive of cirrhosis include (1) an elevated wedged but normal free hepatic vein pressure, (2) angiographic appearance of intrahepatic arteries showing a "tree in winter" look, with "corkscrew" changes of the terminal vessels, (3) absence of hepatopetal collateral circulation, and (4) enlargement of the hepatic artery with distortion of the intrahepatic branches around suspected regenerating nodules.

Course and management. Proper management of patients with portal hypertension caused by cirrhosis cannot be generalized. The need for making a specific etiologic diagnosis is obvious, for certain entities require specific medical therapy (Wilson's disease, galactosemia, fructose intolerance, chronic active hepatitis). This has been reinforced by reports indicating that the liver abnormality may be greatly improved by early institution of specific drug therapy in Wilson's disease.

As in prehepatic portal hypertension, splenomegaly and hypersplenism rarely need specific surgical attention unless they are severe or if hemorrhage occurs.

The management of ascites is discussed in Chapter 24.

Medical management of bleeding from esophageal varices has been discussed under prehepatic portal hypertension. Patients with cirrhosis tolerate gastrointestinal bleeding poorly; should hepatic coma ensue, various maneuvers, many of which are alluded to in Chapter 23, may be useful. Sudden decompensation of liver function may herald ascites also as a consequence of upper gastrointestinal tract hemorrhage.

Surgical treatment for the patients is temporizing at best but may improve the immediate quality of life. In properly selected patients, preferably with quiescent disease, significant and disabling complications of portal hypertension may be treated by portacaval shunting. The conventional proximal splenorenal shunt may be employed in cases of intrahepatic portal hypertension but serves no apparent advantage over a portacaval shunt, while posing some potential disadvantages at least for the pediatric-age patient. The splenorenal shunt is technically somewhat more difficult because the vessels are of relatively small size, and it thereby predisposes to thrombosis of the anastomosis. Secondly, in this procedure the surgeon must sacrifice the spleen and sever "safe" collaterals that arise from the splenic capsule. Furthermore, the caliber of the shunt created by the splenorenal anastomosis enlarges with time and hemodynamically becomes a total portal-bypass channel. Anatomically, the end-to-side portacaval shunt is easier to accomplish and is best for control of esophageal variceal bleeding, whereas the side-to-side type is best for ascites. Generally speaking, the results of end-to-side portacaval shunt and the traditional splenorenal shunt are similar in regard to the immediate postoperative mortality, long-term survival, and the subsequent development of hepatic encephalopathy.

A lower incidence of portal encephalopathy (5% to 18%) is being reported in adult cirrhotics after a selective, distal splenorenal shunt (Warren's procedure). Data in pediatric patients with this particular shunt are unavailable. The procedure is gaining in popularity, especially in treatment of portal hypertension when intrahepatic but presinusoidal causes exist, especially schistosomiasis.

Although long-term survival figures in cirrhotic patients are not improved by any of these surgical maneuvers, episodes of esophageal hemorrhage are definitely eliminated or reduced in most all cases.

Emergency operations done during or immediately after a gastrointestinal bleed have an exceedingly high mortality (up to 50%), whereas elective shunt surgery in cirrhotics carries a 20% mortality figure. Attempts to reduce these impressive figures by careful selection of candidates for portal decompression surgery have been most difficult. Hemodynamic studies of the portal circulation to confirm the presence of hepatofugal flow rather than hepatopetal flow have been unreliable in predicting the final outcome. Recent data suggest that hepatic artery hemodynamics may have prognostic value. A higher cumulative survival rate has been reported if hepatic artery flow increases significantly during intraoperative clamping of the portal vein.

Definite contraindications to conventional splenorenal or portacaval shunts include (1) presence of ascites, (2) history of hepatic or portal encephalopathy, and (3) an established diagnosis of Wilson's disease. Other high-risk markers include active liver disease evidenced by elevated transaminases levels, and the need for multiple blood transfusions (usually associated with prolonged prothrombin time). The increased likelihood of hepatic failure after portacaval shunting correlates best with ongoing activity of liver disease, but other unidentified variables are also important. Patients with Wilson's disease are particularly prone to rapid deterioration of liver function.

The decision to perform a surgical decompression shunt in a child with cirrhosis of the liver remains extremely difficult even in the best of circumstances, since any of the shunt procedures carries with it a sizable mortality both during the operation and in the postoperative period. Besides hepatic failure, aspiration pneumonia and sepsis are not infrequent complications in these poor-risk patients. Although control of distressing and often incapacitating symptoms of portal hypertension can be expected from successful shunt surgery at least in the older child, the patient's overall survival will not be prolonged. Symptoms of postoperative portal encephalopathy can be obviated by use of a protein-restricted diet, at least during the first 4 to 6 postoperative months.

Portal hypertension without cirrhosis

Most patients with intrahepatic portal hypertension but without cirrhosis have a clinical picture indistinguishable from that observed in patients with the "idiopathic" variety of prehepatic portal hypertension. Some are infants or older children who appear in good physical health and by chance are found to have hepatomegaly or an enlarged spleen, or both. Others suddenly present with hematemesis from esophageal varices. Should hepatosplenomegaly be present in such cases, intrahepatic disease is suspected and liver biopsy is subsequently undertaken. The specific diagnosis is established after histologic examination of the tissue.

When splenomegaly is the only clinical abnormality detected during routine physical examination, screening studies to evaluate this sign of portal hypertension eventually lead to splenoportography for pressure measurements and for confirmation of a suspected prehepatic block. The physician's surprise is likely to be substantial when, though splenic pulp pressure is elevated, splenoportography fails to show obstruction of the prehepatic portal venous system. If hematemesis in the face of splenomegaly was the mode of presentation, results of the sequential work-up previously discussed are again similar, and the final diagnosis requires liver biopsy material.

Although a number of entities are recognized as causing intrahepatic but presinusoidal portal hypertension, only one, *congenital hepatic fibrosis,* is of major importance in the pediatric age group. This diagnosis may be immediately suspected if renal disease is also present in the patient or in other family members. Other conditions with similar pathophysiologic consequences that may need occasional consideration include *infiltrative liver diseases* (Gaucher's, Hodgkin's, leukemia, hemangiomatosis), *nodular noncirrhotic regenerative hyperplasia, Felty's syndrome, hepatoportal sclerosis,* and *schistosomiasis.* A similar picture may also be seen in a rare patient with *hereditary telangiectasia* (Rendu-Osler-Weber) or other causes of "forward-flow" portal hypertension.

Congenital hepatic fibrosis

The intrahepatic disorder congenital hepatic fibrosis has a very characteristic pathologic lesion (Fig. 25-15). Broad bands of mature connective tissue are noted in portal and periportal distribution but can also encompass individual hepatic lobules. These fibrous bands contain increased numbers of ectatic and dysplastic branches of the interlobular bile ducts, which have the appearance of large cisterns or flattened, irregularly shaped sacs. These interconnecting bile ducts are lined by cuboid epithelium and the lumens are usually empty. The hepatic lobules may be greatly compressed, rendering it difficult to identify their respective central vein, but regenerative nodules are lacking. The individual hepatocytes are normal, and cholestasis is rarely observed. Chronic inflammatory cells are absent or few in number, except in a rare variant of congenital hepatic fibrosis that is complicated by cholangitis. In these cases intrahepatocytic cholestasis may be observed with

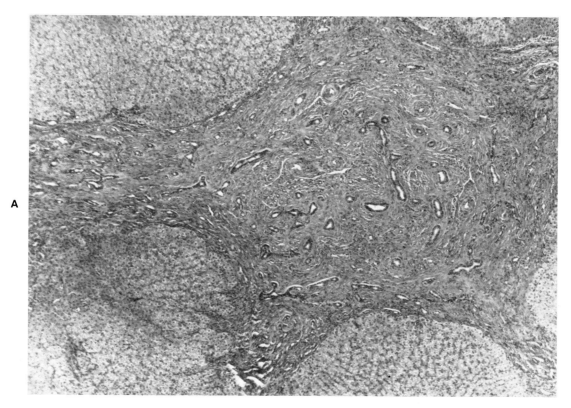

Fig. 25-15. Congenital hepatic fibrosis. **A,** Liver shows extensive hepatic fibrosis containing atypical bile ducts. Surgical liver biopsy comes from a 3-year-old boy who underwent exploratory laparotomy for suspected portal hypertension. At surgery he was believed to have a hamartoma of the liver. An enlarged spleen was removed at operation. At 9 years of age he had hematemesis and melena, and large varices were found roentgenographically. An esophagocologastrotomy was performed. At 18 years of age he had only mild abnormalities of liver function (alkaline phosphatase, 228 IU), and a shunt (portacaval) recently created. **B,** High-power view of the biopsy specimen in **A** to better show the portal fibrosis and atypical bile ducts.

an accompanying acute inflammatory reaction about the dysplastic bile ducts. A reduction in both number and caliber of portal vein branches has also been noted in some cases of congenital hepatic fibrosis.

In half the cases, this entity occurs sporadically; involvement of other family members is lacking. The hepatic lesion is commonly associated with infantile polycystic kidney disease (Potter type I), a condition inherited as an autosomal recessive trait, in which the renal pathologic condition is characterized by cystic tubular dilatation affecting both the cortical and medullary portions of the kidney. In the newborn period and during infancy, the renal lesion dominates the clinical picture with most dying of kidney failure within the first year of life. The hepatic lesion found at autopsy is that of congenital hepatic fibrosis, but the changes are less prominent than those observed in older children. When the hepatic lesion

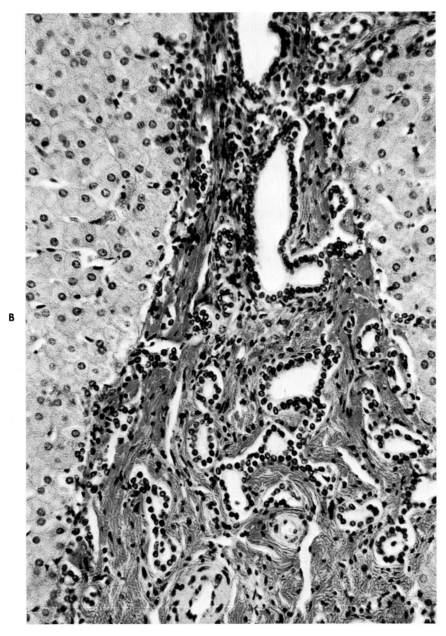

Fig. 25-15, cont'd. For legend see opposite page.

dominates the clinical expression of this disease, asymptomatic hepatomegaly especially involving the left lobe may be found by 1 to 3 years (occasionally younger), and progression of the portal hypertension eventually leads to splenomegaly. Hemorrhage from esophageal varices usually occurs by 5 years of age or later in some. The liver is firm to palpation, with the surface revealing a smooth or finely nodular quality. The liver edge is sometimes irregular suggesting cirrhosis. Asymmetric enlargement of the hepatic lobes may occur because of varying involvement by the disease process, and at times it can be confused with an intrahepatic space-occupying lesion. Abdominal pain is rare but, when present, is usually localized to the right upper quadrant. If symptoms are accompanied by fever, cholangitis may be suspected. Some persons remain completely asymptomatic, with hematemesis not occurring until early adulthood. Since only 10% to 20% of renal tubules are involved in the disease process in the older child, coexisting renal involvement is likewise asymptomatic and often escapes detection by conventional laboratory testing. Occasionally, however, some young children with congenital hepatic fibrosis will show mild to moderate renal abnormalities characterized by increased urea retention and decreased concentrating ability. Later in life, the renal disease may again dominate the clinical picture in cases (up to 25%) that began with primarily hepatic consequences.

That congenital hepatic fibrosis may not represent a distinct entity associated only with infantile polycystic kidney disease has been suggested by the observation that a similar hepatic histopathologic lesion occurs with distinctly different renal lesions, including dysplastic kidneys *(Ivemark's syndrome)*. The hepatic lesion found in the *Meckel's syndrome* (polycystic kidneys, encephalocele, cleft lip and palate, polydactyly) is identical to that of congenital hepatic fibrosis. Although rare, the typical portal lesion of congenital hepatic fibrosis has also been reported in adults with the autosomal dominant form of *polycystic kidney disease*. In addition, some of these patients have von Meyenburg complexes; islands of proliferative dysplastic neoductules in fibrous bands lying within the hepatic lobule.

As mentioned above, some cases of congenital hepatic fibrosis have a cholangiolitic course with intrahepatic microabscess formation indicating a poor prognosis. Cholangiography in these cases shows dilatation of the common duct and major intrahepatic biliary radicals, segmental ductal ectasia, and focal cystic structures along the smaller intrahepatic radicals. Multiple, small gallstones are frequently present in the dilated gallbladder. It is interesting that a somewhat similar clinical course is seen in *Caroli's disease,* a condition in which nonobstructing communicating ectasia and focal cystic dilatation of the intrahepatic biliary tree occur. Both the extensive fibrous tissue bands and portal hypertension characteristic of congenital hepatic fibrosis are absent in Caroli's disease, yet both entities may be associated with a choledochal cyst and renal involvement. The renal abnormality in Caroli's disease occurs in up to 25% of cases and includes both cortical cysts and features of medullary sponge kidneys. Thus it is not surprising that many consider infantile polycystic disease, congenital hepatic fibrosis with renal involvement, and Caroli's disease with renal involvement to be varying expressions of the same pathologic process. Although less precisely, the hepatic lesion in *Jeune's syndrome* (asphyxiating thoracic osteochondrodystrophy and nephropathy) and in *Zellweger's syndrome* (hypotonia with cerebral, hepatic, and renal anomalies) also bears a curious resemblance to congenital hepatic fibrosis.

The diagnosis of congenital hepatic fibrosis is dependent on obtainment of liver tissue preferably by minilaparotomy. Needle liver biopsy alone is not recommended because the pathologic lesion may not be uniform throughout the liver. Some areas may contain minimal amounts of fibrous tissue, whereas in other areas somewhat widened portal zones are seen but without increased numbers of bile ducts, giving the histologic appearance of portal fibrosis or even cirrhosis. Performing a percutaneous liver biopsy using a Truecut needle is advocated by some workers, but the risk of significant bleeding with this device must be kept in mind.

Laboratory studies. When present, abnormalities in liver function studies are usually limited to an elevation of serum alkaline phosphatase or gamma glutamyl transpeptidase (GGT). In occasional patients the transaminases may be elevated from three to five times normal. The BSP test, not surprisingly, shows an abnormality, as in all other causes of portal hypertension. Hypersplenism is evidenced by thrombocytopenia and leukopenia. The urinary abnormality is generally limited to finding a low specific gravity, but elevation of serum urea and creatinine may be noted. The intravenous pyelogram may be abnormal in up to two thirds of cases, with the nephrogram phase showing alternating radiodense and radiolucent streaks radiating from the medulla to the cortex.

Results of other special investigative studies undertaken in congenital hepatic fibrosis may include a normal wedged hepatic vein pressure in most, a suspicion of abnormality of the intrahepatic and extrahepatic bile ducts after an intravenous cholangiogram, and a nonspecific bile-duct abnormality noted by the ^{99m}Tc-DIDA scan. Splenoportography may show an abnormality of the intrahepatic portal venous system characterized by duplication of the venous channels. A recent report noted 16 of 21 children with congenital hepatic fibrosis to have this particular finding, not present in other causes of intrahepatic portal hypertension.

The possibility of other organ malformations besides the liver and kidney should be considered. Musculoskeletal, pulmonary and cardiovascular, central nervous system, and gastrointestinal tract may be involved with minor to severe anomalies, especially in the predominantly renal form (infantile) of the disease.

Clinical course and management. The consequences of portal hypertension, especially that of recurrent hemorrhage from esophageal varices, is the most troublesome complication. Eventually surgery is undertaken to accomplish a portal-systemic shunt. With advancing age a gradual reduction in renal function with uremia and severe hypertension occurs in some. Liver failure secondary to bouts of cholangitis and microabscess formation with septic complications may develop in rare individuals with this variant of congenital hepatic fibrosis.

Prognosis. After a successful portacaval shunt operation has been performed, with alleviation of the threat of hemorrhage from esophageal varices, the majority of patients do reasonably well. Up to 25% will eventually succumb to renal failure. Liver function generally remains intact, except in those cases complicated by cholangitis. Portal encephalopathy does not seem to occur. A long-term follow-up study of pediatric patients with congenital hepatic fibrosis has recently been reported.

Noncirrhotic nodular regenerative hyperplasia, or nodular transformation of liver

Noncirrhotic nodular hyperplasia has been reported with increasing frequency in both the pediatric-age and adult patient. The exact cause is unknown, but the major consequence of this condition is that of intrahepatic portal hypertension. Surprisingly, not all patients have been reported to have splenomegaly despite the presence of portal hypertension. The liver is usually enlarged but not greatly so. Abdominal pain may be present. Liver function tests are reported to be normal with only a prolongation of the BSP test found. When studied, wedged hepatic vein pressures have been normal or elevated. Diagnosis is best made by surgical liver biopsy material, which reveals the nodular appearance of the liver without important perinodular fibrous bands. Reticulum stain preparations are most useful. Microscopically normal-appearing hepatocytes (acidophilic) are found within the majority of the nodules. At other times vacuolated cells containing fat or excess glycogen are present within the nodules, and basophilic hepatocytes are also occasionally noted. The histologic picture is different from that of hepatic adenoma, which is a single lesion, and that of focal nodular hyperplasia and partial nodular transformation of the liver, conditions that usually occur in the perihilar area. In nodular regenerative hyperplasia of the liver, the regenerating nodules tend to compress the juxtaposed normal hepatic parenchyma resulting in mild stromal collapse and reticulum fiber condensation, findings believed to explain the resulting portal hypertension. A few patients with this entity have thrombosis of the portal vein and venules. Other complications reported include hepatic failure and rupture of the liver.

Some workers believe that increased splenic blood flow stimulates the nodular transformation, and indeed regenerative hyperplasia of the liver has been found in congestive heart failure and lymphoproliferative disorders. In adult experiences with this condition, cases of nodular regenerative hyperplasia have been associated with extrahepatic findings, especially rheumatoid arthritis in Felty's syndrome and diabetes mellitus. The role of medications and drugs in producing this entity is strongly considered by some authors.

Hepatoportal sclerosis

Hepatoportal sclerosis, as an entity or group of entities, also included in the category of intrahepatic portal hypertension without cirrhosis, occurs predominantly in adults with rare pediatric cases reported. Signs and symptoms of portal hypertension dominate the clinical picture, and a presinusoidal lesion is suspected when studies reveal an elevated splenic pulp but normal wedged hepatic vein pressure. Liver biopsy material shows minimal portal fibrosis without disruption of the hepatic architecture. The diagnosis may also be suspected from angiographic studies that show a characteristic "withered-tree" appearance of the intrahepatic portal venous arborization. Corrosion casts of the intrahepatic vasculature have confirmed focal obstructive lesions at various bifurcation points at different levels of the intrahepatic portion of the portal vein. Nodularity of the liver is not a feature in this condition. Cases previously called "idiopathic portal hypertension" may have a similar underlying pathologic lesion. In isolated examples of hepatoportal sclerosis, a late sequela has been the sudden deterioration of hepatic function for unknown reasons. Nonselective portocystemic shunts in these patients may be attended by a high incidence of encephalopathy.

Hereditary telangiectasis (Rendu-Osler-Weber disease)

In hereditary telangiectasis arteriovenous shunting may substantially increase portal vein blood flow. Portal hypertension eventually develops as intrahepatic vascular resistance rises, presumably in an effort to decrease venous return to the heart. Liver biopsy material may show only minimal portal fibrosis without cirrhosis. Again, wedged hepatic vein pressures are normal. Diagnosis of Rendu-Osler-Weber disease can be made by the family history, presence of telangiectasia or hemangioma, or the presence of digital clubbing and cyanosis suggestive of arteriovenous shunting.

Schistosomiasis

The pathologic changes produced by the host in response to the ova of *Schistosoma mansoni* and *S. japonicum* gaining access to the portal vein branches is that of perivascular inflammation, with portal and periportal fibrosis in which granulomas may be seen. The liver is enlarged and signs of portal hypertension eventually develop producing splenomegaly or esophageal hemorrhage from varices. Despite the slowly progressive hepatic lesion, cirrhosis does not occur. When studied, wedged hepatic venous pressures are normal or minimally elevated, consistent with a presinusoidal block. The diagnosis can be made from liver biopsy specimens in which ova or debris can be seen in the granulomas. Serologic studies are then confirmatory. The selective distal splenorenal shunt

of Warren is currently considered the operative procedure of choice for treating the portal hypertension.

REFERENCES

Alvarez, F., Bernard, O., Brunelle, F., and others: Congenital hepatic fibrosis in children, J. Pediatr. **99:**370-375, 1981.

Anand, S.K., Chan, J.C., and Lieberman, E.: Polycystic disease and hepatic fibrosis in children, Am. J. Dis. Child. **129:**810-813, 1975.

Baggenstoss, A.H.: Morphologic features: their usefulness in the diagnosis, prognosis and management of cirrhosis. In Popper, H., editor: Cirrhosis, Clin. Gastroenterol. **4:**227-246, 1975.

Boichis, H., Passwell, J., David, R., and Miller, H.: Congenital hepatic fibrosis and nephronophthisis, Q. J. Med. **42:**221-233, 1973.

Carson, J.A., Tunell, W.P., Barnes, P., and Altshuler, G.: Hepatoportal sclerosis in childhood: a mimic of extrahepatic portal vein obstruction, J. Pediatr. Surg. **16:**291-296, 1981.

Case Records of the Massachusetts General Hospital, N. Engl. J. Med. **290:**676-683, 1974.

Dusol, M., Jr., Levi, J.U., Glasser, K., and Schiff, E.R.: Congenital hepatic fibrosis with dilation of intrahepatic bile ducts, Gastroenterology **71:**839-843, 1976.

Hsia, Y.E., Bratu, M., and Herbordt, A.: Genetics of the Meckel syndrome (dysencephalia splanchnocystica), Pediatrics **48:**237-246, 1971.

Ivemark, B.I., Oldfelt, V., and Zetterström, R.: Familial dysplasia of kidneys, liver and pancreas: a probably genetically determined syndrome, Acta Paediatr. **48:**1-11, 1959.

Kerr, D.N., Harrison, C.V., Sherlock, S., and Walker, R.M.: Congenital hepatic fibrosis, Q. J. Med. **30:**91-117, 1961.

Lieberman, E., Salinas-Madrigal, L., Gwinn, J.L., and others: Infantile polycystic disease of the kidneys and liver: clinical, pathological and radiological correlations and comparison with congenital hepatic fibrosis, Medicine **50:**277-318, 1971.

Mikkelsen, W.P., Edmondson, H.A., Peters, R.L., and others: Extra- and intrahepatic portal hypertension without cirrhosis (hepatoportal sclerosis), Ann. Surg. **162:**602-618, 1965.

Murray-Lyon, I.M., Ockenden, B.G., and Williams, R.: Congenital hepatic fibrosis—is it a single clinical entity? Gastroenterology **64:**653-656, 1973.

Nathan, M., and Batsakie, J.G.: Congenital hepatic fibrosis, Surg. Gynecol. Obstet. **128:**1033-1041, 1969.

Mahmoud, A.A.: Schistosomiasis, N. Engl. J. Med. **297:**1329-1331, 1977.

Mall, J.C., Ghahremani, G.G., and Boyer, J.L.: Caroli's disease associated with congenital hepatic fibrosis and renal tubular ectasia, Gastroenterology **66:**1029-1035, 1974.

Odièvre, M., Chaumont, P., Montagne, J.Ph., and Alagille, D.: Anomalies of the intrahepatic portal venous system in congenital hepatic fibrosis, Radiology **122:**427-430, 1977.

Rougier, P., Degott, C., Rueff, B., and Benhamou, J.P.: Nodular regenerative hyperplasia of the liver, Gastroenterology **75:**169-172, 1978.

Shedlofsky, S., Koehler, R.E., DeSchryver-Kecskemeti, K.,

and Alpers, D.H.: Noncirrhotic, nodular transformation of the liver with portal hypertension: clinical, angiographic and pathological correlation, Gastroenterology **79**:938-943, 1980.

Sherlock, S.: Viral hepatitis and cirrhosis. In Popper, H., editor: Cirrhosis, Clin. Gastroenterol. **4**:281-296, 1975.

Sokhi, G.S., Morrice, J.J., McGee, J.O'D., and Blumgart, L.H.: Congenital hepatic fibrosis: aspects of diagnosis and surgical management, Br. J. Surg. **62**:621-623, 1975.

Sommerschild, H.C., Langmark, F., and Maurseth, K.: Congenital hepatic fibrosis: report of two new cases and review of the literature, Surgery **73**:53-58, 1973.

Stromeyer, F.W., and Ishak, K.G.: Nodular transformation (nodular "regenerative" hyperplasia) of the liver: a clinicopathologic study of 30 cases, Hum. Pathol. **12**:60-71, 1981.

ten Bensel, R.N., and Peters, E.R.: Congenital hepatic fibrosis presenting as hepatomegaly in early infancy, J. Pediatr. **72**:96-98, 1968.

Zelman, S.: Liver fibrosis in hereditary hemorrhage telangiectasia, Arch. Pathol. **74**:66-72, 1962.

SUPRAHEPATIC (POSTSINUSOIDAL) PORTAL HYPERTENSION

Occlusion of hepatic veins or suprahepatic portion of the inferior vena cava—Budd-Chiari syndrome

The Budd-Chiari syndrome is extremely rare in pediatric patients. In a large series only 24 of 236 patient affected were less than 20 years of age. Most often (70%) no cause for the disease can be found during life or at autopsy. When present, obstruction of the hepatic venous outflow is caused by compression or invasion by tumor tissue, or thrombi involving the hepatic veins or suprahepatic portion of the inferior vena cava. Enlargement of the caudate lobe in cirrhosis may obstruct the vena cava or hepatic veins. Vena cava bands, webs, or stricture above the hepatic veins are much rarer causes and are congenital. The obstructing membranous band may be the result of an abnormal postnatal obliteration process of the ductus venosus. When thrombotic occlusion of the hepatic vein ostia or suprahepatic portion of the inferior vena cava exists, other predisposing systemic conditions are frequently present, including neoplasms (hepatoma, hypernephroma), leukemia, sickle-cell disease, paroxysmal nocturnal hemoglobinuria, polycythemia, inflammatory bowel disease, allergic vasculitis, and visceral thrombophlebitis migrans. Hepatic vein thrombosis has been also reported as a complication of oral contraceptive medications. Pathologically, the primary lesion shows intimal thickening and fibrous obliteration of the ostium of the major hepatic veins or intrahepatic portion of the inferior vena cava.

A Budd-Chiari–like syndrome can also be associated with constrictive pericarditis and right-atrium myxoma and has also been observed recently in primary pulmonary hypertension. Postoperative obstruction to hepatic venous outflow may occur in the neonate after tense reduction of the intestinal viscera into the small abdominal cavity of patients with either gastroschisis or large omphalocele.

Diagnosis. The diagnosis can be suspected by the clinical story because most patients with portal hypertension secondary to the Budd-Chiari syndrome present with abdominal enlargement (95%) of relatively short duration. The enlargement results from rapidly accumulating ascitic fluid recognized by demonstration of a shifting dullness or a fluid wave. Hepatomegaly (70%) is common but may be difficult to appreciate when tense ascites is present. In such cases these organs can usually be detected by ballottement. Abdominal pain occurs frequently (50%) and splenomegaly and jaundice may be seen in about 25% of cases. Distended superficial abdominal veins or pretibial edema signifies obstruction of the inferior vena cava. Esophageal varices are seldom present except in long-standing disease, and therefore hematemesis is likewise uncommon early in the disease. Absence of hepatojugular reflex may be supportive of the diagnosis.

Useful studies to establish the diagnosis include a series of angiographic and catheterization procedures. A transfemoral venogram of the inferior vena cava and, if possible, wedged hepatic vein pressures and venograms from the wedged position are helpful. Characteristic intrahepatic venous angiographic appearance is described as an interlacing network of fine vessels believed to be hepatic venules. Pressure measurements in the superior vena cava, right atrium, and supradiaphragmatic portion of the inferior vena cava are necessary to rule out cardiac causes of this syndrome such as constrictive pericarditis, myxoma of the right atrium, or heart failure. In the absence of known liver disease echocardiography should always be employed early in the patient presenting with abrupt onset ascites.

Saphenous or femoral vein studies may show complete obstruction of the vena cava, in which case noticeable collateral circulation to the retroperitoneal venous drainage system is commonly observed. Incomplete (functional) obstruction of the infradiaphragmatic portion of the inferior vena cava may result from increased intra-abdominal pressure secondary to ascites (Fig. 25-7). Removal of the ascites and repeat venogram then shows a normal inferior vena cava in the segment in question.

If thrombus occludes the hepatic ostia or intrahepatic portion of the inferior vena cava or both, attempts at obtaining wedged hepatic vein pressures from this site will obviously be unsuccessful even when test injections of dye are used to locate the position of the catheter tip. At times this maneuver may be diagnostic in patients with anatomic lesions that prevent the catheter from entering the hepatic veins.

Open-liver biopsy is recommended to confirm the diagnosis. Elevated intrahepatic venous pressure and resulting liver engorgement may lead to excessive bleeding from the biopsy site, and therefore percutaneous biopsy should not be attempted once the diagnosis is considered in these patients.

Pathology. Depending on the interval between the onset of the disease and liver biopsy, a variety of histopathologic lesions may be found. Early in the disease, pronounced central venous congestion, centrilobular hemorrhage, and necrosis can be seen with minimal inflammatory response (Fig. 25-16). Later, the hepatic cells in these central zones may resemble ghost cells, and thrombi may be found in some of the larger hepatic veins (Fig. 25-16, C). Central veins may show intimal thickening and fibroblastic proliferation.

Management. In general, treatment of the Budd-Chiari syndrome has been disappointing. This is especially true when the disease occurs in association with a thrombophlebitic obliterative process associated with systemic disease. At times, if the precipitating cause is known (tumors, ulcerative colitis, allergic vasculitis, polycythemia, and so on), efforts should be directed toward elimination or treatment of the inciting factor. Otherwise, a portacaval shunt (side to side) is the operation of choice, provided that roentgenologic dye studies show a patent inferior vena cava and obstruction at the level of the hepatic ostia. When obstruction of the inferior vena cava is caused by intraluminal membranes or webs, transcardiac membranotomy has been a successful surgical procedure in both children and adults. If the inferior vena cava is obliterated or constricted, various surgical bypass procedures with prosthetic materials have been employed, including Teflon mesh patching or Dacron graft (azygocaval anastomosis) with occa-

sional success. The presence of pronounced venous collaterals often makes the surgical procedure very difficult. Failure to relieve hepatic venous congestion eventually leads to hepatic failure, coma, and death in all patients.

Veno-occlusive disease. Veno-occlusive disease represents an important cause of postsinusoidal portal hypertension in children living in certain so-called endemic areas. Although affecting people in different parts of the world and called by different names, these entities seem to be related by similarities of the clinicopathologic picture and includes veno-occlusive disease of Jamaica, Indian liver cirrhosis, South African liver disease, and liver cirrhosis of Egyptian children. In many cases occlusion of medium and small hepatic veins has been attributed to ingestion of pyrrolizidine alkaloids. This potential toxin is present in "bush teas" made from the genera *Senecio, Crotalaria, Heliotropium,* and *Cynoglossum.* A similar lesion is found in livestock and experimental animals after they ingest plants containing these alkaloids. Hepatocellular enzymatic conversion of relatively nontoxic pyrrolizidine alkaloids to the pyrrole derivatives yields toxic alkylating substances, which in turn can react with hepatocytes and vascular endothelium, a process that produces hepatic necrosis with or without postsinusoidal obstruction.

Recently, examples of veno-occlusive disease in young infants have been reported in the United States. These cases have been attributed to the ingestion of herbal decoctions employed as a folk remedy particularly in the Mexican-American population. We have seen two similar cases occurring in infants drinking a brew of *gordolobo yerba* (usually *Gnaphalium* but in this case the plant *Senecio longilobus*). Veno-occlusive disease of the liver has also followed chemotherapy of acute leukemia and may be a complication of chemoradiotherapy employed to prepare patients for bone marrow transplantation. Congenital immune deficiency was suggested as predisposing in five infants in Australia who had veno-occlusive disease. Phlebosclerosis and occlusion of the small and medium-sized hepatic veins may be a complication of irradiation therapy of the liver. Some cases are labeled as "idiopathic."

Clinical findings. In children the illness reported from endemic areas is usually ushered in by an acute respiratory infection, and those affected are generally less than 6 years of age. He-

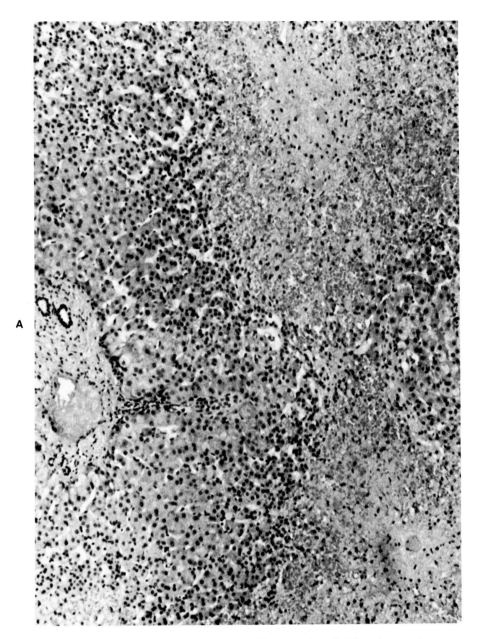

Fig. 25-16. Suprahepatic ("postsinusoidal") portal hypertension. **A,** The microscopic appearance of the liver shows the striking central lobular necrosis and hemorrhage (Budd-Chiari syndrome). This liver biopsy specimen comes from an 11-year-old boy with a protruding abdomen of 10 days' duration. Three days before admission he had complained of abdominal pain and had several episodes of vomiting. One day before admission he experienced difficulty in breathing and had epigastric pain. Past history was unremarkable. Physical examination revealed a slightly thin child with a protuberant abdomen but without obvious icterus. Abdominal examination showed noticeable distention, a definite fluid wave with shifting dullness, and a firm liver edge 10 cm below the right costal margin. The extremities were without edema or clubbing of the digits. A hepatojugular reflex could not be obtained. Initial laboratory data revealed modest abnormalities of the SGOT, serum bilirubin, and prothrombin time.   *Continued.*

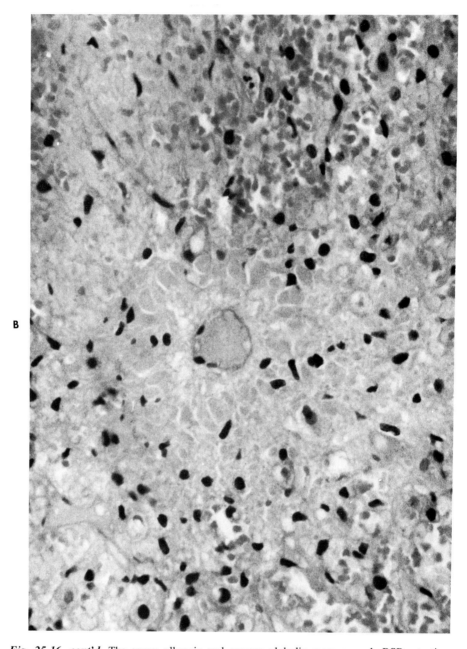

Fig. 25-16, cont'd. The serum albumin and gamma globulin were normal. BSP retention was prolonged. Esophageal varices failed to be demonstrated by roentgenograms, and cardiac catheterization revealed normal pressures in the right atrium and inferior vena cava, whereas wedged hepatic vein pressure was elevated. A liver scan was normal. About 3000 ml of clear ascitic fluid was removed by paracentesis but rapidly reaccumulated. The child was then prepared for surgery. At laparotomy the liver appeared large and congested, and splenomegaly was also apparent. Portal pressure was 20 mm Hg. This liver biopsy section was obtained. **B,** High-power view of a central vein region from **A,** showing severe necrosis and hemorrhage.

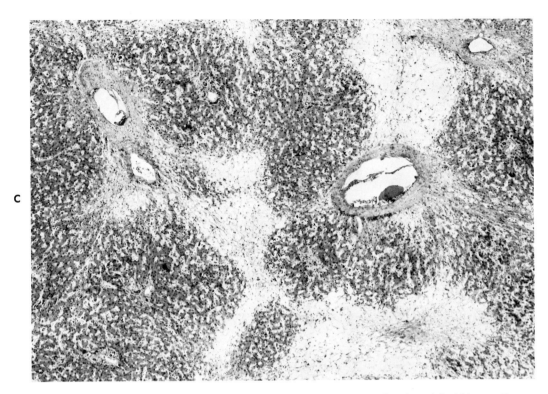

Fig. 25-16, cont'd. **C,** Repeat liver biopsy section taken 3 weeks after the original biopsy. Essentially the same pattern can be seen with exception of loss of red blood cells. This child subsequently died of hepatic decompensation, which occurred over the next 4 weeks.

patomegaly, ascites, and sometimes jaundice develop rapidly, and the acute phase of the disease may be fatal in about 20% of cases. Pyrrolizidine intoxication in young infants may mimic Reye's syndrome where clinical features include pernicious vomiting and altered consciousness. Subacute and chronic forms of this disease also exist (30% of cases) with persistent hepatomegaly and recurrent episodes of ascites in the former, and cirrhosis and esophageal varices as consequences of the latter.

Diagnosis. Diagnosis is easily made on clinical grounds when the signs occur in the young child living in those endemic areas. Splenic pulp pressures are elevated, and the prehepatic portal system is normal. Splenoportography reveals prolonged retention of the contrast medium within the liver. Patency of the major hepatic veins is best determined by retrograde suprahepatic venography. Presumably, wedged hepatic vein pressure should be elevated (postsinusoidal block), and dye injected from this site should be unable to undergo reflux into the sinusoid and presinusoidal areas. However, very few such studies have been performed in children with veno-occlusive disease.

Liver biopsy is used to confirm the diagnosis. Centrilobular congestion, hepatocellular necrosis, subintimal swelling, and occlusion of the small and medium hepatic veins are the typical histologic features early in the disease. Cirrhosis in the chronic form of veno-occlusive disease may be indistinguishable from other forms of liver disease leading to cirrhosis.

Management. There is no specific therapy for this disease. If ingestion of the incriminated alkaloids has provoked this condition, obviously those plants and products derived from such substances should be avoided. About 50% of the patients with the acute disease recover after receiving supportive therapy. Some children continue to have exacerbations, and consequently some 30% develop cirrhosis. The chronic forms may be amenable to portacaval shunting procedures (side to side) but their long-term prognosis remains uncertain.

REFERENCES

Cabrera, J., Brugera, M., Navarro, F., and others: Budd-Chiari syndrome due to a membranous obstruction of the inferior vena cava in a child, J. Pediatr. **96:**435-437, 1980.

Case Records of the Massachusetts General Hospital, N. Engl. J. Med. **273:**156-163, 1965.

Doppman, J., Rubinson, R.M., Rockoff, S.D., and others: Mechanism of obstruction of the infradiaphragmatic portion of the inferior vena cava in the presence of increased intra-abdominal pressure, Invest. Radiol. **1:**37-53, 1966.

Fox, D.W., Hart, M.C., Bergeson, P.S., and others: Pyrrolizidine *(Senecio)* intoxication mimicking Reye syndrome, J. Pediatr. **93:**980-982, 1978.

Griner, P.F., Elbadawi, A., and Packman, C.H.: Veno-occlusive disease of the liver after chemotherapy of acute leukemia, Ann. Intern. Med. **85:**578-582, 1976.

Lyrord, C.L., Vergara, G.G., and Moeller, D.D.: Hepatic veno-occlusive disease originating in Ecuador, Gastroenterology **70:**105-108, 1976.

Mellis, C., and Bale, P.M.: Familial hepatic veno-occlusive disease with probable immune deficiency, J. Pediatr. **88:**236-242, 1976.

Parker, R.G.F.: Occlusion of the hepatic veins in man, Medicine **38:**369-402, 1959.

Rosenberg, L.S., Silverman, A., and Strain, J.E.: Primary pulmonary hypertension presenting as portal hypertension, Am. J. Gastroenterol. **71:**427-431, 1979.

Stillman, A.E., Huxtable, R., Consroe, P., and others: Hepatic veno-occlusive disease due to pyrrolizidine *(Senecio)* poisoning in Arizona, Gastroenterology **73:**349-352, 1977.

Takeuchi, J., Takada, A., Hasumura, Y., and others: Budd-Chiari syndrome associated with obstruction of the inferior vena cava, Am. J. Med. **51:**11-20, 1971.

Taneja, A., Mitra, S.K., Moghe, P.D., and others: Budd-Chiari syndrome in childhood secondary to inferior vena caval obstruction, Pediatrics **63:**808-812, 1979.

Tang, T.T., Davis, S., Keelan, M.H., and others: Hepatomegaly and recurrent ascites in an 11-year-old boy, J. Pediatr. **91:**1015-1020, 1977.

26 *Acute and chronic biliary tract disease*

NONCALCULOUS DISTENTION OF THE GALLBLADDER (ACUTE HYDROPS)

Acute hydrops is defined by (1) the presence of pronounced distention of the gallbladder, (2) the absence of calculi or of any obvious acute infectious disease of the organ, and (3) normal-sized extrahepatic bile ducts. Although acute hydrops was once considered a rare condition, recent awareness that acute hydrops of the gallbladder occurs as an abdominal complication of mucocutaneous lymph node syndrome has resulted in a striking increase in the number of reported pediatric cases. Acute hydrops has been found in neonates and also in older children, though most cases occur in the preschool-age child. A predilection for males has been noted.

The etiology of this condition is not known, but several mechanisms have been proposed, An anatomic abnormality of the cystic duct has been associated in some cases. Narrowing of the cystic duct lumen, twisting of the duct, and even atresia of the duct have been reported as possible causes of this condition. On the other hand, increased mucous secretion by the gallbladder and ineffective emptying may predispose the organ to acute distention that may, in turn, kink the cystic duct. Almost 50% of patients operated upon had noticeable enlargement of the mesenteric lymph nodes, and although obstruction to bile flow did not occur, the temporal relationship of this condition to a preceding infectious illness has been repeatedly observed. In particular, streptococcal and staphylococcal disease may be a forerunner of acute hydrops. Leptospirosal infection has been causative on occasion. A less clear relationship exists in those cases where this condition occurs as a complication of familial Mediterranean fever, leukemia, or the nephrotic syndrome. Direct inflammation of the cystic duct and enlargement of adjacent lymph nodes draining this structure may be important factors leading to distention in some cases. That results of liver function tests are abnormal in some patients has indicated that the cause of acute hydrops of the gallbladder sometimes may be a hepatotropic virus.

Clinical features

The clinical features mimic those of more common surgical conditions of childhood. An acute onset of colicky abdominal pain ushers in the disease, nausea and vomiting are quite common. Because many of the children affected are young, precise localization of the pain is difficult. Older children will often complain of epigastric or right-sided upper abdominal tenderness. In some cases, a history of preceding illness suggesting mucocutaneous lymph node syndrome may be obtained; in others, a more chronic history of recurrent abdominal pain is reported. Pain generally becomes continuous and increases in intensity, suggesting acute appendicitis, or it may be more spasmodic, thereby resembling that of intussusception. Fever is absent or slight and jaundice seldom present. Careful palpation of the abdomen will reveal a mass in the right upper quadrant in more than 50% of cases.

Diagnosis

The diagnosis should be suspected in a young infant or child with a history of recent illness, fever, and rash and presenting with a tender right upper quadrant abdominal pain. When present, abnormal results of screening liver function tests (bilirubin, alkaline phosphatase, gamma glutamyl transpeptidase, and so on) may also suggest acute cholecystitis or complicated choledochal cyst. The gallbladder is not visualized by either oral cholecystography or intravenous cholangiography. The preoperative diagnosis is best made by ultrasonography, which reveals a massively enlarged echofree gallbladder and normal bile ducts. Differential diagnosis of upper abdominal anechoic structures includes choledochal, mesenteric or omental cysts, and rarely a pancreatic pseudocyst. However, a normal gallbladder should be present in all the conditions listed above except for choledocal cysts. Previously, the diagnosis of acute hydrops was seldom suspected until surgery. Acute appendicitis with or without perforation, small bowel obstruction, or intussusception is usually considered. If the diagnosis had not been considered before surgery, a large, distended, edematous gallbladder is an unexpected finding at laparotomy. The color of the bile within the gall bladder may be white, yellow, green, or black, and the material is sterile.

Treatment

Since preoperative diagnosis of acute hydrops is being made with increased frequency, the need for surgical intervention has essentially been eliminated. Treatment of the intercurrent illness when possible, intravenous fluids, supportive care, and then oral alimentation of a low-fat diet generally lead to spontaneous resolution of the hydrops within 2 to 5 weeks. This benign outcome had previously been observed when the diagnosis was confirmed at surgery and a gallbladder-drainage procedure was deferred. Simple aspiration has been used as a form of treatment, especially if obstruction of the cystic duct is not seen by operative cholangiography. Cholecystostomy drainage of the edematous organ has also been successful and is now suggested as the treatment of choice in cases with impending rupture. An equal number of cases have been treated by cholecystectomy.

Pathology

Pronounced edema of the gallbladder wall is seen in most cases. Mild, acute, or chronic inflammation is also present and with variable degrees of fibrosis. Anatomic lesions of the cystic duct (stenosis, hypoplasia) may occasionally be present. The bile is invariably sterile.

Complications and prognosis

Perforation and bile peritonitis are very rare. The prognosis is excellent with conservative treatment or when either simple drainage or removal of the gallbaldder is performed. Normal function of the gallbladder can be demonstrated at a later time after a drainage procedure.

REFERENCES

Bloom, R.A., and Swain, V.A.J.: Non-calculous distension of the gallbladder in childhood, Arch. Dis. Child. **41:**503-508, 1966.

Krensky, A.M., Teele, R., Watkins, J., and Bates, J.: Streptococcal antigenicity in mucocutaneous lymph node syndrome and hydropic gallbladders, Pediatrics **64:**979-980, 1979.

Kumari, S., Lee. W.J., and Baron, M.G.: Hydrops of the gallbladder in a child: diagnosis by ultrasonography, Pediatrics **63:**295-297, 1979.

Magilavy, D.B., Speert, D.P., Silver, T.M., and Sullivan, D.B.: Mucocutaneous lymph node sydrome: report of two cases complicated by gallbladder hydrops and diagnosed by ultrasound, Pediatrics **61:**699-702, 1978.

Mofenson, H.C., Greensher, J., and Molavi, M.: Gallbladder hydrops: complication of Kawasaki disease, N.Y. State J. Med. **80:**249-251, 1980.

Robinson, A.E., Erwin, J.H., Wiseman, H.J., and Kodroff, M.B.: Cholecystitis and hydrops of the gallbladder in the newborn, Radiology **122:**749-751, 1977.

Scobie, W.G., and Bentley, J.F.R.: Hydrops of the gallbladder in a newborn infant, J. Pediatr. Surg. **4:**457-459, 1969.

Slovis, T.L., Hight, D.W., Philippart, A.I., and Dubois, R.S.: Sonography in the diagnosis and management of hydrops of the gallbladder in children with mucocutaneous lymph node syndrome, Pediatrics **65:**789-794, 1980.

ACUTE ACALCULOUS CHOLECYSTITIS

Acute inflammatory disease of the gallbladder remains rare in the preadolescent population and occurs more frequently in the absence of stones than in their presence. The separation of acute cholecystitis from noncalculous distention of the gallbladder is based more on pathologic findings than on the clinical findings. The incidence seems to vary considerably in different countries of the world.

A unifying etiologic mechanism of this disease in the absence of stones is not available. The association of acute cholecystitis with an intercurrent illness has been noted. Bacterial enteric infections (such as typhoid fever, shigellosis, *Escherichia coli*), viral gastroenteritis, scarlet fever, respiratory infections, and pneumonia have been implicated. Parasitic infections with *Giardia* or *Ascaris* have also been found in the gallbladders of some patients. Most often the bile is sterile, though the histologic lesion is suggestive of an acute inflammatory process. Cultures of the bile and gallbladder wall should be taken. Recent reports continue to incriminate a congenital or acquired malformation of the cystic duct as being responsible for the development of acute cholecystitis. Stagnation of bile and mucus within the "obstructed" gallbladder then predisposes the mucosa to bacterial or viral invasion. This explanation is not particularly satisfying, since obstruction to emptying of the gallbladder is rarely seen, even during operative cholangiography. No definite sex ratio exists for this entity in the pediatric population.

Acute gallbladder disease caused by the presence of stones is not so common as one might believe. A more chronic story of vague abdominal pain is likely to be obtained, especially when the pathologic lesion shows chronic cholecystitis with stones. Gallstones within the cystic or common duct are not commonly found, though jaundice is often present in children with this disease. However, common duct stones may become impacted in the ampulla of Vater and produce a clinical picture similar to that of acute or remittent hepatitis.

Clinical features

An acute onset of right-sided abdominal pain, either constant or colicky, is present in all but a rare patient. In the very young child, the pain may be difficult to localize but is usually of greatest intensity in the right upper quadrant. At times, the pain may be greatest in the epigastrium or periumbilical region, especially early in the illness. Palpation of the abdomen reveals signficant tenderness, and voluntary guarding is present. Gentle percussion over the lower rib margin will cause the patient discomfort. If the patient does not voluntarily contract his muscles excessively, a mass may be palpable in the right upper quadrant. Vomiting and nausea may be present in 75% of cases, with jaundice present in about 20%. A history of fatty food intolerance or pain radiating to the right shoulder is rarely elicited in children, in either acute or chronic gallbladder disease. Some fever is usually present.

There is little specificity in the clinical features of acute cholecystitis to permit exact diagnosis preoperatively. Indeed, the findings are usually believed to reflect acute appendicitis, pancreatitis, bowel obstruction, or perforation.

Diagnosis

Laboratory tests are not very helpful. The white blood count is elevated, and there is a predominance of polymorphonuclear cells. Serum bilirubin and amylase levels may be elevated to some degree.

Usually, the diagnosis is made at laparotomy that is performed for other suspected abdominal conditions. The presence of a right upper quadrant tender mass may be suggestive of the diagnosis of acute cholecystitis or acute hydrops. Contrast roentgenography may be necessary to rule out other types of obstructive pain (intussusception). The presence of an extrarenal calcified density in the right upper abdomen, seen on routine roentgenograms of the abdomen, may be useful information.

Diagnosis of acute cholecystitis is seldom possible by oral cholecystography because the gallbladder is not visualized during the acute disease. Nonfilling of the gallbladder by material used for cholecystography is not so useful a diagnostic clue in children as in adults. Ultrasonography is useful for distinguishing between acute hydrops and calculous cholecystitis.

Pathology

A distended, inflamed gallbladder is seen grossly, with inflammatory adhesions to neighboring structures not being uncommon. Varying degrees of acute inflammatory reaction are seen in the mucosa and muscular coats. Fibrosis is minimal or absent. Stones, when present, are either cholesterol or bilirubin in type.

Treatment

Cholecystectomy is the treatment of choice. Operative cholangiography through the cystic or common duct is indicated when stones are present.

Prognosis

The prognosis should be excellent after surgery for patients without underlying hemolytic disease. Transient postoperative dyspepsia may affect some patients.

CHOLELITHIASIS

The incidence of gallstones varies in people throughout the world and within geographic areas of this country indicating ethnic, dietary, and environmental influences. In addition, genetic factors play an important role in the genesis of cholesterol gallstones. In these cases cholesterol stone formation usually occurs, in contrast to the more common calcium bilirubinate stones found in early childhood and associated with hemolytic anemias. The mechanism believed to be responsible for cholesterol gallstone formation involves a disturbance in the concentration of bile salts relative to those of cholesterol and phospholipids (lecithin). The lipid components of bile are kept in micellar solution, provided that the concentration of each remains within a critical range. For each concentration of bile salts (water soluble) and lecithin (amphipathic) there is a critical concentration of cholesterol above which the cholesterol can no

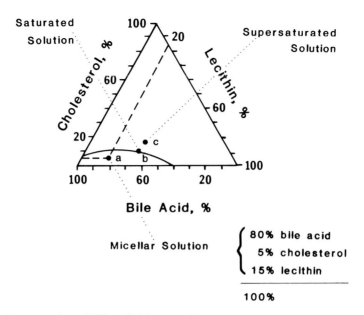

Fig. 26-1. Representation of biliary lipid composition on triangular coordinates. *Solid line,* Approximation of the limits of solubility, as determined by several investigators, for aqueous solutions containing various concentrations of bile acid, lecithin, and cholesterol. *Point A,* A solution composed of 80% bile acid, 5% cholesterol, and 15% lecithin within which cholesterol is solubilized in mixed micelles. *Points B and C,* Solutions that are saturated and supersaturated, respectively, with cholesterol. From LaRusso, N.F.: Practical Gastroenterology **5:**22, 1981.)

longer be held within the confines of the micelle. When cholesterol comes out of solution, its monohydrate form crystallizes. Aggregation of crystals leads to stones (Fig. 26-1).

The concentration of bile acids in bile may be affected by any process that interferes with the enterohepatic circulation (ileal disease and resection, cystic fibrosis, pancreatic insufficiency) or reduces hepatic synthesis of bile acids or lecithin (liver disease), with both events resulting in increased cholesterol saturation of bile. Although less common, gallbladder dysfunction may also reduce the enterohepatic circulation and favor the formation of cholesterol crystals in this organ. The presence of lithogenic bile is an essential factor in the genesis of gallstones. Recent work has attempted to explain why a number of individuals with lithogenic bile do not develop gallstones. Nidation factors such as pH, proteins, mucus, and infection undoubtedly play a role. Other conditions that produce a ''lithogenic'' effect in bile include obesity and the use of oral contraceptive medications (estrogen), both associated with an increased secretion of cholesterol into bile.

A dramatic rise in the incidence of choleli-

thiasis occurs during pregnancy, even in the young teen-ager. Indeed, abnormal gallbladder kinetics have been observed in late pregnancy with incomplete emptying of this structure, an event that may predispose to the precipitation of cholesterol crystals and gallstone formation. Oral contraceptives apparently do not affect gallbladder kinetics in a similar fashion. A positive family history of gallstones, which may reach 50%, is present in some at-risk groups (Pima Indians). The ratio of females to males is striking (4:1 to 10:1) with symptoms beginning at about 8 to 10 years for many patients.

Although hemolytic anemia is reportedly a common cause of cholelithiasis, these patients are often asymptomatic, and stones noted as an incidental finding on roentgenograms taken for other reasons. The incidence of stones in patients with hemoglobinopathies, such as sickle-cell anemia, is now reported to be about 25%, but they are uncommon before 8 to 10 years of age. In some series, investigators report underlying hemolytic disease in all patients with gallstones, whereas other series found less than 20% of cases with a blood disorder as a possible cause. In the absence of an

Table 26-1. Cholelithiasis at Hôpital Sainte-Justine and at Jewish General Hospital, Montreal, 1960 to 1970*

Number	
Males	8
Females	27
Average age (in years)	
Males	9.8
Females	13.9
Predisposing factors	
Obesity in girls	6
Cholecystectomy in parents	5
Hemolytic anemia	4
Admission diagnosis	
Chronic recurrent abdominal pain	30
Acute condition of the abdomen	
With acute cholecystitis	4
With associated pancreatitis	1
X-ray diagnosis	
Gallbladder not visualized	14
Calculi seen	18

*Courtesy H. Blanchard, F. Guttman, and P.P. Collin.

Table 26-2. Pediatric (less than 18 years of age) cases of cholelithiasis at Denver General Hospital,* 1975 to 1981

Number	
Females	20
Males	0
Average age (in years)	17
Predisposing factors	
With Spanish surname	18
Obesity	4
Pregnancy	16
Family history of gallstones	5
Hemolytic anemia	1
Admission diagnosis	
Chronic recurrent abdominal pain	16
Acute condition of abdomen	2
With acute cholecystitis	2
With associated pancreatitis	1
X-ray diagnosis (oral cholecystogram)	
Gallbladder not visualized	11
Calculi seen	9
Ultrasound diagnosis	1

*Forty-eight percent of pediatric admissions are Spanish-surnamed persons.

underlying hemoglobinopathy or hemolytic anemia, gallstones are extremely uncommon in the black population.

Gallstones have been described in the fetus and newborn infant with hemolytic disease (Rh). Hemolysis that occurs in Wilson's disease may lead to gallstone formation, and their discovery may provide the first clue to the underlying diagnosis.

Another association reported with gallstones in nonhemolytic cases include total parenteral nutrition and furosemide treatment in neonates with bronchopulmonary dysplasia. We, and others, have observed gallstones at autopsy in a child dying of Crigler-Najjar syndrome. Malformations of the cystic or common duct, or developmental abnormalities of the gallbladder, may predispose to stone formation. Previous surgery on congenital duodenal anomalies (annular pancreas, duodenal atresia or stenosis) may also predispose to cholecystitis and cholelithiasis. Bacterial contamination of the upper small bowel, or rarely in the gallbladder, may deconjugate bile acids and thereby affect (reduce) the enterohepatic circulation. Gallstones can develop in children with cystic fibrosis (8%). Their bile has been found to be supersaturated with cholesterol, but the judicious administration of pancreatic enzymes partly corrects this anomaly in biliary lipid composition. Metachromatic leukodystrophy has been associated with abnormal gallbladder kinetics, and it predisposes to gallstone formation. Any intestinal condition that results in chronic disease of the terminal ileum (Crohn's ileitis), or necessitates ileal resection (necrotizing enterocolitis, ileal atresia, regional enteritis) will disturb the enterohepatic circulation and predisposes to gallstone formation. An unusual case of gallstones developing in a child with gastroesophageal reflux and hiatal hernia has been reported.

The experience with gallstones in non–cystic fibrotic children from Hôpital Sainte-Justine, Montreal, is summarized in Table 26-1, and a summary of recent cases seen at Denver General Hospital appears in Table 26-2.

In children, the stones are usually found in the gallbladder (Fig. 26-2) and seldom (4% to 6%) occlude either the cystic or the common duct (Fig. 26-3). However, jaundice (65%) in association with other symptoms such as pain and nausea is common.

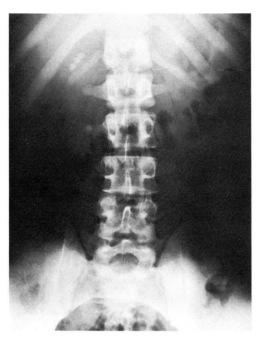

Fig. 26-2. Cholelithiasis. Three stones are seen in the region of the gallbladder and one in the distal portion of the common duct. An 11-year-old boy had a sudden onset of colicky right upper quadrant pain and nausea lasting 3 days. Jaundice then developed, and the patient was hospitalized. Though icterus was present, the slightly enlarged liver was not tender. Abdominal discomfort to palpation was mainly in the epigastrium and right upper quadrant. Laboratory tests revealed moderate elevations of bilirubin and transaminase with normal alkaline phosphatase. Though hematologic assessment was normal, this roentgenogram was ordered.

Clinical features

Intermittent, colicky pain, mild or severe, occurs in more than 95% of patients. Localization to the right upper quadrant or epigastrium without significant radiation to the back or shoulder is common in older children. Radiation of pain to the lower abdomen may cause confusion with acute appendicitis. Multiple attacks are common before diagnosis is made.

A history of nausea and vomiting and fatty food intolerance can be elicited in half the patients. Nonspecific associated complaints include anorexia, fatigue, and listlessness.

Mild to moderate jaundice and abdominal tenderness are the only useful physical signs, since gallbladder enlargement is infrequent in children with cholelithiasis.

Laboratory findings

Laboratory results are seldom useful in diagnosis unless serum bilirubin level is elevated or bile is present in the urine. White blood count is frequently normal or slightly elevated. The peripheral red blood cell smear should be carefully examined for evidence of hemolytic disease. Alkaline phosphatase elevation is most likely to be simultaneously present in the small group with jaundice. Elevated transaminase levels may suggest cholangitis in these patients.

Radiology

Roentgenologic studies are most helpful. Calculi may be seen on routine abdominal films (Fig. 26-2) but usually require cholecystography or ultrasonography for their demonstration (Fig. 26-4 and 26-5). Only 10% to 15% of gallstones contain sufficient calcium to be radiopaque. Rarely, one observes calcium in the wall of the gallbladder (porcelain gallbladder) or in the lumen (milk of calcium bile). With the advent of ultrasonography as a simple and noninvasive technique to evaluate the gallbladder and bile ducts, oral cholecystography has been less frequently employed. The sensitivity of real-time ultrasonography is 98% and specificity between 93% to 97%. This technique can identify stones as small as 2 mm in size and consequently false-negative results are extremely rare. False-positive results, however, are reported to occur in 5% to 10% of cases. When oral cholecystography is employed, one can best prepare the child by giving a single dose on two consecutive days before visualization of the gallbladder by standard roentgenographic technique. Here, false-positive results are extremely rare, but false-negative results may approach 10% of cases. Intravenous cholangiography is seldom necessary for evaluation of pathologic gallbladder conditions because it rarely fills the gallbladder, and common duct stones are extremely rare in the pediatric-age group.

Diagnosis

Although the symptom complex in most children is similar to that in adults, the diagnosis of cholelithiasis is seldom considered, and the reported delay between onset of symptoms and diagnosis is often 1 to 5 years. The physician is more likely to suspect this diagnosis for patients known to have an underlying hemolytic anemia (sickle cell, spherocytosis, others), but this group

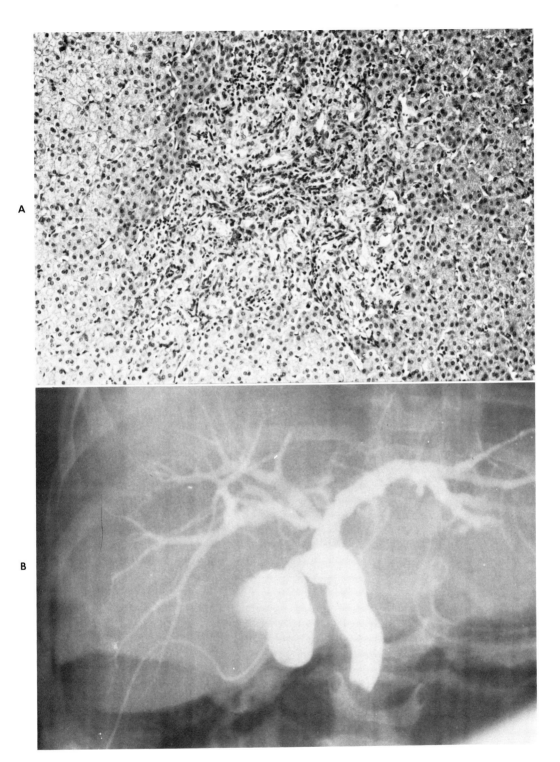

Fig. 26-3. **A,** Needle liver biopsy specimen from a 9-month-old infant with 6 weeks of persistent obstructive jaundice. Bilirubin elevation (10.4 mg/dl) was primarily conjugated (8 mg/dl), and serum alkaline phosphatase was significantly elevated. the histologic lesion is consistent with an extrahepatic obstruction showing proliferating bile ducts and mild portal fibrosis. Centrilobular cholestasis was also present. After this biopsy, barium study of the upper gastrointestinal system revealed extrinsic pressure deformity of the proximal duodenum, suggesting a choledochus cyst. Explorative surgery followed. **B,** Operative cholangiogram in the patient described in **A.** The entire biliary tree (intrahepatic and extrahepatic) is significantly dilated for a child of this age, because of an impacted common duct stone that prevents flow of contrast (and bile) into the duodenum. Removal of the calculus resulted in prompt resolution of the patient's illness.

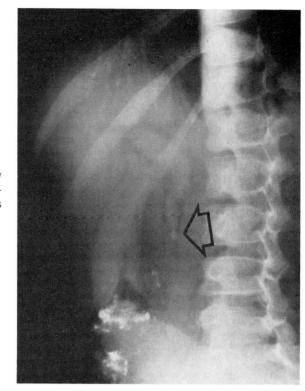

Fig. 26-4. Common duct stone, *arrow,* visualized by an oral cholecystogram in a 5-year-old girl with recurrent colicky upper abdominal pain. No other gallstones were found at surgery.

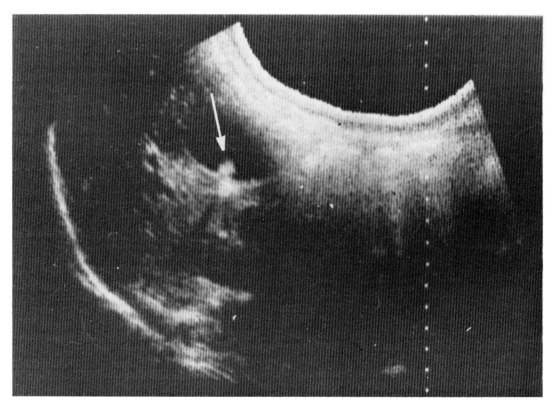

Fig. 26-5. Ultrasound visualization of a solitary gallstone, *arrow,* casting an acoustic shadow in a 13-year-old girl with recurrent epigastric and right upper quadrant abdominal pain. An oral cholecystogram failed to visualize the gallbladder.

represents less than 10% of the patients. Proper roentgenologic studies of the gallbladder are indicated in pediatric patients whose complaints of recurrent abdominal pain of psychophysiologic origin do not fit the classic syndrome described in Chapter 15. Abdominal pain and jaundice obviously will require investigations of the biliary system and liver as well. Indeed, it is not uncommon to suspect viral hepatitis in such patients, especially when jaundice dominates the clinical picture.

Treatment

The approach in the symptomatic patient is surgical, with cholecystectomy, operative cholangiography, and exploration of the common duct when indicated. One must keep in mind the very low yield from exploration of the common bile duct in childhood. The decision to perform elective cholecystectomy even in the absence of symptoms once the gallstones are detected remains controversial. If spherocytosis is present in the patient, staged operative procedures are suggested, with gallbladder removal after splenectomy. Others have done simultaneous cholecystectomy and splenectomy without undue morbidity.

Both a diagnostic and treatment dilemma is posed by the patient with sickle-cell disease who has recurrent abdominal pain, gallstones, or a nonfunctioning gallbladder. In such patients the present trend is toward early elective cholecystectomy, using staged transfusions to better prepare the patient for gallbladder surgery. In such cases the morbidity and mortality in sickle-cell disease patients is similar to that for the general population requiring cholecystectomy.

Prognosis

In nearly all uncomplicated cases, the prognosis is excellent. Common duct stenosis and recurrence of stone formation can occur in 5% of patients. In those unfortunate cases in which common duct obstruction has been lengthy, features of biliary cirrhosis may be found and may persist despite removal of the gallstone.

REFERENCES

Andrassy, R.J., Treadwell, T.A., Ratner, I.A., and Buckley, C.J.: Gallbladder disease in children and adolescents, Am. J. Surg. **132**:19-21, 1976.

Ariyan, S., Shessel, F.S., and Pickett, L.K.: Cholecystitis and cholelithiasis, Pediatrics **58**:252-258, 1976.

Beauregard, W.G., and Ferguson, W.T.: Milk of calcium cholecystitis, J. Pediatr. **96**:876-877, 1980.

Bennion, L.J., Knowler, W.C., Mott, D.M., and others: Development of lithogenic bile during puberty in Pima Indians, N. Engl. J. Med. **300**:873-876, 1979.

Bennion, L.J., and Grundy, S.M.: Risk factors for the development of cholelithiasis in man, parts I, II, N. Engl. J. Med. **299**:1161-1167, 1221-1227, 1978.

Braverman, D.Z., Johnson, M.L., and Kern, F., Jr.: Effects of pregnancy and contraceptive steroids on gallbladder function, N. Engl. J. Med. **302**:362-364, 1980.

Cooperberg, P.L., and Burhenne, H.J.: Real-time ultrasonography, N. Engl. J. Med. **302**:1277-1279, 1980.

Crichlow, R.W., Seltzer, M.H., and Jannetta, P.J.: Cholecystitis in adolescents, Am. J. Dig. Dis. **17**:68-72, 1972.

Crystal, R.F., and Fink, R.L.: Acute acalculous cholecystitis in childhood, Clin. Pediatr. **10**:423-426, 1971.

Hanson, B.A., Mahour, G.W., and Woolley, M.M.: Diseases of the gallbladder in infancy and childhood, J. Pediatr. Surg. **6**:277-283, 1971.

Harned, R.K., and Babbitt, D.P.: Cholelithiasis in children, Radiology **117**:391-393, 1975.

Holt, R.W., Wagner, R., and Homa, M.: Ultrasonic diagnosis of cholelithiasis, J. Pediatr. **92**:418-421, 1978.

Honore, L.H.: Cholesterol cholelithiasis in adolescent females, Arch. Surg. **115**:62-64, 1980.

Isenberg, J.N., L'Heureux, P.R., Warwick, W.J., and Sharp, H.L.: Clinical observations on the biliary system in cystic fibrosis, Am. J. Gastroenterol. **65**:134-141, 1976.

Marks, C., Espinosa, J., and Hyman, L.J.: Acute acalculous cholecystitis in childhood, J. Pediatr. Surg. **3**:608-611, 1968.

Mock, D.M., Perman, J.A., Rosenthal, P., and others: Cholelithiasis in a 2-year-old child with reflux esophagitis and hiatus hernia, J. Pediatr. **96**:878-879, 1980.

Pellerin, D., Bertin, P., Nihoul-Fekete, C., and Ricour, C.: Cholelithiasis and ideal pathology in childhood, J. Pediatr. Surg. **10**:35-41, 1975.

Sarnaik, S., Slovis, T.L., Corbett, D.P., and others: Incidence of cholelithiasis in sickle cell anemia using ultrasonic gray-scale technique, J. Pediatr. **96**:1005-1008, 1980.

Tchirkow, G., Highman, L.M., and Shafer, A.D.: Cholelithiasis and cholecystitis in children after repair of congenital duodenal anomalies, Arch. Surg. **115**:85-86, 1980.

CHOLEDOCHUS CYSTS

Congenital cystic dilatation of the common duct is the most common anatomic aberration of the extrahepatic biliary tree after congenital biliary atresia. Many different names have been used to describe this lesion, but choledochus cyst is the most acceptable. The etiology of this lesion is not completely clear, but most believe it represents a congenital malformation, since other anomalies of the biliary tree are frequently noted during surgical exploration. A double common bile duct, accessory hepatic ducts, double gallbladder, absence of the gallbladder, and atresia of the ducts have been found, as have polycystic kidneys and hypoplastic kidneys. On rare occasions ectatic dilatations (congenital or acquired) of the intrahepatic bile ducts may be found in association with the cystic dilatation of the extrahepatic system. Some believe that a segmental muscular weakness in the wall of the common bile duct is responsible for the dilatation.

Some still favor an acquired distal obstruction about the ampulla as the main predisposing lesion to the development of the cyst. The argument implies that the distal segment may be hypoplastic and therefore requires pressures greater than normal to distend this obstructing region. Proximal distention occurs, and cyst formation develops in the region of weakness. This theory is also supported by those examples in which anomalous insertion of the common bile duct into the distal part of the pancreatic duct has been observed in some cases from choledochal cysts. The reflux of pancreatic juice into this "common channel" is believed responsible for an ongoing inflammatory process, subsequent fibrosis, and stricture of the distal end of the common duct, predisposing to subsequent cyst formation in the proximal segment.

The incidence of choledochus cysts is quite low and accounts for about 5% of cases of so-called gallbladder disease, excluding congenital biliary atresia, in children. About one third of the cases are reported from Japan, where no sex predominance is found. In whites, the incidence is 4 to 1, females to males. More than half the reported cases are diagnosed in patients less than 10 years of age, but less than 5% are symptomatic before 6 months of age. In this very young age group the clinical features are indistinguishable from those of other causes of extrahepatic biliary obstruction (biliary atresia).

Clinical features

The triad of jaundice, pain, and mass is found in less than 10% to 15% of cases. The jaundice may be intermittent, constant, or absent. Abdominal pain is mild, aching, or colicky in nature, often relapsing after intervals of well-being. The pain is generally in the right upper quadrant or may also be noted in the epigastrium. On occa-

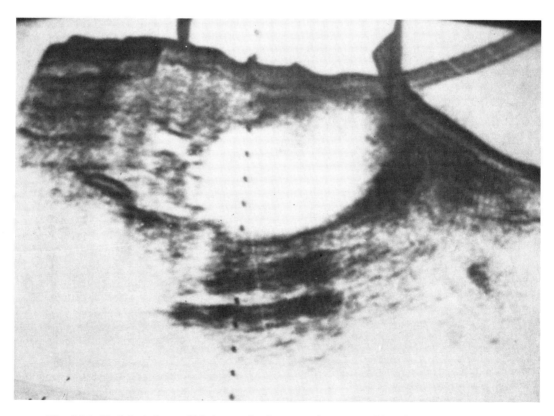

Fig. 26-6. Choledochal cyst. This large echo-free mass demonstrated by ultrasound examination in a 6-week-old infant with persistent cholestasis. A dilated biliary duct is also apparent.

sion it radiates to the back or right shoulder. The mass is palpable in the right upper quadrant, is said to be cystic to palpation, and can be moved laterally but not vertically. Nontender hepatomegaly is commonly present. Associated clinical information, such as vomiting, fevers, acholic stools, dark urine, and pruritus, is elicited from between 25% and 30% of patients. In some cases the symptoms of abdominal pain and vomiting may be attributable to associative pancreatitis, an unusual complication of a choledochal cyst. When the cyst fluid is secondarily contaminated by bacteria, abdominal pain may be severe and mimic other surgical conditions such as acute cholecystitis, perforated appendix, or ruptured ectopic pregnancy, especially in the teen-age female. Some patients are totally asymptomatic, whereas others may present with bile peritonitis from perforation. The sicker the patient appears, the more likely is the possibility that cholangitis is also present.

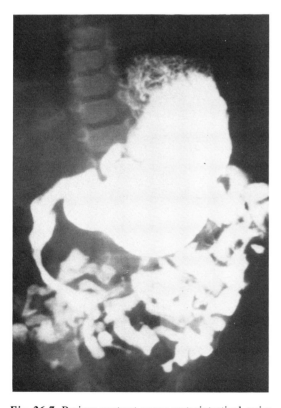

Fig. 26-7. Barium-contrast upper gastrointestinal series in an infant with cholestatic syndrome. Note a large extrinsic mass that widens the duodenal C-loop while also pulling the duodenal bulb downward. A choledochal cyst was found at surgery.

Diagnosis

Before the development of newer radiologic techniques and the availability of ultrasonography, correct diagnosis was seldom made before surgery (in perhaps 25% of cases) despite the frequency of jaundice, abdominal pain, and mass noted at some time in the clinical story. The intermittency of the jaundice and pain and the physician's low index of suspicion contribute to this figure.

The most useful diagnostic studies at present include abdominal ultrasound examination, which usually reveals a large anechoic cystic structure in the right upper quadrant (Fig. 26-6), or barium contrast studies of the upper gastrointestinal tract, which will outline the mass in over 80% of patients. Anteroinferior displacement of the first and second portions of the duodenum is most commonly observed, and the mass effect upon the gastric antrum or duodenal bulb can likewise be seen in many cases (Fig. 26-7). Scanning of the cyst after injection of ^{131}I–rose bengal, or ^{99m}Tc-DIDA at 30 minutes, 6 hours, and 24 hours will confirm the continuity of this structure with the biliary tree. At times percutaneous transhepatic cholangiography provides useful information, especially about the size of the proximal biliary radicals, and will reveal any intrahepatic developmental anomalies of the bile ducts.

In the unusual varieties, where the cyst resides in an intraduodenal or intrapancreatic location, it can best be visualized by upper intestinal endoscopy and retrograde pancreatocholangiography. Although doing so is seldom necessary, the cyst can be filled by contrast material injected intravenously for cholangiography.

Leukocytosis is unusual. The serum bilirubin is slightly raised and of the "mixed" type. Serum cholesterol value is reported elevated in over 50% of cases. In long-standing examples of jaundice associated with choledochal cysts, the prothrombin time is likely to be prolonged. Additional derangement of liver functions (transaminases, alkaline phosphatase, cholesterol) usually signifies hepatic parenchymal involvement. Not infrequently the serum amylase may be elevated. The differential diagnosis includes pancreatic, mesenteric, and echinococcal cysts, retroperitoneal tumors, and, in the neonate, congenital biliary atresia. In the presence of fever and leukocytosis, acute cholecystitis, ruptured appendicitis, and ruptured ectopic pregnancy are often considered in the differential diagnosis. In the teen-age child, the Fitz-Hugh-Curtis syndrome becomes another diagnostic possibility. Persistent "cholestatic" or cholangiolitic hepatitis may have similar biochemical features. Embryonal rhabdomyosarcoma of the biliary tree may cause obstruction, pain, and mass.

Pathology

Three types of extrahepatic and two types of intraheptic cystic dilatation of the bile ducts are described (Fig. 26-8). Type I includes those that begin 2 cm above the entrance into the duodenum and have an abrupt dilatation at both ends of the cyst (Fig. 26-9). The terminal common bile duct is narrow and hypoplastic, whereas the proximal common duct is generally distended; the cystic duct and gallbladder are not affected. The entire common duct may be involved in a cyst of large size, and in such cases the cystic duct may enter directly into the choledochus. These cysts can reach enormous size and contain up to 1 to 2 liters of white to yellow-green colored fluid. On occasion bacteria may be cultured from the cyst fluid. Intracyst contents often include sludgelike material, epithelial debris, and occasionally gravel or more well-formed gallstones. The cyst wall is thickened by accumulation of dense connective tissue, and the inner lining is usually devoid of epithelial covering. Rather, the lumen surface is replaced by granulation tissue and a fibrinous exudate. The gallbladder is normal especially in the older age group.

Type II is a diverticulum type of cyst originating from the midportion of the common duct. This particular variant is more subject to kinking and obstruction.

Type III includes those rare cases of cystic dilatation that occur within the wall of the duo-

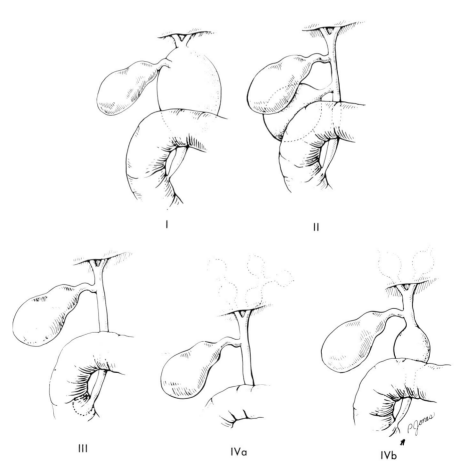

Fig. 26-8. Classification of cystic dilatation of the bile ducts. Types I, II, and III are extrahepatic, whereas type IVa is solely intrahepatic and IVb is mixed intrahepatic and extrahepatic.

denum (choledochocele). They may obstruct bile flow or at times prolapse into the bowel lumen and obstruct the duodenum itself.

Type IV, also known as Caroli's disease (Fig. 26-10), is divided into two subgroups: one where cystic dilatation of the bile ducts occurs only in their intrahepatic location (IVa); the other where cystic dilatations are found in both the extrahepatic and the intrahepatic portions of the bile ducts (IVb).

Since congenital hepatic and renal anomalies have been reported in association with choledochus cysts, biopsy of the liver and intravenous pyelography should be employed in all patients.

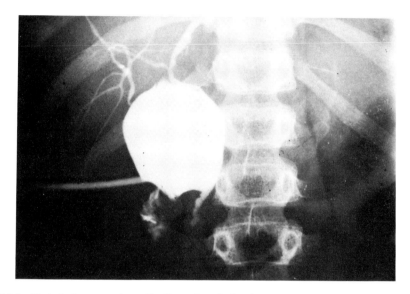

Fig. 26-9. Choledochus cyst (type I). Operative cholangiogram on a young girl with recurrent episodes of colicky right upper quadrant pain. Pruritus was frequently associated with these attacks. Physical examination revealed mild jaundice and a tender mass to the right of the epigastrium. At surgery the large choledochus cyst was found and drained into a loop of jejunum by Roux-en-Y anastomosis.

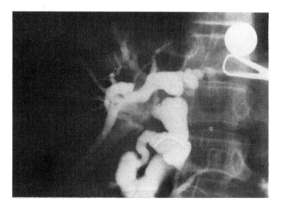

Fig. 26-10. Caroli's disease. Percutaneous transhepatic cholangiogram performed in a 14-year-old girl. Dilated, saccular, intrahepatic bile ducts are present, as well as a saccular dilatation of the common hepatic duct consistent with type IVb disease. The patient had been troubled by postprandial upper abdominal pain and occasional vomiting since 3 years of age. An episode of jaundice was initially believed to be caused by viral hepaitits, but when symptoms and icterus recurred, more definitive diagnostic studies led to the correct diagnosis.

Liver biopsy may show significant intrahepatic canalicular cholestasis, portal fibrosis, and neoductular proliferation. Changes consistent with biliary cirrhosis may be present in the infant with choledochal cyst as early as 6 to 8 weeks of life. Also in the young infant, giant-cell transformation of hepatocytes may be observed. The features in liver biopsy material obtained in the older-age patient are usually mild; however, depending on the degree of obstruction, choledochus cysts may be responsible for features of cholangitis and biliary cirrhosis.

Treatment

Treatment is always surgical, for medical therapy alone will lead to a fatal outcome. Transabdominal tapping of the cyst should be avoided, since this is attended by a high risk of leakage of cyst fluid into the abdominal cavity with resultant bile peritonitis. Removal of the cyst and reconstruction of the normal anatomy is the operative procedure of choice. After cyst removal, a Roux-en-Y choledochojejunostomy or hepaticojejunostomy is gaining favor in experienced hands. Although choledochoduodenostomy or choledochojejunostomy is technically easier to perform, the postoperative morbidity (cholangitis, pancreatitis, stomal stricture) is extraordinarily high (30% to 60%) and frequently requires subsequent surgical reconstruction. Closure of the anastomosis is not suprising when mucosa-lined surface of the intestine is sutured to a nonepithelialized structure as exists in the cyst. Furthermore, failure to remove the cyst leaves the individual with the substantial risk to develop biliary tract adenocarcinoma at a later time.

Complications

Progressive biliary cirrhosis with portal hypertension may evolve with surprising rapidity in the young infant with a choledochal cyst, especially if diagnosis and surgery are delayed. Ascending cholangitis may develop both before and after (10%) surgical reconstruction. Liver abscess formation may be a secondary complication in such patients. Although possible in younger children, choledochal lithiasis and recurrent episodes of pancreatitis are found, especially in the older child (10 to 18 years). Adenocarcinoma of the extrahepatic biliary system occurs in 10 to 20 times greater incidence in patients with choledochal cysts than in the normal population.

Prognosis

With the improvement of surgical techniques in infants and children, the prognosis for survival has improved dramatically, especially in the older child. Before 1953 surgical correction of this entity had a mortality greater than 50%, whereas now the figure is about 10%. Morbidity figures in several large series where surgery was performed by experienced individuals demonstrate that postoperative cholangitis occurred in 10% and stricture of the anastomosis in approximately 5%. In general, patients with choledochal cysts operated upon before 6 months of age have a poorer long-term prognosis, since most of these cases occur in association with other congenital abnormalities of the biliary system including biliary atresia. Eventually the vagaries of biliary cirrhosis and portal hypertension appear in these young infants and children and death results from liver failure, sepsis, or bleeding esophageal varices.

REFERENCES

Barlow, B., Tabor, E., Blanc, W.A., and others: Choledochal cyst: a review of 19 cases, J. Pediatr. **89:**934-940, 1976.

Bass, E.M., and Cremin, B.J.: Choledochal cysts: a clinical and radiological evaluation of 21 cases, Pediatr. Radiol. **5:**81-85, 1976.

Goldberg, P.B., Long, W.B., Oleaga, J.A., and Mackie, J.A.: Choledochocele as a cause of recurrent pancreatitis, Gastroenterology **78:**1041-1045, 1980.

Gots, R.E., and Zuidema, G.E.: Dilatation of the intrahepatic biliary ducts in a patient with a choledochal cyst, Am. J. Surg. **119:**726-728, 1970.

Hermansen, M.C., Starshak, R.J., and Werlin, S.L.: Caroli disease: the diagnostic approach, J. Pediatr. **94:**879-882, 1979.

Kagawa, Y., Kashihara, S., Kuramoto, S., and Maetani, S.: Carcinoma arising in a congenitally dilated biliary tract, Gastroenterology **74:**1286-1294, 1978.

Lilly, J.R.: The surgical treatment of choledochal cyst, Surgery **149:**36-42, 1979.

Murray-Lyon, I.M., Shilkin, K.B., Laws, J.W., and others: Non-obstructive dilatation of the intrahepatic biliary tree with cholangitis, Q. J. Med. **41:**477-489, 1972.

Mittelstaedt, C.A., Volberg, F.M., Fischer, G.J., and McCartney, W.H.: Caroli's disease: sonographic findings, Am. J. Roentgenol. **134:**585-587, 1980.

Norton, L.W.: Caroli's disease: a surgical challenge, Am. Surg. **45:**70-73, 1979.

Rosenfield, N., and Griscom, N.T.: Choledochal cysts: roentgenographic techniques, Radiology **114:**113-119, 1975.

Thomas, C.G., Jr., Zawacki, J.K., Ona, F.V., and Norton, R.A.: Intrapancreatic choledochal cyst, Gastroenterology **71:**1071-1074, 1976.

Todani, T., Watanabe, Y., Narusue, M., and others: Congenital bile duct cysts: classification, operative procedures, and review of 37 cases including cancer arising from choledochal cyst, Am. J. Surg **134:**263-269, 1977.

Todani, T., Narusue, M., Watanabe, Y., and others: Management of congenital choledochal cyst with intrahepatic involvement, Ann Surg. **187:**272-280, 1978.

Valayer, J., and Alagille, D.: Experience with choledocal cyst, J. Pediatr. Surg. **10:**65-68, 1975.

OTHER CONGENITAL OR ACQUIRED ABERRATIONS OF EXTRAHEPATIC BILIARY SYSTEM

Congenital absence of gallbladder. This condition is most likely the result of embryonic maldevelopment. In the pediatric-age group it is most commonly associated with extrahepatic biliary atresia. Later in life it is often found as an isolated abnormality, discovered at surgery for symptoms relating to biliary tract disease. Absence of both the gallbladder and the common duct has also been reported, and in these cases the hepatic duct or ducts insert directly into the duodenum. An atrophic or hypoplastic gallbladder is seen in up to 40% of patients with cystic fibrosis.

Duplication of gallbladder (double gallbladder). This abnormality of embryonic development may be discovered in the course of investigations for right upper quadrant abdominal pain or jaundice. Not infrequently, the cystic duct inserts in an anomalous fashion into the existing biliary drainage system, which predisposes to obstruction and accompanying symptoms. Diagnosis is rarely made before surgical exploration.

Accessory bile ducts. In some patients aberrant bile ducts arise from the liver and enter into the normal ductal structures at any location, or occasionally directly into the duodenum. Such anomalies are more common in patients with choledochal cyst, and it behooves the surgeon to be aware of such a possibility during surgical intervention in these cases.

Congenital stenosis of common duct. Significant narrowing of the distal portion of the common duct, or occasionally at the junction of the common hepatic duct and common bile duct, may be a rare cause of biliary cirrhosis. The cause of this abnormality is seldom found, but a congenital (or acquired) inflammatory process seems likely. Subclinical jaundice may escape detection in many patients, and pruritus and recurrent abdominal pain instead may dominate the clinical picture. Firm, modest hepatomegaly and splenic enlargement are present on physical examination. Ductal dilatation proximal to the obstruction is appreciated by a variety of investigative studies including radioactive technetium scan (DIDA or PIPIDA), ^{131}I–rose bengal, or percutaneous transhepatic cholangiography. Intravenous cholangiography may not visualize the obstruction if jaundice is significant. When present, ultrasound of the bile ducts will show dilatation of the proximal ductal structures but will not precisely define the site of stenosis.

Surgical removal of the stricture and jejunal Roux-en-Y biliary anastomosis should be curative provided that the hepatic changes are not severe. At times choledochotomy permits clearing of intraluminal (sludged) bile accumulated proximal to the stricture, without one having to resort to a biliary-enteric anastomosis.

Duplication cyst of gallbladder and biliary tract. Aberrant gastric tissue in a duplication cyst is capable of producing hydrochloric acid and inducing an inflammatory process in these structures. Abdominal pain, jaundice, hemobilia, and pancreatitis are all possible clinical expressions if a duplication cyst coexists within these biliary tract structures. Preoperative diagnostic studies of value include intravenous cholangiography or percutaneous transhepatic cholangiography. Most often the diagnosis is made during exploratory laparotomy for suspected obstructing biliary tract disease.

Primary sclerosing cholangitis. Primary sclerosing cholangitis is a rare entity in the pediatric-age population, developing in about 1% of individuals with inflammatory bowel disease. Although 50% of all cases occur in association with chronic ulcerative colitis, primary sclerosing cholangitis does not correlate with the extent or duration of the bowel disease. In some, jaundice appears at the same time the symptoms of colitis begin. Sclerosing cholangitis is a progressive process that causes segmental stenosis and eventual obliteration of part or all of the extrahepatic bile ducts. This process may extend into the intrahepatic ducts as well and closely mimic the lesions seen in Caroli's disease. Clinical symptoms usually include recurrent fevers, recurrent right upper quadrant pain and tenderness, low-grade fluctuating jaundice, and pruritus. Laboratory studies are consistent with an obstructive biliary process and include elevated direct-reacting bilirubin, gamma glutamyl transpeptidase (CGT), alkaline phosphatase, and bile acids. Diagnosis is usually confirmed by transhepatic cholangiography or endoscopic retrograde cholangiography. Visualization of the biliary system by intravenous cholangiog-

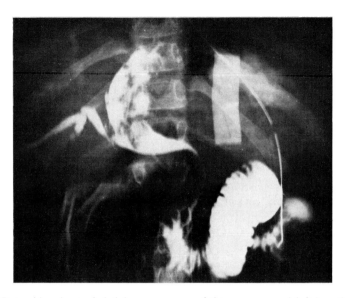

Fig. 26-11. Botryoid embryonal rhabdomyosarcoma of the common and left hepatic ducts. Operative cholangiogram outlines irregular filling defects seen within the dilated distorted bile duct that is partially obstructed. The patient was a 6-year-old boy with several months of severe pruritus followed by the appearance of jaundice. The liver was enlarged and somewhat tender. Ultrasound examination showed the dilated biliary structure, and surgery was undertaken.

raphy is seldom successful in these cases. Roentgenologic features are those of multiple biliary strictures and "beading," with a tapering effect of the intrahepatic biliary radicals. At times the mucosal lining presents an irregular shaggy appearance. Liver biopsy specimens show cholestasis, concentric fibrosis around the interlobular bile ducts, and occasionally features of pericholangitis. Neither medical nor surgical treatment provides any long-term benefit to these unfortunate patients. Temporary improvement has been reported after corticosteroids and cholestyramine. Surgical decompression procedures are palliative at best, and biliary cirrhosis and liver failure eventually ensue within 5 to 10 years. Intrahepatic sclerosing cholangitis has also been reported in association with retroperitoneal fibrosis (Ormond's disease), immune deficiency syndromes, Riedel's thyroiditis, and orbital pseudotumor.

Tumors of biliary tree. The most common pediatric neoplasm of the biliary tract is botryoid embryonal rhabdomyosarcoma. Symptoms are those of biliary obstruction including pruritus, jaundice, right upper quadrant and epigastric abdominal pain, and at times a palpable mass. The intraductal obstruction has been identified preoperatively by ultrasonography, intravenous cholangiography and percutaneous transhepatic cholangiography, or by operative cholangiography (Fig. 26-11). These defects can partially or totally occlude the common duct and may prolapse through the ampulla of Vater where it has the appearance of an intraduodenal filling defect on upper gastrointestinal series or by endoscopy. The tumor is usually locally invasive, but metastases do occur. Upon opening the common duct, one notes that the tumor presents as a soft gelatinous grapelike mass. Despite a large surgical resection (Whipple's procedure), radiation, and drug therapy, the prognosis is extremely grim, with only a single long-term survivor being reported up to now.

REFERENCES

Akers, D.R., and Needham, M.E.: Sarcoma botryoides (rhabdomyosarcoma) of the bile ducts with survival, J. Pediat. Surg. **6:**474-479, 1971.

Akers, D.R., Favara, B.E., Franciosi, R.A., and Nelson, J.M.: Duplications of the alimentary tract: report of three unusual cases associated with bile and pancreatic ducts, Surgery **71:**817-823, 1972.

Cello, J.P.: Cholestasis in ulcerative colitis, Gastroenterology **73:**357-374, 1977.

Chapoy, P.R., Kendall, R.S., Fonkalsrud, E., and Ament, M.E.: Congenital stricture of the common hepatic duct: an unusual case without jaundice, Gastroenterology **80:**380-383, 1981.

Hellstrom, H.R., and Perez-Stable, E.C.: Retroperitoneal fibrosis with disseminated vasculitis and intrahepatic sclerosing cholangitis, Am. J. Med. **40:**184-187, 1966.

McElfatrick, R.R., Ehrichs, E.L., and McLauthlin, C.H.: Congenital absence of the gallbladder and cystic duct, Rocky Mtn. Med. J. **71:**455-458, 1974.

Myers, R.N., Cooper, J.H., and Padis, N.: Primary sclerosing cholangitis, Am. J. Gastroenterol. **53:**527-538, 1970.

Polter, D.E., Gruhl, V., Eigenbrodt, E.H., and Combes, B.: Beneficial effect of cholestyramine in sclerosing cholangitis, Gastroenterology **79:**326-333, 1980.

Pontes, J.F., and Pinotti, H.W.: Anomalies of the gallbladder and biliary system. In Bockus, H.C., editor: Gastroenterology, ed. 3, vol. 3, Philadelphia, 1976, W.B. Saunders Co.

Record, C.O., Eddleston, A.L.W.F., Shilkin, K.B., and Williams, R.: Intrahepatic sclerosing cholangitis associated with a familial immunodeficiency syndrome, Lancet **2:**18-20, 1973.

Warshaw, A.L., Schapiro, R.H., Ferrucci, J.T., Jr., and Galdabini, J.J.: Persistent obstructive jaundice, cholangitis, and biliary cirrhosis due to common bile duct stenosis in chronic pancreatitis, Gastroenterology **70:**562-567, 1976.

Werlin, S.L., Glicklich, M., Jona, J., and Starshak, R.J.: Sclerosing cholangitis in childhood, J. Pediatr. **96:**433-435, 1980.

27 *Exocrine pancreatic insufficiency*

CYSTIC FIBROSIS

The frequency, severity, and chronicity of cystic fibrosis make it one of the most dreaded hereditary disorders of childhood. Historically, the early frustrations in diagnosis and management are suggested by the frequency of changes in the name used to describe the condition. When first described in 1938, it was believed to involve primarily the pancreas (fibrocystic disease of the pancreas), but it soon became apparent that cystic fibrosis is a protean disease capable of producing symptoms and pathologic changes in many parts of the body. Temporary favor was given to the term "mucoviscidosis" when an abnormality in the mucous secretions of exocrine glands was recognized. Later, additional abnormalities were noted in the secretions of non–mucus producing exocrine glands (parotid glands) and eccrine sweat glands as well, and "cystic fibrosis" became the acceptable term.

Although over 40 years have elapsed since cystic fibrosis was first identified as a distinct disease, many challenges remain. Clarification of the basic defect is needed. A reliable screening test that can identify carrier heterozygotes and the homozygote fetus in utero needs to be developed. Specific therapy to halt the progression of pulmonary and hepatic disease awaits discovery. Although 50% of patients with cystic fibrosis can now expect to reach early adulthood, it appears that any further increase in the overall longevity of these patients will require new breakthroughs in understanding the basic pathologic defect.

Incidence

Since 1938, when fibrocystic disease of the pancreas was first separated from the group of conditions lumped together as celiac syndrome, many large surveys pertaining to incidence have been reported. An acceptable incidence figure for this disease in the homozygote state in whites varies from 1:600 to 1:2500. It is rare in American blacks (reported at an incidence of 1:17,000), and essentially nonexistent in African blacks and Mongolians. Variations do occur; in the United

States for example, incidence figures of 1:1500 to 1:10,000 have been reported from different states. It is equally common in Australia (1:2000) but infrequent in Sweden (1:10,000).

This extremely high incidence rate makes cystic fibrosis the most frequently occurring lethal genetic disease for white children. Incidence figures of this nature imply a carrier rate of about 5% for the general population. So staggering are these figures that a heterozygote survival advantage has been suggested. Indeed, both sibships of patients and grandparents of patients are reported to have a larger number of surviving members than controls.

Genetics

Cystic fibrosis is an autosomal recessive disease. As mentioned, the high carrier rate for the mutant gene is believed to imply heterozygote advantage to the individual.

Chromosome studies have not revealed any abnormalities, and linkage with other known loci (ABO blood groups) has not been demonstrated. No sex difference exists. That some families have many affected members and others do not is believed to be attributable to chance alone. Specific organ involvement and severity of disease is generally the same for affected siblings. This is particularly true for the neonatal complication, meconium ileus, and later in life perhaps liver involvement as well.

The discovery of so-called "late onset" cases has also been taken to imply different genetic types of cystic fibrosis, or examples of variable gene penetrance. It is remotely possible that cystic fibrosis is not a single entity but rather a group of closely related genetic abnormalities with similar pathophysiologic consequences. This premise was based upon results of early investigations that attempted to identify in vitro differences (metachromasia) in fibroblasts grown from obligate homozygotes, heterozygotes, and normal individuals. From the observed variations in metachromasia it was concluded that genetic heterogeneity probably exists in phenotypically similar patients.

However, the early enthusiasm for utilizing the quantitative development of intracellular metachromasia in fibroblasts and white blood cells as a means of distinguishing the homozygote cystic fibrotic patient from normals, diminished significantly when the nonspecificity of the technique became obvious. In addition, the technique could not consistently differentiate the heterozygote state, and so it was unsuitable for antenatal diagnosis or genetic counseling.

Attempts to identify the carrier state by a variety of laboratory tools have shown some promise but remain primarily research tools and are not practical for use in screening programs or prenatal diagnosis. In vitro studies using fibroblasts obtained from patients with cystic fibrosis have been handicapped by variables that are inherent to this technique and difficult to control. This explains the frequent inability to reproduce results in other investigative laboratories. A primary concern in any in vitro study is the possibility that the basic defect is not expressed in the particular cell line. However, cystic fibrosis fibroblasts do show certain differences from cells obtained from normals. They are more resistant to the cytotoxic effects of cyclic AMP, dexamethasone, ouabain in potassium-deficient media, and sex steroids, manifesting enhanced survival when compared to control cells. Early results of experiments that studied the incorporation of ^{22}Na into fibroblasts from obligate homozygotes and heterozygotes, and normal individuals after ouabain exposure, showed discriminating quantitative differences among the groups. Fibroblasts from patients with cystic fibrosis and from heterozygotes have been found to accumulate the least cell-associated ^{22}Na, suggesting that these cells have either decreased sodium influx or increased sodium efflux. Such findings are certainly consistent with previous observations that sodium reabsorption in the sweat ducts of patients with cystic fibrosis is impaired. Unfortunately, further studies testing larger numbers of fibroblast strains within the same experimental design failed to confirm earlier findings.

White blood cells from patients with cystic fibrosis have been shown to have reduced cyclic-AMP response to beta-adrenergic stimulation compared to healthy controls. Obligate heterozygotes were found to have an immediate response. Further studies along these lines suggest that the defect appears to be at the beta-receptor coupling site to adenyl cyclase. It is unclear, however, whether the membrane abnormality is a primary or secondary defect in cystic fibrosis patients. White blood cells from cystic fibrosis patients also show an increased calcium uptake, a phenomenon that can be induced in normal white blood cells when they are exposed to the serum of cystic fibrosis patients. A similar enhanced calcium uptake has been noted in the mitochondria of fibroblasts grown in vitro from patients with cystic fibrosis. Once again, heterozygotes show intermediate values. Despite these encouraging observations, the known inherent difficulties in tissue-culture techniques demand that extreme caution be exercised before one applies any methodology to prenatal diagnosis or postnatal heterozygote detection.

Over the years, other forms of methodology have been applied without success in an attempt to separate the asymptomatic heterozygote carriers from normals. A comparison of the sodium concentration in nail clippings from unaffected siblings and parents of patients gave inconsistent results in detection of the carrier state. That two groupings appeared within the unaffected siblings indeed suggested heterozygosity, but, unfortunately, parents could not be distinguished from controls. The application of statistical techniques to four successive sweat-test results was believed by some to permit separation of heterozygotes from controls, but it did not consistently hold true. This study did reinforce the edict that a single determination of sweat chlorides should not be used for genetic counseling.

The early enthusiasm for utilizing either the rabbit tracheal or oyster ciliary bioassay technique for detection of the heterozygote state in cystic fibrosis has been substantially tempered by lack of consistent results, absence of specificity, and the frequent inability to reproduce the results in different laboratories. Other interesting observations have been made in patients with cystic fibrosis and family members over the past 10 years, but none has been able to consistently identify the heterozygote state.

Pathogenesis

The basic defect in cystic fibrosis remains unknown despite extensive research. No single unifying concept providing an explanation for the abnormalities of exocrine gland secretions has been found. Studies of the properties of mucus from patients with cystic fibrosis as well as the eccrine sweat abnormality have also been handicapped by much contradiction. It is unclear, for example, whether the chemical composition—and therefore physiochemical properties—of mucus is primarily abnormal or whether this abnormality is secondary to other events involved in production and secretion of mucus. The physiochemical properties of mucus are affected by many variables, such as ionic strength, pH of the secretion, polymerization, concentration of other macromolecules within the fluid, and electrolytes, which make the study of mucous secretions very difficult. Except for an abnormality in the macromolecular concentration of these secretions in patients with cystic fibrosis, little else can be found abnormal about the mucus. Immunologic and histochemical techniques have given results similar to those of normal mucus.

The hypothesis of hyperpermeable mucus held brief popularity as a mechanism that might best explain the observation that secretions within the ducts tend to lose water and become concentrated. This hyperpermeability was believed to be caused by a serum factor that affects primarily the calcium concentration within the exocrine secretions. However, excess calcium has only been found in submaxillary saliva and not in other exocrine fluids. Calcium does, however, affect the physicochemical properties of mucus secretions. In vitro studies have shown the ability of calcium to polymerize normal glycoproteins, making the mucus more hyperpermeable and viscous. Removal of this ion from cystic fibrosis saliva reverts the abnormal protein pattern to normal. As previously mentioned, white blood cells and fibroblasts from patients with cystic fibrosis do show enhanced uptake of calcium, and the intracellular concentrations of this ion may in turn produce an abnormal biologic fluid. Conceivably this hyperviscoid hypertonic secretion (mucus) may obstruct the exocrine-secreting structure and eventually produce the pathologic lesion seen in most organs (pancreas, lungs, liver, salivary glands). Within the lumen of the ductular structure, inspissated secretions are recognized histologically as eosinophilic concretions.

Whether the reported abnormality in the calcium concentration of certain secretions of patients with cystic fibrosis represents a primary or a secondary disturbance has not been settled. Furthermore, it remains unclear what genetometabolic defect may be responsible for this abnormality in calcium transport.

Another hypothesis implicates a defect in fluid movement both to and from the extravascular space through secretory cells. This defect theoretically could prevent the normal dilution of cellular products to be delivered into the ductular lumen of both mucus- and serum-secreting glands. This highly concentrated material may damage the cells containing this product, especially if discharge of the material is impaired. The abnormalities noted in pancreatic secretory studies in patients with cystic fibrosis support this hypothesis. A concentrated enzyme solution of low volume and low bicarbonate content is obtained from the duodenum after a secretin-pancreozymin test.

The abnormality in the secretions of serous glands, especially the eccrine sweat gland, is different from that seen in other exocrine glands. The increased levels of sodium and chloride in the sweat of patients with cystic fibrosis constitute the most consistent chemical abnormality noted. Normal sweat is delivered as a hypotonic solution, although the primary solution is believed to be isotonic. To explain the abnormality in the final solution (high Na^+ and Cl^-) in patients with cystic fibrosis, a defect in electrolyte reabsorption of sodium and water by the ductular cells has been suggested. A sodium-transport inhibitory factor has been found in the saliva and sweat of patients with cystic fibrosis. It appears to prevent sodium reabsorption along the sweat duct, but the exact site of its action remains unclear. This chemically undefined inhibitory factor also exerts a similar effect in the sweat ducts of normal individuals. The ineffectiveness of cystic fibrosis sweat or serum applied contraluminally (infiltrated through the skin) to alter the sodium concentration of sweat in normal individuals puts to rest the theory that a serum sweat factor exerts its primary effect outside the eccrine secretory cell. It was previously considered that the sweat factor altered the "extraneous mucous coat" and thereby affected extracellular fluid movement both in and out of the cell. The sodium reabsorption–inhibiting factor has been confirmed in not only mixed saliva but also submandibular, sublingual, and submucosal saliva in patients with cystic fibrosis. For unknown reasons parotid saliva does not contain the sodium reabsorption–inhibiting factor. It is interesting that an increase in the sodium and chloride concentration of sweat can be accomplished by iontophoresis of calcium into the skin of normal subjects.

The pathologic lesion seen in the salivary gland correlates well with the type of secretion produced. The predominantly serous fluid–producing parotid gland shows little alteration in morphology, and the secretions contain only slightly higher levels of sodium and chloride than controls do. Submaxillary glands behave more like other mucus-producing glands. They tend to enlarge during life and show histologic abnormalities consistent with the effects of chronic intracellular and luminal obstruction. Studies of sodium and chloride concentrations in submaxillary gland secretions have given conflicting results. The fluid, however, is consistently turbid and high in calcium.

Finally, some workers have sought an abnormality in the autonomic nervous system of patients with cystic fibrosis. Diminished alpha- and beta-adrenergic responses, as well as a suppressed cholinergic response, have been found in some but not all patients with cystic fibrosis. Again, genetic heterogeneity may explain the variable responses of different end organs to autonomic nervous system regulation.

Clinical findings, pathologic lesion, complications, and treatment

The typical patient with cystic fibrosis is easily recognized in the first year of life, since about 90% of affected children have obvious clinical signs and symptoms resulting from both the pulmonary and pancreatic involvement. Early diagnosis of milder forms of this disease is directly related to the development of the sweat test as well as a greater awareness by physicians of the subtle manifestations that can dominate the clinical syndrome.

Pulmonary disease

The production of thick, sticky, dry mucus soon leads the small infant to manifest noisy respirations, intermittent wheezing, and cough. The latter symptom is particularly troublesome during the sleeping hours. Recurrent episodes of bronchitis and pneumonia occur during the first year of life as a primary consequence of obstructing mucous plugs. The role of the reported disturbance of cilial motility in contributing to the pulmonary lesion of cystic fibrosis is at best speculative.

Bronchial or bronchiolar obstruction may lead to a chain of events, the final result being further reduction in functioning lung tissue. These so-called mucoid impactions act as a ball-valve obstruction and produce hyperinflation and localized emphysema. Complete obstruction of the lumen leads to segmental collapse with atelectasis and probably bacterial infection as well. Bronchiectasis of variable degree is always present and is primarily the result of bacterial infection resulting in structural damage to the bronchial and bronchiolar walls. The lesions tend to be more severe in the upper lobes than in the basilar segments. At times one lobe is spared, and the remaining lung parenchyma in that hemithorax is severely affected.

Acute pulmonary lesions can be reversed by vigorous therapy, but slowly and progressively the pulmonary disease continues to compromise the ventilatory capacity of the patient.

Mild tachypnea at rest, intermittent wheezing, and cough continuously plague the patient. Wheezing at times may be so pronounced that patients have been misdiagnosed as being asthmatic; one must keep in mind, however, that both conditions may occur in any one patient.

Physical findings. Typical physical findings mirror the severity of the pulmonary disease. Increased respiratory rate, increased anteroposterior diameter, hyperresonance, depressed diaphragm, and a prolonged expiratory phase are common findings. Overexpansion is also reflected in diminished diaphragmatic excursion. A combination of rhonchi, wheezes, and "sticky" rales can be heard on auscultation. Digital clubbing, with or without cyanosis, develops early in life, coinciding with the advancement of the pulmonary lesion.

Pathology. The pathologic lesion seen in the lungs of patients with cystic fibrosis is consistent with that of chronic obstruction and hyperinflation. The severity of the lesion is age dependent; lungs of newborn infants dying of meconium ileus show no pathologic change. Later one sees mucous plugs occluding small and large bronchi, and acute and chronic inflammatory cells are present in the mucus and epithelial cells. Atelectasis, focal and patchy, subpleural blebs, and "craters" of pus can also be seen in cut sections of lung.

Pulmonary function tests. The consequences of the destructive process on the ventilatory status of the patient are easily recorded by tests of pulmonary function. A high residual lung volume, reduced vital capacity, and reduced maximum expiratory flow volume are characteristic. Serial measurements of pulmonary function in the same child are extremely meaningful in assessing the effectiveness of therapy against progression of the disease. Low values for arterial oxygen tensions can precede the abnormalities of pulmonary function when the latter are measured by conventional means (lung volumes, flow rates, airway conductance, and so on).

Complications. The major complications of obstructive pulmonary disease are pulmonary insufficiency, pulmonary artery hypertension, and cor pulmonale. Eventually, they are responsible for the death of all but a rare patient. Chronic pulmonary infection, hypoxia, and atelectasis contribute to the pulmonary artery hypertension. Hypoalbuminemia, which on occasion develops from other causes (pancreatic insufficiency, liver disease), is an important early finding in cor pulmonale, suggesting an expanded plasma volume.

Other, less common, pulmonary complications that may threaten life are *Staphylococcus* empyema, especially in the infant under 1 year of age, and, in the older child, spontaneous pneumothorax (3%) and severe hemoptysis (1% or 2%). Sudden onset of pain in the chest, accompanied by dyspnea and cyanosis, suggests pneumothorax. Hemoptysis may be the initial symptom in pneumothorax but generally occurs as a consequence of erosive bronchiectasis. Both conditions warrant emergency measures if the patient is to survive, but these events occur in advanced and severe pulmonary disease in which prognosis is predictably poor. Recurrences of pneumothorax are common, and prophylactic surgery or pleural sclerosing agents may be needed.

Lung abscesses in an atelectatic lobe may be the source of intrapulmonary reinfection and require surgical removal to prevent repeated episodes of bronchopneumonia. In selected patients, lobectomy has been successfully performed.

Therapy. Recent studies strongly urge vigorous pulmonary programs in children with cystic fibrosis. The earlier in life the diagnosis is made, the more effective are the treatment efforts. Systematic care, preferably in a supervised home program, and regular evaluation of pulmonary function offer the patient the best possible means of prolonging life.

An active physical therapy program is recommended for the pulmonary complications. Postural drainage techniques can be taught by pulmonary therapists so that parents can perform them at home on the children. Postural drainage after chest percussion should be carried out at least once a day, but especially upon awakening.

In addition, breathing exercises and physical fitness programs can be tailored for each patient. Bronchodilators such as isoproterenol (Isuprel Mistometer, Duo-Medihaler) and aminophylline given by aerosol nebulizers just before postural drainage is also recommended. Spirometric values however are most improved in patients with an underlying asthmatic diathesis. Dense mist, once a cornerstone of therapy in patients with cystic fibrosis, is no longer part of the recommended pulmonary treatment program advocated by cystic fibrosis centers. Controlled studies showed lack of improvement in pulmonary function tests, evaluated before and after the use of this therapeutic regimen.

Bronchial lavage using saline solution in 5% to 10% acetylcysteine (Mucomyst) given through a bronchoscope tube is still employed in selected patients. Complications are potentially devastating, and the presence of a skilled anesthesiologist and pulmonary therapist is necessary. Rapid mobilization of secretions may exceed the ability to remove them through the small bronchoscope tube used for this procedure. Not infrequently, pulmonary function may actually be further impaired for several days after the lavage.

Undoubtedly, antibiotics have been the most important factor in prolonging the life of patients with severe pulmonary disease. There seems to be general agreement that antibiotics should be used only during acute pulmonary infections. These episodes can be recognized by increased cough and sputum production, dyspnea, and sometimes fever.

The choice of drugs can be decided by bacteriologic sensitivities; duration of treatment for acute infections should be 3 weeks. Some disagreement exists about the use of antibiotics on a continuous prophylactic basis, even on a rotational basis. Moderately ill to severely ill patients are sick so much of the time that they are invariably receiving continuous antibiotic drugs anyway. Patients with mild disease probably need antibiotics only for acute exacerbations The choice and combination of drugs must be tailored to the individual patients, sputum flora, and sensitivities when possible. Some agents seem to penetrate the tracheobronchial mucus better than others and consequently are more effective. Dicloxacillin, trimethoprinsulfamethoxazole, chloramphenicol, and ampicillin are effective oral agents. Anti-*Pseudomonas* agents (colistimethate, gentamicin, carbenicillin) are often needed for hospitalized patients. In addition to bone marrow toxicity, chloramphenicol seems to be responsible for optic neuronitis in patients with cystic fibrosis and therefore must be used with caution.

No matter which drugs are used, or in what combination and sequence, all patients eventually develop a tracheobronchial flora in which *Staphylococcus* and *Pseudomonas* predominate. Although these organisms may remain sensitive to available medications, they are never completely eradicated.

Since hypoxia contributes to pulmonary artery hypertension and hastens the progression of the destructive lung disease, these patients should be advised to reside at lower altitudes, preferably at sea level. Chronic oxygen administration at nighttime is of benefit to selected patients, especially those who have recurrent morning headaches believed caused by sleep hypoxia. Oxygen should be administered during all acute exacerbations of the pulmonary disease.

Present data suggests that 50% of patients with cystic fibrosis whose lungs are normal by clinical evaluation after the initial diagnostic and therapeutic efforts are completed have the highest likelihood to survive to early adulthood.

Gastrointestinal disease

The impact of the gastrointestinal disorder in cystic fibrosis is emphasized by the fact that this disease is the leading cause of malabsorption in children. The primary organs that become involved include the pancreas, liver and biliary tract, and both small and large intestines. Secondarily, peptic disease may be the result of advanced pulmonary disease.

The consequences of the pancreatic lesion are well known to most physicians, especially when they occur in the first year of life. However, as more children with cystic fibrosis reach their teens and early adulthood, physician awareness and recognition of late intestinal complications also become mandatory (Table 27-1).

Pancreatic lesion. Probably 80% of patients with cystic fibrosis have pancreatic insufficiency at birth. Before the end of the first year of life an additional 10% of patients develop progressive pancreatic achylia and will require replacement therapy.

The exact mechanism leading to pancreatic insufficiency is not known, but the earliest abnormality reflects a defect in water and electrolyte transport. After secretin and pancreozymin stimulation, the pancreatic juice of patients is abnormal; volume and bicarbonate levels are diminished, and enzyme content may seem relatively

Table 27-1. Gastrointestinal and hepatobiliary manifestations of cystic fibrosis

Organ	Manifestation	All ages (%)	More than 12 years of age (%)
Pancreas	Total achylia	80-90	95
	Partial or normal function	10-20	5
	Pancreatitis	0.1-0.2	?
	Abnormal gamma glutamyl transpeptidase	40	60
	Glucosuria	?	8
	Clinical diabetes	1	1-13
Intestine	Meconium ileus		
	Newborn period	10-15	—
	Equivalent	3-7	24
	Intussusception	1	5
	Rectal prolapse	22	Rare
Gallbladder	Nonvisualizable	23	15
	Microgallbladder	16	18
	Cholelithiasis	0.4	4-12
Liver	Steatosis	15-30	15-30
	Focal biliary cirrhosis	19	25
	Multilobular biliary cirrhosis	2	2-5

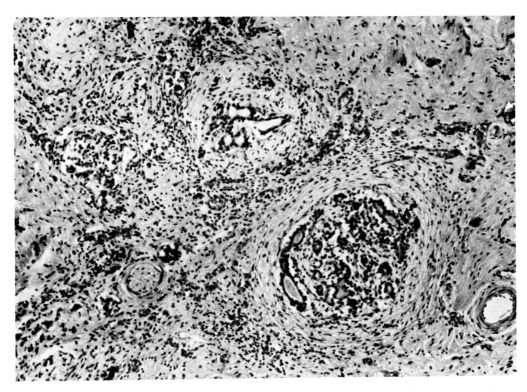

Fig. 27-1. Cystic fibrosis: pancreatic lesion. Autopsy specimen of the pancreas from a 9-year-old child dying of cystic fibrosis and showing extensive fibrous replacement with preservation of small islands of islet cells (upper left). Note the inspissated material in dilated pancreatic ducts.

normal. It is postulated that the lack of adequate diluting fluid from centroacinar and intercalated duct cells may be the most important cause of the pancreatic lesion. Plugging of the small pancreatic ducts by the resulting hyperconcentrated, viscid solution causes destruction distal to the obstruction. Behind the plugs, ductular dilatation and autodigestion of acinar tissue by the proteolytic solution ensue, and progressive inflammation leads to pancreatic fibrosis and exocrine insufficiency (Fig. 27-1).

Clinical features. Malnutrition is evident within the first few months of life. The greatest impact of malabsorption is on fat absorption. The caloric sequestration amounts to 20% to 30% of intake and results primarily from fat malabsorption.

Contrary to traditional impression, children with cystic fibrosis do not consume excessive quantities of calories. In fact, a number of well-designed studies have established that their intake stands 20% below the Recommended Daily Allowance (RDA). It is true however that their appetite is better than that of patients with celiac disease. A third factor contributing to their malnutrition besides malabsorption and insufficient intake is the recent observation that their caloric needs are increased by 30% over the RDA through increased pulmonary and cardiac work and infection.

Steatorrhea is easily recognized by the passage of large foul-smelling stools that appear pale, foamy, and greasy. At times the absence of pancreatic lipase may give rise to other complicating symptoms that can dominate the clinical picture. A hemorrhagic diathesis resulting from vitamin K malabsorption has been the mode of presentation for some patients. Significant gastrointestinal bleeding and skin ecchymoses may temporarily confuse the physician into suspecting a primary hematologic abnormality, nonaccidental trauma, or liver disease. Tetany resulting from hypocalcemia may be another consequence of fat malabsorption; the calcium is saponified by the undigested and malabsorbed fatty acids and lost in the stool. For some reason, vitamin D seems to be relatively unaffected by the pancreatic deficiency, and likewise complication of vitamin A deficiency are seldom seen. Although vitamin E deficiency eventually develops in most patients with cystic fibrosis, its role, if any, in the progression of the disease is not clear. A neurologic syndrome including areflexia, gait disturbance, ophthalmoplegia, decreased proprioceptive and vibratory sensation may be a late consequence of chronic hypovitaminosis E, an important observation now that many (30% to 50%) patients with cystic fibrosis can be expected to live to early adulthood.

In general, the children with cystic fibrosis compensate better for the proteolytic deficiency attending the pancreatic lesion than for the lipase deficiency. Positive nitrogen balance can be achieved by overeating though azotorrhea is usually present. On occasion, hypoproteinemia and edema, often accompanied by anemia, may be an unusual mode of presentation for these infants. A number of children with cystic fibrosis have been reported who developed hypoproteinemia and edema while taking a soybean protein milk product or in others who are exclusively breast-fed. It is not surprising that a number of patients with cystic fibrosis are given a trial on such hypoallergenic formulas. The mild diarrhea, respiratory wheezes, and failure to thrive, seen in some children, are suspected as being allergic responses. Poor weight gain, hypoproteinemia, and edema occur most often in these instances. The mechanism for this is unclear. The impaired absorption of soybean protein compared to cow's milk protein has been blamed upon a trypsin inhibitor previously found in some soy milk preparations. Liver biopsy material in such patients has shown considerable fatty metamorphosis compatible with early nutritional cirrhosis. It is still not clear whether the hypoproteinemia is responsible for the hepatic lesion, or the impaired protein synthesis is secondary to the fatty changes. The low protein content of breast milk (1.5 gm/dl) has also been responsible for precipitating hypoproteinemia and edema occasionally seen in the untreated infant with cystic fibrosis. Iron-deficiency anemia is also a frequent finding in such cases. A greater degree of failure to thrive seems to accompany the affected infants fed either soybean protein milk or breast milk when compared to those receiving a cow's milk formula.

Hypoalbuminemia, with or without edema that develops later in the disease, indicates expansion of the plasma volume resulting from cor pulmonale. Etiologic differentiation of the hypoproteinemia may be difficult if cirrhosis is also present. Patients with cystic fibrosis do not have an exudative enteropathy; except for increased numbers of goblet cells, their intestinal mucosa, as well as lymphatics, are morphologically normal. Mild degrees of villous atrophy may accompany malnutrition.

Progressive destructive changes and fibrosis of the pancreas are believed to result in sufficient disorganization of the islands of Langerhans to affect insulin secretion. As many as 40% to 60% of patients with cystic fibrosis have glucose intolerance. During a glucose tolerance test, serum insulin levels are both lower and delayed in appearance than normal controls regardless of the glucose response. The pattern is similar to that found in adult-onset diabetes. However, serum insulin does rise when tolbutamide or glucagon are given. Impaired glucagon and insulin response has been noted after arginine infusion in patients with cystic fibrosis. Although diabetes mellitus can occur in patients with cystic fibrosis (1%), the disease is characterized by a mild clinical course, partly because of increased insulin sensitivity that exists in these patients.

The pancreatic lesion may also affect iron absorption. Increased iron absorption occurs in untreated patients with pancreatic achylia, and hemosiderosis of the liver may develop. Severe protein depletion may diminish transferrin levels and interfere with iron absorption and transport. Recently, vitamin B_{12} malabsorption has also been demonstrated in cystic fibrosis patients, but clinical evidence indicating a deficiency of this vitamin was lacking. The addition of pancreatic supplements (which often contain vitamin B_{12}), but not vitamin B_{12}–deficient food, is capable of restoring the vitamin B_{12} absorption to near-normal values.

Therapy of pancreatic insufficiency

Drugs. The availability of pancreatic extracts has substantially reduced the morbidity—and for all practical purposes eliminated the mortality—associated with the pancreatic insufficiency of cystic fibrosis. Products currently available for replacement are capable of providing substantial clinical improvement by partially restoring digestion and absorption of fats, proteins, carbohydrates, and vitamins. Although over 15 commercial pancreatic preparations are available, enzyme activities may vary substantially from one product to the next. Pancrease, the newest pancreolipase product, has achieved rapid popularity in the treatment of children with cystic fibrosis. The capsule contains a standardized amount of porcine pancreatic enzyme concentrate in the form of enteric-coated microspheres that are resistant to gastric acid–peptic digestion at pH 5.5, yet quickly solubilize at the intraduodenal pH of 6.0 or greater. Early studies show effectiveness of this product at one third the dosage of previously prescribed pancreolipase preparations. For infants and young children unable to swallow capsules, the contents may be added to liquids or soft foods, but they should not be chewed. One to two capsules per meal, and one taken with snacks, is usually an adequate replacement dosage. An additional advantage of this preparation is the resulting reduced purine intake, thereby lessening the risk of hyperuricosuria and uric acid nephropathy. In some patients, further efficacy of this product (and others as well) may be achieved by the mealtime addition of antacids.

Pancrelipase (Cotazym) comes in a 300 mg capsule or in packets useful for infants and young children with this disease. Some simply remove the powder from the capsule and add it to the food or drink, whereas others add one to two packets of the granules to each 4 to 5 oz of milk. The lipolytic activity of each capsule is said to be sufficient to digest 17 gm of dietary fat, more than enough for an 8 oz feeding.

Viokase is a satisfactory product; its lipase activity is close to that of Cotazym, and protein hydrolysis is said to be more complete than that with other products. Unfortunately, Viokase comes in a tablet so hard that it cannot be chewed. However, it may be obtained in powder form that can be used for small children (1 tsp per 5 oz of milk). Generally speaking, there is little clinical or pharmacologic advantage between Viokase and Cotazym.

Ilozyne, a 400 mg tablet form of pancrelipase, contains the greatest bioactivity of lipase of all available products and is reported capable of digesting 27 gm of fat within 1 hour. This product may be well suited for the older child with cystic fibrosis.

Since lipase is inactivated below pH 4.0, the incomplete effectiveness of replacement therapy is in part attributable to gastric acid–peptic activity or low pancreatic bicarbonate output, conditions that are present in patients with cystic fibrosis. One can do duodenal intubation in patients requiring excessive amounts of pancreatic enzyme replacement (4 to 8 tablets per meal) to determine the pH of duodenal contents, and efforts should be made to raise the intraluminal pH if appropriate. Several agents seem equally effective in producing gastric acid neutrality and allowing for maximum bioactivity of the pancreatic enzyme preparation. Sodium bicarbonate given in tablet form in a dosage of 15 mg/m^2/24 hr along with pancreatic extracts is effective in reducing steatorrhea and subsequently improving weight gain. Similarly, antacids taken simultaneously with pancreatic replacement products will further improve the coefficient of fat absorption, but often without altering the frequency of stooling. Cimetidine, at 20 to 30 mg/kg/day in divided doses, may also be used in refractory cases of persistent steatorrhea and azotorrhea. The combination of cimetidine and sodium bicarbonate added to standard pancreatic replacement therapy has also been employed without significant improvement over that observed when each product was given separately with pancreatic enzymes. Since the long-term consequences of cimetidine in the pediatric age group remain unknown, the potential risks attending the use of this drug may not be justified, especially when other equally effective products are available.

One should recall that the improvement in steatorrhea obtained with pancreatic enzyme replacement and supplemental drug therapy (antacids, sodium bicarbonate, cimetidine) is still incomplete and stools often remain large and offensive. The coefficient of fat absorption achieved in most treated patients is seldom greater than 80% to 85%. Besides the lack of optimum pH values, fat malabsorption may also be caused by diminished intraluminal bile salt concentration and by mucosal dysfunction, the latter characterized by impaired absorption of monoglycerides and certain free fatty acids. The possible role of the observed mucinous covering overlying the absorptive epithelial surface in perpetuating steatorrhea and azotorrhea has not been determined. Excess intake of dietary fat relative to the maximum in vivo bioactivity of replacement enzymes may also be important in perpetuating the malabsorption of fat in patients with cystic fibrosis.

Pancreatin (pancreatic granules) is not acceptable. Although standardized for amylase and trypsin activity, it is not standardized for lipase. Some batches of this product have been found to contain little, if any, of the labile enzyme, lipase.

The dosage of pancreatic extracts required must be individualized. Some patients require less than 600 to 800 mg per meal, whereas others may need three to five times as much. The extracts are best taken with meals and snacks.

Diet. Once the patient is on adequate pancreatic replacement therapy, efforts should be made to assure an adequate caloric intake for maximal growth and weight gain. An optimal nutritional state appears to be extremely desirable in patients with cystic fibrosis. A shortened life survival, at least in some patients with cystic fibrosis, has been attributed to relative malnutrition, especially when weight is disproportionately reduced relative to height. Some workers have noted that optimal nutritional intake, whether achieved orally alone or with parenteral hyperalimentation and oral supplementation, may have a beneficial effect upon the pulmonary disease. Good nutrition prevents linoleic acid deficiency from developing, a condition that may negatively affect oxygen supply to tissues. The mechanism perhaps involves an alteration in prostaglandin synthesis, since linoleic acid deficiency results in an overproduction of prostaglandin $F_{2\alpha}$, a substance known to cause pulmonary bronchoconstriction and pulmonary artery vasoconstriction. In addition, undernutrition may further compromise enterocyte absorptive function and accentuate the malabsorption of fats, proteins, and carbohydrates and perpetuate the malnutrition.

Frequent utilization of the clinic nutritionist is imperative in the long-term management of patients with cystic fibrosis. Despite a reported large appetite, these patients, left to their own dietary devices, will be found to ingest a suboptimal caloric diet that is usually 80% to 90% of the recommended daily allowance. Anorexia is especially prevalent in the face of clinically significant pulmonary disease, and these patients particularly need close monitoring of their nutritional state. High caloric intake, greater than 130% of the recommended daily allowance is suggested, with 20% of the calories as protein, 40% carbohydrate, and 40% as fat. In the newborn or very young infant, Portagen or Pregestimil can be used as formula. These products contain medium-chain triglycer-

ides (C_8 to C_{12}); their absorption, through the portal vein, is relatively independent of pancreatic lipase activity. However, the addition of pancreatic enzyme supplementation is strongly recommended in order to achieve maximum caloric and nutritional benefit, even from these medium-chain triglyceride–containing formulations. Some studies show that steatorrhea is significantly reduced (up to 50%) by the addition of pancreatic enzymes in infants taking Pregestimil, or Portagen alone. Energy supplements in the form of medium-chain triglyceride oil, or glucose polymers such as Polycose, can be added to the diet of the older child. Calorically dense foods should be available for snacks. These extra offerings, however, will require the simultaneous use of pancreatic enzyme supplements. Vitamins A, B, K, and E can be given daily in a water-soluble or -miscible solution at twice the normal dosage (Tri-ViSol, Aquasol-E, Synkayvite). In exceptional patients, a trace-mineral screen may be indicated to ascertain plasma values for zinc, copper, selenium, manganese, and occasionally iron. In the older child troubled by steatorrhea, but without significant pulmonary disease, fat intake may be effectively diminished by use of skim milk in the diet, with supplementation of calories with medium-chain triglyceride oil incorporated into a variety of available recipes (Chapter 29).

Nasogastric enteral alimentation with monomeric or polymeric diets have been successful in terms of improving height and weight parameters. Overnight nutritional programs can be readily carried out at home. However, tolerance for the small mercury-weighted silicone rubber tube (Keofeed) may be difficult for the child with constant coughing or respiratory insufficiency. A temporary program of nutritional rehabilitation with peripheral parenteral nutrition can produce dramatic results by supplying much needed supplemental calories in a child hospitalized with an exacerbation of his disease.

Failure to obtain a therapeutic response, with improvement in the diarrhea, on adequate pancreatic replacement therapy after the addition of alkali, despite an adequate diet, should make one suspect an associated complicating condition. In particular, a substantial number of patients with cystic fibrosis have been shown to have diminished lactase levels. A lactose-free diet has resulted in prompt improvement in some of them.

The coexistence of cystic fibrosis and celiac disease has been reported, which calls for a gluten-free diet.

Hepatobiliary lesion. The observation that the liver of patients with cystic fibrosis may also show pathologic changes was recorded in 1938 by Anderson and subsequently has been shown to occur in 20% to 40% of children with this disease. Symptomatic hepatic disease occurs in 2% to 5% of patients with cystic fibrosis, initially as a neonatal cholestatic syndrome and later as a consequence of portal hypertension secondary to evolving biliary cirrhosis. Since more children with cystic fibrosis are living longer, the physician must be prepared to deal with this complication. Progression to cirrhosis, portal hypertension, and the development of ascites, hypersplenism, and hemorrhage from esophageal varices can tax the patient and physician severely.

Pathogenesis. The mechanism involved in the development of the "diagnostic" hepatic lesion (focal biliary cirrhosis) is believed to be similar to that described for the pancreas. Again, insufficient dilution of the biliary secretory products results in a hyperviscous, hypertonic material that becomes inspissated and plugs the small bile ductular radicles and occassionally the extrahepatic bile ducts as well. The destructive process may start in utero, but overall it seems to be more slowly progressive than is the pancreatic lesion.

Clinical and pathologic features. Prolonged obstructive jaundice in the newborn infant is occasionally associated with cystic fibrosis. When the child is less than 3 months of age, the histologic lesion usually lacks focal findings and rather demonstrates generalized hepatic involvement. Intrahepatocyte and canalicular cholestasis, nonspecific periportal alterations including neoductular proliferation, early fibrosis, and chronic inflammation with preservation of the lobular architecture are typical findings. Giant cells are rarely noted. However, should excess biliary mucus be identified within the intralobular bile ducts, cystic fibrosis may be strongly suspected. Unfortunately, this specific pathologic finding is lacking in over 50% of cases. Either lesion, focal or diffuse, with or without bile-duct plugging, may occur with meconium ileus when the diagnosis of the underlying disease condition is more obvious. In the absence of biliary mucus, extrahepatic biliary obstruction (biliary atresia) may be an important consideration in the differential diagnosis, especially if the cholestasis is clinically complete (acholic stools). Exploration of such a child may reveal obstruction of the common duct by sludged bile. Other causes for neonatal cholestasis have occasionally been identified in patients with cystic fibrosis, particularly cytomegalovirus and nonspecific "giant-cell" hepatitis.

Focal biliary cirrhosis has been found at autopsy in more than 10% of infants with cystic fibrosis dying of nonhepatic causes under the age of 3 months. This pathologic lesion shows eosinophilic concretions plugging small bile ducts and inflammatory foci extending along and about proliferating bile ductules. Minimal increase in fibrous tissue is seen, and the hepatocytes are typically free of bile stasis (Fig. 27-2). This lesion, not withstanding the absence of biliary mucus, is believed to be the forerunner of multinodular biliary cirrhosis, which subsequently develops (Fig. 27-3).

Random liver biopsy specimens obtained after the neonatal period will always reveal variable degrees of fatty metamorphosis, depending primarily, but not entirely, on previous nutrition. Undoubtedly this is the most common hepatic lesion in this disease (Fig. 27-4). Hemosiderosis resulting from increased iron absorption may also be found, especially in untreated pancreatic achylia (Fig. 27-5). Ceroid pigment deposition in hepatocytes of patients with cystic fibrosis may reflect prolonged vitamin E deficiency.

Once the neonatal period is past, a clinically important feature of the liver involvement is the lack of signs and symptoms referable to this organ as it progresses toward biliary cirrhosis. Jaundice does not recur until terminally. The earliest physical sign may be enlargement of the spleen. Clinical signs of hypersplenism include a history of easy bruisability, petechiae, and ecchymoses. A slightly enlarged liver may be mistakenly regarded as secondary to overinflation of the basilar segments of the lungs. In some patients the liver may be impressively enlarged. The nodular quality to the liver's surface and edge may be appreciated by careful palpation. In other children the liver edge may not be palpable and percussion dullness may be absent over the right costal area. Splenomegaly is invariably present in such cases. Massive hematemesis from esophageal varices may be the first indication that cirrhosis and portal hypertension are well advanced but may occur in children less than 10 years of age. Ascites devel-

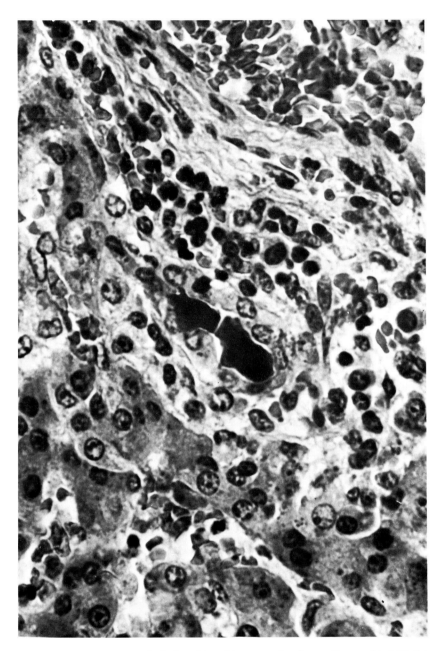

Fig. 27-2. Cystic fibrosis: hepatic lesion. Liver biopsy section from a 3-year-old child dying of pulmonary complications of cystic fibrosis. The liver shows bile duct concretions, mild portal inflammatory change, and fibrosis.

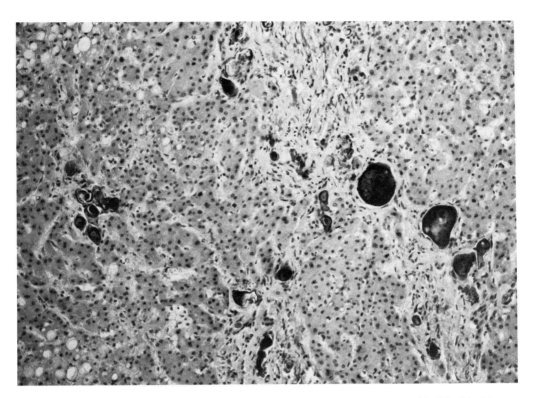

Fig. 27-3. Biliary cirrhosis in cystic fibrosis. Autopsy tissue from a 17-year-old girl with this disease, dying of hepatic failure. Jaundice (cholestatic type) developed without any prodromal illness and progressively increased over several months. Ascites became pronounced, and terminally she lapsed into hepatic coma after hemorrhage from esophageal varices. Advanced biliary cirrhosis, fatty metamorphosis, and laminated concretions of biliary mucus were striking findings in all portal zones.

ops terminally and may be falsely attributed to cor pulmonale.

After the neonatal period the laboratory provides limited help in assessment of the status of the liver disease before extensive cirrhosis is present. Before, advanced liver involvement, serum bilirubin and transaminase levels are invariably normal. The finding of an elevated gamma glutamyl transpeptidase (GGT) at any age, or elevation of the alkaline phosphatase in a pre–teen-age child with cystic fibrosis, is indicative of ongoing focal biliary changes. Prolongation of the BSP clearance test signifies underlying portal hypertension. Serum bile salt levels (glycocholate-RID) are reported to be a better indication of liver disease in cystic fibrosis. Our experience with 119 patients who have had fasting and 90-minute postprandial determinations suggests that a third of the patients have values above the cut-off point (more than 2.1 μmoles/L) for healthy children. On the other hand these patients who have cystic fibrosis with abnormal values cannot be differentiated from the others on the basis of liver size, liver function tests, or Shwachman scores. Six of our patients had values above 2 SD (standard deviations), four are known cirrhotics, and two have not had a biopsy. Of importance is the fact that one child with proved cirrhosis had values within 2 SD. Postprandial values, when the patient was provided with an endogenous load of bile acids to clear from his circulation, appear to be better indicators of liver disease. Longitudinal studies with a histologic backup study will be necessary before the role of this new liver function test is defined.

Hematologic investigations will reveal the features of hypersplenism (leukopenia, thrombocytopenia, anemia) but only late in the disease, when elevated portal hypertension exists. Hematest-positive stools and the presence of hematologic evidence of iron-deficiency anemia may be indicative of gastrointestinal blood loss from esophageal varices.

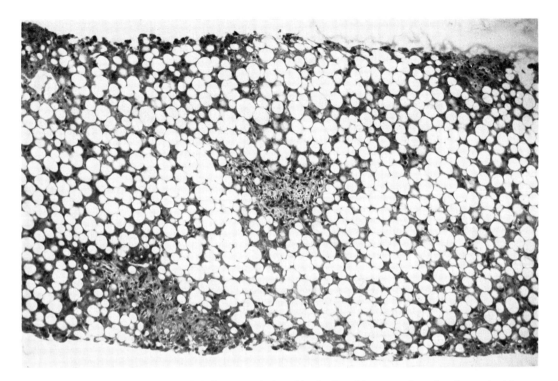

Fig. 27-4. Panlobular macroglobular steatosis found in the liver biopsy section of an 8-month-old infant with chronic diarrhea, failure to thrive, hepatomegaly, edema, and easy bruisability. Sweat chloride was more than 80 mEq/L. The child had been on a soybean-based formula for suspected cow's milk protein intolerance.

Diagnosis and treatment. Premortem diagnosis of advancing liver disease can be made by clinical and laboratory assessment, and only rarely is percutaneous liver biopsy needed to confirm the diagnosis.

The medical management of the neonate with prolonged obstructive jaundice is discussed in Chapter 19. The general medical and surgical management of the complications of portal hypertension caused by cirrhosis are discussed in Chapters 24 and 25. Surgery for bleeding esophageal varices or severe hypersplenism will require construction of a splenorenal or portacaval shunt, usually in association with splenectomy. The procedure is often prolonged and made more difficult by the presence of retroperitoneal edema and fibrosis, similar to that seen in extrahepatic portal hypertension (Clatworthy's sign, Fig. 25-9). Obviously, the patient with cystic fibrosis who has severe pulmonary disease is a poor candidate for any long operative procedure. For most of these patients, surgery is at best temporizing; the progression of the pulmonary and hepatic disease determines the final outcome. In properly selected patients, prophylactic portal systemic shunt surgery has been performed without undue complications. Our policy is to consider shunt surgery after the first bleeding episode attributable to esophageal varices is confirmed. Only patients having Shwachman's scores of 70 points or greater and free of other complicating medical problems (evidence of liver failure, diabetes) are possible candidates. A vigorous preoperative course of pulmonary hygiene is undertaken and continued after surgery. In selected cases shunt surgery can be expected to improve the quality of life. However, a repeatedly observed and discouraging phenomenon in these older children has been the sudden deterioration of pulmonary function, often without known precipitating cause, that progresses rapidly to cor pulmonale. The role of endoscopic sclerosis of esophageal varices, either

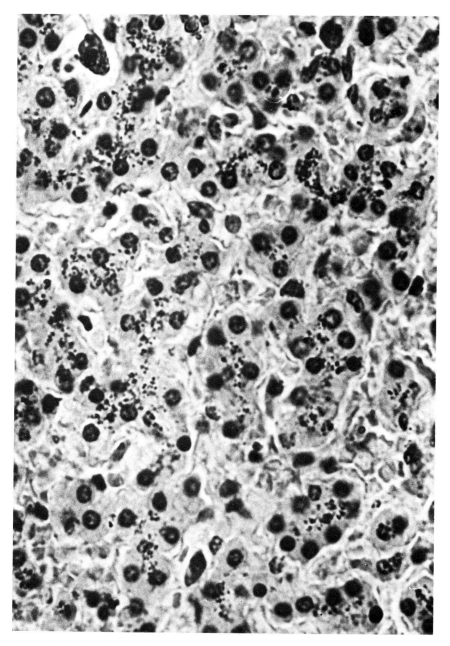

Fig. 27-5. Cystic fibrosis: hepatic lesion. Liver tissue from a 6-week-old child dying of cystic fibrosis before institution of pancreatic replacement therapy. Note the pronounced hemosiderin deposition within the hepatocytes.

before or after esophageal hemorrhage, has promise and needs to be further evaluated as another modality in managing the patient with minimal pulmonary involvement. Up to now, portal encephalopathy has not been reported in patients with cystic fibrosis undergoing portal-systemic shunt surgery. In general, bleeding episodes from varices are poorly tolerated by these patients, and pulmonary and hepatic decompensation may be seen.

Extrahepatic biliary lesion. As many as 30% of children with cystic fibrosis complain of vague abdominal discomfort that at times may be severe. The pain may become localized in the right upper quadrant; if it is associated with fever, leukocytosis, and elevation of bilirubin and alkaline phosphatase, gallbladder disease may be the cause. Cholelithiasis and cholecystitis have been reported in children with cystic fibrosis. The gallbladder bile of patients with cystic fibrosis has been found to be supersaturated with cholesterol with a reduced concentration of bile acids, conditions that predispose to the formation of gallstones. The small, shrunken gallbladder, found in 25% to 30% of children with cystic fibrosis, is believed to represent a primary congenital anomaly rather than a consequence of the disease. A mucocele or mucus hyperplasia of the gallbladder is a common pathologic finding in such cases. Most (80%) of these microgallbladders can be demonstrated roentgenographically after oral or intravenous cholangiography and can function normally despite their small size. Surgical removal of the nonfunctioning gallbladder from patients with right upper quadrant pain but without clinical or laboratory evidence of active gallbladder disease will rarely be of value in alleviating the symptoms.

Intestinal lesions. Meconium ileus is the most familiar of all the intestinal manifestations of cystic fibrosis. Neonatal intestinal obstruction ushers in the disease in 10% to 20% of affected children. The pathogenesis, clinical features, diagnosis, and complications of meconium ileus are discussed in Chapter 3. The treatment is surgical for all patients who cannot be managed medically (Gastrografin enema) and *N*-acetylcysteine given orally. The long-term prognosis for these patients is not believed to be poorer than for those without this complication. However, the anticipated difficulties with nutrition and absorption may be further compounded by removal of significant lengths of nonviable bowel and thereby increase the early morbidity.

Rectal prolapse is most likely to develop within the first 2 years of life and most often before diagnosis. The incidence of this complication in untreated young patients may be as high as 25%. The condition seldom occurs while adequate pancreatic replacement therapy is being received. The mechanism for rectal prolapse is unclear, but it correlates best with conditions in which frequent stooling, excessive straining at stool, and malnutrition exist. Rectal prolapse has also been seen in untreated celiac disease and kwashiorkor, conditions also associated with malnutrition. Hypotonia and diminished perineal muscle tone are found in these debilitated patients. Unless another obvious explanation exists, rectal prolapse in a child is always an indication for a properly performed sweat test.

The sudden appearance of rectal mucosa protruding through the anus is certainly frightening, but it is seldom attended by other problems. The mass may be reduced manually and rarely incarcerates. Decreased numbers of stools and increased sphincter tone result in gradual reduction in frequency of prolapse as the child gets older.

Meconium ileus equivalent refers to symptoms and signs of intestinal obstruction occurring after the neonatal period in children with cystic fibrosis. The incidence is said to be 5% to 7%. It has also been the presenting symptom complex in adults leading to diagnosis of cystic fibrosis. A history of recurrent colicky abdominal pain of varying duration (few hours to several years) is present in essentially all patients. Constipation is present in 50%. A number of underlying causes can be responsible for this clustering of symptoms. One predisposing condition becomes apparent after careful palpation of the abdomen when an often indentable nontender impacted fecal mass is detected in the right lower quadrant or midabdomen.

A combination of events is likely to be responsible for the development of fecal impactions in the terminal ileum, cecum, or ascending colon. Decreased bowel motility, presumably resulting from abnormal deposition of mucus within the intestinal glands and crypts (''mucosis''), evolves with advancing age and permits further inspissation of the stool (Fig. 27-6). This results in more solid or semisolid luminal contents reaching the ileocecal valve. The role of a decreased volume of secretion from the pancreas, biliary system, and intestine is also important in producing the dry or

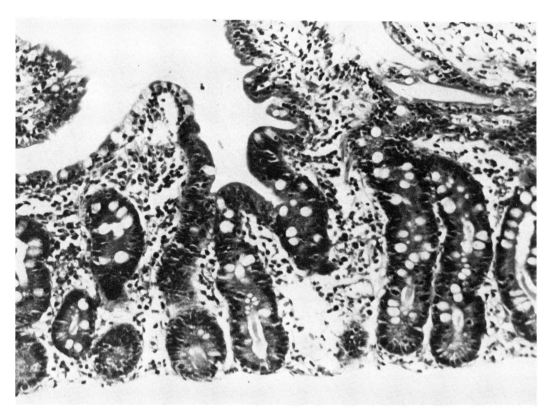

Fig. 27-6. "Mucosis" of the small intestine in cystic fibrosis. Almost every crypt lumen contains an inspissated mucus plug, a finding rarely noted in other intestinal diseases. Goblet cells are not increased, but the villi are somewhat blunted in this 3-year-old child.

puttylike stool. That the propulsive action of the small bowel may be ineffective in delivering this mass into the cecum results in a variety of symptoms and often complications. In the presence of distention, either intestinal obstruction, intussusception, or volvulus may be responsible for the symptom complex.

Emergency attention is needed when intestinal obstruction is present. Three-way abdominal films may show dilated bowel loops with air-fluid levels. A carefully administered barium or Gastrografin enema will permit diagnosis and reduction of either ileoileal, ileocolic, or colocolic intussusception. Inspissated fecal masses attached to the mucosa of the terminal ileum or colon or within the appendix may also act as the lead point in this complication. Inspissated fecal masses and redundant hyperplastic mucosal folds seen in the large bowel may be confused with changes of inflammatory bowel disease (Fig. 27-7). Roentgenographic demonstration of a large-bowel volvulus

requires emergency surgery if immediate reduction is not possible.

In the absence of volvulus or intussusception the fecal impactions causing incomplete obstruction can be treated by vigorous medical regimens. Many of these are often passed during the evacuation phase of the Gastrografin enema. Increased dosage of pancreatic enzymes, mineral oil (2 to 4 oz), and acetylcysteine can be given orally or through a decompression Levin tube. Saline enemas with dissolved pancreatic enzymes (one capsule of Cotazym) and acetylcysteine are also used. Dissolution of the ileocecal impaction occurs, and surgery can be avoided in most cases. The use of new pancreatic preparations such as pancrease has reduced the incidence of meconium ileus equivalent.

The best treatment for these conditions is offered by prophylaxis. Stools should be kept soft and encouraged to be passed daily. Decrease in the frequency of defecation, often noted in older

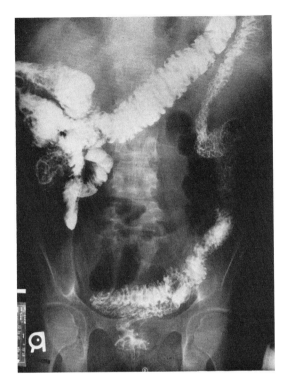

Fig. 27-7. Colonic manifestations of cystic fibrosis. The barium enema shows incomplete filling of the cecum because of inspissated fecal material. The left side of the colon shows loss of haustra and a mucosal pattern resembling the small intestine. The patient was a 24-year-old male with recurrent right lower quadrant pain and a palpable, tender mass. (From Pear, B.L.: Am. J. Roentgenol. **134:**1290, 1980, American Roentgen Ray Society.)

children, reflects better bowel control and decreased intestinal motility. A misinterpretation of this symptom can result in a decrease in pancreatic enzyme replacement to be taken by the patient, which only compounds the problem. As can be seen, both change in symptom and change in treatment are potential contributors to the development of meconium ileus equivalent. Again, patients with asymptomatic fecal masses in the right lower quadrant should be treated vigorously by a medical regimen in an effort to dissolve the mass.

Carbohydrate intolerance, manifested by lactosuria and sucrosuria after oral loads of the respective sugars, was noted in some patients almost simultaneously with the report of congenital lactase deficiency in a patient with cystic fibrosis. Peroral small bowel biopsies subsequently failed to reveal significant histologic changes when the tissue was examined by both light and electron microscopy. However, quantitation of small bowel disaccharidase levels revealed diminished activity in 25% of patients. The histochemical findings did not correlate as well as might be expected with the clinical symptoms of bloating, flatulence, and acid stools. Whether diminished intestinal enzyme content reflects another congenital abnormality of cystic fibrosis or an acquired state is still not known. For some workers, lactase deficiency found in patients with cystic fibrosis is not believed related to the underlying disease entity, since brush-border enzyme activity seemed to parallel the extent of mucosal injury. Furthermore, in children over the age of 5 years, the incidence of lactase deficiency was found to be similar to that noted in healthy non–cystic fibrotic white children. Serial small bowel biopsies starting from early age will be needed to answer this question.

Bile acid malabsorption was indicated in our findings that children with cystic fibrosis excrete abnormal amounts of bile acids in their stools. Because bile acid loss is normal in patients with isolated pulmonary involvement and is significantly improved by pancreatic enzymes, it appears to be dependent on the presence of pancreatic insufficiency and to vary with its severity. Our more current work suggests that a significant interruption of the enterohepatic circulation of bile acids is taking place, leading to altered bile acid kinetics. Although the pathogenesis of bile acid malabsorption in cystic fibrosis remains unknown, the clinical implications may be far reaching and include the following:

1. The defective micellar phase found in cystic fibrosis and in pancreatic insufficiency is secondary not only to a contracted bile acid pool but also to bile acids incapable of forming micelles with the products of lipolysis. In cystic fibrosis, glycoconjugates predominate over tauroconjugates (G:T ratio of 6:1 instead of 2:1 in normals). Because of their pK_a, glycoconjugates precipitate at the low duodenal pH of cystic fibrosis. Therefore, the malabsorption syndrome in cystic fibrosis may not be totally accounted for by pancreatic insufficiency.

2. Since the extent of fecal sequestration of bile acids in cystic fibrosis is comparable to that in infants after an ileal resection, it is likely that a choleretic enteropathy may occur in certain cases. The cathartic effect of large quantities of unabsorbed bile acids reaching the colon is well known.

3. The extensive loss of bile acids has been shown to lead to a contraction of the bile acid pool because the capacity of the liver for compensatory synthesis is exceeded. The relationship between these findings and the high incidence of hepatobiliary disease in cystic fibrosis has been established for cholelithiasis. However, it is tempting to postulate that mucus plugging of the extrahepatic and intrahepatic bile ducts and eventually focal biliary cirrhosis could be caused by alterations of bile acid metabolism.

Other complications (nonpulmonary, nonintestinal)

Nasal polyps. The incidence of nasal polyposis in patients with cystic fibrosis is about 7%, and generally is recognized in patients after 10 years of age. Abnormal formation and secretion of nasal mucus have been considered responsible for the formation of nasal polyps in children. Although most commonly seen in long-standing nasal allergy, this lesion is an indication for a sweat test. Progressive growth of the polyp may cause nasal obstruction and require surgical removal. Recurrences are not uncommon.

Male infertility. Aspermia from mechanical obstruction occurs in over 95% of males with cystic fibrosis and explains the small number of offspring produced by them. Fertility data on 117 males revealed only two who were fertile. The autopsy finding of absence of the vas deferens (and other mesonephric derivatives) in these patients implies a congenital developmental abnormality, but there is also evidence suggesting an acquired phenomenon. The infertility is not related to any hormone deficiency, since levels of testosterone, follicle-stimulating hormone, and luteinizing hormones are normal in these patients. On the contrary, females with cystic fibrosis who survive to the child-bearing age seem capable of becoming pregnant. Eleven such women have had 12 normal children to date. It is curious that most of these women had mild disease and came to diagnosis late (15 years of age and older).

Pancreatitis. Another cause of recurrent abdominal pain, a symptom that may antedate (but frequently postdates) the diagnosis of cystic fibrosis, is relapsing pancreatitis. These rare patients generally have minimal evidence of pancreatic insufficiency, and therefore the diagnosis of cystic fibrosis is delayed, especially if attention is primarily focused on this clinical manifestation. Suf-

ficient clues to proper diagnosis can be found when one pays attention to the entire medical history (pulmonary, nasal polyposis, rectal prolapse, fecal impactions, salt depletion, and so on).

Hypoelectrolytemia and metabolic alkalosis. This derangement of acid-base homeostasis may occur as an acute complication of cystic fibrosis, particularly as part of a heat-prostration syndrome. Infants and young children with cystic fibrosis are especially prone to this complication in the hot weather months, when electrolyte-rich sweat is lost in excessive amounts resulting in hyponatremia, hypokalemia, and hypochloremia. Metabolic alkalosis with dehydration and shock may quickly supervene. Occasionally, a similar serum electrolyte pattern is noted in the absence of pronounced dehydration or hyperpyrexia. In one series, 5 of 11 infants, coming to diagnosis before 1 year of age, manifested hypoelectrolytemia and metabolic alkalosis. Therefore, even in the absence of significant pulmonary or gastrointestinal symptoms, the finding of this electrolyte pattern in a child is considered sufficient cause to order a sweat-chloride determination. Severe hyponatremia and hypochloremia and mild metabolic alkalosis have also been reported in association with inappropriately high levels of antidiuretic hormone released during acute exacerbations of chronic pulmonary disease. Treatment of these patients often requires severe fluid restriction (with or without intravenous hypertonic salt solution) and a diuretic. Simultaneous vigorous treatment of the acute pulmonary condition is mandatory.

Immune-complex phenomenon. The effect of circulating immune complexes as causative in some of the manifestations found in cystic fibrosis has been suggested for some time. During life, circulating pancreatic antibodies are present in patients with cystic fibrosis, and deposits of immunoglobulins have been found about pancreatic acinar tissue examined at autopsy. Some workers believe that the progression of the lung disease may be attributable to an abnormal hyperimmune response or circulating immune-complexes. The observation that hypogammaglobulinemia occurs more frequently in patients with cystic fibrosis with less severe lung disease than age-matched patients with normal or elevated IgG levels is provocative. Occasional examples of cutaneous necrotizing vasculitis and episodic arthritis have also been reported in association with cystic fibrosis.

Diagnosis

It can be seen from the foregoing discussion that cystic fibrosis is truly protean in nature. Its many modes of presentation and complications demand a high degree of awareness if the diagnosis is to be made at any age. An occasional child may be suspected of having cystic fibrosis when the mother complains that he tastes salty when kissed or that she finds salt deposits about the hairline. Excessive salt losses through the sweat glands may result in pronounced dehydration, hyponatremia, hypochloremia, and shock. These observations about "salty babies" with cystic fibrosis eventually led to the development of the most reliable diagnostic test for the disease.

Sweat test

The quantitative pilocarpine iontophoresis sweat test takes advantage of the most consistent chemical abnormality in patients with this disease. Sweat electrolytes are elevated from birth on, a fact that clearly separates those with disease from those without in 98% to 99% of cases. Serial determinations in cystic fibrosis patients always show persistence of the sweat-electrolyte abnormality. No correlation exists, however, between the severity of the disease and the sweat electrolyte abnormality. The test is safe, simple, and reliable if adequate sweat (more than 50 mg) is obtained. Even with the pilocarpine iontophoresis technique, obtainment of an adequate quantity of sweat may be a problem in infants less than 2 to 3 months of age. A rare false-negative sweat test has been noted in the presence of significant hypoproteinemic edema. False-positive results have been reported in malnutrition, Mauriac's syndrome, glycogen storage disease, mucopolysaccharidoses, ectodermal dysplasia, adrenal insufficiency, nephrogenic diabetes insipidus, and hypothyroidism. Fortunately, these conditions are generally recognized by other specific clinical features.

Perhaps only 1% to 2% of patients with cystic fibrosis tested by quantitative pilocarpine iontophoresis will have results that are equivocal, forcing the clinician to make the diagnosis after critical evaluation of other clinical and roentgenologic studies, examination of biopsy material, or analysis of pancreatic secretion and enzyme concentrations.

The introduction of ion-specific electrodes and conductivity tests (Orion, Medtherm) that measure the chloride concentration in pilocarpine-stimulated sweat has resulted in a disturbing increase in the numbers of false-positive test results. In one series this approached 25%. There are both theoretical and technical problems inherent in the use of ion-specific electrodes that are manifest even when testing is performed by experienced technicians. The margin for error escalates rapidly when these techniques are carried out by hospital laboratory personnel on an infrequent basis. Obviously, too much is at stake when one is considering the diagnosis of cystic fibrosis to gamble on the results of "screening" tests. The patient is best referred to a pediatric-oriented central laboratory for proper testing and evaluation of the results. Up to now only the quantitative pilocarpine iontophoresis sweat test, repeated at least twice, should be employed to include or exclude the diagnosis. One should view suspiciously those positive results (chloride greater than 60 mEq/L) in which the sweat *sodium* concentration is disproportionately higher than the chloride value. Such results should always be repeated with careful review of techniques employed in performing the test.

Duodenal drainage

Before the advent of the sweat test, quantitative assessment of exocrine pancreatic function was the primary means of diagnosis of cystic fibrosis. Simple duodenal drainage with determination of pancreatic enzyme concentrations (particularly trypsin) within the duodenal fluid was acceptable. This technique obviously fails to eliminate other conditions associated with partial or complete pancreatic exocrine deficiencies. Furthermore, it fails to indicate the reserve functional capacity of the gland, which may be important in diagnosis. The fact that the electrolyte fraction (water and bicarbonate) in the pancreatic secretions of patients with cystic fibrosis provides a way of separating this entity from other forms of pancreatic insufficiency means that proper technique must be used in order to obtain accurate information. Special duodenal tubes are required, and collections should be taken before and after secretin and pancreozymin stimulation. The method for quantitative assessment of pancreatic function is given in Chapter 32.

The most consistent enzyme deficiency in patients with cystic fibrosis is in lipase secretion, which is usually absent. Amylase and chymotrypsin are abnormally low or absent, but some trypsin can be found after stimulation. Volume is always low, as is bicarbonate production, even in the unusual child (10%) whose pancreatic disease is not revealed by other measurements (fecal fat determinations) or pancreatic function. A recent report has described recurrent acute pancreatitis in patients with cystic fibrosis with normal pancreatic exocrine function.

The Bentiromide test

The Bentiromide test utilizes the oral administration of an investigational drug *N*-benzoyl-L-tyrosyl-*p*-aminobenzoic acid, which is cleaved by pancreatic chymotrypsin in the upper intestinal tract. The liberated para-aminobenzoic acid is then absorbed from the gastrointestinal tract, conjugated in the liver, and excreted into the urine. A 6-hour urine collection period is employed for quantitation of the excreted product. Early data show good correlation of this test with the quantitative fecal chymotrypsin determination. Lack of adequate sensitivity, however, may limit its subsequent usefulness in assessment of pancreatic exocrine function. False-positive results occur in the face of delayed gastric emptying, mucosal disease, and hepatic or renal impairment.

X-ray findings

At times, the diagnosis is first suspected by the radiologist when he sees on the chest roentgenograms chracteristic, but not specific, evidence of hyperaeration and increased peribronchial markings. Later in the disease, more obvious signs of emphysema and patchy atelectasis are superimposed on acute and chronic changes. The tendency toward greater involvement of the upper lobes is often seen in cystic fibrosis. Eventually upper-lobe volume loss occurs and the main pulmonary arteries appear prominent. In far-advanced cases characteristic cystic changes suggesting bronchiectasis or a "honey-combed" lung may be seen. Tension pneumothorax occurs in 2.5% of patients, and empyema may also be noted on occasion.

Unusual pathologic findings

The diagnosis of cystic fibrosis may be strongly suspected on the basis of the histologic appearance of the appendix removed for any reason. The strikingly increased activity of mucus-secreting goblet cells keeps crypt spaces distended and filled with mucus. Eosinophilic casts may be seen either in the lumen or retained in the crypt spaces. The inflammatory component is minimal to subacute, unless acute superimposed disease has occurred. Similar histologic changes have been observed in the colon, and the diagnosis can be suspected by examination of rectal mucosal biopsy material. Again, crypt enlargement and distention by accumulated mucus is typical, and goblet cell numbers may or may not be increased over controls.

Differential diagnosis

When the typical manifestations of cystic fibrosis are present—pulmonary symptoms, malabsorption, and failure to thrive—this condition can be confused with very few entities. Immune deficiency states, particularly in those children with defects of circulating antibodies and delayed hypersensitivity, can mimic completely the major manifestations of cystic fibrosis. In milder forms of cystic fibrosis or where single-organ involvement dominates the clinical picture, the differential diagnosis can be surprisingly large. Milder forms of cystic fibrosis may be mistaken for an allergic disorder, and much time may be lost in diagnosis during manipulations of their environment and diet. When pulmonary symptoms prevail, tracheoesophageal fistula (H type), vascular anatomic lesions, allergy, disorders of sucking and swallowing, and esophageal lesions will often be considered as underlying causes. The entire spectrum of malabsorptive states may be investigated if pancreatic insufficiency, diarrhea, and failure to thrive dominate the early clinical picture. All causes of liver disease and portal hypertension may need evaluation in those unusual cases having this mode of presentation.

Complications

Most complications of cystic fibrosis have been referred to during the discussion of the specific organ involved (pulmonary, pancreatic, intestinal, hepatic). In addition, the social impact of delayed pubescence when accompanied by height and weight retardation needs to be anticipated, since greater numbers of these patients are reaching adolescence. This complication has been treated with androgens with some success on both growth and sexual development; however, improvement in pulmonary function is controversial. Nutritional rehabilitation programs may be necessary.

Prognosis

A child with cystic fibrosis diagnosed now can be expected to live longer and enjoy overall better health than those whose illness was diagnosed 15 to 20 years ago. The mean survival age has increased to 20, whereas in 1960 less than 50% of these children survived 5 years after diagnosis. So many factors are responsible for the improved survival of patients with cystic fibrosis that extrapolation of these data to comparable groups of patients followed in other centers is most difficult.

The sweat test now permits diagnosis before symptoms begin, and institution of therapy (pancreatic and pulmonary) in these children is associated with an improved overall survival. The variability of organ involvement (heterogeneity) and progression of the pulmonary lesion seem to be individually determined phenomena with some predictability in affected siblings.

If one excludes those children with mild disease, prolongation of life can best be attributed to the development of pancreatic replacement therapy, use of antibiotics, and vigorous pulmonary hygiene. Supervised intensive care programs in the home and hospital with these therapeutic measures, as well as aerosol therapy, postural drainage, breathing exercises, prophylactic immunizations, and dietary manipulation to provide a high caloric intake have improved the period of well-being for these children. Finally, intensive pulmonary prophylaxis is likely to improve the chances that these children will achieve more normal height and weight. However, the severity and rate of progression of the pulmonary lesion and the development of cor pulmonale still determine the length and quality of life for most patients. The initial prognosis is poor for infants requiring surgery for meconium ileus, and the long-term prognosis is poor once pneumothorax or hemoptysis occurs.

REFERENCES

Antonowicz, I., Lebenthal, E., and Shwachman, H.: Disaccharidase activities in small intestinal mucosa in patients with cystic fibrosis, J. Pediatr. **92**:214-219, 1978.

Bass, H.N., and Miller, A.A.: Cystic fibrosis presenting with anemia and hypoproteinemia in identical twins, Pediatrics **59**:126-127, 1977.

Beckerman, R.C., and Taussig, L.M.: Hypoelectrolytemia and metabolic alkalosis in infants with cystic fibrosis, Pediatrics **63**:580-583, 1979.

Boyle, B.J., Long, W.B., Balistreri, W.F., and others: Effect of cimetidine and pancreatic enzymes on serum and fecal bile acids and fat absorption in cystic fibrosis, Gastroenterology **78**:950-953, 1980.

Brasfield, D., Hicks, G., Soong, S., and Tiller, R.E.: The chest roentgenogram in cystic fibrosis: a new scoring system, Pediatrics **63**:24-29, 1979.

Breslow, J.L., McPherson, J., and Epstein, J.: Distinguishing homozygous and heterozygous cystic fibrosis fibroblasts from normal cells by differences in sodium transport, N. Engl. J. Med. **304**:1-4, 1981.

Chase, H.P., Long, M.A., and Lavin, M.H.: Cystic fibrosis and malnutrition, J. Pediatr. **95**:337-347, 1979.

Cohen, L.F., di Sant'Agnese, P.A., Taylor, A., and Gill, J.R., Jr.: The syndrome of inappropriate antidiuretic hormone secretion as a cause of hyponatremia in cystic fibrosis, J. Pediatr. **90**:574-578, 1977.

Cox, K.L., and Isenberg, J.N.: Hypersecretion of gastric acid in patients with pancreatic exocrine insufficiency due to cystic fibrosis, Gastroenterology **74**:1022, 1978 (Abstract).

Davis, P.B., Shelhamer, J.R., and Kaliner, M.: Abnormal adrenergic and cholinergic sensitivity in cystic fibrosis, N. Engl. J. Med. **302**:1453-1456, 1980.

Davis, P.B., and di Sant'Agnese, P.A.: A review: cystic fibrosis at forty—quo vadis? Pediatr. Res. **14**:83-78, 1980.

Denning, C.R., Huang, N.N., Cuasay, L.R., and others: Cooperative study comparing three methods of performing sweat tests to diagnose cystic fibrosis, Pediatrics **66**:752-757, 1980.

Deren, J.J., Arora, B., Toskes, P.P., and others: Malabsorption of crystalline vitamin B_{12} in cystic fibrosis, N. Engl. J. Med. **288**:949-950, 1973.

Durie, P.R., Bell, L., Linton, W., and others: Effect of cimetidine and sodium bicarbonate on pancreatic replacement therapy in cystic fibrosis, Gut **21**:778-786, 1980.

Durie, P.R., Newth, C.J., Forstner, G.G., and Gall, D.G.: Malabsorption of medium-chain triglycerides in infants with cystic fibrosis: correction with pancreatic enzyme supplements, J. Pediatr. **96**:862-864, 1980.

Fleisher, D.S., DiGeorge, A.M., Auerbach, V.H., and others: Protein metabolism in cystic fibrosis of the pancreas, J. Pediatr. **64**:349-356, 1964.

Geller, A., Gilles, F., and Shwachman, H.: Degeneration of fasciculus gracilis in cystic fibrosis, Neurology **27**:185-187, 1977.

George, L., and Norman, A.P.: Life tables for cystic fibrosis, Arch. Dis. Child. **46**:139-143, 1971.

Gibson, L.E.: The decline of the sweat test: comments on pitfalls and reliability, Clin. Pediatr. **12**:450-453, 1973.

Goodchild, M.C., Nelson, R., and Anderson, C.: Cystic fibrosis and coeliac disease: co-existence in two children, Arch. Dis. Child. **48**:684-691, 1973.

Graham, D.Y.: Enzyme replacement therapy of exocrine pancreatic insufficiency in man, N. Engl. J. Med. **296**:1314-1322, 1977.

Graham, D.Y.: An enteric-coated pancreatic enzyme preparation that works, Dig. Dis. Sci. **24**:906-909, 1979.

Grand, R.J.: Changing patterns of gastrointestinal manifestations of cystic fibrosis, Clin. Pediatr. **9**:588-593, 1970.

Gurwitz, D., Corey, M., Francis, P.W.J., and others: Perspectives in cystic fibrosis, Ped. Clin. North Am. **26**:603-615, 1979.

Hadorn, B., Johansen, P.G., and Anderson, C.M.: Pancreozymin secretin test of exocrine pancreatic function in cystic fibrosis and the significance of the result for the pathogenesis of the disease, Can. Med. Assoc. J. **98**:377-385, 1968.

Holsclaw, D.S., Rocmans, C., and Shwachman, H.: Intussusception in patients with cystic fibrosis, Pediatrics **48**:51-58, 1971.

Kattwinkel, J., Taussig, L.M., Statland, B.E., and Verter, J.I.: The effects of age on alkaline phosphatase and other serologic liver function tests in normal subjects and patients with cystic fibrosis, J. Pediatr. **82**:234-242, 1973.

Kopel, F.B.: Gastrointestinal manifestations of cystic fibrosis, Gastroenterology **62**:483-491, 1972.

Lemen, R.J., Gates, A.J., Mathé, A.A., and others: Relationships among digital clubbing, disease severity, and serum prostaglandins F$_{2\alpha}$ and E concentrations in cystic fibrosis patients, Am. Rev. Resp. Dis. **117**:639-646, 1978.

L'Heureux, P.R., Isenberg, J.N., Sharp, H.L., and Warwick, W.J.: Gallbladder disease in cystic fibrosis, Am. J. Roentgenol. **128**:953-956, 1977.

Lippe, B.M., Sperling, M.A., and Dooley, R.R.: Pancreatic alpha and beta cell functions in cystic fibrosis, J. Pediatr. **90**:751-755, 1977.

MacLean, W.C., Jr., and Tripp, R.W.: Cystic fibrosis with edema and falsely negative sweat test, J. Pediatr. **83**:86-88, 1973.

Marks, M.I.: The pathogenesis and treatment of pulmonary infections in patients with cystic fibrosis, J. Pediatr. **98**:173-179, 1981.

Matseshe, J.W., Go, V.L.W., and DiMagno, E.P.: Meconium ileus equivalent complicating cystic fibrosis in postneonatal children and young adults, Gastroenterology **72**:732-736, 1977.

Matthews, W.J., Jr., Williams, M., Oliphint, B., and others: Hypogammaglobulinemia in patients with cystic fibrosis, N. Engl. J. Med. **302**:245-249, 1980.

Millis, R.M., Young, R.C., Jr., and Kulczycki, L.L.: Validation of therapeutic bronchoscopic bronchial washing in cystic fibrosis, Chest **71**:508-513, 1977.

Morin, C.L., Roy, C.C., Lasalle, R., and Bonin, A.: Small bowel mucosal dysfunction in patients with cystic fibrosis, J. Pediatr. **88**:213-216, 1976.

Nassif, E.G., Younoszai, K., Weinberger, N.N., and Nassif, C.M.: Comparative effects of antacids, enteric coating, and bile salts on the efficacy of oral pancreatic enzyme therapy in cystic fibrosis, J. Pediatr. **98**:320-323, 1981.

Neutra, M.R., and Trier, J.S.: Rectal mucosa in cystic fibrosis: morphologic features before and after short term organ culture, Gastroenterology **75**:701-710, 1978.

Newman, A.J., and Ansell, B.M.: Episodic arthritis in children with cystic fibrosis, J. Pediatr. **94**:594-596, 1979.

Nousia-Arvanitakis, S., Arvanitakis, C., and Greenberger, N.J.: Diagnosis of exocrine pancreatic insufficiency in cystic fibrosis by the synthetic peptide *N*-benzoyl-L-tyrosyl-*p*-aminobenzoic acid, J. Pediatr. **92**:734-737, 1978.

Oppenheimer, E.H., and Esterly, J.R.: Hepatic changes in young infants with cystic fibrosis: possible relation to focal biliary cirrhosis, J. Pediatr. **86**:683-689, 1975.

Oppenheimer, E.H., and Schwartz, A.: Easy bruisability and terminal coma in a "normal" 5-month-old infant, J. Pediatr. **88**:1049-1053, 1976.

Psacharopoulos, H.T., Howard, E.R., Portmann, B., and others: Hepatic complications of cystic fibrosis, Lancet **2**:78-80, 1981.

Regan, P.T., Malagelada, J.R., DiMagno, E.P., and Go, V.L.W.: Reduced intraluminal bile acid concentrations and fat maldigestion in pancreatic insufficiency: correction by treatment, Gastroenterology **77**:285-289, 1979.

Rosenfeld, R., Spigelblatt, L., and Chicoine, R.: False positive sweat test, malnutrition and the Mauriac syndrome, J. Pediatr. **94**:240-242, 1979.

Rosenstein, B.J., Langbaum, T.S., Gordes, E., and Brusilow, S.W.: Cystic fibrosis: problems encountered with sweat testing, J.A.M.A. **240**:1987-1988, 1978.

Rosenstein, B.J., and Langbaum, T.S.: Incidence of meconium abnormalities in newborn infants with cystic fibrosis, Am. J. Dis. Child. **134**:72-73, 1980.

Roy, C.C., Weber, A.M., Morin, C.L., and others: Abnormal biliary lipid composition in cystic fibrosis, N. Engl. J. Med. **297**:1301-1305, 1977.

Roy, C.C., Delage, G., Fontaine, A., and others: The fecal microflora and bile acids in children with cystic fibrosis, Am. J. Clin. Nutrit. **32**:2404-2409, 1979.

Roy, C.C., Weber, A.M., Morin, C.L., and others: Hepatobiliary disease in cystic fibrosis: a survey of current issues and concepts, Pediatric Gastroenterology and Nutrition. (In press.)

Ryley, H.C., Neale, L.M., Brogan, T.D., and Bray, P.T.: Screening for cystic fibrosis in the newborn by meconium analysis, Arch. Dis. Child. **54**:92-97, 1979.

Schuster, S.R., Shwachman, H., Toyama, W.M., and others: The management of portal hypertension in cystic fibrosis, J. Pediatr. Surg. **12**:201-206, 1977.

Shwachman, H., Kulczycki, L.L., Mueller, H.L., and Flake, C.G.: Nasal polyposis in patients with cystic fibrosis, Pediatrics **30**:389-401, 1962.

Shwachman, H., and Holsclaw, D.: Examination of the appendix at laparotomy as a diagnostic clue in cystic fibrosis, N. Engl. J. Med. **286**:1300-1301, 1972.

Shwachman, H., Lebenthal, E., and Khaw, K.T.: Recurrent acute pancreatitis in patients with cystic fibrosis with normal pancreatic enzymes, Pediatrics **55**:86-95, 1975.

Shwachman, H., Kowalski, M., and Khaw, K.T.: Cystic fibrosis: a new outlook, Medicine **56**:129-149, 1977.

Shwachman, H., Mahmoodian, A., and Neff, R.K.: The sweat test: sodium and chloride values, J. Pediatr. **98**:576-578, 1981.

Shepherd, R., Cooksley, W.G.E., and Cooke, W.D.D.: Improved growth and clinical, nutritional, and respiratory changes in response to nutritional therapy in cystic fibrosis, J. Pediatr. **97**:351-357, 1980.

Solomons, C.C., Cotton, E.K., Dubois, R.S., and Pinney, M.: The use of buffered L-arginine in the treatment of cystic fibrosis, Pediatrics **47**:384-390, 1971.

Stern, R.C., Stevens, D.P., Boat, T.F., and others: Symptomatic hepatic disease in cystic fibrosis: incidence, course, and outcome of portal systemic shunting, Gastroenterology **70**:645-649, 1976.

Stern, R.C., Boat, T.F., Doershuk, C.F., and others: Cystic fibrosis diagnosed after age 13, Ann. Intern. Med. **87**:188-191, 1977.

Taussig, L.M., Belmonte, M.M., and Beaudry, P.H.: *Staphylococcus aureus* empyema in cystic fibrosis, J. Pediatr. **84**:724-727, 1974.

Taussig, L.M., Lobeck, C.C., Di Sant'Agnese, P.A., and others: Fertility in males with cystic fibrosis, N. Engl. J. Med. **287**:586-598, 1972.

Taylor, B., and Sokol, G.: Cystic fibrosis and coeliac disease: report of two cases, Arch. Dis. Child. **48:**692-696, 1973.

Tyson, K.R.T., Schuster, S.R., and Shwachman, H.: Portal hypertension in cystic fibrosis, J. Pediatr. Surg. **3:**271-277, 1968.

Watkins, J.B., Tercyak, A.M., Szczepanik, P., and Klein, P.D.: Bile salt kinetics in cystic fibrosis: influence of pancreatic enzyme replacement, Gastroenterology **73:**1023-1028, 1977.

Wilroy, R.S., Jr., Crawford, S.E., and Johnson, W.W.: Cystic fibrosis with extensive fat replacement of the liver, J. Pediatr. **68:**67-73, 1966.

SHWACHMAN'S SYNDROME (PANCREATIC INSUFFICIENCY AND BONE MARROW DYSFUNCTION)

Physicians, either independently or working in cystic fibrosis clinics, had observed that a few patients who manifested signs and symptoms of pancreatic insufficiency were strikingly free of pulmonary disease. These atypical patients were more puzzling when the sweat test, the most reliable means of diagnosing cystic fibrosis, was found to be normal. Despite normal results of the sweat test, most were treated empirically with pancreatic replacement therapy. The observation that many but not all of these children had an associated neutropenia prompted others to examine patients believed to have primary hematologic abnormalities (cyclic neutropenia, thrombocytopenia, anemia, hypoplastic bone marrow) for evidence of pancreatic insufficiency and indeed found such cases. The number of patients now reported whose symptoms fit into Shwachman's syndrome is still not large with perhaps less than 100 cases reported.

The pathogenesis of this entity is not understood. Symptoms are generally present at a very early age, and the typical histologic lesion in the pancreas has been found in affected infants dying in the first year of life. This would suggest a congenital defect, but some patients may not manifest the symptoms of pancreatic insufficiency until later years. Reports of this entity in siblings support the hypothesis that it represents an inherited lesion with variable penetrance of clinical and pathologic features. Observations made after pancreatic stimulation in these patients indicates that acinar (enzyme) and not ductular (bicarbonate) tissue is primarily affected.

The hematologic findings are less constant than the pancreatic lesion and are more likely to be normal early in the course of the disease. The relationship between these two is unclear, but the frequency with which they occur simultaneously suggests a common source for the pathologic lesions specific for this syndrome. A previous report that serum from patients with Shwachman's syndrome is cytotoxic to their own white blood cells has not been confirmed. Patients with exocrine pancreatic insufficiency from other causes (cystic fibrosis, chronic fibrosing pancreatitis, pancreatectomy) do not have neutropenia, and replacement therapy with pancreatic extracts does not correct the hematologic lesion in Shwachman's syndrome. Although embryologic development of pancreatic exocrine tissue occurs at about the same time as that of myeloid elements, an acquired, in utero insult (infection) that affects these two systems seems unlikely, since the syndrome may occur in siblings of successive pregnancies. Although neutropenia is the most common manifestation of the hematologic abnormality, the pathogenesis of this finding is not completely understood. In vitro studies have shown some patients to have normal granulopoiesis whereas others demonstrate a defect at a stem-cell level. Patients with neutropenia are capable of mounting a leukocytosis response both to infection and after epinephrine stimulation. A recent study demonstrated a polymorphonuclear mobility defect, which may explain the predisposition of some persons with Shwachman's syndrome to have frequent bacterial infection. Hypogammaglobulinemia has been found inconstantly in patients with this condition and most often involves a deficiency of IgA, though IgM and IgG have also been low on occasion.

Clinical and laboratory features

Gastrointestinal. Most patients clinically reveal pancreatic exocrine insufficiency during infancy by passage of frequent, loose, foul-smelling stools. Steatorrhea is suggested by stools that are pale and greasy. Failure to thrive eventually accompanies the complaint of diarrhea, and the child is suspected of having cystic fibrosis. In other patients the manifestations of the pancreatic insufficiency are extremely mild for many years before symptoms become troublesome. In general, the pancreatic manifestations lessen with advancing age despite persistence of pancreatic achylia. We have had experience with nine such patients, one who complained of vague abdominal discomfort unless he took pancreatic extracts. Serum amylase was normal on several occasions.

The sweat electrolytes are invariably normal. Steatorrhea is often present in the younger patient but not constant, and it becomes less severe with age. The D-xylose and glucose tolerance absorption tests are normal. Quantitative assessment of exocrine pancreatic function with secretin-pancreozymin stimulation reveals normal secretory volumes and slightly lowered bicarbonate with diminished or absent enzymes values. As in cystic fibrosis, lipase is the enzyme most often absent or diminished.

Hematologic. Clinical symptoms that can be traced to the hematologic findings are not common. Some patients with anemia and neutropenia may have mild pallor and an increased number of infections that can call attention to this syndrome. Increased bruising and petechiae have been seen in a rare patient.

When a hematologic abnormality is present, the most constant laboratory finding is a diminished white blood cell count that is often variable and rarely constant or cyclic. Neutrophils are most severely affected, with total counts generally less than $1,500/mm^3$. A mild anemia, sometimes present, is typically resistant to iron, folic acid, and vitamin B_{12} therapy. Thrombocytopenia (less than 100,000 platelets/mm^3) is reported in some patients. An elevated fetal hemoglobin level has also been noted in some patients studied.

Discrepant reports of susceptibility to bacterial infections leave this aspect unsettled at present. However, overwhelming infections constitute the leading cause of death in these patients. The reported neutrophil mobility defect may predispose these patients to infections.

Orthopedic. There is a curious association of this syndrome with bone lesions, suggesting metaphyseal dysostosis in the femur, tibia, and ribs in about 10% to 15% of patients. In some, the lesion in the proximal femur is severe enough to

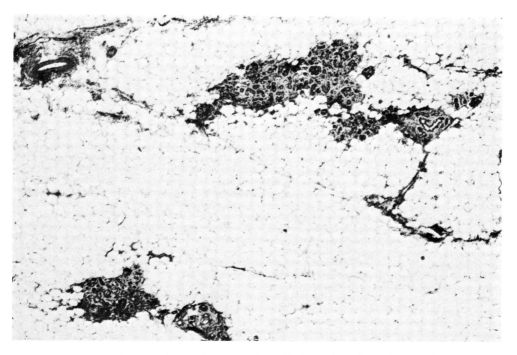

Fig. 27-8. Pancreatic tissue from a 7-year-old boy with Shwachman's syndrome. The pancreas has been almost completely replaced by fatty tissue. Only the islets of Langerhans and some pancreatic ducts are visible. There is no identifiable exocrine tissue and no inflammatory reaction. The child's clinical history of diarrhea, failure to thrive, and persistent neutropenia led to diagnosis at the age of 4 months. At 7 years of age he suddenly developed severe anemia and thrombocytopenia. A repeat bone marrow examination revealed acute myelogenous leukemia, to which he succumbed within 3 months.

disturb the child's gait and create a coxa vara deformity.

Generalized bone changes are not found, and serum calcium, phosphorus, and alkaline phosphatase values are normal.

Growth failure. Growth is sharply retarded, both in height and weight, in most of these patients. Established growth rates are not affected by pancreatic enzyme replacement though weight gain can be improved. Bone age is seldom as retarded as height age. Although repeated infections can affect a child's growth, it does not seem to be a major factor in the growth rate in children with this syndrome. Reports from endocrine studies (growth hormone, thyroid) up to now have shown normal results.

Liver involvement. An occasional case of Shwachman's syndrome has been reported with histologic abnormalities in liver biopsy material, manifested by portal fibrosis and minimal chronic inflammatory changes. Elevated aminotransfer-

ases (SGOT) are noted in such cases and this pathologic lesion may be another rare feature of the syndrome.

Pathologic lesion

Pancreas. The histologic lesion found both during life and at autopsy is consistent with the biochemical abnormality. The gross appearance of the pancreas reveals fatty lobulation, whereas the pancreatogram demonstrates normal duct anatomy. The microscopic lesion is consistent. Scarcity or absence of acinar tissue with preservation of the islets is noted in a gland otherwise replaced entirely by fatty tissue (Fig. 27-8). The absence of inflammatory cells and fibrosis is also striking. The ducts and ductular epithelial cells seem normal, with an occasional plug of inspissated secretion being reported.

Bone marrow. A maturation arrest of the neutrophils just before the mature forms has been most often observed. Hypocellularity of the marrow and

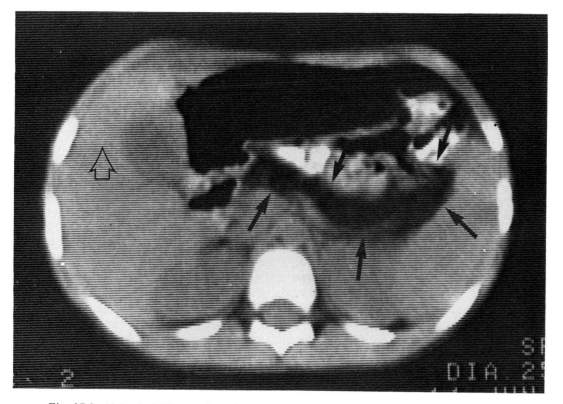

Fig. 27-9. Abdominal CT scan in a 5-year-old child with a previously confirmed diagnosis of Shwachman's syndrome. *Solid arrows,* The pancreas outlined has the radiodensity of fatty tissue, an observation consistent with the known histologic findings in this condition. The normal pancreas has a radiodensity equal to or greater than that of liver tissue, *open arrow.*

increase in the fatty tissue are common. Reduction in the number of megakarocytes is responsible for the thrombocytopenia sometimes noted.

Diagnosis

Pancreatic exocrine insufficiency needs to be considered in all children with diarrhea and failure to thrive. Shwachman's syndrome is probably the most frequent cause of pancreatic insufficiency in childhood after cystic fibrosis. The observation of neutropenia in such infants and children generally leads to the diagnosis. The diagnosis should also be suspected if roentgenograms reveal metaphyseal dysostosis or if laboratory studies reveal thrombocytopenia or an elevated fetal hemoglobin level. Abdominal CT scan clearly reveals the involved pancreas as a lipomatous structure. This may prove to be a specific finding for Shwachman's syndrome (Fig. 27-9).

Quantitative assessment of exocrine pancreatic function by secretin-pancreozymin stimulation (p. 909) and bone marrow studies will confirm the diagnosis. We see no need to undertake an open pancreatic biopsy in the typical case, but pancreatic needle biopsy guided by abdominal CT scanning is now possible.

Differential diagnosis

Once cystic fibrosis has been ruled out by the pilocarpine-iontophoresis sweat test, few causes of exocrine pancreatic insufficiency remain. Exocrine pancreatic insufficiency associated with congenital anomalies constituting a syndrome of congenital aplasia of the alae nasi, deafness, hypothyroidism, dwarfism, absent permanent teeth, and malabsorption is reported. Pancreatic insufficiency has also been associated with the cartilage-hair hypoplasia syndrome in conjunction with Hirschsprung's disease. Rare cases of congenital lipase deficiency, trypsinogen deficiency, and enterokinase deficiency reveal the respective enzyme defect in duodenal drainage fluid after stimulation. The late consequences of chronic relapsing pancreatitis, from whatever cause, are not difficult to recognize from the clinical story. Elevated serum amylase levels and elevated white blood cell count usually are found, whereas exocrine pancreatic insufficiency gradually develops over many years. Diabetes mellitus, a seemingly infrequent complication of Shwachman's syndrome, is commonly found in end-stage pancreatitis, in which islet cells are also affected by the inflammation and resulting fibrosis.

Complications

Retardation of both height and weight, malnutrition, and diarrhea complicate the clinical picture. Death, however, seems related to severe infection rather than to malnutrition. Although most patients have neutropenia, white blood cell phagocytic function seems normal, and only some patients seem to have great susceptibility to infection. Immunoglobulin levels should be checked in patients with an excessive number of infections, since low levels have reported in this condition and may further predispose to bacterial infections. Severe hip involvement with metaphyseal dysostosis may produce coxa vara deformity and seriously affect gait. Anemia and thrombocytopenia are seldom a problem.

Treatment, course, and prognosis

Once the diagnosis is made, pancreatic replacement therapy appropriate for the patient's age is begun. The degree of steatorrhea and frequency of defecation improve. Weight gain follows, but acceleration of the growth may not. Although pancreatic achylia continues, some patients spontaneously overcome the need for pancreatic extracts. The hematologic aspects remain variable or constant and are not affected by therapy. The very young child probably benefits from dietary manipulations, including the use of medium-chain triglycerides (Chapter 29).

At present, even if infections can be promptly treated, the prognosis is still uncertain after the diagnosis is established. In some cases, death occurs from overwhelming infection in a debilitated child before diagnosis can be made. In published reports, 9 of 36 children died in infancy or childhood. We have had 3 deaths in 9 proved cases. Two patients died within the first year of life from infection, and a third died of leukemia at 7 years of age. This latter cause of death has been noted by others as well.

REFERENCES

Aggett, P.J., Harries, J.T., Harvey, B.A.M., and Soothill, J.F.: An inherited defect of neutrophil mobility in Shwachman syndrome, J. Pediatr. **94:**391-394, 1979.

Aggett, P.J., Cavanaugh, N.P.C., Matthew, D.J., and others: Shwachman's syndrome, Arch. Dis. Child. **55:**331-347, 1980.

Bodian, M., Sheldon, W., and Lightwood, R.: Congenital hypoplasia of the exocrine pancreas, Acta Pediatr. Scand. **53**:282-293, 1964.

Brueton, M.J., Mavromichalis, J., Goodchild, M.C., and Anderson, C.M.: Hepatic dysfunction in association with pancreatic insufficiency and cyclical neutropenia: Shwachman-Diamond syndrome, Arch Dis. Child. **52**:76-78, 1977.

Doe, W.F.: Two brothers with congenital pancreatic exocrine insufficiency, neutropenia and dysgammaglobulinaemia, Proc. R. Soc. Med. **66**:1125-1126, 1973.

Goldstein, R.: Congenital lipomatosis of the pancreas: malabsorption, dwarfism, leukopenia with relative granulocytopenia and thrombocytopenia, Clin. Pediatr. **7**:419-422, 1968.

Hill, R.E., Durie, P.R., Gaskin, K.J., and others: Steatorrhea and pancreatic insufficiency in Shwachman's syndrome, Gastroenterology **83**:22-27, 1982.

Hudson, E., and Aldor, T.: Pancreatic insufficiency and neutropenia with associated immunoglobulin deficit, Arch. Intern. Med. **125**:314-316, 1970.

Johanson, A., and Blizzard, R.: A syndrome of congenital aplasia of the alae nasi, deafness, hypothyroidism, dwarfism, absent permanent teeth and malabsorption, J. Pediatr. **79**:982-987, 1971.

McLennan, T.W., and Steinbach, H.L.: Shwachman's syndrome: the broad spectrum of bony abnormalities, Radiology **112**:167-173, 1974.

Saunders, E.F., Gall, G., and Freedman, M.H.: Granulopoiesis in Shwachman's syndrome (pancreatic insufficiency and bone marrow dysfunction), Pediatrics **64**:515-519, 1979.

Schussheim, A., Choi, S.J., and Silverberg, M.: Exocrine pancreatic insufficiency with congenital anomalies, J. Pediatr. **89**:782-784, 1976.

Shwachman, H., Diamond, L.K., Oski, F.A., and Khaw, K.T.: The syndrome of pancreatic insufficiency and bone marrow dysfunction, J. Pediatr. **65**:645-663, 1964.

Woods, W.G., Roloff, J.S., Lukens, J.N., and Krivit, W.: The occurrence of leukemia in patients with the Shwachman syndrome, J. Pediatr. **99**:425-428, 1981.

ISOLATED ENZYME DEFECTS

Congenital isolated defects of exocrine pancreatic secretion are extremely rare. Absence of trypsin, trypsinogen, lipase, or amylase has been reported sporadically. The incompleteness of the studies described in some of these reports, considered in the light of newer findings, raises doubts as to the accuracy of the findings and the actual existence of some of these diagnoses. For example, patients believed to have trypsin or trypsinogen deficiency may actually have congenital enterokinase deficiency. The few patients with congenital lipase deficiency may actually have had Shwachman's syndrome, in that trypsin and amylase were also found to be diminished. In most cases, complete hematologic studies were not reported, and secretin-pancreozymin stimulation tests were not performed. A temporary acquired lipase deficiency has also been described after varicella infection.

Trypsinogen-deficiency disease

Trypsinogen, a pancreatic zymogen, depends on intestinal enterokinase for its primary activation to trypsin (Fig. 27-10). Once formed, trypsin itself is then capable of converting more of the proenzyme trypsinogen to trypsin. In addition, trypsin activates the other proteolytic proenzymes (zymogens), procarboxypeptidase and chymotrypsinogen, which are present in the pancreatic solutions. Absence of trypsinogen or failure to activate it results in complete loss of proteolytic activity from the pancreas.

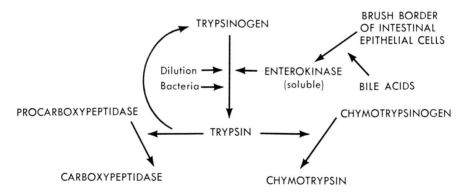

Fig. 27-10. Scheme for the activation of pancreatic zymogens (trypsinogen, chymotrypsinogen, and procarboxypeptidase) in the intestinal lumen. (Modified from Tarlow, M.J.: Arch. Dis. Child. 45:651, 1970.)

The two patients described with trypsinogen-deficiency disease had hypoproteinemia, edema, failure to thrive, and refractory anemia in infancy. Although trypsin was not present in pancreatic juice (amylase and lipase normal), some was noted in the stool. Activation experiments on the duodenal juice with exogenous bovine trypsin demonstrated the presence of procarboxypeptidase and chymotrypsinogen, but trypsinogen was not detected. Sweat chloride determinations were repeatedly normal; steatorrhea was mild. Neutropenia was reported early in the disease.

These infants were successfully treated with a formula containing a protein hydrolysate (Nutramigen) and pancreatic extracts (Viokase, Cotazym).

Congenital enterokinase deficiency

As mentioned previously, enterokinase, an enzyme secreted by the duodenal mucosa, is required to activate the zymogen trypsinogen. If it is absent, trypsinogen is not converted to trypsin, and if trypsin is absent, procarboxypeptidase and chymotrypsinogen are not activated (Fig. 27-10).

Congenital deficiency of enterokinase has now been described in three infants who had failure to thrive, diarrhea, and anemia. They had steatorrhea, but only two infants developed hypoproteinemia. The histologic appearance of duodenal biopsy material and assays of disaccharidase activities were normal in two patients. In their duodenal fluid, trypsin, chymotrypsin, and carboxypeptidase activities could not be detected until enterokinase was added or until their zymogens were incubated with normal duodenal mucosa. Furthermore, enterokinase activity was absent from both duodenal juice and mucosa.

The steatorrhea associated with enterokinase deficiency could very well be secondary to a concomitant deficiency of phospholipase, since its activation also depends on trypsin. Treatment with pancreatic extracts was highly effective because they contain enterokinase.

These cases bear a striking resemblance to those described with trypsinogen deficiency. It has recently been shown that exogenous bovine trypsin may not activate human trypsinogen, the technique used to diagnose trypsinogen deficiency. On the other hand, the addition of enterokinase will promptly activate this same presumably trypsinogen-deficient solution.

Congenital pancreatic lipase deficiency

Isolated pancreatic lipase deficiency has only been sporadically reported. The children may manifest steatorrhea with passage of oily, greasy, bulky stools from early infancy until the time of diagnosis. Failure to thrive is not always a feature of this condition, and abdominal distention and anemia were strikingly absent. Duodenal drainage after pancreozymin-secretin stimulation revealed lipase deficiency or absence of the enzyme.

On the other hand, colipase, the peptide cofactor in pancreatic juice necessary to anchor lipase to the micellar surface, is present in seemingly adequate amounts in the patients studied. Trypsin and amylase are sometimes present in reduced amount. Quantitative fat absorption was not severely abnormal despite the clinical suggestion of steatorrhea. Fat digestion may be facilitated in these patients by the action of lingual, gastric, or intracellular lipases released from sloughed enterocytes. Treatment with pancreatic extract and a low-fat diet partially improved the steatorrhea toward normal values. In a recent report the hematologic status of these patients was normal. The occurrence in siblings, generalized exocrine pancreatic insufficiency, and small stature suggest that these cases may be variants of Shwachman's syndrome.

REFERENCES

Figarella, C., DeCaro, A., Leupold, D., and Poley, J.R.: Congenital pancreatic lipase deficiency, J. Pediatr. **96:**412-416, 1980.

Hadorn, B., Hess, J., Troesch, V., and others: Role of bile acids in the activation of trypsinogen by enterokinase: disturbance of trypsinogen activation in patients with intrahepatic biliary atresia, Gastroenterology **66:**548-555, 1974.

Polonovski, D., and Bier, H.: Pseudotrypsinogen deficiency due to a lack of intestinal enterokinase, Acta Paediatr. Scand. **59:**458-459, 1970.

Rey, J. Frezal, J., Royer, P., and Lamy, M.: L'absence congénitale de lipase pancréatique, Arch. Franc. Pediatr. **32:**5-12, 1966.

Sheldon, W.: Congenital pancreatic lipase deficiency, Arch. Dis. Child. **39:**268-271, 1964.

Tarlow, M.J., Hadorn, B., Arthurton, M.W., and Lloyd, J.K.: Intestinal enterokinase deficiency, Arch. Dis. Child. **45:**651-655, 1970.

Townes, P.L., Bryson, M., and Miller, C.: Further observations on trypsinogen deficiency disease: report of a second case, J. Pediatr. **71:**220-224, 1967.

28 *Pancreatitis*

ACUTE PANCREATITIS

Pancreatitis is not difficult to diagnose in children when it occurs in association with mumps parotitis, immediately after abdominal trauma, or when specific medications known to cause pancreatitis are being taken, but difficulty does arise when these historic points are absent. Lack of personal experience with this disease prevents prompt diagnosis, especially in cases involving more obscure causes, and the difficulty can be further complicated by an atypical mode of presentation that frequently occurs in the younger child. Before the greater application of abdominal ultrasound examination in children with abdominal pain (acute or chronic), few cases came to early diagnosis. Even in large pediatric centers, only one to three cases per year are likely to be seen.

An acute episode of pancreatitis may resolve in one of several ways. The attack may be mild or severe, with complete recovery, or temporary recovery with recurrences, or death. Pancreatitis that becomes recurrent and chronic may also subside spontaneously, but the majority of such cases progress to a disabling state. Familial cases are more likely to be chronic and recurrent.

The number of known causes of pancreatitis is large, though the exact mechanism by which each condition triggers the inflammatory process is not always known. However, once triggered, trypsinogen is activated to trypsin in amounts exceeding the reserve capacity of the trypsin inhibitor in pancreatic secretions. The release of trypsin from its inhibitor autocatalytically activates more trypsinogen to trypsin, which, in turn, can activate other proteolytic proenzymes (chymotrypsinogen, procarboxypeptidase) (Fig. 27-10). Autodigestion of the gland begins and may be focal or may proceed to total autolysis. Fat necrosis of the peripancreatic and retroperitoneal tissues and saponification of calcium often result from released pancreatic lipase (Fig. 28-1). Amylase, also released from the destroyed acinar tissue, may become elevated by way of blood, lymphatic, or peritoneal absorption and be rapidly excreted into the urine.

The role of trypsin as the primary culprit in the progression of pancreatitis has been questioned since excess tryptic activity has not been found in pancreatic tissue or serum from patients with acute inflammatory pancreatic disease. Experimental efforts to reproduce this lesion by intrapancreatic injections of trypsin produced an unusual self-limited inflammation and necrosis with little activation of endogenous trypsin. The intraductal injection of a large amount of trypsin into the dog pancreas produces acute hemorrhagic necrosis. This result is believed to be mediated by the proelastase-activating effect of trypsin. Elastase, which preferentially attacks and digests elastin tissue of blood vessels, is thereby capable of disrupting capillaries and is probably instrumental in cases of hemorrhagic pancreatitis. The pathologic lesion produced experimentally also differs from that of the natural disease. The addition of a trypsin and chymotrypsin inhibitor (Trasylol) does not protect the tissue against producing the atypical reaction in the experimental model.

Attention has focused on the role of activated phospholipase A_2, an enzyme responsible for the conversion of lecithin to lysolecithin. The theory holds that lecithin, present in bile, may regurgitate into the pancreatic duct, where it is then acted on by trypsin-activated phospholipase A_2. Lysolecithins have potent cytolytic properties and act on the phospholipid layers of cell membranes. This could cause their disruption and free the proteolytic zymogens, which are then activated. The newly postulated mechanism of lysolecithin-incited pancreatic injury is intriguing, but it rests on two unconfirmed postulates: the presence of free trypsin to activate phospholipase A_2, and the regurgitation of bile into the pancreatic duct. Furthermore, although recent electron-microscopic studies in the dog confirmed the suspected detergent action of bile or bile acids on the acinar parenchyma, the zymogen granules were not altered in any detectable manner.

Secondary effects are also important in the clinical expression of this disease. Released vasoactive substances (kinins, kallikrein, histamine), by virtue of their effect upon capillary membrane permeability, play an important role in the observed fluid shifts that occur in pancreatitis. Free

843

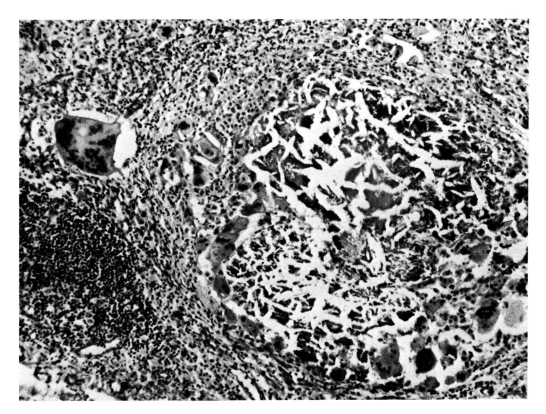

Fig. 28-1. "Acute" relapsing pancreatits. Tissue obtained from the child described in Fig. 28-4 at time of surgery, showing fat necrosis, saponification, and giant cell formation associated with chronic inflammation.

fatty acids may be playing an as-yet unidentified role in either the local tissue injury or in producing some of the systemic effects that occur in cases of pancreatitis particularly when associated with hyperlipidemic states.

Etiology

In contrast to cases in adults where alcoholism and biliary tract disease are the most common causes, most childhood cases of pancreatitis are believed to be caused by drug toxicity, trauma, intercurrent viral infection, genetic cause, or the "idiopathic" category. Since the number of causes of pancreatitis continues to grow, a detailed history is mandatory before one can exclude all of them. A list of suspected causes reported in children follows.

Etiology of pancreatitis

Infectious
 Mycoplasma pneumoniae
 Viral infection
  Mumps
  Epstein-Barr disease

 Coxsackievirus B
 Rubella
 Hepatitis A
 Influenza A
Generalized and systemic disease
 Systemic lupus erythematosus
 Hyperparathyroidism
 Sarcoid disease
 Henoch-Schönlein purpura
 Crohn's disease
 Reye's syndrome
 Cystic fibrosis
 Diabetes
 Uremia
Obstruction or direct injury
 Biliary tract
  Choledochal cyst
  Choledochocele
  Gallstones
 Duplication cyst (duodenum, gastropancreatic)
 Peptic ulcer (penetrating posterior)
 Ascariasis
 Trauma
  Accidental
  Nonaccidental (NAT)

Postsurgical (for peptic ulcer disease)
Duodenal obstruction
  Tumor (lymphoma)
  Stricture
  Annular pancreas
Metabolic
  Hyperlipidemia (types I and V)
  Hereditary pancreatitis
  Alpha-1-antitrypsin deficiency
  Malnutrition (kwashiorkor)
  Rapid refeeding of the malnourished child
Drugs, chemicals, or toxic agents
  Valproic acid
  Alcohol
  Steroids
  Sulfasalazine
  Tetracycline
  Chlorothiazide
  Furosemide
  Borates
  Oral contraceptives
    (estrogen)
  Azathioprine
  Sulfonamides
  Hyperalimentation
  Scorpion bites
Idiopathic

Clinical features

Abdominal pain occurs in at least 75% of cases and is the most common symptom in acute pancreatitis. The pain may develop slowly, be mild and of short duration, or be sudden in onset, severe in intensity, and of prolonged duration. The most intense pain is usually localized in the epigastrium, and in some patients it radiates to the back and upper quadrants as well. The pain is typically constant and may last for 24 to 72 hours. Not infrequently the pain may be precipitated or exacerbated by eating. Nausea and vomiting are very common. In severe cases, the patient may appear pale and sweaty and complain of dizziness. Fever may be low grade or moderate.

On physical examination, the patient is quiet and prefers to lie on his side with his hips slightly flexed. In fulminating cases, shock may be present. Mild scleral icterus may be noted. The abdomen is slightly distended and tender to palpation and percussion, but not rigid. Rebound tenderness may be limited to the upper quadrants or absent altogether. At times the spleen and liver may become enlarged and tender. Bowel sounds are diminished in most cases. An epigastric mass is occasionally palpable in cases of pseudocyst formation. A bluish discoloration around the umbilicus (Cullen's sign) or in the flanks (Grey-Turner's spots) signifies hemorrhagic pancreatitis with ascites. In rare cases, physical signs suggest a left-sided pleural effusion. Indeed, in the younger child, in whom localization of abdominal pain is poor, the presence of unexplained ascites or hemorrhagic pleural effusions should always be suspected to be of pancreatic origin. A nonspecific, nonbacterial "pancreatic pneumonitis" has been described in adults. Mumps pancreatitis is seldom severe and rarely occurs under 5 years of age. Clinical mumps is present in over 50% of these cases.

Laboratory and x-ray findings

The single most important laboratory aid in diagnosis is an elevated serum amylase level that begins to rise within 24 hours after symptoms begin. Serum amylase values greater than three times normal are always significant. Amylase is rapidly cleared by the kidneys, a demonstration of increased permeability to this enzyme during bouts of acute pancreatitis. The serum level peaks and may return to normal within 24 to 72 hours even though pain persists. Greatest elevations, however, are typically present 2 to 12 hours after onset of the disease. A mild-to-moderate elevation of serum amylase may also exist during the convalescent period, and urine amylase values may be abnormal for 24 hours after the serum level is normal. In mild cases of acute pancreatitis or in patients seen later in the clinical disease, urine amylase determinations may provide the needed diagnostic information. Since the renal clearance of amylase increases in pancreatitis (presumably because of decreased renal tubular reabsorption of amylase) but not in other conditions associated with an elevated serum amylase, determination of the amylase-creatinine clearance ratio (ACCR) has been considered a valuable laboratory aid in the diagnosis of this disorder. The reported selectivity of this test in acute pancreatitis is about 95%. The ACCR appears to be more sensitive than either serum or urine amylase determinations alone. It may be calculated by the following formula:

$$\% \frac{C_{\text{amylase}}}{C_{\text{creatinine}}} = 100 \times \left(\frac{U_{\text{amylase}}}{S_{\text{amylase}}} \times \frac{S_{\text{creatinine}}}{U_{\text{creatinine}}} \right)$$

The formula used in this determination has the advantage of being independent of urine volumes and collection times. Values greater than 4% to 5% are abnormal and strongly suggest pancreatic cause for the hyperamylasemia. False-high values

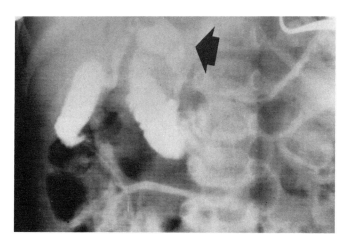

Fig. 28-2. Operative cholangiogram in a 15-month-old girl explored after many episodes of well-documented acute pancreatitis. A nonobstructing type I choledochus cyst, *arrow,* is demonstrated, but reflux into the pancreatic duct did not occur. A sphincterotomy was performed, but recurrent episodes of pancreatitis have continued. Both the family history and an extensive medical work-up were noncontributory.

can occur in diabetic ketoacidosis, in burn patients, and in the face of renal disease.

Because serum lipase determination remains a difficult, prolonged laboratory procedure and may yield false positive results (especially in gallstone disease), it has not achieved the popularity of serum amylase. The virtue of the serum lipase test lies in the slow disappearance of this enzyme from the blood, permitting diagnosis in patients who reach medical care late.

The hematocrit and the hemoglobin level may be elevated in patients who have fulminating pancreatitis caused by hemoconcentration. In severe cases the white blood count is usually elevated, but this is not a constant finding.

Tests of liver function should be obtained because acute biliary tract disease and hepatitis may mimic the clinical picture (Fig. 28-2). Elevation of serum bilirubin and alkaline phosphatase or gamma glutamyl transpeptidase (GGT) is common as a result of spasm or edema of the intra-pancreatic portion of the common duct or the sphincter of Oddi when caused by acute pancreatitis. Although rare chronic fibrosing pancreatitis may produce jaundice as well.

Low serum calcium values (less than 7 mg/dl) may carry a poor prognosis just as the finding of hyperglycemia does, with both results indicating widespread destruction of the gland. Hypocalcemia may occur either early or late in the course of acute pancreatitis. Although some depression

of the serum calcium (total and ionized) is caused by saponification from fat necrosis, neither glucagon, calcitonin, nor gastrin are presently considered responsible for the alterations in calcium metabolism during acute pancreatitis. Parathyroid hormone is appropriately elevated. In severe cases, oliguria or anuria with elevated blood urea nitrogen may also be found.

Ascitic fluid obtained by paracentesis can be very helpful when the diagnosis is less clear. The sterile hemorrhagic fluid generally contains a high amylase content even when serum amylase is not significantly elevated.

Routine abdominal roentgenograms (erect, supine, and decubitus views) may be normal or show dilatation of the transverse colon or an isolated segment of small bowel located in the mid or left upper area of the abdomen (sentinel loop), though this picture is not specific. Rarely will pancreatic calcifications be present early in the course of pancreatitis. Abdominal fluid that is clinically undetectable can be appreciated by these roentgenograms or better still by ultrasound examination.

At present pancreatic ultrasonography is the most reliable noninvasive means available for diagnosing pancreatic inflammatory disease, pancreatic pseudocyst or abscess formation within the gland. The observation that normal pancreatic tissue has an echodensity similar to or greater than that of the left lobe of the liver serves as the basis for assessment of pancreatic disease (Fig. 28-3). De-

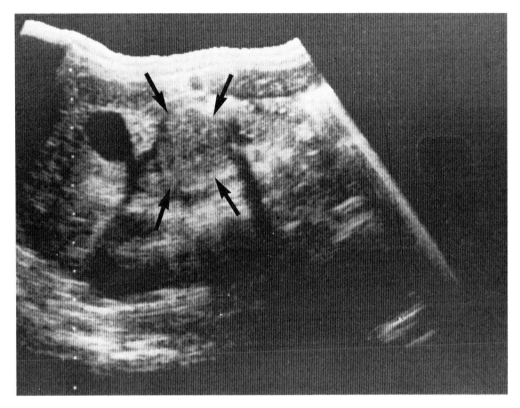

Fig. 28-3. Acute pancreatitis demonstrated by ultrasound in a 3-year-old child subjected to non-accidental trauma. The gland, *arrows*, is greatly enlarged with decreased echodensity relative to the liver. The echo-free structure is the gallbladder.

creased density of the gland relative to hepatic tissue occurs in pancreatitis, presumably because of tissue edema, and thereby permits early diagnosis of this condition by ultrasonography, sometimes before the serum amylase becomes elevated. When the diagnosis of pancreatitis in children is considered, this technique of comparative echodensity evaluation appears to be more reliable than assessment of alterations in the size of the gland. With the availability of ultrasonography, barium studies of the upper intestinal tract are now rarely indicated in assessment of complications of pancreatitis (pseudocyst formation). They may be more useful in ruling out specific causes originating in the intestinal tract (peptic ulcer disease, duodenal Crohn's disease, intraduodenal tumors, and so on).

An oral cholecystogram usually reveals a nonfunctioning gallbladder if obtained during, or shortly after, an attack of pancreatitis. It is likely to be normal when repeated a few weeks later.

If the history suggests one of the many other causes of acute pancreatitis, other appropriate laboratory studies will be needed. In particular, viral studies for mumps or coxsackievirus B, serum lipid profile, alkaline phosphatase and serum calcium and phosphate tests, antinuclear antibody test, and sweat test may be included.

Provocative tests are occasionally used after an episode of acute pancreatitis with the hope of gaining evidence of pancreatic ductal obstruction, but their value remains unsettled. The secretin-pancreozymin stimulation permits evaluation of the rise in pancreatic secretory volume and enzyme and bicarbonate content over basal values. If the ductules are obstructed, no rise occurs, but the serum amylase level may increase after the procedure. This test is sometimes painful when an obstruction to outflow exists.

The morphine-prostigmine test, another provocative test, has has limited use in children. The principle involved is that the prostigmine stimulates pancreatic secretion against a closed, morphine-stimulated sphincter of Oddi. A rise in serum amylase level (threefold) and pain, previously considered positive for pancreatitis, in fact lack specificity and reproducibility. The value of either of these provocative tests is marginal in children with acute pancreatitis, since the diagnosis can usually be suspected from the other parameters discussed previously. Endoscopic retrograde pancreatograms may be of particular value in the older child and teen-ager and are best performed after the acute process has resolved. Repeated attacks of acute pancreatitis call for endoscopic retrograde cholangiopancreatograms. This procedure is not without risk for inducing a relapse, but it is a valuable tool to establish the diagnosis of permanent changes and to help the surgeon who is considering a surgical procedure. We have no experience with this procedure before the teen-age years.

Pathologic lesion

In mild cases, interstitial edema and acute inflammatory cells are present, as well as loss of compactness of acinar tissue and focal areas of necrosis. In more severe cases local and widespread "metastatic" fat necrosis, hemorrhagic changes, and inflammation are found. Occasionally, mucopurulent or eosinophilic concretions are noted in ductular lumens. Recurrent episodes eventually result in pancreatic fibrosis (Fig. 28-4).

Differential diagnosis

Few other conditions in pediatrics can be confused with acute pancreatitis once the diagnosis is entertained. The severity and duration of pancreatic pain best serve to distinguish this diagnosis from the other, more common causes of recurrent abdominal pain of childhood, especially pain having a psychophysiologic cause. Biliary tract disease is relatively rare in children but may be responsible for up to 10% of cases. Peptic disease, with a posterior perforated ulcer, can mimic the entire picture of acute pancreatitis. High small bowel obstruction, particularly with perforation, also causes pain and elevated serum amylase values. A difficult diagnostic problem may be posed by an expanding inferiorly located subhepatic pyogenic or amebic abscess. The diagnosis of pancreatitis is sometimes discovered during abdominal surgery for other suspected causes. Even pneumonia has been reported capable of producing elevated serum amylase values, and abdominal pain is common in children with pneumonia. The serum amylase may also be elevated in acute viral hepatitis and ruptured ectopic pregnancy and in adults with carcinoma of the lung.

Treatment

Medical. Intensity of therapy depends on the condition of the patient and the severity of the attack. All efforts should be made to treat the patient medically and avoid surgery unless there is clear evidence of bowel perforation. The cornerstone of treatment continues to be "rest the gland," thereby preventing intestinal hormone stimulation of the pancreas by secretin and pancreozymin, enzymes normally released in response to intraluminal dietary constituents (especially amino acids and fats) and to gastric acid reaching the duodenum. The patient is given nothing by mouth, and nasogastric suction is started. Intravenous fluids at 1½ to 2 times the maintenance volume, electrolytes, blood, plasma, or salt-poor albumin may be needed to counteract shock. Atropine, 0.01 or 0.02 mg/kg subcutaneously, is helpful in blocking the vagal stimulation of the pancreas and can be used in more severe cases. Pain is best treated with meperidine (Demerol), 1 mg/kg intramuscularly. Both morphine and codeine tend to produce a greater degree of spasm of the duodenum musculature and sphincter of Oddi and therefore are not recommended. If hemorrhagic pancreatitis is suspected, central venous pressure should be monitored and urine output checked closely with an indwelling catheter. Serum electrolytes should be monitored and calcium given when indicated. At times, insulin may also be needed to lower the blood glucose level. Antibiotics (tetracycline, ampicillin) in appropriate dosage are recommended only in severe cases. As soon as the condition of the patient is stable, appropriate roentgenologic studies may be undertaken. Where a known cause for acute pancreatitis is determined and can be eliminated, such treatment obviously should be promptly undertaken.

Once clinical improvement is noticed because of decreased pain and return of bowel sounds, nasogastric suction may be discontinued and the patient fed a high-carbohydrate or bland, low-fat diet, with antacids given 1 and 3 hours postprandially. Oral alimentation may be tried in this clinical setting even when the serum amylase or amylase-creatinine clearance ratio remains somewhat elevated. If pain recurs with oral alimentation, the addition of pancreatic enzymes (Viokase, Cotazym, Pancrease, and so on) to the therapeutic reg-

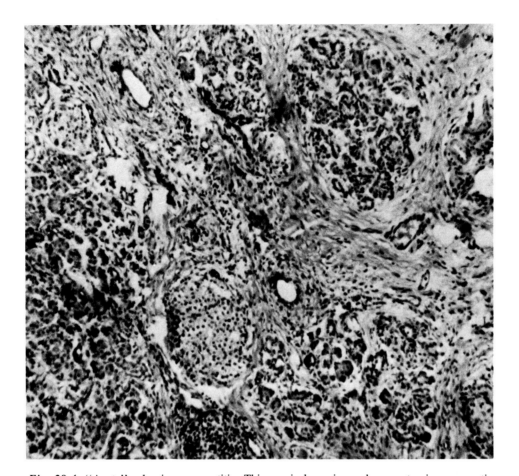

Fig. 28-4. ''Acute'' relapsing pancreatitis. This surgical specimen shows extensive pancreatic fibrosis isolating nests of acini and islets, with minimal inflammatory changes present in this portion of the tissue. This boy's illness began 4 months earlier without known antecedent features such as abdominal trauma, biliary tract disease, or drug ingestion. The family history was negative for similar problems, and there was no history to suggest familial hyperlipidemia. Each episode (five) of pancreatitis was characterized by moderate to severe upper abdominal pain radiating to his back and associated with anorexia and vomiting. The duration of the pain was often more than 24 hours and was alleviated only by meperidine. The initial episodes were treated conservatively. Laboratory tests consistently showed a greatly elevated amylase (more than 2000 Close-Street units) with normal serum calcium and blood glucose levels. Oral cholecystography failed to visualize the gallbladder during an acute episode but did so during an interval of well-being 3 weeks later. A glucose tolerance test and 72-hour stool fat determinations were both within normal limits. A lipid profile revealed a moderate elevation of the prebetalipoprotein fraction on two occasions. After his fifth episode of pancreatitis, it was decided to perform exploratory surgery on this boy with the hope of identifying a cause for his difficulty. The entire length of the pancreas was noted to be studded with small yellow nodules believed to represent saponification of fat (Fig. 28-1). An operative cholangiogram and common duct exploration were normal. On opening of the duodenum, a probe could not be passed into the pancreatic duct through the ampulla of Vater. A distal pancreatectomy was performed, and a probe was then passed retrograde through an exposed duct and appeared at the ampulla of Vater. A sphincterotomy and Roux-en-Y anastomosis to the tail of the pancreas were performed. The abdomen was closed, and the postoperative course was benign. Three months later the patient had a recurrence of the original symptoms.

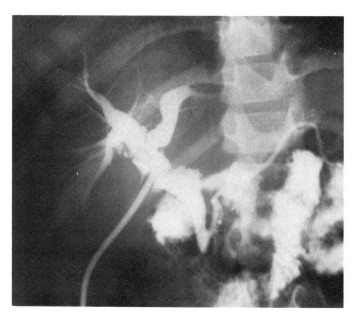

Fig. 28-5. Operative T-tube cholangiogram in a 3-year-old girl with recurrent pancreatitis. The dilated extrahepatic biliary tree is seen, and a normal-sized pancreatic duct is filled in retrograde fashion. A side-to-side choledochoduodenotomy was eventually done because of recurrent attacks, and this child has been free of pain for over 9 years (since 1973).

imen has occasionally been beneficial. Experimental evidence suggests that pancreatic secretion may be inhibited by the intraduodenal presence of trypsin and chymotrypsin. If pain persists after oral alimentation, discontinuation of feeding and reinstitution of nasogastric suction for an additional 24 to 48 hours is usually required.

Surgical. If a diagnosis of acute pancreatitis cannot be made with certainty, signs of peritonitis are present, or perforation or obstruction of bowel exists or is suspected, then surgery is indicated. Surgery can, however, be delayed if acute gallbladder disease is suspected. More often, after opening the abdomen, the surgeon is surprised to find the diagnosis of acute pancreatitis correct and the preoperative diagnosis in error. At this point difficulty arises in deciding what to do, if anything. A cholangiogram should be attempted, since retrograde filling of the pancreatic duct sometimes occurs, providing useful information (Fig. 28-5). The decision to obtain a pancreatogram will depend on the findings at surgery and the condition of the patient. Cholecystectomy has been suggested if acute inflammatory disease of the gallbladder exists. Attempts to drain the pancreas are not indicated during the acute episode because of the possibility of subsequent fistula formation and

breakdown of a surgically created anastomosis. However, drainage of the lesser sac is advised to prevent pseudocyst formation.

In exceptional cases of fulminant hemorrhagic pancreatitis (less than 3%) surgical resection may offer the only chance for survival. In such cases cardiovascular collapse may occur within the first 48 hours, presumably because of circulating vasoactive substances liberated by pancreatic enzymes that gain access to the vascular system, probably through the peritoneal cavity. Recently, peritoneal dialysis has been used in an effort to reduce the concentration of these vasodilating substances with promising results. Surgery is indicated for débridement of necrotic tissue or when abscess formation is suspected, but the timing of such intervention is critical. Partial resections in the face of acute pancreatitis may in fact predispose to pancreatic abscess formation, and, not surprisingly, there is reluctance to intervene surgically if other measures (medical) are available.

Complications

Although hypovolemia and hemoconcentration are common findings early in the course of acute pancreatitis, hypervolemia and congestive heart failure may suddenly develop on the third to fifth

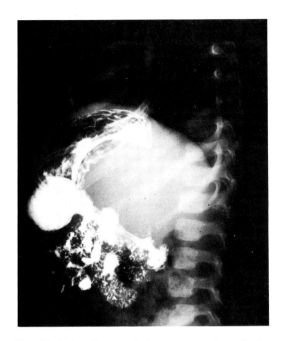

Fig. 28-6. Pseudocyst of the pancreas. Lateral view shows the typical retrogastric mass.

day of therapy. The sudden absorption of fluids from the peritoneal and pleural cavity into the "normalized" circulation is the accepted explanation for this complication. Renal failure from acute tubular necrosis may also play a role in some patients.

Patients who survive the initial episode of acute pancreatitis, especially if it results from trauma, must be followed carefully, for up to 15% will develop an inflammatory mass, be it a pseudocyst, phlegmon, or abscess.

Pseudocyst formation (5%) should be anticipated, the patient's abdomen gently palpated for an epigastric mass, and roentgenologic studies obtained when indicated (Fig. 28-6). Serial ultrasound examinations not only permit early recognition of an evolving pseudocyst but also allow for noninvasive monitoring of its subsequent evolution. Most pseudocysts resolve spontaneously within 4 to 12 weeks. However, those developing a mature fibrous capsule are unlikely to show spontaneous resolution by reabsorption. Recurrent abdominal pain, elevated serum amylase, and intermittent nausea and vomiting are the usual clinical symptoms consistent with this complication of pancreatitis. When surgical drainage of the pseudocyst is indicated, the cyst may be opened

to drain into the stomach, duodenum, or a defunctionalized loop of jejunum via a Roux-en-Y anastomosis.

A solid inflammatory mass that develops after acute pancreatitis is probably a phlegmon, consisting of necrotic tissue mixed with inflammatory exudate and tissue edema. Before ultrasound studies were available, many of these were probably incorrectly considered to be pseudocysts by standard contrast roentgenographic evaluation. This inflammatory mass often resolves spontaneously over 1 to 3 months, but the patient is at risk for development of pancreatic abscess by bacterial seeding into this necrotic tissue.

As mentioned above, pancreatic abscess formation (5%) may follow acute pancreatitis as a result of bacterial seeding of the necrotic tissue. As might be expected, this complication is more likely to occur in severe cases of pancreatitis with extensive necrosis and is usually heralded 10 to 14 days after the initial episode by spiking fevers, chills, and a recurrence of abdominal pain. Surgical drainage is mandatory in all such cases because, untreated, the mortality is probably 100%. Not infrequently, multiple abscesses may be found at surgery. Fistula formation, both internal and external, may develop in patients requiring surgical drainage procedures performed on the inflamed gland. Again, surgery may also predispose to abscess formation in cases operated upon for acute disease.

Splenomegaly developing after an episode of pancreatitis suggests splenic vein thrombosis and may eventually lead to the development of esophageal varices. Occasionally, the inflammatory process causes infarction of the transverse colon with subsequent obstruction. In these considerations either selective angiography or splenoportography will be diagnostic procedures of choice.

Recurrences are the most dreaded complication; the condition may progress to chronic pancreatitis with exocrine and endocrine insufficiency. Fortunately, both are rare events in the pediatric population. Disabling disease with severe recurring pain may lead to narcotic addition and suicide in the older children.

Mortality and prognosis

No correlation exists between the elevation of the serum amylase and the severity of the pancreatic lesion. In acute interstitial pancreatitis, mortality figures for adults are approximately 5%

to 10% if surgery is needed, and 1% in those treated medically. In the fulminating hemorrhagic form of acute pancreatitis, the mortality may be as high as 25% in adults treated medically and 50% to 75% in those coming to surgery. A recent report dealing with a pediatric population found the mortality for acute interstitial pancreatitis to be 17.5%, whereas for acute hemorrhagic pancreatitis it was 86%. Underestimation of the extreme fluid losses that may occur is probably responsible for this high mortality figure. If no precipitating cause can be found for the initial attack, the patient may be expected to have relapses, especially if the family history is positive for pancreatic disease. Surgery in this group is eventually necessary. If underlying renal or hepatic disease exists, the prognosis is much poorer.

REFERENCES

Acosta, J.M., and Ledesma, C.L.: Gallstone migration as a cause of acute pancreatitis, N. Engl. J. Med. **290:**484-487, 1974.

Buntain, W.L., Wood, J.B., and Woolley, M.M.: Pancreatitis in childhood, J. Pediatr. Surg. **13:**143-149, 1978.

Chaves-Carballo, E., Menezes, A.H., Bell, W.E., and Henriquez, E.M.: Acute pancreatitis in Reye's syndrome: a fatal complication during intensive supportive care, South. Med. J. **73:**152-154, 1980.

Cox, K.L., Ament, M.E., Sample, W.F., and others: The ultrasonic and biochemical diagnosis of pancreatitis in children, J. Pediatr. **96:**407-411, 1980.

Das, S.: Pancreatitis in children associated with round worms, Indian Pediatr. **14:**81-83, 1977.

Finch, W.T., Sawyers, J.L., and Schenker, S.: A prospective study to determine the efficacy of antibiotics in acute pancreatitis, Ann. Surg. **183:**667-671, 1976.

Gryboski, J., Hillemeier, C., Kocoshis, S., and others: Refeeding pancreatitis in malnourished children, J. Pediatr. **97:**441-443, 1980.

Izsak, E.M., Shike, M., Roulet, M., and Jeejeebhoy, K.N.: Pancreatitis in association with hypercalcemia in patients receiving total parenteral nutrition, Gastroenterology **79:**555-558, 1980.

Jordan, S.C., and Ament, M.E.: Pancreatitis in children and adolescents, J. Pediatr. **91:**211-216, 1977.

Keating, J.P., Shackelford, G.D., Shackelford, P.G., and Ternberg, J.L.: Pancreatitis and osteolytic lesions, J. Pediatr. **81:**350-353, 1972.

Kotner, L.M., and McFadden, J.C.: Pancreatitis and choledochal cyst with gallstones: an unusual case, J. Arkansas Med. Soc. **71:**299-301, 1975.

Lebenthal, E., and Shwachman, H.: The pancreas: development, adaptation and malfunction in infancy and childhood, Clin. Gastroenterol. **6:**397-413, 1977.

Mallory, A., and Kern, F., Jr.: Drug-induced pancreatitis: a critical review, Gastroenterology **78:**813-820, 1980.

Meneely, R.L., O'Neill, J., and Grishan, F.K.: Fibrosing pancreatitis—an obscure cause of painless obstructive jaundice: a case report and review of the literature, Pediatrics **67:**136-139, 1981.

Michels, V.V., and Beaudet, A.L.: Hemorrhagic pancreatitis in a patient with glycogen storage disease type I, Clin. Genetics **17:**220-222, 1980.

Oderda, G., and Kraut, J.R.: Rising antibody titer to *Mycoplasma pneumoniae* in acute pancreatitis, Pediatrics **66:**305-306, 1980.

Olazabal, A., and Fuller, R.: Failure of glucagon in the treatment of alcoholic pancreatitis, Gastroenterology **74:**489-491, 1978.

Papp, M., Breuer, J.H., Nemeth, E.P., and others: On the lysolecithin content of the pancreas in experimental acute pancreatitis, Gastroenterology **65:**778-787, 1973.

Puppala, A.R., Cheng, J.C., and Steinheber, F.U.: Pancreatitis: a rare complication of Schönlein-Henoch purpura, Am. J. Gastroenterol. **69:**101-104, 1978.

Regan, P.T.: Medical treatment of acute pancreatitis, Mayo Clin. Proc. **54:**432-434, 1979.

Robinson, D.O., Alp, M.H., Grant, A.K., and Lawrence, J.R.: Pancreatitis and renal disease, Scand. J. Gastroenterol. **2:**17-20, 1976.

Seidman E., Deckelbaum, R., Roy, C.C., and others: Chronic relapsing pancreatitis in Crohn's disease. (Submitted to Gastroenterology.)

Steinberg, W.M., Salvato, R.F., and Toskes, P.P.: The morphine-prostigmin provocative test—is it useful for making clinical decisions? Gastroenterology **78:**728-731, 1980.

Traverso, L.W., Tompkins, R.K., Urrea, P.T., and Longmire, W.P., Jr.: Surgical treatment of chronic pancreatitis: twenty-two years' experience, Ann. Surg. **190:**312-319, 1979.

Vennes, J.A.: Transduodenal visualization of the bile and pancreatic ducts, Hosp. Pract., pp. 117-124, 1973.

Waldram, R., Kopelman, H., Tsantoulas, D., and Williams, R.: Chronic pancreatitis, sclerosing cholangitis and sicca complex in two siblings, Lancet **1:**550-552, 1975.

Warshaw, A.L., and Lee, K.H.: The mechanism of increased renal clearance of amylase in acute pancreatitis, Gastroenterology **71:**388-391, 1976.

Warshaw, A.L., and Fuller, A.F., Jr.: Specificity of increased renal clearance of amylase in diagnosis of acute pancreatitis, N. Engl. J. Med. **292:**325-328, 1975.

Weir, G.C., Lesser, P.B., Drop L.J., and others: The hypocalcemia of acute pancreatitis, Ann. Intern. Med. **83:**185-189, 1975.

TRAUMATIC PANCREATITIS

Trauma to the abdomen remains a common cause of acute pancreatitis in the pediatric patient. Blunt trauma to the abdomen and direct injury during an abdominal surgical procedure are included in this category. Nonaccidental trauma (NAT) should also be considered in the differential diagnosis of any young child presenting with otherwise unexplained pancreatitis.

Injury to the pancreas may result from seemingly trivial trauma. Most common blunt injuries to the abdomen in children are the result of auto accidents or falls from a bicycle. For toddlers, push toys, the edge of a coffee table, or a hearthstone may be the offending object. A cumulative survey of childhood pancreatitis puts the incidence for traumatic causes at about 30%. Unless the physician specifically inquires about recent abdominal injury to pediatric patients with abdominal pain, he may not suspect traumatic pancreatitis. The symptoms of acute pancreatitis after blunt injury to the abdomen may start immediately, hours, or even weeks later.

The mechanism by which the pancreas is injured is not completely understood. Its fixed retroperitoneal position is believed to be a liability at times. If a person is slightly flexed, the gland is compressed further by the superior mesenteric vessels against the first and second lumbar vertebrae, and a shock wave traveling through the abdomen can disrupt the small pancreatic vessels or pancreatic tissue itself. At times, the entire tail of the pancreas can be avulsed by seemingly mild trauma. It has been suggested that small, pointed objects such as sticks, ends of bicycle handlebars, and fenceposts may transmit a localized shock wave directly to the pancreas, whereas more diffuse abdominal injury from auto accidents commonly can be expected to cause damage to liver, spleen, or duodenum.

Clinical and laboratory findings

Many signs and symptoms of acute pancreatitis apply to the traumatic form as well. The severity of symptoms is usually proportionate to the violence of the initial pancreatic injury. In mild cases, only transient abdominal discomfort is experienced, and nausea and vomiting are absent or minimal. The initial complaints are often disregarded, but a recurrence within the next few hours or days signifies pancreatic inflammation. Severe pain (usually upper abdominal), nausea, vomiting, pallor, and abdominal distention signify severe injury. The patient's condition may deteriorate rapidly, and shock develops because of massive fluid losses into the abdomen. If there is severe abdominal trauma, it may be difficult to make a clinical diagnosis of pancreatitis, since injury to other underlying structures may mimic these findings. In some cases with delayed symptoms an epigastric mass is palpable (pseudocyst) as the first clinical clue to suggest pancreatic disease.

Abdominal enlargement and shifting dullness are grave findings when they appear early. The digestive action of freed proteolytic enzymes into the retroperitoneal or peritoneal spaces results in a violent inflammatory reaction. Bloody ascitic fluid rapidly accumulates from injured tissues and vessels.

The most helpful laboratory test is the serum amylase determination. Repeated determinations may be indicated whenever abdominal pain develops subsequently to trauma to that portion of the body. Hemoglobin levels, hematocrit, electrolyte levels, serum calcium levels, and glucose values are occasionally needed to further assess the degree of injury and disturbance of body homeostasis.

Three-way films of the abdomen are extremely useful in ruling out associated conditions commonly found after abdominal trauma (perforated viscus, free fluid secondary to capsular tear of spleen or liver).

If the patient has a palpable mass, ultrasound of the abdomen will differentiate an inflammatory phlegmon from a pancreatic pseudocyst.

Pathology

The pancreatic lesion seen grossly may reveal minimal edema, hyperemia, and focal areas of fat necrosis. Total glandular autolysis may be found in severe cases, a result of hemorrhagic necrosis and proteolytic dissolution. Transection usually occurs in the distal end of the gland. Microscopically, variable degrees of edema, hemorrhage, and necrosis are reported in the acute case. Delayed diagnosis reveals a gland with acute and chronic inflammatory cells, necrosis, and fibrosis.

Treatment

The decision as to whether the patient requires immediate surgical intervention or supportive medical management alone must rest on the clinical story and condition of the individual patient. Continued hemorrhage, the possibility of a ruptured viscus, and the patient's deterioration despite adequate blood and fluid replacement are all indications for operative intervention. Many surgeons prefer to use the conservative, nonoperative approach as long as clinical improvement continues. Patients managed medically have a higher incidence of pseudocyst formation and therefore need to be followed closely for several months.

How much to do at the time of laparotomy is not completely agreed on. Active bleeding is controlled, hematomas are evacuated, and the lesser sac is drained. A Roux-en-Y procedure may be performed if a transected portion of pancreas is found at surgery.

Close observations of central venous pressure and urine output, combined with proper replacement of blood, plasma, and electrolytes, are mandatory before, during, and after surgery. Other medical means to reduce stimulation of pancreatic enzymes are useful adjuvants and have been previously discussed (p. 848). Pancreatic pseudocysts may be marsupialized or drained into a neighboring portion of small bowel.

Complications

The most common complication of traumatic pancreatitis is pseudocyst formation (Fig. 28-6) or abscesses, which are less likely to develop if the lesser sac is drained. However, external fistulas are a frequent complication after surgical intervention during the acute stage. Renal shutdown, hypocalcemic tetany, and hyperglycemia may develop during the early phase of the clinical course.

Late complications also include recurrent episodes of pain and progressive pancreatic fibrosis with exocrine and endocrine deficiencies.

Prognosis

Surprisingly the prognosis for the child with traumatic pancreatitis is quite good if the diagnosis is considered early and appropriate supportive measures are promptly begun.

REFERENCES

Hartley, R.C.: Pancreatitis under the age of five years: a report of three cases, J. Pediatr. Surg. **2**:419-423, 1967.

Keating, J.P., Shackelford, G.D., Shackelford, P.G., and others: Pancreatitis and osteolytic lesions, J. Pediatr. **81**:350-353, 1972.

Keeney, R.E.: Enlarging on the child abuse injury spectrum, Am. J. Dis. Child. **130**:902, 1976.

Leistyna, J.A., and Macaulay, J.C.: Traumatic pancreatitis in childhood, Am. J. Dis. Child. **107**:644-648, 1964.

Pena, S.D.J., and Medovy, H.: Child abuse and traumatic pseudocyst of the pancreas, J. Pediatr. **83**:1026-1028, 1973.

HEREDITARY PANCREATITIS (CHRONIC RELAPSING PANCREATITIS)

It would appear that so-called "idiopathic" chronic fibrosing pancreatitis is a very rare entity. A few of the reported cases have had unremarkable clinical symptoms and even negative laboratory studies, coming to diagnosis at laparotomy. The last several years have seen a rapid increase in the number of reported cases of childhood chronic relapsing pancreatitis. The majority of these cases have a definite familial clustering and represent examples of the disease called "hereditary pancreatitis." Thorough investigations of the kindreds of index cases have shown that familial cases have an autosomal dominant pattern of inheritance with complete penetrance but variable expressivity. The number of patients with either proved or suspected hereditary pancreatitis is over 200.

Although all the kindreds reported so far have been whites, no sex preference has been noted. Other familial disease states associated with pancreatitis, such as hyperparathyroidism, hypertriglyceridemia, and cystic fibrosis, were ruled out by proper studies. Although diseases with an autosomal dominant form of inheritance are often associated with structural (anatomic) defects, none has been consistently found in patients with hereditary pancreatitis.

Although many cases are not diagnosed until adulthood, a history of recurrent abdominal symptoms during childhood is frequently present. Attacks of abdominal pain from pancreatic disease tend to be more severe and of longer duration than the episodes triggered by psychophysiologic causes (Chapter 15). Twenty-four to 48 hours of severe pain located in the upper half of the abdomen and radiating to the back is not uncommon. Nausea and vomiting are present and may necessitate hospitalization for correction of dehydration. Laboratory findings are similar to those described for acute pancreatitis from other causes, with elevated serum amylase and lipase levels, hemoconcentration, and leukocytosis. With minimal conservative measures these attacks abate and are followed by pain-free periods that may vary in duration from weeks to years. With successive pain episodes the elevations of serum amylase may become less striking, whereas in advanced cases characterized by significant pancreatic acinar destruction, serum amylase values may be normal during an attack. At this time, evidence of pancreatic insufficiency may be present (steatorrhea, malnutrition), and carbohydrate intolerance may be demonstrable by tolerance tests. Recent data equate these findings with encroachment on the remaining 10% of functioning pancreatic tissue.

In more subtle but advanced cases, pancreatic function can best be assessed by measurement of the volume and bicarbonate response of the gland after secretin (1.5 units/kg) stimulation. Bicarbonate and volume are affected to a greater degree in fibrosing pancreatitis than enzyme production is.

The diagnosis of hereditary pancreatitis is aided by the finding of pancreatic calcifications on routine abdominal roentgenograms obtained during a pain episode. Arranged in a linear fashion in the head of the pancreas, these calcifications are eventually present in 25% to 50% of cases of hereditary pancreatitis and may be noted as early as the second decade of life.

It would appear from recent data that studies of urinary amino acid patterns cannot be relied on to substantiate this diagnosis. The original finding of cystine, arginine, and lysine aminoaciduria occurred in two patients with hereditary pancreatitis who, in addition, suffered from an incomplete form of cystinuria. The diagnosis of chronic fibrosing pancreatitis is not infrequently made at laparotomy, when firm nodular masses are either noted on the surface of the indurated gland or detected by palpation. The pancreatic ductal system, whether viewed by endoscopic retrograde cholangiopancreatography or from an intraoperative pancreatogram, shows distortion in the caliber of both the main pancreatic ducts and abnormal branching. The pathologic lesion seen on biopsy is that of dense interstitial fibrosis, near-total loss of acinar tissue, absence of significant inflammatory reaction, and relative preservation of the islets of Langerhans. Pancreatograms usually reveal ductal dilatation without obvious strictures or stenotic segments.

The treatment of the acute attack is similar to that previously described for other types of acute pancreatitis (p. 848). Restoration of fluid and electrolyte balance and nasogastric suction are the most useful measures. Atropine and meperidine are often used simultaneously to relieve sphincter spasm and to alleviate the pain. Fortunately, these attacks are short lived, and complications (abscesses, pseudocysts, ascites, pleural effusions, shock) are rare in this form of pancreatitis. Surgical procedures, such as sphincterotomies and partial resections, have provided little relief of symptoms for these patients. On the other hand,

surgical drainage of abscesses is mandatory. A pseudocyst may spontaneously regress.

The prognosis for patients with hereditary pancreatitis is not grim during childhood. The severity of the pain episodes determines the degree of disability and absence from school, the latter being a potential problem. Pseudocyst formation does occur (10%) and can be diagnosed by ultrasound examination. Pancreatic insufficiency is a late complication (adulthood) and can be treated with replacement therapy similar to that outlined for cystic fibrosis (Chapter 27). Insulin injections may become necessary in prolonged cases in which diabetes develops. The teen-ager with pancreatitis must be protected from overuse of narcotics in the control of pain episodes, since addiction to drugs is not uncommon; in adults with this disease, suicide has been noted. In this regard, we have had an excellent response with the use of self-hypnosis in controlling the impact of pain episodes in one affected teen-ager.

The increased likelihood that pancreatic carcinoma will develop in patients with hereditary pancreatitis (especially those with pancreatic calcifications) seems well established. The validity of any decision regarding prophylactic total or subtotal pancreatectomy will require careful scrutiny of additional reported cases and the statistical application of life-expectancy figures.

REFERENCES

Castleman, B.: Clinicopathological exercise from case records of the Massachusetts General Hospital, N. Engl. J. Med. **286:**1353-1359, 1972.

Di Magno, E.P., Go, V.L.W., and Summerskill, W.H.J.: Relations between pancreatic enzyme outputs and malabsorption in severe pancreatic insufficiency, N. Engl. J. Med. **288:**813-815, 1973.

Fried, A.M., and Selke, A.C.: Pseudocyst formation in hereditary pancreatitis, J. Pediatr. **93:**950-953, 1978.

Kattwinkel, J., Lapey, A., di Sant'Agnese, P.A., and Edwards, W.A.: Hereditary pancreatitis: three new kindreds and a critical review of the literature, Pediatrics **51:**55-69, 1973.

Whitten, D.M., Feingold, M., and Eisenklam, E.J.: Hereditary pancreatitis, Am. J. Dis. Child. **116:**426-428, 1968.

Williams, T.E., Jr., Sherman, N.J., and Clatworthy, H.W., Jr.: Chronic fibrosing pancreatitis in childhood: a cause of recurrent abdominal pain, Pediatrics **40:**1019-1023, 1967.

Part III

NUTRITIONAL SUPPORT, OSTOMY CARE, SELECTED TESTS AND PROCEDURES

29 *Nutritional support**

The healthy, happy child with a good appetite who is offered a well-balanced diet generally presents no problem in nutritional care. The premature infant, the chronically ill, the adolescent living on pot, pop, and pizza, and the child with a disordered endocrine-metabolic-digestive-absorptive problem can be of significant nutritional concern. It is for the last group of persons that supplemental vitamins or minerals or removal of offending foods or addition of others may be necessary.

In the material to follow, basic nutritional requirements, special diets, supplemental food items, and resources will be presented. It is vitally important to remember, however, that at best these represent general guidelines and not dogma; each patient's needs must be considered and the dietary regimen individualized. Therapeutic diets must be carefully and thoughtfully selected, taught, and evaluated. The child's appetite and acceptance of foods is filled with vagaries and self-assertion. Any diet, no matter how well-defined and reasonable, is of little value if the patient will not accept it. It may be necessary to satisfy the child's appetite with modifications. Although adaptations may not be ideal in dietary treatment, they can be made within certain limits. However, some of the diets, such as the gluten-free diet, require strictness if a clinical response is to occur.

The psychologic impact of any program, no matter how well indicated, warrants understanding by the family and the physician. The child or the adolescent who, for whatever reason, differs from his peer group deserves that his feelings and attitudes be taken into account when a dietary treatment is arranged. This should not prevent the institution of a necessary program. Fortunately, and frequently with the successful response to the dietary regimen, the health of the patient is improved or restored and with it an overall feeling of well-being.

Nutritional care is of great importance during fetal life as well as in the early months of life.

*With the assistance of Lise Bouthillier, B.Sc. (Nutr.), Dietetics Service and Gastrointestinal Unit, Hôpital Sainte-Justine, Montreal.

Evidence, both experimental and clinical, suggests that cell division and myelination of the human brain may be impaired during this critical period with undernutrition. Failure of adequate nutrition during the first year of life may adversely affect both physical and mental development in later years.

There is considerable concern at the present time over drug use and breast feeding. A long list of drugs that are excreted in breast milk has been prepared. The amount of drug excreted by a lactating mother may be very small, but the effects on the nursing infant, though unknown, may be potentially hazardous. Therefore, extreme caution should be exercised in the use of drugs by a lactating mother.

DIETS
Nutritional requirements

The basic nutritional requirements refer to caloric needs, met by protein, carbohydrate, and fat and to vitamins and minerals (Table 29-1). Data on which these requirements are based are increasing, but there is continued need for additional study.

The Ten-State Nutrition Survey and the Nutrition Canada National Survey found that a small percentage of each population surveyed was malnourished or at risk of developing nutritional problems. In these reports the adolescent had the highest prevalence of unsatisfactory nutritional status. Obesity was a major problem in all population groups and constitutes a form of malnutrition that is growing in importance. These reports again serve to emphasize that adequate supervision and counseling about nutritional status is important in the pediatric population. It is obvious that eating habits developed during the early period of life may well carry over into adulthood.

Nutritional problems may result from the unavailability or insufficient intake of food, vitamins, and minerals. They will also develop when there are disturbances in digestion, absorption, or utilization of nutrients. Evaluation of nutritional status should be a regular part of medical

Table 29-1. Recommended daily dietary allowances*

	Age (years)	Weight (kg)	Height (cm)	Energy (kcal)	Protein (gm)	Fat-soluble vitamins			
						Vitamin A activity (μg RE†)	Vitamin D (μg‡)	Vitamin E activity (mg α-TE§)	Vitamin K (μg)
Infants	0.0-0.5	6	60	Kg × 115	Kg × 2.2	420	10	3	12
	0.5-1.0	9	71	Kg × 105	Kg × 2.0	420	10	4	10-20
Children	1-3	13	90	1300	23	400	10	5	15-30
	4-6	20	112	1700	30	500	10	6	20-40
	7-10	30	132	2400	34	400	10	7	30-60
Males	11-14	45	157	2700	45	1000	10	8	50-100
	15-18	66	176	2800	56	1000	10	10	50-100
	19-22	40	177	2900	56	1000	7.5	10	50-100
Females	11-14	46	157	2200	46	800	10	8	50-100
	15-18	55	163	2100	46	800	10	8	50-100
	19-22	55	163	2100	44	800	7.5	8	50-100

*From Recommended Dietary Allowances, revised 1980, Food and Nutrition Board, National Academy of Sciences–National Research Council.
†Retinol equivalent; 1 retinol equivalent = 1 μg of retinol (3.33 IU).

care. A dietary history should always be recorded. Symptoms and signs associated with undernutrition and vitamin deficiencies (Chapters 1 and 2) should be looked for. The ongoing clinical assessment of adequate nutrition includes the regular recording of weights and heights plotted against acceptable standards of growth. Undoubtedly, a personal knowledge of the family and its socioeconomic background, cultural heritage, and psychologic makeup toward food (food faddism) should be taken into account. Hematologic and biochemical data may be useful as additional information.

Infant nutrition

The first 4 to 6 months of life is the period of most rapid growth and development. Nutrient requirements must be met as excesses, and deficiencies or imbalances may have both short-term and long-term consequences. All nutrients needed during that period can be found in one single food, human milk. An inadequate substitute for human milk or the replacement of human milk or formula by solid foods of inferior nutritional value can be detrimental.

Breast milk as a cause of failure to thrive. Breast milk is regarded as the ideal early food for normal healthy infants in terms of the balance of nutrients supplied, their bioavailability, and their immunologic properties. Despite a wider dissemination of information, most doctors and nurses have been brought up in a tradition of bottle feeding and are not familiar with the practical aspects of lactation. Programs for the promotion of breast feeding, for the institution of changes in hospital practices, and for the support of breast feeding mothers during the early weeks of lactation still leave much to be desired. A significant number of mothers still experience breast-feeding failure. They do not produce enough milk to meet their infant's energy requirements. Failure to thrive as a result of inadequate breast feeding is becoming more frequent as an increasing percentage of mothers elect to breast feed.

In a recent study from England, inadequate lactation was recognized in 9 out of 21 cases of failure to thrive admitted over a period of 1 year. Two distinct clinical patterns were recognized:

1. The irritable, fussy, colicky, undernourished infant with poor weight gain.
2. The "contented" underfed babies. These are the most worrisome because often they will not come to the attention of the physician until malnutrition is severe. The mother does not worry because the baby sleeps for long intervals and appears satisfied after brief and widely spaced sessions of suckling.

Water-soluble vitamins							Minerals						
Vitamin C (mg)	Folacin (µg)	Niacin (mg NE‖)	Riboflavin (mg)	Thiamine (mg)	Vitamin B_6 (mg)	Vitamin B_{12} (µg)	Calcium (mg)	Phosphorus (mg)	Iron (mg)	Magnesium (mg)	Zinc (mg)	Copper (mg)	Iodine (µg)
35	30	6	0.4	0.3	0.3	0.5	360	240	10	50	3	0.5-0.7	40
35	45	8	0.6	0.5	0.6	1.5	540	360	15	70	5	0.7-1.0	50
45	100	9	0.8	0.7	0.9	2.0	800	800	15	150	10	1.0-1.5	70
45	200	11	1.0	0.9	1.3	2.5	800	800	10	200	10	1.5-2.0	90
45	300	16	1.4	1.2	1.6	3.0	800	800	10	250	10	2.0-2.5	120
50	400	18	1.6	1.4	1.8	3.0	1200	1200	18	350	15	2.0-3.0	150
60	400	18	1.7	1.4	2.0	3.0	1200	1200	18	400	15	2.0-3.0	150
60	400	19	1.7	1.5	2.2	3.0	800	800	10	350	15	2.0-3.0	150
50	400	15	1.3	1.1	1.8	3.0	1200	1200	18	300	15	2.0-3.0	150
60	400	14	1.3	1.1	2.0	3.0	1200	1200	18	300	15	2.0-3.0	150
60	400	14	1.3	1.1	2.0	3.0	800	800	18	300	15	2.0-3.0	150

‡As cholecalciferol; 10 µg of cholecalciferol = 400 IU of vitamin D.
§α-Tocopherol equivalent; 1 mg of *d*-α-tocopherol = 1 mg of α-TE = 1.49 IU.
‖NE (niacin equivalent) is equal to 1 mg of niacin, or 60 mg of dietary tryptophan.

Table 29-2. Breast-milk volume for energy needs in first 6 months

Age (months)	Weight (kg)	Energy requirements* (kcal/kg)	Volume of breast milk	
			(ml/kg)	(ml/day)
0	3.2	115	170	542
3	5.7	95	137	786
6	7.4	87	123	914

*Lowest current estimated requirements. Adapted from Rowland, M.G.M., and others: Br. Med. Bull. **37**:77, 1981.

Table 29-3. Composition (gm/dl) of breast milk as a function of gestational and postpartum age

	Term milk		Preterm milk	
	Early milk (8 to 11 days)	Mature milk (26 to 29 days)	Early milk (8 to 11 days)	Mature milk (26 to 29 days)
Lactose	6.0 ± 0.2	6.5 ± 0.2	5.6 ± 0.05	6.0 ± 0.1
Protein*	1.7 ± 0.2	1.3 ± 0.1	1.9 ± 0.1	1.4 ± 0.05
Fat	2.9 ± 0.2	3.0 ± 0.1	4.1 ± 0.3	4.0 ± 0.3
Caloric density (kcal/dl)	59 ± 2	59 ± 1	71 ± 2	70 ± 2

Adapted from Anderson, G.H., and others: Am. J. Clin. Nutr. **34**:258, 1981.
*Total nitrogen × 6.25.

Table 29-4. Composition of milk, low birth weight, and infant formulas

	Milk		Low birth weight–infant formulas			
	Whole cow's milk*	Human milk*	SMA "Premie"†	Enfamil Premature‡	Similac Special Care§‖	Similac 24 LBW§
Energy content (kcal/dl)	67	67	81	81	81	81
Major nutrients (gm/dl) Protein concentration	3.2	1.1	2.0	2.4	2.2	2.2
Source	Casein and whey		Demineralized whey and nonfat cow's milk	Demineralized whey and nonfat cow's milk	Nonfat cow's milk	Nonfat cow's milk
Whey/casein ratio	20/80	60/40	60/40	60/40	60/40	20/80
Carbohydrate concentration	4.7	7.1	8.6	8.9	8.6	8.5
Source	Lactose	Lactose	Lactose and glucose polymers	Lactose and glucose polymers	Lactose and glucose polymers	Lactose and glucose polymers
Fat concentration	3.8	3.8	4.4	4.1	4.4	4.5
Source	P/S ratio** 0.04	0.40	Vegetable oils (87%) MCT (13%)	Corn and coco oils (60%) MCT†† (40%)	Corn and copra‡‡ oils (50%) MCT (50%)	Soybean and coco oils (50%) MCT (50%)
Major minerals (per 100 ml) Calcium (mg)	137	34	75	95	144	73
Phosphorus (mg)	91	14	40	48	72	56
Magnesium (mg)	13	3.5	7.0	8.5	10.0	8.0
Copper (mg)	0.01	0.05	0.07	0.08	0.2	0.08
Zinc (mg)	0.39	0.12	0.5	0.5	1.2	0.8
Sodium (mEq)	3.3	0.75	1.4	1.4	1.5	1.6
Potassium (mEq)	3.7	1.3	1.9	2.3	2.6	2.6
Chloride (mEq)	3.1	1.1	1.5	2.0	1.9	2.4
Renal solute load¶ (mOsm/liter)	226	75	175	220	208	153
Oral solute load# (mOsm/kg water)	280	280	268	300	300	290

*See George, D.E., and Lebenthal, E.: In Lebenthal, E., editor: Textbook of gastroenterology and nutrition in infancy, New York, 1981, Raven Press; Lawrence, R.A.: Breast-feeding: a guide for the medical profession, St. Louis, 1980, The C.V. Mosby Co., pp. 44-72.

†Wyeth Laboratories, Philadelphia, Pa.

‡Mead Johnson Laboratories, Evansville, Ind.

§Ross Laboratories, Columbus, Ohio.

‖Similac Special Care is now available at a caloric density of 0.67 cal/ml.

	Normal-infant formulas								
SMA and SMA + iron†	Similac and Similac + iron§	Similac 60/40§	Enfamil and Enfamil + iron‡	Prosobee‡	Isomil§	Pregestimil‡	Nutramigen‡	Portagen‡	RCF (Ross Carbohydrate Free)§
67	67	67	67	67	67	67	67	67	§§
1.5	1.5	1.5	1.5	2.5	2	1.9	2.2	2.5	2
Demineralized whey and nonfat cow's milk	Nonfat cow's milk	Sodium and calcium caseinate	Nonfat cow's milk	Soybean isolate		Casein hydrolysate		Sodium caseinate	Soybean isolate
60/40	20/80	60/40	20/80	—	—	—	—	—	—
7.2	7.2	6.8	7.0	6.8	6.7	9.1	8.8	8.0	§§
Lactose				Sucrose and glucose	Sucrose, corn syrup, corn starch	Corn syrup solids and tapioca starch	Sucrose and tapioca starch	Corn syrup solids and sucrose	CHO should be added
3.6	3.6	3.7	3.8	3.4	3.6	2.75	2.6	3.4	3.6
Vegetable oils and oleo oil	Vegetable oils					Corn oil (60%) MCT (40%)	Corn oil	Corn oil (13%) MCT (87%)	Soybean and coconut oils
44	52	40	57	80	69	63	63	64	70
33	39	20	45	53	50	42	48	48	50
5.3	4.1	4.2	4.8	6.4	5.0	7.4	7.4	13.8	5
0.05	0.04	0.04	0.04	0.06	0.05	0.06	0.06	0.11	0.05
0.37	0.5	0.4	0.43	0.53	0.5	0.42	0.42	0.64	0.5
0.65	1.0	0.7	1.1	1.5	1.3	1.4	1.4	1.4	1.3
1.4	1.7	1.5	1.7	2.3	1.8	1.9	1.8	2.2	1.8
1.1	1.4	0.7	1.4	1.2	1.5	1.7	1.4	1.7	1.5
128	108	90	160	220	124	200	200	152	126
300	290	260	280	252	250	338	443	236	§§

†Most of the renal solute load is provided by excreted nitrogenous products (4 mOsm/gm of dietary protein) and by urinary Na$^+$, K$^+$, and Cl$^-$ (each mEq in the formula = 1 mOsm of renal solute load).

#Osmolality provided by carbohydrates, proteins, and electrolytes.

**Polyunsaturated/saturated fatty acids. Since the lipid source of commercial formulas is vegetable oils with or without saturated medium-chain triglycerides, the P/S ratios vary between 0.32 and 0.70.

††Medium-chain triglycerides.

‡‡Oil extracted from dried decorticated coconut.

§§Variable with the quantity of water and carbohydrate added. It is recommended to add 7 gm/dl of carbohydrates to obtain a calorie density of 67 kcal/dl.

Close monitoring of weight gain in breast-fed babies is important. If test weighing (before and after feeding) suggests that inadequate amounts of milk are being taken, the baby should be carefully examined to rule out other causes of failure to thrive before attempts are made at improving milk production (more frequent feeding, complete emptying of the breasts, and so on).

Perhaps the dogmatic statement that "breast milk should be the sole article of nutrition for the first 6 months" should be reconsidered in the light of recent information suggesting that milk volume, the chief determinant of the infant's total energy intake becomes insufficient by 3 to 4 months to cover needs of a significant number of infants. Table 29-2 shows breast-milk volume estimates necessary to cover such requirements in the first 6 months.

The physician also needs to be aware of the malnourished nursing mother because, in contrast to well-nourished mothers whose milk satisfies the nutritional needs of an infant during the first 6 months, supplementation of the former's infant may be necessary as early as the third month.

Breast milk for low birth weight (LBW) infants. Studies have shown that human milk is inadequate in meeting the nutritional requirements of the small premature infants. The major concern has been based on the protein concentration. Calculations made from information extrapolated from intrauterine growth curves indicate that LBW infants require more protein than human milk can provide. Nutritionally, sodium and calcium needs of LBW infants have also been calculated to be greater and cannot be met by human milk. These observations, however, were based on the composition of term breast milk, but recent work has shown that preterm breast milk has a higher protein and sodium content.

As shown in Table 29-3, preterm milk also has a higher fat content and caloric density than term milk does. Our work in this area shows that gestational age does not change the nitrogen content of preterm milk. The switchover to mature milk values in terms of nitrogen concentration takes place some time between the thirty-sixth and the fortieth week of gestation. Although there is a decrease in nitrogen with postpartum age, our observations suggest that preterm milk contains a third more nitrogen than term breast milk does. Recent evidence indicates that with the major exceptions

of calcium and of vitamin D most of the requirements to achieve intrauterine growth rates can be supplied by the milk of the infant's own mother fed at daily rates of 180 to 200 ml/kg.

Formulas as an alternative to breast milk. The Committee on Nutrition of the American Academy of Pediatrics has recently published revised standards for formulas. These recommendations contain minimum levels for most components necessary to meet the individual infant's nutritional requirements. Upper safety limits are also included when it is pertinent. The nutrient composition of human milk, cow milk, and of various formulas is shown in Table 29-4.

Protein quality is critical, but to a certain extent it can be made up by quantity. Most formulas have a cow's milk base and therefore an amino acid pattern for human infants that is inferior to that of breast milk. The whey-casein ratio of breast milk has been reproduced in a certain number of formulas and represents a distinct improvement. Soybean isolate formulas are satisfactory in terms of nitrogen balance but are contraindicated in LBW infants. Hypophosphatemia is frequent and results from a lowered phosphorus absorption. Despite increased renal conservation of phosphorus, homeostatic control of phosphorus is unduly stressed and may lead to phosphorus-deficiency rickets.

Fat provides about half the calories. The source of fat in most formulas is vegetable oil, which is more soluble than animal fat and therefore more completely absorbed. Despite this, the fat of formulas is still less efficiently absorbed than that of human milk. This has to do with the structure of breast-milk triglycerides, wherein a large proportion of the less-soluble saturated fatty acid, palmitic acid, is in the 2-position of the glycerol molecule, rendering it more soluble as a monoglyceride than as a free fatty acid and therefore more completely absorbed after lipolysis. A further advantage of breast milk is that it contains a bile salt–stimulated lipase. In addition, it is known that human-milk triglycerides are very vulnerable to gastric lipolysis, affected to some extent by gastric lipase but more extensively by swallowed lingual lipase. Since medium-chain triglycerides (MCT) were shown to be extensively absorbed by LBW infants, low birth weight formulas now have 40% to 50% of their fat content as MCT.

Table 29-5. Renal solute load and caloric density of milks and solid foods

	Renal solute load (mOsm/100 gm)	Caloric density (kcal/100 gm)
Milk		
Human	7.0	65-75
Cow's whole	22.8	65
Cow's skim	31.1	36
Formulas	9.1-12.3	67
Infant foods		
Precooked dry cereal		
with milk	—	108
with water	—	52
Vegetables		
Plain	11.1	27-78
Creamed	10.0	42-94
Fruits	5.0	71-136
Dessert and puddings	6.0	96
Meats	57.0	106
Egg yolk	68.8	192

Adapted from Nutrition Committee of the Canadian Pediatric Society: Can. J. Publ. Health **70:**376, 1979.

There are still conflicting views as to the appropriate composition of formulas for LBW infants, but there is evidence that the presently marketed ones (Table 29-4) have distinct advantages and can promote retention rates of nutrients comparable to fetal accretion rates. However, indirect calorimetry measurements do not confirm this and suggest that the accretion rate of fat is much larger and that of protein is smaller than what occurs in utero.

Problems associated with the feeding of solid foods. There are no absolute guidelines for timing the introduction of solids. In most infants, there is no nutritional reason to add solids before 6 months of age. However, some infants are unsatisfied with breast milk or formula alone by 3 to 4 months of age; it is not unreasonable to introduce solids earlier in these babies. By 5 months, most infants have doubled their birth weight and require 35 to 40 ounces of milk to meet their energy needs. The gradual introduction of solids by the age of 6 months appears desirable.

Excessive renal solute load and nutritional imbalance. The renal osmolar load of some baby foods is high. In addition the nutritional value of solid foods is inferior to that of human milk or formula. Yet their caloric density is greater (Table 29-5). Therefore the early introduction of large amounts of solids at the expense of breast milk or formula can lead to problems likely to become clinically manifest when an acute illness leads to large extrarenal losses of water or when a chronic illness is associated with a significant degree of anorexia. There is no convincing evidence that the early feeding of solids plays a role in the etiology of obesity.

Food sensitivity and diarrhea. The early introduction of solid foods is believed to enhance the chance of developing food sensitivities. Despite the lack of solid data, it appears reasonable to recommend that the more allergenic foods (cow's milk, citrus fruits, wheat, and eggs) be withheld for the first 6 to 9 months and for 12 months in infants with a strong family history of allergy. Diarrhea after the introduction of new foods is common; it may last for a few days and then disappear. If it proves to be persistent, the food should be withheld and reintroduced a few months later.

An interesting survey has shown that with the introduction of juices and solids, the incidence of diarrheal episodes doubles whether the infant is breast fed or formula fed. These observations argue in favor of the sound practice of putting off the introduction of solids till 4 to 6 months of age.

REFERENCES

Anderson, G.H., Atkinson, S.A., and Bryan, M.H.: Energy and macronutrient content of human milk during early lactation from mothers giving birth prematurely and at term, Am. J. Clin. Nutr. **34:**258-265, 1981.

Atkinson, S.A., Radde, I.C., Chance, G.W., and others: Macro-mineral content of milk obtained during early lactation from mothers of premature infants, Early Hum. Dev. **4:**5-14, 1980.

Cunningham, A.S.: Morbidity in breast-fed and artificially fed infants, J. Pediatr. **90:**726-729, 1977.

Davies, D.P.: Is inadequate breast-feeding an important cause of failure to thrive? Lancet **1:**541-542, 1979.

George, D.E., and Lebenthal, E.: Human breast milk in comparison with cow's milk. In Lebenthal, E., editor: Textbook of gastroenterology and nutrition in infancy, New York, 1981, Raven Press.

Lawrence, R.A.: Biochemistry of human milk. In Breast-feeding: a guide for the medical profession, St. Louis, 1980, The C.V. Mosby Co., pp. 44-72.

Nutrition Committee of the Canadian Pediatric Society: Statement on infant feeding, Can. J. Publ. Health **70:**376-385, 1979.

Nutrition Committee of the Canadian Pediatric Society: Feeding the low-birth-weight infant, Can. Med. Assoc. J. **124:**1301-1311, 1981.

Rowland, M.G.M., Paul, A.A., and Whitehead, R.G.: Lactation and infant nutrition, Br. Med. Bull. **37:**77-83, 1981.

Sauls, H.S.: Potential effect of demographic and other variables in studies comparing morbidity of breast-fed and bottle-fed infants, Pediatrics **64:**523-527, 1979.

Senterre, J.: Calcium and phosphorus retention in preterm infants. In Stern, L., Oh, W., and Friis-Hansen, B., editors: Intensive care in newborn, II, New York, 1979, Masson Pub. U.S.A., pp. 205-210.

Shenai, J.P., Reynolds, J.W., and Babson, S.G.: Nutritional balance studies in very-low-birth-weight infants: enhanced nutrient retention rates by an experimental formula, Pediatrics **66:**233-238, 1980.

Shenai, J.P., Jhaveri, B.M., Reynolds, J.W., and others: Nutritional balance studies in very-low-birth-weight infants: role of soy formula, Pediatrics **67:**631-637, 1981.

Waterlow, J.C., and Thomson, A.M.: Observations on the adequacy of breast-feeding, Lancet **2:**238-241, 1979.

Therapeutic diets

Many nutritional problems, associated with a wide variety of gastrointestinal disorders, require special formulas or diets. These are designed for patients who have various digestive or absorptive disorders and for children who require supplemental nutritional support. Diet therapy may be employed on a short-term basis, as in postoperative states, or for extended periods of time, as in gluten enteropathy. The approach must be individualized to assure the most satisfactory results.

No bland diets and no low-roughage diets are given here; they are of little therapeutic value in the management of young patients.

Each diet listed is designed to meet the specific medical needs of the patient. Considerable leeway is necessary within the basic plan. It is entirely possible that if dietary therapy is unsuccessful, the diet may be incorrect, it is not being followed, the diagnosis is incorrect, or results are expected too quickly. Regular follow-up care and careful instructions are necessary to assure the maximum benefit of dietary management.

Gluten-free diet

The basic purpose of the gluten-free diet is to exclude the gliadin moiety present in the gluten of wheat (including durum, bulgar, and graham flours) oats, barley, rye, sorghum, triticale, and millet. Most authorities believe that the majority (90%) of celiac patients tolerate moderate amounts of oats once their disease is under control. Since wheat in particular is such a common ingredient in foods, some canned baby foods, and even chewing gum, careful attention to the labeled contents is essential. The diet should initially consist of more carbohydrate and protein than is normally used, in order to compensate for poor absorption. Because of the striking decrease in lactase activity during the acute stage of celiac disease, a lactose-free diet may be necessary in certain cases for at least 6 weeks.

For more detailed information that will be needed for long-term care, reference should be made to a diet manual.

Initially, when absorption is still poor, supplemental minerals and water-miscible preparations of vitamins A, D, E, and K should be given. After the positive clinical response occurs, the supplements should be discontinued.

Generally, bread, cereal, and flour products are the major food items to be eliminated. More specifically, this would include doughnuts, sweet rolls, crackers, muffins, cold and hot cereals, pancakes, cake, pastry, cookies, gravies, sauces made with flour, spaghetti, and noodles. All labels should be checked carefully for gluten, flour, and cereal additives. Other common foods that contain gluten include prepared meats, such as bologna, frankfurters, and luncheon meat, commercial ice cream, and candies with cereal additives.

Monosodium glutamate is now allowed, but the recommendation is to avoid malt (its flavoring is allowed) and hydrolyzed proteins of unknown origin or prepared from wheat, rye, and barley.

Substitutes for the major food items include the following:

Breakfast cereals
  Cereal from rice or corn
  Cornmeal
  Cornflakes
  Soybean
  Puffed Rice
  Rice Krispies
Breads made of
  Arrowroot flour
  Buckwheat flour
  Cornmeal flour
  Soybean flour
  Rice flour
  Potato flour
  Gluten-free wheat starch
  Cornstarch
Bread substitutes
  Potatoes, rice, hominy grits, low-protein wheat-starch pastas
Desserts
  Gelatin with or without fruit
  Tapioca
  Rice pudding
  Custard
  Junket
  Ice cream or sherbet (check labels)
  Cookies, cakes, pastries, and desserts made with gluten-free flours

Favorable response to a gluten-free diet may occur within a week, as evidenced by a decrease in diarrhea, improved appetite, and an overall improvement in attitude and behavior. In some patients clinical improvement may take several months. Because the gluten-free diet provides an inadequate amount of B-complex vitamins, these should be provided daily. Since celiac disease is a lifelong disease, the gluten-free diet should be continued indefinitely.

Resources

Bell, L., Hoffer, M., and Hamilton, J.R.: Recommendations for foods of a questionable acceptance for patients with celiac disease, J. Can. Diet. Assoc. **42:**143-158, 1981.
Gluten-free recipes: Write to 555 Special Foods, Hospital for Sick Children, 555 University Ave., Toronto, Ontario M5G 1X8.
Mayo Clinic diet manual: a handbook of dietary practices by the dietetic staffs of the Mayo Clinic, Rochester Methodist Hospital, and St. Mary's Hospital of Rochester, Minnesota, Philadelphia, 1981, W.B. Saunders Co.

Table 29-6. Lactose content per serving of selected dairy products

Dairy product	Serving	Lactose content (gm)
Milk	1 cup	11
Low-fat milk (2%)	1 cup	9-13
Skim milk	1 cup	12-14
Low-fat yogurts	1 cup	11-15
Ice cream	1 cup	9
Ice milk	1 cup	10
Sherbet	1 cup	4
Cottage cheese	1 cup	5-6
Cheddar cheese	1 oz	0.4-0.6
Processed American cheese	1 oz	0.5
Butter	1 tbs	0.15
Oleomargarine	1 tbs	0

Sheedy, C.B., and Keifetz, N.: Cooking for your celiac child, 1969, Dial Press, Inc., 750 Third Avenue, New York, New York 10017.

Lactose-limited diet

The lactose-limited diet is designed to restrict lactose intake and essentially consists in eliminating all milk and milk products. Lactose is a common ingredient in many food products, but most lactose-intolerant patients tolerate small amounts. Patients with galactosemia need to avoid any significant amount of lactose even as adults. Some gastrointestinal disorders are associated with lactose intolerance (Chapter 9). In these cases, the diet does not need to be too restrictive and depends on the patient's tolerance. Clinical response is usually quite prompt. The duration of the diet is variable and depends on the nature of the intolerance.

After a varying period, small amounts of lactose may be cautiously introduced into the diet. The amount of lactose permitted should not produce symptoms in the previously symptomatic patient who has responded to the diet. Additions to the diet are made according to the patient's tolerance.

All milk and milk products containing large amounts of lactose are eliminated (Table 29-6). Cow's milk–substitute formulas that may be used can be found in Table 39-4. Older persons can use non–dairy creamer type of products. Fruit and vegetable juices may also be beverage substitutes.

Low-lactose milk can be produced by incubation of cow's milk with yeast lactase, which is commercially available. Five to 10 drops of Lact-Aid is added to a liter of milk, which is then placed in the refrigerator for 24 hours. The resultant lactose-hydrolyzed milk offers a reasonable approach for lactase-deficient individuals because 70% to 95% of the 45 gm of lactose present in a liter of milk will be hydrolyzed into glucose and galactose.

Resource

Lact-Aid is available from Sugar Lo Company, P.O. Box 1017, Atlantic City, NJ 08404, or, in Canada, Jan Distributing Co., 302 Cliffwood Rd., Willowdale, Ontario M2H 2E5.

Sucrose-restricted diet

The general principles applicable to the lactose-limited diet are also relevant to a sucrose-free diet. In congenital sucrase and isomaltase deficiency, the diet can include minimal amounts (less than 2%) of sucrose and sucrose-containing foods. In congenital fructose intolerance, the diet should be fructose free, and therefore sucrose must be completely eliminated from the diet. Sucrose can safely be replaced in the diet by glucose (dextrose). Dextrose, purchased at a pharmacy, may be substituted in any recipe for sugar. The diet must be supplemented with vitamin C.

Polymers of glucose such as Caloreen and Polycose may cause problems (cramps, diarrhea) in some patients because a certain percentage of the glycosidic bonds are of the α-1,6 type requiring the disaccharidase activity of isomaltase (dextrinase). In the patient with sucrase-isomaltase deficiency, fructose is well tolerated and constitutes an excellent substitute for sucrose.

Evaporated formulas should not be sweetened except with glucose. Commercial formulas with sucrose can be found in Table 29-4.

Sucrose gives food its sweetness and is found in candies, cookies, and ice cream and naturally in fruit, some vegetables, sugars, and syrups. Foods that taste sweet should be avoided unless artificial sweeteners or dextrose have been used for flavoring.

Fruits and vegetables that are not well tolerated should be excluded.

Evaporated formulas should not be sweetened except with glucose. Commercial formulas with sucrose can be found in Table 29-4.

Substitutions. Generally, the following fruits and vegetables are low in sucrose:

Asparagus	Blackberries
Bamboo shoots	Blueberries
Broccoli	Cherries, fresh
Brussel sprouts	Cranberries
Cabbage	Currants
Cauliflower	Kadota figs, dried
Celery	Lemons
Chard	Loganberries
Chicory	Mulberries
Cucumber	Pears
Eggplant	Raspberries
Green beans	Rhubarb
Lettuce	Strawberries, medium ripe
Lima beans	Tomatoes
Mushrooms	
Parsley	
Peppers	
Potatoes	
Radishes	
Spinach	
Watercress	
Wax beans	

The following foods should be excluded from the diet:

Milk drinks and desserts with added sugar
Sweetened condensed milk
Flavored yogurts
Breakfast cereals, breads, cookies, cakes, and pastries prepared with sugar
Mayonnaise, prepared salad dressings with added sugar
Sugar (cane, beet, granulated, powdered, brown), jam, some honey, jelly, candy, molasses, maple syrups, corn syrup*
Commercially prepared pies, cookies, cakes, diabetic products, ice cream, sherbet
Medicines prepared with syrup
Nuts (except pecans)
Commercial baby foods

Milk protein–free diet

Some infants are intolerant to the protein constituents of cow's milk. For practical purposes, the elimination of specific fractions is not attempted; instead, milk proteins are completely removed from the diet.

A variety of formulas prepared from hydrolyzed casein, vegetable proteins, or meat base (homemade) can be substituted for milk. (See Table 29-4.) These formulas are fortified with all vitamins

*Corn syrup contains a bit of sucrose (7%) and should be used according to patient's tolerance.

and minerals needed for growth, and further supplementation is unnecessary.

Labels should be checked for butter, oleomargarine, cream cheese of any kind, fresh milk, buttermilk, dried milk, condensed milk, evaporated milk, yogurt, casein, lactalbumin, curds, whey, beef, and veal. Dried milk is added to such foods as cold cuts, prepared mixes, and commercial desserts.

After the patient has been symptom free for 3 to 4 months, small amounts of milk may be given and slowly increased, if tolerated. Milk protein should be reintroduced into the diet only with extreme caution. Vomiting, diarrhea, sweating, pallor, a shocklike state, wheezing, and skin eruptions may occur in highly sensitive patients when milk is reintroduced, and the milk should be promptly discontinued.

Resources

Milk free recipes with Prosobee, Mead Johnson Laboratories, Evansville, Indiana 47721, or, in Canada, Mead Johnson, 100 Bld. Industriel, Candiac, Quebec J5R 1J1, or 411 Roosevelt Ave., Ottawa, Ontario K2A 3X9.

Milk free recipes with Isomil, Ross Laboratories, 625 Cleveland Ave., Columbus, Ohio 43216, or, in Canada, Ross Laboratories, 5400 Côte-de-Liesse, Montreal, Quebec H4P 1A5.

Low-protein diet

Nutritional deficiency is a common and often neglected problem in the overall management of children with chronic liver disease. Decreased dietary intake is probably the principal cause of nutritional deficiency though malabsorption is a significant factor in cholestatic conditions. Factors that require investigation include assessment of energy and nutrient needs as well as of the eventual metabolic fate of nutrients once they have been absorbed.

Restriction of dietary protein is indicated in patients who have symptoms of chronic renal insufficiency. Also, protein intake may need to be restricted in patients with severe liver disease at risk for portosystemic encephalopathy. In this type of patient, dietary protein should be limited to 0.5 gm/kg of body weight per 24 hours, gradually increasing to 1 gm/kg/24 hr.

Because the body cannot produce, in sufficient amounts, eight of the 20 amino acids, they must be provided in the diet. These essential amino acids are all found in animal protein in varying proportions. Vegetable proteins are extremely low in one or two of these amino acids. If protein intake is adequate but from poor sources, growth may be impaired. Severe dietary limitations of protein intake will require restricted amounts of milk, cheese, meat, fish, poultry, and eggs, with measured amounts of breads, cereals, and some vegetables. Even fruit can add measurably to the protein intake when protein is severely restricted.

Because restriction of protein intake may result in a negative nitrogen balance and further deterioration of liver function, special mixtures of orally and intravenously administered amino acids have been designed. These preparations contain high concentrations of branched-chain amino acids (leucine, isoleucine, and valine), in addition to arginine and low concentrations of aromatic amino acids (phenylalanine, tyrosine, and tryptophan) and of methionine. Promising results are reported with Hepatic-Aid (McGaw Labs, Glendale, Calif.) and with ketoanalogs of essential amino acids.

Because the diet may be nutritionally inadequate in iron, calcium, B-complex vitamins, and calories, supplementation may be required.

Low-fat diet

A low-fat diet may be indicated in all acute and chronic diseases in which the functions of lipolysis (pancreatic insufficiency), micellar solubilization (liver disease, short bowel syndrome), mucosal absorption (celiac disease, and so on), transport out of the absorptive cell (abetalipoproteinemia or hypobetalipoproteinemia), or transport in the lymphatic system (lymphangiectasis) may be impaired. With acute gastroenteritis, low-fat diets over a few days may be helpful. A reduced fat intake is in order in obesity, since the bulk of dietary calories is provided by lipids. In general, however, a diet that is restricted in fat is unpalatable, dull, and frequently not followed.

A low-fat diet (20 to 30 gm) would include skim milk, lean meat (not more than 4 ounces), bread, cereals, vegetables, fruit, and 1 teaspoon of butter or margarine; it would exclude desserts, gravies, cheese, nuts, olives, bacon, mayonnaise, and salad dressing except as substituted for butter.

Generous servings of green and yellow vegetables should be given to ensure adequate vitamin A. Water-miscible preparations of vitamins E, K,

D (if not in skim milk), and A (if vegetables suggested are not eaten) should be included in the diet. With the restriction of dietary fat, linoleic acid (an essential fatty acid) may be decreased below optimal levels and may need to be supplemented by use of vegetable oil such as corn oil or vegetable margarine.

Medium-chain triglycerides contain fatty acids with 8 to 10 carbons. They are readily absorbed and transported in the portal system without being totally dependent on the presence of bile acids, pancreatic lipase, reesterification mechanisms, and chylomicron formation with lipoproteins. They are indicated and have been shown to be useful in a variety of disorders individually discussed in Part II. Commercial formulas (Portagen and Pregestimil) are available (Table 29-4). Medium-chain triglyceride (MCT) oil does not have any odor or unusual flavor. It has a negligible osmolality and provides 8.3 kcal/gm. One tablespoon weighs 14 gm and provides 116 calories. The primary purpose of MCT oil is to increase the caloric value while improving the palatability of a low-fat diet. The amount of MCT oil used should be small initially and increased gradually to the desired level or to the patient's tolerance. Unpleasant side effects like nausea, vomiting, diarrhea, abdominal distention, or pain may occur with too high levels of intake or too rapid introduction. MCT oil can be added to skim milk, fruit juices, or strained or pureed baby foods. It can also be used for frying or grilling meats. Moderately low heat should be used because MCT oil has a low smoking point. The fat can also be used in place of vegetable oils in recipes for foods such as pastry, biscuits, mayonaise, cream sauce, salad dressings, butter, cookies, cakes, and muffins.

Resource

Recipes using MCT oil and Portagen are available from Mead Johnson Laboratories (see address on p. 869).

Low-sodium diet

The restriction of dietary sodium is important in patients with ascites and edema caused by severe liver disease.

Sodium must be restricted to less than 500 mg (22 mEq) or 250 mg (11 mEq) to be helpful in the management of ascites. The major food sources of sodium would be altered in the following ways to provide the restricted sodium intake:

	500 mg diet	*250 mg diet*
Vegetables	Salt free	Salt free
Bread	Salt free	Salt free
Butter	Salt free	Salt free
Milk	Regular milk, 2 cups	Low-sodium formulas*
Meat	Salt free, 5 ounces	Salt free, 5 ounces

Salt should not be used on any foods or in their preparation, but some patients may wish to use a salt substitute. However, precaution should be taken not to order a salt substitute when there is need for potassium restriction. Most salt substitutes are made from a potassium base. On the other hand, when diuretics or steroids are used in conjunction with low-sodium diets, it may be desirable to order a salt substitute to supply the patient with extra potassium.

Care should be taken not to use water that has been treated in water-softening equipment with sodium compounds. Patients should be cautioned against unprescribed medications. Some alkalizers, antibiotics, cough medicines, laxatives, pain relievers, and sedatives contain sodium.

Foods high in sodium include tomato juice, brains, kidney, smoked meat such as bacon, bologna, frankfurters, luncheon meats, shellfish, cheese, dry cereals, commercial mixes, commercial desserts, spices with salt, and commercial soups.

These diets may be inadequate in iron and in the B vitamins; these should be supplied by preparations that are sodium free if it is necessary.

*Lonalac, 1.2 mEq of sodium per liter, and S-29 (Ross), 0.4 mEq of sodium per liter.

REFERENCES

Bell, L., Hoffer, H., and Hamilton, J.R.: Recommendations for foods of questionable acceptance for patients with celiac disease, J. Can. Diet. Assoc. **42:**2:143-158, 1981.

Cheng, A.H.R., Brunser, O., Espinoza, J., and others: Long term acceptance of low-lactose milk, Am. J. Clin. Nutr. **32:**1989-1993, 1979.

Murray, C.A.: Appendix: Guidelines for pediatric nutritional therapy. In Suskind, R.M., editor: Textbook of pediatric nutrition, New York, 1981, Raven Press.

Welsh, J.D.: Diet therapy in adult lactose malabsorption: present practices, Am. J. Clin. Nutr. **31:**592–596, 1978.

ENTERAL ALIMENTATION

During the past decade, the ability to provide adequate nutritional support and rehabilitation to patients with acute or chronic diseases has improved substantially. Total parenteral nutrition (TPN) has been established as an effective means of providing nutritional requirements as well as fluid and electrolytes in conditions in which gastrointestinal tract function is severely limited or nonexistent for a period of time. Mechanical, metabolic, and catheter-related septic complications of TPN together with the high cost of materials and solutions require that the gastrointestinal tract be used whenever possible for nutritional support. Oral or tube feeding should always be the first choice. Intravenous feeding should be resorted to when enteral alimentation is impossible or inadequate. Enteral alimentation has the following advantages that have been documented experimentally and clinically:

1. The anatomic and functional integrity of the normal intestine and the compensatory adaptation of the remnant bowel after a resection are strongly influenced by the presence of luminal nutrients.
2. The degree of atrophy obtained in the distal small bowel and in the colon with a monomeric diet without fat is comparable to that obtained when the gastrointestinal tract is "put to rest" with total parenteral nutrition.
3. Continuous feeding permits the administration of large amounts of nutrients and calories that could not be done by bolus feeding through lack of appetite, gastric intolerance, abdominal distention, or diarrhea.
4. Both monomeric and polymeric diets decrease gastric emptying time.
5. Elemental diets modestly decrease gastric and pancreatic secretions. As a result, they may be useful in pancreatitis and in the healing of fistulas.
6. Constituents of both monomeric and polymeric diets are more completely absorbed over a shorter length of bowel.

Composition and properties of diets

A spectrum of liquid diets are now available. At one end of the spectrum, there are monomeric diets consisting of amino acids, simple carbohydrates, and minimal essential fat. Some polymeric formulas that primarily consist of liquid forms derived from normal foods, albeit residue free, are at the other end of the spectrum. Table 29-7 lists the composition of the commercially available formulas that we use for enteral alimentation.

The choice of diets depends on the status of the gastrointestinal tract and on the caloric and nutrient requirements of each individual patient. When an otherwise normal gastrointestinal tract is not accessible, we use regular formulas in infants and polymeric diets such as Ensure or Isocal in older children. Palatability is a common problem when chemically defined diets are used as dietary supplements and taken by mouth. Overnight tube feeding is a means of circumventing this problem while providing large amounts of calories.

In most cases, gastrointestinal tolerance for nutrients is limited and requires slow continuous intragastric feeding over a 24-hour period. Osmolality is a concern because hypertonic solutions slow gastric emptying and initial administration of large volumes invariably lead to crampy pain, abdominal distention, vomiting, and diarrhea. The following guidelines should be followed:

1. Initiate enteral alimentation with a monomeric diet (Vital, Vivonex) at a dilution of 0.5 cal/ml and at an initial rate that will provide two thirds of calculated fluid needs.
2. Increases in volume are better tolerated than increases in concentration (osmolality). Tolerance for full volume should be built up over a few days before the concentration is changed.
3. There are theoretical advantages to peptides and to polymers of glucose in terms of osmolality. Small peptides are absorbed faster than amino acids, whereas the long-chain polymers of glucose have a lower osmolality than an equivalent of carbohydrate provided as glucose.
4. The change from a monomeric to a polymeric diet such as Ensure and Isocal should be done gradually because small-bowel absorptive function is influenced by the composition of the diet.

Technical aspects of enteral alimentation

As acceptance of enteral nutritional support gains popularity, the search continues for a feeding tube that combines ease of insertion and patient comfort. Presently available tubes represent a significant advance in terms of patient acceptance and absence of complications. We currently use small-bore (French 10) silicone rubber tubing. It may be left in place for weeks and usually without adverse effects. A feeding tube–placement stylet or an angiocatheter guide wire may facilitate inser-

Table 29-7. Composition (per liter) of chemically defined diets used for enteral nutrition at Hôpital Sainte-Justine

	Carbohydrates (gm)	Protein (gm)	Fat (gm)	Calories (kcal)	Na (mEq)	K (mEq)	Cl (mEq)	Ca^{++} (mg)	P (mg)	Fe (mg)	Osmolality (per kg)
Ensure	145 Corn syrup, sucrose	37.2 Casein, soy	37.2 Corn oil	1060	32.2	32.5	29.9	500	500	9.4	450
Ensure plus	200 Corn syrup, sucrose	55.0 Casein, soy	53.3 Corn oil	1500	46.1	48.6	44.8	634	634	14.3	600
Isocal	132 Corn syrup	34.3 Casein	44.5 Soy oil, MCT†	1060	23.1	33.8	30.3	600	500	9.5	350
Pregestimil*	91 Corn syrup, glucose, tapioca	19 Hydrolyzed casein	28 Corn oil (60%), MCT (40%)	670	14	18.9	16.6	634	423	12.7	338
Vital	185 Glucose, oligosaccharides, polysaccharides, sucrose	42 Peptides, amino acids	11 Sunflower oil (55%), MCT (45%)	1000	17.0	29.9	18.8	667	667	12	460
Vivonex (unflavored)	226.3 Glucose, oligosaccharides	20.4 Amino acids	1.45 Safflower oil	1000	37.4	29.9	50.8	555	555	10	550

*May be prepared at a caloric density of 0.8 cal/ml.

†Medium-chain triglycerides.

tion in difficult cases, but this proves not to be necessary in older children who can be taught to insert the tubes themselves. Equally well tolerated and less likely to crawl up the esophagus is a silicone rubber feeding tube weighted at its distal end with a short column of elemental mercury (Keofeed FR 7). Gravity infusion is unreliable and risky; a constant infusion pump is necessary.

Indications

The place of enteral alimentation in the care of infants and children with intractable diarrhea and Crohn's disease has been discussed in the sections dealing with these disorders. Any chronic illness with associated anorexia, weight loss and malnutrition, burns, glycogen storage disease, infants with failure to thrive, protracted diarrhea and malnutrition, short bowel syndrome, prematurity, gastrointestinal fistulas, pancreatitis, and cystic fibrosis in need of nutritional rehabilitation are some of the clinical indications.

Need for monitoring and complications

Enteral nutrition requires care by a knowledgeable and experienced team who provide appropriate needs while minimizing side effects and preventing complications, which are listed in the following table:

Complications of enteral alimentation

Tube-related problems
Small-bore tubes often ride up the esophagus and may cause esophageal ulceration
Repeated need for reinsertion into the patient with a chronic cough
Risk of aspiration in LBW infants, comatose children, and patients with neuromuscular disorders
Increased risk of otitis media and sinusitis
Gastrointestinal side effects
Occurrence of cramps, vomiting, and diarrhea if full strength and full volume are given from the start
A regimen whereby one fails to account for gastrointestinal tolerance will lead to ongoing gastrointestinal problems
Metabolic complications
Overhydration and dehydration
Hyperglycemia
Azotemia and high ammonia levels
Inadequate calories
Electrolyte, mineral, and trace-metal deficiencies

Jejunostomy feedings

For the past few years interest has increased in the use of early postoperative nutritional support utilizing the small bowel. More recently adults with unresectable cancer of the upper gastrointestinal tract have benefited from the continuous feeding of chemically defined diets through a serosal-tunnel jejunostomy. Technically it is safe and consists in threading for 10 cm down the lumen of the jejunum a silicone rubber catheter (No. 8 French) after creation of a 5 to 7 cm serosal tunnel. Tolerance for a full strength (1 kcal/ml) formula is generally good, though gastric hypersecretion, cramps, diarrhea, and nausea have been reported, especially if the catheter is inserted too close to the ligament of Treitz.

Experience with this technique is limited in infants and children. It would appear to be mainly indicated in older children with severe neurologic or esophagogastric disorder who have a functioning lower gastrointestinal tract. Since both the gastric and duodenal phases of digestion are bypassed, an elemental diet appears essential. Because at home enteral hyperalimentation is the logical alternative to the intravenous route, a feeding jejunostomy that would be free of complications could represent a significant advantage over the currently used nasogastric or nasoduodenal feeding tubes. Improvement in the composition and in the design of catheters is anxiously awaited because the incidence of catheter-related complications (bowel obstruction or perforation) remains a concern, especially when the catheter is left in place on a permanent basis. Jejunostomy feedings are contraindicated in Crohn's disease and in patients who have had a massive intestinal resection.

REFERENCES

Bounous, G.: Protection of the gastrointestinal mucosa by elemental diets, Clin. Invest. Med. **3**:237-244, 1980.

Bury, K.D., Stephens, R.V., and Randall, H.T.: Use of chemically defined, liquid, elemental diet for nutritional management of fistulas of the alimentary tract, Am. J. Surg. **121**:174-183, 1971.

Chrysomilides, S.A., and Kaminski, M.V.: Home enteral and parenteral nutritional support: a comparison, Am. J. Clin. Nutr. **34**:2271-2275, 1981.

Dworkin, L.D., Levine, G.M., Farber, N.J., and others: Small intestinal mass of the rat is partially determined by indirect effects of luminal nutrition, Gastroenterology **71**:626-630, 1976.

Fairclough, P.D., Hegarty, J.E., Silk, D.B.A., and Clark, M.L.: Comparison of the absorption of two protein hydrolysates and their effects on water and electrolyte movements in the human jejunum, Gut **21**:829-834, 1980.

Greene, H.L., McCabe, D.R., and Merenstein, G.B.: Protracted diarrhea and malnutrition in infancy: changes in intestinal morphology and disaccharidase activities during treatment with intravenous nutrition or elemental diet, J. Pediatr. **87**:695-704, 1975.

Greene, H.L., Helinek, G.L., Folk, C.C., and others: Nasogastric tube feeding at home: a method for adjunctive nutritional support of malnourished patients, Am. J. Clin. Nutr. **34**:1131-1138, 1981.

Jones, B.J.M., Payne, S., and Silk, D.B.A.: Indications for pump-assisted enteral feeding, Lancet **1**:1057-1058, 1980.

Koretz, R.L., and Meyer, J.H.: Elemental diets: facts and fantasies, Gastroenterology **78**:393-410, 1980.

Le Leiko, N.S., Murray, C., and Munro, H.N.: Enteral support of the hospitalized child. In Suskind, M., editor: Textbook of pediatric nutrition, New York, 1981, Raven Press.

Morin, C.L., Ling, V.A., and Bourassa, D.: Small intestinal and colonic changes induced by a chemically defined diet, Dig. Dis. Sci. **25**:123-128, 1980.

Nelson, L.M., Russell, R.I., and Lee, F.D.: Elemental diet composition and the structure and function of rat small intestine: comparison of the effects of two diets on morphology and in vivo absorption of water, JPEN **5**:204-206, 1981.

Ricour, C., Duhamel, J.F., and Nihoul-Fekete, M.: Nutrition entérale à débit constant chez l'enfant, Arch. Fr. Pédiatr. **34**:154-170, 1977.

Topper, W.H.: Enteral feeding methods for compromised neonates and infants. In Lebenthal, E., editor: Textbook of gastroenterology and nutrition in infancy, New York, 1981, Raven Press.

PARENTERAL ALIMENTATION

In a few short years, the therapeutic approach to the severe gastrointestinal disorders associated with intractable diarrhea or with major gastrointestinal surgery in neonates and infants has been revolutionized by the advent of total parenteral nutrition (TPN). Some patients may require long-term out-patient parenteral nutrition. Most children in this group have the short bowel syndrome, Crohn's disease, or chronic intestinal pseudo-obstruction, and require parenteral alimentation for months or even years. Infusions are given during the night so that it's possible for the patients to attend school or work.

Indications

Postoperative surgery. Total parenteral nutrition undoubtedly represents the greatest advance in the postoperative care of neonates, and this is where it is having its widest use. Patients with gastroschisis, ruptured omphalocele, midgut volvulus, and multiple small bowel atresias had a high mortality in years past because of their inability to tolerate enteral feedings of sufficient nutrient value to support life.

Parenteral nutrition can carry the malnourished infant over the immediate postoperative period and the adaptation stage of the remaining small bowel after an extensive resection.

Main indications for total parenteral nutrition

Prematurity
Necrotizing enterocolitis
Intractable diarrhea
Major gastrointestinal surgery
Crohn's disease
Chronic intestinal pseudo-obstruction
Chemotherapy and radiation therapy
Pancreatitis
Burns

The ready availability of TPN as a powerful new tool that can ensure growth and development in the absence of a usable gastrointestinal tract leads to the temptation to say that all patients have a right to a trial of hyperalimentation. This is a dangerous pitfall. It is our opinion that TPN is warranted in the infant who has had resection of most of his small bowel only if it is felt that there are reasonable chances that adaptation of the remaining small bowel will eventually permit complete weaning from parenteral alimentation. The situation with regard to intractable diarrhea is somewhat different. Even though TPN in intractable diarrhea may be required for extended periods (more than 1 year), it is cost effective and warranted because in most cases the disease is self-limited.

Enterocutaneous fistulas. In all age groups, TPN has considerably improved the prognosis of gastrointestinal fistulas. It is no longer imperative that early operation be carried out, and some will heal spontaneously. The volume of gastrointestinal secretions, except for gastric secretions, decrease when patients are maintained on nothing by mouth and are receiving intravenous alimentation. A mixture of amino acids and glucose are effective in this regard. Upper tract fistulas close more rapidly and readily; the lower ones, particularly those involving the distal ileum, are more resistant, though some still close spontaneously with TPN.

Because oral nutrition is needed for normal intestinal mucosal growth, for the maintenance of normal absorptive function, and for optimal adaptation of a small bowel remnant, TPN should be supplemented as rapidly as possible with small amounts of oral feeding.

Intractable diarrhea. The use of TPN in intractable diarrhea of early infancy has led to a dramatic improvement in the outcome. The severe malnutrition associated with this disease probably constitutes an important pathogenic component that TPN neutralizes (p. 220). There is good evidence that "bowel rest" and repair of nutritional deficits lead to improvement in intestinal morphology and function. Our results and those of many others suggest that TPN is truly lifesaving in these infants.

Inflammatory bowel disease. The role of TPN in the treatment of chronic inflammatory bowel diseases is not so clear as in the problems mentioned above. Reports available suggest that malnutrition may be corrected, fistulas may heal, and remissions may be achieved. However, there is no evidence that the natural course of these diseases can be altered by such therapy. In certain instances, improvement of nutritional status and bowel rest can be lifesaving in Crohn's disease unresponsive to the usual medical management. TPN can accelerate the healing of fistulas and induce remissions. It is indicated in the preoperative preparation of a cachexic patient. We have had little experience with TPN in chronic ulcerative colitis; it is believed that a good response is achieved in only a small percentage of cases.

Aims

A complete discussion of various regimens and their rationale, shortcomings, and complications is beyond the scope of this section. The foregoing summarizes our own philosophy and approach.

The aim of parenteral nutrition is to provide, intravenously, adequate fluid, electrolytes, calories, nitrogen, vitamins, and trace elements for the repair of nutritional deficits and for maintenance and growth needs. Parenteral alimentation provides total or partial nutrient requirements but should be used *only* when oral feeding is impossible or inadequate.

Importance of monitoring nutrient needs, intake, and excretions

Within reasonable limits excesses of some nutrients are excreted in the urine or gastrointestinal tract and will not accumulate in the body to reach unacceptable and toxic concentrations. On the other hand, some nutrients such as iron, selenium, manganese, copper, vitamin A, and vitamin D may accumulate or be excreted in excess, as milk calcium is, and lead to complications. Similarly excesses or imbalances in carbohydrates, nitrogen,

and fat should be avoided. The risk of an overabundance of nutrients is unique to parenteral alimentation. It is in essence "force feeding," since it bypasses appetite control, gastrointestinal absorption limits, and other metabolic signals of overloading. Deficiencies and excesses are always iatrogenic. To prevent them requires a thorough understanding and expertise in clinical nutrition.

Nutrient-infusate preparation and composition

The stringent requirements for sterility and physiochemical and biologic compatibility of the solutions require a highly qualified and motivated pharmacy department with proper equipment and facilities. The solution must be formulated so that it meets the complete needs of the patient in terms of calories, nitrogen, fatty acids, vitamins, trace elements, and water. It must also be tailored to the route of administration (central versus peripheral) to minimize complications.

Fluid and nutrient needs. In the neonate, as well as in other age groups, tolerance for fluids and calories has to be built up over a period of several days. Edema, electrolyte disorders, hyperglycemia with glucosuria, and hypertonic dehydration may occur unless the rate of perfusion is gradually increased. If protein intake is increased beyond a certain limit, metabolic acidosis, azotemia, and hyperammonemia will occur. Similarly when lipid infusions are used, impaired clearance of fat will lead to complications if quantities perfused are too large (Table 29-8).

Source of nitrogen. Improvements are continually being made in solutions that provide amino acids. Hydrolyzed proteins have been largely abandoned in favor of crystalline amino acids because the former did not deliver optimal proportions of essential amino acids. Furthermore, they contained significant amounts of dipeptides, which are lost in the urine or else bound to dextrose, thereby contributing to an osmotic diuresis. The amino acid composition, electrolyte content, and the osmolarity of the two amino acid solutions Vamin 7% and Travasol 10% are shown in Table 29-9.

Vamin appears to have theoretical advantages over Travasol in terms of the amount of branchedchain amino acids, glycine content, and lower levels of methionine and cystein. Plasma amino acid patterns in neonates and young infants show that Vamin is better suited to needs, but this does not appear to affect nitrogen balance. An amino

Table 29-8. Recommended fluid and nutrient intake per kilogram of body weight

Age group	Water (ml/kg)	Dextrose (gm/kg)	Amino acids (gm/kg)	Lipid (gm/kg)
Neonates	80-150	7-15	2.5	1-3
Infants and young children	120-200	12-30	2.5-4*	1-3
Children and adolescents	80-150	7-15	1.5-3*	1-3

*An intake above 2.5 gm/kg is indicated only when there is documented increased extraurinary losses of nitrogen.

Table 29-9. Composition of two crystalline amino acid solutions

Individual amino acids expressed in grams per 100 gm of amino acids	Vamin 7%	Travasol 10%	Electrolytes, nitrogen osmolarity, and caloric content per liter	Vamin 7%	Travasol 10%
Essential			*Electrolytes* (mEq/L)		
Isoleucine	5.6	4.8	Na	50	70
Leucine	7.6	6.2	K	20	60
Valine	6.1	4.6	Ca	5	—
Total branched chain	19.3	15.6	Mg	3	10
Phenylalanine	7.8	6.2	Cl	55	70
Methionine	2.7	5.8	PO₄	—	60
Threonine	4.3	4.2	Lactate	—	—
Tryptophan	1.4	1.8	Acetate	—	150
Lysine	5.5	5.8	*Nitrogen* (gm/L)	9.4	16.8
Total (essential)	41.0	39.4	*Osmolarity* (mOsm/L)	710	1300
Semiessential			*Calories*	250	400
Tyrosine	0.7	0.4			
Cysteine/cystine	2.0	—			
Histidine	3.4	4.4			
Nonessential					
Alanine	4.3	20.7			
Arginine	4.7	10.4			
Aspartic acid	5.8	—			
Glutamic acid	12.8	—			
Glycine	3.0	20.7			
Proline	11.5	4.2			
Serine	10.7	—			
Total (nonessential)	52.8	56.0			
Essential amino acids as percentage of total amino acids	41.0%	39.4%			

acid mixture modeled after human milk has not been shown to be appropriate. The eventual addition of taurine to amino acid solutions is being examined.

The pathogenesis of abnormal liver function tests and of cholestasis associated with TPN remains unclear. Experimentally, the total amount of nitrogen rather than its source appears to be a critical factor. Qualitative factors may be important. In clinical studies the incidence of liver problems is much higher in premature babies. It is also increased in infants who have had surgery for intestinal obstruction. Duration of TPN and amounts of amino acids perfused are well-documented fac-

Table 29-10. Composition of fat emulsions (per liter) given intravenously

Emulsion	Triglyceride source		Egg-yolk lecithin (gm)	Glycerol (gm)	Fatty-acid profile (%)					
	Soybean (gm)	Safflower (gm)			Oleic	Linoleic	Linolenic	Palmitic	Stearic	Others
Intralipid 10%*	100	—	12	25	26	50	9	10	2.5	2.5
Liposyn 10%*	—	100	12	25	12.9	77.5	—	6.7	2.7	0.2

*Also available as a 20% solution.

tors influencing the incidence of cholestasis. A prospective controlled study has shown that infants receiving a low protein intake (2.3 gm/kg) developed cholestasis later (47 ± 6 versus 27 ± 4 days) than those on a high protein intake (3.6 gm/kg). However, another report suggests that the severity of the underlying liver disease is influenced by neither the duration of TPN or the amounts of amino acids given.

Glucose. Carbohydrates constitute the main source of energy in patients who are fed by central catheter because the glucose concentration may reach 25%. Glucose tolerance is variable and significantly affected by age maturation of metabolic pathways and capacity to secrete insulin. Although premature babies seldom tolerate more than 8 to 12 gm/kg, with time some babies will be able to manage intakes of 20 to 30 gm/kg. Overfeeding with excessive weight gain is not infrequent and should be avoided. Poor tolerance for carbohydrates is common after major surgery and whenever sepsis occurs. In stressed patients (sepsis, severe injury, catabolic states) the careful addition of insulin may improve glucose tolerance. However, young infants may be exquisitely sensitive to small amounts of exogenous insulin. Administration of high glucose concentrations cannot be abruptly decreased or stopped without risk of hypoglycemia. In the premature and small infant, close monitoring of the delivery system is essential to prevent dramatic drops of blood glucose with its complications and sequelae. Within 1 hour of discontinuing parenteral glucose, clinical signs of hypoglycemia may occur.

Fat. Lipids given intravenously provide a large quantity of energy in a small volume of isotonic fluids and thereby make possible TPN through peripheral veins. The preparations available are metabolized as normal exogenous and endogenous fat and are a source of essential fatty acids. Fats are

not lost in the urine or in the feces. The composition of two commercially available preparations is shown in Table 29-10.

The caloric density of Intralipid 10% is 1100 cal/L at an osmolarity of 280 mOsm/L; the corresponding values for Liposyn 10% is 900 cal/L and 340 mOsm/L. Lipid particles bear a close resemblance to chylomicron-rich lymph and are cleared in a manner comparable to chylomicrons. LBW infants clear fat particles at a slower rate than mature infants and children do. Fat-infusion rates that exceed the patient's capacity to hydrolyze the administered triglycerides is associated with a number of complications such as the following:

Displacement of bilirubin from albumin-binding sites
Accumulation of fat in pulmonary capillaries and alveolar macrophages
Infiltration of Kupffer cells
Diminished chemotaxis and bactericidal activity of phagocytes

Present evidence does not suggest that hepatic dysfunction can be secondary to intravenous fat, but the other well-described complications warrant monitoring of fat tolerance. Nephelometry is semiquantitative. Ideally, daily serum triglycerides should be obtained as the intravenous amounts of lipids are being increased, and weekly monitoring is sufficient thereafter.

Although many teams administer lipids through a central catheter, we prefer not to when peripheral veins are easily accessible. Essential fatty acid deficiency can be prevented by the peripheral perfusion of a lipid emulsion once or twice weekly in a dose of 2 to 4 gm/kg. In circumstances when a peripheral vein is not accessible, the lipid emulsion is given through the central catheter. Peripherally fed patients are given fat intravenously on a continuous basis through a Y connector (see discussion on peripheral alimentation).

Table 29-11. Recommended intake of electrolytes and minerals*

	Infants and children (per kg)	Adolescents and adults
Sodium (mmol)†	2-5	75
Potassium (mmol)	2-5	50
Chloride (mmol)	2-5	75
Calcium (mmol)	0.5-2	14
Phosphorus (mmol)	0.5-2	12.5
Magnesium (mmol)	0.05-0.5	10

*These represent the usual maintenance requirements. The range for maintenance and high requirements per kilogram of body weight are given for infants and children.

†mmol = $\dfrac{mEq}{Valence}$; the valence of Na, K, and Cl is 1, whereas that of Ca and Mg is 2.

There is still discussion about the optimal proportions of fat to carbohydrate. A number of comparisons of the nitrogen-sparing effects of intravenously given fat and glucose have been made. In hypercatabolic states a more favorable effect on nitrogen balance can be obtained when nonprotein energy is administered in the form of glucose. As much as 83% of nonprotein energy can come from fat and lead to nitrogen balances that are comparable to those achieved with glucose alone after an initial period of stabilization. In most patients, provided that nitrogen intake is adequate, whether most of the nonprotein energy comes from glucose or from fat probably makes little difference. Fatty livers were commonly the result of essential fatty acid deficiency when a weekly infusion of plasma was the only source of fat.

Electrolytes and minerals. Requirements for electrolytes (Na^+, K^+, Cl^-) vary considerably with the underlying clinical conditions (Table 29-11). Infants with short bowel syndrome, secretory diarrhea, and so on, often have large extrarenal losses, which need to be carefully documented in order to compensate for these ongoing but often variable losses. For example, we see infants with intractable diarrhea requiring up to 12.5 mEq/kg/day of sodium. Maintenance requirements for calcium, phosphorus, and magnesium have not been completely worked out. This explains the wide range of recommendations in Table 29-11. Acute hypocalcemia may lead to tetany, rickets or osteoporosis, a reported complication of TPN when administered on a long-term basis. Hypercalcemia and hypercalciuria (more than 4 mg/kg) need to be contended with also, since nephrolithiasis is a serious problem. It may present early as hematu-

ria. Monitoring of intake, excretion, and serum levels of calcium is essential. Hypophosphatemia is a well-described risk in TPN; it is usually tied to inadequate intakes of phosphorus and vitamin D. Hypophosphatemia leads to depletion of erythrocyte 2,3-diphosphoglycerate as well as phagocyte dysfunction. Magnesium is the fourth most plentiful cation in the body; it is particularly important as a cofactor in enzyme reactions involving ATP. The utilization of high-energy phosphate groups is crucial during protein synthesis and emphasizes the importance of magnesium during periods of anabolism. Serum levels are useful, but urine levels give a better and earlier indication of depletion. Skeletal pain and muscle cramps are prominent symptoms. Magnesium depletion is well described in patients with Crohn's disease or with an ileostomy (Table 29-11).

Trace elements (Table 29-12)

Zinc. Zinc deficiency is associated with growth retardation, impaired wound healing, depressed cellular immunity, skin lesions, and diarrhea. Since the Recommended Daily Dietary Allowance for zinc in adults is 15 mg/day and 20% of ingested zinc is absorbed, 3 mg should be supplied in total parenteral nutrition solutions daily. Appropriate supplementation of TPN solutions with zinc reduces the energy cost of growth and may improve the gain of lean body mass. Requirements in the pediatric age group are high because most infants and children requiring TPN have low stores, are in a catabolic state, or have ongoing large losses of zinc through the gastrointestinal tract. Zinc deficiency may present as severe diarrhea, as in the case of acrodermatitis enteropathica. Clinical zinc deficiency may occur during zinc-supplemented parenteral nutrition. We currently administer 500

Table 29-12. Estimated requirements for trace elements

Trace element	Premature infants (µg/kg)	Infants and children (µg/kg)	Adults (mg)
Zinc	400	100-500	2.5-4
Copper	50	20	0.5-1.5
Chromium	0.3	0.14-0.2	0.01-0.04
Manganese	10	2-10	0.15-0.8
Iodine	8	8	0.2
Selenium	4	4	0.3
Fluorine	57	57	0.9

µg/kg for the first 3 days of TPN; the dosage is then dropped to 300 µg/kg for a period of 3 weeks followed by 100 µg/kg as daily maintenance. In patients who have severe diarrhea, enterocutaneous fistulas, or ileostomies, monitoring of zinc losses is useful. It is reported that 12.2 mg of zinc may be lost in each liter of small-bowel fluid: the figure is 17.1 mg/L of stool or ileostomy output. If oral intake is possible, zinc sulfate tablets providing 50 mg of elemental zinc can be used.

Copper. Copper deficiency may manifest itself by anemia, leukopenia, and neutropenia. Several cases of TPN-induced copper deficiency have been reported. In children copper deficiency may present as osteoporosis. Abnormal collagen metabolism and ascorbic acid metabolism are probably implicated. All children on TPN should receive copper supplementation; an exception are those infants and children with underlying liver disease or with TPN-induced abnormal liver function. The recommended dosage at the moment is 20 µg/kg with a maximum of 400 µg/day in an adult.

Manganese. The nutritional importance of manganese in mammals has been recognized for many years. Clotting and bone defects have been reported in deficiency states. Because manganese is known to potentiate the hepatotoxic potential of certain chemicals, it is best not to add manganese to solutions destined for patients with liver abnormalities. The recommended amount is 10 µg/kg/day.

Chromium. The dominant clinical feature of chromium deficiency developing during TPN administration is glucose intolerance. It is especially likely to occur in long-term or home TPN. The recommended daily intravenous intake in adults is 10 to 20 µg: the corresponding dosage in children is 0.14 to 0.2 µg/kg.

Selenium. Laboratory evidence of selenium deficiency has been demonstrated in adults on intravenous nutrition. Severe muscle pain and a cardiomyopathy (Keshan disease) similar to that seen in certain selenium-deficient areas of China have been described. Selenium has an important role as an antioxidant and may protect cell membranes through prevention of lipid peroxidation. Therefore its action is quite similar to that of vitamin E. Guidelines for essential trace-element preparations for parenteral use by the American Medical Association recommend 100 µg daily in adults.

Fluoride and iodine. Little data are available, and therefore requirements on TPN are unknown. The solution of trace elements currently in use contains 50 µg/ml of fluoride and 5 µg/ml of iodine. The suggested dosage is 1 ml/kg, up to a maximum of 20 ml per day.

As pointed out recently, the need for added trace elements has become greater with sophistication of TPN, with its increased use and duration, and in particular with the introduction of synthetic amino acid solutions.

Although there are commercial sources of trace elements available, the pharmacy department prepares its own. Iron requirements are estimated at 130 µg/kg in premature babies and in infants and at 65 µg/kg in children and adults. It can be added to the TPN solution in the form of iron dextran properly suspended in benzyl alcohol and water. Some prefer to administer iron dextran intramuscularly every 3 weeks; the recommended dosage is 2 mg/kg. The dosage is increased to 6 mg/kg if iron deficiency is documented.

Vitamins. A multivitamin preparation is added routinely to total parenteral nutrient infusates, but the amounts provided are often arbitrary and not based on studies taking into consideration the number of variables affecting needs (Table 29-13). The composition of MVI-12 shown in Table 29-

Table 29-13. Vitamins that can be added to the nutrient infusate and estimated needs*

Vitamin	Composition of vitamin preparation		Recommended amounts of each vitamin		
	MVI-1000 (per 10 ml)	MVI-12 (per 5 ml)	<10 kg (per kg/day)	10-35 kg (daily)	>35 kg (daily)
		Vial 1			
Vitamin C (mg)	1000	100	5	80	45
Vitamin A (IU)	10000	3300	227	2000-3000	5000
Vitamin D (IU)	1000	200	55	400	400
Thiamine (mg)	45	3.0	0.05	1.2	1.0-1.5
Riboflavin (mg)	10	3.6	0.07	1.4	1.1-1.8
Pyridoxine (mg)	12	4.0	0.04	1.0	1.6-2.0
Niacinamide (mg)	100	40.0	0.8	17	12-20
Pantothenic (mg)	26	15.0	1.0	5	5-10
Vitamin E (IU)	10	10	0.6	7-10	12-15
		Vial 2			
Folic acid (μg)	—	400	50	500	400
Vitamin B_{12} (μg)	—	5.0	0.5	5	3
Biotin (μg)	—	60	2-60	20-150	150-300

Prepared with the help of Dr. Andrée M. Weber and Mr. Marjolain Pineault.
*Vitamin K_1 (0.1 mg for children weighing less than 10 kg and 0.2 mg for the other weight groups) is necessary, but it has to be administered separately, since some MVI vitamins cannot be mixed with vitamin K_1.

Table 29-14. Suggested amounts of MVI-1000 and MVI-12 vials 1 and 2

Weight groups	MVI-1000	MVI-12	
		Vial 2	Vial 1
3-10 kg	0.4 ml/kg	0.5 ml/kg	—
10-35 kg	4 ml	5 ml	—
>35 kg	—	5 ml	5 ml

13 supplies all vitamins except vitamin K, which has to be added separately.

Discrepancies between the amounts of vitamins added to infusates and the quantities delivered to the patient have been reported for vitamins A, D, and E. As much as two thirds of vitamin A and one third of both vitamins D and E have been said to adhere to the container and to the intravenous dressing sets and possibly to microfilters. On the other hand 50% of vitamin A can be decomposed by sunlight in 3 hours. The recommendation for 250 IU of vitamin D in LBW infants may have to be revised. Extensive degradation of thiamine has been recorded in the presence of sodium bisulfite.

The formulation of (MVI-12), which is commonly used, is not ideal because the relationship between the concentrations of the 12 vitamins does not correspond to estimated needs. Compromises

can be made, but we prefer to continue using MVI-1000 along with the new preparations MVI-12 vials 1 and 2. Table 29-14 may be useful.

Parenteral nutrition by peripheral veins

The importance of TPN for the acutely and chronically ill infants and children with compromised nutrition because of anatomic or functional disorders of the gastrointestinal tract or with signs of starvation is incontestable. However, TPN is associated with a significant complication rate because a central venous catheter is required for the infusion of a hypertonic glucose solution. Peripheral TPN is an attractive alternative, which has been advocated since the early 1970s. The advantages of this technique in terms of safety and convenience are considerable. Furthermore long-term TPN is feasible through this route if appropriate infusion admixtures are carefully formulated and the team is proficient in the techniques of intravenous infusion and attentive to the importance of close monitoring.

Indications. Although the peripheral route is still being underused, misuse can also be a problem. There is a risk of "hypoalimenting hyperalimentation patients." In one series 37% of peripherally fed neonates and infants lost weight as opposed to 17.5% of those centrally fed. Therefore, if malnutrition and catabolism are not severe and only a small catch-up or brief maintenance is needed, the peripheral vein approach is indicated. The central venous route is preferred when long-term therapy (more than 2 to 3 weeks) can be anticipated and nutritional rehabilitation is required for a moderate to severe degree of malnutrition. Other indications include a repeated history of septic episodes or previously thrombosed central catheters. The most common indication is in LBW infants and in those infants and children who need parenteral supplementation to gastrointestinal nutrition.

Nutrient infusate. The advent of safe lipid emulsions for intravenous use was necessary to make peripheral TPN a realistic approach. Fat not only prevents essential fatty acid deficiency but also constitutes an important source of calories (30% to 50%) and decreases the incidence of thrombophlebitis by keeping the osmolarity of the infusate below 850 mOsm/kg. Because the fat emulsion breaks down when mixed with electrolytes in dextrose and amino acid solutions, it is administered from a separate bottle and reaches the mainline through a Y connector. For the same reason, vitamins, trace elements, and minerals are added to the dextrose–amino acid mixture.

Because concentrations of glucose (10%) and of amino acids (2.5%) should be kept low to protect the vein from phlebitis and tolerance for fat seldom exceeds 3 gm/kg/day, greater fluid intakes are required. It is difficult to deliver more than 70 cal/kg for infants and 40 cal/kg for adolescents while the osmolarity of the infusate is kept around 600 mOsm/L.

Table 29-15 is helpful in calculating osmolarity and caloric density of total parenteral nutrient infusates. We find that close monitoring of these two parameters is particularly important to prolong the "life" of a peripheral vein and to ensure that adequate calories are delivered to the patient.

To the two peripheral vein regimens described

Table 29-15. Osmolarity and caloric density of TPN components

	Osmolarity (mOsm/gm)	Calories (per gm)
Dextrose	5	3.4
Travasol 10%	13	4
Vamin 7%	10	3.6
Intralipid 10%	2.8	11

Table 29-16. Suggested peripheral vein regimens for infants

Component	Quantities/kg/24 hr	
Water	150 ml	200 ml
Travasol 10%	2.5 gm	3.0 gm
Intralipid 10%	2 gm	3 gm
Dextrose	10 gm	15 gm
Calories provided	66	96
Osmolarity of infusate* (mOsm/L)	587	612

*If electrolytes are added to the amino acid solution, the osmolarity will be higher but must never exceed 850 mOsm/L.

in Table 29-16, appropriate supplementation with minerals is necessary and corresponds to the needs previously discussed. Addition of multivitamins and of trace elements is also required if parenteral nutrition is being carried out for a period of more than a few days and if the gastrointestinal tract is being totally bypassed.

Guidelines for administration and monitoring. All aseptic precautions must be observed, and the area over the vessel must be properly prepared before insertion of the butterfly needle or the cannula. The insertion site must be inspected every 8 hours and the dressing changed every 24 hours after a povidone-iodine solution is sprayed on. As a general principle, larger veins have a longer duration of usage than the smaller ones because of high-flow dilution. Although some advocate rotating the insertion site every 48 hours, we believe that a peripheral cannula can be kept in place sometimes for a period of 1 week without evidence of local inflammation. To control adequately the flow rates of both the dextroamino acid mixture and the lipid solution, which are administered through the Y connector, infusion pumps are necessary.

Parenteral nutrition by central catheters

Despite significant advances in the composition, design, insertion techniques, and long-term care of central catheters, several problems relate to their long-term use. Catheter-related complications listed by Heird are as follows:

Disorders related to catheter site
  Arrythmia associated with atrial positioning
  Pneumothorax
  Hemothorax
Disorders related to use of catheter
  Sepsis
  Thrombosis
  Catheter dislodgment or separation
  Perforation of vein with infusion leaks

Although a large study has recently shown that the per diem complication rate of peripheral versus central vein alimentation does not differ, the incidence in the former was only 9% versus 20% for the latter. Furthermore, the most serious complications associated with peripheral vein alimentation was soft-tissue slough (6.7%).

Over the past few years we have exclusively used the Broviac catheters, since the pediatric size has an inner diameter of 0.12 mm whereas the regular size has 0.20 mm. The standard technique involves insertion of the catheter into the external jugular vein through a subcutaneous tunnel starting on the anterior chest wall. Lately we have had good success with threading the catheter into the superior vena cava just above the right atrium through the cephalic, basilic, or axillary veins. Less frequently the catheter is slipped into the inferior vena cava through a small cut down on the femoral vein with the tip of the catheter lying below the origin of the renal veins. The aseptic technique described by Ament and the UCLA group is closely followed. We do not use the transcutaneous subclavian approach.

We have totally dispensed with in-line filters and use a closed plastic bag system for the infusate. Twice-weekly cleansing of the catheter-insertion site followed by a change in tubing and the addition of heparin to the daily infusate (250 units/kg of body weight) appear to have a favorable effect on decreasing the incidence of sepsis and thrombosis. All patients who become febrile during the course of central venous alimentation are carefully examined and cultured. If cellulitis is present at the catheter insertion site or the patient appears toxic, antibiotics given intravenously are immediately started. Catheter removal is carried out if sepsis is documented. In rare instances, when total dependence on TPN exists and no remaining insertion sites are available, we elect to leave the catheter in while treating the patient with aggressive antibiotic therapy, a procedure that sometimes can save the lifeline.

REFERENCES

Adibi, S.A.: Roles of branched-chain amino acids in metabolic regulation, J. Lab. Clin. Med. **95:**475-484, 1980.

Aguirre, A., Fischer, J.E., and Welch, C.E.: The role of surgery and hyperalimentation in therapy of gastrointestinal-cutaneous fistulae, Ann. Surg. **180:**393-401, 1974.

Anderson, B.H., Patel, D.G., and Jeejeebhoy, K.N.: Design and evaluation by nitrogen balance and blood aminograms of an amino acid mixture for total parenteral nutrition of adults with gastrointestinal disease, J. Clin. Invest. **53:**904-912, 1974.

Andrew, G., Chan, G., and Schiff, D.: Lipid metabolism in the neonate. II. The effect of intralipid on bilirubin binding in vitro and in vivo, J. Pediatr. **88:**279-284, 1976.

Benner, J.W., Coran, A.G., Weintraub, W.H., and others: The importance of different calorie source in the intravenous nutrition of infants and children, Surgery **86:**429-433, 1979.

Boeckman, C.R., and Krill, C.E.: Bacterial and fungal infections complicating parenteral alimentation in infants and children, J. Pediatr. Surg. **5:**117-126, 1970.

Bürger, U., Fritsch, U., Bauer, M., and Peltner, H.U.: Comparison of two amino acid mixtures for total parenteral nutrition of premature infants receiving assisted ventilation, JPEN **4:**290-293, 1980.

Cobb, L.M., Cartmill, A.M., and Gilsdorf, R.B.: Early post operative nutritional support using the serosal tunnel jejunostomy, JPEN **5:**397-401, 1981.

Curry, C.R., and Quie, P.G.: Fungal septicemia in patients receiving parenteral hyperalimentation, N. Engl. J. Med. **285:**1221-1224, 1971.

Dahms, B.B., and Halpin, T.C.: Serial liver biopsies in parenteral nutrition-associated cholestasis of early infancy, Gastroenterology **81:**136-144, 1981.

Filler, R.M., and Coran, A.G.: Total parenteral nutrition in infants and children: central and peripheral approaches, Surg. Clin. North Am. **56:**395-412, 1976.

Filler, R.M., Takada, Y., Carreras, T., and Heim, T.: Serum intralipid levels in neonates during parenteral nutrition: the relation to gestational age, J. Pediatr. Surg. **15:**405-410, 1980.

Filler, R.M., Eraklis, A.J., Rubin, V.G., and Das, J.B.: Long-term total parenteral nutrition of infants, N. Engl. J. Med. **281:**589-594, 1969.

Fisher, G.W., Wilson, S.R., Hunter, K.W., and Mease, A.D.: Diminished bacterial defences with Intralipid, Lancet **2:**819-820, 1980.

Forget, P.P., Fernandes, J., and Begemann, P.H.: Utilization of fat emulsion during total parenteral nutrition in children, Acta Paediatr. Scand. **64:** 377-384, 1974.

Fox, H.A., and Krasna, I.H.: Total intravenous nutrition by peripheral vein in neonatal surgical patients, Pediatrics **52:**14-20, 1973.

Greene, H.L., Hambidge, M., and Herman, Y.F.: Trace elements and vitamins. In Bode, H.H., and Warshaw, J.B., editors: Parenteral nutrition in infancy and childhood, New York, 1974, Plenum Publishing Corp., p. 131.

Greene, H.L., Hazlett, D., and Demaree, R.: Relationship between Intralipid-induced hyperlipemia and pulmonary function, Am. J. Clin. Nutr. **29:**127-135, 1976.

Guidelines for essential trace element preparations for parenteral use: a statement by the Nutrition Advisory Group, AMA, J.A.M.A. **241:**2051-2054, 1979.

Hartline, J.V., and Zachman, R.D.: Vitamin A delivery in total parenteral nutrition solution, Pediatrics **58:**448-451, 1976.

Heird, W.C.: Parenteral nutrition. In Lebenthal, E., editor: Textbook of gastroenterology and nutrition in infancy, New York, 1981, Raven Press.

Heird, W.C., and Winters, R.W.: Total parenteral nutrition: the state of the art, J. Pediatr. **86:**2-16,1975.

Jeejeebhoy, K.N., Anderson, G.H., Nakhooda, A.F., and others: Metabolic studies in total parenteral nutrition with lipid in man, J. Clin. Invest. **57:**125-136, 1976.

Keating, J.P., and Teinberg, J.L.: Amino acid–hypertonic glucose treatment for intractable diarrhea in infants, Am. J. Dis. Child. **122:**226-228, 1971.

Kishi, H., Yamaji, A., Kataoka, K., and others: Vitamin A and E requirements during total parenteral nutrition, JPEN **5:**420-423, 1981.

Koop, C.E.: Recent advances in postoperative management of newborn infants, Progr. Pediatr. Surg. **2:**15-28, 1971.

Lloyd-Still, J.D., Schwachman, H., and Filler, R.M.: Protracted diarrhea of infancy treated by intravenous alimentation. I. Clinical studies of 16 infants, Am. J. Dis. Child. **125:**358-364, 1973.

McClain, C.J.: Trace metal abnormalities in adults during hyperalimentation, JPEN **5:**424-429, 1981.

Patel, D., Anderson, G.H., and Jeejeebhoy, K.N.: Amino acid adequacy of parenteral casein hydrolysate and oral cottage cheese in patients with gastrointestinal disease as measured by nitrogen balance and blood aminogram, Gastroenterology **65:**427-437, 1973.

Pollack, P.F., Kadden, M., Byrne, W.J., and others: 100 patient years' experience with the Broviac Silastic catheter for central venous nutrition, JPEN **5:**32-36, 1981.

Postuma, R., and Trevenen, C.L.: Liver disease in infants receiving total parenteral nutrition, Pediatrics **63:**110-115, 1979.

Puri, P., Cuiney, E.J., and O'Donnell, B.: Total parenteral feeding in infants using peripheral veins, Arch. Dis. Child. **50:**133-136, 1975.

Reimer, S.L., Michener, W.M., and Steiger, E.: Nutritional support of the critically ill child, Pediatr. Clin. North Am. **27:**647-660, 1980.

Ryan, J.A., Abel, R.M., Abbott, W.M., and others: Catheter complications in total parenteral nutrition, N. Engl. J. Med. **290:**757-760, 1974.

Shwachman, H., Lloyd-Still, J.D., Khaw, K.T., and Antonowicz, I.: Protracted diarrhea of infancy treated by intravenous alimentation. II. Studies of small intestinal biopsy results, Am. J. Dis. Child. **125:**365-368, 1973.

Sondheimer, J.M., Bryan, H., Andrews, W., and Forstner, G.G.: Cholestatic tendencies in prematures on and off parenteral nutrition, Pediatrics **62:**984-989, 1978.

Strobel, C.T., Byrne, W.J., and Ament, M.E.: Home parenteral nutrition in children with Crohn disease: an effective management alternative, Gastroenterology **77:**272-279, 1979.

Vileisis, R.A., Inwood, R.J., and Hunt, C.E.: Prospective controlled study of parenteral nutrition-associated jaundice: effect of protein intake, J. Pediatr. **96:**893-897, 1980.

Vogel, C.M., Cowin, T.R., and Baue, A.E.: Intravenous hyperalimentation in the treatment of inflammatory diseases of the bowel, Arch. Surg. **108:**460-467, 1974.

Wan, K.K., and Tsallas, G.: Dilute iron dextran formulation for addition to parenteral nutrient solution, Am. J. Hosp. Pharmacy **37:**206-210, 1980.

Weinfield, J., Wilen, S., Yabek, S., and Rodriguez-Torres, R.: Total parenteral hyperalimentation: infants with chronic intractable diarrhea, N.Y. State J. Med. **73:**265-270, 1973.

Wretlind, A.: Development of fat emulsions, JPEN **5:**230-235, 1981.

Ziegler, M., Jakobowski, D., Hoelzer, D., and others: Route of pediatric parenteral nutrition: proposed criteria revision, J. Pediatr. Surg. **15:**472-476, 1980.

Zohrab, W.J., McHattie, J.D., and Jeejeebhoy, K. N.: Total parenteral alimentation with lipid, Gastroenterology **64:**583-592, 1973.

30

JOHN D. BURRINGTON, M.D.*

Pediatric ostomy care and appliances

As more infants survive with complex gastrointestinal and urologic anomalies, the number of children requiring temporary or permanent ostomy appliances is increasing. Medical technology has kept pace, and there is now available a wide variety of appliances, adhesives, and equipment for care of an ileostomy, a colostomy, or an ileal bladder. With the help of an interested physician or enterostomal therapist, every infant or child with an ostomy can be fitted with an appliance that will keep his skin clean, dry, and odor free and will not be visible through his clothes. Although the small stomas on abdomens covered with sensitive skin create special care problems, it is still possible, with proper attention and advice, for most children with ostomies to lead normal lives and enjoy normal activities. Children with ostomies must be seen more often than adults because their rapid growth and varying activities and needs require frequent changes in the appliance. They also need continuing support in adjusting to the special problems of adapting to an ostomy.

The physical and psychologic adjustments to an ostomy can be as monumental for the child as for the adult. Many anticipated difficulties can be avoided if sufficient discussion time with the involved parties precedes the creation of the ostomy. The child (whenever applicable), parents, family physician, surgeon and enterostomal therapist all need to be involved in meaningful discussion. At times, seeing another child who has (or had) an ostomy and talking to his or her parents can be very helpful in alleviating fears and fantasies regarding this problem. This can frequently be arranged through the nearest ostomy society.

ANATOMIC SURGICAL CONSIDERATIONS

Preoperative planning of incisions and stomas must take into consideration the type of appliance

to be worn, the size and shape of the faceplate, the exact level of the belt line, and the possibility of other existing anomalies that might require creation of multiple ostomies.

Necrotizing enterocolitis, idiopathic bowel perforation, imperforate anus, and Hirschsprung's disease are the most common indications for creation of an ostomy in the neonate. Placement of the stoma on such a tiny abdomen (sometimes on infants weighing 1000 gm or less) requires careful planning of both incision and drain sites. To allow adequate surfaces for attachment of the appliance in this age group, the flat area of the abdomen lateral to the navel is an ideal position for placing a temporary stoma.

In the older child requiring a permanent stoma (ulcerative colitis, Crohn's disease, malignant polyposis), the site chosen is usually below the belt line and sufficiently medial to the iliac crest to allow proper appliance fit. Again, a preoperative fitting with the appliance to be utilized is a valuable maneuver. A permanent ostomy must always be a single-end stoma. It should be perfectly round and protrude from the skin 1 cm or less, should not prolapse, and should be placed at least 5 cm from any bony prominence, the navel, or an irregular surgical scar.

After creation of the stoma, the temporary appliance should be carefully tailored and applied before the patient leaves the operating room. Benzoin should be applied to clean dry skin. When this has dried sufficiently to be tacky, a square of skin barrier such as Stomahesive, Hollihesive, or karaya, is cut with a central hole that fits the stoma snugly. A Hollister Karayseal bag or a similar pouch is then carefully applied. The edges of the appliance can then be taped securely with paper tape. A belt is eventually attached to the rings of the appliance.

The surgeon must take time in the operating room to get a tight, secure fit. Nothing is more demoralizing to a child or adolescent to have the appliance work loose on the second or third day and soak him with foul stool.

*Staff Surgeon, Children's Hospital, Denver, Colorado.

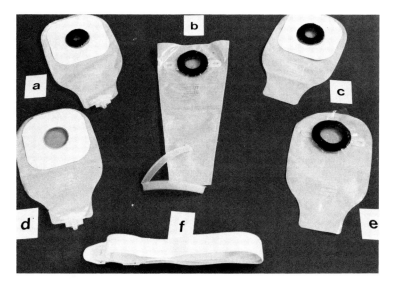

Fig. 30-1. Representative selection of "temporary" ostomy appliances. *a* and *c* (Hollister) combine the sealing properties of a karaya ring with a self-adhering adhesive edge that holds the bag in place. *a* is designed for urinary diversion and *c* for a colostomy. *b* and *e* use karaya rings for a good seal but require a belt, *f,* to support the appliance, since karaya gum is not an adhesive. The urinary bag, *d,* uses only the adhesive edge to obtain a watertight fit. These temporary appliances are suitable only for the immediate postoperative period or in patients with very limited activity.

CHANGING OF APPLIANCE (CHILDREN 10 TO 12 YEARS OF AGE)

Although older children can learn to care for their stomas, the first appliance change should be done by the physician or enterostomal therapist in the presence of one or both parents. This first change needs to be done with great facility and kindness, since it will greatly influence subsequent attitudes. Slowly softening the leading edge of adhesive with the proper solvent while gently working the skin down from the appliance is proper technique. Once the old appliance is removed, the stoma should be plugged with an absorbent cotton ball, a plug of folded toilet tissue, or a tampon. The skin is gently cleansed with water, and when dry, it is usually fitted with a square of a skin barrier cut with a central hole that fits the stoma snugly. A Hollister bag with a karaya ring is then placed over the stoma. If a bag is chosen that has an adhesive square (Fig. 30-1, *A*), the edges should be reinforced with paper tape. We much prefer the appliance with "wings" for attaching a belt (Fig. 30-1, *B*). This permits most of the weight of the bag to be supported by the belt rather than the adhesive. If the stoma is irregular, one can mold the karaya ring to conform by wetting the

index finger and slowly stretching the ring until it provides a snug fit.

The first stools after a major abdominal procedure may be large, loose, and foul, requiring frequent appliance changes to prevent the device from suddenly being pulled loose and tearing the skin.

Elective appliance changes are best done soon after the patient arises, when the bowel is least active. After several changes, the patient and parents should be allowed to attempt a complete change under supervision to prepare them for later responsibilities. Usually, complete responsibility for ostomy care can be taken by children over the age of 10.

MATERIALS

A variety of appliance systems utilizing different adhesive systems are available. Each type has specific advantages that will be familiar to most surgeons and enterostomal therapists.

A representative selection of temporary appliances available in the Hollister line is seen in Fig. 30-1. These rings utilize karaya paste as the adhesive, which is capable of forming a tight seal, even over a very irregular surface. However, since

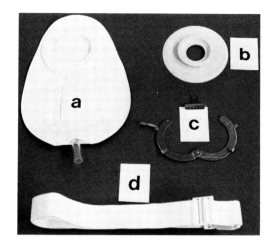

Fig. 30-2. The components of a typical "permanent" appliance (United Surgical System). The rubber disk, *b,* is attached to the skin with any of a variety of adhesives. The appliance, *a,* of light-weight plastic is then placed carefully over the flange on the ring, *b.* The metal collar, *c,* is then closed tightly over the flange of bag, *a,* holding it tightly to the rubber disk or face plate.

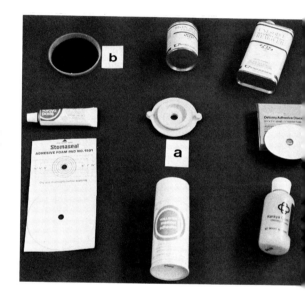

Fig. 30-3. Some adhesive systems available. The rubber face plate, *a,* may be attached to the skin using Skin-Bond cement, Colly-Seel *(b),* and a variety of rubber cements. Unisolve will remove all adhesives except Hollister medical adhesive.

Table 30-1. Comparison of temporary and permanent ostomy systems

	Advantages	Disadvantages
Temporary or disposable	1. Can be tailored to irregular stoma 2. May help heal temporary skin problem 3. Easily disposable when traveling 4. Some types worn without belt 5. Quicker to apply and easier to use 6. Less odor	1. Expensive for long-term use 2. May get skin breakdown from adhesives 3. Karaya ring and Colly-Seels last only 24 to 36 hours 4. Must have additional water-proof tape for swimming
Permanent or reusable	1. More economical once the stoma has stabilized 2. Stays on longer (5 to 10 days)	1. Faceplate cannot be altered 2. Requires more time (40 minutes at first) and privacy to change 3. Most require belt 4. Requires several appliance sets to allow for cleaning 5. Cannot be fitted until 4 to 6 weeks after surgery 6. Generally more difficult to assemble

this material is quite water soluble, it is not very suitable for ileal bladders of ileostomies. All appliances using a karaya gum ring must be supported by a belt, since their adhesive quality is not so good as their sealant property.

Stomahesive has an adhesive back that adheres very well to dry skin, and it is not water soluble. Therefore, we recommend putting the Stomahesive between the skin and the karaya ring.

Components of a typical "permanent" appliance are seen in Fig. 30-2 and are represented by The United Surgical System. Other systems, such as Davol and Marlen, are similar and satisfactory. In these permanent systems, the faceplate is left in place until it begins to loosen, and only the bags are changed on a daily basis. Between changes, one can empty the bag by opening the clamped end.

A sample of the variety of adhesive systems and solvents that are available is shown in Fig. 30-3. An enterostomal therapist, physician, or ostomy society can advise about the unique features of every system. A comparison between the temporary and permanent ostomy ststem is shown in Table 30-1. A list of suppliers of ostomy materials follows:

Hollister, Inc.
211 East Chicago Ave.
Chicago, IL 60611
(312) 642-2000

Marlen Manufacturing & Development Co.
5150 Richmand Rd.
Bedford, OH 44146
(216) 292-7060

Mason Laboratories, Inc. (Colly-Seels)
P.O. Box 194
Willow Grove, PA 19090

Osteolite Co., Inc.
842 E. 18th Ave.
Denver, CO 80218
(303) 861-0256

Perry Products
3803 East Lake St.
Minneapolis, MN 55406
(612) 722-4783

United Surgical
Largo, FL 33540

GENERAL MEDICAL CARE

Occult bleeding from the stoma is common, and the child will generally require a supplemental iron preparation.

Careful attention to fluid intake and output is mandatory, especially in the small infant and in all those patients with ileostomies. Under basal conditions fluid requirements are normally higher in ostomy patients, and therefore episodes of gastroenteritis need to be promptly brought to the physician's attention. Profound, rapid losses of fluids, electrolytes, and bicarbonate can quickly lead to dehydration and acidosis.

Abdominal distention, failure to pass stool for longer than 6 to 12 hours, and sudden onset of diarrhea all suggest obstruction and require prompt attention. Routine abdominal roentgenograms, contrast studies, and surgery may become necessary. Small stomal prolapse (less than 1 to 2 inches) that occurs postprandially may be acceptable if quickly reduced with return of normal color. A problem stoma with chronic prolapse will need revision.

Diet restrictions should be few. Ingestion of large amounts of cold liquids should be avoided, especially in ileostomy patients, since they increase peristalsis. Complete chewing of food is also important in this patient group, since larger, bulkier bits of unchewed food also increase peristalsis and ileostomy drainage. A lactose-free diet may be needed in those conditions associated with secondary lactase deficiency (necrotizing enterocolitis, gastroschisis, postviral enteritis).

An emergency kit or travel kit should be available when the patient plans to be away from home for an extended period. This can be kept in the car or carried in a handbag or small travel case. Facial tissues, premoistened towelettes, spare disposable appliances and bags, cotton balls, and tampons are useful items. Emergency situations may require the use of Lomotil to control the ostomy secretion.

One can treat areas of skin breakdown under the adhesive by dusting with a product such as karaya powder and applying the adhesive directly over them. Corticosteroid spray may also be helpful in reducing the inflammation. Heal-skin, Skinprep spray, Stomahesive, and Reliaseal are all useful in this problem. The last two products are of water-barrier design. If stool can be kept off the raw area for 3 or 4 days, it will most often heal completely.

Two aspirin tablets added to the clean plastic appliance before application will help reduce the odor of the contained stool as effectively as other commercial products such Banish or Ostobon.

The older child with a permanent ostomy should be encouraged to participate in any athletic program appropriate for his size, strength, and abilities. The appliance needs to be emptied before participation and anchored with either a broad-belted athletic supporter, tight elastic panties, or a girdle. A ''pocket'' made of cotton jersey to fit the appliance will prevent the patient from sweating excessively where the plastic rests against the skin. These pockets can be washed as often as necessary.

Prolonged contact between an understanding physician and the child with an ostomy is essential. The support, help, and encouragement of the physician will be called on in many areas for the duration of their association. He will often have to serve as friend, physician, and therapist to his patient with an ostomy and not infrequently as a marriage counselor for the parents.

REFERENCES

Bolinger, B.L.: The adolescent patient. In Broadwell, D.C., and Jackson, B.S., editors: Principles of ostomy care, St. Louis, 1982, The C.V. Mosby Co.

Jeter, K.F.: The pediatric patient: ostomy surgery in growing children. In Broadwell, D.C., and Jackson, B.S., editors: Principles of ostomy care, St. Louis, 1982, The C.V. Mosby Co.

31 *Selected laboratory tests*

BROMSULPHALEIN (BSP) TEST

The Bromsulphalein (sulfobromophthalein) test has been used as a test of liver function for many years. This test is reliable in all patients after 2 to 3 weeks of age when the hepatic clearing capacity for BSP is completely mature. Bromsulphalein is an anionic halogenated phthalein dye that is bound to plasma protein after intravenous injection and is carried to the liver. Within 45 minutes about 95% of the dye is removed from the bloodstream by the liver and excreted into the bile. The remainder is eliminated in the urine (2%) or taken up by muscle tissue. In the liver, BSP is conjugated to glutathione before biliary excretion. BSP is excreted in the urine as a conjugate of glutamic acid, glycine, and cystine and as free dye. This clearing ability of the hepatic cells and the excretion of the dye into the biliary system form the basis on which the BSP test is determined.

Procedure

1. BSP, 5 mg/kg as a 5% solution, is injected intravenously while the patient is fasting.
2. A blood sample is drawn 45 minutes later from a site other than that where the injection was made.
3. The amount of dye remaining in the blood specimen is determined colorimetrically. (Some laboratories use a spectrophotometer and read the results at 580 nm if the patient has hyperbilirubinemia as well as for routine use.)

A two-phase BSP clearance can be done by obtainment of serial samples at 5, 15, 25, 35, and 45 minutes. Plotting these values on semilogarithmic paper gives one both the clearing capacity (K_1 index) and the percent retention at 45 minutes (K_2) (Fig. 31-1). This application of the BSP clearance test permits separation of those conditions with primarily hepatocellular injury, from those with relatively intact hepatic uptake and transport function but abnormal excretory capacity (Fig. 31-2). In some countries the two-phase BSP clearance is utilized in the work-up of the neonatal cholestatic syndrome. The technetium-labeled radionuclide scans have been similarly applied in recent years.

Precautions

Because BSP is extremely irritating to body tissues, great care must be exercised not to inject the dye subcutaneously.

As a general rule, the BSP test is not useful in a patient who is jaundiced.

BSP should not be given within less than 1 week after cholecystography. Iodine and other related halogens may bind the hepatocyte-uptake sites, interfere with BSP transport, and thereby give incorrect retention readings (false-positive results), as barbiturates may when taken within 24 hours of the test.

Results

Most commonly the results of the BSP test are expressed as a percentage of retention at 45 minutes:

1. Newborn infants—up to 15%.
2. Older babies and adults—less than 5%.
3. In patients without jaundice with the following diseases or disorders, abnormal retention of BSP (above 5%) is present:
   a. Cirrhosis
   b. Hepatitis
   c. Biliary tract obstruction
   d. Ascites, portal hypertension
   e. Metastatic lesions of liver
   f. Dubin-Johnson and Rotor syndromes

Interpretation

BSP retention is most useful in following the subsequent course of the patient with hepatitis after jaundice has disappeared. A normal BSP test is helpful in that it implies normal healing of the hepatitis, without residual liver disease. Unless both the early clearance (K_1) and late retention (K_2) values are used, this test is of limited value in differentiating most causes of cholestatic jaundice.

False-negative values may result from an incorrect dosage or from measuring BSP retention in patients with hypoproteinemia.

The results of the BSP retention test can be interpreted in the light of decreased uptake of the dye, as in hepatocellular disease or in heart failure

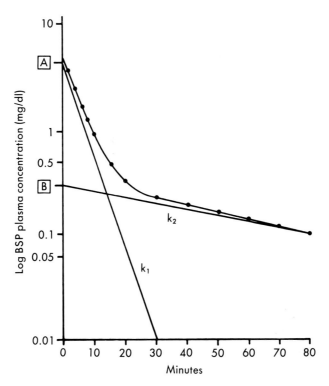

Fig. 31-1. Normal plasma clearance of BSP (Bromsulphalein). Semilogarithmic representation of the remaining plasma BSP at various times after injection shows a double exponential disappearance curve. The K_1 portion of the curve reflects the integrity of the hepatocytes to remove the dye from the plasma. K_2 portion of the curve is primarily dependent on biliary secretion or excretion, or both, after dye removal from the plasma.

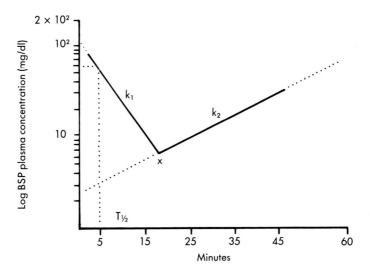

Fig. 31-2. BSP-disappearance curve in a 20-day-old infant with surgical diagnosis of biliary atresia. The K_1 slope is normal. The upward defection of the K_2 portion of the curve is attributable to regurgitation of the excess dye back into the circulation, a consequence of impaired biliary exretion. (From Licastro, R., Neto, V.F., and Rua, E.C.: Argent. Gastroenterol. (São Paulo) **13**:273-277, 1976.)

with a decreased hepatic blood flow. Retention may occur because of impaired conjugation, as in the premature or newborn infant, and lastly because of interference with the transport of BSP out of the hepatic cell or the bile canaliculi. The latter is seen in pediatric patients with bile duct atresia or other forms of obstruction and is rarely caused by Dubin-Johnson or Rotor's syndrome.

REFERENCES

Bianchi, A., and Baker, P.R.: Plasma clearance of Bromsulphalein (BSP) in children with biliary atresia aad other hepatobiliary disorders. World J. Surg., 1981. (Submitted for publication.)

Grausz, H., and Schmid, R.: Reciprocal relation between plasma albumin level and hepatic sulfobromophthalein removal, N. Engl. J. Med. **284:**1403-1406, 1971.

Javitt, N.B.: Clinical and experimental aspects of sulfobromophthalein and related compounds. In Popper, H., and Shaffner, F., editors: Progress in liver disease, vol. 3, New York, 1970, Grune & Stratton, Inc.

Licastro, R., Neto, U.F., and Rua, E.C.: Hepatic sulfobromophthalein clearance in children, Arq. Gastroenterol. **13:**273-277, 1976.

Quarfordt, S.H., Hilderman, H.L., Valle, D., and Waddell, E.: Compartmental analysis of sulfobromophthalein transport in normal patients and patients with hepatic dysfunction, Gastroenterology **60:**246-255, 1971.

SERUM BILE ACIDS

In health, the bulk of the bile acid pool resides either in the gallbladder or in the intestinal lumen. Only small amounts are found normally in portal blood, the hepatocyte, or the peripheral circulation. Bile acid uptake by the liver and secretion by the bile canalicular membrane therefore represent an extremely sensitive and efficient function of the liver.

Liver disease and serum bile acids

In hepatobiliary disease, the levels of bile acids present in the peripheral circulation are greatly augmented. The ratio of trihydroxy to dihydroxy bile acids, which corresponds essentially to that of cholic acid to chenodeoxycholic acid, has been used to assess both the type and the severity of the underlying liver disease. A fall in the ratio is presumably indicative of increasing connective-tissue deposition, decreased functional parenchyma, and increasing necrosis. Our experience with the cholic to chenodeoxycholic acid ratio in differentiating biliary atresia from prolonged neonatal intraheptic cholestasis (neonatal hepatitis) has not been satisfactory. However, a drop in the ratio has been useful in that it is indicative of advanced liver cirrhosis.

Lithocholic acid is a nonpolar bile acid. It can be synthesized by the immature liver through an accessory pathway, but after the first few months of life it is the product of the microbial degradation of chenodeoxycholic acid in the gastrointestinal tract. We and others have shown that lithocholate is hepatotoxic and cholestatic and that conjugation with glycine and taurine does not decrease its toxic potential. Lithocholate has been implicated in the initiation and perpetuation of cholestatic liver disease. Furthermore, in various forms of liver disease, elevated levels of lithocholic are reported. Sulfation has been recognized as an important detoxification pathway for nonpolar bile acids such as lithocholic acid. Of note, however, is our recent observation that sulfated glycolithocholate remains hepatotoxic as opposed to sulfated taurolithocholate. With hepatobiliary disease there are also significant increases in the formation of primary bile acid (cholic and chenodeoxycholic) sulfates. Sulfated bile acids are readily cleared from the serum by the kidney and lost in the stools because they are not reabsorbed.

Radioimmunoassay

Although progress has been slow in establishing the measurement of serum bile acids as a routine liver function test, a breakthrough in methodology recently occurred when bile acid radioimmunoassay became available. The currently marketed glycoconjugate and sulfoglycolithocholate radioimmunoassays by Abbott Laboratories (North Chicago), though lacking specificity, are sensitive, easily performed, and require only small amounts (100 μl) of blood. They have proved to be extremely effective means of assessing the health and disease status of the hepatobiliary system. They are more sensitive indicators of liver dysfunction than the standard liver function tests. The diagnostic value of serum bile acids can be increased in anicteric, biochemically silent forms of liver disease when 90-minute postprandial measurements are taken. Postprandial determinations has also been used to provide an estimate of ileal function.

Results of bile acid radioimmunoassay determinations in infants and children

Our own experience suggests that there is a temporary phase of "physiologic" cholestasis

Table 31-1. Sulfated lithocholate levels in neonatal cholestatic syndromes

	Number of subjects	Sulfated lithocholate (μmoles/L)
Third day of life	52	0.3 ± 0.03
Neonatal cholestasis		
Biliary atresia	19	4.1 ± 0.7
Neonatal hepatitis	23	5.0 ± 0.7
Miscellaneous	8	4.4 ± 1.0
Associated with total parenteral nutrition	13	4.0 ± 1.0

Adapted from Balistreri, W.F., and others: J. Pediatr. **98:**399, 1981.

during the first few weeks of life. The average value ($\overline{X} = 2.05$ μmoles/L) of glycocholate in normal neonates corresponds to the upper limit of normal in other age groups, whereas levels in hyperbilirubinemic ($\overline{X} = 13.4$ mg/dl) LBW newborns were higher ($\overline{X} = 4.72$ μmoles/L). In a group of 55 LBW newborns undergoing phototherapy, there was a very close correlation between the elevation of glycocholate and that of direct-reacting bilirubin but none whatsoever with total bilirubin. A recent report shows that sulfated lithocholate is an excellent marker for neonatal hepatobiliary disease (Table 31-1).

In children and adolescents with cholestatic liver disease there is a semilogarithmic correlation between glycoconjugated bile acids and bilirubin. In practice this means that the glycoconjugate is a much more sensitive index of cholestasis and may be increased ten- to twentyfold before icterus becomes clinically manifest. Discrepancies between bilirubin and glycoconjugate levels are particularly striking in infants and children with paucity of intrahepatic bile ducts (Alagille's and nonsyndromic type). In such cases bilirubin levels may be less than 2 mg/dl, with levels of glycoconjugates in excess of 100 times the normal values.

In patients with chronic liver disease who have no evidence of cholestasis, fasting glycoconjugate levels may pick up a few cases in which other tests are normal, but our experience suggests that postprandial values are more helpful. This latter determination has been particularly useful in the clinically and biologically silent type of liver disease associated with cystic fibrosis. A recent survey of 119 children with cystic fibrosis and normal liver function tests reveals that a third had

fasting or postprandial levels of glycocholate above the upper limit of normal (2.15 μmoles/L in our lab).

REFERENCES

Balistreri, W.F., Suchy, F.J., Farrell, M.K., and Heubi, J.E.: Pathologic versus physiologic cholestasis: elevated serum concentration of a secondary bile acid in the presence of hepatobiliary disease, J. Pediatr. **98:**399-402, 1981.

Davidson, G.P., Corey, M., Morad-Hassel, F., and others: Immunoassay of serum conjugates of cholic acid in cystic fibrosis, J. Clin. Pathol. **33:**390-394, 1980.

Lloyd-Still, J.D., and Demers, L.M.: Serum glycine conjugated bile acids in pediatric hepatobiliary disorders, Am. J. Clin. Pathol. **71:**444-451, 1979.

Roy, C.C., Weber, A.M., Morin, C.L., and others: Hepatobiliary disease in cystic fibrosis: a survey of current issues and concepts, Pediatric Gastroenterology and Nutrition. (In press.)

Samuelson, K., Aly, A., Johanson, C., and Norman, A.: Evaluation of fasting serum bile acid concentration in patients with liver and gastrointestinal disorders, Scand. J. Gastroenterol. **16:**225-234, 1981.

Simmonds, W.J., Korman, M.G., Go, V.L.W., and Hofmann, A.F.: Radioimmunoassay of conjugated bile acids in serum, Gastroenterology **65:**705-711, 1973.

FECAL CHYMOTRYPSIN

The procedure associated with pancreatic drainage is difficult to perform, time consuming, and uncomfortable for the patient. It is therefore hardly suitable as a routine screening test in the investigation of malabsorption. Fecal chymotrypsin determination is advocated as a reliable test of exocrine pancreatic insufficiency and can be applied to the same 72-hour stool collection used for quantitating fecal fat.

Fecal chymotrypsin is a more sensitive index of pancreatic function than trypsin, and, in pediatric patients, studies have pointed out the reliability of fecal chymotrypsin in the diagnosis of the pancreatic insufficiency of cystic fibrosis. Chymotrypsin stability is undoubtedly influenced by motility, bacterial flora, bile, and other factors that lead to varying degrees of binding to mucosal cells and intestinal debris. Despite these objections, which make it, at best, a semiquantitative assessment of pancreatic enzyme secretion, fecal chymotrypsin in milligrams per 72 hours per kilogram provides excellent discrimination between cases of pancreatic and nonpancreatic steatorrhea.

Procedure

The enzyme activity is measured titrimetrically with a pH stat. automatic titrator and the synthetic substrate *N*-acetyl-L-tyrosine ethyl ether (ATEE) or an ultraviolet spectrophotometric method. The acid by-products of the esterolytic activity of chymotrypsin are neutralized by sodium hydroxide, which keeps the pH constant and permits the reaction to continue at this pH. The recorder gives a plot of microliters of titrating solution versus time in seconds. The slope of the line corresponds to the rate of the reaction, which in turn is dependent on enzyme concentration. The technique used in our laboratory is that of Dyck (1967).

Patients are maintained on a normal diet. Use of pancreatic extracts and antibiotics is discontinued at least 5 days before the study is begun. Stools are collected for 72 hours between two nonabsorbable markers, such as charcoal. The specimens are frozen as soon as possible after they are passed, and are pooled in a preweighed paint can. Each determination is carried out in duplicate, and results are expressed in milligrams of chymotrypsin per 72 hours per kilogram of body weight.

Results

Fecal chymotrypsin values expressed in milligrams per kilogram of body weight per 72 hours are as follows:

	Number	Mean ± 1 SD
Cystic fibrosis with steatorrhea	58	0.42 ± 0.37
Nonpancreatic steatorrhea	57	15.3 ± 7.4
Controls	35	6.6 ± 3.9

Interpretation

From these data, it appears that in patients who are suspected of having cystic fibrosis, but who have a normal sweat test, this indirect method of assessing pancreatic exocrine function can be of diagnostic importance. If the chymotrypsin fecal values are low, pancreatic exocrine deficiency is present. Chymotrypsin secretion is depressed earlier and more severely than trypsin and appears to be a more sensitive index of pancreatic exocrine insufficiency than trypsin. Statistically, the overwhelming number of patients with pancreatic exocrine deficiency have cystic fibrosis. It is interesting to note that in children with nonpancreatic steatorrhea, fecal chymotrypsin values are somewhat higher than those in control subjects with fat malabsorption. This is probably related to an increased transit time that decreases the percentage of chymotrypsin being degraded in the lumen.

REFERENCES

Barbero, G.J., Sibinga, M.S., Marino, J.M., and Seibel, R.: Stool trypsin and chymotrypsin, Am. J. Dis. Child. **112:**536-540, 1966.

Bonin, A., Roy, C.C., LaSalle, R., and others: Fecal chymotrypsin: a reliable index of exocrine pancreatic function in children, J. Pediatr. **83:**594-600, 1973.

Dyck, W.P.: Titrimetric measurements of fecal trypsin and chymotrypsin in cystic fibrosis patients with pancreatic exocrine insufficiency, Am. J. Dig. Dis. **12:**310-317, 1967.

TEST FOR SUGARS IN FECES

Patients with deficiencies of intestinal mucosal disaccharidases, the so-called sugar-splitting enzymes, are unable to hydrolyze dietary disaccharides into their respective component monosaccharides. The dietary disaccharides have the following monosaccharide components: lactose is glucose and galactose; sucrose is glucose and fructose; and maltose is glucose and glucose (Table 9-1). If the disaccharides are not absorbed, they pass into the distal ileum and colon, where they are fermented and split by intestinal bacteria into hydrogen and short-chain volatile acids in quantities sufficient to lower the fecal pH to 5.5 or less. An osmotically induced diarrhea also occurs. The sugars are passed in the stools, where most can be detected as reducing substances. The absence of reducing substances in the stools, however, does not rule out the diagnosis of disaccharide intolerance. Sucrose is not a reducing substance and requires special modification in the test for detection. The presence of lactose and maltose can easily be detected by the Clinitest method.

Indications

The test for sugars in the stool is a simple procedure and is indicated in any patient with chronic diarrhea or whenever a child is slow to recover after a diarrheal episode.

Procedure

No special preparation of the patient is necessary, and the test utilizing the Clinitest tablet can be performed in the office, on the wards, or in the laboratory. The stool should be collected in a plastic-lined diaper rather than on an absorbent diaper. Finger-cot specimens or only fresh stool specimens free of urine should be checked for both pH and for the presence of sugars. The clinitest-tablet technique compares very well with chromatography in allowing evaluation of the presence of reducing sugars. Paper chromatography can be useful in determining which type of sugar is present in the stool and should point to the offending sugar. This sugar can then be removed from the diet in a more rational manner.

Technique (with Clinitest tablets)*

1. Place a small amount of liquid stool in a test tube.
2. Dilute it with twice its volume of water.
3. Place 15 drops of this suspension together with a Clinitest tablet in a second test tube.
4. Compare the resulting color with the chart provided for urine testing.

Results

0.25% or less	Negative
0.25% to 0.5%	Suspect
0.5% or more	Abnormal

The test should preferably be carried out as soon as possible after collection, or the stools should be frozen for later testing. If the stool is left at room temperature, bacterial fermentation may diminish the sugar content and lead to falsely low results.

Sucrose is not a reducing sugar, and the test requires the use of 1N hydrochloric acid instead of water, followed by brief boiling.

Sugar detectors specific only for glucose should not be used.

Interpretation

If the results with a Clinitest tablet indicate 0.5% of reducing substances or more (over 1+) in the stool along with an acid pH, a presumptive diagnosis of a carbohydrate intolerance may be made. The most common offending disaccharide is lactose. Further support for the diagnosis can be obtained by a breath test or a disaccharide absorption test. Additional confirmation can be obtained by the disaccharidase analysis of jejunal mucosa obtained by peroral biopsy. Since mucosal enzyme analysis is a time-consuming procedure, it is not indicated in all patients. Some patients with sucrose and isomaltose intolerance may pass enough glucose and fructose in their stools to give a positive Clinitest reaction, possibly as the result of the hydrolysis of sucrose by intestinal bacteria.

Determination of the stool pH and testing for reducing substances can be used as a clinical guide

*Ames Company, Elkhart, Ind.

before the removal of the suspect disaccharide from the diet. As the patient responds to its withdrawal from the diet, the stool pH approaches neutral reaction and the Clinitest result becomes negative (0.25% or less).

REFERENCES

Burke, V., Kerry, K.R., and Anderson, C.R.: Relationship of dietary lactose to refractory diarrhea in infancy, Aust. Paediatr. J. **1:**147-160, 1965.

Krawitt, E.L., and Beeken, W.L.: Limitations of the usefulness of the D-xylose absorption test, Am. J. Clin. Pathol. **63:**261-263, 1975.

Soeparto, P., Stobo, E.A., and Walker-Smith, J.A.: Role of chemical examination of the stool in diagnosis of sugar malabsorption in children, Arch. Dis. Child. **47:**56-61, 1972.

Sunshine, P., and Kretchmer, N.: Studies of small intestine during development: infantile diarrhea associated with intolerance to disaccharides, Pediatrics **34:**38-50, 1964.

TEST FOR DIGESTION AND ABSORPTION
D-Xylose test

D-Xylose, a pentose, is minimally altered by the body after absorption in the upper small bowel. After absorption, xylose enters the systemic circulation through the portal vein and liver and is then excreted in the urine. Apparently the intestinal lacteals and the lymphatic system are not involved in the transport process.

Xylose is primarily absorbed by passive diffusion in the duodenojejunal segment. The amount absorbed, therefore, is dependent on an intact mucosal surface and the absence of diarrhea. Disease processes that alter or compromise the mucosa of the upper small bowel result in decreased absorption and excretion of xylose. Also, a delay in gastric emptying time is a major reason for falsely low serum and urine levels of xylose. Urine excretion values are unreliable in patients with kidney disease and generally in infants and children less than 6 years of age. Since xylose absorption is not dependent on bile salts, pancreatic exocrine secretions, or intestinal mucosal disaccharidases, serum and urine excretion values are normal in malabsorptive disorders other than those associated with mucosal disease. However, the test may have limited usefulness in cases of small intestinal bacterial overgrowth, viral gastroenteritis, and giardiasis.

Indications

The D-xylose test is useful in evaluating the integrity of the upper intestinal mucosa in the following clinical entities:

1. Celiac disease—gluten-sensitive enteropathy
2. Idiopathic steatorrhea
3. Regional enteritis involving the upper small bowel
4. Starvation
5. Short bowel syndrome
6. Blind loop syndrome
7. Milk protein sensitivity

The D-xylose test is a useful means of following the progress of the patient with gluten-sensitive enteropathy. With clinical improvement and restoration of the normal mucosa while the patient is on a gluten-free diet, the serum and urine values of xylose approach and ultimately reach normal levels.

Contraindications

There are no contraindications to the use of the D-xylose test.

Method

After an 8-hour fast, D-xylose is given as a 10% solution at a dose of 14.5 gm/m^2 of body surface (maximal amount 25 gm). Close adherence to this protocol is critical. It is strongly recommended that the test and blood determinations be carried out by the same technician on both in-patients and ambulatory children.

The method for determining D-xylose is that of Roe and Rice with some modification as suggested by Lanzkowsky. When pentoses are heated in acid solution, furfurol is formed and reacts with aniline to yield a colored compound.

Studies have shown that a 1-hour serum-xylose test is a reliable indicator of malabsorption in patients with untreated celiac disease. The test results are reported in children under 30 kg of body weight, or roughly under 8 years of age. The standard test dose of 5 gm of D-xylose is given orally, and the serum xylose is measured exactly 1 hour later. In patients without celiac disease, the 1-hour serum xylose level was above 30 mg/dl. Levels under 30 mg/dl were found in patients with celiac disease. This simplifies the xylose test as a screening procedure. Falsely low levels may result if the patient has not been fasted, has vomited some of the test dose, or has diarrhea. If the results of 25 mg/dl or less are confirmed on a repeat study, a small bowel biopsy is warranted to establish the diagnosis of celiac disease.

Results of serum D-xylose test

The rise in the blood xylose level during the first hour is a reliable index of small bowel func-

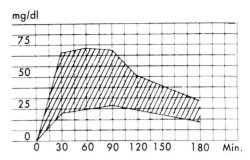

Fig. 31-3. Serum xylose absorption levels. The serum xylose is plotted on the vertical axis and time in minutes on horizontal axis. *Cross-hatched area,* Range of normal absorption at 30-minute intervals. For practical purposes, serum xylose determination at generally 60 minutes provides satisfactory information. A serum D-xylose of 25 mg/dl is considered normal. (Courtesy A. Bonin, biochemist, Hôpital Sainte-Justine, Montreal.)

tion. A normal response is usually associated with a serum level exceeding 25 mg/dl. A more detailed analysis of curves obtained appears in Fig. 31-3.

REFERENCES

Buts, J.P., Morin, C.L., Roy, C.C., and others: One-hour blood xylose test: a reliable index of small bowel function, J. Pediatr. **90:**729-733, 1978.

Christie, D.L.: Use of the one-hour blood xylose test as an indicator of small bowel mucosal disease, J. Pediatr. **92:**725-728, 1978.

Rolles, C.J., Kendall, M.J., Nutter, S., and Anderson, C.M.: One-hour xylose screening test for coeliac disease in infants and young children, Lancet **2:**1043-1045, 1973.

Disaccharide absorption tests

The true incidence of disaccharide intolerance is unknown. Estimates of lactose intolerance, by far the most common statistically, vary according to color, age, and the diagnostic criteria employed.

Estimates of lactase deficiency have been placed at 10% of the white population in the United States with a European ancestry. There is a higher estimated frequency of lactase deficiency in the black population, but the incidence varies widely in different parts of the world. In children, it has been noted that a higher percentage of black children have clinical evidence of milk intolerance. One third of the black children and one tenth of the white children had abnormal lactose absorption curves in a recent study.

Many people are aware of milk intolerance and

report variations in their tolerance to milk. These variations may range from a half glass to as much as a quart. In some patients a glass of milk on one day may be tolerated well, whereas the same amount on another day may result in abdominal distention, flatulence, cramping, and a few watery stools, without any apparent illness associated with the latter response. Studies have been reported in an attempt to assess the threshold level of lactose for symptom production. About 75% of subjects with assay-confirmed lactase deficiency had symptoms with 8 ounces of milk (equivalent to 12 gm of lactose). In addition to increased transit time, colonic fermentation in which volatile fatty acids are formed, an increase in small bowel fluid, and an increase in sodium content all may play a role in producing the symptoms noted in lactase-deficient patients.

Because of these observations, a useful approach is to increase milk intake gradually over several days, carefully recording any symptoms. This procedure may offer a useful diagnostic clue in the patient with recurrent watery diarrhea, recurrent abdominal pain, or the irritable colon syndrome.

Most children with proved milk intolerance have symptoms. The idea that, in adults, lactose intolerance may be secondary to the failure of development of the "adult" lactase enzyme has never been documented. Similarly, there are no data in humans suggesting that lactase decreases on discontinuation of milk or is substrate inducible. It is said that if a sufficient amount of lactose is given, all adults can be shown to have a relative degree of lactase deficiency. Hydrolysis of lactose has been shown to be the rate-limiting step for the intestinal absorption of glucose and galactose given as lactose.

Dietary disaccharides are hydrolyzed into monosaccharides by the specific disaccharidases in the brush border of the upper intestinal mucosa. With a deficiency or absence of the sugar-splitting enzymes, the disaccharides remain in the lumen, lesser amounts of the component monosaccharides are absorbed, and lower serum levels of glucose are found after a loading dose. However it is important to note that up to 30% of healthy subjects with normal lactose activities may have a flat tolerance test after a lactose load. Consequently it is best to use symptoms, acid stools, and excretion of carbohydrates after ingestion of the suspected disaccharides.

Procedure

Oral loads of the disaccharide are given to the patient, and serial serum glucose levels are determined. The following procedures apply to tolerance tests for lactose, sucrose, and maltose, except that the dose for maltose is half the standard dose.

The patient ingests nothing for 8 hours before the test. A fasting serum glucose sample is obtained. The suspected disaccharide is given in the dose of 2 gm/kg as a 10% solution. For maltose, the dose is 1 gm/kg.

Serum glucose is measured at 30, 60, 90, and 120 minutes after the loading dose is given.

A careful record should be kept of the number and character of the stools, the stool pH, and the results of a Clinitest determination for reducing substances on all stools passed during the test and for 8 hours after the test is completed.

Precautions

Because of the danger of shock caused by osmotic water loss into the lumen of the gut, disaccharide absorption tests should be carried out under close supervision, especially in young infants.

Interpretation

In the normal person, the serum glucose level rises more than 30 mg/dl over the fasting level within the test period and usually within 30 minutes if the disaccharide has been instilled intraduodenally. The increase in serum glucose in patients with disaccharide intolerance is usually less than 20 mg/dl. The results graphically shown in Fig. 31-4 were obtained from a patient with lactose intolerance. Lactase deficiency was confirmed in this patient by a jejunal mucosal enzyme assay.

It should be noted in the graph that when lactose was given, the maximum increase in serum glucose was less than 20 mg/dl on two separate tests, and the curve was relatively flat on both occasions. But when a solution of glucose and galactose, the hydrolytic products of lactose, was given in a proportionate dose, the serum glucose curve had a sharp peak and a maximum rise of more than 30 mg/dl. A sucrose tolerance test in the same patient paralleled the findings for glucose-galactose. For routine purposes, a D-xylose absorption test should be ordered to confirm the patient's ability to absorb a monosaccharide. When a maltose-tolerance test was done, a striking increase of serum glucose (more than 70 mg/dl) was

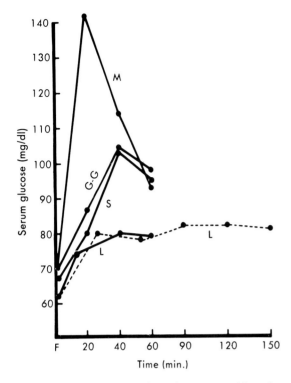

Fig. 31-4. Disaccharide absorption curves. Note the flattened serum glucose curves after ingestion of lactose, *L*, on two separate tests, indicating poor absorption. Normal absorption curves for glucose-galactose, *G-G*, sucrose, *S*, and maltose, *M*, are depicted. This patient has lactose intolerance and lactase deficiency. *F*, Fasting.

also noted. There is a sharp rise in glucose levels after maltose ingestion because hydrolysis of maltose yields two molecules of glucose. These findings then confirm the presence of lactose intolerance and the normal absorption of sucrose and maltose.

Although the study described demonstrates the results in a patient with lactose intolerance, the methods and the results can be used as prototypes for the study of other disaccharides.

Factors other than intestinal disaccharidase that may influence the results of the test are the following: (1) Delayed gastric emptying time. This is a common source of falsely low serum glucose levels. In children who have no symptoms after administration of the disaccharide and have flat serum glucose curves, the absorption test should be repeated after intraduodenal instillation of the disaccharide solution. (2) Rapid peripheral uptake of glucose. A flat curve may also be related to rapid peripheral uptake of absorbed glucose. The

use of capillary instead of venous blood for analysis largely eliminates this problem, since capillary glucose peak levels are higher than venous levels.

An abnormal result of disaccharide absorption test does not distinguish between a primary and a secondary disaccharidase deficiency. A D-xylose or a glucose absorption test should be done as a test of mucosal integrity of the small bowel. When glucose-galactose malabsorption is suspected, 1 gm/ kg of glucose and 1 gm/kg of galactose are given. A flat serum glucose curve indicates malabsorption and should then be followed by a fructose absorption test.

A peak rise in serum glucose of more than 20 mg/dl can occasionally be found in some individuals with clinical and enzymatic evidence of disaccharidase deficiency, whereas some healthy patients may show a flat blood glucose curve after an oral disaccharide tolerance test. A recent report shows that there is a poor correlation between clinical evidence of lactose intolerance, disaccharidase activity and lactose tolerance tests.

REFERENCES

Akesode, F., Lifshitz, F., and Hoffman, K.M.: Transient monosaccharide intolerance in a newborn infant, Pediatrics **51**:891-896, 1973.

Ament, M.E.: Malabsorption syndromes in infancy and childhood, J. Pediatr. **81**:685-697, 867-884, 1972.

Gilat, T., Benaroya, Y., Gelman-Malachi, E., and Adam, A.: Genetics of primary adult lactase deficiency, Gastroenterology **64**:562-568, 1973.

Gracey, M., and Burke, V.: Sugar-induced diarrhea in children, Arch. Dis. Child. **48**:331-336, 1973.

Gray, G.M.: Carbohydrate digestion and absorption, Gastroenterology **58**:96-107, 1970.

Gray, G.M.: Carbohydrate digestion and absorption, N. Engl. J. Med. **292**:1225-1230, 1975.

Harrison, M., and Walker-Smith, J.A.: Reinvestigation of lactose intolerant children: lack of correlation between continuing lactose intolerance and small intestinal morphology disaccharidase activity and lactose tolerance tests, Gut **18**:48-52, 1977.

Simoons, F.J.: New light on ethnic differences in adult lactose intolerance, Am. J. Dig. Dis. **18**:595-611, 1973.

BREATH TESTS IN GASTROINTESTINAL DISORDERS

Pediatric application of the new technique of breath tests to the evaluation of gastrointestinal disease has only recently been reported. Improvement in the technical features of collecting expired air in infants and children, coupled with the availability of stable isotopes, particularly ^{13}C, are largely responsible for this event. In years past, ^{14}C-labeled products had been widely utilized, being incorporated into such substrates as carbohydrates, triglycerides, amino acids, bile acids, and various drugs. The radioactivity of these labeled products has been relatively low (5 μCi), but the long biologic half-life of ^{14}C has always been of concern especially in children. The application of a stable isotope obviates this undesirable aspect but unfortunately requires a much greater degree of sophisticated methodology, including access to a mass spectrometer. Breath-hydrogen analysis is most commonly employed.

The principle utilized in breath-test analysis simply applies what has been known to physiologists for many years; that is, that the end products of many digestive metabolic functions are carbon dioxide and to a certain extent hydrogen, which are gases transported by the bloodstream and eliminated from the body by the lungs. Hydrogen gas is normally present in expired alveolar air in very low concentrations. However, in the face of carbohydrate malabsorption, the unabsorbed moiety is delivered to the colon where it undergoes bacterial fermentation. The hydrogen produced by this fermentation process is then absorbed down a concentration gradient into the blood and eliminated through the lungs to be collected and then quantitated in the expired air by gas liquid chromatography. The major virtue of this test over standard absorption tests is that the product measured is a direct reflection of nonabsorption of the substrate in question, rather than a measurement of a degradation product after absorption, vis-à-vis serial blood glucose levels. In patients with carbohydrate malabsorption, breath hydrogen–excretion rates are two to eight times greater than normal after ingestion of the offending substrate.

Since carbon dioxide is normally present in higher concentrations in expired air, specially labeled substrates are needed to detect abnormal gastrointestinal function. Many such products are available for a variety of metabolic studies. Table 31-2 shows a list of gastrointestinal conditions to which breath hydrogen and carbon dioxide analysis has been applied in recent years. When breath containing [13]CO_2 is being studied, the increase in the ratio of [13]CO_2/[12]CO_2 from the base line determines the significance of the test results.

At present the breath hydrogen test for carbohydrate malabsorption (lactose, sucrose) is the most widely employed. The child is given the substrate (lactose or sucrose at 2 gm/kg) orally after an 8-hour fast, and end-expired tidal air is collected at the nose through a mask or a small nasal prong attached to a 50 ml syringe. End-expired air can also be collected through a small intranasal tube positioned just below the base of the tongue in the posterior oral pharynx. Usually 3 to 5 ml of air are aspirated toward the end of each breath until approximately 30 ml have been collected. Standardization of the breath-sampling techniques is critical in this procedure. Samples are then collected every 30 minutes for 4 hours and the hydrogen concentration is determined by gas liquid chromatography. Recently, portable hydrogen-detecting devices have become available.* Normal individuals expire hydrogen less than 20 ppm, whereas malabsorbers expire greater than 80 ppm.

Interpretation of results should take into consideration known causes of false-positive and false-negative values. False-positive results are almost always caused by upper small bowel contamination, which may, for example, be present in infants during the postinfectious diarrhea state, with partial small bowel obstruction attributable to stenosis or stricture, or in older children with Crohn's disease. False-negative results may be caused by delayed gastric emptying, an important consideration in the child given a hyperosmolar substrate (sugar) to drink. Rapid intestinal transit with prompt colonic evacuation may also give false-negative results. In a few persons (2%), hydrogen-producing colonic bacteria are absent.

The overall reliability of this noninvasive test seems to be quite good. In one study the correlation of breath hydrogen tests in biopsy-proved lactase-deficient patients was 100%.

Pediatric conditions often evaluated by breath hydrogen determination include (1) suspected congenital lactase deficiency; (2) acquired lactase deficiency secondary to gastroenteritis, milk-protein allergy, celiac disease, parasitic infections, malnutrition, late-onset (adult) lactase deficiency; (3) the role of lactose in patients with functional abdominal pain; (4) uncertainty of the mucosal integrity in some patients with the irritable bowel syndrome of childhood; (5) a means of following mucosal repair before dietary rechallenge with the

---

*Quintron Instrument Co., Inc., 3712 W. Pierce St., Milwaukee, WI 53215.

Table 31-2. Breath-test application in children

Function studied	Substrate	Specific breath component measured
Carbohydrate malabsorption		
Lactase deficiency	Lactose	H_2
	^{14}C-lactose	$^{14}CO_2$
Sucrase-isomaltase deficiency	Sucrose	H_2
Fat malabsorption		
Malabsorption screening	^{13}C-trioctanoin	$^{13}CO_2$
	^{14}C-trioctanoin	$^{14}CO_2$
	^{14}C-triolein	$^{14}CO_2$
	^{14}C-tripalmitin	$^{14}CO_2$
Ileal dysfunction and	^{13}C-glycocholate	$^{13}CO_2$
bacterial overgrowth	^{14}C-glycocholate	$^{14}CO_2$
	Glucose	H_2
Hepatic function		
Aminopyrine	^{14}C-aminopyrine	$^{14}CO_2$
	^{13}C-aminopyrine	$^{13}CO_2$
Phenacetin	^{14}C-phenacetin	$^{14}CO_2$
Galactose	^{13}C-galactose	$^{13}CO_2$
	^{14}C-galactose	$^{14}CO_2$
Drug metabolism		
Diazepam	^{14}C-diazepam	$^{14}CO_2$
Levodopa	^{14}C-levodopa	$^{14}CO_2$
Inborn errors of metabolism		
Glycine metabolism	^{13}C-glycine	$^{13}CO_2$
Galactosemia	^{14}C-galactose	$^{14}CO_2$
Carbohydrate metabolism		
Normal	^{13}C-glucose	$^{13}CO_2$
Obesity	^{13}C-glucose	$^{13}CO_2$
Diabetes	^{13}C-glucose	$^{13}CO_2$
	^{14}C-glucose	$^{14}CO_2$
Physiological parameters		
Hydrogen excretion	—	H_2
Methane excretion	—	CH_4
Intestinal transit time	Lactulose	H_2
Intestinal gas syndromes	Foods and juices	H_2, CH_4, CO_2

From Barr, R.G., and others: Pediatrics **62**(3):393-401, 1978, copyright American Academy of Pediatrics.

offending agent. More than likely, if the patient shows no clinical symptoms such as abdominal distention, cramps, or diarrhea after the lactose load required for the breath hydrogen test, he will more than likely tolerate lactose-containing products in normal concentrations. Although little has been published on its use in evaluating children suspected of congenital sucrase-isomaltase deficiency, a recent report using breath-test analysis in this entity failed to document increased breath hydrogen excretion. Variations in bacterial flora and their respective metabolism of the unabsorbed substrate was believed responsible for these surprising findings.

REFERENCES

Barr, R.G., Perman, J.A., Schoeller, D.A., and Watkins, J.B.: Breath tests in pediatric gastrointestinal disorders: new diagnostic opportunities, Pediatrics **62:**393-401, 1978.

Gardiner, A.J., Tarlow, M.J., Symonds, J., and others: Failure of the hydrogen breath test to detect primary sugar malabsorption, Arch. Dis. Child. **56:**368-372, 1981.

Maffei, H.V.L., Metz, G.L., and Jenkins, D.J.A.: Hydrogen breath test: adaptation of a simple technique to infants and children, Lancet **1:**1110-1111, 1976.

MUCOSAL ENZYME ASSAY

Normally, dietary disaccharides are hydrolyzed to their constituent monosaccharides by specific disaccharidases located in the intestinal mucosal cells. This hydrolytic activity is present in the brush border of the intestinal epithelial cells. It is important to note that the dietary disaccharides are not hydrolyzed to any significant extent within the lumen of the intestine by enzymes in the intestinal secretions. The intestinal disaccharidases, particularly lactase, sucrase, and maltase, are located primarily in the upper jejunum. Very low levels of lactase and sucrase activity are found in ileal mucosa. Higher levels of maltase and isomaltase are found in ileal mucosa, but, again, their maximum activity is in the jejunal mucosa.

Indications

Disaccharidase determinations should be obtained whenever a peroral jejunal biopsy is done. This type of documentation is useful before the patient is subjected to long-term, severely restrictive diets such as a lactose- or sucrose-free diet. Infrequently symptoms related to milk intolerance are apparent in patients with other diseases, such as ulcerative colitis, cystic fibrosis, and celiac dis-

ease, in whom confirmatory evidence of lactase deficiency on mucosal analysis will provide a sound basis for use of a lactose-free diet.

The contraindications to a peroral biopsy of small bowel discussed elsewhere apply here.

Procedure

Intestinal mucosal tissue, which should be quickly frozen for subsequent enzyme analysis, is obtained by peroral biopsy. Disaccharidase assays are determined by Dahlquist's method, and the results are expressed in units per gram of wet weight or of protein of intestinal mucosa. In our laboratory one unit of disaccharidase activity is equal to 1 μmol of substrate hydrolyzed per gram of protein.

Results

The enzymes of significance in clinical pediatrics are lactase, sucrase, and maltase. The range of mucosal enzyme activity for these three enzymes is:

Lactase	18.5-93.5
Sucrase	28.0-148.0
Maltase	119.0-461.0

All these enzymes appear to be present in sufficient quantities in the normal infant.

Congenital enzyme deficiencies may exist alone or in combination. Sucrase and isomaltase deficiencies always coexist. Lactase and sucrase deficiencies may coexist in the acquired form. Since there are four different enzymes with maltase activity, the clinical occurrence of maltose intolerance is very rare. Lactase is by far the most common deficiency noted because of its association with other diseases affecting the mucosa of the small bowel.

Patients with monosaccharide (glucose-galactose) intolerance have normal disaccharidase activity. The defect in this disorder appears to be one of transport rather than enzyme deficiency.

Because decreased disaccharidase activity has also been noted in patients with malnutrition, kwashiorkor, and marasmus, nutritional rehabilitation must proceed slowly in such patients and in small increments; otherwise vomiting, diarrhea, and abdominal cramping may occur.

Interpretation

Several precautions are worth mentioning in interpreting mucosal enzyme assay. The peroral specimen must be immediately frozen at $-40°$ C.

In isolated lactase deficiency, the finding of a ratio or 10:1 of sucrase to lactase activity is a more reliable indication of lactase deficiency than a low lactase level is.

Patients with isolated isomaltase-sucrase deficiencies may show an upper normal range of lactase, a moderate decrease in maltase, and very low sucrase activities. The moderate reduction in maltase is related to the relatively small percentage of the starch molecules yielding isomaltose (alpha-dextrins), which remain unhydrolyzed in the absence of the missing disaccharidase, isomaltase.

REFERENCES

Berkel, I., Kiran, O., and Say, B.: Jejunal mucosa in infantile malnutrition, Acta Paediatr. Scand. **59:**58-64, 1970.

Dahlqvist, A.: Specificity of the human intestinal disaccharidases and implications for hereditary disaccharide intolerance, J. Clin. Invest. **41:**463-470, 1962.

Dahlqvist, A.: The intestinal disaccharidases and disaccharide intolerance, Gastroenterology **43:**694-696, 1962.

Meeuwisse, G.W., and Lindquist, B.: Glucose-galactose malabsorption, Acta Paediatr. Scand. **59:**74-79, 1970.

STOOL FAT

Microscopic examination of stools will provide some information of the presence of fat and also on the type of fat present. Neutral fat, which accounts for 20% to 30% of total stool fat in pancreatic insufficiency, stains red with sudan and is identified as globules. In contrast, fatty acids will not stain with sudan and present as fatty acid crystals apparent at high power as refractile crystals under polarized light. However the most accurate way of determining the presence and the degree of steatorrhea is measurement of the fecal fatty acids in a 72-hour stool collection. Determination of fecal fatty acids should be included in the diagnostic evaluation of patients suspected of having a malabsorption disorder.

In normal persons, very little fecal fat is derived from exogenous sources such as unabsorbed dietary fat. Fecal fat content is relatively unaltered by large variations in dietary fat intake. A large percentage of fecal fat found normally is endogenous in origin and is accounted for by desquamated intestinal epithelial cells and bacteria.

Patients with malabsorption also may have increased stool nitrogen. Paralleling the increased fatty acids in the stool of these patients may be a loss of nitrogen, which reflects undigested, unab-

sorbed dietary protein or an endogenous protein loss. Normally, dietary and endogenous proteins are digested by proteolytic enzymes into amino acids that are absorbed. The correlation between high fecal fat content and increased fecal nitrogen is more apparent in patients with disturbances of the digestive phase of absorption, such as in pancreatic exocrine insufficiency. Measurement of fecal fat and fecal nitrogen at times may help to differentiate patients with various forms of malabsorption.

Collection of fecal fat is not a popular activity with either the parents or ward personnel. Some laboratories are reluctant to do the chemical analysis and, for this reason, substitute a variety of screening tests, which, unfortunately, have not been very reliable. Fecal fat determinations should not be ordered indiscriminately, but when accurate assessment is necessary, chemical analysis of a 72-hour specimen should be done.

Indications

Quantitative stool-fat assessment should be carried out whenever failure to thrive does not appear to be secondary to a decreased dietary intake and when gastrointestinal symptoms are compatible with disease and disorders associated with the malabsorption syndromes described in Chapter 10.

Method

Ideally, the patient should be on a normal diet with adequate fat content (35% of diet) and caloric intake for 5 days before the beginning of the test. This diet should be continued, no meals should be omitted, and no medications should be given during the test period. No barium should be ingested for 48 hours before or during the collection. Carmine red in capsules (0.6 to 0.9 gm) or as a 3% solution (10 ml is given at the beginning of the balance period and again 72 hours later. All stools passed from the appearance of the first marker until the appearance of the second marker should be collected and kept in a freezer. The stool containing the first unabsorbable marker is included in the collection; consequently the stool showing the second marker is not part of the collection period. The 72-hour collection is preferred so that daily variation in volume of fecal fat and in colonic function may be eliminated.

In patients who are having profuse diarrhea, a marker is not essential, and a timed 72-hour collection is satisfactory. All stools passed within a

72-hour period are collected in a polyethylene bag opened inside a preweighed plastic container. The can and its contents are then taken to the laboratory for stool-fat analysis. A similar method of collection is used in the hospital for those patients who use a potty chair or a regular commode. Saran Wrap inside the diaper is satisfactory for the young patient, and the stool is then transferred to a suitable container. The modified method of van de Kamer is used to measure the total fecal fatty acid content unless the fat intake is largely made up of medium-chain triglycerides. In this situation, quantitative extraction cannot be achieved, and the method of Jeejeebhoy is used. Fecal nitrogen may be determined by the micro-Kjeldahl method.

Interpretation

There is some variation in the degree of fecal fat that is considered normal in the infant and young child. Premature infants may excrete more fat than full-term newborn infants do. The degree of fecal fat excretion in the premature infant may be related to the fat content and type of fat in his formula (p. 301). With diets that are low in fat and of a vegetable oil source, premature infants excrete lower amounts of fat in the stool.

Normal fecal fatty acid excretion for children over 2 years of age while ingesting a dietary fat intake accounting for 35% of dietary clories is 4.5 gm or less per 24 hours. Schmerling and co-workers reported that fecal fat excretion levels amount to less than 3.5 gm/24 hours for children under 2 years of age.

Coefficient of absorption

Fat absorption and excretion is better expressed as the coefficient of absorption (CA), or the percentage of the dietary fat that is absorbed:

$$\frac{\text{Dietary fat} - \text{Fecal fat}}{\text{Dietary fat}} \times 100 = \text{CA}$$

Within certain limits the coefficient of absorption does not depend on the amount of dietary fat intake but remains rather constant. Its determination requires that a strict record of dietary fat intake by kept. Use of the coefficient of absorption is best reserved for patients whose fecal fat excretion is borderline abnormal.

Coefficient of absorption as related to age

In premature infants	60%-75%
In newborn infants	80%-85%
10 months to 3 years	85%-95%
Older than 3 years	95%

In the pediatric population, the largest amount of fecal fat is excreted by patients with cystic fibrosis, or with pancreatic insufficiency of non–cystic fibrotic origin.

Fecal fatty acid content is the most reliable test available for the study of malabsorption.

REFERENCES

Jeejeebhoy, K.N., Ahmad, S., and Kozak, G.: Determination of fecal fats containing both medium and long chain triglycerides and fatty acids, Clin. Biochem. **3:**157-163, 1970.

Schmerling, D.H., Forrer, J.C.W., and Prader, A.: Fecal fat and nitrogen in healthy children and in children with malabsorption or maldigestion, Pediatrics **46:**690-695, 1970.

The origin of fecal fat (editorial), Lancet **2:**627-628, 1969.

van de Kamer, J.H., ten Bokkel Huinink, H., and Weijers, H.A.: A rapid method for the determination of fat in faeces, J. Biol. Chem. **177:**347-355, 1949.

Walker, B.E., Kelleher, J., Davies, T., and others: Influence of dietary fat on fecal fat, Gastroenterology **64:**233-239, 1973.

Weijers, H.A., and van de Kamer, H.J.: Coeliac disease: criticism of the various methods of investigation, Acta Paediatr. Scand. **42:**24-33, 1953.

SCHILLING TEST

Vitamin B_{12} given orally is normally coupled with intrinsic factor (IF) contained in gastric juice secreted by the stomach, and the vitamin B_{12}–IF complex is then absorbed in the terminal ileum. Only intrinsic factor–bound vitamin B_{12} is absorbed by this route. After parenteral administration or gastrointestinal absorption, cyanocobalamin is bound to plasma proteins and distributed to the liver and blood-forming organs. It is now possible to test simultaneously the absorption of vitamin B_{12} with and without intrinsic factor. The commercial (Dicopac) kit consists of cyanocobalamin cobalt 58 and cyanocobalamin cobalt 57 combined with intrinsic factor; therefore a diagnosis of vitamin B_{12} malabsorption attributable to absent intrinsic factor or to malabsorption syndromes not caused by the lack of intrinsic factor can be made in a single procedure.

Procedure

1. The patient fasts from midnight the night before the test is to be started until 2 hours after the administration of the radioactive vitamin B_{12} capsules.
2. The two capsules in the Dicopac unit dose package, cyanocobalamin Co 57 bound to human gastric juice and cyanocobalamin Co 58, are orally administered simultaneously to the fasting patient.

Table 31-3. Results of 24-hour urine excretion and isotope ratios

Diagnosis	Percentage excreted: mean values percent (usual range)		Cobalt 57 / Cobalt 58 ratio
	Cobalt 57 (B_{12}-IF)	Cobalt (B_{12})	
Normals	18 (10-42)	18 (10-40)	0.7 - 1.3
Pernicious anemia and certain gastric lesions	9 (6-12)	3 (0-7)	>1.7
Malabsorption syndromes not caused by lack of intrinsic factor (IF)	<6	<6	0.7 - 1.3

3. An intramuscular injection of 1 mg of nonradioactive vitamin B_{12} is administered to the patient immediately or up to 2 hours after the administration of the radioactive capsules.
4. The patient is instructed to collect all urine for 24 hours after the administration of the radioactive capsules. The urine is collected in a clean 2-liter bottle, free of radioactivity. The collection should be complete, but an incomplete collection will not necessarily invalidate the entire test.

Calculation and Interpretation

The urinary excretion of each isotope is determined and the ratio calculated to provide information about the relative absorptions and the site of the absorptive defect. This ratio also provides valuable information even if the urinary collection is incomplete (Table 31-3).

REFERENCES

Corcino, J.J., Waxman, S., and Herbert, V.: Absorption and malabsorption of vitamin B_{12}, Am. J. Med. **48**:562-569, 1970.

Pathak, A., Godwin, H.A., and Prudent, L.M.: Vitamin B_{12} and folic acid values in premature infants, Pediatrics **50**:584-589, 1972.

Russell, R.I., and Lee, T.D.: Tests of small intestinal function: digestion, absorption, secretion, Clin. Gastroenterol. **7**:277-315, 1978.

Toskes, P.O., and Deren, J.J.: Vitamin B_{12} absorption and malabsorption, Gastroenterology **65**:662-683, 1973.

TEST FOR OCCULT BLOOD IN STOOL

Bleeding into the gastrointestinal tract may vary from occult blood loss to massive bleeding. A 2+ to 4+ Hematest positive stool may represent blood loss ranging from 3 ml to as much as 80 ml/24 hr. Therefore the degree of positivity of the stool for the Hematest reaction is a reliable indicator not of the amount of blood lost but only of its presence in the stool.

The color imparted to the stool by blood is determined by the site of bleeding within the gastrointestinal tract, the transit time, and the severity of the bleeding. Reportedly, adults can sustain as much as 75 to 200 ml of bleeding in the upper gastrointestinal tract without any change in the color or appearance of the stool. In contrast, rectal and colonic bleeding is more easily detected, since it presents as bright red blood throughout the stool or as streaks on the outside of the stool. In general, a tarry stool indicates hemorrhage from the upper gastrointestinal tract above the ligament of Treitz. The brown-black (coffee grounds) coloration appears when the action of upper intestinal contents produces acid hematin.

The pediatric patient is more likely to ingest products that may make the stool appear to contain blood. A number of foods and medicines containing artificial, nonabsorbable dyes and dietary products, such as beets, Kool-Aid, red licorice, and flavored gelatin, may impart a red color to the stools. Medicinal iron, bismuth, and licorice are known to cause stools to be dark. Therefore it is important to check all suspect stools chemically. Each time a digital rectal examination is done, the stool should be checked for blood. It is possible, however, that a too-vigorous digital examination may cause mucosal trauma, so that a positive result of test for occult blood is obtained.

Chemical determination of occult blood

Ideally, the test for occult blood should yield positive results for amounts undetectable by the naked eye and in excess of the 2 to 4 ml released daily by the gastrointestinal tract. Furthermore, the test should not be affected by iron, meat, or other foods ingested by the patient.

None of the available tests completely fills these requirements, and they are not even semiquantitative. They all depend on the peroxidase activity of blood, which may be appreciably reduced in the gastrointestinal tract by digestive enzymes. Furthermore, hemoglobin can be converted to certain porphyrins that will not be detected by the standard tests for occult blood. High levels of vitamin C in stool may also inhibit the reaction.

Hematest tablet. Hematest tablet (Ames) is currently the most widely used clinical method of testing for occult blood. The tablet contains a mixture of *ortho*-tolidine, strontium peroxide, calcium acetate, and tartaric acid. The addition of water causes the tartaric acid and calcium acetate to react with strontium peroxide to form hydrogen peroxide, which on contact with heme pigment yields oxygen. In turn, the freed oxygen converts *ortho*-tolidine to a blue-colored derivative. The sensitivity of the Hematest procedure is of the order of 1 part of blood in 20,000 parts of fecal material. It will give a weakly positive reaction with as little as 270 mg of hemoglobin (2.7 ml of blood) per 100 gm of stool.

Technique. To minimize false positive reactions, adherence to the following details is necessary. The hands, dropper, and working area must be clean and free of traces of blood.

1. Smear a solid specimen of feces on filter paper. Do not use an emulsion.

2. Place a Hematest tablet so that half the tablet is on the specimen and half on the paper.

3. Place 1 drop of water on the tablet. Wait 10 seconds and flow a second drop on the tablet so that it runs down the sides onto the filter paper.

Interpretation

NEGATIVE. No blue color appears within 60 seconds on the moistened portion of the filter paper around the tablet.

POSITIVE. The moistened area on the filter paper around the tablet turns blue within 60 seconds. The time of appearance and the intensity of the color are related to the amount of blood present. Disregard any color changes on the tablet or color appearing on the filter paper after 1 minute.

Time of appearance of color

Strongly positive: within 15 seconds
Positive: within 15 to 60 seconds
Any color appearing after 1 minute is of doubtful significance and should be disregarded.

Because false-positive reactions are an occasional problem, a positive reaction occurring after 1 minute is an indication to repeat the test. Iron preparations that the patient may be taking, except ferrous fumarate and ferrous carbonate, do not yield false-positive results.

Guaiac slide test (Hemoccult). A simple slide or tape test has been developed for testing for occult blood in the stool. The Hemoccult* slide or tape contains guaiac-impregnated filter paper and is designed to detect fecal blood above 2 to 2.5 ml/100 gm of feces per 24 hours, the range considered normal.

A thin smear of fresh stool is applied to the slide, which is then closed and allowed to dry. The perforated tab on the back is then opened, and a developer contained in the kit is applied. The result is noted 30 seconds later.

Negative: no color change noted
Positive: any trace of blue color considered positive for occult blood and graded 1 +, 2 +, or 3 +

Results show that the guaiac slide test is only one fourth as sensitive as older tests with guaiac. False-positive results may still approach 10% and are probably caused by the presence of (nonhemoglobin) stool peroxidases. However, it is said to be free of the false-negative results occasionally seen with Hematest.

• • •

Testing for occult blood is important in any child with anemia or gastrointestinal complaints. The recognition of occult bleeding depends on results of routine anorectal examination and testing stool specimens as described.

*"Hemoccult" slides, Smith Kline Diagnostics, Division of Smith, Kline & French Laboratories, Dept. E42, 1500 Spring Garden St., Philadelphia, PA 19101.

REFERENCES

Ebaugh, F.G., Jr., Clemens, T., Rodnan, G., and Peterson, R.E.: Quantitative measurement of gastrointestinal blood loss, Am. J. Med. **25:**169-181, 1958.

Glober, G.A., and Peskoe, S.M.: Outpatient screening for gastrointestinal lesions using guaiac-impregnated slides, Am. J. Dig. Dis. **19:**399-403, 1974.

Smith, R.L.: Fecal occult blood tests without dietary restrictions, Br. Med. J. **1:**1336-1338, 1958.

Winawer, S.J.: Fecal occult blood testing, Am. J. Dig. Dis. **21:**885-888, 1976.

Apt-Downey test

The Apt-Downey test is used to differentiate swallowed maternal blood from gastrointestinal bleeding in the infant.

Procedure

A small amount of stool specimen is mixed with tap water (1 part to 5 parts), and the mixture is centrifuged. Then 1 ml of 0.25N sodium hydroxide is added to 5 ml of supernatant pink fluid; after 5 minutes the color is observed.

Interpretation

Brown-yellow color indicates adult hemoglobin. A pink color establishes the presence of fetal hemoglobin.

REFERENCES

Apt, L., and Downey, W.S., Jr.: "Melena" neonatorum, the swallowed blood syndrome: a simple test for the differentiation of adult and fetal hemoglobin in bloody stools, J. Pediatr. **47**:6-12, 1955.

32 *Procedures*

GASTRIC ACIDITY

Free hydrochloric acid is present in the gastric juice of the unfed full-term newborn infant in relatively high concentrations. In the premature infant, the gastric acid output is much less than that of the full-term newborn infant and remains lower for the first few weeks.

The gastric acidity in newborn infants may be high for the first 48 hours whether or not feedings have been taken. Gastric acid is produced by the parietal cells of the stomach, which are present as early as the fourth fetal month and presumably are capable of function after that time. By term the newborn infant has a twofold to threefold increase in parietal cell mass, a higher rate of gastric acid secretion, and a strongly acid pH within 2 hours after birth.

Indications

Gastric acidity should be measured in pediatric patients with (1) intractable ulcer symptoms, (2) suspected Zollinger-Ellison syndrome, or (3) the short bowel syndrome with signs of poor nutrition.

Procedure

Preparation. Patients fast beginning at midnight before the test. Infants younger than 1 year need fast for only 4 to 6 hours. For the test a size 8 to 12 radiopaque polyethylene nasogastric tube is passed, preferably under fluoroscopy, so that the tip lies in the most dependent part of the stomach and along the greater gastric curvature. Once the tube is in place, the infant or small child lies on either his back or left side. Older children and adolescents are allowed to sit if able to do so.

Collection of gastric secretion. Manual suction is carried out with a 20 ml syringe. The stomach contents are aspirated as completely as possible and discarded. Four 15-minute basal collections are then obtained by this method. The aliquots are collected separately in iced containers.

Betazole and pentagastrin stimulation. Betazole (Histalog), 1 mg/kg of body weight, with a maximum dose of 50 mg, is injected subcutaneously. Some degree of flushing of the face may

occur. (As a precautionary measure, an ampule of epinephrine 1:1000 should be kept at hand.) Use of pentagastrin, a synthetic peptide resembling gastrin, is preferable, since it is free of side effects. The dose of pentagastrin is 6 μg/kg of body weight subcutaneously.

Four 15-minute samples of gastric secretion are again collected and saved. All specimens are kept in an ice-filled container and are then taken to the laboratory.

Each 15-minute sample is measured for volume, pH, and titratable acidity. The sum of the total acidity (mEq) in the four 15-minute basal samples corresponds to the *basal acid output* in mEq/hr. The two highest poststimulation 15-minute samples are pooled and multiplied by 2; they correspond to the *peak acid output* in milliequivalents per hour. The rate of acid production is most helpful when one is concerned with detecting hypersecretion.

Results and interpretation

Infant and child respond to betazole and pentagastrin stimulation by putting out concentrations of hydrochloric acid that are comparable to the response expected in the adult. The volume of gastric juice and the total output of acid are lower during the first 4 months of life than they are during early childhood (from 4 to 9 years) and much lower when compared to adult levels (Chapter 7).

There is a considerable degree of overlap between values obtained in controls and those in children with peptic ulcer disease. Our own experience with ulcer patients shows that there is little difference between basal levels in gastric and duodenal ulcers. Poststimulation response is generally higher in children with peptic disease affecting the duodenum but is not of diagnostic value.

The discriminant value of serum gastrin in duodenal ulcers is poor under fasting conditions but improves significantly when obtained 45 to 75 minutes after a meal.

Differentiating between peptic disease and the Zollinger-Ellison syndrome has been greatly facilitated by the availability of gastrin assays. We believe that a high basal acid output (over 10 mEq/hr), a high peak acid output (over 30 mEq/hr), or the failure of the stimulated secretions (peak acid output) to increase at least threefold over basal levels, or all three, constitute indications for gastrin assay in the child. If gastrinemia is then found to be in the equivocal range (200 to 500 pg/ml), a calcium infusion test should be carried out, with the calcium being given intravenously over a 4-hour period at a dose of 15 mg/kg. Gastrin levels are obtained hourly during the infusion. Some workers prefer the secretin provocation test over the calcium infusion test, since it better distinguishes patients with Zollinger-Ellison syndrome from other hyperchlorhydric, hypergastrinemic patients. Pure natural gastrointestinal hormone (GIH secretin, Karolinska Institute, Stockholm) in a dose of 1 to 2 units/kg by intravenous bolus or Boots secretin (Warren-Teed Laboratories, Inc., Columbus, Ohio) 4 units/kg given as an intravenous infusion is recommended. Serum gastrin levels should be determined before and at 5-minute intervals for 30 minutes after the secretin injection. A rise of at least 200 pg/ml over the basal level is consistent with the diagnosis of gastrinoma.

The secretory activity of the fundic glands is low at birth, and this is evidenced by hyposecretion of gastric acid during the first 5 hours of life. Thereafter gastric acid secretion increases sharply but remains low up to the age of 3 months. From age 4 years on, there is a gradual increase in volume and acid concentration approaching adult levels (Chapter 7).

Hyperacidity is found in patients with congenital short bowel syndrome, in whom the values exceed those of normal controls. An increase in both total acid and rate of acid formation and a low pH are found in infants with massive resection of the bowel.

REFERENCES

Agunod, M., Yamaguchi, N., Lopez, R., and others: Correlative study of hydrochloric acid, pepsin, and intrinsic factor secretion in newborns and infants, Am. J. Dig. Dis. 14:400-416, 1969.

Avery, G.B., Randolph, J.G., and Weaver, T.: Gastric acidity in the first day of life, Pediatrics 37:1005-1007, 1966.

Christie, D.L., and Ament, M.E.: Gastric acid hypersecretion in children with duodenal ulcer, Gastroenterology 71:242-244, 1976.

Deren, J.J.: Development of structure and function in the fetal and newborn stomach, Am. J. Clin. Nutr. 24:144-159, 1971.

Euler, A.R., Byrne, W.J., Cousins, L.M., and others: Increased serum gastrin concentrations and gastric hyposecretion in the immediate newborn period, Gastroenterology 72:1271-1293, 1977.

Levant, J.A., Walsh, J.H., and Isenberg, J.I.: Stimulation of gastric secretion and gastrin release by single oral doses of calcium carbonate in man, N. Engl. J. Med. 289:555-558, 1973.

McGuigan, J.E., and Wolfe, M.M.: Secretin injection test in the diagnosis of gastrinoma, Gastroenterology 79:1324-1331, 1980.

Robb, J.D.A., Thomas, P.S., Orszulok, J., Jr., and Odling-Smee, G.W.: Duodenal ulcer in children, Arch. Dis. Child. 47:688-696, 1972.

Rodbro, P., Krasilnikoff, P., and Christiansen, P.M.: Gastric secretion in early childhood, Lancet 2:730-732, 1966.

Schwartz, D.L., White, J.J., Saulsbury, F., and Haller, J.A., Jr.: Gastrin response to calcium infusion: an aid to the improved diagnosis of Zollinger-Ellison syndrome in children, Pediatrics 54:599-602, 1974.

Straus, E., Gerson, C.D., and Yalow, R.S.: Hypersecretion of gastrin associated with the short bowel syndrome, Gastroenterology 66:175-180, 1974.

White, W.D., and Kerrison, J., Jr.: Repeatability of gastric analysis, Am. J. Dig. Dis. 18:7-13, 1973.

^{131}I–ROSE BENGAL TEST

Rose bengal is a red dye that is taken up by the hepatic cells and excreted through the bile into the intestinal tract. The peak concentration is reached in the liver in less than 30 minutes after administration. It is thereafter rapidly excreted into the intestine and is not reabsorbed.

If liver cells are damaged, the rate of uptake by the liver is decreased or excretion into the biliary system is prevented. Obstruction in the intrahepatic or extrahepatic biliary system causes a delay in the excretion of the dye into the intestine. This delay in appearance of the dye varies according to the completeness of biliary obstruction. With complete obstruction, rose bengal dye does not enter the intestinal tract; instead, it is retained in the liver, where its breakdown occurs, and the iodine component of the dye is released into the blood. It is then excreted primarily into the urine. Minute amounts can enter the lumen of the intestinal tract along with intestinal secretions. The amount of rose bengal retained in the liver or excreted in the urine and in the stool reflects hepatocellular dysfunction or obstruction in the biliary system.

These principles have been applied to the study of jaundiced patients. The administration of ^{131}I–rose bengal is followed by the counting of radioactivity in a 3-day collection of urine and feces.

Indications

In pediatrics, the major use of radioactive rose bengal has been in differentiating extrahepatic biliary atresia from neonatal hepatitis (Chapter 19).

Method

1. One day before the test, the patient is given 3 drops of Lugol's solution orally in order to block the uptake of ^{131}I by the thyroid.

2. The dose of ^{131}I–rose bengal is carefully prepared under sterile conditions. A commercially available preparation is diluted with physiologic saline solution to arrive at a dose of 1 mg of dye, containing 1 to 10 microcuries of radioactive substance, in a volume of 1 ml for intravenous injection.

3. Complete urine-free stools are collected in 24-hour intervals for 3 successive days in plastic diaper liners and are transferred to a gallon paint can and saved until counted.

4. Urine is also collected for 3 days. Since it is imperative to prevent contamination of the stool by urine, a plastic pediatric urine collector is used for male patients. In infant girls the urine collector may be affixed to the anus and the urine collected in a metabolic bed.

5. A "standard" dose of rose bengal is prepared, using the same dosage as that given to the patient.

6. Aliquots from the standard and from the total stool and urine collections are assayed in a scintillation counter.

7. The percentage of radioactive rose bengal excreted in the feces and urine is calculated from these counts.

Results

Fecal excretion as percentage of administered dose:

Controls	70 to 97
Extrahepatic atresia of bile ducts	8 or less
Obstructive jaundice with patent bile ducts	5 to 20

Interpretation

When the stool is being collected for monitoring, every precaution must be taken to avoid contamination by urine. False high rates of excretion of ^{131}I–rose bengal may result if urine is mixed with the feces and lead to an erroneous conclusion that the biliary tract is patent. If the test is properly performed and no urine contaminates the stool collection, jaundiced infants who excrete 8% or less of ^{131}I–rose bengal in the stool collection should be considered to have extrahepatic biliary atresia. Additional support for this diagnosis may be obtained from the history, physical examination, and other laboratory data (Chapter 19). If the fecal excretion rate is more than 8%, it is highly unlikely that complete biliary obstruction is present.

In a surprisingly large number of instances, neither neonatal hepatitis nor intrahepatic biliary hypoplasia can be differentiated from extrahepatic atresia by this test. In our experience, roughly one third of infants whose illness was indistinguishable clinically from extrahepatic atresia also excreted less than 8% of the ^{131}I–rose bengal in their feces. It is suggested that the ^{131}I–rose bengal study be repeated 2 to 4 weeks later after the neonate has been treated with phenobarbital and cholestyramine. Separation of those conditions requiring surgery from those needing continued medical management may be accomplished by this technique.

Therefore it would appear that the ^{131}I–rose bengal test may be valuable in differentiating biliary obstruction from hepatitis in 70% to 75% of patients. Although lacking specificity, this test, and radionuclide scans with derivatives of iminodiacetic acids such as DIDA, PIDIDA, or HIDA may add further support for the need to do an operative cholangiogram and open-liver biopsy. Careful evaluation of all the available data preoperatively may save the infant the added risk of anesthesia and surgery if the data suggest hepatitis. (See Chapter 19.)

Misleading results from the test may also stem from contamination of the stool with urine. We also feel that for the most accurate results, aliquots to be counted come from the entire 3-day stool collection, which has been sufficiently homogenized.

REFERENCES

Geppert, L.J., and Brent, R.L.: Radioactive rose bengal: aid in differential diagnosis of infantile jaundice, Am. J. Dis. Child. **94:**544, 1957.

Ghadimi, H., and Sass-Kortsak, A.: Evaluation of the radioactive rose bengal test for the differential diagnosis of obstructive jaundice in infants, N. Engl. J. Med. **265:**351-358, 1961.

Morin, C. Verret, S., and Sass-Kortsak, A.: Radioactive rose bengal: an aid in the differential diagnosis of neonatal obstructive jaundice. Personal communication, 1971.

Poley, J.R., Alaupovic, P., McConathy, W.J., and others: Diagnosis of extrahepatic biliary obstruction in infants by immunochemical detection of LP-X and modified ^{131}I–rose bengal excretion test, J. Lab. Clin. Med. **81**:325-341, 1973.

Sharp, H.L., Krivit, W., and Lowman, J.T.: The diagnosis of complete extrahepatic obstruction by rose bengal I[131], J. Pediatr. **70**:46-53, 1967.

IMAGING OF LIVER AND HEPATOBILIARY SYSTEM WITH IMINODIACETIC ACID DERIVATIVES AND TECHNETIUM 99m

Radionuclide evaluation of both the morphological and the functional components of the liver has progressed significantly with the advent of new radiopharmaceutical agents. Iminodiacetic (IDA) derivatives traverse the pathway (blood $\rightarrow$ liver $\rightarrow$ bile) and are not significantly reabsorbed from the gastrointestinal tract. There is reasonable evidence that IDA compounds share the organic anion pathway utilized by sulfobromophthalein. They are useful for the assessment of hepatobiliary function even in situations where cholestasis (intrahepatic or extrahepatic) is severe.

Several IDA analogs are now available. DIPIDA (diisopropyl IDA) is believed to be the best overall cholescintigraphic IDA analog for the evaluation of hepatobiliary disorders. However two recent studies show that PIPIDA (*p*-isopropyl iminodiacetic acid) may more accurately separate intrahepatic from extrahepatic cholestasis. These observations need to be confirmed in infants suspected of biliary atresia.

REFERENCES

Egbert, R., Lyons, K.P., and Felsher, B.: Reliability of Tc-99m PIPIDA hepatobiliary scintigraphy for the diagnosis of total extrahepatic biliary obstruction, J. Nucl. Med. **22**:P86, 1980 (Abstract).

Harvey, E., Loberg, M., Ryan, J., and others: Hepatic clearance mechanism of Tc-99-m-HIDA and its effects on quantitation of hepatobiliary function: concise communication, J. Nucl. Med. **20**:310-313, 1979.

Joshi, S.N., George, E.A., and Perrilo, R.P.: Quantitative temporal analysis of [99m]technetium *p*-isopropyl-iminodiacetic acid (PIPIDA) as a measure of hepatic function in health and disease, Gastroenterology **81**:1045-1051, 1981.

Pauwels, S., Piret, L., Schoutens, A., and others: Tc-99m-diethyl-IDA imaging: clinical evaluation in jaundiced patients, J. Nucl. Med. **21**:1022-1028, 1980.

Ryoji, O., Klingensmith, W.C., and Lilly, J.R.: Diagnosis of hepatobiliary disease in infants and children with Tc-99m-diethyl-IDA imaging, Clin. Nucl. Med. **6**:297-302, 1981.

PANCREATIC EXOCRINE FUNCTION

The direct evaluation of pancreatic exocrine function has not been so widely used in the pediatric population as it has in the adult population. In part, this has been attributable to technical aspects as well as the reluctance to subject infants and children to duodenal intubation.

Adequate amounts of pancreatic enzymes in an alkaline medium are essential for the digestion and subsequent absorption of dietary fat and protein. Exploration of the exocrine pancreatic function may be essential for an accurate diagnosis in certain patients with various malabsorption syndromes in that the clinical presentations may be quite similar. These patients often present with a history of diarrhea, steatorrhea, failure to thrive, weakness, edema, anemia, and bleeding disorders. Cystic fibrosis is by far the most common cause of diminished pancreatic exocrine function, and in 98% of patients the diganosis is confirmed by the sweat test. Assay of duodenal contents is sometimes necessary in patients with borderline normal sweat test values. The most accurate evaluation of pancreatic exocrine function involves the determination of volume, bicarbonate content, and pancreatic enzymes before and after intravenous stimulation with *secretin* and *cholecystokinin-pancreozymin* (CCK-PZ)

Techniques available

Volume, bicarbonate, and enzyme concentration. Several techniques have been described over the years. In pediatric patients, tests of function were originally designed for the diagnosis of pancreatic achylia in cystic fibrosis. They are based solely on the determination of pancreatic enzyme concentration in duodenal contents. More accurate testing, which can permit differentiation of certain specific types of pancreatic insufficiency, involves assessment of volume output, of bicarbonate content, and of enzymes secreted during a fixed period of time.

To explore the functional capacity of the pancreas, one makes these determinations before and after hormonal stimulation. Because of the rapid destruction of pancreatic enzymes brought about by gastric juice, it is essential that a double-lumen tube be used. Gastric juice has to be suctioned continuously during the aspiration study period. Despite these precautions, the technique is, at best, semiquantitative. In fact, abnormal pancreatic enzyme concentration has been reported from duodenal juice in nonpancreatic conditions such as small bowel and hepatobiliary diseases, malnutrition, and hypoproteinemia. Although it is conceivable that pancreatic insufficiency can coexist with other malabsorptive states, reports based on

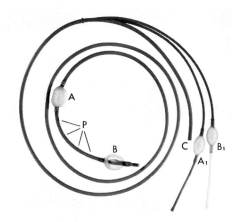

Fig. 32-1. Triple-lumen pediatric duodenal tube. *A* and *B* are occlusive balloons. *A* is inflated first and the tube is withdrawn snugly against the pylorus; then *B* is inflated to prevent duodenal juice from passing into the jejunum. There are multiple perforations, *P*, of central lumen, *C*. *A₁* and *B₁* allow for checking pressure in the occlusive balloons.

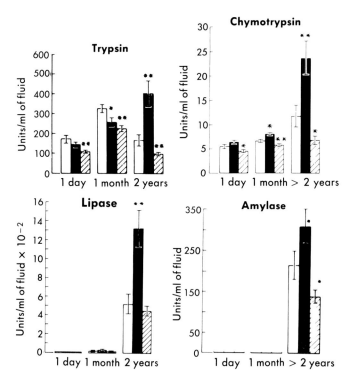

Fig. 32-2. Response of the exocrine pancreas to hormonal stimulation as a function of age. *Open bars,* Basal values; *closed and hatched bars,* response to CCK-PZ and secretin, respectively. (Modified from Lebenthal, E., and Lee, P.C.: Pediatrics **66**(4):556-560, 1980, copyright American Academy of Pediatrics.)

enzyme concentration alone should be interpreted with caution.

More quantitative evaluation requires the use of a specially manufactured triple-lumen pediatric duodenal tube* (Fig. 32-1). It allows isolation of the second and third portions of the duodenum between two inflatable balloons, preventing gastric juice contamination of duodenal juice and losses of the secretions distally. Secretions are quantitatively recovered through the main lumen of the tube. We find that tolerance of children for this tube is poor.

Indications

In the following types of patients, assessment of pancreatic exocrine function may provide useful information: (1) those believed to have cystic fibrosis in whom repeated sweat tests are normal and (2) those suffering other exocrine pancreatic disorders such as enterokinase deficiency, pancreatic insufficiency with neutropenia (Shwachman's syndrome), and chronic pancreatitis. These diseases are discussed in Chapters 27 and 28.

Procedure

The patient is instructed to fast beginning at midnight; for small children, a 4-hour fast is adequate. Diazepam (Valium), 0.1 to 0.2 mg/kg, is given intramuscularly 45 to 60 minutes before the tube is inserted. Cetacaine spray anesthesia to the posterior pharynx is most helpful.

For the collection of duodenal juice, we use a double-lumen pediatric duodenal tube. Gastric juice

*The tube is available in three different sizes from Willy Rusch & Co., Waiblingen, German Federal Republic.

is suctioned continuously through a separate tube.

An initial 10 to 20 ml collection of duodenal juice is made and saved in an iced container. CCK-PZ and, later, secretin, 2 IU/kg of body weight of each, are given slowly intravenously. (If a positive history of porcine allergy is obtained, it is recommended that intradermal skin tests be done for hypersensitivity to both hormones before injection.) Duodenal juice is collected into ice-cooled flasks every 10 minutes for 50 minutes (three 10-minute periods for CCK-PZ and two 10-minute periods for secretin). On each 10-minute sample, the following are determined immediately after collection: (1) volume; (2) bicarbonate concentration; (3) pH; and (4) the enzymes trypsin, chymotrypsin, lipase, and amylase.

Results

The results of the pancreatic response to secretin-pancreozymin stimulation are shown in Fig. 32-2 and in Table 32-1.

Interpretation

Volume and bicarbonate are related primarily to ductular activity, and acinar cells contribute to enzyme secretion. Substantial concentrations of proteolytic enzymes are present at birth in contrast to the low or absent lipase and amylase values. A recent study (Fig. 32-2) alerts one to the lack of response to the secretagogue CCK-PZ during the first month of life.

Patients with cystic fibrosis have a substantial reduction in volume and bicarbonate. They also have a reduction in or absence of enzymes (80% to 90%).

Normal to slightly reduced volume responses,

Table 32-1. Values in duodenal juice after secretin-pancreozymin stimulation (mean values/kg/50 minutes)*

	Controls		Patients with cystic fibrosis	Patients with EPI‡ without cystic fibrosis
	Children†	**Adults**		
Volume (ml/kg/50 min)	3	281	0.8 ± 0.4	1.7-3.9
Bicarbonate (mEq/L)	15	111	1.4 ± 1.5	0-0.04
Lipase (IU)	1464-1424	—	0-341	0-272
Trypsin (mg)	765-788	—	0-450	0.9-321
Chymotrypsin (mg)	880-860	—	0-36	0-165

*Adapted from several sources; see references.
†6 weeks to 13 years of age.
‡Exocrine pancreatic insufficiency.

reduced bicarbonate concentration, and greatly reduced enzyme secretions are found in patients with pancreatic exocrine insufficiency not caused by cystic fibrosis. Low level of lipase or its absence is usually the most striking finding.

Clinical symptoms of pancreatic exocrine insufficiency (steatorrhea, creatorrhea) usually become manifest when 85% to 90% of the gland has been destroyed.

REFERENCES

Brooks, F.: Testing pancreatic function, N. Engl. J. Med. **286:**300-303, 1972.

Dreiling, D.A., and Janowitz, H.D.: The measurement of pancreatic secretory function. In Ciba Foundation Symposium on the Exocrine Pancreas, London, 1962, J. & A. Churchill, Ltd.

Hadorn, B., Zoppi, G., Shmerling, D.H., and others: Quantitative assessment of exocrine pancreatic function in infants and children, J. Pediatr. **73:**39-50, 1968.

Lebenthal, E., and Lee, P.C.: Development of functional response in human exocrine pancreas, Pediatrics **66:**556-560, 1980.

Zoppe, G., Shmerling, H., Gaburro, D., and Prader, A.: The electrolyte and protein contents and outputs in duodenal juice after pancreozymin and secretin stimulation in normal children and in patients with cystic fibrosis, Acta Paediatr. Scand. **59:**692-696, 1970.

TEST WITH ALBUMIN TAGGED WITH CHROMIUM 51
Indications

Low serum levels of protein and albumin are not an uncommon finding and usually accompany diseases of the kidney, liver disorders, malabsorption syndromes, burns, inflammatory bowel disease, inadequate dietary intake, and starvation, among others. There are patients, however, whose hypoproteinemia is not adequately explained as an associated feature of these diseases, and it is for them that further investigation of the cause of the decreased serum albumin is necessary. This search entails consideration of (1) defective or inadequate albumin synthesis, (2) increased or hypercatabolic breakdown of albumin, or (3) loss of albumin, such as occurs in protein-losing enteropathy.

Normally, small amounts of protein are lost into the intestinal tract. The proteins are then digested by proteolytic enzymes into amino acids that are reabsorbed and resynthesized into protein by the liver. Children synthesize albumin at about 0.2 gm/ kg of body weight each day (Table 11-1), of which less than one tenth is lost into the gut. The liver accounts for a further 10% of the albumin degraded daily.

An abnormal loss of proteins into the gastrointestinal tract may be associated with a variety of disorders (Chapter 11). In patients who present with unexplained edema and hypoalbuminemia, an enteric loss of albumin should be considered. Hypoalbuminemia therefore should be thought of as a clinical finding and not as a specific diagnosis.

In patients with protein-losing enteropathy, 8 to 10 gm of albumin per 24 hours may be lost into the gastrointestinal tract. This great rate of loss exceeds the rate of albumin synthesis by the liver and results in hypoalbuminemia. In other patients there may be a decreased rate of synthesis or an increased rate of albumin catabolism, as occurs in some systemic disorders that also result in hypoalbuminemia. To differentiate as clearly as possible the specific cause of the hypoalbuminemia, laboratory investigation is necessary. Apart from the tests needed to rule out kidney and liver disease, techniques to determine albumin loss into the gut as well as albumin turnover may be employed, with isotopically labeled albumin being used.

Choice of radioactive label

^{131}I-albumin is used to evaluate the albumin pool and the rate of degradation of albumin. The albumin tagged with ^{51}Cr is used to measure the enteric albumin loss. Since increased enteric protein loss most often explains the hypoalbuminemia that occurs in several gastrointestinal disease conditions, ^{51}Cr-tagged albumin is most frequently employed. For those patients in whom the cause of the hypoalbuminemia is unclear and complex, the combined use of ^{131}I-albumin and ^{51}Cr-albumin may be necessary.

In the selection of a so-called ideal label for measuring enteric protein loss, certain requirements have been suggested by Waldmann:

1. Labeling of proteins should not alter their survival or distribution.
2. The label should not be absorbed from the gastrointestinal tract.
3. No excretion of label unbound to proteins in the gastrointestinal tract should take place.
4. The label should be easy to detect and quantitate in the stools.
5. It should be safe for the patient.

^{51}Cr-albumin best fits the definition of an "ideal" label for measuring enteric protein loss.

Procedure

^{51}Cr-albumin, 10 to 20 microcuries, is injected intravenously. All stools, free from urine contamination, are collected for a 96-hour period. The composite stool collection is thoroughly homogenized, and an aliquot is then assayed in a scintillation counter. An aliquot of the labeled solution that was given to the patient is used as a standard.

Results and interpretation

^{51}Cr-albumin is excreted into the intestinal tract, and, depending on the site of the enteric protein loss, the label appears in the stool in either the bound or unbound form. An advantage of using radioactive chromium (^{51}Cr) is that the label is not significantly absorbed from or secreted into the gastrointestinal tract. Since some radioactive chromium (^{51}Cr) is excreted in the urine, false-positive values may result if the stool collection is contaminated with urine. Contamination is particularly critical during the first 24 hours of collection because a significantly greater amount of chromium is excreted in the urine during this interval. Since urine excretion of the chromium label is negligible after 48 hours, it is suggested that stools be collected in 24-hour aliquots; the physician should rely on the third and fourth days' fecal excretion of the label in the event of earlier contamination of the stools by urine. Normal persons excrete less than 1% of the administered dose. In patients with protein-losing enteropathy, between 4% and 20% and as much as 40% of the administered dose is recovered in the stool.

CLEARANCE OF ^{51}Cr-ALBUMIN

Calculation of the fraction of the albumin pool cleared into the gastrointestinal tract constitutes a refinement over the technique described above. Stools need to be collected daily for a period of 12 days. A serum sample is obtained 10 minutes after the ^{51}Cr-albumin injection and daily thereafter. To work out the number of milliliters of plasma cleared daily, one divides the counts in the stool within a defined 24-hour period by the counts per milliliter of serum drawn the day before the stool collection.

CLEARANCE OF ALPHA-1-ANTITRYPSIN

Alpha-1-antitrypsin is a low molecular weight glycoprotein that makes up the bulk of the alpha-1-globulin fraction on serum protein electrophoresis. A small amount is normally lost in the stools.

It is not degraded by pancreatic enzymes and is stable upon incubation in stools for 3 days. These properties have been exploited to calculate the milliliters of serum cleared daily of alpha-1-antitrypsin (α_1-AT).

The technique consists of taking blood samples on days 1, 5, and 10 and collecting stools for 10 days. The clearance of serum alpha-1-antitrypsin by the gastrointestinal tract is determined each day by the following formula:

Clearance

$$= \frac{\text{Fecal } \alpha_1\text{-AT concentration} \times \text{Daily fecal volume}}{\text{Average serum } \alpha_1\text{-AT on days 1, 5, and 10}}$$

Results obtained in an adult series with protein-losing enteropathy documented by the clearance of ^{51}Cr-labeled albumin were as follows:

	Number	*Clearance of α_1-AT (ml/day)*
Controls	13	3.1 ± 2.2 (range 0.5-7)
Patients	10	91.7 (range 16.5-218)

REFERENCES

Alper, C.A.: Plasma protein measurements as a diagnostic aid, N. Engl. J. Med. **291**:287-290, 1974.

Alpers, D.H., and Kinzie, J.L.: Regulation of small intestinal protein metabolism, Gastroenterology **66**:471-496, 1973.

Bernier, J.J., Florent, C.H., Desmazures, C.H., and others: Diagnosis of protein-losing enteropathy by gastrointestinal clearance of alpha$_1$-antitrypsin, Lancet **2**:763-764, 1978.

Rothschild, M.A., Oratz, M., and Schreiber, S.S.: Albumin synthesis. In Javitt, N.B., editor: Liver and biliary tract physiology. I, Int. Rev. of Physiol. **21**:249-274, 1980.

Rothschild, M.A., Oratz, M., and Schreiber, S.: Albumin metabolism, Gastroenterology **64**:324-337, 1973.

Shani, M., Theodor, E., Frand, M., and Goldman, B.: A family with protein-losing enteropathy, Gastroenterology **66**:433-445, 1974.

Waldmann, T.A.: Gastrointestinal protein loss in pediatrics. In James, A.E., Wagner, H.N., and Cooke, R.E., editors: Pediatric nuclear medicine, Philadelphia, 1974, W.B. Saunders Co.

Walker, W.A., Lowman, J.T., and Hong, R.A.: Measuring albumin turnover rates in patients with hypoproteinemia, Am. J. Dis. Child. **125**:51-54, 1973.

PERCUTANEOUS LIVER BIOPSY

Microscopic examination of liver tissue can be of considerable assistance in the evaluation of suspected liver disorders. A percutaneous aspiration biopsy of the liver using either the Menghini needle or the disposable Jamshidi (Kormed) needle is especially suited for use in small infants as well as in older children. Liver biopsy is also useful when tissue is needed for enzyme analysis, bacterial or viral culture, study of chemical content, and histochemical and electron-microscopy studies.

Indications

Liver biopsy may be helpful in patients with the following pediatric conditions:

1. Differentiation of cholestatic syndromes of the neonate
2. Prolonged jaundice in other patients
3. Chronic active hepatitis
4. Suspected liver disease (hepatomegaly)
5. Toxic hepatitis
6. Lipid and glycogen storage diseases
7. Portal hypertension
8. Wilson's disease
9. Reye's syndrome

Contraindications

The following are some contraindications and precautions that should be carefully considered before a liver biopsy is attempted:

1. One or more abnormalities in the following test results: prothrombin activity less than 50% of normal (more than 3 seconds over the control); platelet count less than 50,000; bleeding time prolonged more than 7 minutes
2. Significant ascites
3. Extrahepatic cholestasis (suspected)—bilirubin more than 25 mg/dl
4. Suspected hemangioma or hepatoma
5. Small liver—percussion dullness absent
6. Infections of pleura, lung, peritoneum
7. Hepatic vein thrombosis (suspected)

Procedure

Preoperative preparation. Hematocrit and blood count are made. Partial thromboplastin time (PTT), prothrombin time, platelet count, and bleeding time are determined. One unit of blood is typed and cross matched.

The parents and the patient should be given a calm, factual understanding of the procedure and potential risks.

The patient is to take nothing by mouth for at least 4 hours before the procedure.

Preoperative medication. For the patient less than 10 years of age, each 1 ml of solution given contains 12.5 mg of meperidine (Demerol), 6.25 mg of chlorpromazine hydrochloride (Thorazine), and 6.25 mg of promethazine hydrochloride (Phenergan). A dose of 1 ml/10 kg of body weight to a maximum of 1.5 ml per dose is injected intramuscularly.

For patients more than 10 years of age, 2 to 3 mg/kg of secobarbital (Seconal) and 1 mg/kg of meperidine are injected intramuscularly. Up to 0.3 mg/kg of diazepam (Valium) can be given intravenously.

Contents of biopsy tray (Fig. 32-3)

1. Menghini biopsy needle with trocar
2. One 25-gauge ½-inch hypodermic needle
3. One 22-gauge, 1½-inch hypodermic needle
4. One 5 ml Luer-Lok syringe
5. One 10 ml Luer-Lok syringe
6. One 8-inch forceps
7. Ten dressings, 4 by 4 inches
8. Two medicine glasses
9. Three towels
10. One surgical blade
11. One circumcision drape

A disposable tray that comes with a 15-gauge Jamshidi soft-tissue biopsy needle and syringe is now available for Kormed Products (St. Paul, Minnesota). Smaller sizes (19 and 17 gauge) may be ordered individually from the same company.

Operative procedure

Position. The infant may be restrained on a circumcision board or held by assistants. The older patient may assume a supine position with the arms restrained at the sides.

Selection of biopsy site. The upper border of liver dullness is percussed, and the biopsy site selected is at least one intercostal space below, in the anterior to mid-axillary line. Twirling the wooden end of a cotton swab firmly on the skin and then touching the area with tincture of iodine leaves an easily visible landmark.

Selection of needle size. The 1.4 mm Menghini or 17-gauge Jamshidi is routinely used. In situations where the risk of complications is considered to be greater, especially in cases with borderline clotting or bleeding studies or in the very small neonate, it is wise to use the 1.2 mm or 19-gauge needle. The 1.6 mm or 15-gauge one is used only exceptionally; it should be reserved for patients suspected of a metabolic disorder requiring a large core of liver tissue for enzymatic assays.

Technique. The biopsy site is widely scrubbed as in a surgical preparation and the area draped with a sterile circumcision sheet or a disposable Steridrape. The skin, the subcutaneous tissues, and the deeper intercostal muscles are infiltrated with

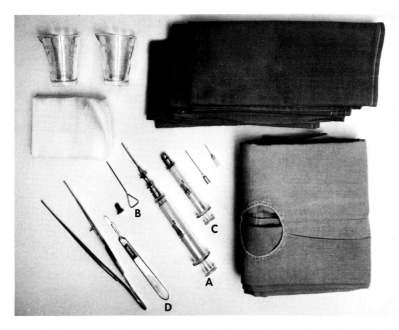

Fig. 32-3. Liver biopsy tray. Contents include Menghini needle, *A*, attached to a 10 ml Luer-Lok syringe; trocar, *B*; scalpel, *D*; 2 ml syringe and hypodermic needles, *C*; and sterile drapes, gauze pads, circumcision drape, and medicine glasses.

1% lidocaine. We do not infiltrate the liver capsule. A very small skin incision is made at the biopsy site. The trocar is then passed several times through the intercostal muscles to form a tract for the biopsy needle. The direction of the trocar should follow an imaginary line that will place the needle at a right angle to the liver. The liver biopsy needle is then attached to a 10 ml Luer-Lok syringe containing 2 to 3 ml of normal saline solution. Before the biopsy is attempted, one always needs to check the system for air leaks by occluding the biopsy needle opening with the gloved fingertip and retracting the plunger of the syringe. If there is a leak in the system, the plunger is easily withdrawn and no suction is felt at the fingertip; the connection of needle and syringe must be adjusted or another syringe employed.

The biopsy needle is then directed through the incision on the superior border of the rib through the tract left by the trocar. The needle is slowly advanced until a "popping" sensation is appreciated as one penetrates through parietal peritoneum and enters the abdomen. Thereafter the liver is soon encountered as the needle is carefully advanced.

Then the needle is withdrawn 2 to 3 mm, flushed with 1 ml of saline solution, and again advanced so as to rest against the liver capsule. With the needle in this portion, maximum suction is developed and maintained when one pulls back on the plunger. An assistant applies continuous counterpressure on the left side of the chest as the operator plunges the needle into the liver and withdraws it immediately on reaching the preset depth, always maintaining syringe suction. The entire time that the needle is in the liver is a fraction of a second.

The core of tissue is gently flushed out of the needle under normal saline solution so as to prevent fragmentation of the specimen. Depending on the studies desired, the biopsy tissue may be divided for microscopic studies and special procedures.

A minimum amount of tissue necessary for evaluation by the pathologist is usually a core longer than 1 cm. A core of this size will most often include several liver lobules with at least one central vein and 3 portal regions.

Failure to obtain a specimen on biopsy may result (1) if suction was not maintained, (2) if the needle was not resting on the capsule when suction and penetration were initiated, (3) if the capsule is too thick and fibrotic, or (4) if a dull needle was used. After these points are rechecked to ensure as far as possible that all is in order, a second attempt can be made to secure a biopsy specimen.

Consultation with an experienced pathologist before the biopsy will result in deriving the most information possible from the biopsy material.

Postbiopsy care

A dressing is securely applied to the biopsy site. The patient should remain fasting and be kept on his right side for several hours. Vital signs are recorded every 15 minutes for 1 hour, then every 30 minutes for 1 hour, and then every hour for 4 hours. Hematocrit is checked at 4-hour intervals until stabilized. Occasional gentle palpation of the abdomen is suggested to check for peritoneal signs.

Complications

Complications are kept to a minimum if careful attention is paid both to the contraindications to using liver biopsy and to procedural details in performing the biopsy. In a recent multicenter survey the incidence of complications associated with 584 liver biopsies was surprisingly high at 4%. Complications reported with a liver biopsy include local pain and infection, breakage of the needle, subcapsular and intraheptic hematoma, hemobilia, capsular bleeding, bile peritonitis, pleural pain and pneumothorax, pneumoscrotum, endotoxic shock, bacteremia, septicemia, penetration of other abdominal organs, arteriovenous fistula, and tumor seeding.

REFERENCES

Menghini, G.: One-second biopsy of the liver—problems of its clinical application, N. Engl. J. Med. **283:**582-585, 1970.

Walker, W.A., Krivit, W., and Sharp, H.L.: Needle biopsy of the liver in infancy and childhood, Pediatrics **40:**946-950, 1967.

SMALL BOWEL BIOPSY WITH THE CAREY CAPSULE

Understanding of the function and morphology of the small bowel mucosa in health and disease has rapidly increased with the development of instruments for peroral biopsies of the small intestine. A number of instruments of various designs can be used; however, in our experience, the Carey capsule* is by far the most satisfactory in terms of size of specimen, ease of use, and safety even

*May be obtained from Precise Products Corp., 7217 W. 27th St., Minneapolis, MN 55426.

in young infants who weigh as little as 3 to 4 kg. However, in some of the smaller infants, a Watson capsule may more easily pass through the upper esophageal sphincter, pylorus, and the junction between the second and third duodenum. Although primarily intended for the small bowel, the Carey capsule can also be used for gastric and esophageal biopsy tissue. The Medi-Tech steerable biopsy apparatus* has recently gained popularity among some pediatric gastroenterologists.

The Carey capsule (Fig. 32-4) consists of two concentric stainless-steel shells. When it is open, sharp-edged holes in each of the halves are superimposed. The capsule is kept open by a small spring that, because of its position, prevents too deep a specimen from being taken. The spring also facilitates taking multiple biopsy specimens, since it permits reopening of the capsule and traps the specimens already taken. With suction through polyethylene tubing (Intramedic, Adam, No. PE 200) with a 50 to 100 ml tight-fitting syringe, mucosa is sucked into the 5.4 mm hole, and the capsule closes instantly. Our recent modification has employed the use of Torcon cardiac catheter tubing, with a matching Amplatz wire guide, and is especially well adapted for the job, since it resists kinking. The size that adapts to the Carey capsule is the JPEP type, 6 F, 100 cm in length, with a 3 cm pulldown zero curve and an outside diameter of 0.059 to 0.061 cm.†

The use of a mercury bag is recommended by the manufacturer. We have dispensed with it and believe that with use of the heavier tubing just recommended, swallowing of the capsule and passage through the esophagogastric junction and the pyloric canal are facilitated, especially in small infants. In view of this modification, the opening in the distal part of the capsule normally reserved for the plastic tube leading to the mercury bag is sealed with epoxy polymer so that an effective vacuum can be created with suction.

Technique

This procedure may be done on an outpatient basis. Platelet count or platelet smear, prothrombin time, partial thromboplastin time, and bleeding times are obtained before biopsy. Aspirin-containing products should be avoided for 2 weeks

*Cooper Scientific Corp., 372 Main St., Watertown, MA 02172.

†This tubing can be obtained from Cook, Inc., Box 489, Bloomington, IN 47401.

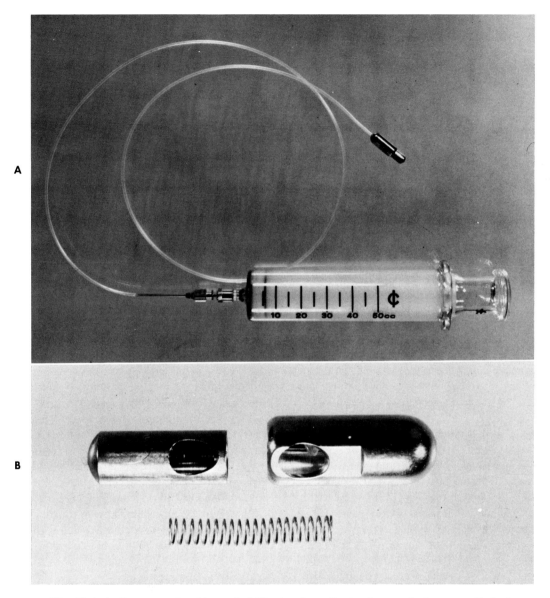

Fig. 32-4. **A**, Carey capsule with attached 50 ml syringe. Suction is created when one pulls back on the plunger. The mucosa is sucked into the 5.4 mm hole, and the capsule closes, cutting the mucosa. **B**, Carey capsule disassembled. The steel spring maintains the two concentric steel shells of the capsule in an open position before the specimen is taken.

before biopsy. It is well to remember that, in generalized malabsorption, often the prolonged prothrombin time responds within a few hours to 5 mg or less of vitamin K injected intramuscularly.

The patient fasts for 4 to 8 hours, depending on age. The posterior part of the pharynx may be anesthetized with a topical anesthetic (Cetacaine) and the sedation used before a liver biopsy (p. 914) is useful in infants and in younger children who are agitated and uncooperative. The routine

oral administration of metoclopramide syrup (0.1 mg/kg) one half hour before shortens the time taken by the capsule to migrate from the stomach to the duodenum. The intramuscular or intravenous route is preferred by some clinicians, and the dosage (0.1 mg/kg) is the same.

The young child is prevented from biting the tube if its "threatened" portion is protected with a short piece of rigid plastic tube used for endotracheal intubation (Foregger 18 F) or, in small infants, if the tube is threaded through a pacifier. During the procedure, several wooden tongue blades tapes together and carefully positioned in the mouth also work to prevent biting down on the tubing.

The older child is more easily able to swallow the capsule if he is sitting on the edge of a bed or a table. Ingesting water sometimes helps stimulate deglutitive movements. In small infants, whose cooperation is impossible to obtain, the capsule is placed at the base of the tongue and gently advanced; swallowing follows shortly thereafter. The patient is then rolled onto his right side, and the capsule is advanced under fluoroscopic control to the area of the pylorus. While the patient is either in this position or supine, gentle advancing force on the tubing is all that is needed to enter the duodenum. Use of excessive force, or against a closed pylorus, causes the capsule to deviate back into the antrum. If the tube does not go out of the stomach easily, air flushed through the capsule may be helpful in locating the pyloric region and stimulates antral contraction. Free draining duodenal juice, with its yellow color and alkaline pH, may be used for cultures (aerobic and anaerobic), examination for *Giardia,* secretory immunoglobulins, bile acid patterns, and pancreatic amylase and trypsin levels. Do not aspirate or the capsule will close and a biopsy specimen of the proximal duodenum instead will inadvertently be obtained.

Fluoroscopic confirmation of the capsule's localization is usually necessary until it is several centimeters distal to the ligament of Treitz. At this time air or saline solution is first flushed through the tubing to ensure that duodenal juice, mucus, and debris are flushed out and that the capsule is fully open. This open position of the capsule can be seen fluoroscopically. Suction is then vigorously applied, and the capsule closes instantaneously. Sometimes a momentary delay is noted before closure occurs. This usually indicates an incomplete mucosal seal at the capsule opening, preventing development of full vacuum when the syringe plunger is withdrawn. After fluoroscopy indicates that the capsule has closed, the tube is pulled back and suction is maintained on the plunger of the syringe. Resistance is usually encountered at the ligament, again at the pylorus, and especially at the gastroesophageal junction; a steady, gentle traction is all that is necessary to retrieve the capsule from the mouth.

If multiple biopsy specimens are desired, the tube is pulled back a few centimeters, and suction is then released. If the capsule does not reopen spontaneously, a few milliliters of saline solution are gently infused through the capsule, causing it to open, and another specimen is taken.

After completion of the biopsy, the hematocrit reading of the patient is checked 4 to 6 hours later. Small infants (less than 10 kg) should also have their abdomen examined for peritoneal signs. In the absence of technical problems a soft diet is given after the procedure.

Handling the specimen

The specimen usually weighs between 5 and 15 mg, wet weight. It should be promptly extracted from its position on the spring after the capsule is disassembled. The intestinal tissue is then positioned villous side up on a small, square slice of absorbable gelatin sponge (Gelfoam) or filter paper. Use of a dissecting microscope (Fig. 10-12) or a hand lens permits a reasonably good assessment of villous morphology and often leads to an immediate diagnosis of the atrophy so typical of celiac disease.

Tissue for morphology is placed in formalin, whereas the portion for intestinal enzymology is quick-frozen on a piece of aluminum foil lying on Dry Ice. A small portion of the tissue sample can be placed in glutaraldehyde for electron microscopy, and another portion can be quick-frozen in isopentane to be evaluated later by immunofluorescent studies. Most specimens taken with the Carey capsule consist of the full-thickness mucosa, lamina propria, and rarely portions of the lamina muscularis mucosae.

Complications

We have used this capsule exclusively since 1964 and have not seen any complications such as gross bleeding, abdominal pain, or perforation. The reason for this good record is that once the mucosa is sucked in, its depth of entry into the capsule is limited by the spring and the capsule closes instantly. Risk of perforation is greatest in the severely hypoproteinemic, edematous patient. Failure to obtain a specimen is rare: we would estimate its incidence at less than 1% of attempts.

Indications and diagnostic value

The major use of intestinal biopsy is in the differential diagnosis of malabsorption syndromes and of other entities responsible for chronic diarrhea, in which histologic lesions may be diagnostic. Recently, a number of other studies have been carried out on the biopsy specimen and already have important clinical applications.

Morphology. The appearance of the intestinal mucosal surface in celiac disease is so characteristic in most cases that examination of a biopsy specimen constitutes the most important single laboratory test. Diseases such as intestinal lymphangiectasis, abetalipoproteinemia, and Whipple's disease also give rise to highly specific lesions. In other mucosal diseases of the small bowel (Chapter 10), the alterations are much less typical. Abnormalities in intestinal biopsy specimens have been noted in a group of patients with acute infectious nonbacterial gastroenteritis. Some characteristic changes noted in the biopsy material from the jejunum consisted of shortening of the villi, crypt hypertrophy, increased cellularity of the lamina propria, and cytoplasmic vacuolation. These changes appeared 12 to 48 hours after ingestion of the Norwalk inoculum in experimental studies.

Enzymology. Homogenates of small bowel mucosa can be used for the diagnosis of disaccharidase insufficiency. Quantitative estimation of disaccharidase activity constitutes, in fact, the most reliable and clear-cut evidence. Increased levels of sucrase and maltase in the intestinal mucosa have been reported in a group of patients with chronic pancreatitis. The mucosal biopsy specimens were essentially morphologically normal. The exact mechanism whereby the disaccharidases, sucrase, and maltase are increased in the mucosa awaits further study. No clinical correlation has been suggested with these levels.

More recently, peptidases and enterokinase have also become the target of some studies, along with a variety of other enzymes such as the glycolytic enzymes.

Transport studies. Incubation of intestinal mucosa with a radioactive substrate placed in an incubation medium has helped the characterization of inborn errors of intestinal transport such as cystinuria and glucose-galactose malabsorption.

Metabolic activity. A further avenue of development for small-bowel biopsies lies in exploration of the in vitro metabolic activity (oxygen consumption, glucose and lipid metabolism, others) of intestinal biopsy specimens from patients with various intestinal disorders.

Intestinal cell kinetics. In vitro incubation of biopsy material with tritiated thymidine can be carried out and permits an estimation of the increased proliferative cell compartments (crypts) in diseases such as gluten enteropathy, in which cell turnover is augmented.

Immunofluorescence. Immunofluorescent studies may be helpful in diseases with immunologic abnormalities. A number of gastrointestinal disturbances are associated with immune-deficiency syndromes. Other entities lead to immune deficiency or are believed to have possible immunologic causes. A more complete discussion can be found in Chapter 12.

Tissue culture studies. Successful culture of small-bowel explants has led to interesting observations concerning the pathogenesis of celiac disease. It is predictable that further advances in this area will lead to clinical applications.

REFERENCES

Ament, M.E.: Prospective study of risks of complication in 6,424 procedures in pediatric gastroenterology, Pediatr. Res. **15**:524, 1981 (Abstract).

Ament, M.E., and Rubin, C.E.: An infant multipurpose biopsy tube, Gastroenterology **65**:205-209, 1973.

Carey, J.B.: A simplified gastrointestinal biopsy capsule, Gastroenterology **46**:550-557, 1964.

Christie, D.L., and Ament, M.E.: A double blind crossover study of metoclopramide versus placebo for facilitating passage of multipurpose biopsy tube, Gastroenterology **71**:726-728, 1976.

Greene, H.L., Rosensweig, N.S., Lufkin, E.G., and others: Biopsy of the small intestine with the Crosby-Kugler capsule, Am. J. Dig. Dis. **19**:189-198, 1974.

Partin, J.C., and Schubert, W.K.: Precautionary note on the use of the intestinal-biopsy capsule in infants and emaciated children, N. Engl. J. Med. **274**:94-95, 1966.

Shwachman, H., Khaw, K.T., and Antonowicz, I.: Diagnosis and treatment: peroral intestinal biopsy, Pediatrics **43**:460-462, 1979.

Townley, R.R.W., and Barnes, G.L.: Intestinal biopsy in childhood, Arch. Dis. Child. **48**:480-482, 1973.

Trier, J.S.: Diagnostic value of perioral biopsy of the proximal small intestine, N. Engl. J. Med. **285**:1470-1473, 1971.

Vanderhoof, J.A., Hunt, L.I., and Antonson, D.L.: A rapid procedure for small intestinal biopsy in infants and children, Gastroenterology **80**:938-941, 1981.

Walker-Smith, J.: Dissecting microscope appearance of small bowel mucosa in children, Arch. Dis. Child. **42**:626-630, 1967.

RECTAL BIOPSY

Histologic examination of the rectal mucosa is very useful in establishing or confirming the diagnosis of several disorders in the pediatric population. Properly done, rectal biopsy is a harmless procedure, and healing of the biopsy site occurs promptly. The patient or parent should be informed, however, that the next stool passed after biopsy has been performed may contain blood. It is dangerous for the patient to undergo a barium enema for 7 days after a rectal biopsy performed with angled cutting forceps, and even then the radiologist always should be informed.

Indications

The indications for doing a rectal biopsy include:

1. Hirschsprung's disease (suspected)
2. Inflammatory bowel disease (suspected)
3. Neural lipidoses
4. Miscellaneous diseases involving the rectal epithelium or the mesenchymal components of the rectal wall in which rectal biopsy may aid in establishing or confirming the diagnosis
5. Immunofluorescent studies

Contraindications

When properly done, there are few contraindications to a rectal biopsy. Patients taking aspirin or those having prolonged bleeding studies should not undergo biopsy until these abnormalities are corrected.

Procedures for biopsy

Sedation with the mixture used for liver biopsy is satisfactory for most patients (p. 914). Before biopsy, a digital examination should be done to rule out any obstruction by feces or tumor.

Direct biopsy. Under direct vision through a proctoscope, a specimen can be obtained with an angled cutting forceps. The specimen is usually taken from the posterior wall of the rectum, below the level of the peritoneal reflection, which corresponds to the superior valve of Houston (8 cm from the anus in the adult). This is the preferred site because, should the very rare complication of perforation occur, it will not lead to peritonitis. In cases of inflammatory bowel disease, and especially when granulomatous colitis is suspected, a specimen may be safely taken from the valves of Houston, which are prominent crescent shelflike folds. Direct pressure for a few minutes with a cotton pledget is sufficient to control any bleeding. When biopsies are required above the peritoneal reflection or in cases where multiple biopsies are necessary, we recommend the use of the much safer flexible crocodile-toothed bi-

opsy forceps employed with our pediatric endoscope.

Suction biopsy. A suction biopsy is a painless procedure through which most infants sleep. No sedation is necessary. The Rubin suction instrument can be used, the overall principle for obtaining tissue being the same as that for small-bowel biopsy. The Rubin tube (Fig. 32-5) is inserted at various levels from the anal margin, starting at 3 cm. It is also possible to pass the suction tube through the sigmoidoscope. Careful insertion of the lightly lubricated biopsy tube causes no discomfort to the patient, nor does the patient feel the excision of the specimen.

The suction tube should be marked in centimeters or inches from the capsule so that the distance from the anal orifice to the biopsy site can be measured. This approach is particularly helpful if more than one biopsy is taken and if the study is being carried out to establish the length of an aganglionic segment.

With the Rubin tube, suction is applied via the lateral arm through a calibrated vacuum gauge by a 50 or 100 ml Luer-Lok syringe attached to the tube. The maximum negative pressure that should be used is 10 inches of mercury.

In suction biopsies, the mucosa is sucked into the capsule and cut with the blade within the capsule.

Failure to obtain tissue may result from failure of the capsule to open or close, use of a dull knife, or aspiration of too large a piece of mucosa into the capsule, thereby incompletely cutting the specimen. After careful rechecking of the biopsy tubes, repeating the attempt is safe and acceptable.

After the specimen is taken, the tube is withdrawn and the biopsy tissue is gently removed. The tissue is then placed with the cut surface down on a piece of filter paper. The tissue is fixed in formalin or frozen in isopentane and sent to the pathologist for morphologic and histochemical studies.

Results

The histologic diagnosis of Hirschsprung's disease is based on the absence of ganglion cells in a full-thickness surgical biopsy specimen of the rectum. If ganglion cells are found in the submucosal tissue obtained by suction tube, the diagnosis of aganglionic megacolon is excluded. However, if extensive examination of the biopsy spec-

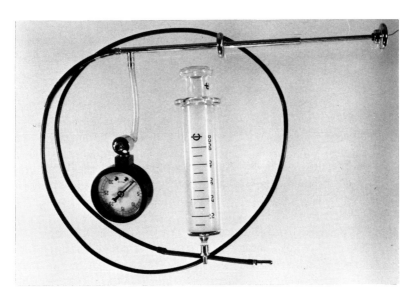

Fig. 32-5. Multipurpose suction biopsy tube with attached pressure gauge. The 50 ml syringe is inserted into the arm of the gauge, and the suction force is measured by the vacuum gauge. The cylindrical knife in the capsule is activated through the pull wire that is secured in the activator handle. Suction applied with the syringe sucks mucosa into the opening in the capsule; the mucosa is cut by the cylindrical knife in the capsule when the activator handle is pulled back.

imen shows no ganglion cells, a full-thickness specimen can be obtained from a valve of Houston, but this is rarely necessary.

Other patients in whom rectal biopsy is helpful are those with diseases known to involve the rectal-colonic tissue such as ulcerative colitis or granulomatous colitis (Crohn's disease) or, less commonly, amebic, *Shigella,* antibiotic-associated, or milk colitis. The presence of crypt abscesses, ulcerations, granulomas, and chronic inflammation in a rectal biopsy specimen is characteristic of inflammatory bowel disease and provides substantive support for the clinical and roentgenologic diagnosis of these diseases.

In the neural lipidoses, characteristic histologic and histochemical changes noted in the myenteric ganglion cells of the rectum consist in ballooning and distention of the cells by stored lipid. These changes are similar to those noted in the central nervous system. Thus rectal biopsy may be indicated in the diagnosis of suspected neural lipidoses and for patients who have unexplained signs of a degenerative nervous system disorder. Based on morphologic and histochemical staining characteristics, the following neural diseases can be diagnosed: (1) Niemann-Pick disease, (2) amaurotic idiocies, such as Tay-Sachs disease, and (3) Hurler's syndrome.

Rectal biopsy should always be done even when sigmoidoscopic findings are absent in a patient suspected of inflammatory bowel disease. Early in the disease of a few patients the mucosa as seen by sigmoidoscopy may appear normal, but findings on biopsy are abnormal. Conversely, sigmoidoscopic appearance may seem abnormal, but microscopic examination of the rectal biopsy material will be normal. In either situation, more reliance should be placed on the pathologist than on the objectivity of the sigmoidoscopist.

As a means of assessing the progress of a patient undergoing therapy, periodic examination of the rectal mucosa can provide valuable information. Not uncommonly, the patient may be doing very well clinically, but rectal biopsy findings indicate that the disease process appears the same or to be worsening.

REFERENCES

Aldridge, R.T., and Campbell, P.E.: Ganglion cell distribution in the normal rectum and anal canal: a basis for the diagnosis of Hirschsprung's disease by anorectal biopsy, J. Pediatr. Surg. **3:**475-490, 1968.

Campbell, P.E., and Noblett, H.R.: Experience with rectal suction biopsy in the diagnosis of Hirschsprung's disease, J. Pediatr. Surg. **4:**410-415, 1969.

Kerner, I., and Morin, C.L.: Utilité de la biopsie rectale par tube à succion en pédiatrie, Union Méd. Can. **100:**1131-1135, 1971.

Martin, L.W., Landing, B.H., and Nakai, H.: Rectal biopsy as an aid in the diagnosis of diseases of infants and children, J. Pediatr. **62:**197-202, 1963.

Morson, B.C.: Rectal biopsy in inflammatory bowel disease, N. Engl. J. Med. **287:**1337-1339, 1972.

ANORECTAL MANOMETRY

Rectal manometry is a useful diagnostic test in the neonate who may have short-segment aganglionosis, in the older child with chronic constipation starting in infancy, and as an investigative tool in other anorectal dysfunctions, such as incontinence.

In 1958 Davidson and Bauer reported on older patients with chronic constipation in whom distal colon motility studies showed abnormality and the rectal biopsy specimens were normal. They considered these patients as having achalasia of the distal rectal segment. Recently, workers using manometric balloon methods have demonstrated an abnormal response of the internal anal sphincter in patients with aganglionosis and in some patients with congenital or acquired anorectal abnormalities.

The pressure-recording device consists of a double balloon fixed to a hollow cylinder. The size of the apparatus can be individualized for use in neonates as well as in adults. The inner balloon (more distal to the operator) is carefully positioned at the internal anal sphincter to reflect reactions of this smooth muscle sphincter. The outer balloon is placed at the external sphincter to respond to reflex reactions of the internal striated muscle sphincter. A third balloon connected to a small catheter is passed through the cylinder and is positioned in the rectum proximal to the inner balloon. The double balloon is connected through transducers to two separate recording channels, one for each component of the double balloon. The test procedure consists of recording the reflex response of the two anorectal sphincters to transient rectal balloon distention. The normal response is reflex relaxation of the internal sphincter, followed immediately by contraction of the external sphincter. In patients with Hirschsprung's disease, the external sphincter contracts normally to rectal distention. However, the internal sphincter either fails to relax or may even contract with this stimulus (Fig. 14-14).

In experienced hands, this manometric procedure permits an accurate diagnosis of Hirschsprung's disease in the neonate at an age when a barium enema may not be diagnostic and without subjecting the patient to the risks associated with rectal biopsy. Anorectal tonometry may be of value as a screening procedure in newborns with the meconium plug syndrome or with difficulty in passing stools, and in the older child with chronic constipation that began in infancy. Experimentally, anorectal manometry is being used as a training or an operant conditioning device in patients with incontinence after rectal surgery. Generally speaking, it would appear that the diagnosis of Hirschsprung's disease is preferentially based on an accurate history, a carefully administered barium enema, and a reliably obtained rectal biopsy sample interpreted by an experienced pathologist. There are no apparent complications or contraindications to rectal manometry.

REFERENCES

Aaronson, I., and Nixon, H.H.: A clinical evaluation of anorectal pressure studies in the diagnosis of Hirschsprung's disease, Gut **13:**138-146, 1972.

Davidson, M., and Bauer, C.H.: Studies of distal colonic motility in children. IV. Achalasia of the distal rectal segment despite presence of ganglia in the myenteric plexus of this area, Pediatrics **21:**746-760, 1958.

Morikawa, Y., Donahoe, P.K., and Hendren, W.H.: Manometry and histochemistry in the diagnosis of Hirschsprung's disease, Pediatrics **63:**865-871, 1979.

Shuster, M.M.: Diagnostic value of anal sphincter pressure measurements, Hosp. Pract., pp. 115-122, April 1973.

Suzuki, H., White J.J., El Shafie, M., and others: Nonoperative diagnosis of Hirschsprung's disease in neonates, Pediatrics **51:**188-191, 1973.

ENDOSCOPY

Direct vision of the lumen of the gastrointestinal tract is an invaluable means for evaluation of the appearance and integrity of the mucosa, detection of lesions, and provision of an access to lesions for biopsy and treatment of some lesions. With the introduction and widespread use of fiberoptic endoscopes, heretofore inaccessible portions of the gastrointestinal tract are readily viewed by the experienced endoscopist. The technique is applicable to the pediatric population and is being increasingly employed by gastroenterologists caring for children.

The indications for endoscopic examination of various areas of the alimentary tract are vomiting of blood, rectal bleeding, inflammatory disorders, biopsy, excision of polyps when possible, and the removal of foreign bodies.

Anoscopy

Digital examination should precede anoscopy to note the sphincteric competence and to check for any masses that may be present. Severe spasm induced by simple digital examination usually signifies low-lying inflammatory bowel disease (proctitis, ulcerative colitis). Anoscopy can precede sigmoidoscopy or colonoscopy. The patient should be placed in the proper position on a specially designed sigmoidoscopy table, and the Sims' left lateral position, knee-chest, or inverted (supine) position can also be used as indicated. A warm, well-lubricated anoscope, with the beveled surface of the tip facing laterally, causes the least discomfort and should be slowly inserted. The general appearance of the mucosa is noted and the area specifically examined for fissures, abscesses, or signs of anal papillitis or cryptitis. Complete viewing of this area requires withdrawal, rotation, and reinsertion of instrument.

Rectosigmoidoscopy

Generally, rectosigmoidoscopy is performed with the infant and young child under sedation (p. 914). In the older child, only mild sedation may be necessary if he is apprehensive. Rarely is medication necessary in the preteen or teen-age patient. Careful explanation of the procedure, a gentle approach, and calm reassurance of the patient during the procedure are most useful. The understandable embarrassment of the patient, particularly a girl, should be considered—privacy, careful draping to preserve modesty, and assurance that if pain should occur the examination will be stopped. Continuation of the procedure after the discomfort has subsided is usually possible without difficulty. Of particular help and assurance to the patient is that the examiner carry on a conversation with the patient on a level in keeping with his age and intelligence.

Indications

The indications for rectosigmoidoscopic examination include the following:

1. Melena or bleeding from the anorectal area
2. Persistent diarrhea
3. Passage of pus and mucus
4. Signs suggestive of chronic inflammatory bowel disease (fistula in ano, hemorrhoids)
5. Obtainment of material for bacteriologic and histologic studies whenever indicated
6. Suspected polyps, tumor, foreign bodies

Contraindications

Contraindications are few in number and include severe necrotizing enterocolitis, toxic megacolon, painful anal lesions, and an uncooperative patient.

Procedure

An organized approach to endoscopic examination of pediatric patients includes preparation of the patient, instruments, examining table, position, and technique.

Sedation, such as that used for liver biopsy, is recommended. Whenever possible, general anesthesia should be avoided, since the risk of bowel perforation is greater in the patient who is asleep.

The patient is prepared psychologically, as previously noted. If he is scheduled for a barium enema, rectosigmoidoscopy can precede the x-ray study provided that a biopsy is not taken; this may save needless enemas. Patients who have ulcerative colitis or acute diarrhea can be examined without the use of cleansing enemas or laxatives. For the more routine examinations, the patient may be given a hypertonic phosphate or saline enema the morning of the examination. Sigmoidoscopy is conducted after the patient has evacuated the lower bowel. Occasionally, when excessive fecal material is encountered during the examination, another enema is given.

Except for the use of smaller-sized instruments such as a ½-inch proctoscope in the newborn or infant under the age of 6 months, the older child and adolescent patient may be examined with the ⅝-inch proctoscope. Fig. 32-6 shows the rectosigmoid junction; the growth of the anal canal and rectum; and the relationship of the size of the examining finger, a proctoscope, and the anatomy.

There are many forms of sigmoidoscopes, varying in length from 6 to 12 inches and having a distal or proximal light source. For routine use, the sigmoidoscope with a light source near the examiner is satisfactory. A distal light source may give a clearer view of the mucosa but is more likely to become covered with fluid or feces, obscuring the view. Recently, the thin flexible fiberoptic sigmoidoscope, 50 cm in length, has been popularized in lieu of rigid proctosigmoidoscopy.

Special proctologic tables are available for both infants and adults. These tables permit the patient to be placed in an inverted position with the head down against a headrest. The tilt table is more comfortable for patient and examiner. If such a

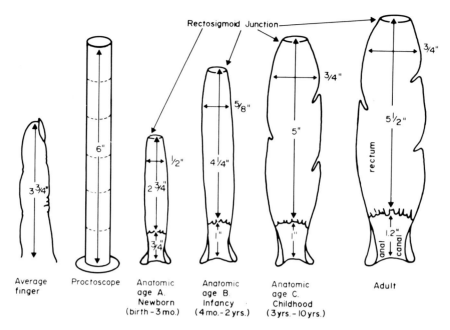

Fig. 32-6. Rectosigmoid junction in various age groups. Note comparative sizes in relation to an average-sized examining finger and a 15 cm long proctoscope. The increase in length of the anal canal and rectum and the increase in width of the rectum at various ages are shown. Note the diameters of ½, ⅝, ¾ inches for proctoscopes at the various ages. (Redrawn from Schapiro, S.: Hosp. Med., pp. 53-72, June 1969.)

table is not available, the examination can be carried out with the patient in the knee-chest position. In emergencies, the examination can be less satisfactorily done with the patient in bed and assuming Sims' position.

With the patient properly positioned and draped, a thorough visual and digital rectal examination should precede endoscopy. In the infant, the examiner's little finger is used; for patients older than 1 year, the well-lubricated index finger can be used. Digital examination prepares the patient for the insertion of an instrument but also provides valuable information. When the buttocks are gently spread, anal fissures and anal anomalies are easily visible. Digital examination provides information as to sphincter tone and the presence of a polyp or an adenoma, rectal prolapse, procidentia, extracolonic masses, and the very rare occurrence in children of hemorrhoids. Stool remaining on the examination finger should always be checked for blood.

The examination then continues, and the well-lubricated, warm proctoscope or sigmoidoscope is gently pressed against the anal opening. The patient is then asked to "strain down"; with obturator held firmly in place, the instrument is easily

passed into the rectum in a direction toward the sacrum; then the obturator is removed. The sigmoidoscope is then slowly passed to a depth of 12.5 cm in the infant and 20 to 25 cm in the older child and the adolescent. It should be advanced only under direct vision and should not be forced. The bowel lumen is often hidden just behind a mucosal fold, which may be gently pushed aside with the tip of the instrument. If spasm or difficulty is encountered, the sigmoidoscope should be withdrawn until the full lumen is again seen, and then a second attempt is made to advance the sigmoidoscope as long as the lumen is in full view. The insufflation of air during sigmoidoscopy is rarely needed and does contribute to the patient's discomfort during the procedure. Before beginning and periodically during the procedure, it is well to inform the patient that he may experience some cramping or even a desire to defecate. Asking the patient to take deep breaths or to pant "like a puppy" can minimize or relieve some of these sensations.

Once the desired depth is reached, the instrument is gradually withdrawn as the examiner carefully looks at all sides of the bowel. If stool or mucus obscures the view, these should be gently removed with a cotton pledget or gentle suction. The color and friability of the mucosa, bleeding sites, petechiae, and ulcers should be noted. Biopsy material should be taken whenever indicated, and the site of the lesion or specimen and its distance from the anus recorded. No special postexamination care is usually necessary.

Complications

Some complications that may occur after sigmoidoscopy include perforation, minimal bleeding from lacerations, and transient abdominal discomfort. Excessive bleeding from the biopsy site should prompt one to check the patient's bleeding status as well as reexamine the biopsy site. Either silver nitrate or electric cautery of the bleeding area will stop the bleeding.

If a perforation is suspected and confirmed by clinical symptoms and roentgenographic examination, prompt surgical intervention is indicated.

REFERENCES

Schapiro, S.: Proctologic conditions in children: a pictorial review, Hosp. Med., pp. 53-72, June 1969.

Turrell, R.: Proctosigmoidoscopy, New Physician, pp. 23-28, Aug. 1960.

Vanderhoof, J.A., and Ament, M.E.: Proctosigmoidoscopy and rectal biopsy in infants and children, J. Pediatr. **89:**911-915, 1976.

Winnan, G., Berci, G., Panish, J., and others: Superiority of the flexible to the rigid sigmoidoscope in routine proctosigmoidoscopy, N. Engl. J. Med. **302:**1011-1012, 1980.

COLONOSCOPY

An increasing experience with colonoscopy is available in the pediatric age group. However, since general anesthesia is believed to be contraindicated with this technique, its usefulness is limited to the older child and adolescent when sedation and analgesia with diazepam (Valium) and meperidine (Demerol) are adequate.

Indications and contraindications are listed in Table 32-2. In the well-prepared patient, the lubricated fiberoptic colonoscope is inserted into the rectum as described for sigmoidoscopy, with the patient in the left lateral position. The colonoscope is always advanced only under direct visual control. Insufflation of small amounts of air is helpful. Difficulties in advancing the colonoscope occur at the sigmoid area, where loop formation may present difficulty. Advancement of the instrument is made only as long as the mucosa is seen slipping by (slide-by maneuver).

Table 32-2. Colonoscopy: indications and contraindications

Indications	Contraindications
Diagnostic colonoscopy	Fulminant ulcerative colitis
Abnormal barium enema	Severe ischemic bowel disease
Unexplained colonic symptoms	Acute radiation colitis
Lower gastrointestinal bleeding	Pregnancy
Suspected cecal or ascending colonic disease	
Operative colonoscopy	
Polypectomy	
Foreign-body extraction	

Modified from Overholt, B.F.: Gastroenterology **68:**1308, 1975.

When further advancement of the scope beyond the junction of the sigmoid–descending colon cannot be accomplished without undue discomfort, the sigmoid-straightening technique may be attempted. This maneuver involves full deflection of the tip of the instrument at this site and slow withdrawal of the scope. This should result in straightening of the sigmoid colon loop over the instrument shaft in an accordion manner. Thereafter the tip is redirected to again visualize the bowel lumen, and the instrument can then be advanced to a greater depth. In difficult cases other maneuvers (alpha or Tajima's maneuver) are occasionally required to successfully pass through the junction of sigmoid–descending colon. A combination of hooking-lifting-telescoping is required to straighten a redundant loop in the transverse colon. Most of these maneuvers will require both an experienced endoscopist and fluoroscopic control. When both are available, the splenic flexure can be reached in 90% of cases and the cecum in 75% to 80%.

The complete examination occurs as the colonoscope is slowly withdrawn, with the mucosa being scanned by changing of the position of the flexible tip. Biopsy specimens, though superficial (mucosa and submucosa only), may be taken and lesions brushed for cytology, the experienced endoscopist is capable of removing polyps and tumors.

The most feared complication is perforation of the bowel, with a reported incidence of less than

2 in 1000, and probably less if polypectomy is not done. Excessive bleeding is rare from biopsy sites unless the patient has a coagulation disorder or has been on aspirin-containing products. Unsuspected serosal tears and retroperitoneal emphysema occasionally have been found at laparotomy and may be more common in pediatric patients undergoing colonoscopy under general anesthesia. Excessive use of air and advancing the scope without clear view of the lumen are likely to cause these difficulties.

REFERENCES

Deyhle, P.: Colonoscopy in the management of bowel disease, Hosp. Pract., pp. 121-128, June 1974.

Gleason, W.A., Jr., Goldstein, P.D., Shatz, B.A., and Tedesco, F.J.: Colonoscopic removal of juvenile colonic polyps, J. Pediatr. Surg. **10:**519-521, 1975.

Livstone, E.M., Cohen, G.M., Troncale, F.J., and others: Diastatic serosal lacerations: an unrecognized complication of colonoscopy, Gastroenterology **67:**1245-1247, 1974.

Morson, B.C.: Rectal biopsy in inflammatory bowel disease, N. Engl. J. Med. **287:**1337-1339, 1972.

Overholt, B.F.: Colonoscopy: a review, Gastroenterology **68:**1308-1320, 1975.

PANENDOSCOPY

Panendoscopy, which permits viewing of the esophagus, stomach, and proximal duodenum, is possible in the pediatric patient. For older children (over 5 years) even an adult fiberoptic flexible endoscope (Olympus GIF-Q) can be used, whereas a pediatric endoscope of smaller diameter (Olypmus GIF-P$_2$) is available for the younger patient. As with colonoscopy, the risks attending this procedure are heightened by the need to employ general anesthesia in the uncooperative younger child.

Sedation is accomplished with intravenous diazepam (Valium), 0.1 to 0.3 mg/kg. If the child becomes excitable, it is better to give meperidine (Demerol), 1 mg/kg intramuscularly or slowly intravenously, rather than to increase the dose of diazepam. With either agent, minimal airway resuscitation equipment should be available (Ambu-Bag). Naloxone (Narcan) can be given intravenously in a dose of 0.02 mg/kg to reverse any narcotic overdosage that produces severe respiratory depression. The oral pharynx should be locally anesthetized with a lidocaine or ethyl aminobenzoate (Benzocaine) derivative (Cetacaine) before passage of the instrument. General anesthesia with endotracheal intubation is usually recommended for neonates, young infants, and preschool age children to obviate respiratory embarrassment during the procedure.

Endoscopy in children should be thought of as an adjunct to good roentgenologic studies should the latter evaluation leave the diagnosis in doubt. Unexplained upper gastrointestinal bleeding (hematemesis) and esophageal conditions (dysphagia, stricture, pyrosis, ingestion of corrosives, foreign body, hiatal hernia, postoperative tracheoesophageal fistula, Mallory-Weiss tears) are acceptable indications for endoscopic examination. Inflammatory conditions of the stomach and duodenum can best be confirmed by endoscopy and biopsy of the lesion. Peptic ulcer disease can be confirmed by this procedure. The value of routine panendoscopy in the evaluation of abdominal pain in a child with normal roentgenographic findings has yet to be determined.

Complications with upper intestinal endoscopy in children are less than 2%. Perforation of the esophagus, stomach, or duodenum or excessive bleeding are exceedingly rare events. The greater morbidity and mortality attend the use of sedative agents or general anesthesia where bronchospasm and transient respiratory arrest may occur. Local phlebitis from diazepam anesthesia given intravenously is not uncommon (1% to 2%).

REFERENCES

Ament, M.E., and Christie, D.L.: Upper gastrointestinal fiberoptic endoscopy in pediatric patients, Gastroenterology **72:**1244-1248, 1977.

Ament, M.E.: Prospective study of risks of complication in 6424 procedures in pediatric gastroenterology, Pediatr. Res. **15:**524, 1981 (Abstract).

Forget, P.P., and Meradji, M.: Contribution of fibreoptic endoscopy to diagnosis and management of children with gastro-oesophageal reflux, Arch. Dis. Child. **51:**60-66, 1976.

Gleason, W.A., Jr., Tedesco, F.J., Keating, J.P., and Goldstein, P.D.: Fiberoptic gastrointestinal endoscopy in infants and children, J. Pediatr. **85:**810-813, 1974.

Graham, D.Y., Klish, W.J., Ferry, G.D., and Sabel, J.S.: Value of fiberoptic gastrointestinal endoscopy in infants and children, South. Med. J. **71:**558-560, 1978.

RETROGRADE ENDOSCOPIC PANCREATOCHOLANGIOGRAPHY

Retrograde endoscopic pancreatocholangiography, or endoscopic retrograde cholangiopancreatography (ERCP), permits cannulation of the sphincter of Vater and subsequent selective injection of contrast material into either the common bile duct or pancreatic duct. This procedure requires fluoroscopic control, and roentgenograms are obtained immediately after injection.

The use of ERCP in children is limited to those rare cases of obstructive jaundice without dilated biliary ducts (sclerosing cholangitis, congenital stricture of common hepatic duct, Caroli's disease, and so on), and relapsing pancreatitis of unknown cause and in patients being readied for pancreatic surgery when knowledge of the ductal anatomy is important. Pancreatic tumors may also be identified by ERCP but are extemely rare in children. Retained common bile duct stones can also be recognized and removed by this technique. Endoscopic papillotomy has been employed in adults to release retained stones in the sphincter of Vater and as a treatment modality for "biliary dyskinesia."

Complications after ERCP are reported at 3% with mortality at 0.2%. Acute pancreatitis and biliary sepsis are most commonly reported.

NONSURGICAL INVASIVE CHOLANGIOGRAPHY

Nonsurgical, percutaneous *transhepatic cholangiography* provides an excellent means for visualization of the hepatobiliary system. This invasive procedure is generally indicated by the results of abdominal ultrasound, CT scan, or radionuclide liver scan (DIDA, PIPIDA, and so on), which show dilatation of the biliary duct system. In this procedure utilizing fluoroscopic visualization, a thin needle is introduced into the liver through the right flank in the locally anesthetized seventh or eighth interspace parallel to the plane of the table. The needle connected to a syringe containing contrast material is slowly withdrawn until a green color appears in the syringe, indicating that a bile duct has been entered. The contrast material is then injected, and proper radiographs are taken. If the intrahepatic duct system is dilated, satisfactory opacification can be obtained in 90% of cases but only in 65% or less if they are not.

Some workers recommend that prophylactic antibiotics be given for 2 days before and 3 days after the procedure. Complications include fever, hypotension, bile leakage, and bile peritonitis in about 8% of the patients reported. This technique has had some limited application in the pediatric patient after portoenterostomy (Kasai's procedure) for biliary atresia.

REFERENCES

Bilbao, M.K., Dotter, C.T., Lee, T.G., and Katon, R.M.: Complications of endoscopic retrograde cholangiopancreatography (ERCP), Gastroenterology **70**:314-320, 1976.

Blustein, P.K., Gaskin, K., Filler, R., and others: Endoscopic retrograde cholangiopancreatography in pancreatitis in children and adolescents, Pediatrics **68**:387-393, 1981.

Okuda, L., Tanikawa, K., Emura, T., and others: Nonsurgical, percutaneous transhepatic cholangiography: diagnostic significance in medical problems of the liver, Am. J. Dig. Dis. **19**:21-36, 1974.

Vennes, J.A., and Silvis, S.E.: Endoscopic visualization of bile and pancreatic ducts, Gastrointest. Endosc. **18**:149-152, 1972.

Index

A

Aagenaes's syndrome, neonatal intrahepatic cholestasis and, 517-518

Abdomen
  acute, etiologic classification of, 340
  contusions of, 120
  distention of, and neonatal intestinal obstruction, 48
  enlargement of, 32-34
    in portal hypertension, 762
    in prehepatic portal hypertension, 770-771
  examination of, 40-42
  injuries to
    acute, 119-122
      in adolescence, 120
      in childhood, 120
      clinical findings in, 120-122
      management of, 122
      in neonatal period, 119-120

Abdominal pain, 30-32
  in celiac disease, 269
  in child 6 to 18 years of age, 32
  chronic recurrent, 32
  in Crohn's disease, 375
  in neonate and infant, 30-31
  in preschool child, 31-32
  psychophysiologic recurrent, 418-429
    diagnostic approach to, 421-428
      differential diagnosis in, 426-428
      history taking in, 422-425
      laboratory findings and roentgenographic studies in, 425-426
      observation in, 421
      physical findings in, 425
    etiology of, 418-421
    treatment and prognosis of, 428-429
  in ulcerative colitis, 354

Abdominoperineal procedure for rectal agenesis, 73
Abdominoperineal repair for anorectal anomalies, 74
Abetalipoproteinemia, 294-297, 728-729
  chronic diarrhea in, 15

Abscess(es)
  amebic, and fever of undetermined origin, 37
  anal, 415
  appendiceal, and secondary peritonitis, 115-116
  of brain, in portal hypertension, 763
  hepatic, and fever of undetermined origin, 37
  intra-abdominal; see Intra-abdominal abscess
  liver; see Liver, abscess of
  pancreatic, in acute pancreatitis, 851
  perianal, in Crohn's disease, 380

Absorption
  defects in; see also Malabsorption; Malabsorption syndromes
    and resection of small intestine, 290-291
    selective, 443-452

Absorption—cont'd
  digestion and
    of dietary constituents, 249-260
    test for, 894-897

Acanthocytes in cirrhosis, 753
ACCR; see Amylase-creatinine clearance ratio

Acetaminophen
  for Crohn's disease, 386
  and fulminating hepatic necrosis, 655
  and gastric damage, 169
  and hepatic coma, 672
  and hepatic necrosis, 661
  and liver damage, 618, 619, 620, 621, 622, 624, 628, 629
  and Reye's syndrome, 636

Acetazolamide, ascites caused by cirrhosis and, 748
Acetylcholine esterase stain and Hirschsprung's disease, 402, 407
Acetylhydrazine and drug-induced liver damage, 618

Acetylcysteine, N-acetylcysteine
  for drug-induced liver damage, 628
  for fecal impaction in cystic fibrosis, 830
  for meconium ileus, 83
    in cystic fibrosis, 829
  for pulmonary disease in cystic fibrosis, 818

Achalasia, 158-161
  anal, 397
  clinical features of, 158-159
  diagnosis of, 159
  differential diagnosis of, 159-161
  prognosis of, 161
  treatment of, 161

Acid reflux test in chalasia, 154-155
Acidity, gastric, procedure to measure, 906-907
Acids and corrosive gastritis, 180

Acrodermatitis enteropathica, 226-228, 451
  chronic diarrhea in, 15

ACTH for ulcerative colitis, 366-367

Actinomycin D
  for hepatocarcinoma, 485
  and liver damage, 620

Activity for ulcerative colitis, 365
Acute hydrops, 797-798
Adenocarcinoma of colon and rectum, 468
Adenoma, villous, 465
Adenomatous polyposis of colon, familial, 461, 462

Adenovirus(es), 511
  and fulminating hepatic necrosis, 655
  and Reye's syndrome, 635
  and viral gastroenteritis, 198

Adolescence, acute abdominal injuries in, 120
Adrenal hypoplasia, congenital, and neonate with diarrhea, 13
Adrenogenital syndrome, salt-losing, and neonate with diarrhea, 13
Aflatoxin B_1 and Reye's syndrome, 635-636